Principles and Practice of Spine Surgery

Principles and Practice of Spine Surgery

edited by

ALEXANDER R. VACCARO, M.D.
The Rothman Institute
Thomas Jefferson University
Philadelphia, Pennsylvania

Professor of Orthopaedic Surgery
Co-chief of the Spine Division
Jefferson Medical College
Thomas Jefferson University

Co-Director of the Delaware Valley
 Regional Spinal Cord Injury Center
Philadelphia, Pennsylvania

RANDAL R. BETZ, M.D.
Chief of Staff and Medical Director
Spinal Cord Injury Unit
Shriners Hospital for Children
Philadelphia, Pennsylvania

Professor of Orthopaedic Surgery,
Temple University School of Medicine
Philadelphia, Pennsylvania

SETH M. ZEIDMAN, M.D.
Assistant Professor of Neurosurgery
Chief of the Division of Complex Spine
University of Rochester School of Medicine and Dentistry
Rochester, New York

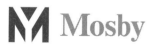

Mosby
An Affiliate of Elsevier

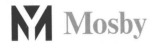

An Affiliate of Elsevier

The Curtis Center
Independence Square West
Philadelphia, Pennsylvania 19106

Principles and Practice of Spine Surgery   ISBN 0-323-01077-6

NOTICE

Medicine is an ever-changing field. Standard safety precautions must be followed, but as new research and clinical experience broaden our knowledge, changes in treatment and drug therapy may become necessary or appropriate. Readers are advised to check the most current product information provided by the manufacturer of each drug to be administered to verify the recommended dose, the method and duration of administration, and contraindications. It is the responsibility of the licensed prescriber, relying on experience and knowledge of the patient, to determine dosages and the best treatment for each individual patient. Neither the publisher nor the editors assume any liability for any injury and/or damage to persons or property arising from this publication.

Library of Congress Cataloging in Publication Data

Principles and practice of spine surgery / edited by Alexander R. Vaccaro, Randal R. Betz, Seth M. Zeidman.
    p. ; cm.
  Includes index.
  ISBN 0-323-01077-6
  1. Spine–Surgery. I. Vaccaro, Alexander R. II. Betz, Randal R. III. Zeidman, Seth M.
[DNLM: 1. Spinal Diseases–surgery. 2. Spine–surgery. 3. Surgical Procedures, Operative–methods. WE 725 P9562 2003]
RD768 .P745 2003
617.5'6059–dc21

          2002033749

Publishing Editor: Richard Lampert
Publishing Services Manager: John Rogers
Senior Project Manager: Beth Hayes
Designer: Mark Oberkrom

EH/CCW
Printed in the United States of America

Last digit is the print number: 9 8 7 6 5 4 3 2

Contributors

Dirk H. Alander, M.D.
Assistant Professor
University of Missouri at Columbia
Columbia, Missouri
*Chapter 36B: Thoracolumbar Trauma: Lower Lumbar
Burst Fractures: L3 to L5*

Todd J. Albert, M.D.
Professor of Orthopaedic Surgery
Jefferson Medical College
Thomas Jefferson University
Co-chief, Spine Division
The Rothman Institute
Philadelphia, Pennsylvania
Chapter 54: Postlaminectomy Cervical Kyphosis

Howard S. An, M.D.
Morton International Professor
Department of Orthopaedic Surgery
Rush-Presbyterian, St. Luke's Medical Center
Chicago, Illinois
Chapter 24: Cervical Degenerative Disc Disease

David Gregory Anderson, M.D.
Assistant Professor
Department of Orthopaedic Surgery
University of Virginia School of Medicine
Charlottesville, Virginia
Chapter 57: Spinal Orthoses

Paul M. Arnold, M.D.
Associate Professor of Neurosurgery
University of Kansas
Kansas City, Missouri
Chapter 29: Prosthetic Vertebral Disc Replacement

Richard A. Balderston, M.D.
Director of Spine Service
Pennsylvania Hospital
Philadelphia, Pennsylvania
*Chapter 40: Degenerative and Isthmic
Spondylolisthesis: Evaluation and Management*

Hugh L. Bassewitz, M.D.
Clinical Assistant Professor
University of Nevada School of Medicine
Desert Orthopedic Center
Las Vegas, Nevada
Chapter 25: Thoracic Degenerative Disc Disease

Gordon R. Bell, M.D.
Vice Chairman
Head of the Section of Spinal Surgery
Department of Orthopaedic Surgery
The Cleveland Clinic Foundation
Cleveland, Ohio
Chapter 1: Developmental Spinal Anatomy

Carlo Bellabarba, M.D.
Assistant Professor of Orthopaedics
University of Washington/Harborview Medical Center
Seattle, Washington
*Chapter 5: Biomaterials and Their Application
to Spine Surgery*
*Chapter 33: Closed Treatment of Cervical Spine
Injuries*

Edward C. Benzel, M.D.
Director of Spinal Disorders
Department of Neurosurgery
The Cleveland Clinic Foundation
Cleveland, Ohio
Chapter 4: Biomechanics of Internal Fixation

Randal R. Betz, M.D.
Chief of Staff and Medical Director
Spinal Cord Injury Unit
Shriners Hospital for Children
Professor of Orthopaedic Surgery
Temple University School of Medicine
Philadelphia, Pennsylvania
Chapter 31: Pediatric Spinal Cord Injury
Chapter 45: Adolescent Idiopathic Scoliosis
*Chapter 46: Neuromuscular Scoliosis: Surgical
Treatment*

K. Craig Boatright, M.D.
Spine Carolina
Asheville, North Carolina
*Chapter 9: Bone Graft and Fusion-Enhancing
Substances: Practical Applications of Gene Therapy*

Scott D. Boden, M.D.
Professor of Orthopaedic Surgery
Emory University School of Medicine
Director, The Emory Spine Center
Atlanta, Georgia
*Chapter 9: Bone Graft and Fusion-Enhancing
Substances: Practical Applications of Gene Therapy*

Michael J. Bolesta, M.D., F.A.C.S.
Department of Orthopaedic Surgery
The University of Texas Southwestern Medical Center
Dallas, Texas
*Chapter 36A: Fractures and Dislocations
of the Thoracolumbar Spine*

Keith H. Bridwell, M.D.
The Asa C. and Dorothy W. Jones Professor of
Orthopaedic Surgery
Chief of Adult and Pediatric Spine Surgery
Washington University School of Medicine
St. Louis, Missouri
*Chapter 41: Adult Deformity: Scoliosis and Sagittal
Plane Deformities*
*Chapter 52B: Complications of Anterior and Posterior
Thoracic and Lumbar Instrumentation*

Brian T. Brislin, M.D.
Department of Orthopaedic Surgery
Thomas Jefferson University
Rothman Institute
Philadelphia, Pennsylvania
Chapter 7: Invasive Spinal Diagnostics
*Chapter 52A: Complications of Anterior and Posterior
Cervical Instrumentation*
Chapter 54: Postlaminectomy Cervical Kyphosis

Russell S. Brummett, II, M.D.
Department of Orthopaedic Surgery
University of Pennsylvania
Philadelphia, Pennsylvania
*Chapter 40: Degenerative and Isthmic
Spondylolisthesis: Evaluation and Management*

Lee M. Buono, M.D.
Department of Neurosurgery
Jefferson Medical College
Thomas Jefferson University
Philadelphia, Pennsylvania
*Chapter 47: Congenital Intraspinal Abnormalities
of the Cervical, Thoracic, Lumbar, and Sacral Spine*

J. Kenneth Burkus, M.D.
The Hughston Clinic
Columbus, Georgia
*Chapter 30: Interbody Fusion Devices: Biomechanics
and Clinical Outcomes*

Rocco R. Calderone, M.D.
Vice Chairman
Department of Surgery
St. John's Regional Medical Center
Oxnard, California
*Chapter 58: Outcomes Assessment in Spine
Surgery*

John J. Carbone, M.D.
Chief, Spine Division
Department of Orthopaedic Surgery
Johns Hopkins Bayview Medical Center
Assistant Professor of Orthopaedic Surgery
The Johns Hopkins University School of Medicine
Baltimore, Maryland
*Chapter 26: Cauda Equina Syndrome Secondary
to Lumbar Disc Prolapse*

Jens R. Chapman, M.D.
Professor of Orthopaedic and Neurologic Surgery
University of Washington School of Medicine
Seattle, Washington
*Chapter 5: Biomaterials and Their Application
to Spine Surgery*
*Chapter 33: Closed Treatment of Cervical Spine
Injuries*

Kazuhiro Chiba, M.D.
Department of Orthopaedic Surgery
Keio University School of Medicine
Tokyo, Japan
*Chapter 12: Natural History and Surgical Treatment
for Ossification of the Posterior Longitudinal
Ligament*

Jeffrey D. Coe, M.D.
The Center for Spinal Deformity and Injury
Los Gatos, California
Chapter 7: Invasive Spinal Diagnostics

Andrew Cree, M.B.B.S. (Hons), F.R.A.C.S.(Orth)
Visiting Medical Officer and Clinical Research Director
Royal Alexandra Hospital for Children
Westmead Hospital
University of Sydney
Sydney, NSW, Australia
Chapter 33: Closed Treatment of Cervical Spine Injuries

Scott D. Daffner
Department of Orthopaedic Surgery
Thomas Jefferson University
Philadelphia, Pennsylvania
*Chapter 6: The Aging Lumbar Spine: The Pain
Generator*

Francis Denis, M.D.
Clinical Assistant Professor
University of Minnesota
Minneapolis, Minnesota
Chapter 37: Sacral Fracture

Denis S. Drummond, M.D.
Emeritus Chief
Division of Orthopaedic Surgery
Children's Hospital of Philadelphia
Professor of Orthopaedic Surgery
University of Pennsylvania School of Medicine
Philadelphia, Pennsylvania
Chapter 42: Pediatric Spondylolisthesis

James M. Ecklund, M.D.
Assistant Chief of Neurosurgery
Walter Reed Army Medical Center
Associate Professor of Surgery
The Uniformed Services University of the Health Sciences
Washington, DC
*Chapter 17: Intradural Intramedullary
and Extramedullary Tumors*

Frank J. Eismont, M.D.
Professor of Orthopaedic Surgery
Chief of the Spine Service
University of Miami School of Medicine
Miami, Florida
Chapter 15: Primary Spinal Tumors

Stephen I. Esses, MD, FRCSC, FACS
Professor
Department of Orthopaedics
Baylor College of Medicine
Houston, Texas
*Chapter 23: Surgical Approaches and Reconstruction
of the Sacrum*

Dapeng Fan, M.D., D.ABNM
Surgical Monitoring Associates
Bala Cynwyd, Pennsylvania
Chapter 8: Surgical Neurophysiologic Monitoring

Jeffrey S. Fischgrund, M.D.
Department of Orthopaedic Surgery
William Beaumont Hospital
Royal Oak, Michigan
Chapter 25: Thoracic Degenerative Disc Disease

Richard R. Frances, M.D., F.R.C.S., Ed.
Assistant Professor
Department of Orthopaedics
The University of Texas
Houston, Texas
*Chapter 23: Surgical Approaches and Reconstruction
of the Sacrum*

Mitchell K. Freedman, D.O.
Instructor of Rehabilitation Medicine
Jefferson Medical College
Thomas Jefferson University
The Rothman Institute
Medical Director of Pain Management and
Rehabilitation Services
Magee Rehabilitation Hospital
Philadelphia, Pennsylvania
Chapter 7: Invasive Spinal Diagnostics
*Chapter 38: Rehabilitation of the Spinal Cord Injury
Patient*

Guy W. Fried, M.D.
Magee Rehabilitation Hospital
Philadelphia, Pennsylvania
*Chapter 38: Rehabilitation of the Spinal Cord Injury
Patient*

Amy Fromal, B.S.
Thomas Jefferson University
Philadelphia, Pennsylvania
Chapter 57: Spinal Orthoses

Walter W. Frueh, MD
Department of Orthopaedic Surgery
Jefferson Medical College
Thomas Jefferson University
Philadelphia, Pennsylvania
*Chapter 47: Congenital Intraspinal Abnormalities
of the Cervical, Thoracic, Lumbar, and Sacral Spine*

Peter G. Gabos, M.D.
Alfred I. duPont Institute
duPont Hospital for Children
Wilmington, Delaware
Chapter 48: Skeletal Dysplasia

Steven R. Garfin, M.D.
Professor of Orthopaedics
Chair of the Department of Orthopaedics
University of California at San Diego Medical Center
San Diego, California
Chapter 14: Tuberculous Infections of the Spine

Kenneth F. Gavin, C.O.
The Rothman Institute
Philadelphia, Pennsylvania
Chapter 57: Spinal Orthoses

Alexander J. Ghanayem, M.D.
Assistant Professor of Orthopaedic Surgery
Chief of the Division of Spine Surgery
Stritch School of Medicine
Loyola University Chicago
Maywood, Illinois
Chapter 16: Metastatic Tumors of the Spine

Jim Giuffre, M.D.
International Spinal Development and Research
Foundation
Las Vegas, Nevada
*Chapter 21: Minimally Invasive Approaches
to the Lumbar Spine*

Jonathan N. Grauer, M.D.
Department of Orthopaedics
Yale University
New Haven, Connecticut
*Chapter 3: Relevant Clinical Biomechanics
of the Spine*

Christopher L. Hamill, M.D.
Clinical Assistant Professor of Orthopaedic Surgery
Department of Orthopaedics
University at Buffalo
State University of New York
Buffalo, New York
*Chapter 27: Lumbar Spinal Stenosis: Nonoperative
and Operative Treatment*

Matthew A. Handling, B.S.
Jefferson Medical College
Thomas Jefferson University
Philadelphia, Pennsylvania
*Chapter 6: The Aging Lumbar Spine: The Pain
    Generator*

Basil M. Harris, M.D., Ph.D.
Jefferson Medical College
Thomas Jefferson University
Philadelphia, Pennsylvania
*Chapter 13: Spinal Infections, Pyogenic
    Osteomyelitis, and Epidural Abscess*
*Chapter 32: Pharmacology and Timing of Surgical
    Intervention for Spinal Cord Injury*
*Chapter 35: Cervical Spine Injuries in the Athlete:
    Return-to-Play Criteria*

Andrea S. Herzka, M.D.
Johns Hopkins University
Johns Hopkins Bayview Medical Center
Baltimore, Maryland
*Chapter 26: Cauda Equina Syndrome Secondary
    to Lumbar Disc Prolapse*

Alan S. Hilibrand, M.D.
Associate Professor of Orthopaedic Surgery
Jefferson Medical College
Thomas Jefferson University
The Rothman Institute
Philadelphia, Pennsylvania
*Chapter 52A: Complications of Anterior and Posterior
    Cervical Instrumentation*

Kiyoshi Hirabayashi, M.D.
Professor of Orthopaedic Surgery
Keio University School of Medicine
Keio Orthopaedic Hospital
Tatebayashi, Gumma
Dean
Keio Junior College of Nursing
Tokyo, Japan
*Chapter 12: Natural History and Surgical Treatment
    for Ossification of the Posterior Longitudinal
    Ligament*

James D. Kang, M.D.
Department of Orthopaedic Surgery
University of Pittsburgh Medical Center
Pittsburgh, Pennsylvania
*Chapter 51: Management of Iatrogenic Neurologic
    Loss Due to Spinal Instrumentation*

Christopher P. Kauffman, M.D.
Department of Orthopaedic Surgery
University of California, San Diego
San Diego, California
Chapter 14: Tuberculous Infections of the Spine

David L. Kirschman, M.D.
University of Kansas Medical Center
Kansas City, Missouri
Chapter 29: Prosthetic Vertebral Disc Replacement

Nitin Khanna, M.D.
Department of Orthopaedic Surgery
Barnes-Jewish Hospital
Washington University
St. Louis, Missouri
Chapter 53: Treatment of Cerebrospinal Fluid Leaks

Gregg R. Klein, M.D.
Jefferson Medical College
Thomas Jefferson University
Philadelphia, Pennsylvania
Chapter 34: Cervical Spine Trauma: Upper and Lower

John P. Kostuik, M.D.
Professor of Orthopaedic Surgery
Chief of the Spine Division
The Johns Hopkins University
Baltimore, Maryland
*Chapter 10: Treatment of Spinal Deformities
    in the Setting of Osteoporosis*

Joseph M. Kowalski, M.D.
Clinical Assistant Professor of Orthopaedic Surgery
University at Buffalo
State University of New York
Buffalo, New York
*Chapter 27: Lumbar Spinal Stenosis: Nonoperative
    and Operative Treatment*

Stephen D. Kuslich, M.D.
Assistant Clinical Professor
Department of Orthopaedic Surgery
University of Minnesota
Emeritus Consultant in Spinal Surgery
St. Croix Orthopaedics
Stillwater, Minnesota
*Chapter 28: Surgical Treatment of Lumbar
    Degenerative Disc Disease: Axial Low Back Pain*

Ranjith Kuzhupilly, M.D.
The Cleveland Clinic
Cleveland, Ohio
Chapter 1: Developmental Spinal Anatomy

Jorge J. Lastra, M.D.
Assistant Professor
Section of Neurosurgery
University of Puerto Rico
San Juan, Puerto Rico
Chapter 4: Biomechanics of Internal Fixation

Mesfin A. Lemma, M.D.
Johns Hopkins University
Johns Hopkins Bayview Medical Center
Baltimore, Maryland
*Chapter 26: Cauda Equina Syndrome Secondary
    to Lumbar Disc Prolapse*

Lawrence G. Lenke, M.D.
Associate Professor of Orthopaedic Surgery
Washington University School of Medicine
St. Louis, Missouri
Chapter 45: Adolescent Idiopathic Scoliosis
Chapter 46: Neuromuscular Scoliosis: Surgical
  Technique

Brenda H. Long, R.N.
Mid-Atlantic Spine
Richmond, Virginia
Chapter 22: Posterior Minimally Invasive Techniques

John E. Lonstein, M.D.
Clinical Professor
Department of Orthopaedic Surgery
Twin Cities Spine Center
Minneapolis, Minnesota
Chapter 43: Congenital Deformities of the Spine

Thomas G. Lowe, M.D.
Assistant Clinical Professor
University of Colorado
Denver, Colorado
Chapter 50: Scheueremann's Disease

John P. Lubicky, M.D., F.A.A.O.S., F.A.A.P.
Professor of Orthopaedic Surgery
Rush Medical College
Chief of Staff
Shriners Hospital for Children
Chicago, Illinois
Chapter 49: Myelomeningocele: Neurosurgical
  Perspectives

Luke Madigan, B.S.
Jefferson Medical College
Thomas Jefferson University
Philadelphia, Pennsylvania
Chapter 13: Spinal Infections, Pyogenic
  Osteomyelitis, and Epidural Abscess

Hallett H. Mathews, M.D.
Clinical Instructor of Orthopaedic Surgery
Medical College of Virginia
Richmond, Virginia
Chapter 22: Posterior Minimally Invasive Techniques

Philip M. Maurer, M.D.
Clinical Assistant Professor
Department of Orthopaedics
Clinical Assistant Professor
Department of Anesthesiology
University of Pennsylvania Health System
Director of Spine Diagnostic and Treatment Center
Department of Orthopaedics
Pennsylvania Hospital
Philadelphia, Pennsylvania
Chapter 7: Invasive Spinal Diagnostics

Christopher Meredith, M.D.
University of Kansas Medical Center
Kansas City, Missouri
Chapter 29: Prosthetic Vertebral Disc Replacement

Sohail K. Mirza, M.D.
Assistant Professor
University of Washington School of Medicine
Seattle, Washington
Chapter 5: Biomaterials and Their Application
  to Spine Surgery
Chapter 33: Closed Treatment of Cervical Spine Injuries

Vert Mooney, M.D.
Medical Director
U.S. Spine and Sport Medical Center
Clinical Professor of Orthopaedics
University of California at San Diego
San Diego, California
Chapter 59: Outpatient Rehabilitation of the Spine
  Patient

Mary Jane Mulcahey, M.S., O.T.R./L.
Director of Rehabilitation Services and Clinical
  Research
Shriners Hospital for Children
Philadelphia, Pennsylvania
Chapter 31: Pediatric Spinal Cord Injury

Peter O. Newton, M.D.
Assistant Clinical Professor of Orthopaedics
University of California at San Diego
San Diego, California
Chapter 44: Thoracoscopic Approach for Pediatric
  Deformity

W. Jerry Oakes, M.D.
Professor of Neurological Surgery
Chief of Pediatric Neurosurgery
University of Alabama
Birmingham, Alabama
Chapter 49: Myelomeningocele: Neurosurgical
  Perspectives

Erin O'Brien, M.D.
The Rothman Institute
Philadelphia, Pennsylvania
Chapter 7: Invasive Spinal Diagnostics

Conor O'Neil, M.D.
Director of Research and Development
Spinal Diagnostics and Treatment Center
Daly City, California
Chapter 7: Invasive Spinal Diagnostics

William M. Oxner, M.D., FRCS
Assistant Professor of Orthopaedic Surgery
Halifax Infirmary Hospital
Halifax, Nova Scotia, Canada
Chapter 51: Management of Iatrogenic Neurologic
  Loss Due to Spinal Instrumentation

Manohar M. Panjabi, Ph.D.
Professor of Biomechanics
Director, Biomechanics Laboratory
Yale University
New Haven, Connecticut
*Chapter 3: Relevant Clinical Biomechanics
of the Spine*

Gregory J. Przybylski, M.D.
Associate Professor of Neurosurgery
Northwestern University
Chief of Neurosurgery
Lakeside Veterans Administration Hospital
Chicago, Illinois
*Chapter 11: Nonoperative and Operative
Management of Spinal Pathology in the Setting
of Paget's Disease*

Thomas J. Puschak, M.D.
Orthopaedics International, Ltd.
Seattle, Washington
*Chapter 2: Relevant Surgical Anatomy of the Cervical,
Thoracic, and Lumbar Spine*

Wolfgang Rauschning, M.D., Ph.D.
Orthopaedic University Hospital
Uppsala, Sweden
*Chapter 2: Relevant Surgical Anatomy of the Cervical,
Thoracic, and Lumbar Spine*

Glenn R. Rechtine II, M.D., F.A.C.S.
Professor of Orthopaedic Surgery
Director of Spine Surgery
Department of Orthopaedics and Rehabilitation
University of Florida College of Medicine
Gainesville, Florida
*Chapter 36A: Fractures and Dislocations
of the Thoracolumbar Spine*

John J. Regan, M.D.
Cedar Sinai Hospital
Los Angeles, California
*Chapter 20: Minimally Invasive Techniques
of the Lumbar Spine*
*Chapter 21: Minimally Invasive Approaches
to the Lumbar Spine*

K. Daniel Riew, M.D.
Assistant Professor of Orthopaedic Surgery
Washington University School of Medicine
St. Louis, Missouri
*Chapter 53: Treatment of Cerebrospinal Fluid
Leaks*

Lee H. Riley III, M.D.
Assistant Professor of Orthopaedic Surgery
Johns Hopkins University
Baltimore, Maryland
*Chapter 55: Management of Postoperative Spinal
Infections*

Michael K. Rosner, M.D.
Walter Reed Army Medical Center
Washington, DC
*Chapter 17: Intradural Intramedullary
and Extramedullary Tumors*

Scott A. Rushton, M.D.
Pennnsylvania Hospital
Philadelphia, Pennsylvania
Chapter 42: Pediatric Spondylolisthesis

Barton L Sachs, M.D., M.B.A.
Associate Professor of Surgery and Rehabilitation
Medicine
Albany Medical College;
Vice President and Chief Medical Officer
Raymedica, Inc.
Albany, New York
*Chapter 19: Minimally Invasive Techniques
of the Thoracic Spine*

Kazuhiko Satomi, M.D.
Department of Orthopaedic Surgery
Keio University School of Medicine
Tokyo, Japan
*Chapter 12: Natural History and Surgical Treatment
for Ossification of the Posterior Longitudinal
Ligament*

Arjun Saxena
Jefferson Medical College
Thomas Jefferson University
Philadelphia, Pennsylvania
*Chapter 47: Congenital Intraspinal Abnormalities
of the Cervical, Thoracic, Lumbar, and Sacral Spine*

Daniel M. Schwartz, Ph.D., D.ABNM
Surgical Monitoring Associates
Bala Cynwyd, Pennsylvania
Chapter 8: Surgical Neurophysiologic Monitoring

Anthony K. Sestokas, Ph.D., D.ABNM
Surgical Monitoring Associates
Bala Cynwyd, Pennsylvania
Chapter 8: Surgical Neurophysiologic Monitoring

Suken A. Shah, M.D.
Assistant Professor
Alfred I. duPont Institute
duPont Hospital for Children
Wilmington, Delaware
*Chapter 47: Congenital Intraspinal Abnormalities
of the Cervical, Thoracic, Lumbar, and Sacral Spine*

Ashwini D. Sharan, M.D.
Assistant Professor of Neurosurgery
Thomas Jefferson University
Philadelphia, Pennsylvania
*Chapter 11: Nonoperative and Operative
Management of Spinal Pathology in the Setting
of Paget's Disease*

Kern Singh, M.D.
Department of Orthopaedic Surgery
Rush Medical Center
Chicago, Illinois
*Chapter 21: Minimally Invasive Approaches
to the Lumbar Spine*

Kush Singh, B.S.
Jefferson Medical College
Thomas Jefferson University
Philadelphia, Pennsylvania
*Chapter 32: Pharmacology and Timing of Surgical
Intervention for Spinal Cord Injury*

Thomas A. St. John
Jefferson Medical College
Philadelphia, Pennsylvania
*Chapter 6: The Aging Lumbar Spine: The Pain
Generator*

Liz Stimson, N.P.
Department of Orthopaedics
University of California at San Diego Medical Center
San Diego, California
Chapter 14: Tuberculous Infections of the Spine

Rajiv V. Taliwal, M.D.
The Rothman Institute
Philadelphia, Pennsylvania
*Chapter 2: Relevant Surgical Anatomy of the Cervical,
Thoracic, and Lumbar Spine*

Bobby K.-B. Tay, M.D.
San Francisco General Hospital
San Francisco, California
Chapter 15: Primary Spinal Tumors

Bret A. Taylor, M.D.
The Rothman Institute
Philadelphia, Pennsylvania
*Chapter 52A: Complications of Anterior and Posterior
Cervical Instrumentation*

John Thalgott, M.D.
Research Director
International Spinal Development & Research Foundation
Las Vegas, Nevada
*Chapter 21: Minimally Invasive Approaches
to the Lumbar Spine*

P. Justin Tortolani, M.D.
Johns Hopkins University
Johns Hopkins Bayview Medical Center
Baltimore, Maryland
*Chapter 26: Cauda Equina Syndrome Secondary
to Lumbar Disc Prolapse*

Louise Toutant, MSN
Nurse Practitioner
Camarillo, California
Chapter 58: Outcomes Assessment in Spine Surgery

Eeric Truumees, M.D.
Section of Spine Surgery
Department of Orthopaedic Surgery
William Beaumont Hospital
Royal Oak, Michigan
*Chapter 39: Soft Tissue Injuries of the Cervical Spine:
Whiplash*

Alexander R. Vaccaro, M.D.
The Rothman Institute
Thomas Jefferson University
Professor of Orthopaedic Surgery
Co-chief of the Spine Division
Jefferson Medical College
Co-Director of the Delaware Valley Spinal Cord Injury
Center
Philadelphia, Pennsylvania
*Chapter 2: Relevant Surgical Anatomy of the Cervical,
Thoracic, and Lumbar Spine*
*Chapter 6: The Aging Lumbar Spine: The Pain
Generator*
Chapter 7: Invasive Spinal Diagnostics
*Chapter 13: Spinal Infections, Pyogenic
Osteomyelitis, and Epidural Abscess*
*Chapter 21: Minimally Invasive Approaches
to the Lumbar Spine*
*Chapter 32: Pharmacology and Timing of Surgical
Intervention for Spinal Cord Injury*
*Chapter 34: Cervical Spine Trauma: Upper
and Lower*
*Chapter 35: Cervical Spine Injuries in the Athlete:
Return-to-Play Criteria*
*Chapter 47: Congenital Intraspinal Abnormalities
of the Cervical, Thoracic, Lumbar, and Sacral
Spine*
Chapter 54: Postlaminectomy Cervical Kyphosis
Chapter 57: Spinal Orthoses

Robert Watkins, M.D.
Spine Surgeon
Los Angeles Spine Surgery Institute
Los Angeles, California
*Chapter 35: Cervical Spine Injuries in the Athlete:
Return-to-Play Criteria*

Bradley E. Weprin, M.D.
Weprin Neurosurgeons for Children
Dallas, Texas
*Chapter 49: Myelomeningocele: Neurosurgical
Perspectives*

Lawrence R. Wierzbowski, AUD., D.ABNM
Surgical Monitoring Associates
Bala Cynwyd, Pennsylvania
Chapter 8: Surgical Neurophysiologic Monitoring

Seth K. Williams, M.D.
Department of Orthopaedics
University of California at San Diego Medical Center
San Diego, California
Chapter 14: Tuberculous Infections of the Spine

Kirkham B. Wood, M.D.
Associate Professor of Orthopaedic Surgery
University of Minnesota
Minneapolis, Minnesota
Chapter 37: Sacral Fracture

Kenneth S. Yonemura, M.D.
Northwest Neuroscience Institute
Seattle, Washington
*Chapter 18: Minimally Invasive Techniques
   of the Cervical Spine*

S. Tim Yoon, M.D., PhD.
Assistant Professor
Department of Orthopaedic Surgery
Emory University
Atlanta, Georgia
Chapter 24: Cervical Degenerative Disc Disease

Seth M. Zeidman, M.D.
Assistant Professor of Neurosurgery
Chief of the Division of Complex Spine
University of Rochester School of Medicine and Dentistry
Rochester, New York
*Chapter 17: Intradural Intramedullary
   and Extramedullary Tumors*
Chapter 56: Failed Back Surgery Syndrome

Acknowledgment

The editors are extremely grateful for the hard work, dedication, tenacity, and creativity of Basil Harris. Without his involvement, the breadth and success of this project could never have been realized.

My family (wife Midge and children Max, Alex, and Juliana) is my strength and support. I cannot thank them enough for their love and encouragement throughout the completion of this text.

A.R.V.

Preface

Principles and Practice of Spine Surgery was conceived as a convenient single volume textbook encompassing the entire breadth of spinal disorders. It is geared primarily for spinal clinicians and clinicians in training, but is sufficiently well detailed to be useful for a busy spinal surgeon at a large tertiary referral center. The text is organized into 10 sections: General Topics, Metabolic Bone Disease, Tumor-Infection, Surgical Techniques, Degenerative Disc Disease, Trauma, Adult Deformity, Pediatrics, Complications, and After Treatment.

The book is designed to update the reader on contemporary issues related to spinal care in a manner that allows for quick reference (text boxes) or more detailed (text) reading.

The summary text boxes throughout the chapter allow the reader to develop a command of the subject material within minutes, and the standard text provides the details desired during more leisure study. The selected reference section provides a launching point for more advanced topic investigation.

This first edition includes the efforts of over 100 authors, each with a unique perspective on contemporary spinal care. Spinal clinicians with background in orthopaedics or neurosurgery, both in academics and private practice, share their research and experiences in the management of various adult and pediatric spinal disorders. Scientists and engineers in research and industry have contributed their expertise on subjects such as anatomy, biomechanics, and electrophysiologic monitoring.

We thank the authors for their outstanding contribution. Without them this work would not have been meaningful or even possible.

Alexander R. Vaccaro, M.D.
Basil M. Harris, M.D., Ph.D.
Seth M. Zeidman, M.D.
Randal R. Betz, M.D.

Contents

Principles and Practice of Spine Surgery

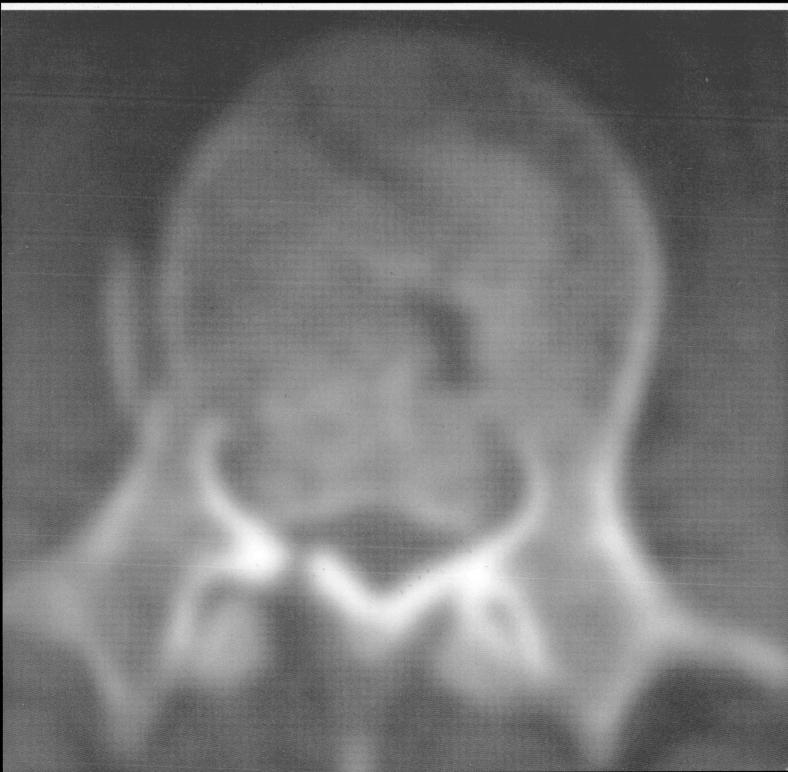

Developmental Spinal Anatomy

Ranjith Kuzhupilly, Gordon R. Bell

THE PREEMBRYONIC PERIOD (WEEKS 0 TO 3)

The preembryonic period, which begins at fertilization and continues for approximately 3 weeks, is characterized by the development of the bilaminar germ disc. After the fertilized ovum reaches the 16-cell stage through mitosis, the inner cell mass cavitates to form the blastocyst by day 4 (Figure 1-1 and Plate 1-1). During the second week, the blastocyst is embedded in the endometrial stroma. The inner cell mass, which by this stage is concentrated at one pole of the blastocyst, will give rise to the embryo proper and is called the *embryoblast*. The embryoblast forms the bilaminar germ disc by differentiating into the cuboidal hypoblast layer adjacent to the blastocyst cavity and the columnar epiblast layer dorsal to it, which in turn cavitates to form the amniotic cavity. The bilaminar germ disc is converted to the trilaminar germ disc during the next stage, the embryonic period.[13]

THE EMBRYONIC PERIOD (WEEKS 3 TO 8)

The third week of gestation is characterized by the processes of gastrulation and neurulation. *Gastrulation* is the process of the formation of all three embryonic germ layers: ectoderm, mesoderm, and endoderm.[13] *Neurulation*, which is initiated in the latter half of the third week, is a process of folding that converts the neural plate, a thickening of the ectoderm overlying the notochord, to the neural tube[9] (Figure 1-2 and Plate 1-2). Gastrulation is heralded by the formation of the primitive streak on the surface of the epiblast. The primitive streak is a linear proliferative zone of uncommitted cells that forms within the epiblast. At the cephalic end of the primitive streak is a slightly elevated area called the *primitive node*, which surrounds the primitive pit. The epiblast cells then migrate toward the streak and invaginate underneath it to form the endoderm. Other cells that come to lie between the endoderm and epiblast form the mesoderm, and the superficial epiblast cells form the ectoderm. The endoderm at the cephalic edge thickens to form an oval area of vesicular cells called the *prechordal plate*. The cells that migrate from the cranial end of the streak form the paraxial mesoderm. The cells that migrate from the midregion of the streak form the intermediate mesoderm, and the cells that migrate from the caudal part form the lateral plate mesoderm. Each of these three germ layers gives origin to specific tissues and organs under the influence of various stimulatory and inhibitory genes and the proteins elaborated by them.[9,13]

Notochord

From the primitive pit, a rod-like process of cells called the *notochordal process* moves cranially up to the prechordal plate by day 20. The notochordal process, which is the precursor of the skeletal axis, becomes canalized and caudally breaks through the ectodermal surface at the primitive node. The tube then opens ventrally starting at the level of the pit and proceeds cephalad. The

---

PREEMBRYONIC PERIOD

- Weeks 0 to 3
- Embryoblast forms the bilaminar germ disc, which then forms the trilaminar germ disc

---

EMBRYONIC PERIOD

- Weeks 3 to 8
- Most active period:
  - Formation of organ systems
  - Developmental anomalies occur during this period
- Gastrulation: formation of endoderm, mesoderm, and ectoderm
- Neurulation: process of folding that results in formation of neural tube
- Formation of notochord, neural crest, and somites
- Formation of the three brain vesicles:
  - Prosencephalon (future forebrain)
  - Mesencephalon (future midbrain)
  - Rhombencephalon (future hindbrain)
- Development of cervical and cephalic flexure

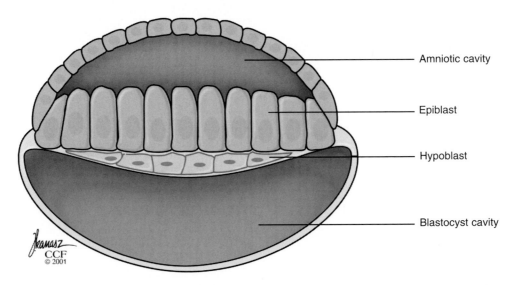

Figure 1-1. (See Plate 1-1.) Formation of bilaminar germ disc from the embryoblast. The epiblast is adjacent to the amniotic cavity, and the hypoblast is adjacent to the blastocyst cavity. *(Courtesy Cleveland Clinic, Division of Education, © 2001.)*

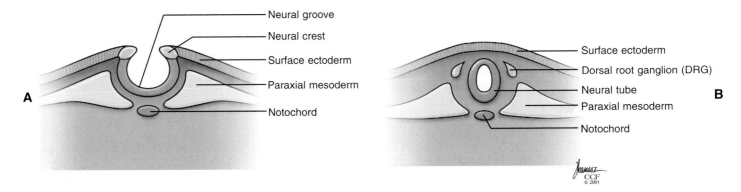

Figure 1-2. (See Plate 1-2.) Formation of neural tube and dorsal root ganglion (axial view). **A,** Elevation of ectoderm creates neural folds that invaginate and ultimately fuse to form a neural tube. **B,** Neural crest cells form from lateral edges of these neuroectodermal cells, migrate toward the underlying mesoderm, and give rise to cranial nerve ganglia, spinal ganglia, and dorsal root ganglia (DRG). *(Courtesy Cleveland Clinic, Division of Education, © 2001.)*

yolk sac therefore transiently communicates with the amniotic cavity through the opening at the pit called the *neurenteric canal* (Figure 1-3 and Plate 1-3). After the tube opens, it is converted to a central ventral bar of mesoderm called the *notochordal plate*, which detaches from the endoderm by day 22 to 24 and becomes entirely contained within the mesoderm. It then forms a solid cylinder of cells to form the definitive notochord.[13]

Neurulation

At the initiation of neurulation, the notochord and prechordal mesoderm cause the overlying ectoderm to thicken and to form the neural plate. This tongue-shaped structure elongates gradually toward the primi-tive streak, and by the end of the third week, the lateral edges of this plate become elevated to form the neural folds, which surround the neural groove. The neural folds fuse in the midline in the region of the embryo's future neck. The fusion gradually proceeds cephalad and caudad, thereby forming the neural tube. The two ends of the neural tube communicate with the amniotic cavity through openings called *neuropores*. The cranial neuropore closes by approximately day 25, and the caudal neuropore closes by approximately day 27. Neurulation is then completed. The closed neural tube has a narrow caudal portion representing the future spinal cord and a broad cephalic portion, with a number of dilatations called *brain vesicles*, representing the future brain. The primary brain vesicles are the *proencephalon* (the future

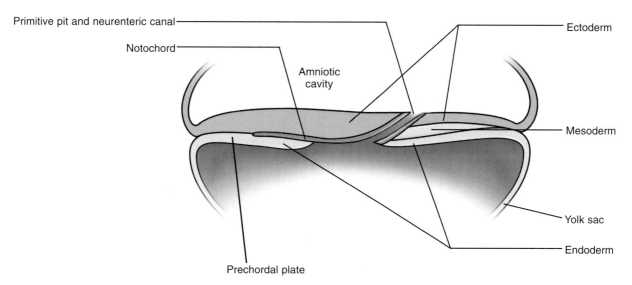

Primitive pit and neurenteric canal

Notochord

Amniotic cavity

Ectoderm

Mesoderm

Yolk sac

Endoderm

Prechordal plate

Figure 1-3. (See Plate 1-3.) Sagittal representation showing initial stages of formation of notochord. The notochordal process becomes canalized and breaks through the caudal aspect of the ectoderm. This allows transient communication between the yolk sac and the amniotic cavity through the neurenteric canal. *(Courtesy Cleveland Clinic, Division of Education, © 2001.)*

forebrain), the *mesencephalon* (the future midbrain), and the *rhombencephalon* (the future hindbrain). Two flexures develop: the cephalic flexure, in the region of the midbrain structure, and the cervical flexure, at the junction of the hindbrain structure and the spinal cord.[10,13]

Neural Crest

As the neural folds elevate and meet in the midline as described earlier, the cells at the lateral border, or "crest," of the folds migrate to enter the underlying mesoderm. These neuroectodermal cells undergo transition from epithelial to mesenchymal cells to form what are called the *neural crest cells* (see Figure 1-2 and Plate 1-2). The neural crest cells give rise to cranial nerve ganglia, spinal or dorsal root ganglia, the sympathetic chain and preaortic ganglia, parasympathetic ganglia, Schwann cells, glial cells, and leptomeninges (arachnoid and pia mater). In addition, they also give rise to the "C" cells of the thyroid, adrenal medulla, melanocytes, connective tissue and bones of face and skull, conotruncal septum in the heart, and odontoblasts and dermis in the face and neck.[13]

Paraxial Mesoderm

Along the length of the notochord, the mesenchyme becomes organized into three zones: the medial paraxial mesoderm, a narrower intermediate mesoderm, and the flattened lateral plate mesoderm. By the beginning of the third week, the paraxial mesoderm is organized into segments called *somitomeres*. The segmentation proceeds cephalocaudally. In the cephalic region, the somitomeres, in association with neural plate segmentation, form neuromeres, which contribute most of the head

mesenchyme. By day 20, somitomeres organize into somites, starting in the cervical region and proceeding at a rate of three pairs per day. By the end of week 5, there are 42 to 44 pairs of somites: 4 occipital, 8 cervical, 12 thoracic, 5 lumbar, 5 sacral, and 8 to 10 coccygeal. The first occipital and last five to seven coccygeal somites disappear, and the remainder form the axial skeleton.[9,10,13]

DEVELOPMENT AND OSSIFICATION OF VERTEBRAE

By the beginning of the fourth week, the somite undergoes further specialization into the sclerotome, myotome, and dermatome. The sclerotome develops first, through central cavitation of each newly formed somite, which then becomes filled with a loose population of core cells. The somite then ruptures medially, and the core cells, together with some cells from the ventromedial wall of the somite, remain adjacent to the notochord and neural tube (Figure 1-4 and Plate 1-4). This group of cells is called the *sclerotome*. The ventral portion of the sclerotome surrounds the notochord and represents the future vertebral body, whereas the dorsal portion surrounds the neural tube and represents the future posterior elements of the vertebrae. The concomitant expansion of the dorsolateral body wall involves cells from the dorsolateral aspect of the somite, which form the dermomyotome (Figure 1-4 and Plate 1-4). The dermomyotome differentiates into the spindle-shaped cells of the myotome medially and the epithelial cells of the dermatome laterally. The dermatomes give rise to the dermis of the neck, back, and ventral and lateral trunk. The myotomes further split into a dorsal epimere and a ventral hypomere. The epimeres form the deep epaxial muscles of the back, such as the erector

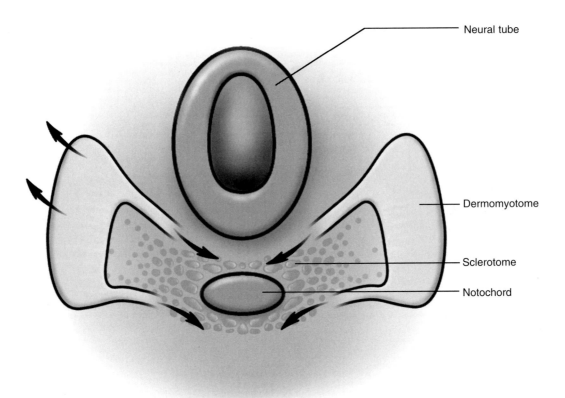

Figure 1-4. (See Plate 1-4.) Conversion of somite to sclerotome and dermatomyotome (axial view). The paraxial mesoderm organizes into segments called *somitomeres*, which subsequently become *somites* beginning by approximately day 20. Each somite undergoes further specialization into the sclerotome, myotome, and dermatome by the beginning of the fourth week. A portion of the *sclerotome* surrounds the notochord and becomes the vertebral body and posterior elements. The dorsolateral aspect of the somite forms the *dermomyotome*, which differentiates into the *myotome* medially and the *dermatome* laterally. The dermatomes give rise to the dermis of the neck, back, and ventral and lateral trunk, and the myotomes form the deep back muscles and abdominal muscles. *(Courtesy Cleveland Clinic, Division of Education, © 2001.)*

spinae, and the hypomeres form the lateral and ventral body wall of the thorax and abdomen, including the intercostals, the external oblique, the internal oblique, the tranversus abdominis, and the rectus abdominus muscles. Thus, each somite forms its own dermatome, myotome, and sclerotome with its own segmental nerve supply.[1,9,13]

The loose mesenchymal tissue of the sclerotome forms a cylindrical column called the *perichordal tube* that surrounds the notochord. Each sclerotome is divided into a cranial and a caudal part by a sclerotomic fissure (Figure 1-5 and Plate 1-5). The mesenchyme adjoining the fissure undergoes rapid cell proliferation to form dense cell aggregates called *dense perichordal discs*. Thus, each perichordal disc is flanked cranially and caudally by less dense, or "loose," cell aggregates (Figure 1-6 and Plate 1-6). The cranial half of one segment then fuses with the caudal half of the adjoining segment to form a loose perichordal disc, which gives rise to the primordium of the vertebral body, or centrum. Chondrogenesis begins at the center of the loose perichordal disc by constricting the notochordal tissue passing through it, which eventu-

ally disappears. The notochordal cells, however, remain at the center of the dense perichordal discs, which is the precursor of the future intervertebral disc.[9,12,13]

The segmental nerve, which originally lay at the center of the sclerotome, comes to lie between adjacent centra and opposite the intervertebral disc, in the fully developed vertebral column, whereas the segmental vessels ultimately come to lie over the middle of the centrum[1,9,12,13] (see Figure 1-5 and Plate 1-5).

A rapid cell proliferation at the ventrolateral aspect of the sclerotome results in the formation of the rib primordium, or costal process. Caudal to this, the cells of the remaining part of the sclerotome form the membranous precursor of the neural arch elements. The neural arch anlagen thus forms in the caudal part of the caudal hemisclerotome. The neural arch primordium contributes substantially to the formation of the vertebral body, especially in the cervical region, where it may contribute as much as half the body mass. In the precartilaginous stage, the sclerotome that aligns itself along the notochord and the neural tube form the membranous vertebral column. Chondrification results in a

---

DEVELOPMENT AND OSSIFICATION OF VERTEBRAE

- Formation of sclerotome, myotome, and dermatome from somite.
- Each typical vertebra is ossified by three primary ossification centers: Two for the neural arch and one for the centrum.
- Secondary ossification centers develop by the fifteenth or sixteenth year of life.
- Two primary curvatures (thoracic and pelvic) and two secondary curvatures (cervical and lumbar) develop.
- Primary curves are kyphotic; secondary curves are lordotic.

---

cartilaginous vertebral column, and endochondral ossification produces the definitive bony vertebral column. Each centrum is chondrified from a pair of centers, which appear at the sixth week and coalesce shortly thereafter. Each half of the neural arch is chondrified from a center at its base, which extends ventrally to the pedicles and dorsally to the laminae. The laminar centers meet in the midline by the fourth month. The costal processes chondrify separately. As chondrification and subsequent ossification proceed, a cartilaginous connection, known as the *neurocentral synchondrosis*, demarcates the ossified neural arch from the ossified centra. The neurocentral synchondrosis is ossified late in fetal life, beginning with the upper lumbar vertebrae. It is situated anterior to the pedicles and lies within the vertebral body, being most medially located in the cervical and sacral regions. This may on occasion lead to difficulty in differentiating from a traumatic defect of the axis in early childhood.[9,12,14,15,18]

Intervertebral Disc and Notochord

After the notochord is ensheathed in perichordal mesenchyme, a series of undulations, or "chordaflexures," appear that are related to the dense and loose perichordal discs. This is thought to be due to a differential rate of transverse growth between the dense and loose perichordal disc areas. As a result, fusiform enlargements appear in the areas encircled by the dense perichordal discs. As the loose perichordal disc areas undergo chondrification and develop into the early vertebral bodies, the expanded notochordal segments within the developing intervertebral discs are drawn farther apart, stretching the chord tissue into a "mucoid streak" that eventually disappears before the formation of the definitive vertebral body (see Figure 1-6). The notochord is, therefore, a major contributor to the nucleus pulposus, which constitutes 15% of the fully developed disc. The notochord cells may remain viable up to 5 years of age. They have also been shown to remain viable within the discs of the sacrum in specimens 22 to 45 years old.[9,13,16,18,20]

Toward the end of the embryonic period, the developing disc shows an external fibrous zone, an intermediate fibrocartilaginous zone, and an internal hyaline zone adjacent to the notochord. The more peripheral layers of the annulus are embedded into the outer rim of the cartilaginous plate, with the most external lamellae showing fibrous attachments to the longitudinal ligaments. Toward the end of the first decade of life, the circumferential portion of the cartilaginous plate becomes ossified to form the ring apophysis, with outer annular fibers becoming deeply incorporated in this structure. Before the ring apophysis fuses with the vertebral body by the end of the second decade, the vessels that supply nutrition to the plate and, via diffusion, to the intervertebral disc enter through the interval between the ring apophysis and the vertebral body. The plexus of vessels found within the connective tissues surrounding the annulus play an important role in disc nutrition in both fetal and adult life. The deeper portions of the disc probably never vascularize and therefore depend on diffusional nutrition. This is mediated by radially arranged specialized vascular glomeruli, which enter the cartilaginous end of the 30-week-old vertebra at its periphery and are directed toward the developing disc.[12,17,18]

Ossification of Vertebrae

Each typical vertebra has three primary ossification centers: one for the centrum and one for each half of the vertebral arch (Figure 1-7 and Plate 1-7). At approximately the ninth week, the chondrous centrum is invaded by pericostal vessels, which produce ventral and dorsal vascular lacunae to support the ossification. Thus the single ossification center for the centrum initially shows dorsal and ventral components, which later unify into a single ossification center. These centers usually appear first in the lower thoracic and upper lumbar regions and develop more rapidly in the caudal than in the cranial vertebrae. The centrum occasionally ossifies from two centers. When one of these is suppressed, a wedge-shaped hemivertebrae may develop.[18]

The vertebral arch ossification centers appear first in the cervical region by approximately the eighth week. Two such centers appear, one for each half of the neural arch. The arch segments and the centra fuse at the site of the neurocentral synchondrosis, anterior to the pedicles. In the first year of life, the neural arch elements unite, initially in the lumbar region and then in the thoracic and cervical regions. In the upper cervical region, the centra unite with the arches by the third year, whereas in the lower lumbar region, union is not completed until the sixth year.[18]

By the fifteenth or sixteenth year of life, secondary centers of ossification appear at the tips of the transverse processes and within the spinous process. Two annular epiphyseal discs for the circumferential parts of the upper and lower surfaces of the body also develop. These fuse with the rest of the vertebra by the middle of the third decade. The costal articular facets are extensions of the annular epiphyseal discs. In the bifid spinous process of the seventh cervical vertebra, there are two such secondary centers. The lower cervical and upper lumbar vertebrae may show an additional costal

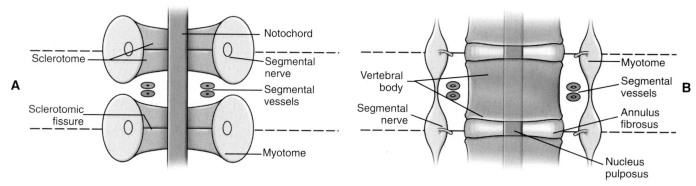

Figure 1-5. (See Plate 1-5.) Coronal representation of formation of the vertebral column from adjacent sclerotome segments. **A,** Each sclerotome is divided by sclerotomic fissure into a cranial and a caudal portion. The cranial half of one sclerotome segment fuses with the caudal half of the adjoining segment, ultimately giving rise to the primordium of the vertebral body (centrum). **B,** Some of the notochordal tissue eventually disappears, whereas other notochordal cells remain and become the precursor of the intervertebral disc. The segmental nerve, which was originally located at the center of the sclerotome, comes to lie between adjacent centra, opposite the intervertebral disc. The segmental vessels come to lie over the middle of the centrum. *(Courtesy Cleveland Clinic, Division of Education, © 2001.)*

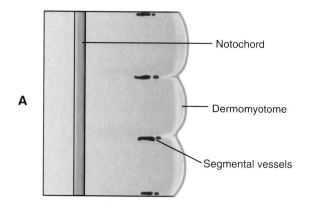

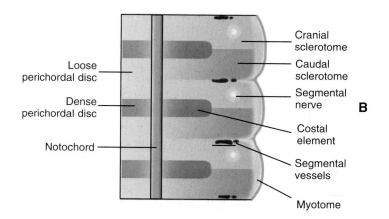

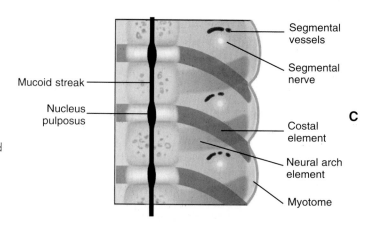

Figure 1-6. (See Plate 1-6.) Schematic representation of mammalian vertebrae development. **A,** Notochord is surrounded by axial mesenchyme with the segmental vessels located between adjacent sclerotomes. The dermomyotome forms from the dorsolateral aspect of the somite. **B,** Differentiation of axial mesenchyme into *dense* perichordal disc, which becomes the intervertebral disc, and *loose* perichordal disc, which becomes the centrum. The costal element is located lateral to the future intervertebral disc. Note the relationship of the segmental vessels to the future centrum: they originally lie between adjacent sclerotomes but ultimately come to lie at the mid-point of the centrum, which is composed of cranial and caudal portions of adjacent sclerotomes. **C,** Differentiation of notochord into the mucoid streak and the nucleus pulposus. The notochordal cells at the center of the dense perichordal disc persist as the precursor of the future intervertebral disc (nucleus pulposus). *(Courtesy Cleveland Clinic, Division of Education, © 2001.)*

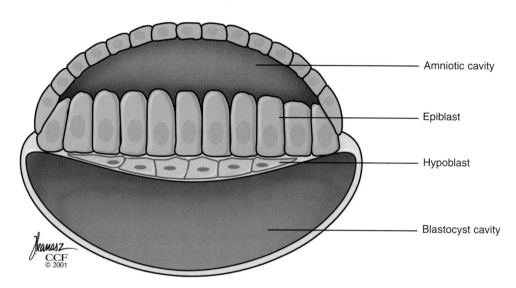

Plate 1-1. Formation of bilaminar germ disc from the embryoblast. The epiblast is adjacent to the amniotic cavity, and the hypoblast is adjacent to the blastocyst cavity. *(Courtesy Cleveland Clinic, Division of Education, © 2001.)*

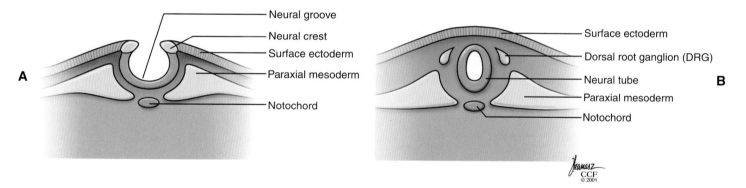

Plate 1-2. Formation of neural tube and dorsal root ganglion (axial view). **A,** Elevation of ectoderm creates neural folds that invaginate and ultimately fuse to form a neural tube. **B,** Neural crest cells form from lateral edges of these neuroectodermal cells, migrate toward the underlying mesoderm, and give rise to cranial nerve ganglia, spinal ganglia, and dorsal root ganglia (DRG). *(Courtesy Cleveland Clinic, Division of Education, © 2001.)*

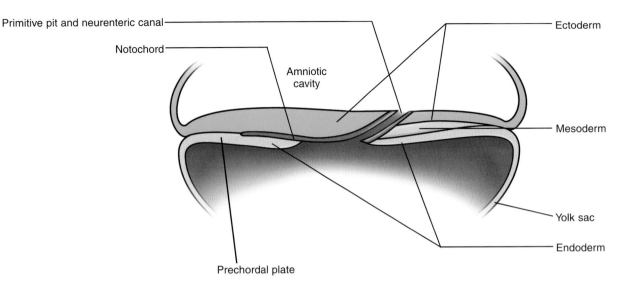

Plate 1-3. Sagittal representation showing initial stages of formation of notochord. The notochordal process becomes canalized and breaks through the caudal aspect of the ectoderm. This allows transient communication between the yolk sac and the amniotic cavity through the neurenteric canal. (*Courtesy Cleveland Clinic, Division of Education, © 2001.*)

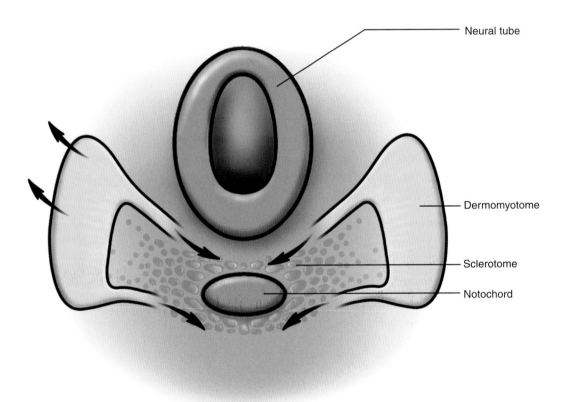

Plate 1-4. Conversion of somite to sclerotome and dermatomyotome (axial view). The paraxial mesoderm organizes into segments called *somitomeres*, which subsequently become *somites* beginning by approximately day 20. Each somite undergoes further specialization into the sclerotome, myotome, and dermatome by the beginning of the fourth week. A portion of the *sclerotome* surrounds the notochord and becomes the vertebral body and posterior elements. The dorsolateral aspect of the somite forms the *dermomyotome*, which differentiates into the *myotome* medially and the *dermatome* laterally. The dermatomes give rise to the dermis of the neck, back, and ventral and lateral trunk, and the myotomes form the deep back muscles and abdominal muscles. (*Courtesy Cleveland Clinic, Division of Education, © 2001.*)

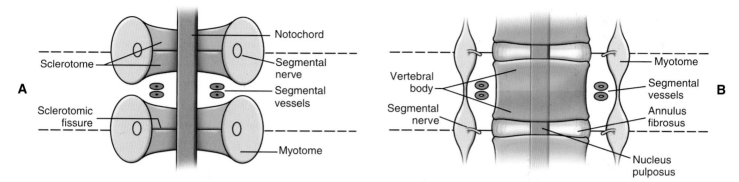

Plate 1-5. Coronal representation of formation of the vertebral column from adjacent sclerotome segments. **A,** Each sclerotome is divided by sclerotomic fissure into a cranial and a caudal portion. The cranial half of one sclerotome segment fuses with the caudal half of the adjoining segment, ultimately giving rise to the primordium of the vertebral body (centrum). **B,** Some of the notochordal tissue eventually disappears, whereas other notochordal cells remain and become the precursor of the intervertebral disc. The segmental nerve, which was originally located at the center of the sclerotome, comes to lie between adjacent centra, opposite the intervertebral disc. The segmental vessels come to lie over the middle of the centrum. *(Courtesy Cleveland Clinic, Division of Education, © 2001.)*

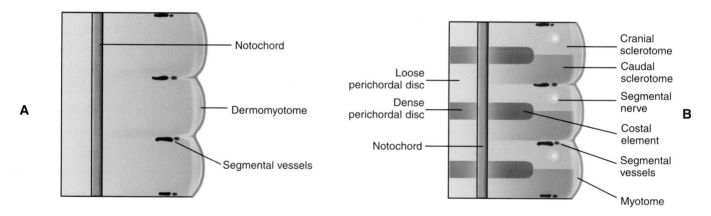

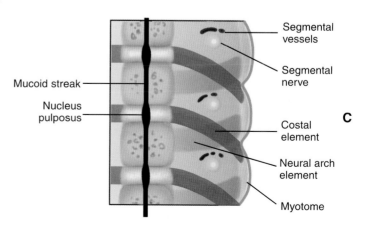

Plate 1-6. Schematic representation of mammalian vertebrae development. **A,** Notochord is surrounded by axial mesenchyme with the segmental vessels located between adjacent sclerotomes. The dermomyotome forms from the dorsolateral aspect of the somite. **B,** Differentiation of axial mesenchyme into *dense* perichordal disc, which becomes the intervertebral disc, and *loose* perichordal disc, which becomes the centrum. The costal element is located lateral to the future intervertebral disc. Note the relationship of the segmental vessels to the future centrum: they originally lie between adjacent sclerotomes but ultimately come to lie at the mid-point of the centrum, which is composed of cranial and caudal portions of adjacent sclerotomes. **C,** Differentiation of notochord into the mucoid streak and the nucleus pulposus. The notochordal cells at the center of the dense perichordal disc persist as the precursor of the future intervertebral disc (nucleus pulposus). *(Courtesy Cleveland Clinic, Division of Education, © 2001.)*

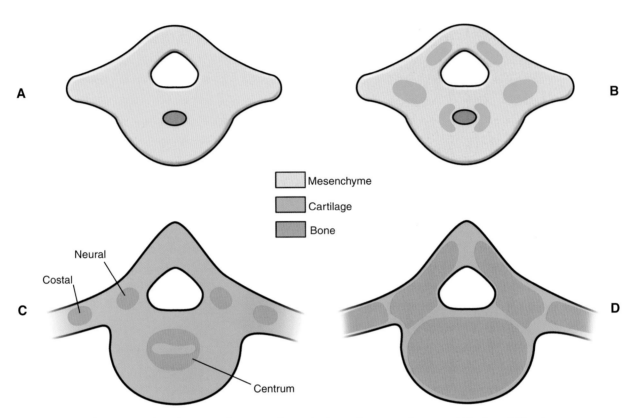

A

B

Mesenchyme

Cartilage

Bone

Neural

Costal

C

Centrum

D

Plate 1-7. Developmental stages of a typical vertebra: membranous **(A)**, chondrification **(B)**, ossification **(C)**, and at birth **(D)**. The sclerotome that surrounds the notochord forms the membranous vertebral column. This is converted to a cartilaginous model via the process of chondrification, in which the cartilaginous centrum is formed by two centers and each half of the neural arch is formed by one center. Each costal process is chondrified separately. *(Courtesy Cleveland Clinic, Division of Education, © 2001.)*

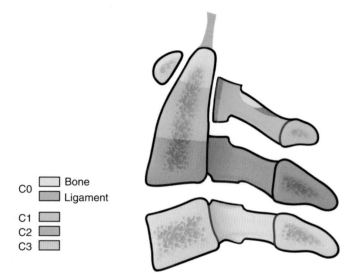

C0 ☐ Bone
☐ Ligament

C1 ☐
C2 ☐
C3 ☐

Plate 1-8. Formation of the atlantoaxial complex. Three sclerotome segments contribute to the formation of the atlantoaxial complex: the proatlas (C0), the atlas (C1), and the axis (C2). The *proatlas* (C0) forms the tip of the odontoid process, the anterior arch of C1, the dorsal aspect of the superior facet of C1, the upper portion of the transverse ligament, the apical odontoid ligament, and the retroarticular ligaments. The *atlas* (C1) sclerotome forms the remainder of the posterior arch of C1 and the remaining inferior portion of the odontoid, which represents the body (centrum) of the atlas. The *axis* (C2) sclerotome forms the posterior arch, the body, and the lateral masses of C2. *(Courtesy Cleveland Clinic, Division of Education, © 2001.)*

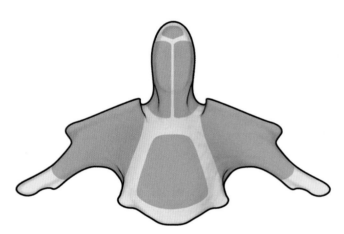

Plate 1-9. The ossification centers of the axis. The arch is formed from two primary ossification centers and the centrum from a single center. The dens is ossified from two laterally placed ossification centers that unite just before birth. The tip of the odontoid is ossified by a separate center that appears in the second year of life and unites with the remaining portion of the odontoid by the twelvth year. *(Courtesy Cleveland Clinic, Division of Education, © 2001.)*

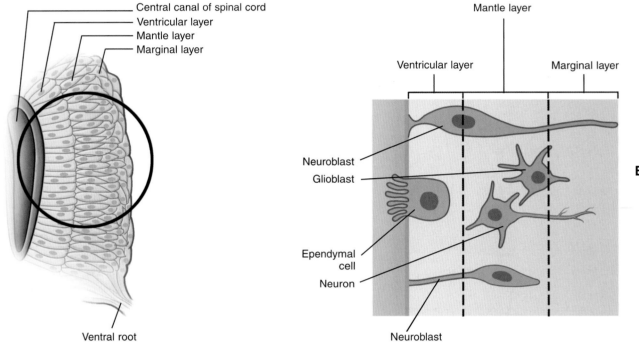

Central canal of spinal cord
Ventricular layer
Mantle layer
Marginal layer

A

Ventral root

Mantle layer

Ventricular layer

Marginal layer

B

Neuroblast
Glioblast

Ependymal
cell

Neuron

Neuroblast

Plate 1-10.   Schematic representation of the development of the central nervous system (**B** represents the enlarged circular area of **A**). Neuroepithelial cells surrounding the neural tube proliferate to form the deep *ventricular layer*, which gives rise to neurons, glial cells, and ependymal cells. These cells migrate peripherally to form the *mantle layer*, which forms the gray matter. Neuronal processes from these cells grow peripherally to form the *marginal layer*, which has no cell bodies and gives rise to the white matter of the central nervous system. (*Courtesy Cleveland Clinic, Division of Education, © 2001.*)

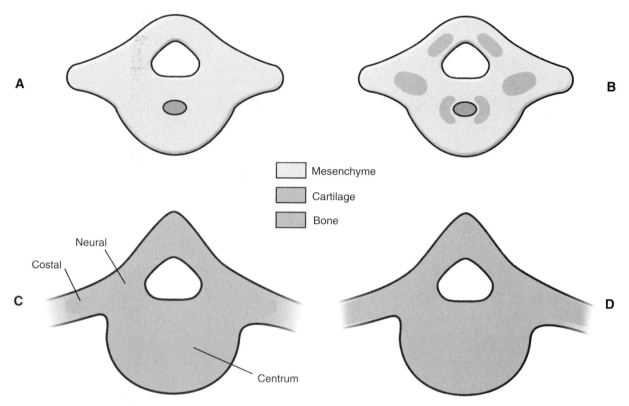

Mesenchyme
Cartilage
Bone

Neural
Costal
Centrum

Figure 1-7. (See Plate 1-7.) Developmental stages of a typical vertebra: membranous **(A)**, chondrification **(B)**, ossification **(C)**, and at birth **(D)**. The sclerotome that surrounds the notochord forms the membranous vertebral column. This is converted to a cartilaginous model via the process of chondrification, in which the cartilaginous centrum is formed by two centers and each half of the neural arch is formed by one center. Each costal process is chondrified separately. *(Courtesy Cleveland Clinic, Division of Education, © 2001.)*

center of ossification, which may produce additional ribs.[18]

The occipital region, the atlantoaxial complex, the sacrum, and the coccyx are the exceptions to the above description. The occipital region is of somitic origin and is derived from four occipital myotomes. The atlanto-axial complex has a complex multisegmental origin (Figures 1-8 and 1-9 and Plates 1-8 and 1-9). The C0 sclerotome, or proatlas, gives rise to the tip of the odontoid process, the anterior arch of the atlas, the dorsal part of the superior atlas facet, the upper half of the transverse ligament, the apical odontoid ligament, and the retroarticular ligaments. The C1 sclerotome, or atlas, gives rise to the remainder of the atlas and the inferior major part of the odontoid process, which is considered to represent the body or centrum of the atlas. The atlas shows an ossification center in each lateral mass at about the seventh week that gradually extends into the posterior arch, where they unite between the third and fourth years. A separate center appears in the anterior arch toward the end of the first year, which unites with lateral masses between the sixth and eighth years. The vertebral arch of the axis is ossified from two primary centers appearing at the seventh or eighth week and the centrum from a center appearing at the fourth or fifth month. The dens is ossified from two laterally placed

centers appearing at the sixth month and uniting just before birth (see Figure 1-9 and Plate 1-9). At the tip of the odontoid process, a center appears at the second year and unites with the main mass by the twelvth year. The base of the odontoid is separated from the body of the axis by a cartilaginous disc, the circumference of which is ossified, although the center remains cartilaginous until advanced age. The proximal aspect of the odontoid occasionally fails to unite with the rest of the axis and may persist as an "os odontoideum." The most caudal occipital somite, the ante-proatlas, occasionally forms the third condyle at the basion or anterior midline point of the foramen magnum to articulate with the tip of the odontoid. A more frank separation of this ante-proatlas segment may in fact result in the formation of a true occipital vertebra proximal to the C1 segment.[12,18]

In the sacrum, the central centers for the proximal three sacral segments appear by week 9, whereas the centers for the fourth and fifth segments do not appear until the twenty-fourth week. The neural arch has bilateral ossification centers similar to a typical vertebra. Between the twenty-fourth and thirty-second week, six additional ossification centers appear anterolateral to the anterior sacral foramina of the upper three sacral segments, and these give rise to the sacral alae. The alae represent the costal elements of a typical vertebra.

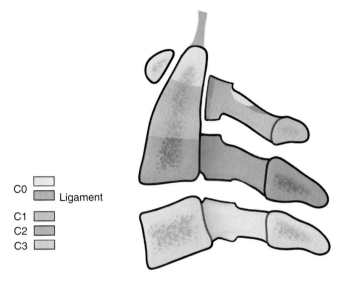

C0 ☐
☐ Ligament
C1 ☐
C2 ☐
C3 ☐

Figure 1-8. (See Plate 1-8.) Formation of the atlantoaxial complex. Three sclerotome segments contribute to the formation of the atlantoaxial complex: the proatlas (C0), the atlas (C1), and the axis (C2). The *proatlas* (C0) forms the tip of the odontoid process, the anterior arch of C1, the dorsal aspect of the superior facet of C1, the upper portion of the transverse ligament, the apical odontoid ligament, and the retroarticular ligaments. The *atlas* (C1) sclerotome forms the remainder of the posterior arch of C1 and the remaining inferior portion of the odontoid, which represents the body (centrum) of the atlas. The *axis* (C2) sclerotome forms the posterior arch, the body, and the lateral masses of C2. *(Courtesy Cleveland Clinic, Division of Education, © 2001.)*

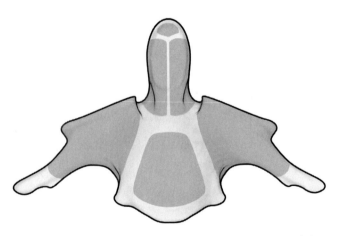

Figure 1-9. (See Plate 1-9.) The ossification centers of the axis. The arch is formed from two primary ossification centers and the centrum from a single center. The dens is ossified from two laterally placed ossification centers that unite just before birth. The tip of the odontoid is ossified by a separate center that appears in the second year of life and unites with the remaining portion of the odontoid by the twelfth year. *(Courtesy Cleveland Clinic, Division of Education, © 2001.)*

DEVELOPMENT OF THE NERVOUS SYSTEM

- Central nervous system development
  - Ventricular layer (formation of neuroblasts, glioblasts, and ependymal cells)
  - Mantle layer (formation of gray matter)
  - Marginal layer (formation of white matter)
- Peripheral nervous system development
  - Spinal neural crest cells form dorsal root ganglia, postganglionic parasympathetic neurons, sympathetic chain ganglia, and other supportive structures (e.g., pia mater, arachnoid and glial cells)

Between the eighteenth and twentieth years, lateral epiphyseal plates appear on the articular surfaces of the sacral alae. By the middle of the third decade, the entire sacrum is usually fused.[12,18]

The coccyx lacks neural arch elements and forms a single ossific center for each of the bodies. The first of these appears before the age of 5 years, and the next three ossify over the ensuing 5-year intervals.[18]

Curvatures of the Spine

When viewed in profile, the spine has two *primary curves*: the thoracic curvature and the pelvic curvature. These are concave ventrally during fetal life and maintain their kyphotic alignment after birth. The thoracic curve extends from the 2nd to the 12th thoracic vertebrae and is caused by the greater height of the posterior parts of the vertebral bodies. The pelvic curve extends from the lumbosacral joint to the apex of the coccyx.[18]

The cervical and lumbar curves on the other hand are *secondary*, or compensatory, curves and are lordotic (convex ventrally). The cervical curve, which is the least pronounced, extends from the atlas to the second thoracic vertebra and develops late in intrauterine life. The lumbar curve extends from the 12th thoracic vertebra to the lumbosacral junction and is caused by both the greater height of the anterior part of the intervertebral discs and the shape of the vertebral bodies. The lumbar curve appears at about 12 to 18 months of age when the child begins to walk and is required to align the center of gravity of the trunk above the legs.[18]

DEVELOPMENT OF THE NERVOUS SYSTEM
Central Nervous System

The proliferation of the layer of neuroepithelial cells surrounding the neural tube gives rise to neurons, some glial cells, and the ependymal cells that line the central canal of the spinal cord and the ventricles of the brain. This layer is called the *ventricular layer*, the most central (deepest) portion of which contains neuroblasts, which are precursors of the neurons of the central nervous system and are formed on day 24. These migrate peripherally to form the mantle layer outside the ventricular layer, which develops into the gray matter. Neuronal processes grow more peripherally from these to form the

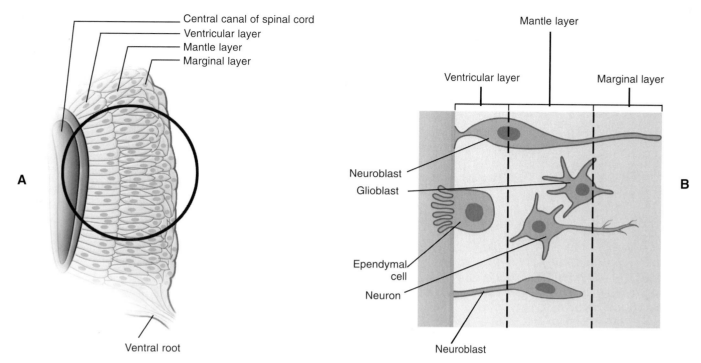

Figure 1-10. (See Plate 1-10.) Schematic representation of the development of the central nervous system (**B** represents the enlarged circular area of **A**). Neuroepithelial cells surrounding the neural tube proliferate to form the deep *ventricular layer*, which gives rise to neurons, glial cells, and ependymal cells. These cells migrate peripherally to form the *mantle layer*, which forms the gray matter. Neuronal processes from these cells grow peripherally to form the *marginal layer*, which has no cell bodies and gives rise to the white matter of the central nervous system. (*Courtesy Cleveland Clinic, Division of Education, © 2001.*)

marginal layer, which has no neuronal cell bodies and gives rise to the white matter of the central nervous system[9,10] (Figure 1-10 and Plate 1-10).

Once neuroblast production ceases, the neuroepithelial cells form glioblasts, which then develop into the different types of glial cells, such as astrocytes and oligodendrocytes. Finally, the neuroepithelial cells differentiate into the ependymal cells.

Differential thickening of the lateral walls of the spinal cord results in the formation of a longitudinal groove on either side of the cord, called the *sulcus limitans*. This separates the dorsal part of the developing spinal cord, called the *alar plate*, from the ventral part, called the *basal plate*. The alar plate and basal plate are associated with afferent and efferent functions, respectively, in the fully developed spinal cord. The alar plate gives rise to the dorsal columns of the spinal cord, and the basal plate gives rise to the ventral and lateral gray columns.[9,10]

The spinal cord initially occupies the entire length of the vertebral canal, but due to the relatively more rapid growth of the bony canal and dura, the spinal cord comes to rest farther proximally (ascensis spinalis). Thus, by 6 months of fetal age, it is at the level of the first sacral vertebra; by birth, it is at the second or third lumbar level; and by adulthood, it usually terminates at the inferior border of the first lumbar vertebra. As a result of this differential growth of the spinal cord, the nerve roots run obliquely from the cord to the corresponding level of the vertebral column. The roots inferior and distal to the conus medullaris form the cauda equina.[9,10]

The pia mater extends distally from the conus medullaris to the first coccygeal segment and represents the line of regression of the embryonic spinal cord. The dura and arachnoid terminate at the level of the second sacral vertebra in adults.[9,10]

Peripheral Nervous System

The dorsal root ganglia are derived from the spinal neural crest cells. These cells form small clumps in the space between the neural tube and the somites dorsally before differentiating into segmental dorsal root ganglia. There is some experimental evidence that the differentiation of these ganglia is mediated by brain-derived neural growth factor, a protein secreted by the adjacent neural tube. Dorsal root ganglia develop bilaterally at each segmental level except the first cervical and the second and third coccygeal levels, resulting in 7 cervical, 12 thoracic, 5 lumbar, and 1 coccygeal pair.[9,10]

Postganglionic parasympathetic neurons, as well as peripheral motor neurons supplying the gut tube from esophagus to the rectum, are derived from the occipito-cervical and sacral neural crests.[9,10]

Spinal cord neural crest cells that migrate to an area ventral to the future dorsal root ganglia form a series of condensations before developing into the ganglia of the sympathetic chain. In the cervical region, three ganglia develop; in the coccygeal region, one ganglion develops; and in the thoracic, lumbar, and sacral regions, the number of ganglia corresponds to the number of somites. One pair of preaortic ganglia originates from the cervical neural crest. Ganglia formed in association with the mesenteric arteries and renal arteries are developed from the thoracic and lumbar neural crest cells. The development of these ganglia may be mediated by insulin-like growth factor.[9,10]

Spinal neural crest cells also give rise to support and protective structures, such as the pia and arachnoid of the spinal cord and the glial cells of the ganglia. Some of these cells also give rise to Schwann cells, which form the myelin sheaths of peripheral nerves.[9,10]

APPLIED EMBRYOLOGY AND CLINICAL IMPLICATIONS
Neural Tube Closure Defects

A failure of the neural tube to close normally is called *spinal dysraphism*. Dysraphism may involve either the cranial or caudal neuropore and therefore may result in either cranial or lumbosacral defects. Neural tube defects usually occur during the third week of development. A failure in distal closure causes the vertebral neural arches to be underdeveloped or unfused in the midline. This may result in an open vertebral canal, which is called *spina bifida*. The mildest variant of this condition is *spina bifida occulta*, whereby the vertebral arches of a single vertebra fails to fuse, but there is normal differentiation of the underlying neural tube. Spina bifida occulta is more common in the lumbosacral spine. The defect is sometimes associated with an overlying sacral tuft of hair, angioma, pigmented nevus, or dimple. Spina bifida occulta may represent a normal variation and occurs at the L5 to S1 level in approximately 10% of the population.[2,9,10]

The more severe cases of spinal dysraphism are collectively called *spina bifida cystica* and occur in approximately 1 in 1000 births. When the dura and arachnoid protrude through the vertebral canal, a meningocele results. If neural tissue is included in the protrusion, it is called a *meningomyelocele*. Meningomyeloceles are more common in the lumbar and sacral areas, and the spinal cord and the spinal nerves of the involved segments may not develop normally. This may result in severe anomalies of the pelvic organs and legs. Spina bifida cystica is sometimes associated with hydrocephalus.[2,9,10]

A defect in cranial neuropore closure results in an exposed mass of dorsal undifferentiated neural tissue called exencephaly, anencephaly, or craniorachischisis. *Exencephaly* refers to the presence of exposed brain tissue of the embryo. This abnormal tissue undergoes degeneration, resulting in a spongy, vascular mass consisting mainly of hindbrain structures. This condition is referred to as *anencephaly*. Anencephalic embryos usually die at term or shortly after birth. The entire spectrum of closure defects involving the cranial neuropore is also referred to as *craniorachischisis*. A closure defect occurring

---

> ### APPLIED EMBRYOLOGY
>
> - Skeletal anomalies
>   - C1 ring and odontoid anomalies
>   - Basilar impression
>   - Occipitocervical synostosis
>   - Congenital spinal deformity
>   - Defects in formation
>   - Defects in segmentation
>   - Limbic vertebrae
>   - Accessory ribs
> - Neural tube closure defects (spinal dysraphism)
> - Hydrocephalus
> - Herniation of the brain
> - Chiari malformation
> - Chordoma

distally in the spinal cord is called *rachischisis* or *myeloschisis*. This is often not fatal, although neural dysfunction results. Failure of the neural tube to close in the occiput and upper cervical spine is called *inionschisis*.[3,9-11]

In more severe closure defects, the neural tube may not only fail to fuse but may also fail to differentiate or separate from the surface ectoderm. This can result in a condition called *craniorachischisis totalis*, in which the brain and the spinal cord are exposed and degenerate. This usually results in spontaneous abortion.[9,10]

Neural tube defects have been found to be associated with use of the antiepileptic drug valproic acid and with maternal diabetes and hypothermia. Valproic acid is thought to interfere with folate metabolism, and folate administration during pregnancy reduces the risk of neural tube defects.[2,9,10]

Severe neural tube defects are associated with high α-fetoprotein levels in the amniotic fluid and may be detected with amniocentesis. The fetal vertebral column can also be assessed at 8 to 12 weeks with ultrasound for neural tube closure defects of a severe nature.[9,10]

Hydrocephalus

Disruption of the normal flow of cerebrospinal fluid through the central nervous system may result in obstructive hydrocephalus. In congenital aqueductal stenosis, the cerebral aqueduct is severely narrowed, commonly from fetal viral infection (e.g., cytomegalovirus) or infection with the protozoan *Toxoplasma gondii* or less commonly as an X-linked recessive trait. The cerebral aqueduct is the narrow channel of communication between the third ventricle and the fourth ventricle of the brain. Narrowing at this level results in the dilatation of the more proximal lateral and third ventricles. If the apertures of the fourth ventricle are blocked, all of the ventricles are dilated.[10]

Herniation of the Brain

Occasionally, fully differentiated brain and meninges protrude through an unossified gap in the cranium, resulting in a meningoencephalocele. If the ventricular cisternae are also included in this herniation, it is called a *meningohydroencephalocele*.[10]

Chiari Malformation

This condition is associated with abnormally small posterior cranial fossae and herniation of the cerebellum through the foramen magnum into the vertebral canal. There may be an associated hydrocephalus where there is interference with absorption of cerebrospinal fluid. This condition occurs in 1 in 1000 births and may also be associated with spina bifida with meningomyelocele and spina bifida with myeloschisis.[10]

Chordoma

These neoplasms develop from the remnants of the notochord and may arise anywhere along the tract of the original notochord, although they are more common in the caudal and cephalic ends. One third of these arise in the base of the skull and nasopharynx, and the remainder are nearly exclusively in the lumbosacral area. These usually appear in the fourth decade of life, are slow growing, are locally invasive, and can metastasize.[10]

Babinski Response

In the adult, the Babinski response is an abnormal clinical finding that typically signifies spinal cord compression. In infants, however, it may be present as a normal finding. This is thought to be due to the immaturity of their developing nervous system, which, at birth, has not completed the myelination process. Thus, this response in infants is mediated by a different mechanism from that of the pathologic reflex seen in later life and is not considered clinically significant until the end of the second year.[7]

Accessory Ribs

Accessory ribs may develop from the costal processes of lower cervical or upper lumbar vertebrae. An extra lumbar rib typically causes no clinical symptoms, whereas a cervical rib, which occurs in 0.5% to 1% of the population and arises from the seventh cervical vertebra, may cause pressure on the brachial plexus and subclavian artery. In these cases, a cervical rib is rudimentary and may be present as only a fibrous band.[9,12]

Basilar Impression

Basilar impression is a deformity of the base of the skull characterized by cephalad migration of the proximal cervical spine that results in pressure on the brain stem from the odontoid. Primary basilar impression is a congenital anomaly, which may be associated with conditions such as occipitocervical synostosis, hypoplasia of the atlas, bifid posterior arch of atlas, odontoid anomalies, and Klippel-Feil syndrome.[8]

Occipitocervical Synostosis

Occipitocervical synostosis is a congenital union between the atlas and the base of the occiput. This may range from complete incorporation of the atlas into the base of the occiput to a fibrous band uniting one small area of the atlas to the occiput. It is sometimes associated with basilar impression.[8]

Anomalies of the C1 Ring

Dubousset reported the congenital absence of the facet of C1, called a *hemiatlas*, leading to severe progressive torticollis. Tomograms and computed tomography scans are useful for diagnosis of this condition. Dubousset also found an increased incidence of vertebral vessel anomalies associated with this condition.[4,8]

Anomalies of the Odontoid

Odontoid anomalies include *aplasia* (complete absence) to *hypoplasia* (partial absence) to *os odontoideum*. Os odontoideum is an oval or round ossicle with a smooth cortical border located either in the normal position of the odontoid (orthotopic) or adjacent to the foramen magnum, where it may fuse to the clivus (dystopic). It is often difficult to distinguish an os odontoideum from a remote nonunion of an odontoid fracture. However, the radiologic gap between the odontoid and the body of the axis is generally wider and more proximal with an os odontoideum. Any of these may lead to C1 to C2 instability.[6,8]

The gap between the odontoid process and the body of the axis may be confused with a persistent neurocentral synchondrosis if it is situated at the base of the odontoid. In this situation, demonstration of movement between the odontoid and the body of the axis confirms the diagnosis of os odontoideum.[6,8]

Odontoid anomalies with ligamentous laxity are also more common in Down syndrome, Morquio's syndrome, and Klippel-Feil syndrome.[6,8]

Congenital Spinal Deformity

Congenital scoliosis may be due to a defect in either formation or segmentation and is commonly due to a combination of the two. The centrum of a vertebra may arise from bilateral, rather than a single, primary ossification center. If one of these centers is hypoplastic, a wedge-shaped hemivertebra will occur and can lead to scoliosis. Fully segmented and semisegmented hemivertebrae are more prone to progressive scoliosis than an unsegmented hemivertebra. A "free" hemivertebra with healthy discs above and below is considered fully segmented, whereas a hemivertebra that is fused to one of its adjacent vertebrae is considered semisegmented, and a hemivertebra that is fused to both its adjacent vertebrae is considered unsegmented. If the entire body is absent or hypoplastic and the posterior elements are normal, congenital kyphosis will result.[8,10,18,19]

Segmentation defects may be purely lateral, posterolateral, posterior, anterior, or circumferential. The circumferential failure of segmentation may lead to loss of segmental motion or decreased height but causes no deformity. A unilateral segmentation defect (unilateral bar) may lead to progressive scoliosis, a posterolateral defect in segmentation causes lordoscoliosis, a posterior defect causes lordosis, and an anterior defect in segmentation leads to kyphosis.[8,10,18]

The Klippel-Feil syndrome is a condition characterized by a short neck, low hairline, and restricted neck movements due to congenital fusion of one or more vertebrae. The number of cervical vertebrae may be less than normal, and there may segmentation defects at several cervical levels. A failure of segmentation occurs between the ages of 3 and 8 weeks. The cervical nerve roots, as well as the intervertebral foramina, may be small, and there commonly are other associated defects in the genitourinary, cardiopulmonary, and nervous systems. Sprengel's deformity, which is characterized by a high-riding scapula with an occasional bony bridge between the scapula and cervical spine, occurs in 25% to 35% of cases.[8,10]

Limbic Vertebrae

Limbic bones are sometimes seen on the anterosuperior and less often on the anteroinferior aspects of the vertebral bodies, especially in the lumbar vertebrae. This is thought to represent a form of anterior disc extrusion separating a small fragment of bone from the involved vertebral body and is often associated with Scheuermann's disease. They are to be distinguished from "intercalary" bones in the anterior spinal ligament, which represent osteophytes, and from "tear drop" fracture fragments. Limbic vertebrae are visible on lateral films, and discography shows the passage of contrast medium into the radiolucent line of separation.[5]

THE FETAL PERIOD

The final phase of intrauterine development from the ninth week to birth is known as the fetal period. Further maturation of all the organ systems and rapid growth of the body takes place during this time. The embryonic period is the most active period, and all of the organ systems are formed during this period. As a result, most of the developmental anomalies that were described occur during the embryonic period. However, the fetal period is the time when prenatal screening techniques can usually detect birth defects.[13]

FETAL PERIOD

- Week 9 to birth
- Characterized by maturation and growth of organ systems
- Prenatal screening can detect birth defects

SELECTED REFERENCES

Campbell RL, Dayton DH, Sohal GS: Neural tube defects: a review of human and animal studies on the etiology of neural tube defects, *Teratology* 34:171-187, 1986.

Chaurasia BD: Calvarial defects in human anencephaly, *Teratology* 29:165-172, 1984.

Dubousset J: Torticollis in children caused by congenital anomalies of the atlas, *J Bone Joint Surg Am* 68:178-188, 1986.

Fielding JW, Hensinger RN, Hawkins RJ: Os odontoideum, *J Bone Joint Surg Am* 62:376-383, 1980.

Hensinger RN: Congenital anomalies of the cervical spine *Clin Orthop Rel Res* 264:16-36, 1991.

Moore KL, Persaud TVN, Schmitt W, eds: *The developing human: clinically oriented embryology*, ed 6, Philadelphia, 1998, WB Saunders.

Winter RB: Congenital spinal deformity. In Lonstein JE et al., eds: *Moe's textbook of scoliosis and other spinal deformities*, ed 3, Philadelphia, 1995, WB Saunders, pp. 257-294.

REFERENCES

1. Bell GR: Anatomy of the lumbar spine: developmental to normal adult anatomy. In Weisel SW et al., eds: *The lumbar spine*, vol 1, ed 2, Philadelphia, 1996, WB Saunders, pp. 43-52.
2. Campbell RL, Dayton DH, Sohal GS: Neural tube defects: a review of human and animal studies on the etiology of neural tube defects, *Teratology* 34:171-187, 1986.
3. Chaurasia BD: Calvarial defect in human anencephaly, *Teratology* 29:165-172, 1984.
4. Dubousset J: Torticollis in children caused by congenital anomalies of the atlas, *J Bone Joint Surg Am* 68:178-188, 1986.
5. Epstein BS, ed: *Diseases of invertebral discs: the spine, a radiological text and atlas*, ed 4, Philadelphia, 1976, Lea & Febiger.
6. Fielding JW, Hensinger RN, Hawkins RJ: Os odontoideum, *J Bone Joint Surg Am* 62:376-383, 1980.
7. Green M, ed: *Pediatric diagnosis: interpretation of symptoms and signs in children and adolescents*, ed 6, Philadelphia, 1998, WB Saunders, pp. 112-137.
8. Hensinger RN: Congenital anomalies of the cervical spine, *Clin Orthop Rel Res* 264:16-36, 1991.
9. Larsen WJ, ed: *Human embryology*, ed 2, New York, 1997, Churchill Livingstone.
10. Moore KL, Persaud TVN, Schmitt W, eds: *The developing human: clinically oriented embryology*, ed 6, Philadelphia, 1998, WB Saunders.
11. Muller F, O'Rahilly R: Cerebral dysraphia (future anencephaly) in a human twin embryo at stage 13, *Teratology* 30:167-177, 1984.
12. Parke WW: Development of the spine. In Herkowitz HN et al., eds: *Rothman-Simeone's the spine*, 4th ed. Philadelphia, 1999, WB Saunders, p. 3-27.
13. Sadler TW, ed: *Langman's medical embryology*, ed 8, Philadelphia, 2000, Lippincott Williams & Wilkins.
14. Smith JT, Skinner SR, Shonnard NH: Persistent synchondrosis of the second cervical vertebra simulating a hangman's fracture in a child, *J Bone Joint Surg Am* 75:1228-1230, 1993.
15. Swischuk LE: Anterior displacement of C2 in children: physiologic or pathologic? *Paediatr Radiol* 122:759-763, 1977.
16. Walmsley R: The development and growth of the intervertebral disc, *Edinb Med J* LX:341-363, 1953.
17. Whalen JL et al.: The intrinsic vasculature of developing vertebral end plates and its nutritive significance to the intervertebral discs, *J Paediatr Orthop* 5:403-410, 1985.
18. Williams PL, Warwick R, eds: *Gray's anatomy*, ed 36, New York, 1980, Churchill Livingstone, pp. 72-419.
19. Winter RB: Congenital spinal deformity. In Lonstein JE et al., eds: *Moe's textbook of scoliosis and other spinal deformities*, ed 3, Philadelphia, 1995, WB Saunders, pp. 257-294.
20. Wolfe HJ, Putscher WGJ, Vickery AL: Role of the notochord in human invertebral disk. I. Fetus and infant, *Clin Orthop* 39:205-215, 1965.

Relevant Surgical Anatomy of the Cervical, Thoracic, and Lumbar Spine

Thomas J. Puschak, Alexander R. Vaccaro, Wolfgang Rauschning, Rajiv V. Taliwal

Techniques of instrumentation for the cervical, thoracic, and lumbosacral spine have evolved dramatically in the past three decades. Lateral mass screws and pedicle screws can be coupled with plates or rods to stabilize fusions in the posterior occipitocervical and subaxial cervical regions. Recently transarticular screw fixation of the atlantoaxial joint has gained favor for C1 to C2 stabilization. In the thoracic spine, transpedicular fixation is being used more frequently for reconstruction of traumatic and neoplastic spinal injuries, as well as for deformity correction. In the lumbosacral spine, the use of pedicle screws for stabilization of degenerative, traumatic, and neoplastic conditions has become ubiquitous. There has also been a proliferation of interbody fusion devices for anterior and posterior use in the thoracic and lumbar spine. Comprehensive knowledge of spinal anatomy, especially with regard to the relationships of the bony anatomy and adjacent neurovascular and visceral structures, is needed to minimize surgical complications.

POSTERIOR OCCIPITOCERVICAL ANATOMY
Occiput

Internal fixation for occipitocervical fusion was initially described using wires.[55,67] More recently various authors have described the use of plates, rods, and screws.[36,53,57-60] The latter techniques provide more rigid fixation and are useful in the treatment of instability due to trauma and rheumatoid arthritis, as well as the treatment of multilevel degenerative disease. Thorough knowledge of the bony anatomy of the occiput and its relationship with the dural venous sinuses is needed to safely place screws in the occiput.

The occiput is a flat bone, which acts as the bony protection for the cerebellum and posterior fossa. It is adjacent to the foramen magnum, where the spinal cord and brain stem join and exit the cerebrum. The posterior border of the foramen magnum is called the *opisthion*, and the anterior border is called the *basion*. The convex

> ## OCCIPUT
>
> - External occipital protuberance (inion): Thickest region of occiput
> - Inion thickness: 11 to 17 mm
> - External occipital crest: Midline from inion to foramen magnum
> - Transverse occipital landmarks: Supreme, superior, and inferior nuchal lines
> - Ideal screw placement: Along external occipital crest below inion

occipital condyles border the foramen magnum laterally and articulate with the superior articular facets of the atlas. The thickest part of the occiput is the external occipital protuberance, or inion, which is located in the center of the occiput and is a good landmark for the placement of wires or screws (Figure 2-1). According to Ebraheim et al., the thickness of the inion ranges from 11 to 17 mm and decreases in a radial fashion.[10] The zone extending 2 cm lateral to the inion is usually thicker than 8 mm and is mainly cortical bone with little diploic bone.[10] The external occipital crest runs from the external occipital protuberance caudally to the foramen magnum. Transverse occipital landmarks extend laterally from the inion and external occipital crest and are known as the supreme, superior, and inferior nuchal lines. The supreme nuchal line is not present in all persons. The thickness of the occiput decreases caudally from the superior to the inferior nuchal lines. Ebraheim et al. describe the relationship of the dural sinuses to the external occipital landmarks and note that the projection of the confluence of the sinuses (i.e., torcular Herophili or simply torcular) on the surface of the occiput runs laterally 12 mm above and 5 mm below the inion.[10] They also report that the transverse dural sinus is more centered about the external occipital protuberance. The transverse sinus extends 7 mm superior and

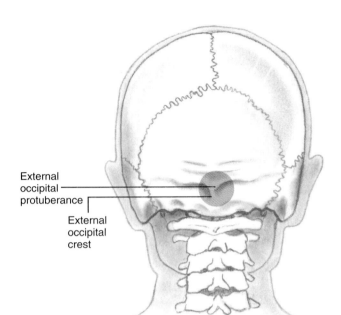

Figure 2-1. Posterior view of the skull. *(Redrawn from Hollinshead WH, Rosse C: Textbook of anatomy, ed 9, New York, 1985, Harper & Row.)*

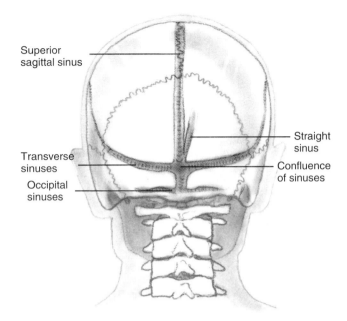

Figure 2-2. The relationship between the occipital calvarium and venous sinuses. *(Redrawn from Ebraheim NA, Lu J, Biyani A, Brown JA: An anatomic study of the thickness of the occipital bone. Implications for occipitocervical instrumentation, Spine 21[15]:1725-1729, 1996.)*

inferior to the external protuberance as it projects laterally (Figure 2-2).

The ideal placement of occipital screws is along the external occipital crest below the inion. Ebraheim et al. suggest that 8-mm screws can be safely placed 2 cm lateral to midline at the level of the inion; 1 cm from midline, 1 cm below the inion; and 0.5 cm from midline, 2 cm below the inion.[10] The surgeon should minimize directing the most cranial screw cephalad to avoid penetrating the transverse dural sinus.

Atlantoaxial Joint

Posterior fusion of the C1 to C2 articulation has long been used for the treatment of atlantoaxial instability arising from trauma, inflammatory arthritides, os odontoideum, and various other diseases. Several wiring techniques have been described for fixation of the atlantoaxial joint.[6,35] Postoperative immobilization in a halo is often required following wiring procedures. Magerl and Seeman described the transarticular screw fixation technique that provides more-rigid fixation of the atlantoaxial joint and may decrease the amount of postoperative external immobilization needed.[47] This technique may also be used in conjunction with occipitocervical plating. Due to the narrow anatomic constraints associated with placement of the transarticular screw, the cervical spinal cord and vertebral artery are potentially at risk. Anatomic variations including a narrow C2 isthmus, anomalous vertebral arteries, or erosion of the C2 lateral mass may prevent safe placement of transarticular screws.[47,51,61,63] Comprehensive knowledge of the bony anatomy and course of the vertebral artery is imperative to safely expose the posterior

---

VERTEBRAL BODY

- Groove: Located anteriorly on superior surface of posterior ring of atlas, along with first cervical spine nerve
- Distance from midline to medial edge of vertebral artery groove: 8 to 18 mm
- Dissection on superior atlas: 8 mm from midline
- Dissection on posterior arch: 12 mm from midline

---

atlas and axis and is critical for the safe placement of transarticular screws.

The vertebral arteries ascend in the transverse foramina of the cervical vertebrae, exit the transverse foramen of the atlas, and run medially in the vertebral artery groove. They eventually merge to become the basilar artery. The vertebral artery groove is located anteriorly on the superior surface of the posterior ring of the atlas. It extends from the transverse foramen to the medial edge of the posterior ring. The vertebral artery lies in the groove along with the first cervical spinal nerve. The structures in the groove are posterior to the lateral mass of the atlas, lateral to the spinal canal, and anterior to the atlantooccipital membrane. The distance from midline to the medial edge of the vertebral artery groove ranges from 8 to 18 mm.[26] During posterior exposure of the atlas and axis, Ebraheim et al. recommend that dissection along the superior atlas edge be limited to 8 mm from the midline and that dissection along the posterior arch be carried no further than 12 mm lateral to midline[26] (Figure 2-3; see also Plate 2-1).

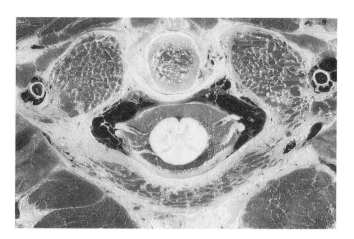

Figure 2-3. (See Plate 2-1.) Axial section of the atlas through the lateral masses and the posterior arch. The midportion of the odontoid process displays articular cartilage anteriorly and also posteriorly where it articulates with the transverse ligament. Lateral to the dens there is loose areolar vascular tissue. The lateral masses are composed of strong cancellous bone, whereas the arches contain more cortical bone. The vertebral arteries are about to enter the transverse foramina of the atlas. They are surrounded by a rete of veins, which is continuous with the venous sinusoids, which surround the nerve roots in the root canals (periradicular venous plexus) and with the wide sinusoids that surround the thecal sac (epidural veins, internal vertebral venous plexus). These venous compartments display black on cadaveric sections because they are filled with cruor mortis. Note that these epidural veins constitute wide vascular compartments with relatively few septa rather than a serpiginous rete of veins. The thecal sac is oval and renders ample space for the spinal cord, which clearly displays the anterior median fissure and the posterior median sulcus. A great number of rootlet filaments emerging from the anterolateral and posterolateral sulcus stepwise merge intrathecally to larger dorsal and ventral roots. *(Courtesy Wolfgang Rauschning.)*

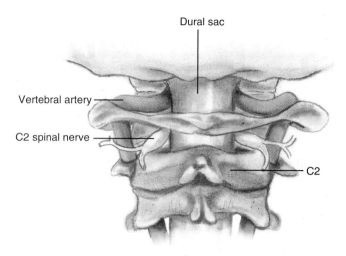

Figure 2-4. Posterior view of the relationship of the vertebral artery to the upper cervical spinal elements. *(Redrawn from Ebraheim NA et al.: The quantitative anatomy of the vertebral artery groove of the atlas and its relation to the posterior atlantoaxial approach, Spine 23[3]:320-323, 1998.)*

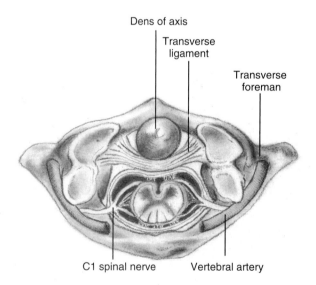

Figure 2-5. Transaxial view of the course of the vertebral artery in relationship to the superior border of the atlas. *(Redrawn from Ebraheim NA et al.: The quantitative anatomy of the vertebral artery groove of the atlas and its relation to the posterior atlantoaxial approach, Spine 23[3]:320-323, 1998.)*

The C2 pedicle lies anterior to the articular process and is often confused with the isthmus of the pars interarticularis when described in the literature. The transarticular screw traverses the isthmus of C2 and enters the posterior aspect of the C1 to C2 joint on its way to the lateral mass of the atlas. Paramore, Dickman, and Sonntag reported an 18% incidence of high-riding transverse foramina, at least on one side, preventing placement of transarticular screws.[51] Taitz and Arensburg noted a 33% incidence of erosion of the C2 transverse foramen.[63] Angiography has shown that the vertebral artery takes an oblique course through the axis.[4] As it enters the lateral mass of C2 inferiorly, it courses approximately 45 degrees laterally before it exits to enter the transverse foramen of the atlas, forming a groove within the axis. Solanki and Crockard reported that the vertical depth of this groove is inversely related to the internal height of the C2 lateral mass as well as the length and width of the C2 pedicle.[61] They quantified this groove by CT scan and found that if the ver-

tical depth of the groove exceeds 5 mm, the height of the lateral mass and pedicle width of C2 are both less than 2 mm, making it impossible to safely pass a 3.5-mm screw (Figures 2-4 and 2-5). Recently Mandel et al. reported that if the C2 isthmus is less than 5 mm in height or width as identified on CT scan, the placement of a 3.5-mm transarticular screw becomes technically difficult and dramatically increases the chances of penetration of the vertebral artery groove[48] (Figure 2-6). They also noted that approximately 10% of the population has anatomy prohibitive of placing a transarticular screw on at least one side. In light

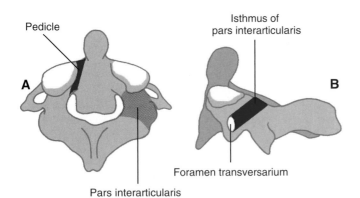

Figure 2-6. Schematic illustration of the C2 vertebral body. **A,** Pedicle and pars interarticularis. **B,** Foramen transversarium and isthmus of pars interarticularis. *(Redrawn from Mandel IM et al.: Morphologic considerations of C2 isthmus dimensions for the placement of transarticular screws, Spine 25[12]:1542-1547, 2000.)*

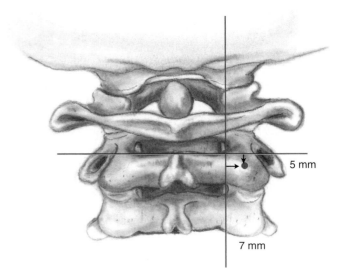

Figure 2-7. Posterior view of the axis illustrating the starting point of a C2 pedicle screw. *(Redrawn from Ebraheim NA et al.: Anatomic consideration of C2 pedicle screw placement, Spine 21[6]:691-695, 1996.)*

of these anatomic findings, preoperative CT scans with sagittal reconstruction are extremely valuable to determine if screw placement is safe and possible. The medial and superior borders of the C2 isthmus should also be identified at the time of surgery to aid in visual identification of the C2 pedicle and proper screw trajectory.

Another potential complication of transarticular screw fixation is hypoglossal nerve injury caused by a misdirected or too-long screw. Ebraheim et al. report that the hypoglossal nerve takes a vertical course anterior to the lateral part of the C1 lateral mass and C1 to C2 joint.[31] That study also reported that the optimal screw length for the transarticular technique is 38 mm; however, this number my vary depending on the individual's anatomy. To avoid risking injury to the hypoglossal nerve, the surgeon must take care not to past-point with the drill and must select an appropriate length screw based on the individual patient's anatomy.

C2 Pedicle

Transpedicular fixation of the axis has been described for treatment of traumatic spondylolisthesis of the axis (hangman's fracture).[56] Pedicle screw fixation at C2 can also be used as part of an occipitocervical plating or as a rostral anchor in posterior cervical fusions that extend up to the axis. The C2 pedicle lies posteromedial to the transverse foramen, and the superior articular process covers it laterally. Xu et al. have reported that the C2 pedicle projection lies 5 mm caudal to the superior C2 lamina edge and 7 mm lateral to the lateral border of the spinal canal.[68] The pedicle axis is directed 30 degrees medial to the sagittal plane and 20 degrees rostral to the axial plane. The inferior pedicle width is approximately 3 mm less than the width of the superior pedicle.[23] The lateral wall of the pedicle, which is adjacent to the transverse foramen, is very thin compared with the medial wall. Because the inferior pedicle is narrow and the lateral wall is thin, to avoid vertebral artery injury by

> ### ANATOMIC CONSTRAINTS TO C2 PEDICLE OF TRANSARTICULAR SCREW PLACEMENT
>
> - There is an 18% incidence of high-riding transverse foramina on one side, preventing transarticular screw placement.
> - In 10% of population, anatomy precludes placement of transarticular screw.
> - Medial and superior border of C2 isthmus should be palpated before screw placement.
> - Avoid potential for hypoglossal nerve injury from overpenetration of C1 lateral mass.

penetrating the transverse foramen, direct C2 pedicle screws to the superior medial portion of the pedicle. As in the placement of transarticular screws, the surgeon should identify the superior and medial borders of the C2 isthmus at the time of screw placement to increase the accuracy of placement[21] (Figures 2-7 to 2-9).

POSTERIOR SUBAXIAL CERVICAL ANATOMY

Posterior fusion of the subaxial spine has been advocated for the treatment of cervical instability due to trauma, degenerative disease, tumor, and iatrogenic etiologies. Wertheim and Bohlman described the triple-wire technique for posterior cervical fixation, and posterior wiring has been the gold standard for internal fixation of the posterior subaxial cervical spine.[67] In the past decade, plating with the use of lateral mass screw fixation has become a popular method of posterior cervical stabilization. Lateral mass plating does not rely on the posterior laminar, making it a good fixation option for patients with previous posterior decompressions and

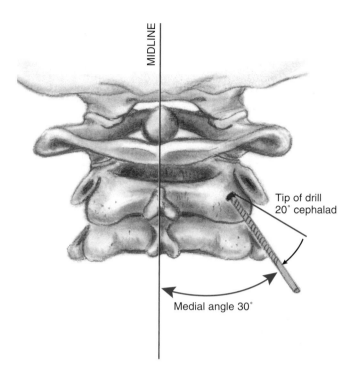

Figure 2-8. The trajectory of C2 pedicle screw insertion. *(Redrawn from Ebraheim NA et al.: Anatomic consideration of C2 pedicle screw placement, Spine 21[6]:691-695, 1996.)*

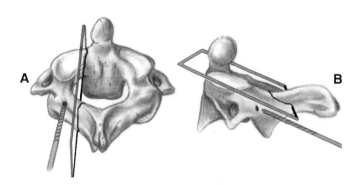

Figure 2-9. Drawing of posterior aspect of C2 with the direction of the drill bit parallel with medial border and superior aspect of the pedicle. **A,** Posterosuperior view. **B,** Lateral view. *(Redrawn from Ebraheim NA et al.: Anatomic consideration of C2 pedicle screw placement, Spine 21[6]:691-695, 1996.)*

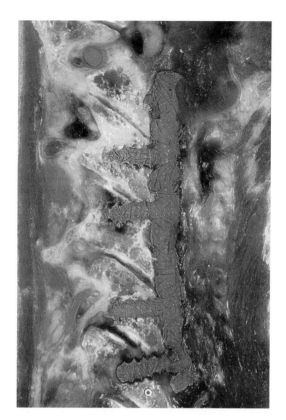

Figure 2-10. (See Plate 2-2.) Posterior screw-plate fixation of a breast cancer metastasis that had caused severe pain in a 57-year-old woman who died 6 months after surgery. The plate was removed from the frozen specimen and the screw tracts and the plate cavity were filled with a blue casting medium. This slide is a sagittal cryosection through the articular pillar from C3 to C6. Three screws traverse the facet joints. At C4 and C6 the screws have poor purchase in the metastatic bone; the lowest screw erodes the bone. The 18-mm-long screws (11 mm effective screw length) are oriented sagittally in the articular mass and point toward the nerve roots, ganglia, and segmental arteries.

for those with anomalous or deficient posterior elements. The Magerl and Roy-Camille techniques of insertion are most commonly used; however, numerous techniques have been described[2,38,57,60,72] (Figures 2-10 and 2-11; see also Plates 2-2 and 2-3).

Transpedicular fixation of the subaxial cervical spine is another method of fixation that is less commonly used than lateral mass fixation. It is a newer technique that has recently been described by Jeanneret, Gebhard, and Magerl[39] and Abumi and Kaneda[1] in separate studies. At this time the indications for this technique are limited but include reconstruction after correction of cervical kyphosis.

Thorough knowledge of the anatomy of the cervical lateral mass and pedicle, as well as their relationship with the exiting cervical nerve roots and vertebral artery, is needed to safely place screws into the subaxial cervical spine (Figure 2-12; see also Plate 2-4).

Cervical Lateral Mass

The lateral masses are present from C2 to C7. The lateral mass at C2 is not considered part of the articular pillars

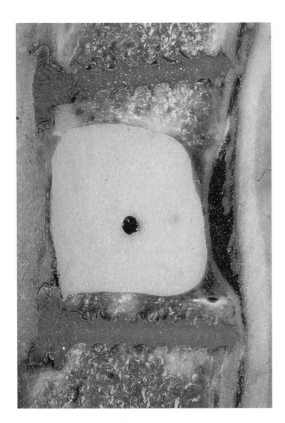

Figure 2-11.   (See Plate 2-3.) Breast cancer metastasis of C6 with a pathologic fracture in a 45-year-old woman with intractable pain. The corpectomy defect was filled with methylmetha-crylate and secured with a nonlocking Oroszco screw-plate. This paramedian sagittal close-up section 2 years postoperatively shows that the cement in the C6 vertebrectomy defect is firmly bonded to the remodeled endplates. There is no recurrence of the metastasis after two years. Note also the anterior bulging of the thickened dura and the sharp outlines and the blue cast of the screw tracts. The screws have transgressed the posterior vertebral wall with one tread. Their tips are covered by a thick layer of coalesced periosteum and dura. The epidural space is obliterated. The segmental nerves are lying free in the subarachnoid space and the spinal cord is not compressed. (*Courtesy Wolfgang Rauschning.*)

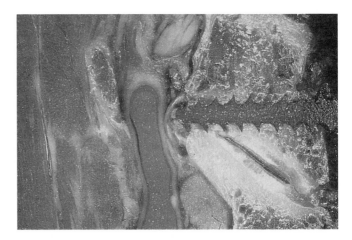

Figure 2-12.   (See Plate 2-4.) Articular pillar anatomy in a 72-year-old man who had been operated on by posterior screw-plate fixation using a small AO/ASIF DC plate and 3.5-mm cancellous screws. Before in situ freezing of the spine and removal of the specimen, the arteries had been injected with red contrast medium. The implants were extracted from the specimen and the screw tracts and plate cavities were filled with a blue casting medium. This screw has violated the inferior articular process of C5: its tip lies in the upper portion of the facet joint stopping short of the vertebral artery. Note also the C5 root sheath and the C6 dorsal root ganglion. (*Courtesy Wolfgang Rauschning.*)

CERVICAL LATERAL MASS

- Mass is the bony junction between the superior and inferior articular processes.
- Superior articular facet is oriented 35 degrees in sagittal plane; it increases gradually to 55 degrees at C7.
- Sulcus at junction of lateral mass and lamina represents projection of center to medial border of vertebral artery.
- Cervical root (dorsal ramus) is located anterior to superior articular process.

---

because the superior articular process is more anterior than the inferior articular process. The lateral mass is the bony junction between the superior and inferior articular processes. The superior process at C2 is oriented 35 degrees cephalad in the sagittal plane, and this increases gradually to 55 degrees at C7.[64] There is a sulcus at the junction of the lamina and facet, known as the medial facet line, which defines the border between the lateral mass and lamina. Ebraheim, Xu, and Yeasting note that this sulcus roughly represents the projection of the center to medial border of the vertebral artery on the posterior cervical spine.[13]

Understanding the relationship of the cervical nerve roots and vertebral artery to the lateral mass is the key to safe placement of lateral mass screws. The spinal roots exit the cervical neuroforamen above their respective pedicle and lie anterior to the superior articular process (Figure 2-13; see also Plate 2-5). The nerve branches into its smaller dorsal and larger ventral rami at the anterolateral corner of the superior articular process. The dorsal ramus takes a posterior course along the anterolateral corner of the base of the superior articular process and divides into a medial and lateral branch (Figure 2-14). The medial branch innervates the joint capsule and deep muscles of the neck. The lateral branch also innervates the deep muscles as well as the skin of the posterior neck. The distance between the dorsal ramus and the antero-lateral corner of the superior facet ranges from 5 to 7 mm.[25] The surgeon must take care not to place screws at the anterolateral tip of the superior articular process to

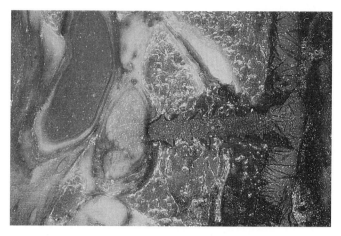

Figure 2-13. (See Plate 2-5.) Sagittal close-up section at C6 to C7 showing a screw that transgresses and partially fractures the inferior articular process of C6. Both ganglia are accommodated in deep furrows at the anterior surface of the articular masses. This recessing of the ganglia allows the vertebral artery to take a straight course toward the transverse foramen of C6. The plate snugly fits on the inferior articular process of C6, whereas at C7 there is a considerable gap between the plate and the articular mass. The tip of the screw is in direct contact with the C7 ganglion. Note that the motor root is located at the lower pole of the dorsal root ganglion. At C7 the vertebral artery swings anteriorly and laterally because it normally runs outside the transverse foramina of C7. (*Courtesy Wolfgang Rauschning.*)

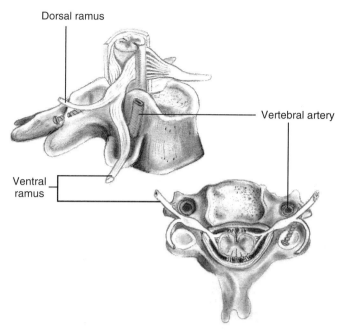

Figure 2-14. The dorsal ramus of the cervical nerve is potentially at risk for injury from overpenetration of its superior articular process during lateral mass screw placement. (*Redrawn from Ebraheim NA et al.: The anatomic location of the dorsal ramus of the cervical nerve and its relation to the superior articular process of the lateral mass, Spine 23[18]:1968-1970, 1998.*)

avoid injuring the dorsal ramus. The ventral ramus is larger and runs anterior, lateral, and inferior along the posterior ridge of the transverse process. The ventral rami lie 1 to 2 mm anterior to the ventral cortex of the lateral mass[24] and combine to form the cervical plexus, which becomes the brachial plexus. The average distance from the posterior center of the lateral mass to the nerve roots superior and inferior to it is 5.5 mm.[69] The average distance from the posterior center of the lateral mass to the lateral dural edge is 9 mm.[69] The distance from the surface of the posterior midpoint of the lateral mass to the spinal nerve measured in a course 15 degrees lateral to the sagittal plane is 16 mm from C3 to C6 and 8 mm at C7.[29]

The distance from the posterior midpoint of the lateral mass to the transverse foramen ranges from 9 to 12 mm[13] (Figure 2-15). From C3 to C5, the lateral border of the vertebral artery lies approximately 5 to 6 degrees medial to the posterior midpoint of the lateral mass.[13] At C6 the lateral border of the artery lies 6 degrees lateral to the posterior midpoint of the lateral mass[13] (Figures 2-16 to 2-18). Lateral mass screws started at the posterior midpoint of the lateral mass, which are directed at least 10 degrees lateral to the sagittal plane, should not be in danger of injuring the vertebral artery. Preoperative CT or MRI scans should be used to identify bony and arterial anomalies.

The Magerl and Roy-Camille techniques are the most commonly used methods of lateral mass screw

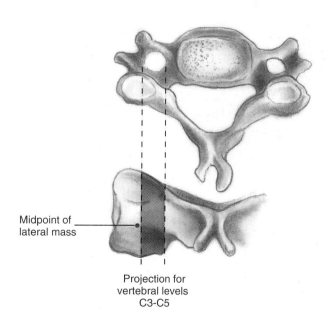

Figure 2-15. The relationship between the center of the cervical artery mass and the boundaries of the foramen transversarium. (*Redrawn from Ebraheim NA, Xu R, Yeasting RA: The location of the vertebral artery foramen and its relation to posterior lateral mass screw fixation, Spine 21[11]:1291-1295, 1996.*)

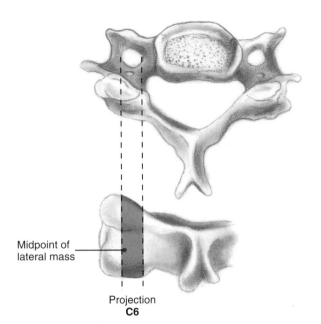

Midpoint of lateral mass

Projection
C6

Figure 2-16. The relationship between the posterior midpoint of the lateral mass and the vertebral artery foramen at C6. Note superimposition of the posterior midpoint of the lateral mass over the vertebral artery foramen. *(Redrawn from Ebraheim NA, Xu R, Yeasting RA: The location of the vertebral artery foramen and its relation to posterior lateral mass screw fixation, Spine 21[11]:1291-1295, 1996.)*

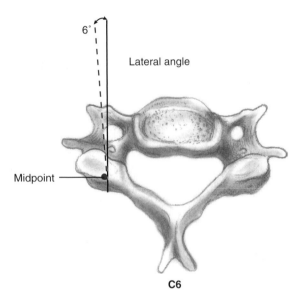

6° | Lateral angle

Midpoint

C6

Figure 2-17. The relationship between the posterior midpoint of the lateral mass and the vertebral artery foramen at C6. Note that the angle between the parasagittal plane and the line connecting the posterior midpoint of the lateral mass with the lateral limit of the vertebral artery foramen is directed lateral to the sagittal plane. *(Redrawn from Ebraheim NA, Xu R, Yeasting RA: The location of the vertebral artery foramen and its relation to posterior lateral mass screw fixation, Spine 21[11]:1291-1295, 1996.)*

insertion. The Magerl technique has been associated with a higher incidence of nerve injury, whereas the Roy-Camille technique has been associated with facet penetration.[38] The surgeon must be cautious to place screws as laterally and superiorly as possible when using the Magerl technique to avoid injuring the dorsal ramus. When using the Roy-Camille technique, the surgeon must be careful with choice of screw length to avoid penetration of the facet joint. Safe screw lengths tend to be longer in the Magerl technique than the Roy-Camille technique due to the more oblique trajectory of the screw. Because the lateral mass of C7 is smaller, the surgeon can start the screw more inferiorly and direct it more laterally and superiorly to try to get a longer screw length. If the C7 lateral mass is too small, a C7 pedicle screw may be considered. It is also imperative for the surgeon to be familiar with the instrumentation system being used to avoid placing a wrong-sized screw. The measurement listed on the screw is not always the working length of the screw.

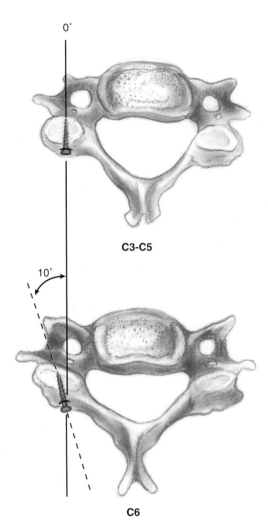

0°

C3-C5

10°

C6

Figure 2-18. Safety angulations for lateral mass screw placement at C3 to C5 and C6. *(Redrawn from Ebraheim NA, Xu R, Yeasting RA: The location of the vertebral artery foramen and its relation to posterior lateral mass screw fixation, Spine 21[11]:1291-1295, 1996.)*

Cervical Pedicles

Xu et al. reported that between C3 and C7, the average pedicle height and width are 6.5 mm and 5 mm, respectively.[71] They noted that there is no space between the pedicle and the nerve root superior or between the pedicle and the dura medially from C3 to C7. The space between the pedicle and the inferior nerve root averages 1.5 mm. The lateral cortex of the pedicle tends to be thinner than the medial cortex. The projection of the axis of the pedicle is 2 mm inferior to the superior facet and 5 mm medial to the lateral edge of the lateral mass from C3 to C6.[30] At C7 the projection of the pedicle is 1 mm inferior to the middle of the transverse process and 2 mm medial to the lateral border of the lateral mass.[30]

Jeanneret recommends that the starting point for cervical pedicle screws be 3 mm inferior to the superior facet in the center of the lateral mass, angling 45 degrees

---

CERVICAL LATERAL MASS SCREW PLACEMENT

- Distance from posterior midpoint of lateral mass to spinal nerve measured in a course 15 degrees lateral to sagittal plane is 16 mm from C3 to C6 and 8 mm at C7.
- Distance from posterior midpoint of lateral mass to transverse foramen is 9 to 12 mm.
- C6 to C5 lateral border of vertebral artery lies about 5 to 6 degrees medial to posterior midpoint of lateral mass. At C6 the lateral border of artery lies 6 degrees lateral to midpoint of lateral mass.
- Screws started at midpoint of lateral mass and aimed 10 degrees lateral to sagittal plane should pose no risk of injury to vertebral artery.

CERVICAL PEDICLE SCREWS

- Between C3 and C7, average pedicle height and width are 6.5 mm and 5 mm, respectively.
- Space between pedicle and inferior nerve root averages 1.5 mm.
- Pedicle projection is 2 mm inferior to superior facet and 5 mm medial to lateral edge of lateral mass from C3 to C6. At C7 it is 1 mm inferior to midline of transverse process and 2 mm medial to lateral border of lateral mass.

PEDICLE SCREW INSERTION RECOMMENDATIONS

- Jeanneret: Starting point 3 mm inferior to superior facet in center of lateral mass angling 45 degrees medially
- Abumi: Starting point slightly lateral to lateral mass midpoint just below superior facet angling medially 30 to 45 degrees

---

medially.[39] Abumi recommends that the starting point be slightly lateral to the midpoint of the lateral mass and just below the superior facet, angling medially by 30 to 45 degrees.[1] To enhance the accuracy of screw placement and minimize complications, laminoforaminotomies should be performed so that the borders and trajectory of the pedicle can be visualized.

ANTERIOR CERVICAL ANATOMY

Since the 1950s anterior cervical decompression and arthrodesis have been an effective and widely used treatment for radiculopathy and myelopathy caused by cervical spondylosis, cervical stenosis, trauma, and tumor.[3,5,9,54] The anatomic structures potentially at greatest risk during anterior decompression are the vertebral artery and recurrent laryngeal nerve. Injury of the sympathetic trunk during dissection of the longus colli muscles for retractor placement can result in Horner's syndrome. Understanding the location and course of these structures is key to avoiding iatrogenic injuries (Figure 2-19; see also Plate 2-6).

Vertebral Body

The cervical vertebral body is unique due to the uncinate processes. The uncinate processes are bony ridges on the superior lateral surface of the body. The superior surface is concave, and the inferior surface of the adjacent vertebra is convex. The uncinate process articulates with the inferior surface of the adjacent vertebra, forming the uncovertebral joint of Luschka.

Anterior plating of the cervical spine is widely used for stabilization after anterior cervical fusion. Injury to the cervical spinal cord during drilling or screw placement is a potential complication of this technique. Ebraheim reported on the dimensions of the cervical vertebral bodies and noted that the mean depths of the superior end plates increase from C3 to C7.[27] They also note that the average depth at midbody in the midline and at 5 mm lateral to the midline is 14 mm. In addition to these guidelines, the surgeon should use measurements of vertebral body depth on preoperative CT scans or MRI scans as well as direct measurements at the time of surgery after decompression to choose safe screw lengths. An intraoperative radiograph should be obtained after hardware placement to ensure that the screws do not extend into the spinal canal.

Recurrent Laryngeal Nerve

The recurrent laryngeal nerve can potentially be injured during the anterior cervical approach by inadvertently cutting it while ligating the inferior thyroidal artery or by excessively or continuously retracting it with the midline structures. The resultant dysphagia, dysphonia, and vocal cord paralysis may be transient or permanent.

The recurrent laryngeal nerve is a branch of the vagus nerve. The right side loops around the subclavian artery, and the left side loops around the aortic arch prior to ascending into the neck. Ebraheim et al. describe the

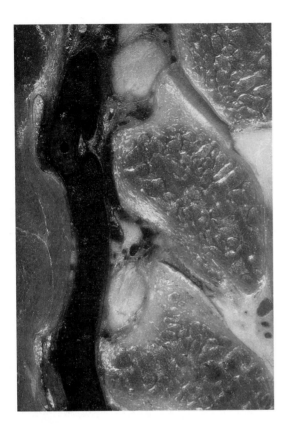

Figure 2-19. (See Plate 2-6.) Sagittal section through the lateral portion of the articular pillar of a normal midcervical spine. The articular masses, composed of superior and inferior articular processes and a virtual pars interarticularis, are roughly rhomboid and carry obliquely sloping articular facets dorsosuperiorly and ventroinferiorly. Circumferentially meniscoid synovial folds (tags) project into the zygapophyseal or facet joints. Anterior to the upper articular process, deep notches accommodate the root sleeve, ganglion portion of the root, and the postganglionic cervical spinal nerve. This section also displays the vertebral artery (black) in the transverse foramina of the vertebrae.

RECURRENT LARYNGEAL NERVE

- Nerve is at risk during ligation of inferior thyroidal artery or continuous retraction of midline structures.
- Right side: Nerve ascends superomedially making a 25-degree angle with the sagittal plane. It lies 6.5 mm anterior and 7 mm lateral to tracheoesophageal groove.
- Left nerve (direct course): Nerve ascends 5 degrees off sagittal plane; it is located deep within tracheoesophageal groove.

course of the nerves as the nerves ascend in the neck.[21] On the right the nerve ascends superomedially, making a 25-degree angle with the sagittal plane. It lies 6.5 mm anterior and 7 mm lateral to the tracheoesophageal groove. The left nerve takes a more direct course in the neck, ascending 5 degrees off of the sagittal plane, and is deep within the tracheoesophageal groove. Due to the more indirect course, the recurrent laryngeal nerve on the right is in particular danger if the inferior thyroidal artery is not ligated far enough laterally and if the midline structures are retracted too vigorously or too continuously.

Vertebral Artery

The vertebral artery arises from the posterior superior aspect of the subclavian artery on the right and from the brachiocephalic artery on the left. Occasionally, on the left, it arises directly from the aortic arch. It ascends posteriorly to enter the transverse foramen at C6 and then continues cephalad through the remaining transverse foramina of the other cervical vertebrae. In the intertransverse space, the vertebral artery and nerve roots are surrounded by a fibroligamentous band[22] that is adherent to the lateral aspect of the uncovertebral joint. The vertebral artery ascends in a slightly posterior and medial direction from C6 to C3.[43] The mean distance from the medial edge of the longus colli to the medial edge of the vertebral artery decreases from 11.5 mm at C6 to 9 mm at C3.[45] Thus, the vertebral artery tends to lie more anterior and lateral at C6, and posterior and medial at C3. Between C3 and C6, the average distance between the lateral border of the vertebral body and the transverse foramen is 2 mm[18] (Figure 2-20; see also Plate 2-7).

To avoid injury to the vertebral artery during anterior decompressions, the surgeon should be aware of its course. Preoperative review of CT and MRI scans will identify anomalous arteries or unusually vertebral morphology. The medial borders of the longus colli and lateral edge of the vertebral body are reliable intraoperative landmarks to locate the vertebral artery. Care should also be taken with wide decompressions at the higher levels, because the vertebral artery tends to be more posterior and medial. Also, the surgeon should be careful to free the fibroligamentous band from the uncus with an angled 4-0 curette prior to removal of uncovertebral osteophytes to minimize arterial laceration.

Vertebral Vein

Lu et al. describe three classic patterns of the vertebral vein: a single or double vein, a venous plexus, or absence of the vein.[46] The vertebral vein descends in the transverse foramina and lies anteromedial or anterolateral to the vertebral artery. At C7 usually only the vertebral vein occupies the transverse foramen. Eventually the vertebral vein empties into the brachiocephalic vein. The vertebral vein is also encased in the fibroligamentous band that is attached to the uncus. Therefore, attention to dissecting the fibroligamentous band from the uncovertebral joint prior to performing anterior

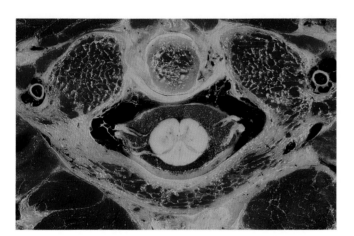

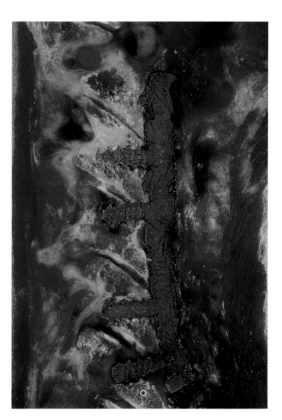

Plate 2-1.   Axial section of the atlas through the lateral masses and the posterior arch. The midportion of the odontoid process displays articular cartilage anteriorly and also posteriorly where it articulates with the transverse ligament. Lateral to the dens there is loose areolar vascular tissue. The lateral masses are composed of strong cancellous bone, whereas the arches contain more cortical bone. The vertebral arteries are about to enter the transverse foramina of the atlas. They are surrounded by a rete of veins, which is continuous with the venous sinusoids, which surround the nerve roots in the root canals (periradicular venous plexus) and with the wide sinusoids that surround the thecal sac (epidural veins, internal vertebral venous plexus). These venous compartments display black on cadaveric sections because they are filled with cruor mortis. Note that these epidural veins constitute wide vascular compartments with relatively few septa rather than a serpiginous rete of veins. The thecal sac is oval and renders ample space for the spinal cord, which clearly displays the anterior median fissure and the posterior median sulcus. A great number of rootlet filaments emerging from the anterolateral and posterolateral sulcus stepwise merge intrathecally to larger dorsal and ventral roots. *(Courtesy Wolfgang Rauschning.)*

Plate 2-2.   Posterior screw-plate fixation of a breast cancer metastasis that had caused severe pain in a 57-year-old woman who died 6 months after surgery. The plate was removed from the frozen specimen and the screw tracts and the plate cavity were filled with a blue casting medium. This slide is a sagittal cryosection through the articular pillar from C3 to C6. Three screws traverse the facet joints. At C4 and C6 the screws have poor purchase in the metastatic bone; the lowest screw erodes the bone. The 18-mm-long screws (11 mm effective screw length) are oriented sagittally in the articular mass and point toward the nerve roots, ganglia, and segmental arteries.

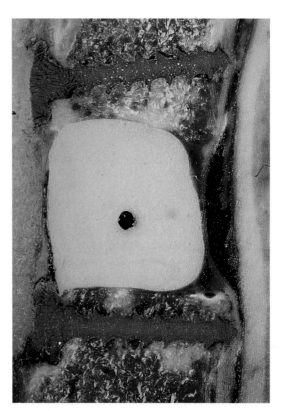

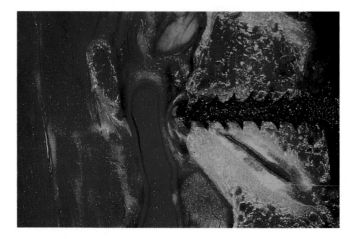

Plate 2-3. Breast cancer metastasis of C6 with a pathologic fracture in a 45-year-old woman with intractable pain. The corpectomy defect was filled with methylmethacrylate and secured with a nonlocking Oroszco screw-plate. This paramedian sagittal close-up section 2 years postoperatively shows that the cement in the C6 vertebrectomy defect is firmly bonded to the remodeled endplates. There is no recurrence of the metastasis after two years. Note also the anterior bulging of the thickened dura and the sharp outlines and the blue cast of the screw tracts. The screws have transgressed the posterior vertebral wall with one tread. Their tips are covered by a thick layer of coalesced periosteum and dura. The epidural space is obliterated. The segmental nerves are lying free in the subarachnoid space and the spinal cord is not compressed. (Courtesy Wolfgang Rauschning.)

Plate 2-4. Articular pillar anatomy in a 72-year-old man who had been operated on by posterior screw-plate fixation using a small AO/ASIF DC plate and 3.5-mm cancellous screws. Before in situ freezing of the spine and removal of the specimen, the arteries had been injected with red contrast medium. The implants were extracted from the specimen and the screw tracts and plate cavities were filled with a blue casting medium. This screw has violated the inferior articular process of C5: its tip lies in the upper portion of the facet joint stopping short of the vertebral artery. Note also the C5 root sheath and the C6 dorsal root ganglion. (Courtesy Wolfgang Rauschning.)

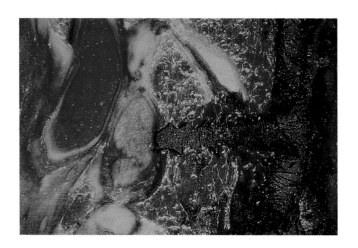

Plate 2-5. Sagittal close-up section at C6 to C7 showing a screw that transgresses and partially fractures the inferior articular process of C6. Both ganglia are accommodated in deep furrows at the anterior surface of the articular masses. This recessing of the ganglia allows the vertebral artery to take a straight course toward the transverse foramen of C6. The plate snugly fits on the inferior articular process of C6, whereas at C7 there is a considerable gap between the plate and the articular mass. The tip of the screw is in direct contact with the C7 ganglion. Note that the motor root is located at the lower pole of the dorsal root ganglion. At C7 the vertebral artery swings anteriorly and laterally because it normally runs outside the transverse foramina of C7. (Courtesy Wolfgang Rauschning.)

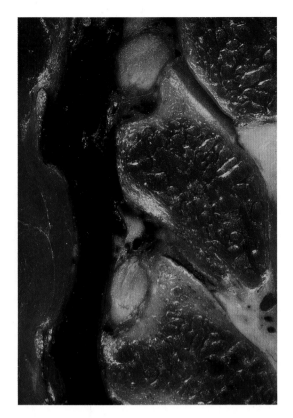

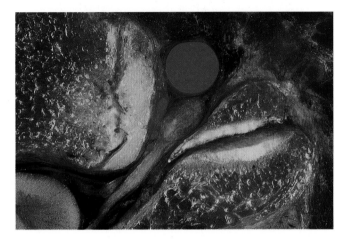

Plate 2-6. Sagittal section through the lateral portion of the articular pillar of a normal midcervical spine. The articular masses, composed of superior and inferior articular processes and a virtual pars interarticularis, are roughly rhomboid and carry obliquely sloping articular facets dorsosuperiorly and ventroinferiorly. Circumferentially meniscoid synovial folds (tags) project into the zygapophyseal or facet joints. Anterior to the upper articular process, deep notches accommodate the root sleeve, ganglion portion of the root, and the postganglionic cervical spinal nerve. This section also displays the vertebral artery (black) in the transverse foramina of the vertebrae.

Plate 2-7. Close-up view of a severely degenerated upper cervical spinal segment displaying advanced uncovertebral spondylosis and slight facet joint arthrosis. The sclerotic uncinate process is oriented in the sagittal plane and osteophytes project laterally toward the vertebral artery and posteriorly into the root canal. Medially in the canal the motor root and the radicular arteries are encroached on. The cylindric (darker) dorsal root ganglion is buttressed in the notches at the anterior surface of the superior articular processes. Note the location of the vertebral artery immediately anterior to the ganglion. The epidural and periradicular veins are small in this specimen. The orientation of the uncinate process and its relationships to the radicular structures and its contribution to neurovascular compromise is essential for surgical decompression such as uncoforaminotomy. Most degenerated specimens displayed significant "anterior" encroachment emanating from the uncovertebral region. Facet joint osteophytes were usually small and rarely projected into the root canals. *(Courtesy Wolfgang Rauschning.)*

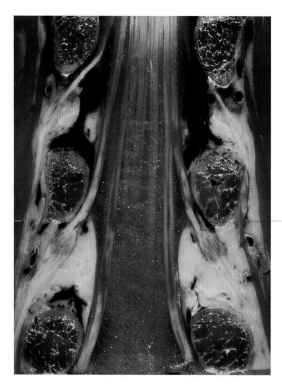

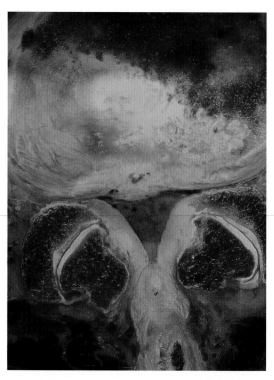

Plate 2-8.   Coronal section through the pedicles of L2, L3, and L4. This section through the midpedicle level shows the serpentiginous course of the nerve roots in a thecal sac of normal width. The shallow (axillary) pouches of the root sleeves lie immediately below the pedicles, where the roots snugly follow the pedicles. The cancellous and cortical bone and the cross-sectional shape of the pedicles vary within wide ranges. At L2 to L3 large veins lie lateral to the dura; at L3 to L4 the dura is bordered by fat interspersed with smaller veins. At L2 to L3 the section is closer to the base of the pedicles and therefore shows the ventral internal venous plexus, whereas at L3 to L4 the posterior, less-vascularized portion of the foramen is displayed. At two levels the entire course of the "roots" can be followed. This root-complex consists of the still intrathecal roots, the root sheath (or root sleeve), the dorsal root ganglion and the ventral root, and the postganglionic lumbar nerve. The long, cylindric lumbar ganglia take a steep and obliquely-inferiorly directed course toward the upper lateral corner of the inferiorly adjacent or caudally adjacent pedicle. The segmental arteries are located lateral to the ganglion and close to the inferior-lateral margin of the pedicle. The lumbar nerve curves around the lateral aspect of the pedicle below, firmly held by the deep portions of the iliopsoas muscle.

Plate 2-9.   Severe degenerative spinal stenosis at the L4 to L5 level in a 70-year-old with a history of intermittent claudication and occasional radicular leg pain. The central and lateral stenosis is most pronounced at this motion segment level and is almost exclusively caused by soft tissues. Anteriorly, the circumferentially "ballooning" disc narrows the thecal sac anteriorly and also completely obliterates the retrodiscal portion of the root canals (neuroforamina). The facet joints, especially the superior articular processes, are moderately hypertrophied, rendering a ball-and-socket configuration of the facet joints. Note the effusion posteriorly of the left facet joint and the sclerotic meniscoid tag posteriorly into the right facet joint. The thecal sac is severely compressed posterolaterally by the thick ligamentum flavum and assumes a triangular slit-shaped configuration in which the roots of the cauda equina are tightly packed without any cerebrospinal fluid surrounding them. The two ligamenta flava are continuous posteriorly with the thick and degenerative interspinous ligament. (Courtesy Wolfgang Rauschning.)

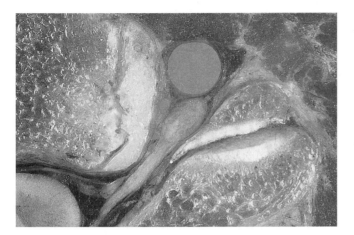

Figure 2-20. (See Plate 2-7.) Close-up view of a severely degenerated upper cervical spinal segment displaying advanced uncovertebral spondylosis and slight facet joint arthrosis. The sclerotic uncinate process is oriented in the sagittal plane and osteophytes project laterally toward the vertebral artery and posteriorly into the root canal. Medially in the canal the motor root and the radicular arteries are encroached on. The cylindric (darker) dorsal root ganglion is buttressed in the notches at the anterior surface of the superior articular processes. Note the location of the vertebral artery immediately anterior to the ganglion. The epidural and periradicular veins are small in this specimen. The orientation of the uncinate process and its relationships to the radicular structures and its contribution to neurovascular compromise is essential for surgical decompression such as uncoforaminotomy. Most degenerated specimens displayed significant "anterior" encroachment emanating from the uncovertebral region. Facet joint osteophytes were usually small and rarely projected into the root canals. (Courtesy Wolfgang Rauschning.)

foraminotomies will minimize vertebral venous bleeding as well.

Sympathetic Trunk

Horner's syndrome, which consists of ipsilateral ptosis, miosis, anhidrosis, and enophthalmos, can occur after anterior cervical approaches from injury to the sympathetic ganglia cephalad to the inferior half of the stellate ganglion or from postganglionic injuries. Ebraheim et al. have described the location and course of the sympathetic trunk in the anterior cervical spine.[32] The longus colli muscles lie on the anterior aspect of the atlas and transverse processes of C3 to C6. These muscles diverge caudally. The sympathetic trunks lie in the loose fascia anterior to the longus colli muscles. The superior cervical ganglion is located at the C2 to C3 level. The middle cervical ganglion is smallest and is usually located opposite of C6. It may be absent in up to 50% of patients or fused to the inferior portion of the superior cervical ganglion. The stellate ganglion lies lateral to the longus

colli between the base of the transverse process of C7 and the neck of the first rib. The sympathetic trunk connects all of these ganglia and is located approximately 10 mm lateral to the medial border of the longus colli. The trunk converges medially toward C6.[32] Extensive lateral mobilization and transverse sectioning of the longus colli should be avoided to reduce the risk of injuring the sympathetic chain. The careful placement of blunt-tipped retractors under, rather than on, the mobilized muscle may also minimize this complication.

ANTERIOR THORACOLUMBAR ANATOMY

A variety of pathologic conditions involving the anterior aspects of the thoracic and lumbar vertebrae can best be approached by anterior decompression and fusion. A number of fixation systems and interbody fusion devices are available for stabilization of the anterior thoracolumbar spine. An understanding of the anatomy of this area of the spine and the surrounding structures is needed to place these devices safely.

Thoracic Spine

The anterior transthoracic approach to the spine is often used for the treatment of fractures, tumors, infection, deformity, and herniated thoracic discs resulting in myelopathy. The thoracic region of the spine has an inherent stability due its articulation with the rib cage. The vertebrae between T2 and T8 have similar topographic characteristics. The T1 vertebra shares similarities with the cervical vertebrae such as bilateral superior uncinate processes, and the T11 and T12 vertebrae represent a transition toward the characteristics of the lumbar spine, especially with regard to the facet joint morphology. In the axial plane, the thoracic bodies are heart shaped with similar anterior-posterior and transverse diameters and gradually increase in size from T1 to T12. The pressure of the aorta flattens the surface of the left side of the bodies. Each vertebra has a superior and inferior costal articulation bilaterally. The ribs articulate with the superior facet of the same number vertebral body and the inferior facet of the vertebra above.

Over the past two decades a number of fixation devices have been developed for anterior thoracolumbar spine stabilization. Most of these are systems consisting of plates or rods connected to screws that are directed into the vertebral body in the coronal plane. Placement of the plates should be centered on the lateral aspect of the body. If the plate is too anterior, there is risk of injury of the great vessels, and the screws may enter the contralateral foramen. If the plate is too far posterior, the screws may enter the spinal canal. Ebraheim et al. recommended that the screws be perpendicular to the lateral plane of the vertebral body and enter the spine in the anterior or middle part of the body to avoid inadvertently angling posteriorly toward the spinal canal.[15] Screws started in the posterior portion of the vertebral body must be directed anteriorly to avoid penetration of the spinal canal. Care must also be taken in choosing the screw length to avoid overpenetration.

Lumbar Spine

The lumbar vertebral bodies tend to be kidney shaped in the axial plane due to the anterior-posterior diameter being smaller than the transverse diameter and the concave shape of the posterior body. The anterior body height is greater than the posterior body height, leading to the overall lordosis of the lumbar spine. The size of the vertebral bodies increases in the caudal direction. Ebraheim et al. noted that the average depth increases from 26 mm to 30 mm from L1 to L4, while the average width increases from 36 mm to 44 mm over the same levels.[28] When placing anterior plating devices in the lumbar spine, the surgeon should follow the same precautions described in anterior plating of the thoracic spine.

Anterior lumbar interbody fusion has recently become a common procedure for the treatment of various conditions in the lower lumbar spine. A number of interbody devices, including cylindric cages and carbon fiber rectangular cages, are available along with the more traditional iliac crest bone grafts or allograft struts. Placement of these devices requires total or subtotal discectomy for preparation of the disc space. Thorough knowledge of the vascular and visceral anatomy adjacent to the L4 to L5 and L5 to L1 discs is needed to safely place these devices.

The bifurcation of the aorta into the common iliac arteries and the confluence of the common iliac veins into the inferior vena cava occur slightly cephalad to the L4 to L5 disc space. The arterial bifurcation is anterior to the venous confluence. Ebraheim et al. reported on the dimensions of the trigone that the common iliac vessels make.[14] They noted that the average distance or width between the left common iliac vein and right common iliac artery is 55 mm and that the average height measured from the apex of the trigone to the sacral promontory is 35 mm. They also noted that approximately 7 mm of the medial edge of the left common iliac vein is uncovered. The surgeon must be aware of the medial-

lying left common iliac vein during anterior approaches to the lower lumbar spine. In order to adequately expose the L4 to L5 disc, the great vessels must be mobilized. The aorta and vena cava are tethered to the spine by the lumbar vessels, which should be identified and ligated to reduce the risk of traction laceration of the great vessels. Care must also be taken to identify and mobilize the ureter at the L4 to L5 disc level. The anterior approach to L5 to L1 does not require as much mobilization of the great vessels; however, the middle sacral artery traverses the disc space and should be identified and ligated to avoid troublesome bleeding.

Retrograde ejaculation is a potential complication of anterior lumbar interbody fusion due to injury of the presacral parasympathetic plexus, which lies anterior to the sacrum and lower lumbar spine. The soft tissues should be incised sharply in the midline and dissected bluntly to mobilize the nerves laterally in order to minimize the occurrence of retrograde ejaculation.

POSTERIOR THORACOLUMBAR ANATOMY

The posterior approach to the thoracolumbar spine has been used to treat a variety of disorders such as deformity, trauma, infection, tumor, and degenerative disease. Direct decompression of the neural elements can be achieved by laminectomy. Instability can be effectively addressed by performing a posterior fusion. Posterior fixation has undergone a dramatic evolution from the original Harrington hook and rod constructs to the modern segmental screw and rod fixation systems. Pedicle screw fixation has become the most common technique of posterior lumbar stabilization. Numerous studies have shown the biomechanic advantages of pedicle screw fixation in the lumbar spine over the use of hooks and wires.[7,34,40] Other studies have reported on the safety of this technique in both children and adults.[37,52] Recently there has been an increase in the use of pedicle screws in the thoracic spine. Transpedicular fixation of the thoracic spine may allow better correction of deformity,[37,62] does not rely on intact posterior elements, and may allow instrumentation of fewer segments than traditional instrumentation systems because of the increased rigidity of the construct. Comprehensive knowledge of the thoracic pedicle morphology is needed to minimize injuring the spinal cord, great vessels, and pleura. Although transpedicular fixation of the lumbar spine has been proved safe, thorough knowledge of lumbar anatomy and pedicle morphology is needed to avoid iatrogenic injury.

Thoracic Pedicle

The thoracic pedicles are oval shaped, with larger superior-inferior dimensions than transverse widths. Vaccaro et al. reported that average pedicle heights range from 8 to 15 mm and tend to gradually increase from T4 to T12 and that the average width ranges from 3 to 10 mm.[65] The narrowest transverse diameters usually occur between T4 and T6. Cinotti et al. reported on a series in which 35% of thoracic pedicles had diam-

> **THORACIC PEDICLE**
>
> - Larger superior-inferior dimensions than transverse widths create oval shape.
> - Average height is 8 to 15 mm; average width is 3 to 10 mm.
> - Diameter is less than 5 mm in 35% of pedicles.
> - Transverse plane angulation at T4 is around 15 degrees medially; it becomes more parallel to sagittal plane from T5 to T12. At T12, path may be diverged.
> - Entry point is 7 to 8 mm medial to lateral edge of superior facet and 3 to 4 mm superior to midline of transverse process of T1 and T2. Between T3 and T12, point lies 5 mm medial to lateral edge of superior facet and 5 mm superior to midline of transverse process.

> **LUMBAR PEDICLE**
>
> - Pedicle insertion angle: L1 axis is approximately 7 degrees medial in transverse plane. Medial inclination increases to 18 degrees at L5.
> - Screw insertion site set in relation to transverse process.
> - Pedicle axis projects 2 to 4 mm superior from L1 to L3, at midline at L4, and 1.5 mm inferior to midline at L5.

eters less than 5 mm, most occurring between T4 and T8.[8] The T1 and T2 pedicles have slightly larger dimensions than the middle thoracic pedicles. The transverse plane angulation of the pedicle at T4 is approximately 15 degrees medial and gradually becomes more parallel to the sagittal plane from T5 to T12.[65] In some studies pedicles at T12 have been found to be divergent. The medial pedicle cortex is the thickest. Ebraheim et al. reported that the distance between the superior and inferior pedicle cortex and the adjacent exiting nerve root is approximately 2 mm.[17] They noted that there is no epidural space between the dura and the medial edge of the pedicle. In another study Ebraheim et al. reported that the projection point or entry for the thoracic pedicle is 7 to 8 mm medial to the lateral edge of the superior facet and 5 mm superior to the midline of the transverse process.[20] Vacarro et al. noted that caudal to T9, there is a gradual transition of the pedicle toward the center of the transverse process.[65]

Accuracy of the starting point for thoracic pedicle screws is crucial due to the narrow dimensions of the pedicles and the proximity of vital adjacent structures.[66] Preoperative planning should include CT scans to identify the pedicle dimensions and any anatomic variations. The surgeon should be careful not to start the screw too medially, to avoid penetrating the spinal canal and to avoid directing the screw into the great vessels. Open laminotomy is also helpful in minimizing screw misdirection by enabling direct visualization of the medial cortex.[70]

Lumbar Pedicle

The pedicles in the lumbar spine tend to be short and medially inclined. Pedicle heights vary in individuals, and the widths tend to increase from L1 to L5. The L1 pedicle axis is directed approximately 7 degrees medial in the transverse plane. This medial inclination gradually increases at each lumbar level and is approximately 18 degrees at L5.[64] Ebraheim et al. reported that the average distance from the lumbar pedicle to the superior

and inferior adjacent nerve roots and lateral dural edge are 5 mm, 1.5 mm, and 1.5 mm, respectively[16] (Figure 2-21; see also Plate 2-8). The projection point or entry of the lumbar pedicle is at the junction of the superior articular process and transverse process. When present, the mamillary process can aid in identification of the starting point. In relation to the midline of the transverse process, the pedicle axis projects 2 to 4 mm superior from L1 to L3, is at the midline at L4, and is 1.5 mm inferior to the midline at L5[12] (Figure 2-22).

As in the thoracic spine, preoperative imaging is helpful in identifying pedicle morphology and anatomic variations. Laminotomy or laminectomy is helpful by allowing direct visualization of the medial pedicle cortex. Also, intraoperative radiographs or fluoroscopy may aid in the placement of screws. The surgeon should be aware of the close relationship that the thecal sac and exiting nerve roots have with the medial and inferior walls of the lumbar pedicles (Figure 2-23; see also Plate 2-9).

SACRAL ANATOMY

The sacrum is the triangular base of the spine and comprises five fused vertebrae. Each sacral vertebra is separated from the adjacent vertebrae by a transverse line known as the linea transversaria. The sacral promontory is the superior anterior border of the first sacral body. The bilateral sacral alae are actually lateral masses that represent the fusion of vestigial costal elements and transverse processes. There are four intervertebral foramina bilaterally on both the ventral and dorsal sacral surfaces. The laminae fuse posteriorly, giving rise to the spinous tubercle.

Screw fixation of the sacrum is often used in instrumentation of the lumbosacral spine (Figure 2-24). There are several techniques of screw placement at S1 and S2 based on anatomic and biomechanic considerations. Screws can be placed medially toward the sacral promontory or laterally toward the ala and may have unicortical or bicortical purchase. Each technique has various proponents and potential pitfalls.[33,41,49] Potential complications from misdirected bicortical screws are injury to the lumbar nerve roots, iliac vessels, or sympathetic chain and perineal pain from sacral nerve root irritation. Esses et al. recommend placement of screws superior to the first sacral foramen directed toward the promontory parallel to the superior S1 endplate.[33]

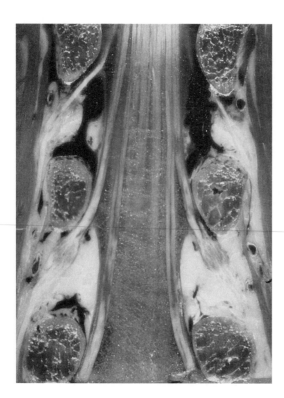

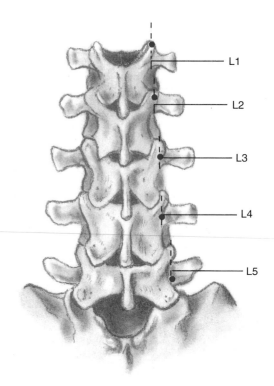

Figure 2-21. (See Plate 2-8.) Coronal section through the pedicles of L2, L3, and L4. This section through the midpedicle level shows the serpentiginous course of the nerve roots in a thecal sac of normal width. The shallow (axillary) pouches of the root sleeves lie immediately below the pedicles, where the roots snugly follow the pedicles. The cancellous and cortical bone and the cross-sectional shape of the pedicles vary within wide ranges. At L2 to L3 large veins lie lateral to the dura; at L3 to L4 the dura is bordered by fat interspersed with smaller veins. At L2 to L3 the section is closer to the base of the pedicles and therefore shows the ventral internal venous plexus, whereas at L3 to L4 the posterior, less-vascularized portion of the foramen is displayed. At two levels the entire course of the "roots" can be followed. This root-complex consists of the still intrathecal roots, the root sheath (or root sleeve), the dorsal root ganglion and the ventral root, and the postganglionic lumbar nerve. The long, cylindric lumbar ganglia take a steep and obliquely-inferiorly directed course toward the upper lateral corner of the inferiorly adjacent or caudally adjacent pedicle. The segmental arteries are located lateral to the ganglion and close to the inferior-lateral margin of the pedicle. The lumbar nerve curves around the lateral aspect of the pedicle below, firmly held by the deep portions of the iliopsoas muscle.

Figure 2-22. The starting point for pedicle screw insertion in relationship to the contiguous transverse process. (*Redrawn from Ebraheim NA et al.: Projection of the lumbar pedicle and its morphometric analysis, Spine 21[11]:1296-1300, 1996.*)

SACRAL PEDICLE SCREEN INSTRUMENTATION

- Recommended insertion trajectory: superior to first sacral foramen directed toward promontory parallel to S1 endplate
- Sacral ala screws: Angled 30 to 40 degrees laterally to avoid neurovascular injury

---

Ebraheim et al. reviewed the course of the L4, L5, and S1 nerve roots across the ala and recommended angling S1 ala screws 30 to 40 degrees laterally to avoid iatrogenic nerve injury.[30] Licht, Rowe, and Ross reported that medial direction of S1 screws places the left common iliac vein and sympathetic chain at risk.[41] Screws at S2 and S3 directed medially may also injure the sympathetic chain. They also noted that lateral direction of S1 screws places the lumbosacral plexus at greater risk and that lateral direction of a screw at S2 may injure the S1 nerve root. The surgeon must be aware of the relationship of the neurovascular structures to the anterior border of the sacrum, especially when placing screws with bicortical purchase (Figure 2-25).

PERTINENT ANATOMY OF THE ILIAC CREST

Autogenous bone grafting remains the gold standard for spinal fusion. The anterior and posterior iliac crests are the most frequent bone graft harvest sites used for spinal surgery. Both sites have anatomic considerations the surgeon must be aware of to avoid complications.

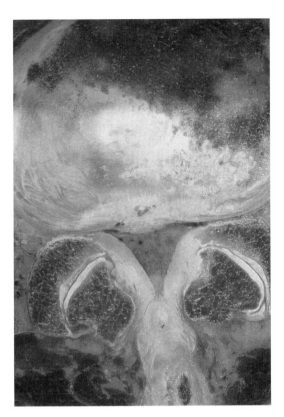

Figure 2-23. (See Plate 2-9.) Severe degenerative spinal stenosis at the L4 to L5 level in a 70-year-old with a history of intermittent claudication and occasional radicular leg pain. The central and lateral stenosis is most pronounced at this motion segment level and is almost exclusively caused by soft tissues. Anteriorly, the circumferentially "ballooning" disc narrows the thecal sac anteriorly and also completely obliterates the retrodiscal portion of the root canals (neuroforamina). The facet joints, especially the superior articular processes, are moderately hypertrophied, rendering a ball-and-socket configuration of the facet joints. Note the effusion posteriorly of the left facet joint and the sclerotic meniscoid tag posteriorly into the right facet joint. The thecal sac is severely compressed posterolaterally by the thick ligamentum flavum and assumes a triangular slit-shaped configuration in which the roots of the cauda equina are tightly packed without any cerebrospinal fluid surrounding them. The two ligamenta flava are continuous posteriorly with the thick and degenerative interspinous ligament. *(Courtesy Wolfgang Rauschning.)*

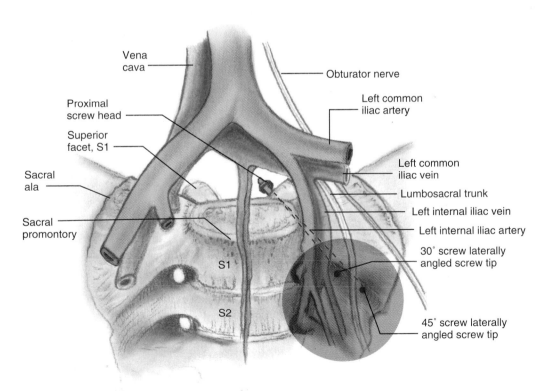

Figure 2-24. Vascular anatomy at risk for laterally angled S1 sacral screws. *(Redrawn from Mirkovic S et al.: Spine 16[6]:S289-S294, 1991.)*

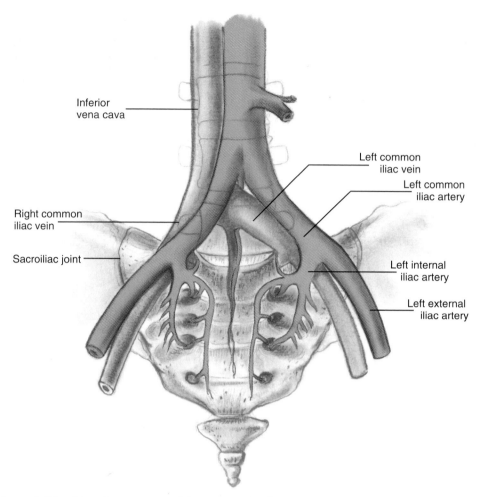

Figure 2-25.   Vascular anatomy of the anterior lumbosacral spine. *(Redrawn from Esses SI et al.: Surgical anatomy of the sacrum: a guide for rational screw fixation, Spine 16[6]:S283-S288, 1991.)*

Anterior Iliac Crest

The anterior crest is often harvested for anterior spinal fusions. It is approached through an oblique incision paralleling the crest posteriorly from the anterior-superior iliac spine. Injury to the lateral femoral cutaneous nerve, also known as meralgia paresthetica, is a well-described complication of anterior iliac bone graft harvesting that is very difficult to treat. The nerve usually courses along the lateral border of the psoas major, crosses the ilium, and runs toward the anterior-superior iliac spine. Its course is variable and must be understood to minimize injury. Murata et al. described the course of the lateral femoral cutaneous nerve.[50] They found that the nerve varies both in its relationship with the anterior-superior iliac spine and in its course across the iliacus muscle. In their series the nerve ran under the inguinal ligament 58% of the time, and an additional 29% crossed at the anterior-superior iliac spine (ASIS).[50] Eleven percent of the time, the nerve crossed the anterior crest within 2 cm posterior to the ASIS, and 2% of the time, it crossed greater than 2 cm posterior to the ASIS.[50] The incision and dissection of the anterior iliac crest should remain at least 2 cm lateral to the anterior-

superior iliac spine to minimize the risk of meralgia paresthetica. The surgeon must also be careful to leave the anterior-superior iliac spine intact to preserve the appearance of the region and to avoid detaching the inguinal ligament and causing an iatrogenic inguinal hernia (Figure 2-26).

Posterior Iliac Crest

The posterior crest is often harvested for posterior spinal fusions and can be approached through a separate skin incision or through the same incision used for the posterior approach to the lumbar spine. Cancellous bone

---

LATERAL FEMORAL CUTANEOUS NERVE

- Relationship to anterior-superior iliac spine (ASIS)[50]
  - Courses under inguinal ligament in 58%
  - Crosses anterior-superior iliac spine in 29%
  - Crosses 2 cm posterior to ASIS in 11%
  - Crosses more than 2 cm posterior to ASIS in 2%

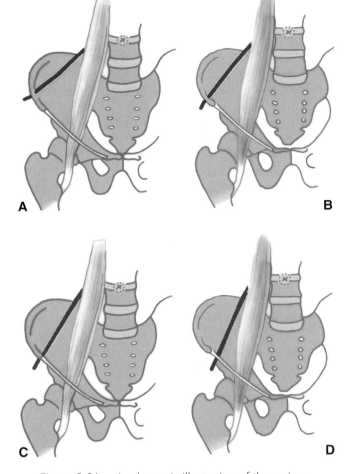

A B

C D

Figure 2-26. A schematic illustration of the various courses of the lateral femoral cutaneous nerve in relationship to the anterior-superior iliac spine. **A,** Type A nerves crossed over the iliac crest more than 2 cm posterior to the anterior-superior iliac spine. **B,** Type B nerves crossed over the iliac crest within two centimeters posterior to the anterior-superior iliac spine. **C,** Type C nerves crossed at the anterior-superior iliac spine. **D,** Type D nerves crossed under the inguinal ligament and anterior to the anterior-superior iliac spine. *(Redrawn from Murata Y et al.: The anatomy of the lateral femoral cutaneous nerve, with special reference to the harvesting of iliac bone graft, J Bone Joint Surg Am 82A[5]:746-747, 2000.)*

CLUNEAL NERVES

- Nerves arise from posterior primary rami of L1, L2, and L3.
- Medial branch of superior cluneal nerve lies approximately 7 cm from posterior-superior iliac spine.
- Medial, intermediate, and lateral branches of cluneal nerve perforate thoracolumbar fascia 8 cm inferior, 2 cm superior, and 12 cm superior to the superior crest border.

---

rior iliac spine. The medial, intermediate, and lateral branches of the nerve perforate the thoracolumbar fascia. These points of perforation lie 6 cm inferior to crest for the medial branch, 2 cm superior for the intermediate branch, and 12 cm superior for the lateral branch. To avoid injury to the cluneal nerves, the incision should not be carried more than 8 cm anterolateral to the posterior-superior iliac spine.

Laceration of the superior gluteal artery during posterior iliac crest bone graft harvesting is a potentially life-threatening complication. The superior gluteal artery is a branch of the internal iliac artery and exits the pelvis through the sciatic notch. It stays along the bone proximal to the piriform muscle. The artery can be lacerated by an osteotome if the graft is taken too close to the sciatic notch. Inadvertent placement of a retractor in the sciatic notch may also injure the artery. Several techniques can be employed to minimize injury to the superior gluteal artery.[42] At the level of the posterior-superior iliac spine, the dissection should not be carried inferior to the insertion of the gluteus maximus. Retractors should not be placed in the sciatic notch. While using an osteotome, the surgeon should engage the cutting edge in only the outer cortex and should direct the instrument cephalad to avoid slipping toward the sciatic notch.

SELECTED REFERENCES

Ebraheim NA et al.: An anatomic study of the thickness of the occipital bone. Implications for occipitocervical instrumentation, *Spine* 21(15):1725-1729, 1996.

Ebraheim NA et al.: Anatomic considerations of anterior instrumentation of the thoracic spine, *Am J Orthop* 26(6):419-424, 1997.

Ebraheim NA et al.: Anatomic considerations for anterior instrumentation of the lumbar spine, *Orthopedics*, 22(10):935-939, 1999.

Ebraheim NA et al.: Anatomic relationship of the cervical nerves to the lateral masses, *Am J Orthop* 28(1):39-42, 1999.

Esses SI et al.: Surgical anatomy of the sacrum: a guide for rational screw fixation, *Spine* 16(6 Suppl):S283-S288, 1991.

Heller JG et al.: Anatomic comparison of the Roy-Camille and Magerl techniques for screw placement, *Spine* 16(6 Suppl):S552-S557, 1991.

Jeanneret B, Gebhard JS, Magerl F: Transpedicular screw fixation of articular mass fracture-separation: results of an anatomical study and operative technique, *J Spinal Disord* 7:222-229, 1994.

Lu J, Ebraheim NA: The vertebral artery: surgical anatomy, *Orthopedics* 22(11):1081-1085, 1999.

Magerl F, Seeman P: Stable posterior fusion of the atlas and axis by transarticular screw fixation. In *Cervical spine*, vol 1, New York, 1987, Springer-Verlag, p322.

Roy-Camille R, Saillant G, Mazel C: Internal fixation of the lumbar spine with pedicle screw plating, *Clin Orthop* 203:7-17, 1986.

---

can be harvested between the iliac table, or corticocancellous strips can be taken by stripping the gluteal muscles off of the outer table of the ilium.

During the superficial approach, the surgeon must be aware of the course of the cluneal nerves. These nerves arise from the posterior primary rami of L1, L2, and L3 and supply sensation to the gluteal area. Injury can result in annoying numbness in the region or painful neuromas. Lu et al. describe the relationship of the superior cluneal nerve to the posterior iliac crest.[46] They note that the medial branch of the superior cluneal nerve lies approximately 7 cm from the posterior-supe-

Xu R et al.: The anatomic relation of lateral mass screws to the spinal nerves: a comparison of the Magerl, Anderson, and An techniques, *Spine* 24(19):2057-2061, 1999.

REFERENCES

1. Abumi K, Kaneda K: Pedicular screw fixation for nontraumatic lesions of the cervical spine, *Spine* 22:1853-1863, 1997.
2. Anderson PA et al.: Posterior cervical arthrodesis with AO reconstruction plates and bone graft, *Spine* 16(6 Suppl):S72-S79, 1991.
3. Bailey RW, Badgley CE: Stabilization of the cervical spine by anterior fusion, *J Bone Joint Surg Am* 42:565-594, 1960.
4. Bland JH: *Disorders of the cervical spine: diagnosis and medical management*, Philadelphia, 1987, WB Saunders.
5. Bohlman HH et al.: Robinson anterior cervical discectomy and arthrodesis for cervical radiculopathy: long-term follow-up of one hundred and twenty-two patients, *J Bone Joint Surg Am* 75(9):1298-1307, 1993.
6. Brooks AL, Jenkins EB: Atlanto-axial arthrodesis by the wedge compression method, *J Bone Joint Surg Am* 60:279, 1978.
7. Chang KW et al.: A comparative biomechanical study of spinal fixation using the combination spinal rod-plate and transpedicular screw fixation system, *J Spinal Disord* 1:257-266, 1988.
8. Cinotti G et al.: Pedicle instrumentation in the thoracic spine, *Spine* 24(2):114-119, 1999.
9. Cloward RB: The anterior approach for removal of ruptured cervical disks, *J Neurosurg* 15:602-617, 1958.
10. Ebraheim NA et al.: An anatomic study of the thickness of the occipital bone. Implications for occipitocervical instrumentation, *Spine* 21(15):1725-1729, 1996.
11. Ebraheim NA et al.: Anatomic consideration of C2 pedicle screw placement, *Spine* 21(6):691-695, 1996.
12. Ebraheim NA et al.: Projection of the lumbar pedicle and its morphometric analysis, *Spine* 21(11):1296-1300, 1996.
13. Ebraheim NA, Xu R, Yeasting RA: The location of the vertebral artery foramen and its relation to posterior lateral mass screw fixation, *Spine*, 21(11):1291-1295, 1996.
14. Ebraheim NA et al.: The quantitative anatomy of the iliac vessels and their relation to anterior lumbosacral approach, *J Spinal Disord* 9(5):414-417, 1996.
15. Ebraheim NA et al.: Anatomic considerations of anterior instrumentation of the thoracic spine, *Am J Orthop* 26(6):419-424, 1997.
16. Ebraheim NA et al.: Anatomic relations between the lumbar pedicle and the adjacent neural structures, *Spine* 22(20):2338-2341, 1997.
17. Ebraheim NA et al.: Anatomic relations of the thoracic pedicle to the adjacent neural structures, *Spine* 22(14):1553-1556, 1997.
18. Ebraheim NA et al: Location of the vertebral artery foramen on the anterior aspect of the lower cervical spine by computed tomography, *J Spinal Disord* 10(4):304-307, 1997.
19. Ebraheim NA et al.: Morphometric evaluation of lower cervical pedicle and its projection, *Spine* 22(1):1-6, 1997.
20. Ebraheim NA et al.: Projection of the thoracic pedicle and its morphometric analysis, *Spine* 22(3):233-238, 1997.
21. Ebraheim NA et al.: Vulnerability of the recurrent laryngeal nerve in the anterior approach to the lower cervical spine, *Spine* 22(22):2664-2667, 1997.
22. Ebraheim NA et al.: Anatomic basis of the anterior surgery on the cervical spine: relationships between uncus-artery-root complex and vertebral artery injury, *Surg Radiol Anat* 20(6):389-392, 1998.
23. Ebraheim NA et al.: Quantitative anatomy of the transverse foramen and pedicle of the axis, *J Spinal Disord* 11(6):521-525, 1998.
24. Ebraheim NA et al.: Safe lateral-mass screw lengths in the Roy-Camille and Magerl techniques: an anatomic study, *Spine* 23(16):1739-1742, 1998.
25. Ebraheim NA et al.: The anatomic location of the dorsal ramus of the cervical nerve and its relation to the superior articular process of the lateral mass, *Spine* 23(18):1968-1971, 1998.
26. Ebraheim NA et al.: The quantitative anatomy of the vertebral artery groove of the atlas and its relation to the posterior atlantoaxial approach, *Spine* 23(3):320-323, 1998.
27. Ebraheim NA et al.: The vertebral body depths of the cervical spine and its relation to anterior plate-screw fixation, *Spine* 23(21):2299-2302, 1998.
28. Ebraheim NA et al.: Anatomic considerations for anterior instrumentation of the lumbar spine, *Orthopedics* 22(10):935-939, 1999.
29. Ebraheim NA et al.: Anatomic relationship of the cervical nerves to the lateral masses, *Am J Orthop* 28(1):39-42, 1999.
30. Ebraheim NA et al.: The lumbosacral nerves in relation to dorsal S1 screw placement and their locations on plain radiographs, *Orthopedics* 23(3):245-247, 2000.
31. Ebraheim NA et al.: The optimal transarticular C1-2 screw length and the location of the hypoglossal nerve, *Surg Neurol* 53(3):208-210, 2000.
32. Ebraheim NA et al.: Vulnerability of the sympathetic trunk during the anterior approach to the lower cervical spine, *Spine* 25(13):1603-1606, 2000.
33. Esses SI et al.: Surgical anatomy of the sacrum: a guide for rational screw fixation, *Spine* 16(6 Suppl):S283-S288, 1991.
34. Gaines RW et al.: Improving quality of spinal internal fixation: evolution toward "ideal immobilization": a biomechanical study, *Orthop Trans* 11:86-87, 1987.
35. Gallie WE: Fractures and dislocations of the cervical spine, *Am J Surg* 46:495, 1939.
36. Grob D et al.: Posterior occipitocervical fusion: a preliminary report of a new technique, *Spine* 16:S17-24, 1991.
37. Hamill CL et al.: The use of pedicle screw fixation to improve correction in the lumbar spine of patients with idiopathic scoliosis, *Spine* 21:1241-1249, 1996.
38. Heller JG et al.: Anatomic comparison of the Roy-Camille and Magerl techniques for screw placement, *Spine* 16(6 Suppl):S552-S557, 1991.
39. Jeanneret B, Gebhard JS, Magerl F: Transpedicular screw fixation of articular mass fracture-separation: results of an anatomical study and operative technique, *J Spinal Disord* 7:222-229, 1994.
40. King AG, Tahmoush KM, Thomas KA: Biomechanical testing of pedicle screws versus lamina hooks as distal anchors for scoliosis instrumentation, *Proceedings of the 32nd Annual Meeting of the Scoliosis Research Society*, St. Louis, Sept 25-27, 1997.
41. Licht NJ, Rowe DE, Ross LM: Pitfalls of pedicle screw fixation in the sacrum: a cadaver model, *Spine* 17(8):892-896, 1992.
42. Lim EVA, Lavadia WT, Roberts JM: Superior gluteal artery injury during iliac bone grafting for spinal fusion: a case report and literature review, *Spine* 21:2376-2378, 1996.
43. Lu J, Ebraheim NA: The vertebral artery: surgical anatomy, *Orthopedics* 22(11):1081-1085, 1999.
44. Lu J et al.: Anatomic considerations of superior cluneal nerve at posterior iliac crest region, *Clin Orthop* 347:224-228, 1998.
45. Lu J et al.: Anatomic considerations of the vertebral artery: implications for anterior decompression of the cervical spine, *J Spinal Disord* 11(3):233-236, 1998.
46. Lu J et al.: Cervical venous structure in the inter-transverse and intra-transverse foraminal region: an anatomic study, *Am J Orthop* 29(3):196-198, 2000.
47. Magerl F, Seemann P: Stable posterior fusion of the atlas and axis by transarticular screw fixation. In *Cervical spine*, vol 1, New York, 1987, Springer-Verlag, p. 322.
48. Mandel IM et al.: Morphologic considerations of C2 isthmus dimensions for the placement of transarticular screws, *Spine* 25(12):1542-1547, 2000.
49. Mirkovic S et al.: Anatomic consideration for sacral screw placement, *Spine* 16(6 Suppl):S289-294, 1991.
50. Murata Y et al.: The anatomy of the lateral femoral cutaneous nerve, with special reference to the harvesting of iliac bone graft, *J Bone Joint Surg Am* 82(5):746-747, 2000.
51. Paramore CG, Dickman CA, Sonntag VKH: The anatomic suitability of the C1-C2 complex for posterior transarticular screw fixation, *J Neurosurg* 85:221-224, 1996.
52. Puschak TJ, Kling TF, Lindseth RE: Safety of pedicle screw fixation in the pediatric spine, *Proceedings of the 16th Annual Meeting of the Mid-America Orthopaedic Association*, Acapulco, April 22-26, 1998.
53. Ransford AO, Crockard HA, Pozo JL: Craniocervical instability treated by contoured loop fixation, *J Bone Joint Surg Br* 68:173-177, 1986.
54. Robinson RA, Smith GW: Anterolateral cervical disc removal and interbody fusion for cervical disc syndrome, *Bull Johns Hopkins Hosp* 96:223-224, 1955 (abstract).

55. Robinson RA, Southwick WO: Indications and techniques for early stabilization of the neck in some fracture dislocations of the cervical spine, *South Med J* 53:565-579, 1960.

56. Roy-Camille R, Saillant G, Bouchet T: Technique du vissage des pedicules deC2. In Roy-Camille, ed: *Journees d'Orthopedie de la Pitie: Rachis Cervical Superieur*, Paris, 1986, Masson pp. 41-43.

57. Roy-Camille R, Saillant G, Mazel C: Internal fixation of the unstable cervical spine by a posterior osteosynthesis with plates and screws. In the Cervical Spine Research Society Editorial Committee, ed: *The cervical spine*, ed 2, Philadelphia, 1989, JB Lippincott, pp. 390-403.

58. Sakou T, Kawaida H, Morizino Y: Occipitoatlantoaxial fusion utilizing a rectangular rod, *Clin Orthop* 239:136-144, 1989.

59. Sasso RC et al.: Occipitocervical fusion with posterior plate and screw instrumentation: a long-term follow up study, *Spine* 19:2364-2368.

60. Smith MD, Anderson P, Grady MS: Occipitocervical arthrodesis using contoured plate fixation: an early report on a versatile fixation technique, *Spine* 18:1984-1990, 1993.

61. Solanki G, Crockard HA: Peroperative determination of safe superior transarticular screw trajectory through the lateral mass, *Spine* 24(14):1477-1482, 1999.

62. Suk SI et al.: Segmental pedicle screw fixation in the treatment of thoracic idiopathic scoliosis, *Spine* 20:1399-1405, 1995.

63. Taitz C, Arensburg B: Vertebral artery tortuosity with concomitant erosion of the foramen of the transverse process of the axis: possible clinical implications, *Acta Anat (Basel)* 141:104-108, 1991.

64. Vaccaro AR: Spine Anatomy. In Garfin SR, Vaccaro AR, eds: *Orthopaedic knowledge update: spine*, Chicago, 1997, American Academy of Orthopaedic Surgeons.

65. Vaccaro AR et al.: Placement of pedicle screws in the thoracic spine. I. Morphometric analysis of the thoracic vertebrae, *J Bone Joint Surg Am* 77(8):1193-1199, 1995.

66. Vacarro AR et al.: Placement of pedicle screws in the thoracic spine. II: An anatomical and radiographic assessment, *J Bone Joint Surg Am* 77(8):1200-1206, 1995.

67. Wertheim SB, Bohlman HH: Occipitocervical fusion: indications, technique and long-term results in thirteen patients, *J Bone Joint Surg Am* 69:833-836, 1987.

68. Xu R et al.: Morphology of the second cervical vertebra and the posterior projection of the C2 pedicle axis, *Spine* 20:259-263, 1995.

69. Xu R et al.: The location of the cervical nerve roots on the posterior aspect of the cervical spine, *Spine* 20(21):2267-2271, 1995.

70. Xu R et al.: Anatomic considerations of pedicle screw placement in the thoracic spine: Roy-Camille technique versus open-lamina technique, *Spine* 23(9):1065-1068, 1998.

71. Xu R et al.: Anatomic relation between the cervical pedicle and the adjacent neural structures, *Spine* 24(5):451-454, 1999.

72. Xu R et al.: The anatomic relation of lateral mass screws to the spinal nerves: a comparison of the Magerl, Anderson, and An techniques, *Spine* 24(19):2057-2061, 1999.

Relevant Clinical Biomechanics of the Spine

Jonathan N. Grauer, Manohar M. Panjabi

The spine is a complex series of articulating vertebrae that have innate stability, provide protection to the neural elements, and allow segmental motion to occur in a controlled fashion. The first two chapters of this text illustrated the anatomy of the cervical, thoracic, and lumbar spine. The purpose of this chapter is to define biomechanical concepts that are useful in clinical spine practice. This requires precise use of terminology and application of principles. Once a background is established, the intact and unstable spine will then be contrasted.

DEFINITION OF TERMS

The goal of clinical biomechanics is to describe in vivo situations, understand pathology, and guide treatment in the clinical arena. However, there are clear limitations to the type of experiments that can be performed in vivo. Many biomechanical studies are thus performed in the cadaveric laboratory. Results from such studies are then confirmed clinically.

Sagittal, *coronal*, and *axial planes* are clinical terms. A more precise, less ambiguous Cartesian coordinate system is generally used in the laboratory. Figure 3-1 demonstrates a global coordinate system that is used to describe the body as a whole. Similar coordinate systems can be based on any definable body part to describe motions of one anatomic structure relative to another.

Studies generally divide the spine into functional spinal units (also called motion segments). This base unit is composed of two adjacent vertebral bodies, the intervertebral disc, facets, and ligaments and is the smallest specimen whose mechanical properties can be extrapolated to longer spinal segments.

Kinematics is the study of motion without addressing the inciting forces. These motions are determined by the anatomic geometry of the osseous and ligamentous structures and the interplay of their mechanical properties. Rotations and translations occur around the x, y, and z axes. Motions can be described as a main motion in the plane being studied and secondary, or coupled, motions in the other two planes. As such, each vertebral body has six degrees of freedom: three rotational and three translational (black arrows in Figure 3-2). An example of a kinematic study is that of describing the rotational and translational motions of the head relative to the torso during whiplash trauma.

For each motion in a plane, be it rotational or translational, an instantaneous axis of rotation can be described. This is a line in the body or a hypothetical extension of it that does not move and is perpendicular to the plane of the body's motion. Of note, the axis of rotation may be dynamic. Further, alterations in such axes of rotation have been correlated with underlying pathologies both in the laboratory and clinically.

Each three-dimensional motion can be considered in terms of a helical axis of rotation concept. This is done by considering rotation around and translation along a single axis. This notion can be useful in the mathematic

---

DEFINITIONS

- Motion segments: Functional spinal units
- Functional spinal unit
  - Comprises two adjacent vertebral bodies, intervertebral disc, facets, and ligaments
  - Is smallest specimen whose mechanical properties can be extrapolated to longer spinal segments
- *Kinematics*: The study of motion without addressing inciting forces
- Motions
  - Main: Motion in plane being studied
  - Secondary, or coupled: Motions in other two planes
- Degrees of freedom: Each vertebral body has size—three rotational and three translational
- *Kinetics*: The study of motions produced by defined loads
- Loads: Forces or moments
  - Force: Applied to a point on an object, a force translates the point
  - Moment: Equal and opposite parallel forces separated by a defined distance acting on an object

analysis of motions in the laboratory but has been less extrapolated to the clinical scenario due to its less intuitive nature.

Kinetics is the study of motions produced by defined loads. Such loads can be forces or moments (outlined arrows in Figure 3-2). A force applied to a point on an object translates the point. A moment involves equal and opposite parallel forces that are separated by a defined distance acting on an object. Moments offer the experimental advantage of distributing forces equally along the length of a column to which they are applied. As with kinematics, resulting main and coupled motions can be studied (see black arrows in Figure 3-2). To return to the whiplash example, kinetics explains the motions of the cervical spine during whiplash trauma as a function of the acceleration loads applied.

To facilitate three-dimensional motion analysis in the laboratory, optical, magnetic, and electronic motion monitoring systems have been developed. These modalities complement plain and/or fluoroscopic radiographs such as those used clinically. Other highly precise monitoring systems such as roentgen stereometric analysis have also been developed for specific applications to maximize three-dimensional sensitivity. Some of these modalities are limited to the laboratory, whereas others have been used in clinical research or practice.

FUNCTIONAL BIOMECHANICS OF THE SPINE

Physiologic flexibility testing studies document the load-displacement behavior of functional spinal units under the application of pure moments (Figure 3-3). As pure moments are applied in a stepwise fashion, motion responses are monitored and load-displacement curves are generated (Figure 3-4, *A*). It becomes readily apparent that the resulting plots are nonlinear. This is because the spine, which is flexible at low loads, stiffens with increasing loads.

In order to characterize the spine's response to loading, two parameters have been described: range of motion (ROM) and neutral zone (NZ). ROM is the displacement of a motion segment from one extreme to the other when physiologic moments are applied in any of the six degrees of freedom. NZ is the central portion of the ROM for which no significant resistance is met.[2] NZ is thus a measure of spinal laxity.

An image of a ball in a bowl has been used as an analogy to clarify the NZ and ROM concepts (Figure 3-4, *B*).[1] The load-displacement curve is transformed into a bowl by flipping the extension portion of a flexion/extension curve around the displacement axis. An imaginary ball moves easily within the bottom of the bowl (NZ) but requires greater effort to push it up the sloping sides of the bowl (ROM). These motion parameters exist for each

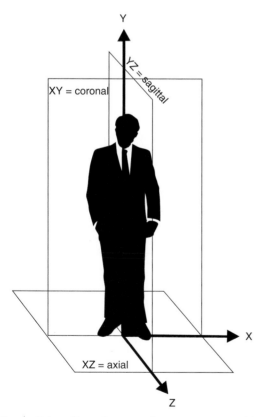

Figure 3-1. Cartesian coordinate system used in mathematic descriptions of the body. *XY* plane is the coronal plane, *XZ* is the axial plane, and *YZ* is the sagittal plane. *(Redrawn from White AA III, Panjabi MM: Clinical biomechanics of the spine, ed 2 Philadelphia, 1990, JB Lippincott.)*

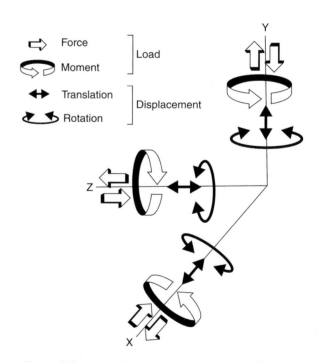

Figure 3-2. A motion segment is composed of two adjacent vertebral bodies and the intervertebral disc, facets, and ligaments. This can be loaded with forces or moments. Resultant displacements are translations and/or rotations. *(Redrawn from White AA III, Panjabi MM: Clinical biomechanics of the spine, ed 2 Philadelphia, 1990, JB Lippincott.)*

of the three planes of motion: flexion/extension, lateral bending, and axial rotation.

Stiffness testing offers a similar but different means of testing the physiologic properties of a motion segment. Rather than applying a defined pure moment, segments are displaced predetermined intervals. The load to achieve this displacement, as well as the distribution of motion within multilevel specimens, is determined. The

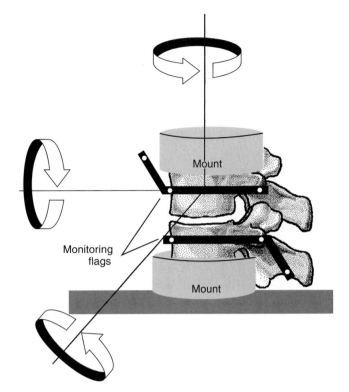

Figure 3-3. Flexibility testing is performed by applying pure moments. Resultant displacements are monitored with motion monitoring flags applied to each vertebra.

FUNCTIONAL BIOMECHANICS

- Physiologic flexibility testing studies document load-displacement behavior of functional spinal units under application of pure moments
  - Resulting plots nonlinear
  - Spine, flexible at low loads, stiffens with increasing loads
- Parameters characterizing spine's response to loading
  - Range of motion (ROM): Displacement of a motion segment from one extreme to the other when physiologic moments are applied in any of six degrees of freedom
  - Neutral zone (NZ)
    - Central portion of ROM for which no significant resistance is met
    - Measure of spinal laxity
  - Motion parameters exist for each of three planes of motion: Flexion/extension, lateral bending, and axial rotation

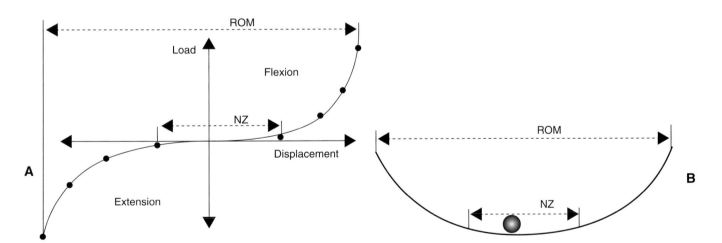

Figure 3-4. **A,** Nonlinear response of a spine segment loaded in flexion (positive load) and extension (negative load). Range of motion *(ROM)* is the total displacement observed under physiologic loading. Neutral zone *(NZ)* is the component of the ROM before the change in stiffness is observed. **B,** A ball-in-a-bowl analogy is shown. The ball can move easily in the bottom of the bowl but encounters increased resistance at the limits of motion. *(Redrawn from Panjabi MM. Low back pain and spinal instability. In Weinstein J, Gordon S, eds, Low back pain: a scientific and clinical overview. Rosemont, Ill, American Academy of Orthopaedic Surgeons, 1996.)*

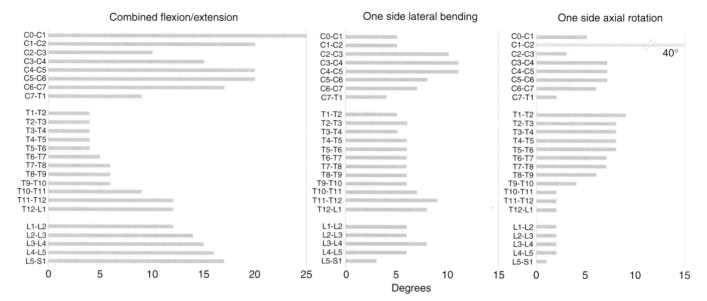

Figure 3-5. A composite of the values for rotatory range of motion at the different levels of the spine in the traditional planes of rotation. *(Redrawn from White AA III, Panjabi MM: Clinical biomechanics of the spine, ed 2, Philadelphia, 1990, JB Lippincott.)*

greatest advantage of such testing is the ability to analyze interdependency of motion at multiple levels. In other words, a change in stiffness at one level will affect an adjacent level's motion, unlike with the flexibility testing. This is because an adjacent level will be exposed to greater or lesser forces depending on if the level of primary interest becomes more or less stable. This is in contrast to the previously described flexibility testing, where pure moments distribute equally along the length of the segments being tested, irrespective of the segmental stiffnesses.

Testing protocols such as those described have been used to define baseline motions for each level of the human spine and serve as benchmarks from which changes can be studied (Figure 3-5).[6]

BIOMECHANICAL AND CLINICAL INSTABILITY

Biomechanical instability is noted when supraphysiologic motions are observed with physiologic loading. This laboratory diagnosis may be due to factors such as traumatic injury, degenerative changes, or postoperative destabilization. Many such variables have been studied in controlled experiments.

The effective stabilization of lumbar spinal ligaments was studied in a transection model.[3,5] Specimens loaded in flexion were most affected when ligaments were sequentially transected from posterior to anterior. Specimens loaded in extension were most affected when ligaments were sequentially transected from anterior to posterior. It was thus suggested that specific instabilities could be anticipated with the rupture of specific spinal ligaments.

Another study looked at the destabilizing effect of sequentially increasing flexion/compression injuries.[4]

INSTABILITY

- **Biochemical instability:** Noted when supraphysiologic motions are observed with physiologic loading
- **Clinical instability:** Loss of spine's ability to maintain patterns of displacement under physiologic loads so there is no major deformity or progression of deformity, no initial or additional neurologic deficit, and no incapacitating pain; requires mechanical instability plus propensity to progress or involvement of neurologic component
- **Acute instability:** Occurs after sudden catastrophic failure of sufficient number of spinal constraints
- **Chronic instability:** Occurs after disease process leaves sufficient constraints ineffective to prevent significant displacement or deformity of spine or neurologic injury over a more prolonged period of time

---

This study confirmed the burst fracture hypothesis of Denis, which suggested that the middle column disruption of burst fractures was a crucial predictor of spinal stability.

The role of muscles in stabilizing the spine has been more difficult to quantitate. The cross-sectional area of the muscles around the spine, and the relative length of moment arms over which the muscles act, provide significant potential stability to the spine.

The extrapolation of biomechanical instability to clinical instability is controversial. White and Panjabi[6] defined clinical instability as the loss of the spine's ability to maintain patterns of displacement under physiologic loads so that there is no major deformity or progression of deformity, no initial or additional neurologic deficit, and no incapacitating pain. It follows from this definition that clinical instability requires mechanical instability plus a propensity to progress or involvement of a neurologic component.

It can be seen from this working definition that two classes of instability arise: acute, after trauma or surgery; and chronic, after disease or partial injury to the stabilizing constraints on the spine. Acute instability occurs after sudden catastrophic failure of a sufficient number of spinal constraints. Chronic instability occurs after a disease process leaves sufficient constraints ineffective to prevent significant displacement or deformity of the spine or neurologic injury over a more prolonged period of time.

Each region of the spine has distinct stability characteristics, which makes it difficult to generalize for the entire spine. These differences correspond to variations in vertebral anatomic geometry, neurologic structure and pathways, exogenous load application, and local motor controls. Thus biomechanical characteristics of the cervical, thoracic, and lumbar spine will be considered independently in the following sections.

REGIONAL BIOMECHANICAL CHARACTERISTICS OF THE SPINE
Cervical Spine

The cervical spine is more mobile than the other regions of the spine (see Figure 3-5). The C0 (occiput) to C1 and C1 to C2 levels are, in particular, specifically suited to their anatomic location. Flexion/extension is greatest at C0 to C1, but this parameter is relatively evenly distributed over the cervical levels. Conversely, most of the axial rotation takes place between C1 and C2, and very little between C0 and C1. Lateral bending is more in the middle region, and only half as much as in the end levels. Due to the natural lordosis and facet architecture, there is also significant motion coupling in this spinal region. For example, axial rotation to one side is coupled with lateral bending to the same side.

The first systematic approach to the analysis of clinical stability was in the cervical spine.[6] This was initiated from ligament transection experiments[3] and modified with the results of multiple other laboratory experiments and clinical observations. A checklist of factors to diagnosis clinical instability was developed (Table 3-1). This helped provide the clinician with a systematic approach to the assessment of clinical instability.

Injury to the anterior elements, including the posterior longitudinal ligament and all the anatomic structures anterior to it, is worth two points. Injury to the posterior elements, including all of the anatomic structures posterior to the longitudinal ligament, is worth two points. Positive stretch test, increase in disc height of more than 1.7 mm with distraction of the head, is worth two points. Sagittal plane displacement of more than 3.5 mm, relative sagittal plane angulation of more than 11 degrees, and spinal cord injury are also worth two points each. If only neutral posture radiographs are available, then relative angulation of more than 11 degrees is worth two points. Abnormal disc narrowing, developmentally narrow spinal canal, nerve root injury,

---

BIOMECHANICAL CHARACTERISTICS

CERVICAL SPINE
- More mobile than other regions of spine
- Flexion/extension greatest at C0 to C1, but relatively evenly distributed over cervical levels
- Most axial rotation takes place between C1 and C2, very little between C0 and C1
- Lateral bending more in middle region, and only half as much as in end levels
- Natural lordosis and facet architecture lead to significant motion coupling in cervical spine

THORACIC SPINE
- Least mobile region of spine because of stability provided by costovertebral articulations and rib cage
- Lateral bending evenly distributed between vertebral segments
- More axial rotation in upper thoracic spine
- More flexion/extension in lower thoracic spine

LUMBAR SPINE
- Less still than thoracic spine in flexion/extension—trend that continues as one moves toward sacrum
- Minimal rotation
- Primarily constrained anatomically by more coronally oriented facet joints

---

Table 3-1	Checklist for the Diagnosis of Clinical Instability in the Cervical Spine

Element	Point Value*
Anterior elements destroyed or unable to function	2
Posterior elements destroyed or unable to function	2
Positive stretch test	2
Radiographic criteria	4
Flexion-extension radiographs	
Sagittal plane translation >3.5 mm or 20% (2 pt)	
Sagittal plane rotation >20 degrees (2 pt)	
OR	
Resting radiographs	
Sagittal plane displacement >3.5 mm or 20% (2 pt)	
Relative sagittal plane angulation >11 degrees (2 pt)	
Abnormal disc narrowing	1
Developmentally narrow spinal canal (diameter <13 mm)	1
Spinal cord injury	2
Nerve root injury	1
Dangerous loading anticipated	1

Modified from White AA III, Panjabi MM: *Clinical biomechanics of the spine*, ed 2, Philadelphia, 1990: JB Lippincott.
*A point value total of 5 or more indicates clinical instability.

Table 3-2	Checklist for the Diagnosis of Clinical Instability in the Thoracic and Thoracolumbar Spine (T11 to L1)	
Element		**Point Value***
Anterior elements destroyed or unable to function		2
Posterior elements destroyed or unable to function		2
Radiographic criteria		4
Sagittal plane displacement >2.5 mm (2 pt)		
Relative sagittal plane angulation >5 degrees (2 pt)		
Spinal cord or cauda equina damage		2
Disruption of costovertebral articulations		1
Dangerous loading anticipated		1

Modified from White AA III, Panjabi MM: *Clinical biomechanics of the spine,* ed 2, Philadelphia, 1990, JB Lippincott.
*A point value total of 5 or more indicates clinical instability.

Table 3-3	Checklist for the Diagnosis of Clinical Instability in the Lumbar and Lumbosacral Spine (L1 to S1)	
Element		**Point Value***
Anterior elements destroyed or unable to function		2
Posterior elements destroyed or unable to function		2
Radiographic criteria		4
Flexion-extension radiographs		
Sagittal plane translation >4.5 mm or 15% (2 pt)		
Sagittal plane rotation		
>15 degrees at L1 to L2, L2 to L3, and L3 to L4 (2 pt)		
>20 degrees at L4 to L5 (2 pt)		
>25 degrees at L5 to S1 (2 pt)		
OR		
Resting radiographs		
Sagittal plane displacement >4.5 mm or 15% (2 pt)		
Relative sagittal plane angulation >22 degrees (2 pt)		
Cauda equina damage		3
Dangerous loading anticipated		1

Modified from White AA III, Panjabi MM: *Clinical biomechanics of the spine,* ed 2, Philadelphia, 1990, JB Lippincott.
*A point value total of 5 or more indicates clinical instability.

and anticipated exposure to dangerous loading are worth one point each. If the sum of the points is five or more, then the spine is considered to be clinically unstable.

Thoracic Spine

The thoracic spine is the least mobile region of the spine due to the stability provided by the costovertebral articulations and the rib cage (see Figure 3-5). Lateral bending is evenly distributed between the vertebral segments, while there is more axial rotation in the upper thoracic spine and more flexion/extension in the lower thoracic spine. This is consistent with the lower thoracic spinal region as a transitional segment between the biomechanics of the upper thoracic spine and the lumbar region.

Thoracic instability is a less common entity, but it has a separate checklist due to the differences in anatomy at these levels (Table 3-2). Anterior or posterior element injury, sagittal plane displacement of more than 2.5 mm, relative sagittal plane angulation of more than 5 degrees, and spinal cord or cauda equina damage are worth two points each. Disruption of costovertebral articulations and anticipated exposure to dangerous loading are worth one point each. As with the cervical spine, if the sum of the points is five or more, then the spine is considered to be clinically unstable.

Lumbar Spine

The lumbar spine is less stiff than the thoracic spine in flexion/extension—a trend that continues as one moves toward the sacrum (see Figure 3-5). This might play a part in accounting for the higher incidence of disc disease in the L4 to L5 and L5 to S1 disc levels. Of note, there is minimal rotation in the lumbar spine. This is primarily due to the anatomic constraints of the more coronally oriented facet joints in this region.

A stability checklist was also developed for the lumbar spine (Table 3-3). Anterior or posterior element injury is worth two points each. The intervertebral translations and rotations given in Table 3-3 are measured on either flexion/extension or resting radiographs (two points each if abnormal). Damage to the cauda equina is given three points, and the anticipated exposure to high loading on the spine is given one point. If the sum of the points is five or more, then the spine is considered to be clinically unstable.

CONCLUSIONS

This chapter defined biomechanical terminology that can be applied to the spine. The difference between kinematics and kinetics was highlighted. After presenting means of testing functional mechanics of the spine, normal intervertebral motions were provided. This led to a precisely defined explanation of biomechanical and clinical instability.

There are multiple ways in which one can develop an unstable spine. However, identifying such a scenario makes a clinician consider immobilization and/or surgical intervention. Checklists can assist in this process and are presented here as tools. Nevertheless, a patient must always be assessed on an individual basis and a treatment plan formulated with all information that is available.

SUGGESTED REFERENCES

Panjabi MM: The stabilizing system of the spine. II. Neutral zone and instability hypothesis, *J Spinal Disord* 5:390-397, 1992.
Panjabi MM et al.: Validation of the three-column theory of thoracolumbar fractures: a biomechanical investigation, *Spine* 20: 1122-1127, 1995.

White AA III, Panjabi MM: *Clinical biomechanics of the spine*, ed 2, Philadelphia, 1990, JB Lippincott.

REFERENCES

1. Panjabi MM: Low back pain and spinal instability. In Weinstein J, Gordon S, eds: *Low back pain: a scientific and clinical overview*, Rosemont, Ill, American Academy of Orthopaedic Surgeons, 1996.
2. Panjabi MM: The stabilizing system of the spine. II. Neutral zone and instability hypothesis, *J Spinal Disord* 5:390-397, 1992.
3. Panjabi MM, White AA III, Johnson RM: Cervical spine biomechanics as a function of transection of components, *J Biomech* 8:327-336, 1975.
4. Panjabi MM et al.: Validation of the three-column theory of thoracolumbar fractures: a biomechanical investigation, *Spine* 20:1122-1127, 1995.
5. Posner I et al.: A biomechanical analysis of the clinical stability of the lumbar and lumbosacral spine, *Spine* 7:374-389, 1982.
6. White AA III, Panjabi MM: *Clinical biomechanics of the spine*, ed 2, Philadelphia, 1990, JB Lippincott.

Biomechanics of Internal Fixation

Jorge J. Lastra, Edward C. Benzel

BRIDGING AND MULTISEGMENTAL FIXATION IMPLANTS
Hardware Components

Bridging and multisegmental fixation spinal implants are composed of a combination of components that cannot function alone. Therefore they differ from abutting implants (i.e., struts) that function alone in the intervertebral space. Bridging implant components include the following items: anchors (penetrating and gripping), longitudinal members (rods and plates), cross-connectors (cross-fixators), and accessories (e.g., washers).

Anchors

Anchors affix to a single spinal level. Anchors include penetrating and gripping types (implants). Penetrating types (implants) penetrate the bone. These are sub-divided into those with pullout resistance (e.g., screws) and those without pullout resistance (e.g., nails, spikes, and staples). Gripping types (implants—hooks and wires) do not penetrate the bone surface but instead provide a "grip" of the spine.

Penetrating implants
Screws are penetrating implants with pullout resistance characteristics. An understanding of screw anatomy is essential to minimize the incidence of failure. Components of the screw include the head, core, thread, and tip (Figure 4-1). The head resists translational loads along the long axis of the screw. It should be designed to abut the underlying surface of a plate or bone so that forces are truly applied along the axis of the screw.

The core of a screw is important regarding screw fracture, bending resistance, and torsion resistance. The strength of a screw is proportional to the cube of its core diameter (D). This is calculated by the equation defining the section modulus (Z):

$$Z = \frac{\pi D^3}{32}$$

Z is equivalent to strength. Therefore the difference in strength between screws with a core diameter of 5 mm and 6 mm is nearly twofold.

The thread of the screw contributes to pullout resistance. The thread depth and the pitch are important factors in thread design (see Figure 4-1). The pitch is the distance from a point on one thread to the corresponding point on an adjacent thread. The distance a screw advances axially in one turn is the lead. This is equal to the pitch. The thread depth is the screw's outer diameter minus the inner diameter (core) divided by 2.

Pullout resistance is in general proportional to the volume of bone between threads. The volume of bone between the threads is increased by increasing the thread depth and the distance between threads (pitch) (Figure 4-2, *A*, *B*, and *C*). Another method of altering the

---

BRIDGING AND MULTISEGMENTAL SPINAL IMPLANTS

- Anchors
  - Penetrating: Screws, nails, spikes, staples
  - Gripping: hooks, wires
- Longitudinal members: Rods and plates
- Cross-connectors: Cross-fixators
- Accessories: Washers and rod sleeves

ANCHORS

- Screw types
  - Cortical (machine-type)
  - Cancellous (wood-type)
  - Self-tapping (variant of machine-type)
- Gripping implants
  - Do not penetrate bone interface
  - Provide greater functional surface area of contact (advantageous in osteoporotic patients)
  - Hooks: Used for lamina, pedicle, transverse process fixation
  - Wires: Used individually or as multiple strands

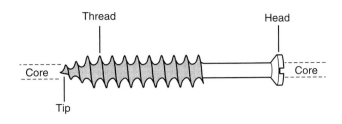

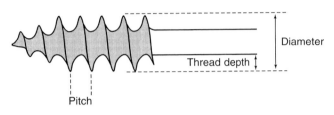

Figure 4-1. Anatomy of a screw.

volume of bone between threads is by changing the thread shape (Figure 4-2, *D*). An increase in the depth of the screw penetration and the use of triangulation also increase pullout resistance (Figure 4-2, *E* and *F*).[4]

The three types of screws are (1) machine (cortical), (2) self-tapping machine, and (3) wood (cancellous) (Figure 4-3). The self-tapping machine screw is a variant of both a machine screw and a screw tap.

Machine (cortical) screws have shallow threads to minimize bone compression during screw insertion. They are used in relatively incompressible bone. Pretapping is used in cortical bone to avoid pathologic bone compression and microfracture by the screw. Pretapping may increase pullout resistance in cortical bone. Tapping carves threads into the walls of the screw hole for the cortical screw. This is performed by the cutting edges of the screw tap.

Two fundamental elements for the adequate function of a screw tap are the tapered tip and the full-length flute (see Figure 4-3, *A*). The tapered tip helps to place the screw in the desired orientation by directing the screw down the predrilled hole in the bone. The full-length flute gathers bone debris carved from the wall of the hole drilled by the screw tap. This process is enhanced by periodically loosening the screw by approximately one-quarter to one-half turn during tightening. This permits the bone debris to collect in the flute. Tapping is desirable prior to placing machine screws because compression during screw insertion causes microfractures that decrease bone integrity if a screw tap is not used.

Self-tapping machine screws have a leading edge flute that allows debris to accumulate within the boundaries of the flute (see Figure 4-3, *B*). They have a short flute (approximately three threads) that cannot accommodate all debris from the drill. Therefore a larger drill hole is often used in order to facilitate debris accumulation.

Cancellous (wood) screws are used in softer material (see Figure 4-3, *C*). Compression of cancellous bone by the screw during insertion increases its density and its pullout resistance. Tapping cancellous bone therefore

weakens the implant-bone interface and decreases pullout resistance.

Other screw types are the lag screw and screws that change configuration within the bone (Figure 4-4, *A* and *B*, and *C*).

Gripping implants

Gripping implants do not penetrate the bone interface but instead provide a "grip" of the spine. These include hooks and wires. They provide a greater functional surface area of contact with the cortical bone interface than do penetrating implants. Therefore they provide a particular advantage in osteoporotic patients.[7] Hooks are used for lamina, pedicle, and transverse process fixation. The correct placement of hooks is critical. A note of caution: a pedicle hook inserted too deeply may cut into the pedicle and diminish the construct integrity (Figure 4-5, *A*). Conversely, hook insertion to insufficient depth results in an improper engagement of the pedicle, reducing its ability to augment torsional stability (Figure 4-5, *B*). The mode and magnitude of force application to the spine by a hook and the integrity of the bone to which it is applied are also critical.

Wires can be used individually or as multiple strands. The use of two wires doubles the contact surface with bone, thereby increasing the pull-through resistance. Some of this pull-through resistance is diminished if the wires are twisted.

Twisting appears to be the optimal method of wire-to-wire affixation. The use of more than two full twists, however, adds no additional security. Commercial wire tighteners provide more consistent twists with a concomitant diminished surface injury.[14] Wires are sensitive to notching (injury to the surface of an implant that adversely affects its structural integrity). Titanium is particularly prone to the ill effects of notching (notch sensitive).[15] The braiding of multiple small strands of wire into a cable greatly reduces the danger posed by this phenomenon.

Longitudinal Members

Longitudinal members include plates and rods. They are connected to other implant components (anchors and cross-members) via the use of a variety of component-to-component connectors: (1) three-point shear clamps,

---

LONGITUDINAL MEMBERS

- Plates and rods connected to other implant components via various component-to-component connectors
  - Three-point shear clamps
  - Lock screw connectors
  - Circumferential grip connectors
  - Constrained bolt-plate connectors
  - Semiconstrained component-rod connectors
  - Constrained screw-plate connectors
  - Semiconstrained screw-plate connectors
  - Axially dynamic connectors

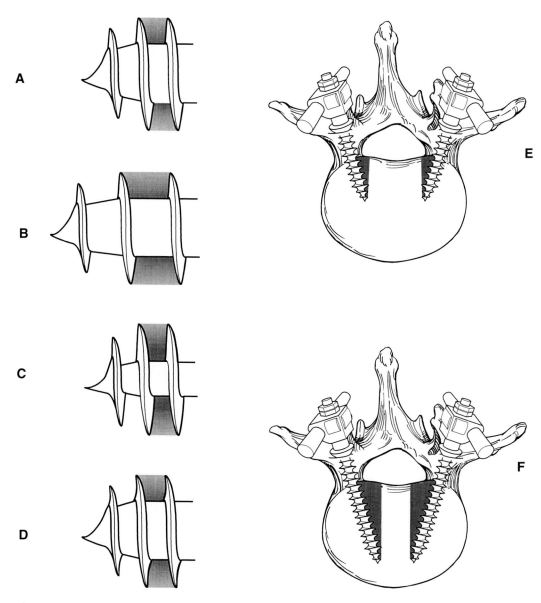

Figure 4-2. **A,** Screw pullout resistance is mainly a function of the volume of bone (hatched area) between the screw threads. **B,** The pitch affects the pullout resistance by altering the thread distance. **C,** The thread depth affects pullout resistance by altering the thread width. **D,** The thread shape affects the pullout resistance by altering the volume of bone directly. **E,** The triangulation of the pedicles provides additional resistance to pullout. Pullout resistance is proportional not only to volume of bone between screw threads, but also to the triangular area defined by the screw, the perpendicular, and the posterior vertebral body surface (shaded area). **F,** Screw length contributes significantly to pullout resistance when the screws are triangulated. The shaded area increases with longer screws or with increase in the screw angle. The triangulation effect requires cross-connectors.

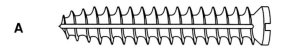

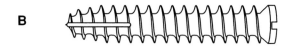

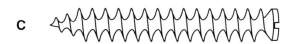

Figure 4-3. **A,** A screw tap has a tapered tip and the full-length flute. **B,** A self-tapping screw has a leading-edge flute that does not extend the length of the screw. **C,** Wood screws do not have a tapered tip.

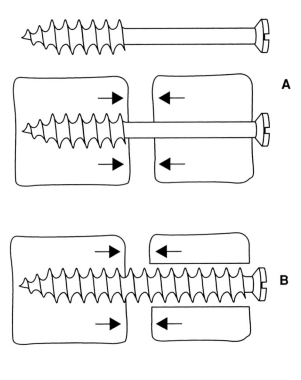

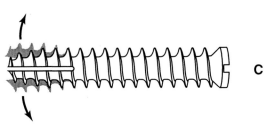

Figure 4-4. **A,** A lag screw approximates the distal bone to the proximal fracture. **B,** The same could be accomplished with drilling of the proximal bone with a regular screw. This principle is used in odontoid screw fixation. **C,** Depiction of a screw that changes configuration within the bone, which may prevent pullout.

(2) lock screw connectors, (3) circumferential grip connectors, (4) constrained bolt-plate connectors, (5) semiconstrained component-rod connectors, (6) constrained screw-plate connectors, (7) semiconstrained screw-plate connectors, and (8) axially dynamic connectors (Figure 4-6).[4]

Three-point shear clamps
Three-point shear clamps provide significant resistance to axial, torsional, and bending-moment force application. They rely on the force applied to the interface and the friction between components (Figure 4-7).

Lock screw connectors
Lock screw connectors use a set screw mechanism to oppose the rod to the other half of the component system (Figure 4-8). They provide one half of the pincer mechanism required for security. The other half of the pincer mechanism is usually provided by either a three-point shear clamp or a circumferential grip connector. The lock screw connector may be applied end-on or tangentially (see Figure 4-6, *B*). An appropriately designed tangential set screw provides a biomechanical advantage.

Circumferential grip connectors
Circumferential grip connectors may be used to provide both halves of the pincer mechanism, or truly circumferential force application (Figure 4-9). More commonly, only one half of the pincer is provided, such as with a lock screw.

Constrained bolt-plate connectors
Constrained bolt-plate connectors are very rigid. These are the strongest connectors available. They are stiff and

do not yield, except in failure. These connectors are available either screw-plate or screw-rod systems (see Figure 4-6, *D*).

Semiconstrained component-rod connectors
Semiconstrained component-rod connectors (see Figure 4-6, *F*) are less stiff than constrained bolt-plate connectors and allow some movement. These connectors allow some toggling of the component on the rod (Figure 4-10). Toggling, fretting, and loosening at the component-rod interface are potential complications.

Constrained screw-plate connectors
Constrained screw-plate connectors rigidly fix the screw to the plate or rod using a variety of strategies: (1) expansion heads, (2) cam locks, (3) screw head securing mechanisms, (4) locking plates, and (5) screws with a modified pitch close to the head to lock the screw to the plate. The last strategy does not bring the plate to the bone.

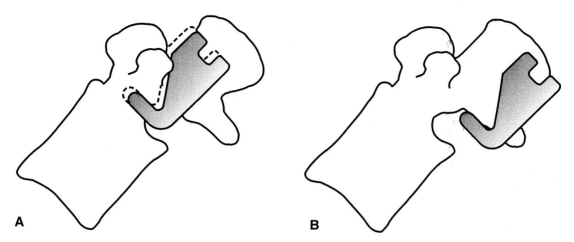

Figure 4-5. **A,** Pedicle hook inserted too deeply may cut into the pedicle and fail. **B,** Pedicle hook inserted to insufficient depth results in an improper engagement of the pedicle with high probability for failure.

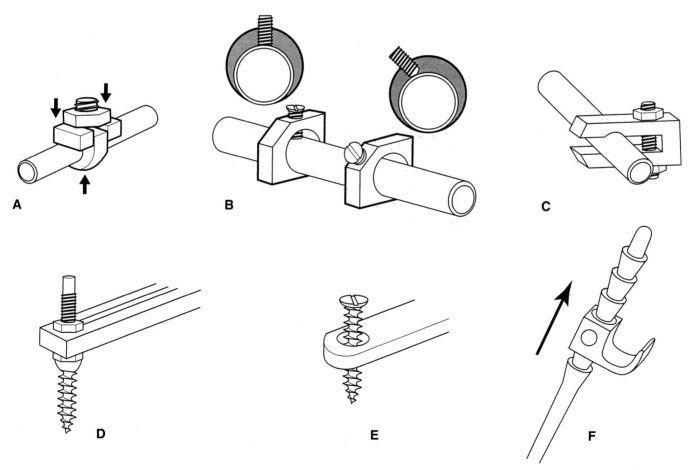

Figure 4-6. The six fundamental component-to-component locking mechanisms. **A,** Three-point shear clamps. **B,** Lock screw connectors. End-on *(left)* or tangential *(right)* application. **C,** Circumferential grip connector. **D,** Constrained bolt-plate connector. **E,** Semiconstrained screw-plate connector. **F,** Semiconstrained component-rod connector with an exaggerated depiction of allowed toggle.

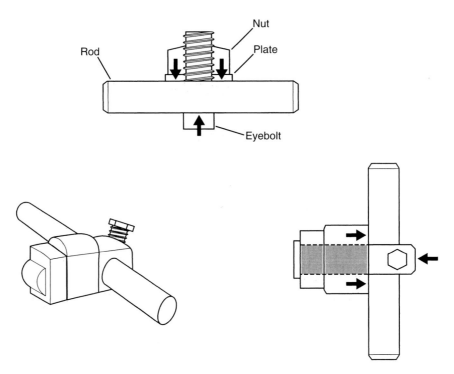

Figure 4-7. Three-point shear clamps.

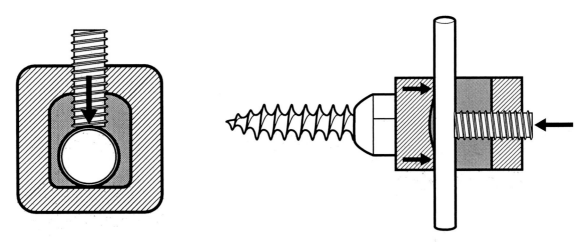

Figure 4-8. Lock screw connector.

Despite the strength of rigid fixation, it occasionally fails because it does not permit subsidence of the spine. Subsidence of the spine or of a fusion may be defined as "settling," or loss of vertical height. Three phenomena of normal aging that directly affect the subsidence of the spine are (1) disc interspace height loss, (2) symmetric vertebral body collapse (axial deformation, or deformation along the neutral axis), and (3) angular deformation (kyphosis, or deformation about an axis of rotation) (Figure 4-11).[4] Therefore the spine "collapses" during aging. The spine seems to want to deform. This is related to the inevitable and obligatory effect of gravity and repetitive loading. This repetitive axial impulse loading is associated with ambulation. Rigid implants may retard this process, but they do not eliminate this process from occurring.[10] When rigid implants indeed do impede subsidence, the harmful effects of stress shielding may become manifest.

Usually, constrained screw-plate fixation failure is a result of one of three mechanisms: (1) construct failure, (2) implant failure, or (3) failure of the construct to allow bone graft–vertebral body margins to "see" adequate stresses, resulting in failure to fuse. Construct failure often occurs when too much is asked of the implant. An

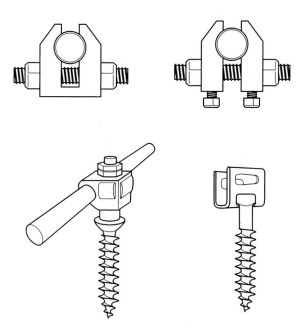

Figure 4-9. Circumferential grip locking system.

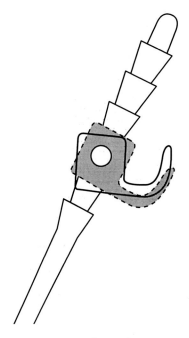

Figure 4-10. Semiconstrained component-rod connector with an exaggerated depiction of allowed toggle.

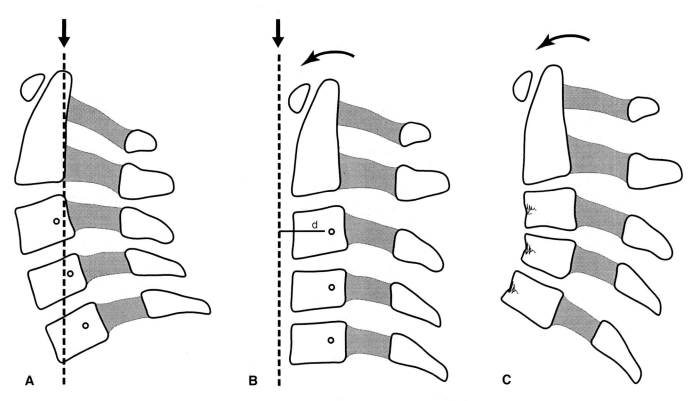

Figure 4-11. **A,** Cervical spine lordotic curvature results, in part, because of a nonpathologic situation where the dorsal vertebral body height is less than the ventral height. **B,** Ventral disc interspace height loss via the typical degenerative process results in the loss of lordotic posture. **C,** The loss of lordotic posture causes the creation and elongation of the moment arm applied to the spine, d, leading to ventral vertebral body compression, and further possible exaggeration of a pathologic kyphotic posture may then ensue.

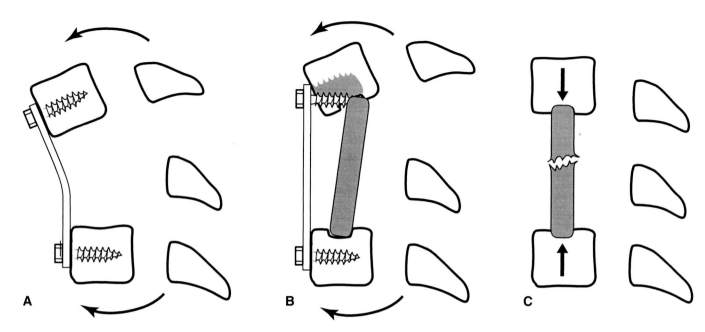

Figure 4-12. Examples of construct failure: **A,** implant failure (plate bending), **B,** "kick-out" of the implant, and **C,** bone graft fracture.

excessive load at the screw–vertebral body interface or an excessive mismatch between the integrity of the native vertebral bone and the construct is usually a causative factor. This may result in implant failure, "kick-out" of the implant or the bone graft (strut), and/or bone graft fracture (Figure 4-12).

Implant failure occurs when the implant itself fails via screw or plate fracture. Implant fracture occurs at the point of maximum stress application. The point of fracture of screws with a fixed inner diameter (core) with a constrained screw-plate fixation construct is usually at the screw-plate interface. This can be altered by modifying the shape of the core (Figure 4-13). The point of failure of a ramped inner diameter screw is somewhere between the tip of the screw and the plate. By altering the diameter of the core, the section modulus is altered exponentially (to the third power). This changes the point of maximum stress in the screw. Stress equals the bending moment applied (M) divided by Z (strength), or M/Z. Therefore increasing the inner diameter of a screw increases its strength by a power of three. This finding is relevant because of the fact that an implant always fails at the point of maximum stress application.[9]

A plate, although bulky, is no stronger than its weakest point. Plates also fail at the point of maximum stress application (Figure 4-14).

Constrained systems do not allow high stresses to be applied to the bone graft. This directly increases the possibility of pseudarthrosis according to Wolff's law. Wolff's law dictates that bone is formed where stresses are present for both tensile and compressive forces, and it is absorbed where such stresses are not present.[16] Therefore constrained systems, to one degree or another, shield stress.

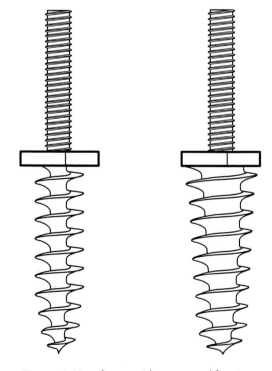

Figure 4-13. Screw with core modification (ramped/conical inner diameter).

Semiconstrained screw-plate connectors

Semiconstrained screw-plate connectors are less stiff and allow some movement at the component-to-component interface. The screw is usually used to approximate the plate to the bone. However, the screw is not rigidly affixed to the plate (see Figure 4-6, *E*). This permits the toggling

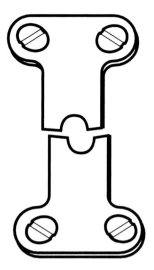

Figure 4-14. Plates fracture at the point of maximum stress application.

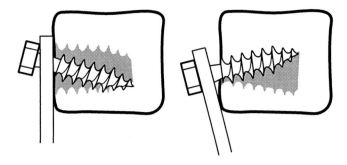

Figure 4-15. Semiconstrained screw-plate systems allow toggling of the screw in the plate, with the possibility of screw-bone failure.

of the screw on the plate (Figure 4-15). Therefore truly rigid fixation is not achieved. Examples of this type of connector are lateral mass fixators, Caspar plates, and dynamic compression plates. Dynamic compression plates use a teardrop-shaped hole in the plate to cause the plate to slide when the screw is tightened.

Axially dynamic connectors

Axially dynamic spine stabilization (e.g., DOC Ventral Cervical Stabilization System by DePuy-AcroMed or Advanced Biomechanical Concept [ABC] by Aesculap) permits some axial deformation but at the same time limits its extent and controls the type of deformation allowed (controlled dynamism) (Figure 4-16). Semiconstrained systems allow some degree of dynamism (uncontrolled dynamism). However, they cause degradation of the screw-bone interface (see Figure 4-15).

Controlled dynamism is achieved by an implant that permits the spine to deform (subside) in a predetermined manner (usually axially, along the axis of the spine). If an implant resists subsidence, normal settling does not occur. If the implant does not fail, it will increase the possibility of a pseudarthrosis because of the diminished compression forces (stresses) applied to the bone graft. A construct may fail and then permit subsidence of the spine and subsequent fusion.

Dynamic constructs include absorbable implants (initially not dynamic) and implants that themselves deform (initially dynamic). Absorbable implants allow spinal deformation only after the implant is absorbed. Hence, they are absorbed usually after 1 or 2 months and permit only late subsidence. On the other hand, deformable implants permit immediate axial and/or angular deformation after insertion. After surgery, subsidence occurs early.[5] Therefore absorbable implants do not effectively function as dynamic implants that enhance fusion.

Intermediate points of fixation should be considered in order to avoid failure with constructs.

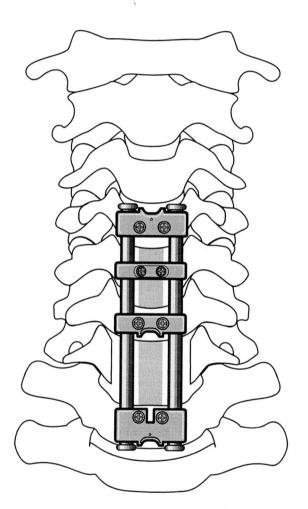

Figure 4-16. Axially dynamic spine stabilization.

Cross-Connectors

Cross-connectors provide the fixation of parallel or bilaterally placed fixation devices to each other in a rigid or semirigid manner. This effectively creates a quadrilateral frame and substantially increases stiffness and stability. Cross-fixation is particularly advantageous in long constructs where it limits torsional stresses that can result

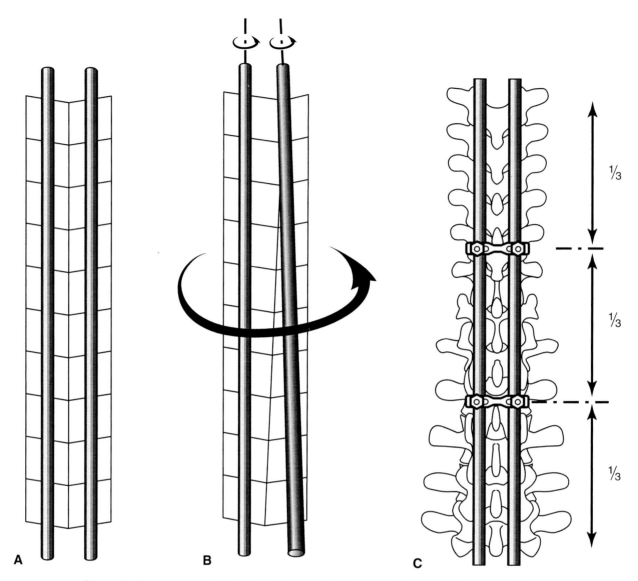

Figure 4-17. **A, B,** Cross-fixation resists torsional stresses that result in rotation of one rod about the other. **C,** Two cross-fixation points should be used in long constructs at the junctions of the terminal thirds of the construct with the middle third.

CROSS-CONNECTORS

- Provide fixation of parallel or bilaterally placed fixation devices: Rigid or semirigid
- Increase stiffness and stability
- Long constructs: Increase torsional rigidity; place approximately at junctions of terminal thirds of rod with middle third
- Short constructs: Diminish parallelogram deformation phenomenon, possibility of sagittal plane translation, and pullout failure when used with triangulated screws

in a twisting of the rods about each other (Figure 4-17, *A* and *B*).

Cross-fixators in long constructs should be placed approximately at the junctions of the terminal thirds of the rod with the middle third (Figure 4-17, *C*). Cross-fixation is of substantial clinical significance with regard to shorter constructs as well. It diminishes the parallelogram deformation phenomenon (Figure 4-18), the possibility of sagittal plane translation, and pullout failure when used with triangulated screws. Of note, the triangulation effect is not achieved when rigid cross-fixation is not used. When hook-bone interfaces fail, they usually fail at one interface at a time. Rigid cross-fixation minimizes the chance of failure by requiring multiple hook-bone interfaces to fail simultaneously, which is much less likely.

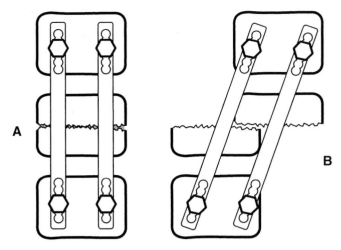

Figure 4-18. Lateral translational deformation may be prevented with a cross-fixation and toe-in configuration of pedicle screws. Before **(A)** and after **(B)** lateral translation.

Accessories

Accessories include washers and rod sleeves. Sleeves around the rod may function as spacers for spinal extension, enhancing force application and increasing extension (Figure 4-19).

ABUTTING IMPLANTS (STRUTS)

Struts are structures placed between two vertebral bodies with the usual goal being that the bone graft becomes an integral part of the fusion mass. They function as a spacer. A strut may be a bone graft, a cage filled with bone, or rarely an inert material (e.g., metal or ceramic). Several interbody struts have been used. These include tricortical bone grafts, rectangular and cylindrical bone grafts, bone dowels, threaded bone dowels, carbon fiber implants (cages), and threaded interbody fusion cages (TIFC).[1,6,7,11-13] The goal of the strut is to provide structural support and to sustain the axial load until the bone graft remodels and fusion is achieved. Autologous cancellous bone is rich in osteogenic substrates, but it lacks substantial mechanical strength and exhibits a low resistance to axial loading. Therefore the structural support can be obtained by using a hard outer shell surrounding the cancellous bone, such as cortical bone, a metal shell, or other materials such as carbon fiber.

Cages are of two types—flat faced and round faced—based on the nature of the surface presented to the graft bed. Flat-faced cages present a flat surface to the graft bed (Figure 4-20), and round-faced cages present a round surface to the graft bed (Figure 4-21). The graft bed is composed of either an endplate or a vertebral body cancellous bone. Theoretically, struts will adequately resist axial loads and, to a lesser extent, the rotational and translational forces impinging on the spinal segment in question (Figure 4-22, *A* and *B*). The larger the surface area of contact and the closer the strut approximates the edge of the vertebra, the greater the resistance to the subsidence. Obviously, a strut with

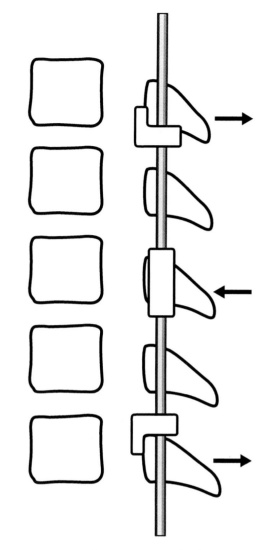

Figure 4-19. Depiction of a sleeve.

STRUTS

- Can be bone grafts, cages filled with bone, or (rarely) inert material such as metal or ceramic
- Provide structural support and sustain axial load until bone graft remodels and fusion is achieved

---

a large surface area of contact that approximates the vertebral body wall circumferentially is ideal.

IMPLANT PROPERTIES

Failure of an implant can be immediate or delayed. Immediate failure occurs when the application of a load to the implant exceeds the static strength of the implant. This rarely occurs.

Delayed (fatigue) failure occurs because of the cumulative damage related to cyclical loading. Implants

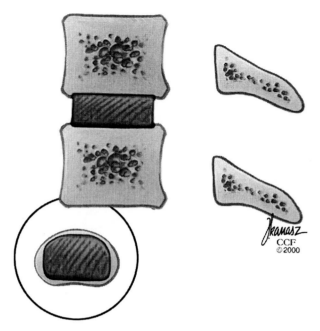

Figure 4-20. Depiction of a flat-faced cage. *(Courtesy Cleveland Clinic Foundation, 2000.)*

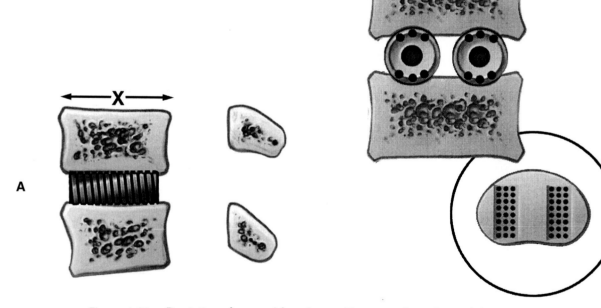

A   **B**

Figure 4-21. Depiction of a round-faced cage. The cage abuts the endplates, as depicted in a lateral view **(A).** Surface area of contact with the endplate, however, may be suboptimal **(B).** *(Courtesy Cleveland Clinic Foundation, 2000.)*

usually fail after cyclical loading and implant fatigue. Of note, the average spine undergoes about 3 million cycles per year.

Resistance to implant material injury or deformation depends on (1) implant composition, (2) implant morphology, (3) structural characteristics, and (4) material implant treatment and preparation.

Implant Composition

Metallurgy is the study of metals and their material—properties, shaping, and treatment by heating and/or cooling. An element is a simple substance that cannot be separated into simpler components by routine chemical means. An alloy is a metal made by mixing and melding two or more elements and other substances.

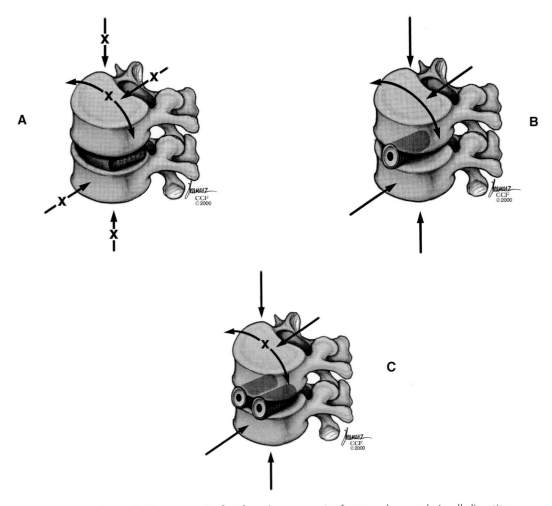

Figure 4-22. **A,** Theoretically, flat-faced cages resist forces adequately in all directions. **B,** A single, round-faced cage does not resist forces adequately. **C,** Two round-faced cages resist forces better, but still do not prevent translation adequately. *(Courtesy Cleveland Clinic Foundation, 2000.)*

Elements that are commonly used for spinal implants include aluminum, titanium, vanadium, chromium, manganese, iron, cobalt, nickel, zirconium, niobium, and molybdenum. Of these, titanium is the only element used in a pure (unalloyed) form in spinal implants. Contaminant elements commonly found in implants include hydrogen, oxygen, carbon, and nitrogen. These contaminants exist in implant materials because they are difficult to eliminate, or because they stabilize certain phases of the element or the alloy.

Titanium is available in four different grades. The grades are classified according to the degree of contamination. Grade 1 is the most pure, and grade 4 is the least pure (most contaminated). Often the contamination is desired because it changes the implant characteristics (e.g., as oxygen contamination increases, the implant strength increases). Grade 1 is less able to tolerate stretch (tensile force application) than grade 4. Grades 2, 3, and 4 have tensile strength similar to that of 316 stainless steel.

The modulus of elasticity (stiffness, stress/strain) and the density do not change significantly from grade to grade. Stainless steel has a greater modulus of elasticity than titanium. Therefore it is stiffer. The modulus of elasticity is defined as stress divided by strain. Stress is the force applied to an object (load/area). Strain is the response of the object to the force (length deformation/unit length). Modulus of elasticity is a constant that is characteristic of a given material. The greater the modulus of elasticity, the stiffer the implant. Ultimate tensile yield strength is the highest stress (load) tolerable before failure. The 0.2% tensile yield stress is defined as the load that causes a 0.2% deformation. Titanium's density and modulus of elasticity do not change from grade to grade, but its ultimate tensile yield strength and 0.2% tensile yield stress depend largely on its grade.

Alloys commonly used for spine surgery applications include 316 stainless steel, cast Co-Cr-Mo, Ti-6Al-4V, Ti-13 niobium-13 zirconium, Vitallium, and 22-13-5 stainless steel (22Cr-13Ni-5Mn).

The ductility of an object is a measure of its deformability. A ductile object is one that can permanently deform before failure. Brittle objects fail without permanent deformation.

Implant Morphology

The size and shape of an implant affect its resistance to failure. For example, the greater the diameter, the greater the resistance to failure.

Surface Characteristics

An implant's performance is affected by its surface characteristics through (1) corrosion, (2) material properties, and (3) construct-construct interface friction.

Corrosion

Corrosion is the degeneration of a metal by oxidation or a similar process, leading to metal weakening. Corrosion rarely affects spinal stability. Bone fusion usually occurs first. There are three types of corrosion: (1) crevice, (2) fretting, and (3) galvanic.

Crevice corrosion occurs within crevices and small cavities on a metal surface, usually at the junction of two similar metals. Titanium is more resistant than 316 stainless steel to this process.

Fretting corrosion occurs via a repetitive friction mechanism. A protective passive surface film is mechanically disrupted at the metal-metal interface. Wire-rod interfaces are less resistant than hook-rod interfaces to this process. The protective passive film is a layer that covers the metal, protecting it from corrosion. Titanium is much more resistant to corrosion than 316 stainless steel owing to titanium's characteristic development of a surface film (layer of oxide).

Anodizing is an electrolytic process that increases the thickness of a naturally occurring surface layer of oxide. The surface film is reformed to varying degrees if the metal is scratched or abraded. Also, even a trace amount of iron in titanium decreases the stability of the protective film. This is due to the anodic breakdown potential. As the iron content of a metal is increased, the corrosion rate is increased.

Material Properties

Material properties are affected by the surface characteristics of an implant. For example, the fatigue resistance of a metal may be enhanced by the process of shot peening.[8] Shot peening is a surface treatment wherein small pellets are shot against the surface of a metal, thus creating a compression deformation of the surface. Shot peening augments the number of cycles required to cause failure. The TSRH rod, which has a matte surface, is an example.

Component-to-Component Interface Friction

A knurled rod may be used to increase friction at the component-to-component interface (e.g., CD rod). The combination of the rough surface of the knurled rod and the set screw attachment mechanism creates a high-friction component-to-component interface (Figure 4-23).

Material Treatments

Metals can undergo a variety of structural alterations to improve resistance to failure. These include work hardening, annealing, and cold working. In addition, metal properties can be changed by adding or not removing contaminants.

Work hardening is the permanent deformation of a metal. Work hardening increases the metal's yield strength (hardness) and decreases the metal's ductility (malleability).

Annealing alters the microstructure of the material. With annealing, the material is heated and cooled by a specific predetermined cycle, making the metal softer and weaker.

Cold working deforms the material at room temperature, making the metal harder and stronger. This increases the metal's tensile strength.

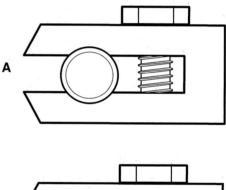

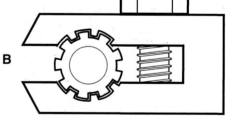

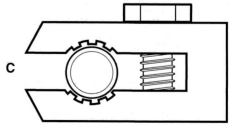

Figure 4-23. **A,** The two opposing surfaces of a component-component interface must match to optimize its security, as depicted. **B, C,** Opposing surfaces do not match, decreasing security.

Osteointegration

Osteointegration is defined by the direct bonding of bone to an implant. Titanium has the greatest osteointegration capacity of all currently used metals. Ceramics and biologic glasses have an even greater osteointegration potential. Osteointegration results in a smoother, more even, distribution of the load between the implant and the bone.[2]

MECHANISMS OF LOAD BEARING BY INSTRUMENTATION CONSTRUCTS: MODES OF FORCE APPLICATION

An understanding of the forces applied to the spine by spinal implants is imperative for the planning and application of an implant strategy. These forces are often extremely complex. Spinal instrumentation techniques usually apply forces to the spine by one of or a combination of six basic mechanisms. These mechanisms are (1) simple distraction fixation, (2) tension band fixation, (3) three-point bending fixation, (4) fixed moment arm type of cantilever beam fixation, (5) nonfixed moment arm type of cantilever beam fixation, and (6) applied moment arm type of cantilever beam fixation.

Simple Distraction Fixation

Simple distraction generally applies a force in line with the instantaneous axis of rotation (IAR). The IAR is usually located in the interbody region. This region is the neutral axis (Figure 4-24). Distraction provides effective resistance of axial loads without applying bending moment if the distraction is performed in line with the IAR (Figure 4-25, *A*). If distraction ventral to the IAR is performed, the result is spine extension (Figure 4-25, *B*). Distraction dorsal to the IAR results in spine flexion and kyphosis (Figure 4-25, *C*). Distraction applied to the spine at a finite perpendicular distance from the IAR causes a bending moment to be applied to the spine, which may not be desirable.

OSTEOINTEGRATION

- Definition: Direct bonding of bone to implant
- Greatest potential: Ceramics and biologic glasses
- Greatest capacity of all currently used metals/alloys: Titanium

---

MECHANISMS OF LOAD BEARING

- Simple distraction fixation
- Tension band fixation
- Three-point bending fixation
- Fixed moment arm cantilever beam fixation
- Nonfixed moment arm cantilever beam fixation
- Applied moment arm cantilever beam fixation

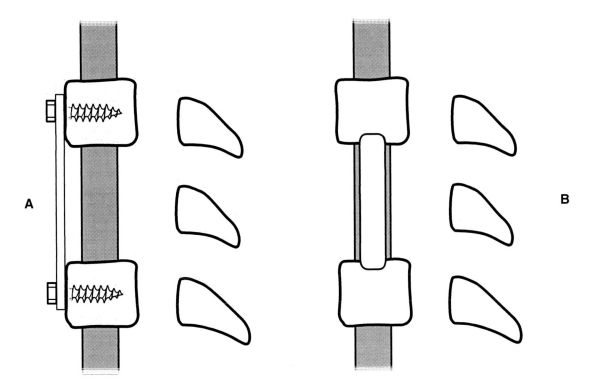

A   B

Figure 4-24.   The neutral axis is depicted by the gray area. This region may be buttressed by a rigid plate **(A)**, by an interbody strut **(B)**, or by both.

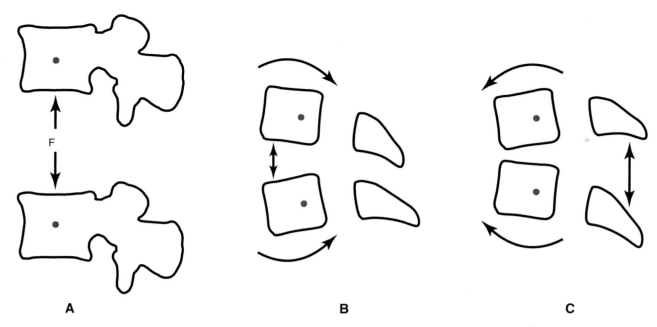

A   **B**   **C**

Figure 4-25.   **A,** Distraction applied in line with the instantaneous axis of rotation (IAR) does not cause a bending moment. **B,** Distraction ventral to the IAR causes extension of the spine. **C,** Conversely, distraction dorsal to the IAR causes flexion of the spine.

Tension Band (Compression) Fixation

Tension band fixation applies compression at the application sites (Figure 4-26). This can be achieved with wires, clamps, springs, or rigid constructs. Tension band fixation is usually utilized dorsally, but it can be applied ventrally. Dorsally applied bending moments result in extension, and ventrally applied bending moments result in flexion of the spine (Figure 4-27).

The forces applied by a tension band fixation construct are described by the following equation:

$$Mtbf = Ftbf \times Diar - tbf$$

Mtbf is the bending moment, Ftbf is the compression force applied at the upper and lower termini of the construct at the instrument-bone interface, and Diar − tbf is the perpendicular distance from the IAR to the tension-band fixation applied-force vector (Figure 4-28).[3] Bending moments increase—and hence fixation improves—with an increased distance from the application of force to the IAR. Bending moment and integrity of fixation are not improved by lengthening tension band fixation constructs.

Three-Point Bending Fixation

Three-point bending fixation consists of similar forces in which a fulcrum applies a force vector that is opposite to the direction of the terminal force vectors. This mechanism is usually applied with an accompanying distraction force application (Figure 4-29). Three-point bending forces can be compared with the force vectors at work when a person is standing on the end of a springboard

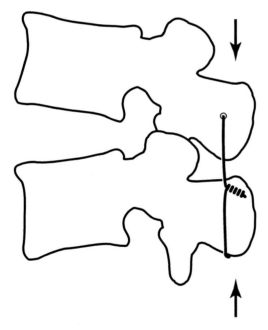

Figure 4-26.   Depiction of tension band fixation.

(Figure 4-30, *A*). The three-point bending forces are defined by the following equation:

$$M = D_1 \times D_2 \times F_{3PB}/D_{3PB}$$

D_1 and D_2 are the distances from the fulcrum to the terminal hook-bone interfaces, D_{3PB} is the sum of D_1 and D_2,

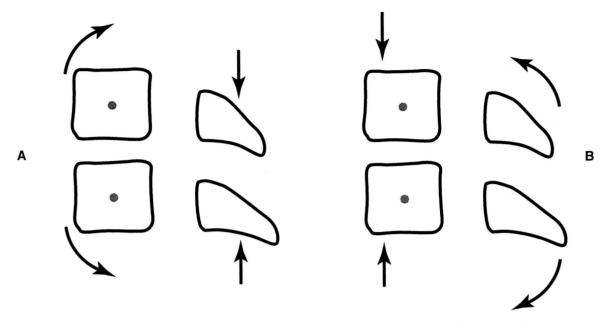

Figure 4-27. **A,** Tension band fixation dorsal to the instantaneous axis of rotation (IAR) causes spine extension. **B,** Conversely, tension band fixation ventral to the IAR causes spine flexion.

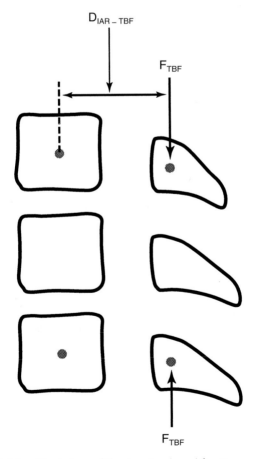

Figure 4-28. Depiction of the tension band fixation equation.

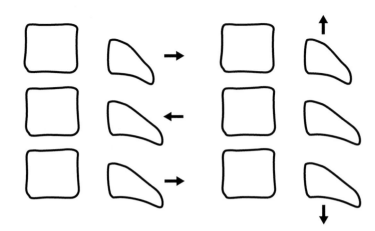

Figure 4-29. Three-point bending is nearly always applied with distraction.

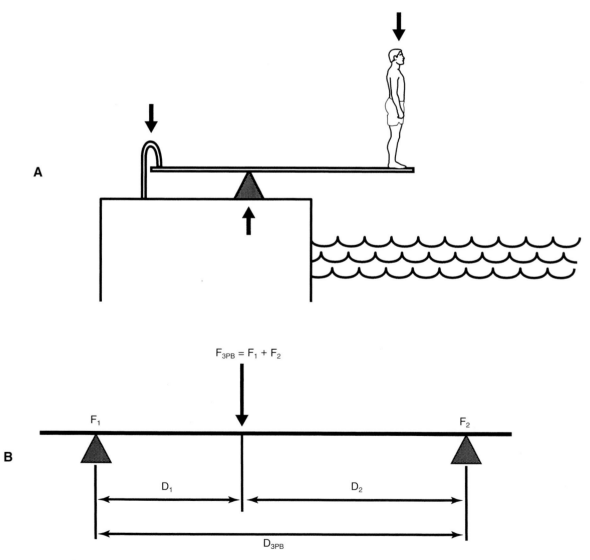

$$F_{3PB} = F_1 + F_2$$

Figure 4-30. **A,** A model of three-point bending depicted by a person standing on the end of a springboard. **B,** A similar and more graphical model is also depicted. *Arrows* depict force vectors. F_{3PB}, F_1, F_2, D_1, and D_2 are defined in the text.

and F_{3PB} is the ventrally directed force applied at the fulcrum (Figure 4-30, *B*).[3,16]

Three-point bending forces are affected by the length of the construct and not by the distance from the IAR. Therefore multiple spinal segments (five or more) are necessary to effectively apply this technique. Of note, the application of dorsal distraction forces to a lordotic spine may result in inadvertent flexion (Figure 4-31).

Cantilever Beam Fixation

A cantilever is a large projecting bracket or beam supported at only one end (Figure 4-32). Cantilever beam fixation usually bears a load over a space where support cannot be placed or is not desired. Three types of cantilever beam fixation are applied clinically: fixed moment arm, nonfixed moment arm, and applied moment arm.

Fixed Moment Arm

Fixed moment arm cantilever beam fixation rigidly buttresses the spine and usually can bear an axial load without the assistance of other structures. This form of fixation results in significant stress at the point of maximum stress application (Figure 4-33).

Nonfixed Moment Arm

Nonfixed moment arm cantilever beam fixation does not effectively bear an axial load without the assistance of other structures (e.g., vertebral body, interbody strut). It assists the already present axial load–supporting structures with their job (Figure 4-34, *A*). Toggling of the screw is allowed (Figure 4-34, *B*). The maximum stress is therefore located at the point of maximum bending moment application, in the mid-portion of the screw (see Figure 4-34, *B*). Consequently, this technique is appropriately used only when axial load–resisting capabilities of the spine are present. Because of their biomechanical characteristics of nonfixed moment arm beam fixation, the ability to resist screw pullout is diminished. Lateral mass screw fixation is an example of this technique. Incidentally, it may augment stability by pulling the bone to the underside of the plate (Figure 4-35).

Applied Moment Arm

Applied moment arm cantilever beam fixation applies a bending moment, either in flexion or in extension. This form of fixation can be accomplished by a variety of techniques (Figures 4-36 and 4-37).

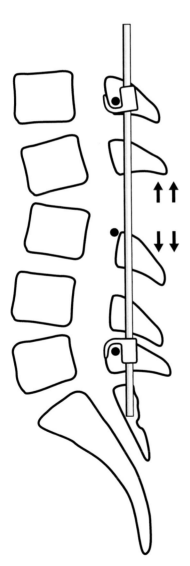

Figure 4-31. The application of three-point bending with distraction in the lordotic lumbar spine may result in spine kyphosis.

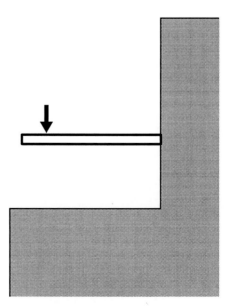

Figure 4-32. Depiction of a cantilever (projecting beam supported at one end only).

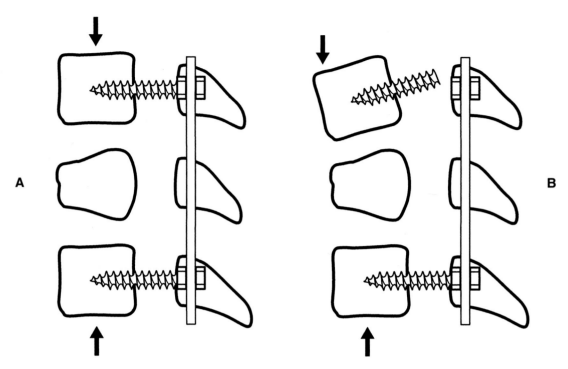

Figure 4-33.   **A,** Fixed moment arm cantilever beam fixation bears the axial load of the spine. **B,** This structure may result in significant stresses at the point of maximum stress application and hence failure.

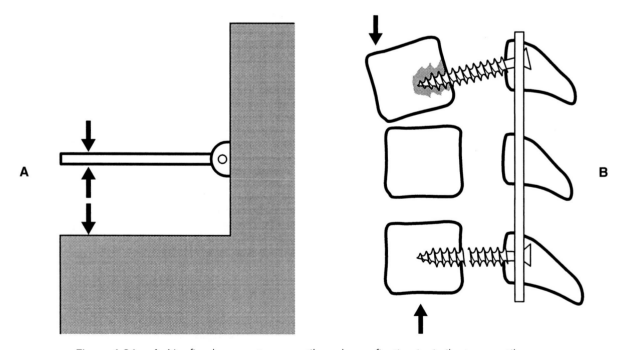

Figure 4-34.   **A,** Nonfixed moment arm cantilever beam fixation is similar to a cantilever beam fixed to a wall with a hinge. **B,** This construct may fail with toggling of the screw and pullout or fracture of the screw at the point of maximum stress application. Notice the difference in location of screw fracture between fixed and nonfixed moment arm cantilever beam fixation constructs.

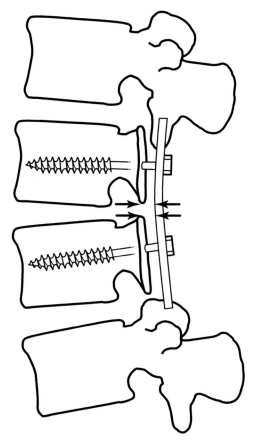

Figure 4-35. Technique of pulling the bone to the underside of the plate.

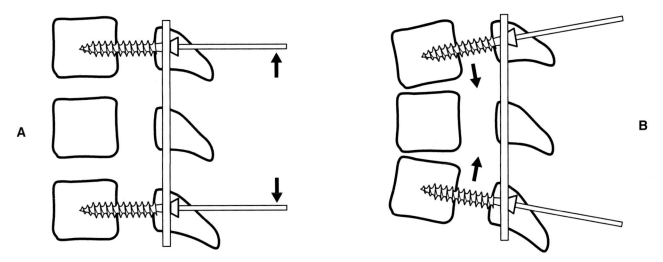

Figure 4-36. Flexion of a neutral spine **(A)** obtained with dorsal distraction using applied moment arm cantilever beam fixation **(B)**.

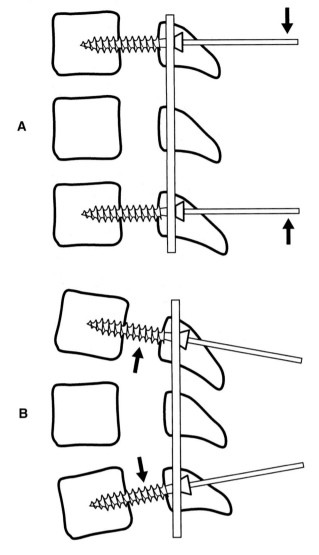

Figure 4-37. Extension of the neutral spine **(A)** obtained with dorsal compression using applied moment arm cantilever beam fixation **(B).**

SELECTED REFERENCES

Benzel EC: Biomechanics of lumbar and lumbosacral spine fractures. In Rea GL, ed: *Spinal trauma: current evaluation and management*, Park Ridge, Ill, 1993, American Association of Neurological Surgeons.

Benzel EC: *Biomechanics of spine stabilization: principles and clinical practice*, ed 1, New York, 1995, McGraw Hill.

Benzel EC, ed: *Spinal instrumentation*, Park Ridge, Ill, 1994, American Association of Neurological Surgeons.

White AA, Panjabi MM: *Clinical biomechanics of the spine*, ed 2, Philadelphia, 1990, JB Lippincott.

REFERENCES

1. Abitbol JJ, Heim SE: Threaded femoral cortical dowels for the treatment of lumbar degenerative motion segment pain: a radiological analysis and early clinical experience, *Proceedings of the 12th annual meeting of the North American Spine Society*, New Orleans, Oct 22-25, 1997, p. 101.

2. Bennett GT: Materials and material testing. In Benzel EC, ed: *Spinal instrumentation*, Park Ridge, Ill, 1994, American Association of Neurological Surgeons.

3. Benzel EC: Biomechanics of lumbar and lumbosacral spine fractures. In Rea GL, ed: *Spinal trauma: current evaluation and management*, Park Ridge, Ill, American Association of Neurological Surgeons, 1993.

4. Benzel EC: *Biomechanics of spine stabilization: principles and clinical practice*, ed 1, New York, 1995, McGraw Hill.

5. Benzel EC et al.: Controlled intervertebral settling in multiple level ventral cervical fusion procedures with a dynamic stabilization implant. Poster presented at the annual meeting of the American Association of Neurological Surgeons Spine Section, Rancho Mirage, Calif, Feb 11-14, 1998.

6. Brantigan JW, Steffe AD, Geiger JM: A carbon fiber implant to aid interbody lumbar fusion: mechanical testing, *Spine* 16(6):277-282, 1991.

7. Brooke NSR et al.: Preliminary experience of carbon fiber prostheses for treatment of cervical spine disorders, *Br J Neurosurg* 11(3):221-227, 1997.

8. Coe JD et al.: Influence of bone material density on the fixation of thoracolumbar implants: a comparative study of transpedicular screws, laminar hooks, and spinous process wires, *Spine* 15:902-907, 1990.

9. Collins JA: *High cycle fatigue in failure of materials in mechanical design: analysis, prediction, prevention*, New York, 1981, Wiley.

10. Graham RS et al.: Determination of the loss of height during settling of cervical fusion bone grafts. Presented at the annual meeting of the American Association of Neurological Surgeons annual Spine Section meeting, Rancho Mirage, Calif, Feb 11-14, 1998.

11. Kitchel SH: Threaded cortical bone dowels: biomechanical properties and early clinical results. *Proceedings of the 12th annual meeting of the the North American Spine Society*, New Orleans, Oc 22-25, 1997, pp. 29-30.

12. Ray CD: Spinal interbody fusions: a review, featuring new generation techniques, *Neurosurg Q* 7(2):135-156, 1997.

13. Ray CD: Threaded titanium cages for lumbar interbody fusions, *Spine* 22(6):667-680, 1997.

14. Schultz RS, Boger JW, Dunn HK: Strength of stainless steel surgical wire in various fixation modes, *Clin Orthop Rel Res* 198:304-307, 1985.

15. Senderi GJ et al.: A biomechanical evaluation of MRI compatible wire for use in cervical spine fixation. Presented at the annual meeting of the Cervical Spine Research Society, 1992.

16. White AA, Panjabi MM: *Clinical biomechanics of the spine*, ed 2, Philadelphia, 1990, JB Lippincott.

Biomaterials and Their Application to Spine Surgery

Carlo Bellabarba, Sohail K. Mirza,
Jens R. Chapman

Exciting advances in the field of biomaterials are likely to revolutionize the way in which we treat spinal disorders. Since the initial use of stainless steel as a fixation device, our understanding of spinal pathomechanics and the mechanical and physiologic effects of spinal instrumentation have inspired a progression toward implants made of more biocompatible and versatile materials. Developments in the fields of polymer chemistry, ceramics, and metallurgy have changed the landscape of spinal instrumentation, as has the recognition that the complementary properties of various substances can be exploited through the use of composite materials.

However, the demands placed on biomaterials are such that no currently available spine implant is ideally suited to the challenge of meeting the necessary mechanical requirements while integrating itself unobtrusively into this rigorous physiologic and biomechanical milieu. The ideal implant would be completely biocompatible and nonferromagnetic, would provide just the necessary degree of stability for the appropriate period of time without disturbing its environment, would be invisible to standard imaging techniques, and would disappear when its presence is no longer required. It would consist of plentiful materials that are inexpensive and easily manufactured or processed. None of the various currently available implant materials described here are capable of meeting all of these criteria, and the relative merits and disadvantages of each are discussed.

OVERVIEW OF CHEMICAL BONDING

On the most basic of levels, biomaterials are distinguished by the nature of the chemical bonds between their respective atoms, as these seemingly esoteric details provide the basis for understanding the individual properties of each material.

Metallic Bonding
Stainless Steel, Titanium, and Tantalum

Metals consist of tightly arranged positively charged atomic nuclei associated with surrounding free electrons. The freedom these atoms are permitted in their association with each other (i.e., the lack of directionality of this bond) accounts for both the high density of these materials and their ductility, or ability to deform without fracture. It also allows additional elements to be incorporated into the metal's crystalline structure. The relatively free flow of surrounding electrons accounts for the high electrical and thermal conductivity.

Covalent Bonding
Polymers and Biologic Molecules

The bonds that compose these long chains of carbon-based molecules differ from the previously-mentioned metallic bonds in that they are highly directional, as electrons are held in fixed orbits between neighboring nuclei and therefore have a preferred orientation. This restriction imparted on electron flow hampers their conductive abilities, making these materials effective insulators.

Equally as important in establishing the properties of materials made of these polymers are the van der Waals forces, which are weak hydrogen bonds that link the individual chains to each other. These weaker bonds allow the individual chains to displace with respect to each other, accounting for the plastic deformation seen when these materials are stressed.

Polymers are generally organized into a backbone with side chains, the structure and complexity of which have a profound influence on their physical properties, with the molecular weight of the polymer chain having the most influence.[122]

Ionic Bonding
Ceramics

Ceramics are defined as highly structured molecules composed of positively charged ions that "share" negatively charged nonmetal ions (usually oxygen). Because, as with covalent bonds, the ionic bond imposes a fixed position and orientation to its shared electrons, these bonds are highly directional and the molecules are generally not conductive. This arrangement results in molecules composed of a three-dimensional crystal lattice, with more random molecular orientation seen in glassy materials.

METALS

The three metallic alloys most commonly used in orthopedic surgery are titanium, stainless steel, and cobalt-chrome. Tantalum has also shown promise as a potential interbody implant. The application of cobalt chrome is mainly in the field of arthroplasty.

Stainless Steel

Stainless steel is among the most frequently used biomaterials in internal fixation devices. It combines cost effectiveness with favorable mechanical properties and acceptable resistance to corrosion, and it has withstood the test of time, having been successfully implanted in humans for decades.[50]

Commercial stainless steel is available in a multitude of grades and alloys, the majority of which are unsuitable as implants, mainly because of unfavorable corrosion properties. Corrosion is undesirable because it degrades the mechanical properties of the implants and releases metal ions into the surrounding tissues with potentially unwanted metabolic effects. Stainless steel types 316 and 316L are those with biomedical implant

---

METALS

- Stainless steel
  - High modulus of elasticity, therefore stress shielding
  - Susceptible to corrosion
  - High signal artifact on magnetic resonance imaging
  - Metal sensitivity
- Titanium
  - Lower modulus of elasticity, so less stress shielding
  - High corrosion resistance
  - Less signal artifact on magnetic resonance imaging
  - More biocompatible than stainless steel
- Tantalum
  - Maintains strength with high porosity
  - Can mimic infrastructure of cancellous bone
  - Promotes osseointegration
  - Interbody fusion device with no need for bone graft
  - Magnetic resonance imaging artifact similar to titanium
  - Superb biocompatibility

---

application. Type 316L is an iron-based alloy that contains 17% to 20% chromium, 10% to 14% nickel, 2% to 4% molybdenum, less than 2% manganese, less than 0.75 % silicone, and less than 0.03% carbon. Chromium protects against corrosion by producing a regenerating oxide film that prevents perforation and electrical conduction. Nickel and molybdenum also protect against corrosion. Minimizing the amount of carbon in the alloy is essential to its resistance to corrosion because carbon can bond to chromium and form chromium carbide precipitates, resulting in areas of local chromium depletion and loss of its protective effects.[112]

Crevice corrosion is particularly difficult to avoid with stainless steel fixation products. Implants undergo a passivation process as a final step in manufacturing, whereby immersion in a nitric acid solution enhances corrosion resistance by removing embedded iron products from the machining operation and by forming a dense oxide film on the implant surface.[154] Crevice corrosion occurs with the close juxtaposition of two implanted stainless steel components. This results in an intervening fluid layer with a lower oxygen tension than that in the surrounding fluid, establishing a battery that degrades this protective passive film, facilitating corrosion.[25,50,110,112]

In addition to its potentially problematic corrosive properties, another disadvantage of stainless steel is that its modulus of elasticity (approximately 200 GPa) is approximately 12 times that of cortical bone (and 80% greater than that of titanium), leading to the potential for local stress shielding of bone.[50]

The physical properties of stainless steel and other alloys depend not only on the composition of the alloy but also on the manufacturing process. The lowest strength (and highest ductility) is achieved through *annealing*, which is therefore appropriate for the manufacture of implants such as reconstruction plates and cerclage wires, in which malleability is an important characteristic. The *cold-worked* condition is of intermediate strength and is the standard method for manufacturing screws, plates, rods, and intramedullary nails. The *cold drawn* condition is the highest strength, and it is used for implants that require a high yield strength (i.e., resistance to permanent bending), such as Schanz screws, certain spinal fixation rods, and Kirschner wires.

Implant-quality stainless steel is nonmagnetic and therefore does not experience movement or generate heat in surrounding tissues during magnetic resonance imaging (MRI). Signal artifact adjacent to stainless steel implants, however, severely limits the ability to visualize these areas.[57,87,104,120] In the spine, the need to accurately image adjacent to hardware is of critical diagnostic importance. Stainless steel artifact, therefore, has been a major contributor to the development of spinal implants made of alternative materials.[104,163]

Another disadvantage of stainless steel is the issue of metal sensitivity,[155] which can cause local and remote inflammatory responses and increased pain at the implant site with bony resorption and implant failure. This potential problem has motivated the development of various forms of nickel-free stainless steel that are currently under investigation for potential biomedical use.[50] Nitrogen replaces nickel in these materials, which contributes to their increased strength and resistance to corrosion. Both the biocompatibility and the mechanical properties of nickel-free stainless steel appear favorable, although its increased strength and toughness adversely affect its ability to be machined, which poses challenges to manufacturers. In addition, nickel-free stainless steel may not eliminate the problem of metal allergy because (1) minute amounts of nickel (less than 0.1%) remain, which may be sufficient to trigger the immune system, and (2) other components of stainless steel, such as chromium, have also been shown to produce cutaneous metal sensitivity.[48,155]

Titanium

Titanium is the ninth most abundant element and the fourth most abundant structural metal in the earth's crust.[4] It has become the preferred metal for use in spine implant design for three main reasons. (1) It has outstanding biocompatibility (i.e., resistance to corrosion and inflammatory tissue response).* (2) It has favorable ferromagnetic properties, which cause less image artifact during MRI.[139,144] (3) Compared with stainless steel, it has a modulus of elasticity closer to that of bone, thus minimizing the stress-shielding effect.[10]

The excellent biocompatibility of titanium is reflected by the rarity of known allergic reactions to titanium and its alloys[105] and by the favorable response of tissues to titanium surfaces. A passive film of titanium dioxide forms on the surface of titanium when exposed to oxygen. This film regenerates immediately when damaged and protects the implant against fretting corrosion. Similar protective films of variable thickness can be added electrochemically through an "anodizing"

---

*References 3, 108, 121, 142, 160, 161.

process, which can also be exploited for the color coding of titanium implants.[128]

Studies have suggested that the improved biocompatibility of titanium may protect against postoperative infection.[3,121] In vitro testing in cell culture and organ culture assays and in vivo testing with subcutaneously placed implants have also corroborated this enhanced biocompatibility.[142,160,161] Tissue response to titanium implants has been shown to be less exuberant than that to stainless steel implants and is typified by a thin, uniformly oriented fibrous tissue layer without the reactive tissue that has been observed adjacent to stainless steel implants[160] (Figure 5-1). The absence around titanium implants of the reactive, fluid-filled capsule commonly formed around stainless steel may also be in part a function of the rough surface texture of titanium, which may stabilize soft tissue motion by promoting its attachment to the implant,[128] although comparison of tissue ingrowth characteristics of standard titanium surfaces with that of mechanically and chemically polished titanium surfaces has not corroborated this theory.[130] This same tissue adherence phenomenon may help prevent the propagation of infection.[74,75] The ability of surrounding tissues to anchor to titanium is the basis for the success of porous-coated and fiber-metal implants in joint arthroplasty[62,80] and may prove useful in achieving interbody fusions without bone graft[107] and in anchoring prostheses to bone in the nascent field of disc replacement.[5,31,55,173]

The two main forms of titanium that are used in implants are *commercially pure titanium*, which is mainly used in porous-coated and fiber-metal arthroplasty components, and a *titanium-aluminium-vanadium alloy (TAV, Ti-6Al-4V)*, in which strength is enhanced at the expense of ductility by limiting the oxygen concentration much more than in commercially pure titanium. The use of titanium alloys is therefore limited in implants where significant contouring is required. These two types can be combined without apparent consequence; studies have shown that the use of commercially pure titanium

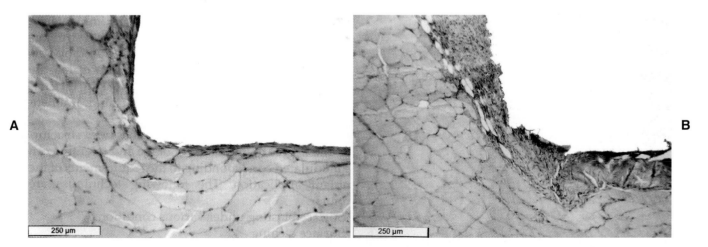

A   250 μm   **B**   250 μm

Figure 5-1. Histologic sections through soft tissue in contact with titanium **(A)** and stainless steel **(B)** implants showing how the tissue response and formation of reactive fibrous tissue capsule are far more abundant adjacent to stainless steel. *(From Pohler, OEM: Unalloyed titanium for implants in bone surgery, Injury 31(suppl 4): D7-D13, 2000.)*

in conjunction with titanium alloys does not cause galvanic corrosion.[49]

Although TAV is the most commonly used titanium alloy implant, other titanium alloys have also been developed with structural variations that influence their mechanical properties in ways that may make them better suited for specific uses. Ti-15Mo (TM) and Ti-15Mo-5Zr-3Al (TMZA) are newer titanium alloys with a structural variation that imparts lower strength but higher ductility and higher resistance to notch sensitivity.[49] This latter property may be an important advantage in implants that are subjected to repeated bending, such as spinal rods and internal fixation plates.

One additional disadvantage of titanium and its alloys is their susceptibility to wear, which has limited the use of titanium as a bearing surface in total joint replacement.[118,119] In the spine, pseudarthrosis has been associated with findings of wear debris and a macrophage cellular response similar to that seen around joint prostheses.[165]

Tantalum

Tantalum is an inert metal with favorable corrosion properties, high strength, and high ductility, which have led to its extensive use in the electronic and biomedical industries.[6,30,71,152] It is also extremely biocompatible,[35,91] and it is nonferromagnetic.[6,45,91] Its unique potential in orthopedic reconstructive procedures lies in its ability to be manufactured with a highly porous infrastructure that mimics that of cancellous bone (Figure 5-2), allowing its favorable mechanical properties to be combined with the ability to promote osseointegration. Osseointegration has previously been demonstrated using nonporous tantalum implants in dental and orthopedic applications for periods of up to 8 to 12 years.[2] Its superb biocompatibility and suitable mechanical properties have led to its standardization as a surgical implant material.[6]

The key to the potential of tantalum as a reconstructive material in orthopedics is its ability to tolerate a higher porosity while maintaining acceptable mechanical properties. This is a distinct advantage over the porous ceramic materials that are subsequently discussed, in which a limitation to achieving the ideal porosity for bioactivity and osseointegration is the associated decrease in the structural integrity of the material.[43,158] Tantalum implants are able to accommodate 75% to 80% porosity, and studies have shown that the majority of the porous structure of tantalum has been osseointegrated within 16 weeks of implantation.[8,9] Perhaps more important, from a clinical standpoint, is the speed with which shear strength of the construct develops. Even at 4 weeks, the bone-tantalum interface has a minimum shear fixation strength that is substantially higher than has been obtained with other porous materials that have less volumetric porosity. This early shear strength can best be attributed to the higher volume fraction available for ingrowth than is seen in fiber metal coatings (40% to 50% porosity) and sintered-beaded coatings (30% to 35% porosity), meaning that for any given percentage of bony ingrowth, a greater volume of bone is present within the porous tantalum, thus giving a proportionate increase in interface strength.[8,9] It is possible that the surface microtexture of the struts forming the porous material also contributes to the overall osteogenic response.[27,72,79,99]

Because of its high porosity, the structural stiffness of tantalum is relatively low, approaching that of subchondral bone, a property that could be advantageous in bone remodeling. Unlike sintered beads, fiber metal, or porous materials used to coat implants with plasma spray (discussed later), its high structural integrity allows it to be formed in bulk for the filling of bone defects or other reconstructive applications that require either standard or customized implant shapes and sizes. Its porous geometry may also be advantageous for use in a composite material, in combination with other osteoconductive or osteoinductive agents.

The radiographic characteristics of tantalum implants have also been compared with those of titanium in vitro, with evidence that tantalum creates either less[109] or an equivalent amount of[164] artifact on MRI and greater amounts of artifact on computed tomography (CT),[109,164] suggesting only a limited role for CT in spinal imaging after tantalum implantation.

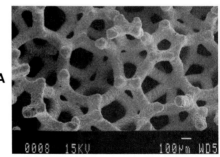
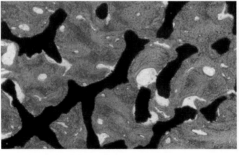
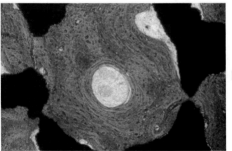

A **B**

Figure 5-2. Scanning electron micrographs of tantalum showing the cellular structure formed by the tantalum struts **(A)** and intimate interface between tantalum and vascularized bone 1 year after implantation **(B)**. *(From Bobyn, J.D., et al., Characteristics of bone ingrowth and interface mechanics of a new porous tantalum biomaterial, J Bone Joint Surg Br 81B:907-914, 1999.)*

Metal Failure

Fatigue is the main mode of failure of current metallic implants. All metals have an endurance limit. If the stress to which the implant is subjected is kept below the endurance limit, fatigue failure will not occur, and an infinite number of loading cycles can be endured. However, a finite number of loading cycles above the endurance limit can be tolerated before failure of the implant will occur. Under the latter circumstances, the only way to avoid implant failure is to unload the implant (e.g., progressive healing of a fracture or fusion of a spinal segment) or to remove the implant. Both the endurance limit and the fatigue life can be affected by extrinsic implant defects such as notches or bends, which act as stress risers. Fatigue failure can be objectively identified through electron microscopic techniques, which demonstrate characteristic concentric striations extending from the point of crack initiation.[112]

POLYMERS
Nonabsorbable Polymers

Nonabsorbable polymers with current biomedical applications, either alone or with other materials in composite implants, include polyethylene, polymethylmethacrylate (PMMA), and polyaryletherketones (polyetheretherketone [PEEK] and polyetherketoneetherketoneketone [ULTRAPEEK]).

Advantages of polymer biomaterials are their ease and flexibility of manufacturing, relatively low cost, and availability in a wide range of properties.[56] Minimum requirements of polymeric implants are that they be biocompatible, have long-term stability (low water absorption and high resistance to aging), and have sufficient stability to tolerate autoclaving or gamma irradiation.

Ultra-High Molecular Weight Polyethylene

Although its application in the spine has been limited, the emergence of total disc replacements may make the use of ultra-high molecular weight polyethylene (UHMWPE) more commonplace.[5,31,55,173]

NONABSORBABLE POLYMERS

- Ultra-high molecular weight polyethylene
  - Linear arrangement of ethylene monomers
  - Subject to creep, abrasion, and wear
  - Component of most artificial discs
- Polymethylmethacrylate
  - Exothermic polymerization of methylmethacrylate
  - Historically used for anterior column reconstruction
  - More recently used in vertebroplasty/kyphoplasty
  - Mixing under vacuum maximizes mechanical properties
- Polyaryletherketones
  - PEEK and ULTRAPEEK
  - Matrix component of composite cages
  - High wear resistance
  - Excellent thermal stability

Polyethylene has the simplest possible carbon chain construct, being linear and almost completely devoid of branching, a property that enhances its crystallinity.[56] The main problems with UHMWPE are its limited longevity, with eventual creep, abrasion, and the production of wear debris that has been shown to severely compromise fixation of implants.[7,134,146,151] New technologies are being investigated to address the problem of wear. Crosslinking of the polyethylene molecules has shown the most encouraging potential,[54,103] with 80% to 90% less particulate wear debris noted than in conventional UHMWPE.[56] Poor thermoplastic stability does not permit UHMWPE components to be sterilized by standard autoclave methods, requiring the use of gamma irradiation, which must be done in a vacuum to avoid free radical formation.

Polymethylmethacrylate

The application of PMMA in spine surgery has traditionally been restricted to the reconstruction of anterior column defects, particularly in surgery for vertebral metastases.[34,83] However, with the growing popularity of vertebroplasty, a discussion of its properties merits inclusion in this forum.

The acrylic bone cement consists of a polymerized powder and a liquid monomer (methylmethacrylate [MMA]), which, when mixed, induce an exothermic polymerization of PMMA. The mixing and application techniques are critical to the compressive strength of the final construct. Increased porosity creates stress risers and reduces strength. Mixing under vacuum and avoiding air bubbles during application help maximize the compressive strength.[56,111]

One disadvantage of PMMA that may be particularly problematic is the exothermic nature of PMMA polymerization, which generates temperatures of up to 80° C. Contact with neural elements through posterior positioning of PMMA in anterior spinal reconstruction or through leakage into the spinal canal during vertebroplasty can theoretically lead to thermal injury to the spinal cord or nerve roots[101,162] (Figure 5-3).

Polyaryletherketones

PEEK and ULTRAPEEK are members of the polyaryletherketone (PAEK) family. PEEK was first developed in 1978 for use in wire insulation. Its favorable mechanical properties, including a high wear resistance, combined with its effectiveness as a thermal and electrical insulator, have given it a wide range of electronic, automotive, and biomedical applications.[56] The medical grade version of PEEK, approved for long-term implantation, is known as PEEK-Optima LT. Because of a high melting temperature (334° C), it can be subjected to repeated standard autoclaving sterilization. It is also stable to ionizing radiation.

The opportunity to manipulate the mechanical properties of PEEK by fiber reinforcement is also an attractive feature of this material (see *Composites* below), as is the similarity of its modulus of elasticity to that of bone.

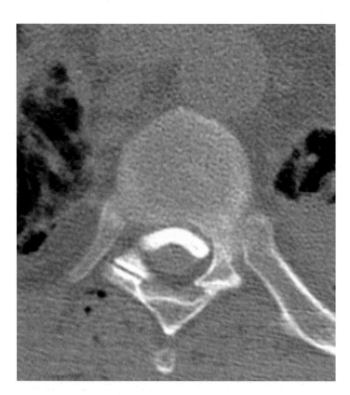

Figure 5-3. Computed tomography scan showing extrusion of polymethylmethacrylate into the spinal canal during vertebroplasty, resulting in canal compromise and paralysis.

These principles are the basis for the design of carbon fiber interbody fusion cages.[19-23]

Bioabsorbable Polymers

Interest in bioabsorbable polymeric materials has been steadily increasing. As with other materials for implantable devices, they have to satisfy several biologic and technical requirements. The versatility that would be required of the optimal bioabsorbable implant is indeed formidable. This material would be required to degrade at the appropriate rate (over 1 to 2 years) to maintain adequate strength until its stabilizing role has been fulfilled, gradually transferring increasing load to bone, and then to degrade at a rate that allows the body to suitably metabolize its degradation products. These same products of degradation cannot be toxic or carcinogenic or cause adverse inflammatory reactions. The material must be able to withstand either the extremes of temperature or irradiation required for effective sterilization before implantation. In light of all these requirements, it is hardly surprising that the ideal bioabsorbable implant has yet to be developed.

An effective bioabsorbable implant would eliminate the potential for various implant-related complications such as stress shielding, corrosion, release of wear debris, stress concentration at screw holes, and the occasional need for implant removal.[70] Bioabsorbable materials have had limited use to date in spinal fixation, mainly because of their relatively low strength and the

---

BIOABSORBABLE POLYMERS

- Insufficient strength for thoracolumbar spine stabilization
- Promising role in cervical spine stabilization
- Polyglycolic acid
  - Metabolized to glycine
  - Degrades in 4 to 6 weeks
  - Inflammatory soft tissue reaction
  - Formation of sterile cysts
- Poly-L-lactic acid
  - Metabolized to L-lactate
  - Degrades in 6 to 12 months
  - Less stiff than polyglycolic acid
  - Generates less inflammatory tissue reaction than polyglycolic acid

---

rapid degradation of mechanical properties once implanted[44] (Table 5-1). Their lower modulus of elasticity (approximately 3% that of stainless steel) is favorable from the standpoint of stress shielding; however, currently available bioabsorbable implants have a tensile strength that is far less than that of stainless steel at the time of implantation.[70] Although these issues have also limited their usefulness in other facets of orthopedics, the magnitude of the forces across particularly the thoracic and lumbar spines cannot be acceptably supported by currently available bioabsorbable implants.[46] Three-dimensional porous scaffolds in various geometric forms do, however, have a potential application in the manufacture of tissue-engineered implants in the future.[70]

Because of its different biomechanical characteristics, there may be a role for bioabsorbable implants in the cervical spine. Indeed, reports have emerged that suggest a possible role for bioabsorbable plate and screw fixation in the cervical spine.[28]

Polyhydroxy Acids (Polyglycolic and Polylactic Acids)

Most of the biocompatibility criteria cited earlier can effectively be met only by materials that will degrade into molecules already present in vivo, which can be safely excreted by cellular metabolic pathways. Polyglycolic and poly-L-lactic acid both meet this criterion and have been the most extensively used of bioabsorbable polymers. Although generally insoluble, polyglycolic acid (PGA), which has been extensively evaluated as the first widespread synthetic absorbable suture material,[85] is known to be biocompatible and is slowly hydrolyzed in water to glycolic acid. Glycolic acid is eventually converted to the naturally occurring amino acid, glycine, which is then either used in catabolic processes or metabolized via the Krebs cycle.

Similarly, polylactic acid, which has also traditionally been used as a suture material, becomes hydrolyzed within the body to lactic acid, which then becomes similarly metabolized. Only the *levo*-isomer of lactic acid,

Table 5-1	Tensile Strength and Elastic Modulus of Common Biomaterials	
Biomaterial	Tensile Strength (MPa)	Elastic Modulus (MPa)
Cancellous bone	10-20	490
Cortical bone	80-150	15,000
Poly-L-lactide solids	70	4,000
Polyglycolide solids	57	6,500
Titanium	550	100,000
Titanium alloy	900	110,000
Stainless steel	600-1,500	190,000
PMMA	30	2,200
UHMWPE	40	800-2,700
Alumina bioceramics	595	420,000
Zirconia bioceramics	1,000	210,000
Carbon fibers	2,500-7,000	250
Nonreinforced PEEK	100	3,700

PMMA, Polymethylmethacrylate; UHMWPE, ultra-high molecular weight polyethylene; PEEK, polyetheretherketone.

however, is recognized by cellular metabolic pathways, requiring that implants be made specifically of poly-L-lactic acid (PLLA).

Degradation of the implants occurs through hydrolysis of the ester bonds linking the monomers, which leads to implant fragmentation and loss of strength. The rate of degradation can be affected both by changes in the implant's structure and by the environment in which they are placed. Structural factors that delay degradation include a higher molecular weight, higher mass, increased chain orientation and side chain bulk, and increased crystallinity, whereas environmental factors that prolong degradation include those that subject the implant to lower stresses and decreased vascularity.[70] Although PLLA is less stiff than PGA, it degrades over 6 to 12 months,[61] whereas PGA has the distinct disadvantage of being degraded over 4 to 6 weeks.[12,13,15,16]

Tissue Reaction

Tissue reaction to bioabsorbable implants depends mainly on the degradation rate and toxicity of degradation products, but it also depends on factors such as implant shape and mass and the stress and/or presence of micromotion at the implant-tissue interface.[70] Soft tissue reactions are generally more severe in response to PGA than PLLA and consist, in response to the former, of a fibrous capsule with a high concentration of mononuclear and polymorphonuclear inflammatory cells, as well as lymphocytes and occasional giant cells. Lymphocytic and plasmacytic infiltration is unusual in the milder tissue reactions occasionally seen with PLLA implants.[41,61,70,117] Sterile cyst formation has also been reported adjacent to bioabsorbable implants and is more commonly seen with PGA.[14,136]

CERAMICS

Ceramics are defined as nonmetallic inorganic molecules of highly varied composition, linked by ionic bonds.[82] They are highly biocompatible, probably

because of their high oxidation states. The main types with biomedical application are the inert bioceramics (alumina $[Al_2O_3]$ and zirconia $[ZrO_2]$), bioactive calcium phosphates (beta tricalcium phosphate [B-TCP] and, calcium hydroxyapatite [HA]),[67] and bioactive glasses (Bioglass 45S5 and Apatite wollastonite).[100,171] The bioactivity of a material is a measure of its ability to bond biologically to bone. Inert ceramics stimulate only a minor fibrous reaction and are used mainly as bearings in total joint replacements. Bioactive ceramics are used as coatings to enhance fixation of a device or as bone-graft substitutes because of their osteoconductive properties.[82]

Ceramic implants, particularly the bioactive types, are unique among others discussed in that their purpose is often not simply to enhance the ability of biologic materials to achieve fusion but rather to eliminate the need for bone grafting altogether. This important distinction deserves careful emphasis considering the complications associated with bone graft harvest,[170] including reports of chronic donor site pain in up to 25% of patients[153] and the problems inherent in the use of allograft bone.[29] Because of their porous structure and their resulting ability to promote ingrowth of bone, ceramics have the potential to replace autologous bone, particularly as an interbody structural graft. However, although the degree of porosity of a given ceramic material correlates directly with its ability to promote ingrowth of bone (i.e., higher bioactivity), its compressive strength varies inversely with the degree of porosity.[43] The challenge has therefore been to determine the molecular structure that can achieve the optimal compromise between strength and ability to promote ingrowth.*

The development of calcium phosphate cements, such as Norian SRS, has also increased the level of enthusiasm for the potential application of these materials to spine surgery.†

---

*References 17, 38, 40, 127, 147, 172.
†References 36, 73, 102, 115, 122, 123, 140.

CERAMICS

- Nonmetallic, highly oxidized inorganic molecules
- Brittle
- Inert bioceramics
  - Alumina and zirconia
  - Modulus of elasticity 300 times that of bone
  - Susceptible to fracture
  - Limited role as interbody strut
- Bioactive calcium phosphates
  - Hydroxyapatite and beta-tricalcium phosphate
  - Osteoconductive
  - Promising as bone graft substitute
  - Positive results as interbody implant in cervical spine
  - Hydroxyapatite
    - Structure similar to apatitic component of bone
    - Able to bond directly to bone
    - Has preferable osseointegrative properties to beta-tricalcium phosphate
    - Nondegradable
  - Beta-tricalcium phosphate
    - Degraded by osteoclasts and dissolution
  - Calcium phosphate cements
    - Multitude of promising applications
    - Harden through precipitation of soluble calcium phosphate compounds
    - Degrade slowly
- Bioactive glasses
  - Bioglass 45S5 and apatite wollastonite
  - Osseointegrative properties exceed those of hydroxyapatite
  - Limited clinical use due to extreme brittleness

Inert Bioceramics

Alumina and zirconia ceramic implants have a fine-grained polycrystalline microstructure and are manufactured through the use of pressing and sintering techniques at high temperature. The inert bioceramics are known to have low reactivity levels compared with metals, polymers, and bioactive ceramics[67,116] but are somewhat limited in their application because of their inherent brittleness. Although alumina ceramic has been used in interbody struts after corpectomy,[86] its main orthopedic application is in arthroplasty,[18] because of its scratch resistance and exceedingly low coefficient of friction. The Young's modulus of alumina is 300 times greater than that of cancellous bone and 190 times higher than PMMA. Because of its brittleness and susceptibility to fracture, its application in spinal implants may be limited. Improvements in the manufacturing process, however, have made fracture of both alumina and newer-generation femoral head prostheses made of the stronger and tougher zirconia (ZrO_2) a less common occurrence.[82]

Bioactive Calcium Phosphates

Bioactive ceramics are osteoconductive, acting as a scaffold to enhance bone formation on their surface, and are used either as a coating on various substrates* or to fill bone defects.[82] The first in vivo use of tricalcium phosphate (TCP) was by Albee and Morrison in 1920.[1] Additional testing subsequently evaluated the ability of calcium phosphate to heal nonunions[81] and the effect of HAs on bone healing.[132] However, elucidation of the characteristics of these materials and their clinical applicability did not progress significantly until the 1970s.† To this day, the standard calcium orthophosphonates (CaPs) used in biomedical applications are B-TCP and HA.

Calcium phosphates are prepared, like other ceramic materials, through a process of thermal consolidation, or sintering, which allows for modification of the porosity of the material, a factor with vital implications to the biologic and mechanical properties of the resulting implant. They can be manufactured as either blocks or granules. Subtle differences in the composition and structure of calcium phosphate compounds may have a profound effect on their in vivo behavior.[11] The excellent biocompatibility afforded by their similarity to the mineral component of bone has made calcium phosphate ceramics an excellent bone substitute. Combining B-TCP with HA allows the adjustment of porosity and biodegradability, thus allowing the bioactivity to be adjusted as desired.[148]

Most calcium phosphates used in vivo are CaPs, which contain the Po_4^{3-} orthophosphonate group. These can be divided into two broad categories: (1) low-temperature CaP, which is obtained by precipitating from solution at room temperature; this class includes the calcium phosphate cements, the most commonly known of which is Norian SRS; and (2) high-temperature CaP, which is obtained through a thermal reaction; the majority of remaining CaP materials (e.g., ProOsteon) belong in this category.

Low-Temperature CaP

Until the discovery of calcium phosphate cements, these had little biomedical application except as a necessary step in the manufacturing of high-temperature CaP. The most commonly used low-temperature CaPs are octocalcium phosphate (OCP), a naturally occurring precursor in the formation of apatitic calcium phosphates in teeth and bones,[26] and precipitated hydroxyapatite (PHA), which has the distinction of being very similar to the apatite present in bone. PHA, or a carbonated form thereof (carbonate-apatite), is the main end product of the curing reaction in most of the calcium phosphate cements (e.g., Norian SRS, BoneSource, Cementek, alpha-BSM). Because most low-temperature CaP compounds are either naturally occurring or similar to a naturally occurring substance, a high degree of biocompatibility is one of their main advantages.

---

*References 76, 84, 88, 97, 106, 114, 135, 141, 168.
†References 42, 65, 66, 95, 133, 138.

High-Temperature CaP

The traditional CaPs used in medicine (B-TCP, HA) belong in this category. B-TCP has been extensively used as a bone substitute and is considered resorbable because it is susceptible to osteoclast-mediated degradation[53] and standard dissolution. The alpha-isomer of TCP has the same chemical composition as B-TCP but a different crystalline structure, which renders it more soluble in water. This solubility, combined with its ability to transform to PHA, makes it an ideal component of calcium phosphate cements.

HA $Ca5(PO_4)3OH$ is the high-temperature form of PHA. Its properties include the highest solubility in water and highest biocompatibility of the CaPs. Bioactive calcium phosphate ceramics such as calcium HA have been studied for more than 20 years. They have been shown to be biocompatible, nontoxic, and capable of bonding directly to bone, mainly because of the similarity of synthetic calcium HA to the apatitic mineral component of human bone.[60,92-95] Most bone graft substitutes are made of HA (e.g., ProOsteon), which is essentially nonresorbable, because degradation of HA takes decades to occur.[11]

The application of calcium HA can be expanded to plasma-sprayed coatings that can be applied to various fixation devices,[32,64,137] including pedicle screws, to enhance osseointegration of the implant and thus fixation strength.* HA-coated bioabsorbable (PLLA) implants are also under investigation.[167] In this scenario, thinner coatings (25 to 50 µm) are advantageous because they have the least effect on the mechanical properties of the substrate metal and they are less susceptible to delamination and fatigue.[39,98] Stable fixation of the construct is, however, a prerequisite for osseointegration because micromotion of even 100 µm has been associated with formation of a reactive fibrous membrane at the bone-implant interface.[59,60,149] Nevertheless, it has been shown that continuous loading may allow an HA-coated implant to replace a motion-induced fibrous membrane with bone.[150]

Biphasic calcium phosphate (B-TCP/HA composite). B-TCP and HA have also been combined as a composite material (biphasic calcium phosphate [BCP]) to maximize the osseointegrative potential of HA and the degradation properties of B-TCP. The usual combination is an approximate mixture of 60:40 HA/B-TCP.

Tetracalcium phosphate [$Ca4(PO_4)2O$]. Tetracalcium phosphate (TetCP), which has the most basic structure of any CaP, is the most soluble CaP below pH 5, yet it is poorly degradable. It deserves mention because it is the main component of many CPCs (e.g., BoneSource, Cementek).

The fine balance required between achieving sufficient porosity to promote bony ingrowth and maintaining sufficient structural integrity to prevent implant collapse is well illustrated by in vivo studies using various animal models. These have demonstrated almost universal implant fracture when using porous HA blocks for cervical interbody fusion, with loss of disc height and graft extrusion in up to 39% of cases.[38,172] Anterior plating does not appear to influence the incidence of fracture or disc space collapse with these porous implants, but it has been shown to decrease the rate of anterior extrusion and increase osseointegration of the ceramic block.[172] Conversely, use of a dense HA implant showed minimal graft collapse despite fracture but a lower fusion rate (30%).[40,127] Promising results have been shown using HA interbody fusion spacers in the porcine lumbar spine.[169]

Biomechanical studies in cadaveric porcine cervical spines have shown HA/B-TCP with 40% porosity to have equivalent properties to tricortical autograft.[156] Toth and coworkers[158] attempted to determine the ideal compromise between porosity and strength of a ceramic implant by comparing 50:50 HA/B-TCP ceramics of 30%, 50%, and 70% porosity with structural autograft in a caprine model. Interestingly, although the degree of bony ingrowth was directly related to their porosity, all three ceramic implants had less graft collapse and higher fusion rates than did the autograft.

The few clinical studies have suggested good results when using HA for anterior cervical fusion after discectomy in lieu of autograft,[145,157] although additional investigation is warranted.

Guigui et al.[77,78] suggested that a biphasic ceramic (65:35 HA/B-TCP) is equally as effective as an autograft in achieving posterolateral lumbar arthrodesis in a sheep model. The use of HA in conjunction with an osteoinductive medium such as demineralized bone matrix also gave comparable fusion rates to autologous graft in a rabbit model.[129]

These results suggest that the use of calcium phosphate ceramics as bone graft substitutes for instrumented posterior spinal fusion is justified, thus avoiding the potential morbidity associated with iliac crest bone graft harvesting.[47]

Calcium Phosphate Cements. Since their discovery for dental applications in the 1980s by Brown and Chow, many forms of CPCs have been designed[51] (Table 5-2). CPCs are essentially composed of an aqueous solution and one or more CaPs, which, on mixing, precipitate into less soluble CaPs whose enlarging crystal structures then become enmeshed. Because, unlike with PMMA, there is no polymerization reaction but simply a precipitation of crystals, there is little release of heat, making its use in the spine attractive.[123] There are two broad categories of CPCs based on their end products: apatite CPC (most common) and brushite CPC. All apatite CPCs have PHA or a carbonated form thereof (Norian SRS) as the end product. Because they have lengthy setting times, apatite CPCs minimize the liquid content, thus increasing viscosity, which gives the advantage of ease of manipulation but the disadvantage of being difficult to inject. Biocompatibility of this material is excellent, although inflammatory reactions may occur when the CPC does not set.[124] It biodegrades slowly, with a 30% degradation noted 2 years after implantation in a rabbit model.[37]

In contrast to apatite CPCs, brushite CPC can be initially very liquid and still set rapidly. It is slightly less

---

*References 76, 84, 88, 97, 106, 114, 135, 141, 168.

Table 5-2	Main Forms of Apatite Calcium Phosphate Cements		
Cement Name	**Company**	**Components**	**End Product**
alpha-BSM	ETEX	ACP, DCPD	PHA
Biobone	Merck BmbH		
Embarc	Lorenz Surgical		
Norian SRS	Norian (Synthes)	Alpha-TCP, CaCO$_3$, MCPM	CAP
Norian CRS			
BoneSource	Leibinger	TetCP, DCP	PHA
Cementek	Teknimed	Alpha-TCP, TetCP, MCPM	PHA
Biocement D	Merck GmbH	Alpha-TCP, DCP, CaCO$_3$, PHA	CAP
Biopax	Mitsubishi Materials	Alpha-TCP, TetCP, DCPD	PHA
Fracture Grout	Norian (Synthes)	TetCP, CaCO$_3$, H$_3$PO$_4$	PHA

Modified from Bohner M: Calcium orthophosphonates in medicine: from ceramics to calcium phosphate cements. *Injury* 31(suppl. 4):37-47, 2000.

ACP, amorphous calcium phosphate = $Ca_3(PO_4)_2 \cdot nH_2O$
DCPD, dicalcium phosphate dihydrate = $CaHPO_4 2H_2O$
Alpha-TCP, alpha-tricalcium phosphate = $\alpha\text{-}Ca_3(PO_4)_2$
MCPM, monocalcium phosphate monohydrate = $Ca(H_2PO_4)_2 \cdot H_2O$
TetCP, tetracalcium phosphate = $Ca_4(PO_4)_2O$
DCP, dicalcium phosphate = $CaHPO_4$
PHA, precipitated hydroxyapatite = $Ca_{10-x}(HPO_4)_x(PO_4)_{6-x}(OH)_{2-x}$
CAP, carbonate-apatite = $Ca_{8.8}(HPO_4)_{0.7}(PO_4)_{4.5}(CO_3)_{0.7}(OH)_{1.3}$

strong than apatite CPC, and unlike apatite CPCs, its mechanical properties in vivo deteriorate, probably secondary to the higher solubility of its end product, dicalcium phosphate dihydrate (DCPD).[90] Although brushite CPC is biocompatible, inflammatory reactions may occur, particularly when used in large quantities.[58] Brushite CPCs degrade faster than apatite, in part because, in addition to osteoclastic degradation, they also undergo simple dissolution.[11,125] Although this rapid degradation gives the theoretical disadvantage of resulting in the formation of immature bone, this is preventable by adding B-TCP granules to the cement paste, which anchor to bone and degrade less rapidly, thus encouraging mature bone formation.[125]

Bioactive Glasses

The most extensively studied bioactive glass used for orthopedic applications is Bioglass 45S5, which is composed of 45% SiO$_2$, 24.5% CaO, 6% P$_2$O$_5$, and 24.5% Na$_2$O. The bonding mechanism of bioactive glasses to bone is thought to consist of a series of surface reactions that form a hydroxycarbonate apatite layer at the glass surface. Although the osseointegrative properties of this material have been shown to exceed those of HA,[126] their extreme brittleness and disadvantageous mechanical properties have limited their clinical use.[82]

Apatite wollastonite glass ceramic, which has osteoconductive properties similar to those of Bioglass 45S5 but has superior mechanical strength, has been successfully used clinically and shows potential for expanded applications in spine surgery.[82,100]

COMPOSITE MATERIALS

Composites are formed by one or more materials that have different and complementary physical properties, which impart greater versatility than would be possible with each individual component. This allows the components of a composite material to be tailored to a specific need. They are normally composed of a matrix phase, with a second phase used for reinforcement.[63] A biologic example is bone, which must combine compressive strength through its inorganic matrix component, with tensile strength, provided by its collagen fiber polymers. Several composite materials have already been discussed. However, in medical technology, composite materials refer mainly to a *polymer matrix* reinforced with *pyrolytic carbon fibers* as a reinforcement. One can exploit this process to optimize mechanical properties by tailoring anisotropic material properties to the desired function. This design, however, must be based on a thorough understanding of the loads to which the implant will be subjected. Loads directed perpendicular to the orientation of reinforcing fibers would have to be accommodated by an effectively unreinforced matrix, which normally has mechanical properties far inferior to those of the reinforcing fibers (Table 5-3). These materials also come at the price of a complicated manufacturing process that must effectively adhere the fibers to the matrix. In fact, the properties of composites are highly influenced not only by the specific material components but also by the interface between the individual materials. Debonding because of shear forces between fiber and matrix is a frequent reason for failure in composite materials.[63]

Table 5-3	Strength of Common Components of Composite Materials	
Material		**Strength (MPa)**
Matrix material		
Polyamide (PA)		50
Polysulfone (PSU)		85
Polyetheretherketone (PEEK)		90
Reinforcing fiber material		
Glass fibers		1500-4500
Carbon fibers		2500-7000
SIC or Si_3N_4 fibers		2700-3500

From Gasser B: About composite materials and their use in bone surgery, *Injury* 31(suppl. 4):48-53, 2000.

COMPOSITE MATERIALS

- Polymer matrix (e.g., PEEK, ULTRAPEK) with carbon-fiber reinforcement
- Fiber reinforcement can be directional
- Complicated manufacturing process
- Delamination of individual components a potential problem
- Radiolucent
- Modulus of elasticity similar to bone
- Positive clinical results as interbody fusion cage

Carbon Fiber Polymer Matrix

In medical applications, composite materials usually consist of carbon fiber in a thermoplastic polymer matrix, such as PEEK, ULTRAPEK, polyurethane (PUR), or various epoxy resins (EP).[63] The fiber reinforcement structure can impart anisotropic (directional) or isotropic (nondirectional) properties to the material, according to the specific need.

The quest to develop a radiolucent interbody implant with the ability to provide immediate segmental stability while allowing unobstructed radiographic visualization of the fusion led to the proliferation of composite devices consisting of the above-mentioned combination of nonabsorbable polymer (PEEK, ULTRAPEK) with carbon fiber reinforcement.[19,20,22,23] These cages were originally machined from blocks of composite consisting of 68% long fiber pyrolytic carbon in PEEK. Later versions of the cage were made from a composite of similar long fiber carbon in ULTRAPEK.[19] They were designed to substitute for the insufficient mechanical properties of structural allograft or autograft more commonly used in lumbar interbody fusions at the time,[21] allowing the polymer to provide structural support while the autograft with which it was packed could optimize the fusion milieu. Structural features included ridges to resist displacement and load-bearing struts. With the subsequent development of metallic implants, however, its proponents now cite the ability to visualize the fusion on standard radiographs as the main advantage to this category of device. Additional advantages are the excellent bio-

compatibility of the material, a higher ultimate strength than that of metals used in orthopedic implants, and an elastic modulus far closer to that of bone (approximately 17 GPa), thus minimizing the stress-shielding effect.[96,166]

Clinical results of these composite devices have been reported to be favorable. In 1993, Brantigan and Steffee reported a 100% fusion rate using a carbon fiber cage in 28 levels 2 years postoperatively.[19] Brantigan et al. also documented a 100% partial- to complete-fusion rate within 6 months in a caprine lumbar spine model.[22] A report of 23 consecutive patients undergoing post-corpectomy reconstruction using an ULTRAPEK/carbon fiber composite cage showed excellent results.[33] Nonunion with subsequent cage fragmentation and release of particulate debris into surrounding tissues has, however, been reported.[159]

Other Composite Materials

A polyetherurethane/bioglass composite (PU-C), stabilized with an anterior plate of carbon fiber–reinforced PEEK (CF-PEEK), has been shown to provide high primary stability with anterior instrumentation alone in metastatic disease.[143]

Biocompatible osteoinductive polymer (BOP) is a composite material of *N*-vinylpirrolydone and MMA inside a matrix of polyamide fibers and calcium gluconate that was introduced in 1992 as a bone graft substitute for use in anterior cervical interbody fusion. Although some preliminary studies were promising,[24,113,131] citing results equivalent to those of autologous bone graft, enthusiasm was tempered by reports of poor osseointegration and an unacceptable rate of implant-related complications.[52,68] More recent investigations have corroborated these latter findings, emphasizing a high incidence of postoperative disc space collapse, implant displacement, and a low fusion rate.[89]

CONCLUSIONS

A multitude of implants are currently available for the treatment of spinal disorders. A comprehension of their basic material properties and how these correlate to their potential clinical uses allows the clinician to intelligently select the appropriate implant for each specific condition.

SELECTED REFERENCES

Bannon BM et al.: Titanium alloys for biomaterial application: an overview. In Luckey HA, Kubli F, eds: *Titanium alloys in surgical implants*, America Society for Testing and Materials, 1983, pp. 12-13.

Bobyn JD et al.: Characteristics of bone ingrowth and interface mechanics of a new porous tantalum biomaterial, *J Bone Joint Surg Br* 81(5):907-914, 1999.

Bostman OM, Pihlajamaki HK: Adverse tissue reactions to bioabsorbable fixation devices, *Clin Orthop* 371:216-227, 2000.

Brantigan JW et al.: Lumbar interbody fusion using the Brantigan I/F cage for posterior lumbar interbody fusion and the variable pedicle screw placement system: two-year results from a Food and Drug Administration investigational device exemption clinical trial, *Spine* 25(11):1437-1446, 2000.

Clark CR, Keggi KJ, Panjabi MM: Methylmethacrylate stabilization of the cervical spine, *J Bone Joint Surg Am* 66(1):40-46, 1984.

Delecrin J et al.: A synthetic porous ceramic as a bone graft substitute in the surgical management of scoliosis: a prospective, randomized study, *Spine* 25(5):563-569, 2000.

Disegi JA: Titanium alloys for fracture fixation implants, *Injury* 31(suppl. 4):14-17, 2000.

Disegi JA, Eschbach L: Stainless steel in bone surgery, *Injury* 31(suppl. 4):2-6, 2000.

Gasser B: About composite materials and their use in bone surgery, *Injury* 31(suppl. 4):48-53, 2000.

Hamadouche M, L Sedel: Ceramics in orthopaedics, *J Bone Joint Surg Br* 82(8):1095-1099, 2000.

Ibanez J et al.: Results of the biocompatible osteoconductive polymer (BOP) as an intersomatic graft in anterior cervical surgery, *Acta Neurochir* 140(2):126-33, 1998.

Rokkanen PU et al.: Bioabsorbable fixation in orthopaedic surgery and traumatology, *Biomaterials* 21(24):2607-2613, 2000.

Schulte M et al.: Vertebral body replacement with a bioglass-polyurethane composite in spine metastases: clinical, radiological and biomechanical results, *Eur Spine J* 9(5):437-44, 2000.

Shimazaki K, Mooney V: Comparative study of porous hydroxyapatite and tricalcium phosphate as bone substitute, *J Orthop Res* 3(3):301-10, 1985.

Swiontkowski MF et al.: Cutaneous metal sensitivity in patients with orthopaedic injuries, *J Orthop Trauma* 15(2):86-89, 2001.

Thalgott JS et al.: Anterior interbody fusion of the cervical spine with coralline hydroxyapatite, *Spine* 24(13):1295-1299, 1999.

Toth JM et al.: Evaluation of porous biphasic calcium phosphate ceramics for anterior cervical interbody fusion in a caprine model, *Spine* 20(20):2203-2210, 1995.

Wang JC et al.: MR parameters for imaging titanium spinal instrumentation, *J Spinal Disord* 10(1):27-32, 1997.

REFERENCES

1. Albee FM, Morrison H: Studies in bone growth, *Ann Surg* 71:32-38, 1920.
2. Alberius P: Bone reactions to tantalum markers: a scanning electron microscopic study, *Acta Anat (Basel)* 115(4):310-318, 1983.
3. Arens S et al.: Influence of materials for fixation implants on local infection: an experimental study of steel versus titanium DCP in rabbits, *J Bone Joint Surg Br* 78(4):647-651, 1996.
4. Bannon BM et al.: Titanium alloys for biomaterial application: an overview. In Luckey HA, Kubli F, eds: *Titanium alloys in surgical implants*, America Society for Testing and Materials, 1983, pp. 12-13.
5. Bao QB et al.: The artificial disc: theory, design and materials, *Biomaterials* 17(12): 1157-1167, 1996.
6. Black J: Biological performance of tantalum, *Clin Mater* 16(3):167-173, 1994.
7. Bobyn JD: Polyethylene wear debris, *Can J Surg* 34(6):530-531, 1991.
8. Bobyn JD et al.: Characteristics of bone ingrowth and interface mechanics of a new porous tantalum biomaterial, *J Bone Joint Surg Br* 81(5):907-914, 1999.
9. Bobyn JD et al.: Tissue response to porous tantalum acetabular cups: a canine model, *J Arthroplasty* 14(3):347-354, 1999.
10. Bobyn JD et al.: Producing and avoiding stress shielding: laboratory and clinical observations of noncemented total hip arthroplasty, *Clin Orthop* 274:79-96, 1992.
11. Bohner M: Calcium orthophosphates in medicine: from ceramics to calcium phosphate cements, *Injury* 31(suppl. 4):37-47, 2000.
12. Bostman OM: Absorbable implants for the fixation of fractures, *J Bone Joint Surg Am* 73(1):148-153, 1991.
13. Bostman OM: Osteolytic changes accompanying degradation of absorbable fracture fixation implants, *J Bone Joint Surg Br* 73(4):679-682, 1991.
14. Bostman OM, Pihlajamaki HK: Adverse tissue reactions to bioabsorbable fixation devices, *Clin Orthop* 371:216-227, 2000.
15. Bostman OM et al.: Absorbable polyglycolide screws in internal fixation of femoral osteotomies in rabbits, *Acta Orthop Scand* 62(6):587-591, 1991.
16. Bostman OM et al.: Impact of the use of absorbable fracture fixation implants on consumption of hospital resources and economic costs, *J Trauma* 31(10):1400-1403, 1991.
17. Bouler JM et al.: Macroporous biphasic calcium phosphate ceramics: influence of five synthesis parameters on compressive strength, *J Biomed Mater Res* 32(4):603-609, 1996.
18. Boutin P: Total arthroplasty of the hip by fitted aluminum prosthesis: experimental study and 1st clinical applications, *Rev Chir Orthop Reparatrice Appar Mot* 58(3):229-246, 1972.
19. Brantigan JW, Steffee AD: A carbon fiber implant to aid interbody lumbar fusion: two-year clinical results in the first 26 patients, *Spine* 18(14): p. 2106-7, 1993.
20. Brantigan JW, Steffee AD, Geiger JM: A carbon fiber implant to aid interbody lumbar fusion: mechanical testing, *Spine* 16(suppl. 6):S277-S282, 1991.
21. Brantigan JW et al.: Compression strength of donor bone for posterior lumbar interbody fusion, *Spine* 18(9):1213-1221, 1993.
22. Brantigan JW et al.: Interbody lumbar fusion using a carbon fiber cage implant versus allograft bone: an investigational study in the Spanish goat, *Spine* 19(13):1436-1444, 1994.
23. Brantigan JW et al.: Lumbar interbody fusion using the Brantigan I/F cage for posterior lumbar interbody fusion and the variable pedicle screw placement system: two-year results from a Food and Drug Administration investigational device exemption clinical trial, *Spine* 25(11):1437-1446, 2000.
24. Brotchi JL et al.: The use of a synthetic graft, the biocopolymer B.O.P., in the anterior cervical spine: experience in 100 cases, *Rachis* 1:367-372, 1989.
25. Brown SA, Simpson JP: Crevice and fretting corrosion of stainless-steel plates and screws, *J Biomed Mater Res* 15(6):867-878, 1981.
26. Brown WS, Lehr J, Frazier A: Octocalcium phosphate and hydroxyapatite: crystallographic and chemical relations between octocalcium phosphate and hydroxyapatite, *Nature* 196:1050-1055, 1962.
27. Brunette DM: The effects of implant surface topography on the behavior of cells: *Int J Oral Maxillofac Implants* 3(4):231-246, 1988.
28. Brunon J et al.: Anterior osteosynthesis of the cervical spine by phusiline bioresorbable screws and plates: initial results apropos of 5 cases, *Neurochirurgie* 40(3):196-202, 1994.
29. Burchardt H: Biology of bone transplantation, *Orthop Clin North Am* 18(2):187-196, 1987.
30. Burke GL: The corrosion of metals in tissues, and an introduction to tantalum, *Can Med Assoc* 43:125-128, 1940.
31. Buttner-Janz K, Schellnack K, Zippel H: Biomechanics of the SB Charite lumbar intervertebral disc endoprosthesis, *Int Orthop* 13(3):173-176, 1989.
32. Capello WN et al.: Hydroxyapatite in total hip arthroplasty: clinical results and critical issues, *Clin Orthop* 355:200-211, 1998.
33. Ciappetta P, Boriani S, Fava GP: A carbon fiber reinforced polymer cage for vertebral body replacement: technical note, *Neurosurgery* 41(5):1203-1206, 1997.
34. Clark CR, Keggi KJ, Panjabi MM: Methylmethacrylate stabilization of the cervical spine, *J Bone Joint Surg Am* 66(1):40-46, 1984.
35. Cochran KWD, Mazur M, DuBois KP: Acute toxicity of zirconium, columbium, strontium, lanthanum, cesium, tantalum, yttrium, *Arch Ind Hyg* 1:637-650, 1950.
36. Cohen MS, Whitman K: Calcium phosphate bone cement: the Norian skeletal repair system in orthopedic surgery, *AORN J* 65(5):958-962, 1997.
37. Constantz BR et al.: Histological, chemical, and crystallographic analysis of four calcium phosphate cements in different rabbit osseous sites, *J Biomed Mater Res* 43(4):451-461, 1998.
38. Cook SD et al.: Evaluation of hydroxylapatite graft materials in canine cervical spine fusions, *Spine* 11(4):305-309, 1986.
39. Cook SD et al.: Hydroxylapatite coating of porous implants improves bone ingrowth and interface attachment strength, *J Biomed Mater Res* 26(8):989-1001, 1992.
40. Cook SD et al.: In vivo evaluation of anterior cervical fusions with hydroxylapatite graft material, *Spine* 19(16):1856-1866, 1994.
41. Cutright DE, Hunsuck EE: Tissue reaction to the biodegradable polylactic acid suture, *Oral Surg Oral Med Oral Pathol* 31(1):134-139, 1971.
42. Cutright DE et al.: Reaction of bone to tricalcium phosphate ceramic pellets, *Oral Surg Oral Med Oral Pathol* 33(5):850-856, 1972.
43. Daculsi G, Passuti N: Effect of the macroporosity for osseous substitution of calcium phosphate ceramics, *Biomaterials* 11:86-87, 1990.

44. Daniels AU, Chang MK, Andriano KP: Mechanical properties of biodegradable polymers and composites proposed for internal fixation of bone, *J Appl Biomater* 1(1):57-78, 1990.

45. Davis PL et al.: Potential hazards in NMR imaging: heating effects of changing magnetic fields and RF fields on small metallic implants, *Am J Roentgenol* 137(4):857-860, 1981.

46. Deguchi M et al.: Biomechanical evaluation of translaminar facet joint fixation: a comparative study of poly-L-lactide pins, screws, and pedicle fixation, *Spine* 23(12):1307-1312, discussion p. 1313, 1998.

47. Delecrin J et al.: A synthetic porous ceramic as a bone graft substitute in the surgical management of scoliosis: a prospective, randomized study, *Spine* 25(5):563-569, 2000.

48. Deutman R et al.: Metal sensitivity before and after total hip arthroplasty, *J Bone Joint Surg Am* 59(7):862-865, 1977.

49. Disegi JA: Titanium alloys for fracture fixation implants, *Injury* 31(suppl. 4):14-17, 2000.

50. Disegi JA, Eschbach L: Stainless steel in bone surgery, *Injury* 31(suppl. 4):2-6, 2000.

51. Driessens FC et al.: Osteotransductive bone cements, *Proc Inst Mech Eng* 212(6):427-435, 1998.

52. DuBuisson AL, Stevenaert A: Soft cervical disc herniation: a retrospective study of 100 cases, *Acta Neurochir* 125:115-119, 1993.

53. Eggli PM, Schenk R: Porous hydroxyapatite and tricalcium phosphate cylinders with two different pore size ranges implanted in the cancellous bone of rabbits, *Clin Orthop* 232:127-138, 1981.

54. Endo MM et al.: Comparative wear and wear debris under three different counterface conditions of crosslinked and non-crosslinked ultra high molecular weight polyethylene, *Biomed Mater Eng* 11(1):23-35, 2001.

55. Enker P et al.: Artificial disc replacement: preliminary report with a 3-year minimum follow-up, *Spine* 18(8):1061-1070, 1993.

56. Eschbach L: Nonresorbable polymers in bone surgery, *Injury* 31(suppl. 4):22-27, 2000.

57. Fishman EK et al.: Metallic hip implants: CT with multiplanar reconstruction, *Radiology* 160(3):675-681, 1986.

58. Flautre B et al.: Volume effect on biological properties of a calcium phosphate hydraulic cement: experimental study in sheep, *Bone* 25(suppl. 2):35S-359S, 1999.

59. Friedman RJ: Advances in biomaterials and factors affecting implant fixation, *Instr Course Lect* 41:127-136, 1992.

60. Friedman RJ et al.: Current concepts in orthopaedic biomaterials and implant fixation, *Instr Course Lect* 43:233-255, 1994.

61. Fuchs M et al.: Degradation of and intraosseous reactions to biodegradable poly-L- lactide screws: a study in minipigs, *Arch Orthop Trauma Surg* 118(3):140-144, 1998.

62. Galante J et al.: Sintered fiber metal composites as a basis for attachment of implants to bone, *J Bone Joint Surg Am* 53(1):101-114, 1971.

63. Gasser B.: About composite materials and their use in bone surgery, *Injury* 31(suppl. 4):48-53, 2000.

64. Geesink R, Hoefnagels N: Eight years results of HA-coated primary total hip replacement, *Acta Orthop Belg* 63(suppl. 1):72-75, 1997.

65. Getter L et al.: A biodegradable intraosseous appliance in the treatment of mandibular fractures, *J Oral Surg* 30(5):344-348, 1972.

66. Getter L et al. Three biodegradable calcium phosphate slurry implants in bone, *J Oral Surg* 30(4):263-268, 1972.

67. Giannini S et al.: Bioceramics in orthopaedic surgery: state of the art and preliminary results, *Ital J Orthop Traumatol* 18(4):431-441, 1992.

68. Godard JJ, Farhad O, Steimle R: Biocopolymer (BOP) intervertebral implant for arthrodesis: a study of 45 cases, *Chirurgie* 117:398-404, 1991.

69. Gogolewski S: Resorbable polymers for internal fixation, *Clin Mater* 10(1-2):13-20, 1992.

70. Gogolewski S: Bioresorbable polymers in trauma and bone surgery, *Injury* 31(suppl. 4):28-32, 2000.

71. Gold JP et al.: Safety of metallic surgical clips in patients undergoing high-field- strength magnetic resonance imaging, *Ann Thorac Surg* 48(5):643-645, 1989.

72. Goldberg VM et al.: Biology of grit-blasted titanium alloy implants, *Clin Orthop* 319:122-129, 1995.

73. Goodman SB et al.: Norian SRS cement augmentation in hip fracture treatment: laboratory and initial clinical results, *Clin Orthop* 348:42-50, 1998.

74. Gristina AG: Biomaterial-centered infection: microbial adhesion versus tissue integration, *Science* 237(4822):1588-1595, 1987.

75. Gristina AG et al.: Adhesive colonization of biomaterials and antibiotic resistance, *Biomaterials* 8(6):423-426, 1987.

76. Guglielmino E et al.: Improvements in bio-mechanical adhesion of screws used in medical field: first application in spinal surgery, *Biomed Mater Eng* 5(1):1-7, 1995.

77. Guigui P et al.: Experimental model of posterolateral spinal arthrodesis in sheep. I. Experimental procedures and results with autologous bone graft, *Spine* 19(24):2791-2797, 1994.

78. Guigui P et al.: Experimental model of posterolateral spinal arthrodesis in sheep. II. Application of the model: evaluation of vertebral fusion obtained with coral (Porites) or with a biphasic ceramic (Triosite), *Spine* 19(24):2798-2803, 1994.

79. Hacking SA et al.: The osseous response to corundum blasted implant surfaces in a canine hip model, *Clin Orthop* 364:240-253, 1999.

80. Hahn H, Palich W: Preliminary evaluation of porous metal surfaced titanium for orthopedic implants, *J Biomed Mater Res* 4(4):571-577, 1970.

81. Haldeman KM: Influence of a local excess of calcium and phosphorus on the healing of fractures, *Arch Surg* 29:385-396, 1934.

82. Hamadouche M, Sedel L: Ceramics in orthopaedics, *J Bone Joint Surg Br* 82(8):1095-1099, 2000.

83. Harrington KD: The use of methylmethacrylate for vertebral-body replacement and anterior stabilization of pathological fracture-dislocations of the spine due to metastatic malignant disease, *J Bone Joint Surg Am* 63(1):36-46, 1981.

84. Hasegawa K, Yamamura S, Dohmae Y: Enhancing screw stability in osteosynthesis with hydroxyapatite granules, *Arch Orthop Trauma Surg* 117(3):175-176, 1998.

85. Herrmann JB, Kelly RJ, Higgins GA: Polyglycolic acid sutures: laboratory and clinical evaluation of a new absorbable suture material, *Arch Surg* 100(4):486-490, 1970.

86. Hosono N et al.: Vertebral body replacement with a ceramic prosthesis for metastatic spinal tumors, *Spine* 20(22):2454-2462, 1995.

87. Hueftle MG et al.: Lumbar spine: postoperative MR imaging with Gd-DTPA, *Radiology* 167(3):817-824, 1988.

88. Hulshoff JE et al.: Mechanical and histologic evaluation of Ca-P plasma-spray and magnetron sputter-coated implants in trabecular bone of the goat, *J Biomed Mater Res* 36(1):75-83, 1997.

89. Ibanez J et al.: Results of the biocompatible osteoconductive polymer (BOP) as an intersomatic graft in anterior cervical surgery, *Acta Neurochir* 140(2):126-133, 1998

90. Ikenaga M et al.: Biomechanical characterization of a biodegradable calcium phosphate hydraulic cement: a comparison with porous biphasic calcium phosphate ceramics, *J Biomed Mater Res* 40(1):139-144, 1998.

91. Issa TK, Bahgat MA, Linthicum FH Jr, Tissue reaction to prosthetic materials in human temporal bones, *Am J Otol* 5(1):40-43, 1983.

92. Jarcho M: Biomaterial aspects of calcium phosphates: properties and applications, *Dent Clin North Am* 30(1):25-47, 1986.

93. Jarcho M: Calcium phosphate ceramics as hard tissue prosthetics, *Clin Orthop* 157:259-278, 1981.

94. Jarcho M, O'Connor JR, Paris DA: Ceramic hydroxylapatite as a plaque growth and drug screening substrate, *J Dent Res* 56(2):151-156, 1977.

95. Jarcho M et al.: Tissue, cellular and subcellular events at a bone-ceramic hydroxylapatite interface, *J Bioeng* 1(2):79-92, 1977.

96. Jenkins GM, Grigson CJ: The fabrication of artifacts out of glassy carbon and carbon-fiber- reinforced carbon for biomedical applications, *J Biomed Mater Res* 13(3):371-394, 1979.

97. Kawagoe K et al.: Augmentation of cancellous screw fixation with hydroxyapatite composite resin (CAP) in vivo, *J Biomed Mater Res* 53(6):678-684, 2000.

98. Kester MAM, Taylor SK: Influence of thickness on the mechanical properties and bond strength of HA coatings applied to orthopaedic implants, *Trans Orthop Res Soc* 16:550, 1991.

99. Kieswetter K et al.: Surface roughness modulates the local production of growth factors and cytokines by osteoblast-like MG-63 cells, *J Biomed Mater Res* 32(1):55-63, 1996.

100. Kokubo T et al.: CaP-rich layer formed on high-strength bioactive glass-ceramic A-W, *J Biomed Mater Res* 24(3):331-343, 1990.

101. Konno S et al.: The European Spine Society AcroMed Prize 1994: Acute thermal nerve root injury, *Eur Spine J* 3(6):299-302, 1994.

102. Kopylov P et al.: Norian SRS versus external fixation in redisplaced distal radial fractures: a randomized study in 40 patients, *Acta Orthop Scand* 70(1):1-5, 1999.

103. Kurtz SM et al.: Advances in the processing, sterilization, and crosslinking of ultra- high molecular weight polyethylene for total joint arthroplasty, *Biomaterials* 20(18):1659-1688, 1999.

104. Laakman RW et al.: MR imaging in patients with metallic implants, *Radiology* 157(3):711-714, 1985.

105. Lalor PA et al.: Sensitivity to titanium: a cause of implant failure? *J Bone Joint Surg Br* 73(1):25-28, 1991.

106. Lapresle P, Missenard G: Hydroxylapatite-coated Diapason screws: first clinical report, *J Spinal Disord* 8(suppl. 1):S31-S39, 1995.

107. Leong JC, Chow SP, Yau AC: Titanium-mesh block replacement of the intervertebral disk, *Clin Orthop* 300:52-63, 1994.

108. Leventhal G: Titanium: a metal for surgery, *J Bone Joint Surg Am* 33:475, 1951.

109. Levi AD et al.: The radiographic and imaging characteristics of porous tantalum implants within the human cervical spine, *Spine* 23(11):1245-1250, discussion p. 1251, 1998.

110. Levine DL, Staehle RW: Crevice corrosion in orthopedic implant metals. J Biomed Mater Res, 1977. 11(4): p. 553-61.

111. Lewis G, Nyman JS, Trieu HH: Effect of mixing method on selected properties of acrylic bone cement, *J Biomed Mater Res* 38(3):221-228, 1997.

112. Litsky AS, Spector M: Biomaterials. In Simon SR, ed: *Orthopaedic basic science*, Rosemont, Ill, 1994, American Academy of Orthopaedic Surgeons, pp. 447-486.

113. Lozes et al.: Discectomies of the lower cervical spine using interbody biopolymer (BOP), *Acta Neurochir* 96:88-93, 1989.

114. Magyar G, Toksvig-Larsen S, Moroni A: Hydroxyapatite coating of threaded pins enhances fixation, *J Bone Joint Surg Br* 79(3):487-489, 1997.

115. Mahr MA et al.: Norian craniofacial repair system bone cement for the repair of craniofacial skeletal defects, *Ophthal Plast Reconstr Surg* 16(5):393-398, 2000.

116. Marti A: Inert bioceramics (Al2O3, ZrO2) for medical application, *Injury* 31(suppl. 4):33-36, 2000.

117. Matlaga BF, Salthouse TN: Ultrastructural observations of cells at the interface of a biodegradable polymer: polyglactin 910, *J Biomed Mater Res* 17(1):185-197, 1983.

118. McKellop HA, Rostlund TV: The wear behavior of ion-implanted Ti-6Al-4V against UHMW polyethylene, *J Biomed Mater Res* 24(11):1413-1425, 1990.

119. McKellop HA et al.: In vivo wear of titanium-alloy hip prostheses, *J Bone Joint Surg Am* 72(4):512-517, 1990.

120. Mechlin M et al.: Magnetic resonance imaging of postoperative patients with metallic implants, *Am J Roentgenol* 143(6):1281-1284, 1984.

121. Melcher GA et al.: Infection after intramedullary nailing: an experimental investigation on rabbits, *Injury* 27(suppl. 3):SC23-SC26, 1996.

122. Mermelstein LE, McLain RF, Yerby SA: Reinforcement of thoracolumbar burst fractures with calcium phosphate cement: a biomechanical study, *Spine* 23(6):664-670, discussion pp. 670-671, 1998.

123. Mirza AJ et al.: Vertebroplasty with a cavitation drill, University of Washington Orthopaedic Research Report, 2001 pp. 27-30.

124. Miyamoto Y et al.: Histological and compositional evaluations of three types of calcium phosphate cements when implanted in subcutaneous tissue immediately after mixing, *J Biomed Mater Res* 48(1):36-42, 1999.

125. Ohura K et al.: Resorption of, and bone formation from, new beta-tricalcium phosphate- monocalcium phosphate cements: an in vivo study, *J Biomed Mater Res* 30(2):193-200, 1996.

126. Oonishi H et al.: Quantitative comparison of bone growth behavior in granules of Bioglass, A-W glass-ceramic, and hydroxyapatite, *J Biomed Mater Res* 51(1):37-46, 2000.

127. Pintar FA et al.: Fusion rate and biomechanical stiffness of hydroxylapatite versus autogenous bone grafts for anterior discectomy: an in vivo animal study, *Spine* 19(22):2524-2528, 1994.

128. Pohler OE: Unalloyed titanium for implants in bone surgery, *Injury* 31(suppl. 4):7-13, 2000.

129. Ragni P, Lindholm TS: Interaction of allogeneic demineralized bone matrix and porous hydroxyapatite bioceramics in lumbar interbody fusion in rabbits, *Clin Orthop* 272:292-299, 1991.

130. Rahn B: *Cultured cells contacting implant material of different surface treatment, in biomaterials*, London, 1982, John Wiley and Sons, pp. 39-44.

131. Ramos JA et al.: The use of biocompatible osteoinductive polymer (BOP) in orthopaedic surgery, *Rev Mex Ortop Traum* 4:106-108, 1990.

132. Ray RD, Gloyd P, Mooney G: Bone regeneration, *J Bone Joint Surg Am* 34(3):638-647, 1952.

133. Rejda BV, Peelen JG, de Groot K: Tri-calcium phosphate as a bone substitute, *J Bioeng* 1(2):93-97, 1977.

134. Revell PA et al.: The production and biology of polyethylene wear debris, *Arch Orthop Trauma Surg* 91(3):167-181, 1978.

135. Rocca M et al.: Biomaterials in spinal fixation: an experimental animal study to improve the performance, *Int J Artif Organs* 23(12):824-30, 2000.

136. Rokkanen PU et al.: Bioabsorbable fixation in orthopaedic surgery and traumatology, *Biomaterials* 21(24):2607-2613, 2000.

137. Rorabeck CH et al.: The Nicolas Andry award: comparative results of cemented and cementless total hip arthroplasty, *Clin Orthop* 325:330-344, 1996.

138. Roy DM, Linnehan SK: Hydroxyapatite formed from coral skeletal carbonate by hydrothermal exchange, *Nature* 247(438):220-222, 1974.

139. Rupp RE, Ebraheim NA, Wong FF: The value of magnetic resonance imaging of the postoperative spine with titanium implants, *J Spinal Disord* 9(4):342-346, 1996.

140. Sanchez-Sotelo J, Munuera L, Madero R: Treatment of fractures of the distal radius with a remodellable bone cement: a prospective, randomised study using Norian SRS, *J Bone Joint Surg Br* 82(6):856-863, 2000.

141. Sanden B et al.: Improved extraction torque of hydroxyapatite-coated pedicle screws, *Eur Spine J*, 9(6):534-537, 2000.

142. Schroeder A, Pohler O, Sutter F: Tissue reaction to an implant of a titanium hollow cylinder with a titanium surface spray layer, *SSO Schweiz Monatsschr Zahnheilkd* 86(7):713-727, 1976.

143. Schulte M et al.: Vertebral body replacement with a bioglass-polyurethane composite in spine metastases: clinical, radiological and biomechanical results, *Eur Spine J* 9(5):437-444, 2000.

144. Scuderi GJ et al.: A biomechanical evaluation of magnetic resonance imaging-compatible wire in cervical spine fixation, *Spine* 18(14):1991-1994, 1993.

145. Senter HJ, Kortyna R, Kemp WR: Anterior cervical discectomy with hydroxylapatite fusion, *Neurosurgery* 25(1):39-42, discussion pp. 42-43, 1989.

146. Shanbhag AS et al.: Quantitative analysis of ultrahigh molecular weight polyethylene (UHMWPE) wear debris associated with total knee replacements, *J Biomed Mater Res* 53(1):100-110, 2000.

147. Shima T et al. Anterior cervical discectomy and interbody fusion: an experimental study using a synthetic tricalcium phosphate, *J Neurosurg* 51(4):533-538, 1979.

148. Shimazaki K, Mooney V: Comparative study of porous hydroxyapatite and tricalcium phosphate as bone substitute, *J Orthop Res* 3(3):301-310, 1985.

149. Soballe K et al.: Tissue ingrowth into titanium and hydroxyapatite-coated implants during stable and unstable mechanical conditions, *J Orthop Res* 10(2):285-299, 1992.

150. Soballe K et al.: Hydroxyapatite coating converts fibrous tissue to bone around loaded implants, *J Bone Joint Surg Br* 75(2):270-278, 1993.

151. Sochart DH: Relationship of acetabular wear to osteolysis and loosening in total hip arthroplasty, *Clin Orthop* 363:135-150, 1999.

152. Soulen RL, Budinger TF, Higgins CB: Magnetic resonance imaging of prosthetic heart valves, *Radiology* 154(3):705-707, 1985.

153. Summers BN, Eisenstein SM: Donor site pain from the ilium: a complication of lumbar spine fusion, *J Bone Joint Surg Br* 71(4):677-680, 1989.

154. Svare CW, Belton G, Korostoff E: The role of organics in metallic passivation, *J Biomed Mater Res* 4(3):457-467, 1970.

155. Swiontkowski MF et al.: Cutaneous metal sensitivity in patients with orthopaedic injuries, *J Orthop Trauma* 15(2):86-89, 2001.

156. Takahashi T et al.: Biomechanical evaluation of hydroxyapatite intervertebral graft and anterior cervical plating in a porcine cadaveric model, *Biomed Mater Eng* 7(2):121-127, 1997.

157. Thalgott JS et al.: Anterior interbody fusion of the cervical spine with coralline hydroxyapatite, *Spine* 24(13):1295-1299, 1999.

158. Toth JM et al.: Evaluation of porous biphasic calcium phosphate ceramics for anterior cervical interbody fusion in a caprine model, *Spine* 20(20):2203-2210, 1995.

159. Tullberg T: Failure of a carbon fiber implant: a case report, *Spine* 23(16):1804-1806, 1998.

160. Ungersbock A, Pohler OE, Perren SM: Evaluation of the soft tissue interface at titanium implants with different surface treatments: experimental study on rabbits, *Biomed Mater Eng* 4(4):317-325, 1994.

161. Ungersbock A, Pohler OE, Perren SM: Evaluation of soft tissue reactions at the interface of titanium limited contact dynamic compression plate implants with different surface treatments: an experimental sheep study, *Biomaterials* 17(8):797-806, 1996.

162. Wang GJ et al.: The safety of cement fixation in the cervical spine: studies of a rabbit model, *Clin Orthop* 139:276-282, 1979.

163. Wang JC et al.: MR parameters for imaging titanium spinal instrumentation, *J Spinal Disord* 10(1):27-32, 1997.

164. Wang JC et al.: A comparison of magnetic resonance and computed tomographic image quality after the implantation of tantalum and titanium spinal instrumentation, *Spine* 23(15):1684-1688, 1998.

165. Wang JC et al.: Metal debris from titanium spinal implants, *Spine* 24(9):899-903, 1999.

166. Williams DFM et al.: Potential of polyetheretherketone (PEEK) and carbon fiber reinforced PEEK in medical applications, *J Mater Sci Lett* 6:188-190, 1987.

167. Yasunaga T et al.: Bonding behavior of ultrahigh strength unsintered hydroxyapatite particles/poly(L-lactide) composites to surface of tibial cortex in rabbits, *J Biomed Mater Res* 47(3):412-419, 1999.

168. Yerby SA, Toh E, McLain RF: Revision of failed pedicle screws using hydroxyapatite cement: a biomechanical analysis, *Spine* 23(15):1657-1661, 1998.

169. Ylinen P et al.: Lumbar spine interbody fusion with reinforced hydroxyapatite implants, *Arch Orthop Trauma Surg* 110(5):250-256, 1991.

170. Younger EM, Chapman MW: Morbidity at bone graft donor sites, *J Orthop Trauma* 3(3):192-195, 1980.

171. Yuan H et al.: Bone induction by porous glass ceramic made from Bioglass(R) (45S5), *J Biomed Mater Res* 58(3):270-276, 2001.

172. Zdeblick TA et al.: Anterior cervical discectomy and fusion using a porous hydroxyapatite bone graft substitute, *Spine* 19(20):2348-2357, 1994.

173. Zeegers WS et al.: Artificial disc replacement with the modular type SB Charite III: 2- year results in 50 prospectively studied patients, *Eur Spine J* 8(3):210-217, 1999.

The Aging Lumbar Spine: The Pain Generator

Thomas A. St. John, Matthew A. Handling,
Scott D. Daffner, Alexander R. Vaccaro

Age-related changes in the lumbar spine manifest as a pathologic, symptomatic disease process in some patients. The degenerative changes that occur in the various components of the spine are reviewed here along with various mechanisms that might cause these changes. Clinical expressions of these changes are considered in association with their potential pain generators.

The precise cause and sequence of age-related changes in the spine remain unknown. The spectrum of changes seen in the normal aging spine anatomically, biochemically, biomechanically, and radiographically may also occur, to an exaggerated extent, in the pathologically degenerated spine.[9] Disc degeneration implies a decline of the physical and chemical properties of the entire anulus fibrosus and nucleus pulposus or a portion of it, with pathologic changes evident at the cellular and molecular level.[41] Normal changes associated with aging occur within the intervertebral disc, which at times may result clinically in low back pain, mechanical instability, disc herniation, and/or nerve compression.

THE INTERVERTEBRAL DISC

The intervertebral disc performs many roles as a functional member of the spinal unit. Physically, it acts as a focus of motion between two vertebral bodies. As a result of its intrinsic viscoelasticity, it functions to absorb and distribute loads applied to the spinal column. It has been suggested that the anulus is the principal stabilizing element of the spine, playing a more critical role in motion stabilization than the facet joints, the posterior ligaments, or even the ligamentum flavum.[79] With increasing age, the intervertebral discs undergo dramatic changes in volume, shape, structure, and composition, which have consequences on their ability to perform their native function of load transfer and stability.

Age-Related Changes in Anatomy and Morphology

The intervertebral disc is a fibrocartilaginous complex that serves as the major structural link between the bodies of adjacent vertebrae. The 23 discs of the average spinal column make up 22% of the length of the spine, 20% of the length in the thoracic area, and up to 33% of the length in the lumbar area. The morphology of the intervertebral disc changes in shape and size (becomes larger) in a linear fashion as one goes from the cervical to the lumbar region; however, its internal structure remains remarkably consistent.[68] Each intervertebral disc is made up of a gelatinous nucleus pulposus surrounded by a laminated anulus fibrosus. The anulus fibrosus forms the outer boundary of the intervertebral disc. It is composed of concentric layers of fibrocartilaginous tissue and fibrous proteins that run obliquely from one vertebra to another. Typically, there are 12 concentric lamellae, which enclose the nucleus. Anteriorly, the lamellae are distinct and can be separated. With aging, these layers become more indistinct. Posteriorly, they tend to merge and cannot be easily dissected, even in the young specimen. In a single lamella, the fibers are parallel to each other but are tilted with respect to the axis of the spine by approximately 65 degrees.[39] The direction of the tilt alternates with each adjacent lamella. The layers of collagen fibers of the anulus fibrosus slant in alternate directions, thus crossing each other at different angles, which vary with the degree of intradiscal pressure placed on the nucleus propulsus.[10] Fiber tilt is thought to be essential to disc morphology, conveying the ability to withstand compression, twisting, and flexion.[39] These angles do not change as the spine ages (Figure 6-1).

> ### ANATOMY OF THE SPINAL COLUMN
>
> - 33 Vertebrae
> - 23 Intervertebral discs
>   - Inner nucleus propulsus
>   - Outer anulus fibrosus
> - Facet joints
> - Cartilagenous end plates
> - Spinal ligaments

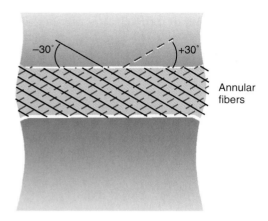

Figure 6-1. The directions of annular fiber tilt, showing the alternating pattern of the crossing annular fibers.

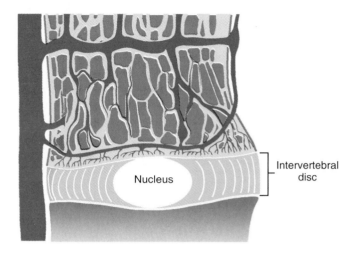

Figure 6-2. The microvascular anatomy of the intervertebral disc and vertebral end plate.

There is no definitive structural interface between the nucleus and the anulus, and this region is called the *transition zone*.[43] This zone becomes increasingly difficult to identify with advancing age. The nucleus pulposus is situated posterocentrally within the disc and occupies approximately 40% of the disc cross-sectional area. It consists of collagen fibrils that are randomly arranged in a hydrated matrix of proteoglycans, similar in composition to the embryonic notochordal tissue of which it is a remnant. This structural organization gives the nucleus the quality of a highly viscous gel. With aging, the nucleus becomes more fibrotic, less capable of drawing in water, and therefore less functional.

Discs are situated between the cartilaginous end plates of two vertebrae. These vertebral end plates, initially composed of hyaline cartilage and then later of calcified cartilage, form the superior and inferior boundaries of the intervertebral disc. Collagen fibers of the lamellae in the outer anulus attach directly to bone through Sharpey's fibers. The collagen fibers from the inner anulus fibrosus attach to the cartilaginous end plates. There are no connections between the nucleus and the end plates. Furthermore, the end plates do not have any direct fibrous attachment to bone. Therefore, this junction (end plate/vertebral body) is a region susceptible to failure, especially when exposed to shear forces.[68]

At birth, the intervertebral disc vascularity is prominent, with the greatest concentration of blood vessels in the posterior lamellae of the anulus fibrosus. Vessels can be identified penetrating the anulus and even the nucleus from the end plates (Figure 6-2). Over time, vascularity diminishes to such a significant degree that by skeletal maturity, the normal disc no longer contains blood vessels, except at the very periphery.[27] The adult intervertebral disc is the largest avascular structure in the human body. This loss of vasculature may indeed mark the beginning of the degenerative process.

As aging progresses, the disc volume and shape go through predictable changes. The primary alterations include loss of disc height, protrusion of the central disc

---

AGE-RELATED CHANGES IN THE INTERVERTEBRAL DISC

- Loss of disc height
- Protrusion of the central disc into the vertebral body
- Bulging/buckling of the anulus fibrosus

---

into the vertebral body, and buckling or bulging of the anulus. All discs eventually develop similar age-related changes; however, within the same person, the rate is not the same for each disc.[12] For instance, in some people, the degenerative process in one or more discs may advance at a rapid degree, while the remaining discs retain a relatively normal morphology.

Throughout the aging process, the outer anulus fibrosus remains roughly the same size, but the inner anulus expands at the expense of the nucleus.[14] Myxomatous degeneration occurs first in the inner portions of the anulus, causing disruption of the annular fibers. This leads to the development of clefts and fissures, which may extend into the periphery. Collections of gas are sometimes seen within these clefts and are identified radiographically as a vacuum sign. Macroscopically, the disc becomes brown and yellowish and assumes a disorganized structure. In all parts of the disc, the concentration of viable cells decreases, particularly in the nucleus.[92,93] These normal age-related changes eventually affect the structural integrity of the disc, making it less effective at responding to normal compressive and tensile loads and increasing the potential for injury such as disc herniation.

Changes in disc tissue structure and composition precede and accompany the changes in gross morphology of the disc.[12] The changes in disc size, vascularity, and structural organization begin during the growth and development stage, before any overt disc degeneration. In this sense, age-related changes in the disc begin shortly after birth.[72]

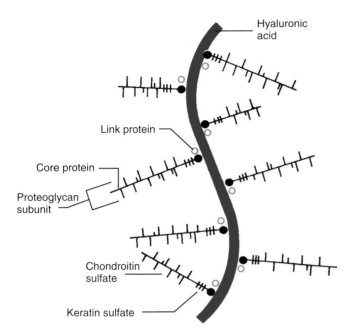

Figure 6-3. A proteoglycan molecule, showing the various subcomponents, including the hyaluronic acid backbone, link protein, and chondroitin sulfate and keratin sulfate side chains.

Biochemistry

Like other connective tissues in the body, the intervertebral disc consists of a small population of cells and an abundant extracellular matrix.[12] Disc cells synthesize macromolecules, which in turn create the framework of the disc. The primary structural components of the disc macromolecular framework are proteoglycans and collagens.[12,21] Proteoglycans exist in the form of monomers and as larger aggregates. The monomer subunits consist of a protein core to which multiple glycosaminoglycans, such as keratin sulfate and chondroitin sulfate, are attached. The aggregates consist of multiple proteoglycan monomer subunits attached to a long hyaluronic acid filament via link proteins (Figure 6-3).

Proteoglycans interact with water to help the tissue become stiff and resist compression, whereas collagen helps provide the tissue with tensile strength. The structural integrity and the mechanical properties of the disc depend on these macromolecules and their interactions with water. The nucleus pulposus is able to hold its fluid pressure mainly due to the presence of negatively charged glycosaminoglycan chains.[12] Due to the fact that mature discs are avascular, nutrients and waste products must be transported through the disc matrix.[41] The nutritional supply routes are from the peripheral parts of the anulus and the central part of the vertebral end plate. A high osmotic pressure within the disc plus the hydrostatic pressure acting on the disc allows diffusion, and thus solute transport, to occur.[16] This, however, requires high intrinsic water content.

The main consequence of disc degeneration is the loss of these hydrostatic properties. At birth, the nucleus is composed of approximately 88% to 90% water,

> ### BIOCHEMICAL CHANGES OF THE AGING DISC
>
> - Loss of a clear transition between the nucleus and anulus
> - Increase in the collagen content
> - Loss of negatively charged proteoglycan chains
> - Reduction in the number of proteoglycan aggregates[9]
> - Reduction of water content

whereas by the age of 70 years, water content has dropped to 65% to 70%.[34] There is a decrease in the osmotic swelling pressure of the disc and a twofold increase in creep under compression from age 30 to 80 years.[50] This age-related decrease in the ability of the disc to imbibe water and thus distribute load occurs because of changes in the macromolecular organization of proteoglycans and collagen.[60] The gradual reduction with age in water content of the nucleus occurs after proteoglycan fragmentation, with subsequent ingrowth of collagenous tissue.[67] Although collagen is mainly responsible for the tensile strength of the disc, proteoglycans are the main factors that resist compression and provide resilience to the disc tissue.[35]

The mucopolysaccharide/protein complexes in young discs are large molecules that are made up of chondroitin sulfate A and C side chains, which are strongly hydrophilic macromolecules. After skeletal maturity, these macromolecules begin to break down into smaller molecules. Newer macromolecules are produced that consist of chondroitin sulfate B and keratin sulfate, which are smaller and have less water-binding capabilities.[67] As the hydrostatic pressure of the nucleus pulposus decreases with age, it becomes more fibrotic, less turgid, and less capable of redistributing compressive loads to the inner layers of the anulus. A larger portion of the load is therefore taken up directly through the anulus, which may lead to bulging and perhaps nerve compression.[67]

Changes in the anulus fibrosus have also been observed with aging. The number of viable cells decreases, along with a general reduction in cellular metabolic activity.[9] As with the nucleus, the major biochemical change is a decrease in proteoglycans. Larger collagen fibrils form as the disc matures. Some investigators have postulated that these larger diameter fibrils may be less strong than their narrow counterparts and thus more likely to fail.[40]

In addition, characteristic changes occur in the vertebral end plates with skeletal maturity. Calcification of the cartilaginous end plates combined with a loss of vascularity can have a detrimental effect on disc nutrition, which is dependent on the diffusion of nutrients across the end plates.[9]

The biochemical changes in the aging disc include the loss of a clear transition between nucleus and anulus; an increase in collagen content; the loss of negatively charged proteoglycan chains, which decrease the affinity of the nucleus for water; and reduced numbers of proteoglycan aggregates.[34,73] This series of biochemical events, combined with an increasingly inefficient mechanism of disc nutrition, results in the inability of the intervertebral disc to function as a perfect gel.[9] The initiating event for these changes is unknown. Kang et al. showed, however, that herniated discs produce increased levels of various enzymes and cytokines that are capable of degrading the extracellular macromolecular matrix.[46] The role that these degradative chemicals play in disc degeneration has yet to be elucidated.

Disc Mechanics

Knowledge of both the anatomy and biomechanics of the intervertebral discs is important in helping to identify the structures that may be responsible for pain generation as the normal spine proceeds through the aging process. For the spine to function efficiently, it must confer a skeletal scaffolding to the muscles of the body and have inherent strength and flexibility. The spinal column is divided into a series of functional units. A particular functional unit is composed of two vertebral bodies, with facet joints posteriorly and an intervening intervertebral disc anteriorly.[10] The anterior column of the spine is a weight-bearing structure that provides flexibility and shock absorption to the spinal column.[10] The posterior spinal column functions to house and protect the neural elements and, through the geometry and morphology of the facet joints, guides the movement of the spinal functional unit. Individually, intervertebral discs provide a very strong articulation between two adjoining vertebrae, providing significant stability to the spine and allowing the uniform transmission of load. Compressive pressure placed on the disc is dissipated circumferentially in a passive manner. Although the major function of the nucleus pulposus is to resist and redistribute compressive forces within the spine to the anulus fibrosus, the anulus functions to withstand tension.

All of the spinal elements function collectively to provide flexibility, protection of the neural elements, and structural support to the skeleton. With spinal degeneration, several of these roles are significantly altered, leading in some cases to instability, pain, deformity, and loss of neurologic function.[32] Although spinal motion segment instability is not fully understood, it is thought to result in the clinical expression of low back pain.[32] A disturbance in any one component of the spinal unit, such as a decrease in the water content of the nucleus or a tear in the anulus, may affect the mechanical function of the other components. For instance, if the ability of the disc to share in load distribution is impaired, there may be a detrimental effect on the facet joints, leading to further degenerative changes.[32]

Historically, focus has been on the intervertebral disc as the site where the degenerative cascade is initiated. It has been proposed that degenerative changes occur first in the intervertebral disc, which eventually result in secondary changes to facet and ligamentous morphology and function due to altered load sharing.[15] Experimental evidence from animal models of disc degeneration has supported this view. Using a rabbit model in one study and a canine model in another study, disc degeneration was produced by either direct mechanical injury to the disc or injection of chymopapain into the disc tissue.[11,33,54] Secondary facet degeneration was observed in both models after initial intervertebral disc degeneration.[11,33,54] In addition, Panjabi et al., using in vitro biomechanical testing, described a cascade of secondary changes that occurred in the facet joints as a result of disc injuries.[71]

This theory of spinal degeneration, however, is not universally accepted. Some researchers have shown evidence that facet degeneration occurs independent of disc degeneration.[63,95] Furthermore, biomechanical studies have found that torsional stresses, which occur when the facets are asymmetrically oriented, may be the primary force responsible for initiating and producing disc injury.[24] Animal models of torsional instability have been developed to help study the effects of force application on changes to the intervertebral disc. Sullivan et al.[88] and Cauchoix et al.[17] observed disc degeneration using this model both radiographically and histochemically, respectively.

Frymoyer suggested that determination of the relative importance of the intervertebral disc and facets in initiating the degenerative process is not as productive as visualizing the spinal unit as a "three-joint complex," in which both the facets and discs play a contributory role.[27] Using this three-joint concept proposed by Kirkaldy-Willis,[49] the progression of spinal degeneration has been described as occurring in three stages. In stage I, early changes in the biochemistry and physiology of the three-joint complex may be responsible for the production of clinical symptoms. Stage II is heralded by an increase in spinal segment motion, producing sympto-

---

SPINAL FUNCTIONAL UNITS

- Two vertebral bodies
- Intervertebral disc
  - Functions to provide flexibility for the spinal column and as a weight-bearing structure
- Facet joint/posterior elements
  - Functions to house and protect spinal cord[10]

THREE STAGES OF PROGRESSION OF SPINAL DEGENERATION

- Stage I: Changes in the physiology and biochemistry of the three-joint complex may produce clinical symptoms
- Stage II: Increase in spinal segment motion, producing symptomatic instability
- Stage III: Osteophyte formation, which may lead to stiffness within the spinal segment[49]

matic instability.[49] Stage III describes the process of osteophyte formation, which may mechanically decrease the degree of instability present, leading to stiffness within the spinal segment.

The unstable spinal segment, with its altered ability to load share and to distribute stress, may attempt to stabilize itself through the formation of osteophytes along the vertebral body rim and the articular facets, which narrow the spinal canal.[9] This may decrease the clinical manifestation of spinal instability but may lead to the anatomic presence of spinal stenosis. Also, hypertrophy of the joint capsule and ligaments due to continuous stretch on these structures may further compromise the space available for the neural elements.[9]

All of these changes have the cumulative effect of reducing spinal canal dimensions. The intervertebral disc further contributes to this process by diffusely bulging into the spinal canal and neuroforamen, which is the mechanical consequence of the biochemical changes occurring in the aging disc. Also, the loss of disc height reduces the foraminal space for the exiting neural structures.[9] Changes generally occur gradually, allowing the patient to acclimate to the smaller volumetric canal area and remain asymptomatic for a long period of time. Occasionally, however, patients with congenitally narrow canals experience severe symptoms of stenosis with an acute disc protrusion due to their inability to tolerate even small decreases in canal dimensions.

Mechanisms of Age-Related Changes

Buckwalter identified several mechanisms that may contribute to age-related changes in the intervertebral disc, including a decline in cell nutrition, fewer viable cells, cell senescence, posttranslational modification of matrix proteins, accumulation of degraded matrix macromolecules, and fatigue failure of the matrix.[12]

Cells in the center of the intervertebral disc rely primarily on diffusion of nutrients through the extracellular matrix from blood vessels on the periphery of the anulus and within the vertebral bodies. Several factors contribute to a decrease in the efficacy of this process. During early growth and development, disc volume expands, causing an increase in the distance to the peripheral blood supply. Furthermore, with skeletal maturity, much of the remaining vasculature atrophies, increasing the reliance of disc nutrition on the diffusion process. Calcification of the cartilage end plates, however, can hinder nutrient delivery and waste removal.[21] Over time, there is an accumulation

of degraded matrix macromolecules, as well as decreased water content, which will further compromise cell nutrition.

In addition to declining nutrient delivery from compromised diffusion, cell metabolism becomes adversely affected by a drop in pH levels.[12] Lactate levels rise secondary to increased lactate production, low oxygen tension, and reduced lactate clearance, thus decreasing the pH. This eventually may lead to cell death. In the discs of infants, only 2% of cells in the nucleus show morphologic signs of necrosis, whereas in the young adult disc, there may be more than 50% cell necrosis, and even 80% among the elderly.[12]

Among the cell population that does not undergo necrosis, there may be a decline in cellular functions, which further contributes to age-related degeneration. Although this has not been proven, Buckwalter notes that many normally differentiated cell populations become senescent as a result of changes in gene expression.[12] In addition, several investigators have described posttranslational protein modifications of matrix macromolecules, which cause connective tissue matrices to lose their elasticity and strength.[14,61] An example of this would be an increase in collagen cross-linking with age, which occurs through nonenzymic glycation. Increased cross-links alter the mechanical properties of the disc. Moreover, glycation products are thought to stimulate cells to release cytokines and proteases, which further add to tissue breakdown.[61] Over time, as matrix tissue breaks down and is turned over, there is an inevitable accumulation of breakdown products, which may alter tissue properties, such as diffusion of nutrients as well as mechanical performance.[13] Furthermore, accretion of degraded matrix molecules can hinder the assembly of new macromolecules.[81]

During the course of normal spinal motion, the intervertebral disc, as part of its function to dissipate load, undergoes repetitive deformations in disc volume and shape. With age, these repetitive deformations may eventually lead to fatigue failure of the disc matrix, seen as fissures, cracks, or myxoid degeneration, or on the microscopic level as fragmentation of macromolecules or disruption of collagen.[12]

MECHANISMS OF AGE-RELATED CHANGES

- Decline in cell nutrition
- Decrease in number of viable cells
- Cell senescence
- Posttranslational modification of matrix proteins
- Accumulation of degraded matrix macromolecules
- Fatigue failure of the matrix[13]

SUMMARY OF AGE-RELATED CHANGES

- A decline in cell nutrition brings about a series of events, including
  - Decreased concentration of viable cells
  - Cell senescence
  - Accumulation of degraded matrix molecules
- Continued aging results in
  - Posttranslational modifications of collagen
  - Decreased water content, and
  - Compromised cellular function
- These changes make the disc tissue more vulnerable to progressive fatigue failure and less able to function under the demands of repetitive deformation.[12]

A final mechanism for age-related changes to the intervertebral disc involves an autoimmune etiology, as suggested by several investigators. With anular tears, the disc material that was previously avascular becomes exposed to the bloodstream and consequently the immune system. This may in turn result in a cellular immune response, which can theoretically contribute to biochemical changes and/or biomechanical failure, resulting in further tissue degeneration.[52,66] This mechanism, however, has yet to be proved.

Clinical Manifestations of the Aging Disc

The age-related changes outlined here occur gradually over time and do not necessarily lead to symptoms in the majority of patients. In fact, disc abnormalities are commonly seen in asymptomatic subjects (Figure 6-4). In an imaging study by Boden et al., degeneration at one or more lumbar levels was observed in 35% of subjects between the ages of 20 and 39, and in nearly all patients older than 60.[7] Similarly, Powell et al. found magnetic resonance imaging (MRI) signal intensity abnormalities in 30% of asymptomatic pregnant women younger than 30 years of age and in 50% between the ages of 40 and 50.[77] Some authors have suggested that a "dark disc" on MRI represents the earliest stage in the process of degenerative disc disease, whereas others propose that it is an expression of the normal aging process.[25,65,90]

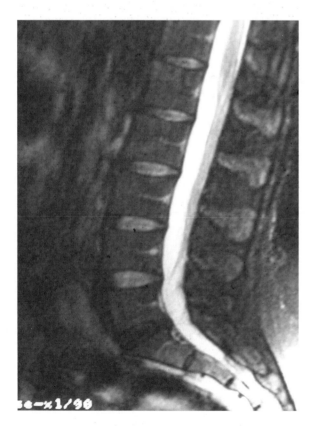

Figure 6-4. Sagittal magnetic resonance image (T2) showing advanced disc degeneration at the L5 to S1 level.

A great deal of research has been done to characterize the continuum of the aging process as it relates to the relationship of a normal aging disc and a symptomatic degenerated disc. Many studies have examined possible etiologic causes for symptomatic degenerative disc disease expression, including physical loading conditions experienced during postural loading and work and leisure activities, as well as the effects of vibration and degree of aerobic conditioning.[29,42,89] Several physical and psychosocial risk factors have been postulated as contributing factors for low back pain; these include repetitive lifting or pulling, exposure to prolonged industrial or vehicular vibrations, and several anatomic factors such as obesity, sagittal malalignment, and pregnancy.[28,29,48,70] A beneficial effect of exercise has been noted secondary to its contribution to improved disc nutrition.[96,99] On the other hand, cigarette smoking has been shown to have a deleterious effect on disc health.[99] One study showed that 57% of patients with disc disease were smokers versus 37% of a control population.[85] Interestingly, a retrospective cohort study on identical twins found that genetic factors had the greatest correlation with disc degeneration.[6]

The greatest challenge faced by clinicians is the need to distinguish the cause of symptomatic spinal disease with imaging and diagnostic modalities that may be expressing findings consistent with the normal aging process. Other nonorganic influences must also be considered such as the patient's psychosocial history in regard to job dissatisfaction, stress, drug addiction, and Worker's Compensation status.[26] Furthermore, one must consider an individual's perception and response to painful stimuli.[9]

Disc Herniation

As the intervertebral disc ages, the anulus fibrosis begins to fibrillate and radial fissures develop, which may extend toward its periphery. The nucleus pulposus, no longer able to be contained by the anulus, may herniate into these radial clefts, most commonly in a posterolateral direction, as a result of torsional stresses.[27] Regardless of whether a disc herniation occurs, degenerative changes such as decreasing water content and increasing collagen will continue to progress normally. In the elderly population, the degenerated disc may become desiccated and fibrotic, making herniation an

> **PHYSICAL AND PSYCHOSOCIAL RISK FACTORS FOR LOW BACK PAIN**
>
> - Repetitive lifting or pulling
> - Exposure to prolonged industrial or vehicular vibrations
> - Obesity
> - Sagittal malalignment
> - Pregnancy
> - Cigarette smoking
> - Lack of exercise

unlikely event, perhaps explaining why most herniations occur between the ages of 30 and 50, while the nucleus still has good turgor.[9]

Herniation of the nucleus can occur anteriorly, posteriorly, or laterally to the disc space. The posterior anulus tends to be weakest adjacent to midline, where it lacks reinforcement from the strong fibers of the posterior longitudinal ligament (PLL), helping to explain the frequency of posterolateral disc herniations.[9] When the nuclear material has violated the anulus but not the PLL, the herniation is considered to be contained. However, if the PLL fibers are also torn, the disc fragment is then said to be extruded. A free or sequestered fragment of nucleus may then enter the spinal canal (Figure 6-5).

The site of a disc protrusion as well as its direction will determine a patient's clinical manifestation, if any, of pain, weakness, or sensory and reflex changes (Figure 6-6). Lumbar disc herniations generally cause radicular complaints. A cauda equina syndrome may occur in the lumbar region with large midline disc herniations that significantly compress several spinal nerve roots.[8]

No nerves are present within the substance of a normal mature intervertebral disc.[98] However, the posterior anulus and the PLL are the most highly innervated structures in the functional spinal unit. Branches of the sinuvertebral nerve ramify through the tissues in and around the PLL (Figure 6-7). This highly innervated region is also the most common site of disc herniation, undoubtedly helping to explain the production of low

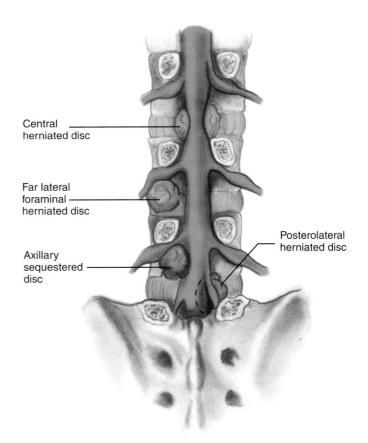

Figure 6-6. Different locations of possible disc herniations.

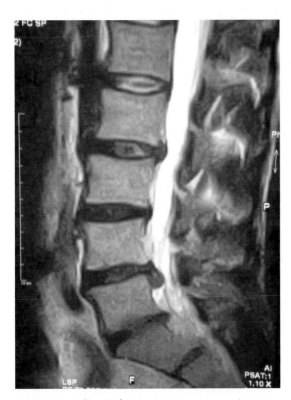

Figure 6-5. Sagittal magnetic resonance image (T2) showing a free extruded disc fragment at the L4 to L5 level.

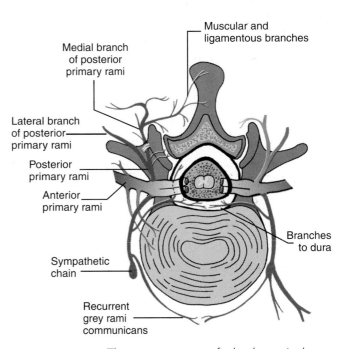

Figure 6-7. The neuroanatomy of a lumbar spinal unit.

LOCATIONS OF DISC HERNIATION

- Posterolateral disc herniation: Produces symptoms in the distribution of the nerve root below
- Far lateral disc herniation: Produces symptoms corresponding to the exiting nerve root
- Axillary disc herniation: Produces symptoms corresponding to the exiting nerve root
- Central disc herniation: Affects crossing nerve roots or produces a cauda equina syndrome if large disc

CLINICAL PRESENTATIONS OF PATIENTS WITH SPINAL STENOSIS

- Low back pain
- Claudication pain
- Radiculopathy
- Cauda equina syndrome

back pain associated with disc herniations. Furthermore, large herniations, in addition to producing tension on the nerve roots, can compress the nerve against bone and/or ligamentum.[9] In response to even small amounts of tension, as well as an autoimmune response to exposed nuclear material, inflammatory changes may occur in the environment of the nerve root, which becomes irritated, edematous, and cordlike.[9] Although nerve roots are not normally sensitive to mechanical stimulation, nerve roots that are chronically inflamed will produce radicular symptoms in response to physical manipulation.[98] This has been shown experimentally by placing sutures or an inflatable balloon in proximity to a nerve root in patients who had undergone surgery for disc herniation and then mechanically stimulating the disc postoperatively.[55,87] Chronic and long-standing inflammation of the nerve root can lead to eventual fibrosis with perhaps a limited potential for return to normal nerve function.[98]

Segmental Instability

Spinal instability, defined as abnormal motion between two or more vertebrae beyond physiologic constraints, is commonly caused by chronic disc degeneration, with concomitant arthritic changes to the facet joints and attenuation of supporting spinal ligamentous structures. Abnormal spinal motion over time results in deformation of the facet joints and continued failure of the structural properties of the intervertebral disc. A definitive characterization of degenerative instability is lacking. However, radiographic evidence of instability may include vertebral retrolisthesis, spondylolisthesis, disc space narrowing, malalignment of the spinous processes, and rotational deformity of the pedicles.[69] On flexion-extension radiographs, various authors have cited lumbar vertebral translation of 3 to 4 mm or more, or angular displacement of 10 degrees to 15 degrees, as objective evidence of excessive vertebral motion.[69] As with stenosis, instability may result in chronic and repetitive nerve root compression and irritation. Although instability can occur at a single level, degeneration is commonly diffuse and may involve multiple levels.[9]

Segmental instability may occur iatrogenically, after a decompressive laminectomy procedure. Studies have shown that the removal of 50% or more of the facet joints bilaterally at a single lumbar level may result in instability.[69] Also, instability may occur adjacent to a prior long-standing fusion. Typically, this "transition syn-

drome" occurs at the segment above the fusion, with a retrolisthesis of the junctional level.[69] Risk factors for breakdown at adjacent levels include imbalance in the sagittal plane, particularly with loss of lordosis of the fused segment, with compensatory hyperextension of the spine above.[69] Abnormal stresses are transferred to the junctional level, which can lead to facet and disc degeneration and ligament hypertrophy.

Spinal Stenosis

Spinal stenosis is thought to arise as a result of degenerative changes occurring simultaneously between the disc, facet joints, and ligaments, leading to narrowing of spinal canal dimensions. Initially, the most common complaint in patients with early symptomatic lumbar stenosis is chronic back discomfort. Eventually, claudication-type symptoms may develop with progression of the disease process. Pain and discomfort typically are experienced in the upper thighs and buttocks and are related to ambulation. A patient's complaint of pain and lower extremity weakness is often alleviated with forward lumbar flexion and aggravated by standing, walking, or spine extension. With flexion, the spinal canal dimensions increase, whereas with extension it decreases, thus exacerbating the symptoms. Claudication pain arises secondary to mechanical irritation of the spinal nerves, which are entrapped by hypertrophied spinal elements and have poor excursion due to the stenosis. Furthermore, nerve root ischemia is often present due to vessel stenosis within the vasonervosum of the cauda equina.[9]

Patients with symptomatic spinal stenosis may also present with radiculopathy, similar to that seen with a disc herniation. In extreme cases of spinal stenosis, patients may present with symptoms of cauda equina syndrome that involve bladder dysfunction and/or perineal and rectal pain.[69] Overlap of these symptom patterns is not uncommon. On examination, the clinical picture of a patient with spinal stenosis is typically benign, with the absence of any significant neurologic deficits. The clinician must use care to distinguish the symptoms of neurogenic claudication from those of vascular claudication, which often coexist in this patient population.

Discogenic Back Pain

A particular diagnostic and treatment challenge for the spinal care physician is in the evaluation of a patient with severe chronic low back pain who has no signs of nerve impingement, either radiographically or on physical examination. Leg pain may or may not accompany

"INTERNAL DISC DISRUPTION"

- Term introduced by Henry Crock
- Describes a pain syndrome that results when the internal structure and metabolic function of the intervertebral disc become altered, while the external appearance of the disc remains normal[99]

the back pain, but it is typically less severe when present. The pathogenesis of this pain syndrome is thought in the majority of cases to involve pathologic degeneration of the intervertebral disc. Henry Crock introduced the term "internal disc disruption" (IDD) in 1970 to describe a situation in which the internal structure and metabolic function of the disc become altered.[18] The disc is rendered painful by these internal changes, whereas its external appearance remains essentially normal.[84]

Radiographs may often show minimal changes that are typical of the degenerated disc, such as disc space narrowing, end plate sclerosis, and osteophyte formation. The pathologic feature of IDD involves radial tears through the anulus fibrosus. It is thought that the affected disc then releases certain proteins (i.e., neuropeptides) that are noxious to the surrounding neural elements.[99] The pathophysiology of discogenic pain is complex and not completely understood. However, it has been suggested that mechanical loading of a disrupted anulus may sensitize the surrounding nociceptors, which are then further irritated by released chemical mediators.[4,44,82] The ability of material from the nucleus pulposus to stimulate an inflammatory response was substantiated by McCarron et al., using a canine model, whereby they injected homogenized autogenous nucleus pulposus into the canine lumbar epidural space.[58] A classic acute inflammatory response was observed on gross, as well as microscopic inspection.[58]

Patients with IDD typically complain of a deep-seated lower back pain, which is aggravated by activity.[99] The pain may refer into the lower extremity; however, it does not follow a dermatomal distribution, nor are there typical features of radiculopathy.[47,99] There often is a remote history of a traumatic event. Physical examination tends to be nonspecific, with normal neurologic findings and negative root tension signs. Furthermore, a study that attempted to identify clinical features that were reliably present in patients with IDD was unsuccessful.[84] No conventional clinical test or combination of tests was found to reliably identify patients with IDD.[84]

MRI plays a limited role in establishing the diagnosis of IDD. Although MRI reliably shows the changes that occur in the degenerated intervertebral disc, it does not necessarily help to establish which disc is symptomatic. Anular tears can be observed using spin-echo or T2 weighted images enhanced with gadolinium.[80] Furthermore, patients with chronic low back pain are frequently noted to have a "high-intensity zone" on T2 weighted lumbar magnetic resonance images,[2] which initially was thought to correlate with IDD. Never-

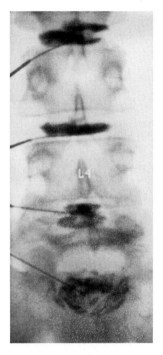

Figure 6-8. A lumbar discogram showing injection of dye at multiple levels.

theless, attempts to establish this high-intensity zone (or HIZ lesion) as a pathoanatomic sign for IDD have been controversial. Although some authors have reported the HIZ sign to be diagnostic of the painful intervertebral disc, others have found the interobserver reliability and the positive predictive value to be unacceptably low.[2,78,83,86]

Discography plays an important role in establishing the diagnosis of discogenic back pain (Figure 6-8). Evidence of disc degeneration may or may not be present on discography, and as such, it is not a test of disc degeneration. Rather, its use lies in determining whether the intervertebral disc has become symptomatic, regardless of its morphology.[97] The key portion of a discogram is the patient's subjective pain response. A positive study should reproduce the patient's chronic pain pattern, and multiple discs should be injected to provide for intrapatient controls. Postdiscography computed tomography scanning can be used to diagnose radial tears within the anulus. However, it is currently unclear whether the routine use of postdiscography computed tomography is necessary to establish the diagnosis of IDD.[99]

FACET JOINTS

The apophyseal facet joints of the spine are typical diarthrodial joints, which are subjected to the same degenerative processes seen in other joints of the body. The concept that facet joints could be a source of pain was introduced in the 1940s by Badgley, who demonstrated the neural innervations to the facet joint complex, through cadaveric dissection.[5] The current understanding of facet joint arthropathy and its contribution to the generation of pain in the aging spine continue to evolve.

Anatomy and Cartilage Nutrition

The facet joints of the vertebrae arise from the junction of the pedicles and the laminae. There is both a superior articular process that articulates with the vertebrae above and an inferior articular process that articulates with the vertebrae below. The facet joints of the spine share the same anatomic characteristics as any diarthrodial joint found elsewhere in the body.[27] They contain synovial fluid and are lined with hyaline articular cartilage overlying subchondral bone. Each joint is enclosed in a fibrous capsule. The joint capsules and soft tissue structures along the anterolateral surfaces of the anulus have encapsulated nerve endings, which are capable of producing pain.[98]

The function of the facet joints is to restrain excessive mobility of the motion segment, as well as to help distribute axial loads over a broader area.[62] Their articulations help to prevent anterior movement of the superior vertebrae on the inferior vertebrae. The joints also allow limited flexion and extension as well as varying degrees of lateral flexion and rotation. The normal configuration of the intervertebral disc, facet joints, ligaments, and the joint capsule has been compared with a tripod.[31] On account of this configuration, the spinal motion segment can accommodate the various motions mentioned above without any significant alteration in the intervertebral disc space that is available.

Hyaline articular cartilage is composed of water, proteoglycans, collagen, and chondrocytes. Approximately 75% of cartilage is made up of water, which plays a major role in joint lubrication and joint nutrition.[27] The interaction of water with proteoglycans is responsible for the mechanical properties of cartilage compressibility and allows for nutrient diffusion as well. Proteoglycans make up approximately 50% of the dry weight of cartilage.[27] With normal aging, the concentration of chondroitin sulfate decreases, with a concomitant increase in keratin sulfate.[56] In the osteoarthritic facet, the concentration of keratin sulfate is decreased, and there is an increase in the ratio of chondroitin 4–sulfate to chondroitin 6–sulfate. In addition, there is an overall decrease in proteoglycan aggregates, and the glycosaminoglycan chains become shorter.[27]

Articular cartilage is avascular and, as a result, must rely on diffusion from the surrounding environment for nutrition. The primary source of nutrients comes from the synovial fluid, with little, if any, contribution from subchondral bone.[27] Loading of the cartilage through normal activity provides a mechanism by which fluid is pumped in and out of the tissue, allowing for nutrient delivery through diffusion.[27] Conversely, excessive loads, as well as joint immobilization, can have a harmful effect on articular cartilage. Abnormal loading is thought to promote subchondral microfractures, which can lead to stiffening of the overlying cartilage, subjecting it to additional stresses.[27] Immobilization, on the other hand, causes degeneration through a decrease in nutrient delivery brought about by decreased pumping of synovial fluid in and out of the cartilage.[91]

Pathologic Changes With Degeneration

Osteoarthritis is characterized by the gradual deterioration of articular cartilage. There is no known etiology of osteoarthritis, but chronic or repeated strain or injury to a joint contributes to the development and progression of the process. An abnormal position of the facet joints as a result of trauma can lead to early degeneration of the articular cartilage.

There are two major pathologic responses that occur during osteoarthritis. The first is the deterioration of the cartilage with progressive loss of the hyaline cartilage down to the subchondral bone.[27] Some unknown initial insult, which might involve biomechanical, biochemical, inflammatory, or immunologic events, causes the release of enzymes that are capable of degrading cartilage proteoglycans and collagen.[27,57,74-76] The breakdown of these macromolecules results in structural abnormalities within the articular cartilage. Subsequently, focal erosions occur, leading to the formation of fissures within the deteriorating cartilage.[27] The second pathologic response that occurs is the proliferative response that cartilage undergoes, in an attempt to repair itself. The changes seen when this occurs are the development of osteochondrophytic spurs, subchondral bone cyst formation, and sclerosis of subchondral bone.[27] It is the failure of the proliferative process to keep up with the degenerative process that leads to the clinical expression of osteoarthritis.[27]

Cartilage tissue is not innervated and thus is insensitive to pain. The development of pain from an osteoarthritic facet joint must therefore result from nociceptors within the joint capsule, the synovial membrane, or the periosteum of the joint facets.[51] Neurophysiologic studies have shown that mechanical stimuli can activate these nociceptors.[36] Possible mechanisms for mechanical stimulation include pressure on denuded subchondral bone, intramedullary hypertension, subchondral microfractures, capsular distention, and periosteal elevation secondary to osteophyte formation.[27]

With disc degeneration, loss of disc space height leads to foraminal narrowing with subsequent altered facet joint contact forces, with or without subluxation. This abnormal joint space loading contributes to the etiology of facet joint arthritis with resultant hypertrophic changes, osteophyte formation, and thickening of the ligamentum flavum.[38] This is manifested macroscopically as facet joint capsule thickening with sub-

---

PATHOLOGIC CHANGES IN CARTILAGE WITH OSTEOARTHRITIS

- First: Cartilage matrix degradation, which results in focal erosions and fissures down to the subchondral bone
- Second: Proliferative response of the cartilage, which results in osteochondrophytic spurs, bone cyst formation, and sclerosis of subchondral bone[27]

sequent encroachment on the neural elements. Spinal stenosis due to facet joint hypertrophy, often in association with intervertebral disc bulging and ligamentum flavum inbuckling may occur centrally within the spinal column, along the nerve root as it courses anteromedial to the facet joint, or within the intervertebral foramen.[31] In addition to mechanical irritation of the nerve roots, there may also be chemically induced noxious stimuli, which is caused by inflammatory reactions within the synovium and/or joint capsule.[62]

Facet Syndrome

Facet joint syndrome remains a poorly defined clinical entity. Symptoms are thought to include localized neck or back pain, with possible radiation into the extremities, low back stiffness, paralumbar tenderness, and the absence of neurologic deficits.[27,53,64] Early in the process, radiographs may reveal minimal changes or appear normal altogether.[20] The diagnosis must be made clinically and is confirmed by the injection of a local anesthetic into the joint under fluoroscopic guidance.[22,62] A pathoanatomic study of patients suspected of having facet syndrome identified histologic changes in the articular cartilage of the facet joints characteristic of chondromalacia.[20] Nevertheless, other studies have been unable to identify a consistent clinical picture for patients with this disorder, leading some investigators to question the value of this diagnosis.[45,62] The extent to which primary facet joint arthropathy causes symptoms may be related more to its contribution to spinal stenosis, both centrally and in the neuroforamen.[27]

LIGAMENTS AND BONE

The ligaments of the spine, like the facet joints, function to limit extremes of motion between adjacent vertebrae. They typically are subjected to tensile loads and contain high concentrations of elastin.[59] With age, the tensile properties of ligaments become diminished,[19] and it is known from studies on nonspinal ligaments that there is an increase in the relative concentration of collagen compared with elastin.[27]

The changes that ligaments undergo with aging are thought to be similar to the macroscopic changes that occur with prolonged joint immobilization.[27] These include disorganization of ligament fibrillar organization, increases in collagen degradation, reduced collagen cross-links, and decreases in the concentration of proteoglycans, with a concomitant loss of water.[59] These changes result in weakening of the ligaments as measured by energy absorption to failure.[59]

The manner in which ligaments may contribute to symptomatic degeneration remains poorly defined. Fraying, partial rupture, necrosis, cyst formation, and crystal deposition (calcium pyrophosphate) have all been observed to occur in the aging interspinal ligaments.[15] Symptoms may occur from these processes, as a result of painful bursae, known as Baastrup's disease.[15] Furthermore, thickening and/or buckling of

the ligaments, particularly the ligamentum flavum, is thought to play a significant role in spinal stenosis by decreasing the space available for the neural elements.[8] Ossification of the spinal ligaments may also occur, causing symptoms of compression. This entity is prevalent in particular ethnic groups (i.e., Asians), and it is thought to involve a genetic predisposition.[94]

As with the intervertebral discs, facet joints, and ligaments, aging and degeneration cause characteristic changes to occur in bone. There is a significant decrease in vascularity of the vertebral end plate, by skeletal maturity, which has important implications for nutrient delivery to the intervertebral disc.[27] With continued aging, sclerosis of the end plates is observed, leading to an increase in end plate stiffness.[27] This effectively reduces the contribution of the end plate to force dissipation, allowing greater stress to be transferred to the intervertebral disc.[27]

Several mechanisms are thought to exist whereby aging bone may be a possible source of symptomatic degeneration. First, subacute microfractures of the end plates has been implicated as a source of low back pain.[37] Schmorl's nodes are an example of end plate failure; however, they are found with equal frequency among those with and without low back pain.[30] Second, bone may play a role in the development of degenerative spondylolisthesis, secondary to fatigue fractures of the lamina.[23] This may be a contributing factor to spinal stenosis. Finally, an increase in vertebral body interosseous pressure has been observed with spinal degeneration.[3] It has been suggested that one mechanism for osteoarthritic pain is that the increased pressure activates perivascular nociceptors, causing the sensation of pain.

CONCLUSIONS

The aging spine and symptomatic spinal degeneration may be two points on a continuum, which are distinguished only by the extent of their pathology. The contributions that the different spinal components make to symptomatic disease are beginning to be understood through studies that examine the relationship between the age-related biochemical changes and the mechanical properties of the spine. Nevertheless, a complete understanding of when physiologic aging becomes a pathologic process awaits a more thorough identification of the various pain generators within the spine.

SELECTED REFERENCES

Battie MC et al.: 1995 Volvo Award in Clinical Sciences: determinants of lumbar disc degeneration—a study relating lifelong exposures and magnetic resonance imaging findings in identical twins, *Spine* 20(24):2601-2612, 1995.

Boden SD et al.: Abnormal magnetic resonance scans of the lumbar spine in asymptomatic subject, *J Bone Joint Surg Am* 72:403-408, 1990.

Boden SD et al.: The pathophysiology of the aging spine. In *The aging spine*, Philadelphia, 1991, WB Saunders, pp. 21-38.

Buckwalter JA: Spine update: aging and degeneration of the human intervertebral disc, *Spine* 20:1307-1314, 1995.

Crock HV: Internal disc disruption: a challenge to disc prolapse fifty years on, *Spine* 11:650-653, 1986.

Frymoyer JW, Moskowitz RW: Spinal degeneration: pathogenesis and medical management. In Frymoyer JW, ed: *The adult spine: principles and practice,* New York, 1991, Raven, pp. 611-634.

Holm S: Pathophysiology of disc degeneration, *Acta Orthop Scand Suppl* 251:13-15, 1993.

Jackson RP, Jacobs RR, Montesano PX: 1988 Volvo Award in Clinical Sciences: racet joint injection in low-back pain—a prospective statistical study, *Spine* 13:966-971, 1988.

Kirkaldy-Willis WH: *Managing low back pain,* New York, 1983, Churchill Livingstone.

Mooney V: Facet joint syndrome. In Jayson MIV, ed: *The lumbar spine and back pain,* Edinburgh, 1992, Churchill Livingstone, pp. 291-306.

Mooney V: Where is pain coming from? *Spine* 12:754-759, 1987.

Naylor A: The biomechanical changes in the human intervertebral disc in degeneration and nuclear prolapse, *Orthop Clin North Am* 2:343-358, 1971.

Pearce RH: Morphologic and chemical aspects of intervertebral disc aging. In Buckwalter JA, Goldberg VM, Woo SL-Y, eds: *Musculoskeletal soft tissue aging: impact on mobility,* Rosemont, Ill, 1993, American Academy of Orthopaedic Surgeons, pp. 363-379.

Silveri CP, Simeone FA: Lumbar disc disease. In An HS, ed: *Principles and techniques of spine surgery,* Baltimore, 1998, Williams and Wilkins, pp. 425-441.

Tertti M et al.: Disc degeneration in magnetic resonance imaging: a comparative biochemical histologic and radiographic study in cadaver spines, *Spine* 16:629-634, 1991.

Videman T et al.: The long-term effects of physical loading and exercise lifestyles on back-related symptoms, disability, and spine pathology among men, *Spine* 20:699-709, 1995.

Zdeblick TA et al.: Discogenic back pain. In Rothman RH, Simeone FA, eds *The spine,* Philadelphia, 1999, WB Saunders, pp. 749-765.

REFERENCES

1. Akeson WH et al.: Biomechanics and biochemistry of the intervertebral discs: the need for correlation studies, *Clin Orthop Rel Res* 129:133-140, 1977.

2. Aprill C, Bogduk N: High-intensity zone: a diagnostic sign of painful lumbar disc on magnetic resonance imaging, *Br J Radiol* 65:361-369, 1992.

3. Arnoldi CC: Intravertebral pressures in patients with lumbar pain: preliminary communication, *Acta Orthop Scand* 43:109-117, 1972.

4. Ashton IK et al.: Substance P in intervertebral discs: binding sites on vascular endothelium of the human annulus fibrosus, *Acta Orthop Scand* 65:635-639, 1994.

5. Badgley CE: I. The importance of the lumbosacral joint in low back pain with sciatic radiation. II. A new theory to explain radiation of pain. Presented at the annual meeting of the American Academy of Orthopaedic Surgeons, St. Louis. 1936.

6. Battie MC et al.: 1995 Volvo Award in Clinical Sciences: determinants of lumbar disc degeneration—a study relating lifelong exposures and magnetic resonance imaging findings in identical twins, *Spine* 20(24):2601-2612, 1995.

7. Boden SD et al.: Abnormal magnetic resonance scans of the lumbar spine in asymptomatic subject, *J Bone Joint Surg Am* 72:403-408, 1990.

8. Boden SD et al.: Clinical syndromes and physical examination of the lumbar spine. In *The aging spine,* Philadelphia, 1991, WB Saunders, pp. 101-125.

9. Boden SD et al.: The pathophysiology of the aging spine. In *The aging spine,* Philadelphia, 1991, WB Saunders, pp. 21-38.

10. Borenstein DG, Wiesel SW, Boden SD: *Low back pain: medical diagnosis and comprehensive management,* Philadelphia, 1995, WB Saunders.

11. Bradford DS et al.: Chymopapain, chemonucleolysis, and nucleus pulposus regeneration: a biochemical and biomechanical study, *Spine* 9:135-147, 1984.

12. Buckwalter JA: Spine update: aging and degeneration of the human intervertebral disc, *Spine* 20:1307-1314, 1995.

13. Buckwalter JA, Roughley PJ, Rosenberg LC: Age-related changes in cartilage proteoglycans: quantitative electron microscopic studies, *Microsc Res Techn* 28:398-408, 1994.

14. Buckwalter JA et al.: Soft-tissue aging and musculoskeletal function, *J Bone Joint Surg Am* 75:1533-1548, 1993.

15. Bywaters EGL: The pathological anatomy of idiopathic low back pain. In White AA III, Gordon SL: *American Academy of Orthopaedic Surgeons symposium on idiopathic low back pain,* St. Louis, 1982, Mosby, pp. 144-177.

16. Cassar-Pullicino VN: MRI of the aging and herniating intervertebral disc, *Eur J Radiol* 27(3):214-228, 1998.

17. Cauchoix J, Yaacubi E, Romero CG: An experimental model of lumbar degenerated discs in rabbits. Presented at the tenth meeting of the International Society for Study of the Lumbar Spine, Montreal, Canada. 1984.

18. Crock HV: Internal disc disruption: a challenge to disc prolapse fifty years on, *Spine* 11:650-653, 1986.

19. Dumas GA, Beaudoin L, Drouin G: *In site* mechanical behavior of posterior spinal ligaments in the lumbar region: an *in vitro* study, *J Biomech* 20:301-310, 1987.

20. Eisenstein SM, Parry CR: The lumbar facet arthrosis syndrome: clinical presentation and articular surface changes, *J Bone Joint Surg Br* 69:3-7, 1987.

21. Eyre D et al.: The intervertebral disk: basic science perspectives. In Frymoyer JW, Gordon SL, eds: *New perspectives on low back pain,* Park Ridge, Ill, 1989, Academy of Orthopaedic Surgeons, pp.147-207.

22. Fairbank JC et al.: Apophyseal injection of local anesthetic as a diagnostic aid in primary low back pain syndromes, *Spine* 6: 598-605, 1981.

23. Farfan HF: The pathological anatomy of degenerative spondylolisthesis: a cadaver study. *Spine,* 5:412-418, 1980.

24. Farfan HF, Huberdeau RM, Dubow HI: Lumbar intervertebral disc degeneration: the influence of geometrical features on the pattern of disc degeneration—a post mortem study, *J Bone Joint Surg Am* 54:492-510, 1972.

25. Fischgrund JS, Montgomery DM: Diagnosis and treatment of discogenic low back pain, *Orthop Rev* 22:311-318, 1993.

26. Frymoyer JW, Cats-Baril WL: An overview of the incidence and costs of low back pain, *Orthop Clin North Am* 22(2):263-271, 1991.

27. Frymoyer JW, Moskowitz RW: Spinal degeneration: pathogenesis and medical management. In Frymoyer JW, ed: *The adult spine: principles and practice,* New York, 1991, Raven, pp. 611-634.

28. Frymoyer JW et al.: Epidemiologic studies of low back pain, *Spine* 5:419-423, 1980.

29. Frymoyer JW et al.: Risk factors in low back pain: an epidemiological survey, *J Bone Joint Surg Am* 65:213-218, 1983.

30. Frymoyer JW et al.: Spine radiographs in patients with low-back pain: an epidemiologic study in men, *J Bone Joint Surg Am* 66:1048-1055, 1984.

31. Garfin SR et al.: Spinal stenosis. In Rothman RH, Simeone FA, eds: *The spine,* Philadelphia, 1992, WB Saunders, pp. 791-875.

32. Goel VK, Weinstein JN: Role of mechanics in lumbar spine disease. In Goel VK, Weinstein JN, eds: *Biomechanics of the spine: clinical and surgical perspective,* Boca Raton, 1990, CRC Press, pp. 1-5.

33. Gotfried Y, Bradford DS, Oegema TR Jr: Facet joint changes after chemonucleolysis-induced disc space narrowing, *Spine* 11:944-950, 1986.

34. Gower WE, Pedrini V: Age-related variations in protein polysaccharides from human nucleus pulposus, annulus fibrosus, and costal cartilage, *J Bone Joint Surg Am* 51:1154-1162, 1969.

35. Greenwald RA, Moy WW, Seibold J: Functional properties of cartilage proteoglycans, *Semin Arthritis Rheum* 8:53-67, 1978.

36. Grigg P, Schaible HG, Schmidt RF: Mechanical sensitivity of group III and IV afferents from posterior articular nerve in normal and inflamed cat knee, *J Neurophysiol* 55:635-643, 1986.

37. Hansson T, Roos B: Microcalluses of the trabeculae in lumbar vertebrae and their relation to the bone mineral content, *Spine* 6:375-380, 1981.

38. Herkowitz HN et al.: Surgical management of cervical disc disease. In Rothman RH, Simeone FA, eds: *The spine,* Philadelphia, 1992, WB Saunders, pp. 597-654.

39. Hickey DS, Hukins DWL: Relation between the structure of the annulus fibrosus and the function and failure of the intervertebral disc, *Spine* 5:106-116, 1980.

40. Hickey DS, Hukins DWL: Aging changes in the macromolecular organization of the intervertebral disc: an X-ray diffraction and electron microscopic study, *Spine* 7:234-242, 1982.

41. Holm S: Pathophysiology of disc degeneration, *Acta Orthop Scand Suppl* 251:13-15, 1993.

42. Hulshof C, Veldjuijzen van Zanten B: Whole body vibration and low back pain: a review of epidemiologic studies, *Int Arch Occup Environ Health*, 59:205-220, 1987.

43. Inoue H, Takeda T: Three dimensional observation of collagen framework of lumbar intervertebral discs, *Acta Orthop Scand* 46:949, 1975.

44. Ito S, Yamada Y, Tsuboi S: An observation of ruptured annulus fibrosus in lumbar discs, *J Spinal Disord* 4:462-466, 1990.

45. Jackson RP, Jacobs RR, Montesano PX: 1988 Volvo Award in Clinical Sciences: facet joint injection in low-back pain—a prospective statistical study, *Spine* 13:966-971, 1988.

46. Kang JD et al.: Herniated lumbar intervertebral discs spontaneously produce matrix metalloproteinases, nitric oxide, interleukin-6, and prostaglandin E2, *Spine* 21:271-277, 1996.

47. Karasek M, Bogduk N: Twelve month follow-up of a controlled trial of intradiscal thermal anuloplasty for back pain due to internal disc disruption, *Spine* 25(20):2601-2607, 2000.

48. Kelsey JL, Hardy RJ: Driving motor vehicles as a risk factor for acute herniated lumbar intervertebral disc, *Am J Epidemiol* 102:63-73, 1975.

49. Kirkaldy-Willis WH: *Managing low back pain*, New York, 1983, Churchill Livingstone.

50. Koeller W et al.: Biomechanical properties of human intervertebral discs subjected to axial dynamic compression: influence of age and degeneration, *J Biomech* 19:807-816, 1986.

51. Kramer J: *Intervertebral disc disease: causes, diagnosis, treatment, and prophylaxis*, New York, 1990, Thieme, p. 60.

52. LaRocca H: New horizons in research on disc disease, *Orthop Clin North Am* 2:521-531, 1971.

53. Lippitt AB: The facet joint and its role in spinal pain: management with facet joint injections, *Spine* 9:746-750, 1984.

54. Lipson SJ, Muir H: Experimental intervertebral disc degeneration: morphologic and proteoglycan changes over time, *Arthritis Rheum* 24:12-21, 1981.

55. Macnab I: The mechanism of spondylogenic pain. In Hirsch C, Zotterman Y, eds: *Cervical spine*, Oxford, 1972, Pergamon, pp. 88-95.

56. Mankin HJ, Lippiello L: Biochemical and metabolic abnormalities in articular cartilage from osteoarthritic human hips, *J Bone Joint Surg Am* 52:424-434, 1970.

57. Martel-Pelletier J et al.: Neutral proteases capable of proteoglycan digesting activity in osteoarthritic and normal human articular cartilage, *Arthritis Rheum* 27:305-312, 1984.

58. McCarron RF et al.: The inflammatory effect of nucleus pulposus: a possible element in the pathogenesis of low back pain, *Spine* 12:760-764, 1987.

59. Miller EJ, Gay S: The collagens: an overview and update, *Meth Enzymol* 144:3-41, 1987.

60. Mitchell PEG, Hendry NGC, Billewicz WZ: The chemical background of intervertebral disc prolapse, *J Bone Joint Surg Br* 43:141-151, 1961.

61. Monnier VM et al.: Post-translational protein modification by the Maillard reaction: relevance to aging of the extracellular matrix molecules. In Buckwalter JA, Goldberg VM, Woo SL, eds: *Musculoskeletal soft tissue aging: impact of mobility*, Rosemont, Ill, 1993, American Academy of Orthopaedic Surgeons, pp. 49-50.

62. Mooney V: Facet joint syndrome. In Jayson MIV, ed: *The lumbar spine and back pain*, Edinburgh, 1992, Churchill Livingstone, pp. 291-306.

63. Mooney V: Where is pain coming from? *Spine*, 12:754-759, 1987.

64. Mooney V, Robertson J: The facet syndrome, *Clin Orthop* 115:149-156, 1976.

65. Nachemson A:Lumbar discography: were are we today? *Spine* 14:555-557, 1989

66. Naylor A:The biomechanical changes in the human intervertebral disc in degeneration and nuclear prolapse, *Orthop Clin North Am* 2:343-358, 1971.

67. Nixon J: Intervertebral disc mechanics: a review, *J R Soc Med*, 79(2):100-104, 1986.

68. Oegema TR Jr: Biochemistry of the intervertebral disc *Clin Sports Med* 12(3):419-439, 1993.

69. *Orthopaedic knowledge update 6*, Beaty JH, ed, Rosemont, Ill, 1999, American Academy of Orthopaedic Surgeons.

70. Ostgaard HC, Andersson GBJ, Karlson K: Prevalence of low back pain during pregnancy, *Spine* 16:549-552, 1991.

71. Panjabi MM, Krag MH, Chung TQ: Effects of disc injury on mechanical behavior of the human spine, *Spine* 9:707-713, 1984.

72. Pearce RH: Morphologic and chemical aspects of intervertebral disc aging. In Buckwalter JA, Goldberg VM, Woo SL-Y, eds: *Musculoskeletal soft tissue aging: impact on mobility*, Rosemont, Ill, 1993, American Academy of Orthopaedic Surgeons, pp. 363-379.

73. Pedrini-Mille A et al.: Proteoglycans of human scoliotic intervertebral disc, *J Bone Joint Surg Am* 65:815-823, 1983.

74. Pelletier JP et al.: Collagenase and collagenolytic activity in human osteoarthritic cartilage, *Arthritis Rheum*, 26:63-68, 1983.

75. Pelletier JP et al.: Collagenolytic activity and collagen matrix breakdown of the articular cartilage in the Pond-Nuki dog model of osteoarthritis, *Arthritis Rheum* 26:866-874, 1983.

76. Pelletier JP et al.: The role of synovial membrane inflammation in cartilage matrix breakdown in the Pond-Huki dog model of osteoarthritis, *Arthritis Rheum* 28:554-561, 1985.

77. Powell MC et al.: Prevalence of lumbar disc degeneration observed by MRI in symptomless women, *Lancet* 2:1366-1367, 1986.

78. Ricketson R, Simmons JW, Hauser BO: The prolapsed intervertebral disc: the high-intensity zone with discography correlation, *Spine* 21:2758-2762, 1996.

79. Rolander SD: Motion of the lumbar spine with special reference to the stabilizing effect of posterior fusion, *Acta Orthop Scand Suppl* 90:1-144, 1966.

80. Ross JS, Modic MT, Masaryk TJ: Tears of the annulus fibrosus: Assessment with Gd-DTPA-enhanced MR imaging, *Am J Neuroradiol* 19:1251-1254, 1989.

81. Roughley PJ, White RJ, Poole AR: Identification of a hyaluronic acid-binding protein that interferes with the preparation of high buoyant-density proteoglycan aggregates from adult human articular cartilage, *J Biochem* 231:129-138, 1985.

82. Saal JS, Saal JA:Management of chronic discogenic low back pain with a thermal intradiscal catheter: a preliminary report, *Spine* 25(3):382-388, 2000.

83. Schellhas KP et al.: Lumbar disc high-intensity zone, *Spine* 21:79-86, 1996.

84. Schwarzer AC et al.: The prevalence and clinical features of internal disc disruption in patients with chronic low back pain, *Spine* 20(17):1878-1883, 1995.

85. Silveri CP, Simeone FA: Lumbar disc disease. In An HS: *Principles and techniques of spine surgery*, Baltimore, 1998, Williams and Wilkins, pp. 425-441.

86. Smith BMT et al.: Interobserver reliability of detecting lumbar intervertebral disc high-intensity zone on magnetic resonance imaging and association of high intensity zone with pain and annular disruption, *Spine* 23(19):2074-2080, 1998.

87. Smyth MJ, Wright V: Sciatica and the intervertebral disc: an experimental study, *J Bone Joint Surg Am* 40:1401-1418, 1958.

88. Sullivan JD, Farfan HF, Kahn DS: Pathologic changes with intervertebral joint rotational instability in the rabbit, *Can J Surg* 14:71-79, 1971.

89. Svensson HO, Andersson GBJ: Low back pain in 40-47 year old men: work history and work environment factors, *Spine* 8:272-276, 1983.

90. Tertti M et al.: Disc degeneration in magnetic resonance imaging: a comparative biochemical histologic and radiographic study in cadaver spines, *Spine* 16:629-634, 1991.

91. Thompson RC Jr, Bassett CAL: Histological observations on experimentally induced degeneration of articular cartilage, *J Bone Joint Surg Am* 52:435-443, 1970.

92. Trout JJ, Buckwalter JA, Moore KC: Ultrastructure of human intervertebral disc. II. Cells of the nucleus pulposus, *Anat Rec* 204:307-314, 1982.

93. Trout JJ et al.: Ultrastructure of human intervertebral disc. I. Changes in notocordal cells with age, *Tissue Cell* 14:359-369, 1982.

94. Tsuyama N: Ossification of the posterior longitudinal ligament of the spine, *Clin Orthop* 84:71-84, 1984.

95. Vanharanta H et al.: A comparison of CT/discography, pain response and radiographic disc height, *Spine* 13:321-324, 1988.

96. Videman T et al.: The long-term effects of physical loading and exercise lifestyles on back-related symptoms, disability, and spine pathology among men, *Spine* 20:699-709, 1995.

97. Walsh TR et al.: Lumbar discography in normal subjects: a controlled, prospective study, *J Bone Joint Surg Am* 72:1081-1088, 1990.

98. Weinstein JN: Anatomy and neurophysiologic mechanisms of spinal pain. In Frymoyer JW, ed: *The adult spine: principles and practice*, Raven Press, 1991, New York, pp. 611-634.

99. Zdeblick TA: Discogenic back pain. In Rothman RH, Simeone FA, eds: *The spine*, Philadelphia, 1999, WB Saunders, pp. 749-765.

Invasive Spinal Diagnostics

Mitchell K. Freedman, Brian T. Brislin,
Alexander R. Vaccaro, Conor O'Neil,
Jeffrey D. Coe, Philip M. Maurer, Erin O'Brien

If surgery or other interventional treatment is being considered for a patient with spinal pain and the source of pain is unclear despite a thorough clinical evaluation and appropriate imaging studies, electrodiagnostics and/or diagnostic injections may be indicated. There are two aspects to the validity of any diagnostic test, the rationale for the test, and the clinical utility. The rationale for a test is its scientific basis, including both its plausibility and limitations. The clinical utility of a test is the ability of the test to definitively diagnose the pathologic lesion responsible for a disease (diagnostic utility) and to establish prognosis or predict response to treatment (predictive utility). Prior to performing a diagnostic injection for spinal pain, the validity of the injection should be carefully considered.

RATIONALE FOR DIAGNOSTIC INJECTIONS

The rationale for the use of diagnostic injections is that the injection of a pathologic lesion of a spinal structure results in a characteristic change in pain sensation. There are two types of pain response seen with diagnostic injections: analgesic and provocative. The pain that results from the mechanical and/or chemical stimulus of an injection is known as the *provocative response*. The pain relief that occurs after the injection of local anesthetic is known as the *analgesic response*. Biologically, the rationale for both types of pain responses as indicators of tissue pathology is plausible. Pain is a perception and as such results from electrical activity in specific areas of the cerebral cortex.[104] One of the determinants of electrical activity in the cortical areas responsible for pain perception is the signal coming in to the cortex from the periphery. Pathologic lesions in spinal structures lead to injury and inflammation, which result in firing of free nerve endings. Free nerve endings in tissues that respond to noxious stimuli are known as *nociceptors*, and the process responsible for converting a noxious stimulus into electrical activity in the cortex is known as *nociception*. Pathologic lesions also cause sensitization of nociceptors, leading to the commonly experienced phenomenon of tenderness. The rationale for the provocative response is that if a tissue is tender, pain may be reproduced by irritating the sensitive area. The rationale for the analgesic response is that the pain resolves after anesthetic blockade because the nociceptor is anesthetized and the signal that leads to the perception of pain in the cerebral cortex is eliminated.

Although biologically plausible, the rationale for both analgesic and provocative responses as indicators of tissue pathology has limitations. A fundamental limitation of the rationale for diagnostic injections is that although the pain response to an injection can define the state of activity of nociceptors in a particular structure, it cannot, by itself, define the pathologic lesion responsible for pain. To diagnose the pathologic lesion responsible for pain, the injection response must be correlated with imaging studies and the clinical examination. As an example, radicular pain is usually secondary to either a herniated nucleus pulposus or lateral spinal stenosis. A nerve root injection will reveal only if a particular nerve is irritated, not the etiology of the pathology. The primary utility, then, of a nerve root injection is to determine if a pathologic lesion seen on imaging studies is the source of the patient's pain.

Diagnostic injections must be specific for the structure being investigated; that is, only nerve endings in the target structure should be provoked or anesthetized. As a corollary, the injection must adequately provoke or anesthetize the nerve endings in the target structure. For this reason, to ensure precision and specificity, diagnostic injections must be performed under fluoroscopic guidance, with contrast enhancement. Although the primary purpose for performing diagnostic injections with contrast enhancement is to ensure specificity, in some circumstances the contrast-enhanced images from the injection will either confirm findings seen on other imaging studies or demonstrate pathology not seen on other imaging studies. Specific injection techniques are only available for certain components of the spine, namely, the discs, synovial joints, nerves, and, to a certain extent, the epidural space. Injections have the potential to diagnose pathologic lesions of these structures; however, it is not possible, using precision injection techniques, to diagnose other pathologic lesions that may be responsible for pain, such as myofascial pain, dural irritation, and instability.

A basic principle of sensory physiology is that the intensity of a perception is dependent on the intensity of the stimulus being applied. In the case of deep somatic tissues such as bones, joints, and muscles, it has been demonstrated that even normal tissues can hurt if sufficient pressure is applied. This has lead to the concept of the pain threshold, that is, a tissue is defined as pathologic not because it hurts when provoked but rather because the threshold for pain is decreased. To determine whether the pain threshold of a particular tissue is decreased, there must be a norm for comparison. This has important implications for provocative responses, as responses that are not referenced to the intensity of the stimulus and to established normative values might not be valid.[84]

The potential for placebo responses must be considered in evaluating analgesic responses to diagnostic injections. A number of studies have established that inert injections (e.g., of normal saline) can lead to analgesic responses in patients with spinal pain.[66,95] For this reason, an analgesic response to a single injection cannot be considered diagnostic. Given that placebo responses are to some extent determined by positive beliefs and expectations on the part of the patient, patient education may be important in preventing placebo responses.[102] The patient should be clearly informed that the injection is strictly for diagnostic purposes and that any potential benefit to them will accrue only if they are able to make a decision about whether their pain has decreased. The physician should not display any bias as to the value of one result over another. If a patient does report pain relief after an injection, it is important to determine whether this represents a placebo response. There are several strategies for doing so. The duration of the analgesic response should be compared with the duration of action for the local anesthetic that is injected. If an analgesic response is due to the effect of local anesthetic on activated nociceptors, the pain relief should last as long as the duration of action of the local anesthetic. Comparative local anesthetic blocks can be considered, in which on separate occasions the same structure is anesthetized using local anesthetics with different durations of action. If, on each occasion, the pain relief lasts as long as the duration of action of the local anesthetic use, the responses are considered unlikely to be placebo responses. Comparative local anesthetic blocks have been compared with saline controls for medial branch blocks in the cervical region and have been found to be valid.[5,82,84,86]

Although control injections theoretically represent the most reliable way to exclude placebo responses, there are drawbacks associated with their use. Placebo responses have been shown to increase with repeated administration; therefore, even with a control injection, there is a concern about an increase in the placebo response with repeated administration (if an active treatment follows a control injection, a placebo response is still possible). Saline injections pose ethical and practical (billing) problems. Control injections involve considerable additional time and expense; they may only be justified in certain situations (the results of the test are being used for presurgical planning). In some circumstances, an active injection of one structure can serve as a fortuitous control for an injection of another structure. If a patient has a negative response to an active injection of one structure, this could be considered as the control for subsequent injections.[61,102]

Another major limitation of the rationale for diagnostic injections results from plasticity in the central nervous system. The central nervous system does not function as a hard-wired system but rather in different modes or states. One state is normal sensibility, in which pain perception is highly correlated with tissue injury, as is seen with acute pain. The rationale for diagnostic injections is most plausible in this state. The nervous system can also function in a sensitized state. Allodynia is a sensitized state, in which a low-intensity stimulus acting via low-threshold afferents generates pain. In this state, the nervous system may not be able to distinguish between noxious and nonnoxious stimuli. Hyperalgesia also occurs, in which noxious stimuli result in a pain response that is augmented in amplitude and duration (i.e., pain thresholds are decreased).

There are several mechanisms that can result in sensitization. One important mechanism that has been well studied is localized sensitization of the dorsal horn. Tissue injury results in a continuous barrage of input to dorsal horn cells, which leads to sensitization of these cells. As a result, not only injured tissue but also surrounding normal tissue exhibits allodynia and hyperalgesia. In this circumstance, what formerly were nonnoxious stimuli, such as touch or pressure, may be perceived as pain, and pain thresholds for noxious stimuli may be lowered, in the absence of tissue pathology.

In the presence of localized sensitization of the dorsal horn, it is also possible that an anesthetic injection of an injured nerve or structure may not produce complete pain relief. Anesthetizing an adjacent normal nerve or structure may relieve pain, and provoking a normal structure or nerve may reproduce a patient's clinical pain.[45,76,98] An example of this effect is provided in a recent study by Caragee et al.,[11] who reported on a population of patients that might be expected to have local sensitization of the dorsal horn (secondary hyperalgesia). The patients had iliac crest bone graft pain but no low back pain. One would expect that the dorsal horn cells that receive afferent innervation from the iliac crest

---

DIAGNOSTIC INJECTIONS

- Used to identify pain secondary to
  - Facet joint pathology
  - Intervertebral disc pathology
  - Epidural space/nerve root pathology
  - Sacroiliac joint pathology
- Confounding factors
  - Placebo
  - Sensitization of dorsal horn cell from nociceptors
  - Chronic pain
  - Somatization disorders

would be sensitized; therefore, these dorsal horn cells would also respond to nonnoxious stimuli from other structures that project to these same cells. Just as touching an area of skin with secondary hyperalgesia causes pain, one would expect that stimulating a structure, such as the intervertebral disc, that projects to the sensitized dorsal horn cell would also cause pain. In fact, Carragee et al.[11] demonstrated pain responses to disc injections in a significant number of these individuals. The deep somatic receptive fields of the neurons of the dorsal horn responsible for processing nociceptive signals are large, and the same receptive field could be expected to include discs, iliac crest, sacroiliac joint, and other structures. Therefore, the ability of the nervous system to determine which one of these tissues is being stimulated is limited. In the presence of local sensitization of the dorsal horn or more generalized sensitization of the nervous system, one could expect that any sensation produced in the receptive field may be interpreted as pain.[11]

Although localized sensitization of the dorsal horn is perhaps the best-studied mechanism of sensitization, there are other mechanisms as well. In the presence of chronic pain secondary to tissue injury, generalized sensitization of the nervous system can affect receptive fields remote from any area of tissue injury. The mechanism associated with this may be that chronic pain and its attendant disability are associated with negative emotions such as fear, anger, and anxiety, as well as depression, all of which may be associated with generalized sensitization of the nervous system. In addition, there may be constitutional differences between individuals, which may be the mechanism behind diffuse musculoskeletal pain disorders such as fibromyalgia.[15]

Regardless of the mechanism, nervous system sensitization is characterized by a change in the way that nociceptive signals arising in the periphery are processed in the central nervous system.[98] The mechanism of sensitization can be primarily sensitization of the dorsal horn or a more generalized sensitization of the nervous system.[12,15] In this condition, the rationale for diagnostic injections may not be valid, as pain responses to injections may not reflect activity of the actual nociceptors, which are injected.[76,98]

As part of this process, it is important to recognize that pain is a complex phenomenon that is composed of two separate but related components: a sensory component and an affective component. The sensory component of pain results from injury or irritation of tissue by a pathologic lesion. It allows the brain to perceive the presence of noxious stimuli and to characterize them in terms of their location, quality, and intensity. However, in addition to being a sensory experience, like vision or hearing, pain has a strong affective component. The affective component of pain consists of the negative emotions (fear, anxiety, anger) and depression that accompany pain. Although the emotional and psychologic distress associated with pain is most likely a result of tissue injury, it may be influenced by preexisting psychologic, cognitive, and social factors.[27] Identifying the affective component of pain is important for several reasons. One reason is that the affective component may sensitize sensory pathways, which may invalidate the results from any diagnostic injections that may be performed. Moreover, psychologic distress has been shown to negatively affect outcomes from treatment; therefore, the implications of psychologic distress on eventual treatment, regardless of any results on diagnostic injections, should be considered.[92] As an example, patients with somatization disorders are probably not good candidates for spinal fusion for axial pain. Therefore, discography is not a clinically useful test in those individuals and should be performed only in exceptional circumstances. Patients with chronic pain and abnormal psychometric testing may be more likely to have abnormal discograms.[12]

CLINICAL UTILITY

The clinical utility of a diagnostic test has two components: the diagnostic utility and the predictive utility. The *diagnostic utility* is the ability of the test to definitively diagnose the pathologic disorder responsible for pain, and the *predictive utility* is its ability to predict the response to treatment. To establish the diagnostic utility of a test, it is necessary to have a gold standard against which the test result can be compared.[35] If there is a gold standard for definitively diagnosing a particular pathologic disorder, then the result from a diagnostic test can be compared with the gold standard, allowing the sensitivity and specificity of the test to be defined. The sensitivity and specificity, in conjunction with the clinical findings, can then be used to calculate the odds that a particular disorder is present. Without a gold standard, typically obtained from biopsy, surgery, or long-term follow-up, the sensitivity and specificity of the test, and therefore its ability to definitively diagnose a disorder, cannot be determined.

The pathologic lesions responsible for radicular pain, primarily disc herniations and stenosis, have well-defined gold standards for the diagnosis including magnetic resonance imaging (MRI), computed tomography (CT)-myelography, and surgical exploration. Therefore, the sensitivity and specificity of diagnostic injections for radicular pain (i.e., selective nerve root injections) can be calculated. Unfortunately, in contrast to radicular pain, the pathologic lesions for axial pain have not been well defined. Therefore, no gold standards exist, and there is no way to determine the sensitivity and specificity of diagnostic injections performed for axial pain, such as disc and synovial (facet, sacroiliac) joint injections.

CLINICAL USE OF DIAGNOSTIC TESTS

- Diagnostic utility: Ability of a test to definitively diagnose the pathologic disorder responsible for pain
- Predictive utility: Ability of a test to predict the response to treatment

The ultimate criterion for a diagnostic test is whether the patient's condition can be improved as a result of the study. Although the diagnostic utility of many injections, particularly injections for axial pain, cannot be precisely defined, it is important to remember that if a test can predict the response to treatment and is reliable and reproducible, it may be clinically useful.[48,49,87]

Effective treatments for spinal pain may include both surgery and minimally invasive pain management procedures.[18,20,53,87,88] Traditionally, the indication for surgery has been loss of neurologic function. Increasingly, surgery is performed for pain without neurologic loss, essentially becoming a pain management procedure. The tissue injury that accompanies surgery may lead to adverse consequences. Therefore, if surgery is being considered for patients with chronic pain, the predictive utility of a test should be well defined.

DIAGNOSTIC STRATEGIES

There are a number of disorders that can cause spinal pain. Establishing which of these disorders is responsible for pain in an individual patient can be challenging. Advanced imaging studies such as CT and MRI frequently demonstrate structural lesions that are potential causes of spinal pain, but there also is a high incidence of anatomic abnormalities in asymptomatic individuals, making it difficult to be certain that a structural lesion is actually a source of pain.[7,42,79] Furthermore, on occasion individuals in pain will have normal anatomy, at least as demonstrated on conventional imaging studies.[111]

Patients with pain from a spinal etiology may present with deep somatic pain or neurogenic pain. These sensations may be caused by pathology in different structures. There are several clinical characteristics that can help to differentiate between somatic and neurogenic pain. Usually, somatic pain is perceived in the back or neck, leading to the term *axial pain*, whereas neurogenic pain is perceived in the leg or arm, leading to the term *radicular pain*. Somatic pain is deep, "achy," and poorly localized, whereas neurogenic pain is sharp, lancinating, and well localized. There may be specific areas of weakness and/or paresthesias in the extremity. A positive straight leg raise may be present. Somatic pain has no accompanying neurologic complaints and a negative straight leg raise.

The pathophysiologic mechanisms responsible for each of these syndromes are very different. Somatic pain results from irritation of nociceptors in the somatic structures of the spine (vertebrae, facet joint, sacroiliac joint, intervertebral disc, and myofascial structures), whereas neurogenic pain presumably results from irritation of the nerve roots. The nerve can be injured at the level of the ventral or dorsal segmental root proximal to the foramen, the spinal nerve traversing the foramen, or the dorsal or ventral rami distal to the foramen. Defining the pain syndrome as specifically as possible allows one to limit the number of lesions that could be causing symptoms. Only lesions that can result in the pain syndrome exhibited by the patient should be considered, regardless of findings on diagnostic tests. If a patient complains of axial pain, the diagnostic strategy should focus on workup of the somatic structures previously mentioned. Visceral pathology must be considered as well. If a patient complains of neurogenic pain, the diagnostic strategy should focus on lesions such as disc protrusions and stenosis. Somatic pain and neurogenic pain frequently coexist in the same patient. When they do, it is important to recognize them as separate processes, because the diagnostic strategy will be different for each.

In addition to defining the potential lesions that can be responsible for pain, it is important to determine which segment of the spine is likely to be affected. The spine is a series of repeating segments. Although both the vertebral column and spinal nerves are organized segmentally, the spinal nerves have a high degree of somatotopic representation in the cerebral cortex, whereas the somatic components that constitute the vertebral column do not. For that reason, radicular pain patterns are more characteristic of the level of involvement, even though discrimination between adjacent roots may be challenging.

Prevalence studies have been conducted for lumbar axial spine, demonstrating that the prevalence is 31% for disc lesions, 14% for facet lesions, and 15% for sacroiliac lesions. In 29% of patients, no pain source was identified.[2] Similar studies have not been performed in the cervical spine, with the exception that the prevalence of facet joint lesions in patients with whiplash is roughly 60%.[65] Thus, in the absence of all other data, lumbar disc pathology appears to be the most common

---

PAIN

- Axial (somatic)
  - Confined to the trunk or proximal extremity
  - Poorly localized
  - "Achey"
  - Tension signs *not* present
- Radicular (neurogenic)
  - Radiates down extremity
  - Well localized
  - "Sharp, lancinating"
  - Patient may complain of paresthesias or specific weakness in an extremity
  - Tension signs generally present

INDICATIONS FOR DIAGNOSTIC INJECTION

- Provocative test to identify whether a given structure is the source of pain
- Identify whether a specific disc, facet joint, or sacroiliac joint is responsible for discomfort in the presence or absence of structural abnormalities seen on anatomic studies
- Identify whether a given nerve root is responsible for discomfort

cause of lumbar pain, whereas facet lesions are the most common cause of neck pain in patients with whiplash injury. In the case of radicular pain, younger patients are more likely to have a herniated nucleus pulposus, whereas an older patient is more likely to have spinal stenosis.[30]

Diagnostic injections are functional procedures that can further delineate whether the area in question is responsible for pain. Injections can be useful if the imaging study does not correlate with all other information. Typically, this occurs as one of two scenarios. One common scenario is that there are multiple pathologic lesions on imaging studies, and the clinical information is not sufficiently localizing. In this case, an injection may determine which of the lesions is the cause of the patient's symptoms. The second common scenario is that structures that are likely sources of pain based on clinical criteria are normal or show only nonspecific abnormalities on imaging, in which case an injection is needed to assess for occult pathology (pathology not identified on imaging). Precision diagnostic injections can be performed on discs, synovial joints, and nerves. If an injection is indicated for a patient with axial pain, disc, facet, and/or sacroiliac joint injections are appropriate. If the patient has neurogenic pain, which may result from irritation of a spinal nerve, it should be investigated with selective nerve root injections. Fully characterizing the source of a patient's pain may take several injections. In general, an injection evaluation should commence at the most likely level, targeting the structure that is most likely to be responsible for pain based on clinical and epidemiologic criteria.

The question arises as to which structure should be investigated first. Although occult pathology is a possibility, more often a structure that is actually a source of pain should exhibit some pathologic changes on imaging studies. All other factors being equal, it is reasonable to initiate investigations at the site of the most obvious pathology. It may be necessary to inject multiple structures. In deciding which structure to inject first, it is important to take two other factors into consideration: the clinical utility of the injection and the risk. Consider the example of a patient with only low back pain. Epidemiologic studies suggest that the disc is more commonly injured than the facet joint. If making a diagnosis were the primary consideration, the appropriate strategy would be to inject discs first and facet joints second if the disc injection had negative results. However, the implications of the results from the injection on treatment must also be considered. Radiofrequency rhizotomy is a minimally invasive treatment option available for treating

facet pathology.[104] The treatment options for discogenic pain at this time may be considered to be spinal fusion or intradiscal electrothermal therapy, both of which are much more invasive. With facet injections, there may be some chance of therapeutic benefit if a steroid is added to the anesthetic. There is no direct therapeutic benefit from discography; therefore, in this circumstance, it would be reasonable to inject facet joints first rather than the discs. Furthermore, although the risk of complications with discography is low, when they do occur they can be catastrophic. This is another reason to proceed with the less invasive facet joint injections first.

In summary, for patients with spinal pain whose pathology is not evident based on history and physical examination or imaging studies, diagnostic injections may be clinically useful. The injections that are available are disc, facet joint, sacroiliac joint, and nerve injections. The order of injection selection is based on clinical evaluation, risk-benefit ratio, and whether the test will lead to a change in treatment. For instance, if a patient refused to consider fusion or intradiscal electrothermal therapy, discography should not be performed.

Discography
Lumbar Discography

Discography is a provocative clinical test. The majority of the information obtained from a discogram is provided by the provocative response after injection of the disc with contrast medium. A lesser degree of information can then be obtained by injecting the disc with analgesic to alleviate pain initially caused by the provocative injection. However, in addition to provoking pain, injection of contrast medium into the disc may demonstrate pathology that is not otherwise revealed on conventional imaging studies. Prior to the introduction of sophisticated imaging studies such as CT and MRI, lumbar discography was often used primarily as a radiologic imaging study to complement myelography.[64] Several studies have confirmed the accuracy of lumbar discography as a radiologic test in demonstrating both disc herniations and disc degeneration.[5,10,35] With the advent of MRI and in particular the use of gadolinium enhancement in evaluating postoperative patients, the utility of lumbar discography purely as a radiologic study is diminished. However, both cadaver and clinical studies have demonstrated that discography is slightly more sensitive than MRI in detecting disc pathology, particularly when postdiscography CT scanning is added.[2,35,90] Interpretation of the radiologic images obtained at the time of discography is important. The images should be reviewed to confirm that the needle was placed into the nucleus and that the subsequent dye injection filled the nucleus. Annular injections, injections into the space between the annulus and the nuclear cavity, and venous uptake are all possible and may invalidate the results.[66,70] A variety of classification schemes have been developed to describe annular pathology as visualized by discography.* Regardless of

---

BASIS FOR ORDER OF SELECTION
OF DIAGNOSTIC INJECTIONS

- Clinical examination
- Risk-benefit ratio of treatment
- Will test(s) lead to change in treatment?

---

* References 64, 70, 75, 82, 83, 90, 92, 98.

the exact classification scheme that is used, it is important to note the degree of annular degeneration, the presence of annular fissures, and whether the annulus is competent or incompetent. If a patient has a convincing pain response but no evidence of a radial annular fissure on discography, postdiscography CT scanning should be considered. On occasion, a disc that is normal on plain discography is disrupted on CT discography.[90] In addition to annular pathology, both Schmorl's nodes and end plate disruptions should be noted, because they may be clinically significant.[46,69]

The rationale for provocative discography is that the pain provoked during disc injection results from irritation of sensitized nerve endings in the disc. The sensitization of these nerve endings is a result of disc pathology. For this rationale to be valid, the injection must selectively affect the nerve endings in the annulus of the disc being studied. The nerve endings in the lumbar disc are in the end plates and middle and outer annuli.[109] Although pathologic processes involving the end plate can occur, the innervated portion of the disc that is most commonly injured is the annulus.[46,69] A number of authors have suggested that the pain provoked at discography may be from stimulation of structures other than the annulus, including the end plates or vertebral body, the dorsal root ganglion, or facet joints (via transmission of mechanical stimulation).[37,40,107] Despite these hypotheses, there is good evidence that the provocative response resulting from discography is related to stimulation of nerve endings in the outer annulus, rather than other factors.[72,102] Although relatively unusual, painful end plate disruptions can also occur.[46]

Discography appears to be specific for stimulation of the disc, but there are a number of potential limitations. It is possible that there may be sensitized nerve endings within the disc that are not stimulated by disc injection. Discogenic pain is believed to be a result of annular fissures originating in the nucleus and extending to the outer annulus, which is where the majority of the discs' nerve endings reside. During discography, contrast medium is injected into the nucleus. If there are no fissures, the contrast medium will be confined to the nucleus. However, histologic studies have demonstrated that there can be middle or outer annular abnormalities that are not contiguous with the nucleus.[35] In such cases, an injection into the nucleus could lead to a false-negative result.

In the absence of a gold standard for axial pain, a number of studies have investigated the ability of discography to provoke back pain in asymptomatic subjects, in an effort to better define the potential for false-positive results. The premise of discography is that reproduction of a patient's typical clinical symptoms during the injection identifies the disc as the source of pain. The rationale for its use is that the results can help to discriminate among the various structures that may be responsible for axial pain. Therefore, to establish its validity, the criteria for a truly positive disc must be determined in the relevant population, which are patients who have back pain.

Holt, in 1968, reported a 36% rate of positive discography in asymptomatic subjects, leading him to discredit the use of the test.[44] There were several methodologic flaws with Holt's study. The most notable flaws were that all of his subjects were prisoners, that he used a highly irritating contrast medium, and, most important, that he did not include a positive pain response as a criterion for a positive injection (i.e., the criterion for a positive result was based primarily on radiologic images).

Holt's findings were subsequently refuted in a well-designed study by Walsh et al., who demonstrated a 0% rate of positive discography in asymptomatic volunteers.[106] These authors studied 10 asymptomatic subjects and 7 patients with chronic low back pain. The criteria for a positive result differed between the two groups. For both groups, a positive result required a 3/5 pain intensity (using a pain thermometer), two types of pain behavior (as assessed by videotape review), and structural degeneration. For the patients with chronic low back pain, a positive result also required that the provoked pain be similar to their usual pain. Obviously, it was not possible to evaluate the similarity of pain in asymptomatic subjects, because they had no pain prior to the injection. Among the asymptomatic subjects, 5 of 10 had at least one structurally abnormal disc; however, none satisfied the criteria for a positive test. Thus, the false-positive rate in these asymptomatic volunteers was 0%. Among the patients with chronic low back pain, all seven had at least one structurally abnormal disc and six of seven patients had at least one disc that satisfied the criteria for a positive result. Overall, 13 discs were structurally abnormal, with 7 being positive and 6 being negative for pain. Of note, two of the seven had at least one disc that was structurally abnormal and was associated with intense, but atypical, provoked pain, as well as pain behaviors. In each case, the test result was considered to be negative, given that the provoked pain was different from the patient's typical pain.

DISCOGRAPHY

- Rationale
  - Pain provoked by irritating sensitized nerve endings in the disc
  - Nerve endings in end plates and annulus
- Limitations
  - Some sensitized nerve endings in disc not stimulated
  - Injection into nucleus; if no fissures extend into annulus, pain may not be reproduced during discography
  - Asymptomatic patients with chronic pain or somatization disorder may have painful discs
- Complications
  - Infection: 0 to 1.3% of patients
  - Nerve root irritation
  - Allergic reaction
  - Retroperitoneal hemorrhage
  - Increase in pain in patients with chronic pain

The study by Walsh et al. was important for several reasons. First, using strict criteria for a positive test, including postinjection review of videotaped responses, there was excellent interrater reliability. Diagnostic tests that rely on an observer's interpretation are not clinically useful unless there is good interobserver reliability; the same test applied to the same patient should always produce the same result.[90] Thus their study established reproducible criteria for a positive result from discography. Second, by demonstrating a 0% false-positive rate in asymptomatic subjects, Walsh et al. effectively refuted Holt's assertion that the false-positive rate of discography was so high as to make it useless. Third, they demonstrated that patients with chronic low back pain were capable of developing different types of pain in response to provocation discography. According to their criteria, only provoked pain that was similar to the patient's typical symptoms constituted a positive test. Atypical provocative pain, even if intense and accompanied by pain behaviors, constituted a negative test.

The asymptomatic subjects studied by Walsh et al. were healthy volunteers, with an average age of 23. Caragee et al. recently expanded on the study by Walsh et al. of asymptomatic subjects by studying a cohort of subjects who did not have low back pain, but whose clinical background was closely matched to that of patients with low back pain who typically present for discography.[12] Thirty subjects with no history of low back pain were recruited: 10 had previous cervical surgery with good results, 10 had the same surgery but had persistent chronic cervical pain, and 10 had primary somatization disorders. Lumbar discography was performed and interpreted according to the protocol of Walsh et al. Four somatization patients dropped out prior to beginning the study, and two stopped the study after only one or two discs were injected and therefore were not included in the study analysis.

Among the subjects with good results from previous cervical surgery, 7 of 10 had at least one disc that had an outer annular rupture (10 of a total of 30 discs), whereas only 1 of 10 had a positive result. The patient with a positive test had a high Zung depression score. Of the subjects with chronic pain, 5 of 10 patients had at least one disc that had an outer annular rupture (11 of a total of 32 discs), with 4 of 10 having at least one positive disc. Of the discs with significant structural abnormalities, seven were positive and four were negative. Among the subjects with somatization disorder, one of four had at least one disc that had an outer annular rupture (6 of a total of 13 discs). Of the six discs with significant structural abnormalities, two were positive and four were negative. Based on these data, Caragee et al. concluded that in individuals with normal psychometrics and without chronic pain, the rate of false-positive results is very low if strict criteria are applied and that the rate of false-positive results increases with increased annular disruption.

The study by Caragee et al. is important for a number of reasons. First, it confirms the finding by Walsh et al. that in subjects without a history of low back pain and without psychosocial risk factors, provocation of a significant pain response with discography is unusual,

with an incidence of 0% versus 10% in the study by Caragee et al. It also confirms the finding by Walsh et al. that although discs in this population are often structurally abnormal (combining the studies, 12 of 20 had at least one structurally abnormal disc), they are no more likely to be positive than is a structurally normal disc. More important, Caragee et al. reveal that in subjects without a history of low back pain but with a history of chronic pain or a somatization disorder, provocation of a significant pain response with discography is common, with an incidence of 40% in the chronic pain group and of 75% in the somatization disorder group. Furthermore, the more disrupted the annulus, the greater is the chance of a positive response.

The study by Caragee et al. is a powerful reminder of the importance of psychosocial factors in modulating pain, while also demonstrating the potential of false-positive responses with discography. However, in assessing the importance of this information, it is necessary to reconsider the premise of discography.

The data of Walsh et al. on patients with chronic low back pain demonstrated that it is common for patients undergoing discography to have intense pain that is very different in location and character from their clinical symptoms. In their study, the criteria for a positive test in the chronic low back pain population required that provoked pain be similar to the patient's clinical symptoms. Unfortunately, without a gold standard for axial pain, the validity of incorporating measures of familiarity of pain into the criteria for a positive test cannot be precisely defined.[90] Caragee et al.[11,12] clearly demonstrated the potential for false-positive responses with discography. However, given the premise of discography and the fact that patients with chronic low back pain frequently have intense but atypical pain during discography, it is difficult to know the significance of any pain response in an asymptomatic subject.

The addition of pressure monitoring to provocative discography provides the potential to predict outcome and improves interobserver reliability and therefore reproducibility. Assessment of the response to discography requires measuring pain before and after the injection. There are three components to pain: intensity, location, and character. If the location and character provoked at discography are similar to or exactly the same as the patient's clinical symptoms, they satisfy the criteria for concordant pain. The intensity of pain is measured both by the patient's self-report, for example, using a numerical rating, and by observed pain behaviors. However, the intensity of provoked pain is dependent on the intensity of the stimulus. In simple terms, the harder one pushes on the syringe, the more likely the disc is to hurt. By measuring intradiscal pressures, intensity of the stimulus can be quantified, allowing more reliable comparisons between patients and discographers. Although it is possible to estimate injection pressures manually, the use of a controlled inflation syringe with digital pressure readout provides a precise value.

If a disc is normal structurally and does not elicit a pain response, it is considered by some to serve as a control disc. A control injection may be helpful in the decision of whether a pain response at another disc is a true-positive result or reflects an exaggerated reaction to nociception. However, a more valid control would probably be a structurally abnormal disc. Although the significance of the results from control injections have not been formally validated, clinical experience suggests that if at least one structurally abnormal disc does not hurt, pain provoked at another disc is more likely to be a true-positive result.

The primary indication for provocative discography is to determine whether a patient with chronic spinal pain for whom aggressive efforts at conservative care have failed can be helped with spinal fusion or with other invasive treatments, such as IDET. In contrast to the surgical treatment of radiculopathy, the surgical treatment of axial pain is controversial, in that studies have demonstrated a wide disparity in outcome.* This disparity has been attributed to a number of factors, including type of fusion (interbody vs. intertransverse, instrumented vs. noninstrumented), approach (anterior vs. posterior vs. 360 degree), surgeon variability, and methodologic differences. The results from discography have been an important part of the preoperative evaluation in most of these studies, but typically the criteria for a positive test have not been strictly defined. The validity of the criteria used to define a positive discogram is another variable that has the potential to affect surgical outcome.

In an effort to develop criteria for discography that can be used to predict surgical outcome, Derby et al. reported on a cohort of patients who underwent provocative discography under pressure monitoring. They hypothesized that pain at discography that occurs at low pressures below the typical weighted values implies a highly sensitized annulus, presumably a result of chemical irritation of the annulus by enzymes and breakdown products involved in the inflammatory process, whereas pain that occurs at higher pressures is more likely to be a result of chronic mechanical stimulation of nociceptors in the annulus.[18]

Looking at all surgical cases combined, there was no significant difference in outcome between patients undergoing interbody versus intertransverse fusion, with both groups having approximately a 50% favorable outcome. However, among patients classified as having a chemically sensitive disc, there was a highly significant difference in outcome between patients undergoing interbody versus intertransverse fusion. Within that group, 89% of the interbody fusion patients had a favorable outcome, whereas only 20% of the intertransverse fusion patients had a favorable outcome. Patients with chemically sensitive discs who did not have surgery of any kind had an 88% unfavorable outcome. Based on these data, it appears that there may be a subset of patients with degenerative disc disease who have chemically sensitive discs and who have outcomes with surgery that rival those of patients undergoing partial disc excision for herniated nucleus pulposus. The

---
*References 16, 26, 33, 57, 63, 74, 80, 99.

> ## THE POSITIVE DISCOGRAM
>
> - Concordant pain: Pain that mimics normal discomfort in location and character
> - Control disc: Nonpainful structurally normal or abnormal disc
> - Positive results: Low-pressure injection reproduces pain and implies chemical irritation of annulus; chemically sensitive discs seem to respond to interbody fusion

surgery performed must be an interbody fusion, presumably because the disc is completely excised, therefore removing the source of the noxious stimulus. If these results stand up to long-term follow-up and are replicated by other investigators, the use of pressure-controlled discography will be validated as a diagnostic test to predict which patients will benefit from surgical fusion.[18]

There are some who do not believe that discography is necessary prior to fusion; they believe that the diagnosis of discogenic pain can be made on the basis of clinical and radiographic criteria. There are substantial data suggesting that the clinical examination is of minimal use in discriminating between potential axial pain generators.[93,95] A possible exception to this is a McKenzie mechanical assessment, which may be able to predict the results from discography.[21] There have been several studies demonstrating that MRI cannot reliably predict which discs are painful on discography, at least to the level of confidence required to rely solely on MRI for surgical decision-making.[78,99,111] A high-intensity zone in the posterior annulus, as visualized on MRI, was recently proposed as a marker for painful discs.[3] However, the prevalence of a high-intensity zone in asymptomatic individuals is too high for clinical use.[14] If a patient undergoes a fusion for lumbar axial pain without preoperative discography, both the patient and the surgeon should be aware that the level adjacent to the planned fusion may be a source of clinical symptoms, regardless of the findings on MRI.

Complications.   There are two approaches to the lumbar disc: posterior and lateral.[1] The posterior approach necessitates a dural puncture and therefore should be avoided. Disc puncture is typically performed with a 22- or 25-gauge needle (Figures 7-1 and 7-2). There is some evidence that the use of an introducer needle can reduce the risk of infection, although this is not a universal practice.[28] This is rarely encountered, but a variety of complications are possible with discography, including neural injury, bleeding, and intradural leakage of injected substances.[37,67,101] There have been case reports of disc herniations resulting from discography.[32,34] Although studies in dogs have had conflicting results on the potential for disc injury during discography, the weight of evidence in humans suggests that this is not a significant problem.[34,47,50,52]

The most significant risk associated with discography is infection. The rate of discitis reported in the literature

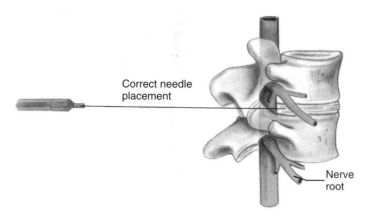

Figure 7-1. Approach to discogram is lateral to the superior articular process.

is as high as 1.3% per disc, and serious morbidity has resulted.[28,36,51] However, practice audits at centers performing a large volume of discography have demonstrated infection rates as low as 0 of 10,000 (R. Derby, P. Maurer, personal communication). There is experimental evidence that prophylactic antibiotics, both intravenous and intradiscal, can prevent discitis.[29,60,78] As a result, many practitioners routinely administer prophylactic antibiotics, particularly to high-risk patients such as those with diabetes. Other complications associated with discography include nerve irritation from the needle, allergic reactions to iodinated contrast agents, retroperitoneal hemorrhage, subarachnoid puncture, and chemical meningitis. Patients with chronic pain may have exacerbation of low back pain for 1 year or longer.*

Cervical Discography

Cervical discography is comparable in many ways to lumbar discography. The underlying premise of both is the same: injection of the disc replicates the clinical noxious stimulus responsible for the patient's symptoms, and reproduction of the patient's clinical symptoms during the injection confirms the disc as the source of pain. Both are subject to the confounding variables of nervous system plasticity and psychologic factors. Similar to lumbar discography, cervical discography is a provocative clinical test rather than a radiologic imaging test.

A major difference between lumbar and cervical discography is the relationship between pain provocation and disc morphology. In the lumbar spine, discs have varying degrees of disruption of the outer annulus. The pain resulting from lumbar discography has been shown to be directly related to the degree of fissuring of the outer annulus.[72,103] This finding provides a link between disc pathology and provoked pain, supporting circumstantial evidence suggesting that internal disc disruption is an important cause of axial low back pain.[7] Obviously, it would not have been possible to make this observation if all lumbar discs had the same degree of annular disruption.

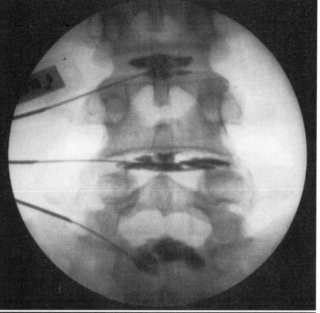

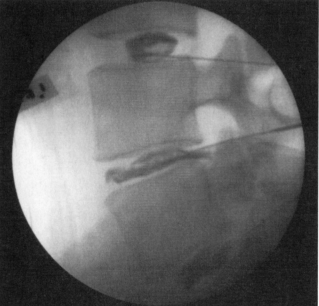

Figure 7-2. Anteroposterior **(A)** and lateral **(B)** radiographs demonstrating lumbar provocative discography at the L3 to L4, L4 to L5, and L5 to S1 levels.

CERVICAL DISCOGRAPHY

- Positive discogram does not reliably give a specific diagnosis
- May predict success with anterior fusion
- Complications: Puncture of carotid artery, hematoma, spinal cord compression, and discitis

---

*References 13, 24, 29, 31, 58, 60, 78.

Morphologically, cervical discs are very different from lumbar discs. Although both have a peripheral annulus fibrosus and a central nucleus, the cervical disc also has posterolateral uncovertebral joints. These are not true joints but rather are clefts in the annulus, which communicate with the nucleus in the majority of individuals by early adulthood.[77] As a result of these clefts, if contrast agent is injected into a cervical disc, the majority of them will demonstrate "annular tears." Some cervical discs hurt when injected, but others do not. Because they all have annular disruption, however, it is not possible to correlate provoked pain with underlying pathology.[91] Bogduk and Aprill studied patients with axial neck pain with the use of both zygapophyseal joint injections and discography.[3] Using 100% pain relief as the criterion for a positive z-joint, they discovered that 41% had a positive disc and a positive z-joint at the same level. If z-joint blocks were both highly sensitive and specific, this result would be an indication that there is a high false-positive rate associated with discography; that is, if the z-joint block is a true-positive, the disc must be a false-positive. However, the z-joint blocks in this study were not controlled, which in other studies have been shown to have a false-positive rate of 27%.[53] This would suggest a 14% false-positive rate for discography, if the response to z-joint blocks were used as the gold standard to judge discography.[6]

At the present, the mechanisms responsible for cervical discogenic pain are unknown. Therefore, although a positive discogram in the lumbar spine can be used to diagnose a specific pathologic syndrome, a positive discogram in the cervical spine does not reliably provide a specific diagnosis. Ideally, a diagnostic test will reveal the underlying target disorder that is responsible for pain.[89] The fact that cervical discography cannot do so compromises its clinical utility and constitutes a significant difference between cervical and lumbar discography.

Diagnostic Utility. As with lumbar discography, a number of studies have been conducted on cervical discography in asymptomatic individuals.[91,97] Holt, in 1964, reported a 100% rate of positive discography in asymptomatic subjects. As in his study on lumbar discography, all of his subjects were prisoners and he used a highly irritating contrast medium. In contrast to his lumbar study, a positive pain response, rather than a radiologic abnormality, was the criterion for a positive result.[43] Shinomiya et al. reported a 50% rate of positive discography in patients without neck pain. However, this was a group of patients with spondylitic myelopathy, which is not the population under consideration for cervical discography.[97]

Schellhas et al., in a well-designed study, used nonirritating contrast medium to perform cervical discography on a group of volunteers recruited from the community as well as on a series of patients with chronic neck pain.[91] They found that the majority of discs, in both subjects and patients, including those that appear normal on MRI, had annular tears on discography. However, discs from asymptomatic subjects, even if morphologically abnormal, were associated with low-level pain responses. Among patients with chronic neck pain, there was a group who had intense pain with disc injection.[91]

The results from the study of Schellhas et al.[91] refute the findings of Holt[43] and of Shinomiya et al.,[97] which suggested that the degree of pain provocation with discography was unrelated to the presence of neck pain. Schellhas et al.'s findings demonstrated that most cervical discs are morphologically abnormal and are associated with some discomfort on injection but that there is a definite severe concordant pain response in symptomatic patients that does not occur in asymptomatic subjects. The study by Schellhas et al. complements the study by Walsh et al.[106] in the lumbar spine, demonstrating that although pain can occur during the injection of discs in asymptomatic subjects, this occurs at low levels of intensity. Schellhas et al. evaluated interobserver reliability for the morphologic evaluation of MRI and discograms but did not assess the interobserver reliability of the pain response, as did Walsh et al. The importance of psychosocial factors was not addressed in the study by Schellhas et al., but presumably they are as important with cervical discography as they are with lumbar discography.

Predictive Utility. As in the lumbar spine, the surgical treatment of axial neck pain is controversial. However, there is evidence that 70% to 80% of patients selected for anterior spinal fusion on the basis of discography can achieve satisfactory outcomes.[56,86,108] Although the results from discography played an important part in surgical decision-making in these studies, the criteria for a positive test are not strictly defined. Unlike the lumbar spine, pressure-controlled discography has not been used in the cervical spine. There is some information on the normative values for intradiscal pressures in the cervical spine, but it is technically difficult to measure pressures accurately at the time of cervical discography.[81] At the present, there is no way to reproducibly measure the stimulus applied to the cervical disc.

Complications. The cervical disc is approached via a right anterolateral approach.[1] There are a number of potential complications that can occur.[17,38,62,110] As the needle is advanced to the disc, puncture of the carotid artery or deeper vessels of the neck can lead to bleeding complications and possible airway compromise. If the needle is advanced too far posteriorly, it may puncture vessels in the anterior epidural space, potentially resulting in hematoma formation and spinal cord compression. Puncture of the spinal cord itself is possible, with the obvious consequences, particularly if contrast agent is injected into the cord. Acute quadriplegia has been reported after cervical discography, presumably related to posterior displacement of disc tissue with injection and resultant spinal cord compression.[62]

In addition to the risks associated with needle placement, infectious complications related to cervical discography are potentially devastating. If the needle passes through the hypopharynx or esophagus, there is a potential for enteric organisms to be introduced into the disc. Discitis may lead to epidural abscess, with resultant quadriplegia.[17] Because of the potentially catastrophic adverse effects associated with discitis in the cervical spine, some consider diabetes mellitus to be an absolute contraindication to cervical discography. Prophylactic antibiotics, either intravenous or intradiscal, should be strongly considered for all patients.

Summary of Cervical Discography.   At this point, cervical discography must be considered an art rather than a science. We do not really know what underlying disorder are being diagnosed with this test, nor can the results of surgery be reliably predicted. Given the potential complications associated with cervical discography, it should be performed only by individuals who have a detailed understanding of the anatomy of the cervical spine and are skilled in performing and interpreting diagnostic spinal injections of other structures, most notably the lumbar disc. Because virtually all cervical discs have annular tears, the role of CT discography in the cervical spine is limited. There are no published data suggesting that postdiscography CT provides clinically useful information.

Although retrospective studies suggest that anterior interbody fusion may be an effective treatment for discogenic neck pain, at the present, there are no criteria that can be used to reliably predict outcome from surgery. Understanding that clinically useful criteria for the interpretation of cervical provocative discography have not been defined, experienced discographers consider the following characteristics to suggest a symptomatic disc: concordant or exact pain (exact is more significant), intensity greater than 6/10, pain 1 minute after injection of at least 50% of the maximum intensity, two or more pain behaviors in response to injection, low intradiscal pressure at pain provocation (as estimated by manual pressure), and a negative control injection.

Synovial Joint Injections

The current method of diagnosing the sacroiliac and/or facet joints as the cause of pain is based on the resolution of pain after anesthetic injections. There is no gold standard anatomic study or surgery to verify that these joints are indeed the source of a given patient's pain. The history and physical examination also do not reliably diagnose facet dysfunction in the cervical or lumbar spine.[8,96] When assessing somatic pain, there may be considerable overlap in referral patterns among sacroiliac dysfunction, facet induced pain, and discogenic pain in the lower back[22,25,73] (Figures 7-3 and 7-4). Cervical

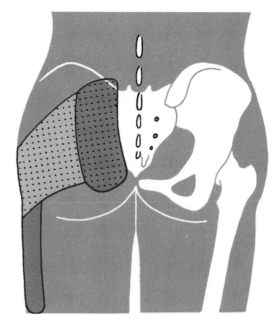

Figure 7-3.   Characteristic patterns of pain referral secondary to sacroiliac dysfunction. *(From Fartin JD et al.: Sacroiliac joint: pain referral maps upon applying a new injection arthrography technique. I. Asymptomatic volunteers, Spine 19(19):1475-1482, 1994.)*

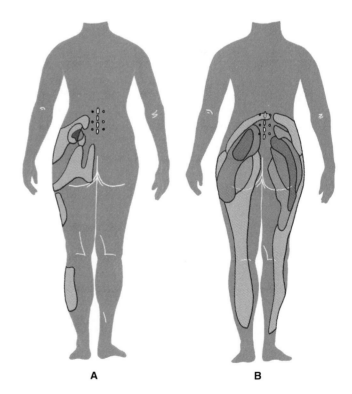

A **B**

Figure 7-4.   Facet pain referral patterns produced by intraarticular injections of hypertonic saline in asymptomatic and symptomatic patients. **A,** Normal. **B,** Abnormal. *(Redrawn from Mooney V, Robertson J: Facet joint syndrome, Clin Orthop 115:149-156, 1976.)*

SYNOVIAL JOINT INJECTIONS

- Sacroiliac joints and facet joints can cause low back pain
- Single blocks of facet joint: False-positive responses in up to 38% of patients
- Double or triple block paradigms minimize false-positive findings
- Relief obtained
  - Lidocaine: 50% to 75% pain relief for 30 to 60 minutes
  - Bupivicaine: Relief for 2 to 3 hours
  - Saline: No relief

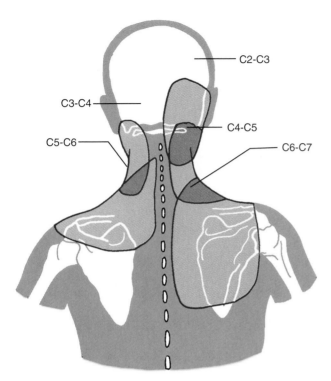

Figure 7-5.   Composite map depicting referral of pain from stimulation of cervical zygapophyseal joints in asymptomatic population. *(Redrawn from Dwyer A, Aprill C, Bogduk N: Cervical zygapophyseal joint pain patterns: study in normal volunteers, Spine 15(6):453-457, 1990.)*

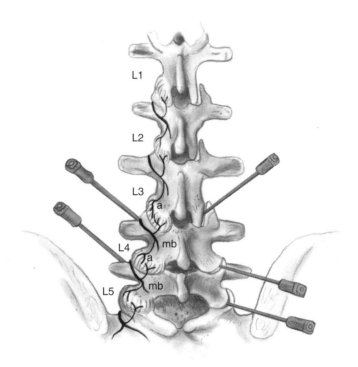

Figure 7-6.   Posterior view of the lumbar spine demonstrating the location of the zygoapophyseal joints *(a)* and their innervation by the medial branches of the dorsal rami. On the left, needle position for the L3 and L4 medial branch blocks used to anesthetize the L4 to L5 "z" joint are shown. On the right, the needle positions are shown for intraarticular joint injections. *(Redrawn from Mooney V, Robertson J: Facet joint syndrome, Clin Orthop 115:149-156, 1976.)*

facet joints also create characteristic patterns of pain (Figure 7-5). Sclerodermal pain patterns derived from noxious stimulation of spinal muscles and ligaments can also cause confusing clinical presentations. Hip pathology must be considered as a part of the differential diagnosis when there is groin or anterior thigh pain.

The sacroiliac joint and the facet joints can be injected for diagnostic or therapeutic purposes. A diagnostic block of the medial branch is performed when an ablative procedure is being considered. Percutaneous radiofrequency denervation of both the cervical and lumbar zygapophyseal joints has been shown to provide extended pain relief in the appropriate patient.[65,66,104] To date, there are no controlled studies of percutaneous radiofrequency ablation of the sacroiliac joint.

Several facet joints are usually injected at one time. The selection of the specific facet joint to be evaluated is based on the pattern of the patient's pain complaints. In the lower back, it may be unclear as to whether the sacroiliac joint or the facet joint should be evaluated. A given facet joint is evaluated by intraarticular injection or by blocking the medial branch of the dorsal ramus at the level of the specific joint and at the level above it.

Technique

The medial branch of the dorsal ramus is blocked at the base of the superior articular process and the adjacent transverse process. Fluoroscopic guidance is mandatory.

The "Scotty dog" is visualized via an oblique view. The needle is placed via a posterior lateral approach. For an intraarticular injection, a similar approach is used except that the needle is placed directly into the targeted facet joint (Figure 7-6).

Sacroiliac joint injections also require fluoroscopic guidance. The fluoroscope is angled so as to superimpose the anterior and posterior joint planes. The needle is placed posteriorly into the inferior aspect of the joint.

Single blocks of the facet joint provide false-positive responses up to 38% of the time.[93] Double- or triple-block paradigms minimize false-positive findings. Similar results would be expected in the sacroiliac joint. Lidocaine (2%) should provide relief of at least 50% to 75% of the patient's discomfort for 30 to 60 minutes. A longer-acting agent such as 0.5% bupivacaine should provide 50% to 75% pain relief for at least 2 to 3 hours. On occasion a third block is performed with saline, which should not provide any relief. Small volumes of fluid should be used.[4,68,85,94] Immediately after the injection, the patient should be evaluated at rest and with activity to evaluate whether the pain has changed as a result of the injections. Pain may occur as the local anesthetic is injected into the joint. This may also help to substantiate that the joint injected is a cause of pain.

Complications from lumbar facet joints injections are rare. Chemical meningitis with the use of local anesthetics has been reported in facet joint injection.[100] Bleeding, infection, and allergic reactions are possible with all joint injections.

Selective Epidural Injections
Lumbar Selective Epidural Injection

As is the case with the intervertebral disc, spinal nerves can be injected with contrast agent, local anesthetic, or other substances. Both the provocative response (pain occurring in response to a mechanical and/or chemical stimulus) and the analgesic response provide clinically useful information.

Nerve root blocks were first developed to diagnose the source of radicular pain when imaging studies suggested possible compression of several roots.[22,39,41,55,59] Early studies on selective nerve root injections described an extraforaminal approach, in which a needle is advanced at right angles to the spinal nerve outside the neural foramen. Localization of the needle adjacent to the nerve relies on leg pain provocation, presumably resulting from penetration of the nerve by the needle.[39,55,59]

A selective epidural injection is a variation of the selective nerve root injection. As the nerve roots leave the dura to enter the foramen and form the spinal nerve, they carry an extension of the dura with them, which becomes the epineurium of the spinal nerve. The epineurium is in turn enveloped by an epiradicular membrane, which is an extension of the anterior and posterior epidural membranes.[54] The injection of contrast agent into the epiradicular membrane outlines the nerve root, dorsal root ganglion, spinal nerve, and ventral ramus. Proximally, contrast will flow around the dural sac at the takeoff of the nerve root. If injected outside the epiradicular membrane, contrast agent spreads diffusely in the epidural fat and therefore is of limited diagnostic value (Figure 7-7).

A selective epidural injection differs from a selective nerve root injection in that the goal is to inject into the epiradicular tissues. The spread of injected solutions depends on the anatomy of the epiradicular membrane, which is an extension of the epidural space, leading to use of the term *selective epidural injection*. There are two major advantages of a selective epidural technique over a selective nerve root technique. First, with a selective epidural injection, a foraminal approach is used and contact with the nerve is less likely, minimizing the potential for neural injury. Rather than relying on leg pain provocation from needle contact, needle localization is confirmed with contrast-enhanced images demonstrating an outline of the nerve (Figure 7-8). Second, a selective epidural approach ensures that the injection incorporates all the sites where pathology can affect the nerve, from the disc level in the subarticular zone extending lateral to the extraforaminal zone. If the pathology that causes a patient's symptoms is a paramedian disc herniation but the nerve is injected in the extraforaminal zone, as with a classic selective nerve

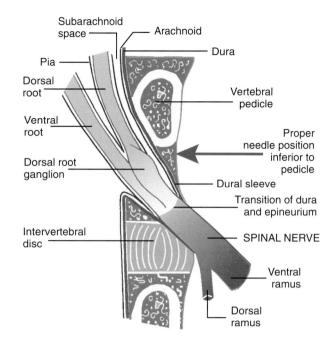

Figure 7-7. The needle placed for a selective epidural steroid injection should be just inferior to the pedicle, at the dorsal and ventral roots for the spinal nerve. *(Redrawn from Bogduk N: Clinical anatomy of the lumbar spine and sacrum, ed 3, New York, Churchill Livingstone, 1997 p. 143.)*

SELECTIVE EPIDURAL INJECTIONS

- Transforaminal approach
  - From 80% to 100% relief with or without activity after injection
  - Provocative pain at onset of injection consistent with foraminal pathology
  - Provocative pain later in injection consistent with paramedian disc herniation
  - Evaluate patient 1 to 2 weeks after injection if steroid was injected
- False-positive results
  - Psychologic factors
  - Placebo response
  - Injection not specific to a given nerve root; injected fluid may spread to adjacent roots or their nociceptive structures
  - Central regulation of pain may cause aberrant responses
- Clinical
  - Positive responses may support clinical impression that nerve root is source of pain
  - Negative response may be more clinically significant than positive response
  - Patients with 1 year of pain that responds to steroid injected near symptomatic nerve root have 85% positive surgical outcome

root injection, the portion of the nerve from which the pain originates may not be anesthetized, potentially leading to a false-negative result.

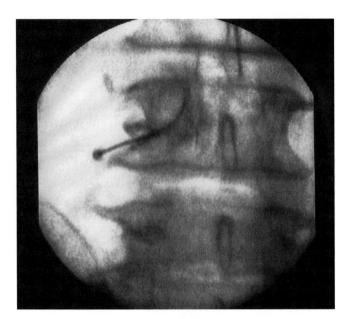

Figure 7-8. Transforaminal selective epidural injection at the L4 to L5 level with contrast outlining the L4 nerve root.

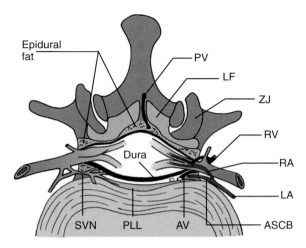

Figure 7-9. A transverse section through the vertebral canal and intervertebral foramina to demonstrate the relations of the lumbar nerve roots. The roots are enclosed in their dural sleeve, which is surrounded by epidural fat in the intervertebral foramina. Radicular veins (RV) and radicular arteries (RA) run with the nerve roots. Anteriorly, the roots are related to the intervertebral disc and posterior longitudinal ligament (PLL), separated from them by the sinuvertebral nerves (SVN), elements of the anterior internal vertebral venous plexus (AV), and the anterior spinal canal branches (ASCB) of the lumbar arteries (LA). Posteriorly, the roots are separated from the ligamentum flavum (LF) and zygoapophyseal joints (ZJ) by elements of the posterior internal venous plexus (PV) and epidural fat that lodges in the recess between the ligamentum flavum of each side. (Redrawn from Bogduk N: Clinical anatomy of the lumbar spine and sacrum, ed 3, New York, Churchill Livingstone, 1997 p. 143.)

Diagnostic Utility. The selective epidural injection is performed to assess radicular pain. It has two components. The first is the provocative pain response resulting from contrast agent injection, and the second is the analgesic response resulting from injection of local anesthetic and/or a corticosteroid. In the evaluation of provoked pain, it is important to compare the location and character of the provoked response with the patient's typical symptoms. Furthermore, the onset of provoked pain should be related to the location of the leading edge of the contrast solution when pain begins.[19] Normal epidural tissue is not painful when gently stimulated by contrast solution. In the absence of scar tissue, pain provocation indicates that the tissue stimulated is irritated. For example, early pain provocation of pain, when contrast agent is still in the foramen, suggests foraminal stenosis or a foraminal disc herniation. Late pain provocation when the contrast agent approaches the disc above is consistent with a paramedian disc herniation.

Immediately after the injection, the effect of the local anesthetic on the patient's symptoms should be assessed, both at rest and in response to mechanical stimulation. Studies on selective nerve root injections have used the criterion for a positive analgesic response of 80% to 100% relief.[76,98] The significance of lesser degrees of pain relief in response to an injection is uncertain. If a corticosteroid is included in the injection solution, the patient should be reevaluated 1 week later because the degree of pain relief at that interval can also provide important information.

There are a number of factors that can lead to false-positive and false-negative results from selective epidural injections. Psychologic factors and placebo responses may affect the outcome.[76,98] Selective epidural injections do not provide a selective nerve root block.

Pain-sensitive structures that may be affected include the dura of segmental nerve roots, the posterior longitudinal ligament, and the outer aspect of the lumbar intervertebral disc. The sinuvertebral nerve and the medial branch of the dorsal ramus and the structures they innervate will be anesthetized as well (Figure 7-9). Medication covers more than one spinal level when 2 ml of fluid is injected. North et al. questioned the sensitivity and specificity of diagnostic injections. Confounding issues include inhibition of afferent information from joints as well as superficial structures, which may generate pain or are sites of referred pain.[76] Central regulation of pain may also alter with peripheral nerve blocks. A negative response to a selective epidural injection may be more clinically significant than a positive response to selective epidural injection. In general, information obtained from diagnostic selective epidural injections should support the rest of the clinical and diagnostic evaluation. It should not be the only factor used for diagnosis.

Clinical Utility. Selective epidural injection may have a clinical use for prognostication of surgical outcome, despite this lack of specificity. Derby et al. found that patients with pain that was present for longer than 1 year had a response to steroid injection that predicted surgical outcome. A positive response to steroid injected into the symptomatic root had an 85% positive surgical outcome, whereas a negative response had a 95% poor surgical outcome.[20] Individual studies have also investigated the predictive value of pain provocation, immediate pain relief from local anesthetic injection, and prolonged pain relief from corticosteroid injection in the evaluation of patients with radiculopathy.[20,22]

The following protocol should be used to interpret the response to selective nerve root injections: If a patient has concordant or exact provoked pain in response to injection of contrast, complete pain relief after the injection of local anesthetic, and a prolonged steroid response (>1 week), the injected nerve root is mediating the patient's symptoms. A good result can be expected from surgical decompression of the nerve root, assuming a correctable lesion is demonstrated on imaging studies. If a patient has discordant pain, incomplete immediate pain relief, and no prolonged steroid response, the injected nerve is probably not mediating the patient's symptoms. If an intermediate response occurs, a number of different possibilities exist. The patient may still have symptoms arising from a single nerve root, may have symptoms from multiple roots, or may not have radicular pain. If the clinical situation is highly suggestive of radiculopathy, it may be reasonable to repeat the selective nerve root injection at an adjacent nerve.

The usefulness of a selective epidural injection is primarily related to the associated provocative and analgesic pain responses. However, the contrast-enhanced images from the injection can reveal pathologic findings.[19,22] Two examples of this are a perpendicular nerve root sign, resulting from up-down foraminal stenosis, and obstruction to proximal flow of the contrast agent, which can occur with foraminal stenosis, disc herniations, and scar tissue. Such findings tend to confirm findings evident on MRI or CT-myelography.

Complications. Nonpositional headaches, transient increase in low back pain or leg pain, facial flushing, vasovagal reaction, and hyperglycemia are potential complications. Dural punctures are infrequent. Allergic reactions to medications may occur. Systemic effects of corticosteroids include fluid retention and congestive heart failure as well as suppression of the secretion of adrenal glucocorticoids for up to 3 months. Cushinoid syndrome has been reported. Epidural hematoma, infection, and nerve root damage are rare.[9]

Cervical Selective Epidural Steroid Injection

As in the lumbar spine, the epineurium of each cervical spinal nerves root is enveloped by an epiradicular membrane, which is an extension of the anterior and posterior epidural membranes.[54] As a result, selective epidural injections may be performed in the cervical spine and, given the analogous innervation of the cervical and lumbar spines, may be used to accomplish the same goal: to determine the nerve root responsible for radicular pain.[71]

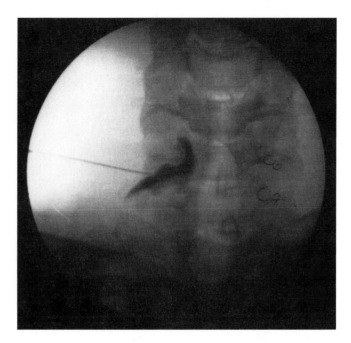

Figure 7-10. Posteroanterior view of fluoroscopically guided, contrast-enhanced cervical transforaminal epidural steroid injection at the C7 level.

Cervical selective nerve root injections are performed using an anterolateral approach, with the radiologic landmark being the base of the superior articular process as viewed in an oblique projection of the spine and the midpoint of the lateral mass as viewed in the anteroposterior projection. Care must be taken to keep the needle tip posterior to the vertebral artery at all times; the needle should not pass medial to the foramen (Figure 7-10).

Unlike in the lumbar spine, there is no information on the diagnostic or predictive value of pain provocation, immediate pain relief from local anesthetic injection, or prolonged pain relief from use of a corticosteroid in the evaluation of a patient with cervical radiculopathy. Nevertheless, the responses to these injections are commonly interpreted using the same criteria as in the lumbar spine. There have been no studies correlating pathology with the contrast-enhanced images from selective cervical epidural injections; the primary reason to use contrast agent with fluoroscopically guided injections is to ensure that the injectate is confined to the target nerve root.

Complications. Very few complications have been reported with cervical selective epidural injection. Empirically, one would expect possible complications to include bleeding with the potential for spinal cord injury, nerve root damage, and allergic reactions to iodinated contrast agents. One of the authors (M.F.) has seen the occurrence of transient paresthesias induced in a patient with cervical stenosis and a spinal cord syrinx created by injection directly into the spinal cord.

SELECTED REFERENCES

Derby R et al.: The ability of pressure controlled discography to predict surgical and non-surgical outcome, *Spine* 24(4):364-371, 1999.

Donelson R et al.: A prospective study of centralization of lumbar and referred pain: a predictor of symptomatic discs and anular competence, *Spine* 22(10):1115-1112, 1997.

Gunzburg R et al.: A cadaveric study comparing discography, magnetic resonance imaging, histology, and mechanical behavior of the human lumbar disc, *Spine* 17(4):417-426, 1992.

Hitselberger WE, Witten RM: Abnormal myelograms in asymptomatic patients, *J Neurosurg* 28(3):204-206, 1968.

Hsu KY et al.: Painful lumbar endplate disruptions: a significant discographic finding, *Spine* 13(1):76-78, 1988.

Malmivaara A et al.: Plain radiographic, discographic, and direct observations of Schmorl's nodes in the thoracolumbar junctional region of the cadaveric spine, *Spine* 12(5):453-457, 1987.

North RB et al.: Specificity of diagnostic nerve blocks: a prospective, randomized study of sciatica due to lumbosacral spine disease, *Pain* 65(1):77-85, 1996.

Schellhas KP et al.: Cervical discogenic pain: prospective correlation of magnetic resonance imaging and discography in asymptomatic subjects and pain sufferers, *Spine* 21(3):300-311, discussion 311-312, 1996.

Shinomiya K et al.: Evaluation of cervical diskography in pain origin and provocation, *J Spinal Disord* 6(5):422-426, 1993.

Siddall PJ, Cousins MJ: Spinal pain mechanisms, *Spine* 22(1):98-104, 1997.

Turner JA et al.: The importance of placebo effects in pain treatment and research, *JAMA* 271:1609-1614, 1994.

Walsh TR et al.: Lumbar discography in normal subjects: a controlled, prospective study, *J Bone Joint Surg Am* 72(7):1081-1088, 1990.

REFERENCES

1. Aprill C: Diagnostic disc injection. In Frymoyer JW: *The adult spine*, New York, 1991, Raven, pp. 403-442.
2. Aprill C: The role of automatically specific injections in the sacroiliac joint. Presented at the First Interdisciplinary World Congress on Low Back Pain and Its Relation to the Sacroiliac Joint, San Diego, Calif, Nov 5-6, 1992.
3. Aprill C, Bogduk N: High-intensity zone: a diagnostic sign of painful lumbar disc on magnetic resonance imaging, *Br J Radiol* 65:361-369, 1992.
4. Barnsley L, Lord S, Bogduk N: Comparative local anesthetic blocks in the diagnosis of cervical zygapophyseal joint pain, *Pain* 55:99-106, 1993.
5. Bernard TN Jr: Using computed tomography/discography and enhanced magnetic resonance imaging to distinguish between scar tissue and recurrent lumbar disc herniation, *Spine* 19(24):2826-2832, 1994.
6. Bogduk N: Pain: zygapophyseal blocks and epidural steroids. In Cousins MJ, Bridenbaugh PO, eds: *Neuroblockade in clinical anesthesia and management*, ed 2, Philadelphia, 1989, Lippincott, pp. 935-954.
7. Bogduk N: *Clinical anatomy of the lumbar spine and sacrum*, ed 3, New York, 1997, Churchill Livingstone, p. 143.
8. Bogduk N, Marsland A: The cervical zygapophysial joints as a source of neck pain, *Spine* 13(6):610-617, 1988.
9. Botwin KP et al.: Complications of fluoroscopically guided transforaminal lumbar epidural steroids, *Arch Phys Med Rehabil* 81(8):1045-1050, 2000.
10. Brodsky AE, Binder WF: Lumbar discography: its value in diagnosis and treatment of lumbar disc lesions, *Spine* 4(2):110-120, 1979.
11. Caragee E et al.: False positive findings on lumbar discography: reliability of subjective concordance assessment during provocative disc injection, *Spine* 24(23):2542-2552, 1999.
12. Caragee E et al.: The rates of false positive lumbar discography in select patients without low back symptoms, *Spine* 25(11):1373-1381, 2000.
13. Caragee E et al.: Can discography cause long-term back symptoms in previously asymptomatic patients? *Spine* 25(14):1803-1808, 2000.
14. Caragee E, Paragioudakis SI, Khurana S: Lumbar high intensity zone fred discography in subjects without low back problems, *Spine* 25(23):2987-2992, 2000.
15. Clauw DJ: The pathogenesis of chronic pain and fatigue syndromes, with special reference to fibromyalgia, *Med Hypoth* 44:369-378, 1995.
16. Colhoun E et al.: Provocation discography as a guide to planning operations on the spine, *J Bone Joint Surg Br* 70B(2):267-271, 1988.
17. Connor PM, Darden BV II: Cervical discography complications and clinical efficacy, *Spine* 18(14):2035-2038, 1993.
18. Derby R et al.: The ability of pressure controlled discography to predict surgical and non-surgical outcome, *Spine* 24(4):364-371, 1999.
19. Derby R et al.: Precision percutaneous blocking procedures for localizing spinal pain. II. The lumbar neuraxial compartment, *Pain Digest* 3:175-188, 1993.
20. Derby R et al.: Response to steroid and duration of radicular pain as predictors of surgical outcome, *Spine* 17(6 Suppl):S176-S183, 1992.
21. Donelson R et al.: A prospective study of centralization of lumbar and referred pain: a predictor of symptomatic discs and anular competence, *Spine* 22(10):1115-1122, 1997.
22. Dooley JF et al.: Nerve root infiltration in the diagnosis of radicular pain, *Spine* 13(1):79-83, 1988.
23. Dwyer A, Aprill C, Bogduk N: Cervical zygapophyseal joint pain patterns: a study in normal volunteers, *Spine* 15(6):453-457, 1990.
24. Erlacher PR: Nucleography, *J Bone Joint Surg Br* 34:204-210, 1952.
25. Fartin JD et al.: Sacroiliac joint: pain referral maps upon applying a new injection arthrography technique. I. Asymptomatic volunteers, *Spine* 19(19):1475-1482, 1994.
26. Fluke MM: The treatment of lumbar spine pain syndromes diagnosed by discography: lumbar arthrodesis, *Spine* 20(4):501-504, 1995 (letter; comment).
27. Fordyce WE, ed: *Back pain in the workplace*, Seattle, 1995, IASP Press, pp. 11-25.
28. Fraser RD, Osti OL, Vernon-Roberts B: Discitis after discography, *J Bone Joint Surg Br* 69B(1):26-35, 1987.
29. Fraser RD, Osti OL, Vernon-Roberts B: Iatrogenic discitis: the role of intravenous antibiotics in prevention and treatment—an experimental study, *Spine* 14(9):1025-1032, 1989.
30. Frymoyer JW: Back pain and sciatica, *N Engl J Med* 18(5):291-300, 1988.
31. Gardner WJ et al.: X-ray visualization of the intervertebral disk with a consideration of the morbidity of disk puncture, *Arch Surg* 64:355-364, 1952.
32. Gill K: New-onset sciatica after automated percutaneous discectomy, *Spine* 19(4):466-467, 1994.
33. Gill K, Blumenthal S: Functional results after anterior lumbar fusion at L5-S1 in patients with normal and abnormal MRI scans, *Spine* 17(8):940-942, 1992.
34. Grubb S, Lipscomb H, Guilford W: The relative value of lumbar roentgenograms metrizamide myelography, and discography in the assessment of patients with chronic low-back syndrome, *Spine* 12(3):282-286, 1987.
35. Gunzburg R et al.: A cadaveric study comparing discography, magnetic resonance imaging, histology, and mechanical behavior of the human lumbar disc, *Spine* 17(4):417-426, 1992.
36. Guyer RD et al.: Discitis after discography, *Spine* 13(12):1352-1354, 1988.
37. Guyer RD, Ohnmeiss DD: Lumbar discography: position statement from the North American Spine Society Diagnostic and Therapeutic Committee, *Spine* 20(18):2048-2059, 1995.
38. Guyer RD et al.: Complications of cervical discography: findings in a large series, *J Spinal Disord* 10(2):95-101, 1997.
39. Hauesien DC et al.: The diagnostic accuracy of spinal nerve injection studies: their role in the evaluation of recurrent sciatica, *Clin Orthop* 198:179-183, 1985.
40. Heggeness MH, Doherty BJ: Discography causes end plate deflection, *Spine* 18(8):1050-1053, 1993.
41. Herron LD: Selective nerve root block in patient selection for lumbar surgery: surgical results, *J Spinal Disord* 2(2):75-79, 1989.
42. Hitselberger WE, Witten RM: Abnormal myelograms in asymptomatic patients, *J Neurosurg* 28(3):204-206, 1968.
43. Holt E Jr: Fallacy of cervical discography, *JAMA* 188:799-801, 1964.
44. Holt EP Jr: The question of lumbar discography, *J Bone Joint Surg Am* 50(4):720-726, 1968.
45. Hogan Q, Abram S: Back pain: beguiling physiology (and politics), *Regional Anesth* 22(5):395-399, 1997 (editorial).

46. Hsu KY et al.: Painful lumbar endplate disruptions: a significant discographic finding, *Spine* 13(1):76-78, 1988.

47. Inufusa A et al.: Effect of annular puncture on the adolescent canine intervertebral disc. Presented at the 12th annual meeting of the North American Spine Society, New York, Oct 22-25, 1997.

48. Jaeschke R, Guyatt G, Sackett DL: Users' guides to the medical literature. III. How to use an article about a diagnostic test. A. Are the results of the study valid? Evidence-Based Medicine Working Group, *JAMA* 271(5):389-391, 1994.

49. Jaeschke R, Guyatt GH, Sackett DL: Users' guides to the medical literature. III. How to use an article about a diagnostic test. B. What are the results and will they help me in caring for my patients? The Evidence-Based Medicine Working Group, *JAMA* 271(9):703-707, 1994.

50. Johnson RG: Does discography injure normal discs? An analysis of repeat discograms, *Spine* 14(4):424-426, 1989.

51. Junila J, Niinimaki T, Tervonen O: Epidural abscess after lumbar discography: a case report, *Spine* 22(18):2191-2193, 1997.

52. Kahanovitz N et al.: The effect of discography on the canine intervertebral disc, *Spine* 11(1):26-27, 1986.

53. Karasek M, Bogduk N: Twelve month follow up of a controlled trial of intradiscal thermal anuloplasty for back pain due to internal disc disruption, *Spine* 25:2601-2607, 2000.

54. Kikuchi S: Anatomical and experimental studies of nerve root infiltration, *Nippon Seikeigeka Gakkai Zasshi* 56(7):605-614, 1982.

55. Kikuchi S et al.: Anatomic and clinical studies of radicular symptoms, *Spine* 9(1):23-30, 1984.

56. Kikuchi S, MacNab L, Moreau P: Localisation of the level of symptomatic cervical disc degeneration, *J Bone Joint Surg Br* 63B(2):272-277, 1981.

57. Knox BID, Chapman TM: Anterior lumbar interbody fusion for discogram: concordant pain, *J Spinal Disord*; 6(3):242-244, 1993.

58. Konings J, Veldhuizeu AG: Topographic anatomic aspects of lumbar disc puncture, *Spine* 13:958-961, 1988.

59. Krempen JF, Smith BS: Nerve-root injection: a method for evaluating the etiology of sciatica, *J Bone J Surg Am* 56(7):1435-1444, 1994.

60. Lang R et al.: Penetration of ceftriaxone into the intervertebral disc, *J Bone Joint Surg Br* 76A(5):689-691, 1994.

61. Lasagna L: Further studies on the pharmacology of placebo administration, *J Clin Invest* 37:533-537, 1958.

62. Laun A, Lorenz R, Agnoli AL: Complications of cervical discography, *J Neurosurg Sci* 25(1):17-20, 1981.

63. Lee CK, Vessa P, Lee JK: Chronic disabling low back pain syndrome caused by internal disc derangements: the results of disc excision and posterior lumbar interbody fusion, *Spine* 20(3):356-361, 1995.

64. Lindblom K: Diagnostic puncture of intervertebral disks in sciatica, *Acta Orthop Scand* 17:237-238, 1948.

65. Lord SM: Chronic cervical zygapophyseal joint pain after whiplash: a placebo controlled prevalence study, *Spine* 21(15):1737-1745, 1996.

66. Lord SM et al: Percutaneous radiofrequency neurotomy for chronic zygapophyseal joint pain, *NEJM* 1996; 335(23):1721-1726.

67. MacMillan J, Schaffer JL, Kambin P: Routes and incidence of communication of lumbar discs with surrounding neural structures, *Spine* 16(2):167-171, 1991.

68. Maigne JY, Aivaliklis A, Pfefer F: Results of sacroiliac joint double block and value of sacroiliac pain provocation tests in 54 patients with low back pain, *Spine* 21(16):1889-1892, 1996.

69. Malmivaara A et al.: Plain radiographic, discographic, and direct observations of Schmorl's nodes in the thoracolumbar junctional region of the cadaveric spine, *Spine* 12(5):453-457, 1987.

70. McCutcheon ME, Thompson WC: CT scanning of lumbar discography: a useful diagnostic adjunct, *Spine* 11(3):257-259, 1986.

71. Mendel T, Wink CS, Zimny ML: Neural elements in human cervical intervertebral discs, *Spine* 17(2):132-135, 1992.

72. Moneta GB et al.: Reported pain during lumbar discography as a function of anular ruptures and disc degeneration: a re-analysis of 833 discograms, *Spine* 19(17):1968-1974, 1994.

73. Mooney V, Robertson J: Facet joint syndrome, *Clin Orthop* 115:149-156, 1976.

74. Newman MH, Grinstead GL: Anterior lumbar interbody fusion for internal disc disruption, *Spine* 17(7):831-833, 1992.

75. Ninomiya M, Muro T: Pathoanatomy of lumbar disc herniation as demonstrated by computed tomography/discography, *Spine* 17(11):1316-1322, 1992.

76. North RB et al.: Specificity of diagnostic nerve blocks: a prospective, randomized study of sciatica due to lumbosacral spine disease, *Pain* 65(1):77-85, 1996.

77. Oda J, Tanaka H, Tsuzuki N: Intervertebral disc changes with aging of human cervical vertebra: from the neonate to the eighties, *Spine* 13(11):1205-1211, 1988.

78. Osti OL, Fraser RD, Vernon-Roberts B: Discitis after discography: the role of prophylactic antibiotics, *J Bone Joint Surg Br* 72(2):271-274, 1990.

79. Paajanen H et al.: Magnetic resonance study of disc degeneration in young low back pain patients, *Spine* 14(9):982-985, 1989.

80. Parker LM et al.: The outcome of posterolateral fusion in highly selected patients with discogenic low back pain, *Spine* 21(16):1909-1916, discussion 1916-1917, 1996.

81. Pospiech J et al.: Intradiscal pressure recordings in the cervical spine, *Neurosurgery* 44(2):379-384, discussion 384-385, 1999.

82. Quinnell RC, Stockdale HR: An investigation of artifacts in lumbar discography, *Br J Radiol* 53(633):831-839, 1980.

83. Quinnell RC, Stockdale HR: The use of in vivo lumbar discography to assess the clinical significance of the position of the intercrestal line, *Spine* 8(3):305-307, 1983.

84. Quinnell RC, Stockdale HR, Willis DS: Observations of pressures within normal discs in the lumbar spine, *Spine* 8(2):166-169, 1983.

85. Revel M et al.: Capacity of the clinical picture to characterize low back pain relieved by facet joint anesthesia, *Spine* 23(18):1972-1976, discussion 1977, 1998.

86. Riley LH Jr, et al.: The results of anterior interbody fusion of the cervical spine: review of ninety-three consecutive cases, *J Neurosurg* 30(2):127-133, 1969.

87. Saal JS, Saal JA: Management of chronic discogenic low back pain with a thermal intradiscal catheter: a preliminary report, *Spine* 25:382-388, 2000.

88. Saal JA, Saal JS: Intradiscal electrothermal treatment for chronic discogenic low back pain: a prospective outcome study with minimal 1-year follow-up, *Spine* 25:2622-2627, 2000.

89. Sackett DL et al.: *Clinical epidemiology: a basic science for clinical medicine*, ed 2, Boston, 1991, Little, Brown.

90. Schellhas K: Venous opacification during discography: therapeutic implications. Presented at the 4th annual meeting of the International Spinal Injection Society, Vancouver, BC, Canada, Aug 16, 1996.

91. Schellhas KP et al.: Cervical discogenic pain: prospective correlation of magnetic resonance imaging and discography in asymptomatic subjects and pain sufferers, *Spine* 21(3):300-311, discussion 311-312, 1996.

92. Schofferman J et al.: Childhood psychological trauma correlates with unsuccessful lumbar spine surgery, *Spine* 17(6):138-144, 1992.

93. Schwarzer AC et al.: The false positive rate of uncontrolled diagnostic blocks of the zygapophyseal joint, *Pain* 58:195-200, 1994.

94. Schwarzer AC, Aprill CN, Bogduk N: The sacroiliac joint in chronic low back pain, *Spine* 20(1):31-37, 1995.

95. Schwarzer AC et al.: The relative contributions of the disc and zygapophyseal joint in chronic low back pain, *Spine* 19(7):801-806, 1994.

96. Schwarzer AC et al.: Clinical features of patients with pain stemming from the lumbar zygapophyseal joints: is the lumbar facet syndrome a clinical entity? *Spine* 19(10):1132-1137, 1994.

97. Shinomiya K et al.: Evaluation of cervical diskography in pain origin and provocation, *J Spinal Disord* 6(5):422-426, 1993.

98. Siddall PJ, Cousins MJ: Spinal pain mechanisms, *Spine* 22(1):98-104, 1997.

99. Simmons JW et al.: Awake discography: a comparison study with magnetic resonance imaging, *Spine* 16(6 Suppl):S216-S221, 1991.

100. Thomson SJ, Lomay DM, Collett BJ: Chemical meningism after lumbar facet joint block with local anesthetic and steroids, *Anesthesia* 46:563-564, 1991.

101. Troisier O: An accurate method for lumbar disc puncture using a single channel intensifier, *Spine* 15(3):222-228, 1990.

102. Turner JA et al.: The importance of placebo effects in pain treatment and research, *JAMA* 271:1609-1614, 1994.

103. Vanharanta H et al.: The relationship of pain provocation to lumbar disc deterioration as seen by CT/discography, *Spine* 12(3):295-298, 1987.

104. van Kleef M et al.: Randomized trial of radiofrequency lumbar facet denervation for chronic low back pain, *Spine* 24(18):1937-1949, 1999.

105. Videman T, Malmivaara A, Mooney V: The value of the axial view in assessing discograms: an experimental study with cadavers, *Spine* 12(3):299-304, 1987.

106. Walsh TR et al.: Lumbar discography in normal subjects: a controlled, prospective study, *J Bone Joint Surg Am* 72(7):1081-1088, 1990.

107. Weinstein J, Claverie W, Gibson S: The pain of discography, *Spine* 13(12):1344-1348, 1988.

108. Windsor RE et al.: Injection technique: principles and practice of lumbar discography, *Phys Med Rehab* 6(4):743-770, 1995.

109. Yoshizawa H et al.: The neuropathology of intervertebral discs removed for low back pain, *J Pathol* 132:95-104, 1980.

110. Zeidman SM, Thompson K, Ducker TB: Complications of cervical discography: analysis of 4400 diagnostic disc injections, *Neurosurgery* 37(3):414-417, 1995.

111. Zucherman J et al.: Normal magnetic resonance imaging with abnormal discography, *Spine* 13(12):1355-1359, 1988.

Surgical Neurophysiologic Monitoring

Daniel M. Schwartz, Lawrence R. Wierzbowski,
Dapeng Fan, Anthony K. Sestokas

Continuous monitoring of spinal cord function during corrective spine surgery has become commonplace in many academic and community hospitals. The evolution of improved surgical techniques and significant engineering advances in spinal instrumentation not only has broadened the surgical candidate population, but also has heightened the risk for iatrogenic spinal cord and/or spinal nerve root injury. Hence the need for intraoperative neurophysiologic monitoring (IONM) has grown substantially in recent years.

In general the primary goal of IONM is to reduce the point prevalence of iatrogenic neurologic sequelae associated with manipulation of neural elements or tracts. For corrective spine surgery, techniques are now available to monitor the sensory and motor spinal cord tracts, spinal nerve roots, and peripheral nerves from the time of anesthesia induction to that of emergence.[15] It no longer is necessary to augment IONM during spine surgery with a temporally limited wake-up test, nor is it compulsory to infer changes in motor function from alterations in a single sensory modality (upper extremity somatosensory evoked potential

[SSEP]), which may not be monitorable in selected patient populations.

INTRAOPERATIVE MONITORING DURING CERVICAL SPINE SURGERY

With improved surgical technique, understanding of biomechanics, and internal fixation devices, the number of patients undergoing corrective cervical spine surgery today has grown by an order of magnitude over that in the past decade. Patients such as those with cervical myelopathy, cervical instability, and ankylosing spondylitis are clearly at high risk for both surgical and nonsurgical intraoperative neural injury. Consequently IONM must begin immediately following induction for monitoring asleep intubation to prevent spinal cord compression secondary to neck extension.

The strategy for monitoring asleep intubation should include recording of upper extremity SSEPs and transcranial electrical motor evoked potentials (TcMEPs). The ulnar nerve is preferred over the more popular median nerve as a stimulation site for upper extremity SSEPs because its lower spinal nerve root entry at C7 to T1 facilitates protection of the entire cervical neuraxis, which may be at risk during intubation. TcMEPs should be recorded over distal hand (e.g., first dorsal interosseous or abductor pollicis brevis) and leg (e.g., tibialis anterior, gastrocnemius) muscles for all cervical spine surgeries; however, if the surgical level includes C5, then it is imperative also to record TcMEPs from the deltoid muscle in order to guard against increased susceptibility to C5 spinal nerve root injury.

Once postinduction baseline responses are obtained, the anesthesiologist is directed to commence with intubation under monitoring guidance. A TcMEP should be recorded immediately upon gaining airway access and prior to taping of the endotrachial tube.

(**Caveat:** Because TcMEPs are recorded over muscle, it is imperative that the neuromuscular junction not be entirely blocked. It is preferable to intubate following administration of a short-acting depolarizing muscle relaxant [i.e., succinylcholine chloride]. This also will

---

MULTIMODALITY INTRAOPERATIVE NEUROPHYSIOLOGIC MONITORING (IONM) DURING SPINE SURGERY

- Used to reduce the point prevalence of iatrogenic neurologic sequelae
- IONM techniques are now available to monitor:
  - Ventral motor spinal cord tracts—transcranial electrical motor evoked potentials (TcMEPs)
  - Dorsal sensory spinal cord tracts—ulnar nerve (UN) and posterior tibial nerve (PTN) Somatosensory Evoked Potentials (SSEPs)
  - Spinal motor nerve root function—spontaneous (sp) and electrically stimulated (st) electromyography (EMG)
  - Spinal sensory nerve root function—dermatomal evoked potentials (dEPs)

ensure recording of uncompromised TcMEPs following positioning.) When it is clear that there are no significant time-locked changes in TcMEP amplitude following intubation, ulnar nerve SSEPs should be recorded once again prior to positioning of the patient.

Because of their sensitivity to impending brachial plexopathy, ulnar nerve SSEPs should be rerecorded immediately after application of countertraction of the shoulder(s) with adhesive tape for anterior positioning or after the patient is turned prone.[12] If the unilateral ulnar nerve SSEP is noted to change ≥30% following shoulder taping, then the tape should be released immediately and reapplied with less countertraction. To ensure corticospinal tract integrity, TcMEPs also should be reelicited following positioning or the application of weight for neck traction. If a significant change in TcMEPs is noted, it is imperative first to raise the patient's mean arterial blood pressure (MAP) to ≥90 mm Hg to improve perfusion to the spinal cord. If the change is secondary to weight placement, then the weight must be removed. In these situations we have yet to see a lack of improvement in TcMEPs within a few minutes of weight release. Following recovery, the amount of weight should be titrated to a tolerable amount.

Should TcMEP amplitude changes be due to turning the patient from supine to prone, and response amplitude does not show any signs of improvement within 15 minutes of raising MAP, then spinal cord injury dosage of methylprednisolone should be infused to reduce the exacerbating effects of spinal cord edema. Reevaluation of TcMEPs with intermittent SSEP testing should be conducted over the next 20 minutes. If improvement in TcMEP amplitude of at least 30% is not noted, then we recommend not proceeding with surgery. In this case the patient should be turned supine and monitoring continued throughout emergence from anesthesia. (**Caveat:** It is important to remember that for the most part changes in neurophysiologic signals represent precursors to irreversible anatomic injury; therefore prompt intervention is the key to prevention of neurologic sequelae.) When the decision is made to bring the patient back to the operating room for a second attempt (usually ≥48 hours), it is critical to keep MAP high (≥90 mm Hg) both prior to and following positioning to ensure adequate spinal cord perfusion pressure.

Assuming no untoward changes in neurophysiologic homeostasis with positioning, multimodality monitoring during cervical spine surgery may proceed as follows. When surgery involves the upper cervical spine (i.e., C1 to C4), SSEPs need only include responses to upper extremity stimulation; however, below C4 it is imperative to include lower extremity (posterior tibial or peroneal nerve) SSEPs to monitor the entire neuraxis. In the latter situation, upper extremity SSEPs act to complement their lower extremity counterparts, both as a cross-check of proximal cervical spinal cord integrity and as protection against impending brachial plexus injury. TcMEPs should be used as the primary measure of spinal cord integrity unless severe myelopathy precludes recordable responses. (**Caveat:** There is a minority of severely myelopathic patients for whom TcMEPs simply are unrecordable, regardless of changes in stimulation or recording parameters. By comparison, there are many more such patients who present either with unmonitorable or poorly defined SSEPs, which would preclude any monitoring at all if TcMEPS were not available.)

For anterior procedures TcMEPs should be recorded following placement of vertebral body distracters, because decompression approaches the posterior longitudinal ligament and because it involves the spinal cord dura. TcMEPs also should be recorded prior to and following application of weight or neck extension (i.e., water-ski maneuver) for vertebral body distraction, impaction of interbody fusion graft, and placement of internal fixation devices that either may give rise to spinal cord compression or produce concussive injury.

Posterior decompressive and stabilization procedures seem to pose increased risk for neurologic injury to both the spinal cord and the spinal nerve roots (C5 to C6) and warrant more frequent TcMEP recordings. In addition to the potential for injury during laminectomy/foraminotomy in patients with cervical spondylitic myelopathy, there is high risk of both compressive and

---

IONM MONITORING FOR SPINAL CORD AND BRACHIAL PLEXUS PROTECTION DURING INTUBATION AND POSITIONING FOR CERVICAL SPINE SURGERY

- Postinduction preintubation baseline TcMEPs
- Postintubation TcMEPs, ulnar and posterior tibial nerve SSEPs
- Postpositioning TcMEPs and SSEPs
- TcMEPs and SSEPs during and following weight application
- Ulnar nerve SSEPs following shoulder taping

INTERVENTIONAL STEPS WHEN TcMEP AND/OR SSEP AMPLITUDE(S) DECREASE DURING INTUBATION AND POSITIONING FOR CERVICAL SPINE SURGERY

- During or following intubation
  - Neck flexion
- Following shoulder taping
  - Release the tape and reapply after ulnar nerve SSEP amplitudes improves
- Following neck hyperextension or weight application
  - Neck flexion and reposition
  - Release weight
  - Raise MAP to 90 mm Hg
  - Consider terminating surgery if no amplitude recovery within 20 minutes
- Following prone positioning
  - Reposition head
  - Reposition supine if no amplitude recovery
  - Consider terminating surgery if no amplitude recovery within 20 minutes

vascular injury in those with upper cervical spine instability due to fracture or degenerative disease. The potential for vascular injury in these cases is due in part to the proximity of the vertebral and anterior spinal arteries. For these patients it is important to use SSEPs not only because they augment TcMEPs in detecting compressive injury, but also because of their sensitivity to compromised spinal cord and brainstem blood flow. Although compromise of spinal cord blood supply by direct injury to the vertebral artery is relatively rare, changes in neurologic function due to inadequate spinal cord perfusion are not. In our experience the vast majority of intraoperative changes identified in this surgery are due primarily to inadequate blood pressure, which leaves the spinal cord with insufficient reserves to withstand the surgical manipulations needed for corrective management.[13,15] It is our clinical philosophy to have anesthesia maintain MAP at 75 mm Hg or greater once the exposure is completed. In this way, lower blood pressures during exposure reduce blood loss, whereas higher ones during corrective surgical maneuvers provide a vascular safety margin when the spinal cord is placed under surgical stress.

In addition to iatrogenic spinal cord injury, spinal nerve root palsy remains an unsolved complication after laminectomy or laminoplasty for cervical myelopathy. The cause of the iatrogenic radiculopathy has been attributed to the posterior migration of the spinal cord after decompression causing stretching and edema of the affected nerve roots, most commonly C5 and C6. Although most patients recover spontaneously after transient nerve root palsy, some patients need further surgical intervention, including foraminotomy, durotomy, or additional anterior decompression to relieve the tethered nerve roots. Until recently this complication has gone undetected intraoperatively due to the relative insensitivity of SSEPs and dermatomal evoked potentials (dEPs) to such decompression-induced nerve root injuries. We have added TcMEP and spontaneous electromyographic recordings from deltoid and biceps muscles whenever the C5 and C6 nerve roots are at risk for iatrogenic injury.

There has been ongoing debate as to the value of dEPs in IONM. After a decade of recording intraoperative dEPs to assess the adequacy of cervical or lumbar spinal nerve root decompression, we have concluded that successful recording is dependent on two factors: (1) use of a total intravenous anesthetic[14] and (2) careful patient selection. Because these cortical dEPs are quite fragile, any concentration of nitrous oxide or potent inhalational agent precludes reliable recording. Moreover, dEPs are only of potential value in patients who are undergoing surgical decompression for acute ($\leq$6 months) radicular symptoms. In patients with myelopathic signs or those with longer-standing radicular symptoms, dEPs become much more difficult both to record and to interpret owing to axonal changes. Technically the level of electrical stimulation must be held low so as not to spread either to another dermatome or to a mixed nerve. Excessive averaging also will result in such amplitude degradation that the results will be uninterpretable.[10]

INTRAOPERATIVE MONITORING DURING THORACIC SPINE SURGERY

In contrast to cervical spine surgery, there is almost universal agreement about the need for IONM during thoracic spine surgery. Spinal cord protection clearly is of paramount importance during single-stage anterior, posterior, or combined anterior/posterior spinal fusion.

Many of the principles described for IONM during cervical spine surgery also hold for thoracic spine procedures. In particular, it no longer is adequate or acceptable to monitor the thoracic spinal cord solely on the basis of lower extremity mixed nerve SSEPs. Patients undergoing corrective spine surgery to address scoliotic deformities, fractures, and neoplastic and degenerative disease are at risk for diverse causes of iatrogenic injury to the spinal cord at different times during these procedures, thereby mandating a multimodality approach to IONM.

Iatrogenic spinal cord injury during thoracic spine surgery often occurs as a result of mechanical or ischemic insult. Mechanical injury can result from direct spinal cord contusion or concussion during placement or adjustment of instrumentation. Ischemic injury usually results from inadequate spinal cord perfusion secondary to vascular compromise and/or hypotension. Stretching of spinal cord vascular supplies following the application of distractive and compressive forces for scoliosis correction is a primary factor leading to spinal cord shock. Because these injuries can produce differential loss of sensory and motor function, the key to successful intraoperative monitoring is careful measurement and cross-checking of function with SSEPs and TcMEPs following each critical maneuver or event. Prior to surgery, monitoring should be used to guard against spinal cord and brachial plexus injury associated with patient positioning, as described previously. Upper extremity SSEPs should be rechecked periodically during long surgical procedures to identify and prevent impending brachial plexus and/or peripheral nerve

---

IONM STRATEGY DURING CERVICAL SPINE SURGERY

- C1 to C4
  - Combined TcMEPs, and SSEPs for monitoring spinal cord motor and sensory tracts
- C5 to C7
  - Combined TceMEPs, and SSEPs for monitoring spinal cord motor and sensory tracts
  - TcMEPs and spontaneous EMG (spEMG) from deltoid and biceps muscles for monitoring C5 to C6 nerve roots
  - C5 to C8 dermatomal evoked potentials (dEPs) for monitoring C5 to C8 sensory nerve root only in cases with limited acute (i.e., 6.0 mo) radicular symptoms

injury.[14] Upper extremity SSEPs and TcMEPs can also serve as controls to exclude technical and global physiologic explanations for changes in corresponding lower extremity recordings.

Anterior thoracic spine surgery includes discectomy, vertebrectomy, and spinal cord decompression and fusion with interbody strut bone graft or cage. Because the ventral spinal cord is at increased risk from this surgical approach, TcMEPs should be recorded frequently from anterior tibialis and/or gastrocnemius and one other lower extremity muscle group, such as the foot flexors.

The spinal cord is at increased risk for ischemic injury during anterior procedures if segmental arteries are ligated. Although there is still some debate about the need for monitoring during segmental artery ligation,[18,26] our experience together with that of others[15,20] suggests that monitoring is extremely important in light of the potential consequences of ischemic injury to the spinal cord. As the main source of arterial blood to the spinal cord, anterior segmental arteries supply the ventral two thirds of the cord. Occlusion of major feeder vessels, such as the artery of Adamkiewicz, can cause spinal cord infarction resulting in paraplegia. The only way to identify these nutrient feeder vessels reliably is to test them provacatively prior to ligation.

We routinely monitor segmental artery ligation using TcMEPs, owing to their sensitivity to ischemic spinal cord injury.[7,13,15] A new baseline TcMEP is usually obtained prior to test clamping. The segmental artery is temporarily clamped for 3 minutes, and TcMEPs are rerecorded. If TcMEPs show amplitude degradation >50% on one or both sides with no clinical changes in the upper extremity muscle responses, the clamp is released immediately and further manipulations are interrupted until there is full recovery. Figure 8-1 presents data recorded during anterior/posterior spinal fusion for correction of scoliosis, in which lower extremity muscle TcMEPs almost disappeared bilaterally after clamping of the T11 segmental artery. Twenty seconds after the clamp was released TcMEPs showed improvement, and after 4 minutes they had recovered fully. This type of provocative testing is especially warranted when the patient undergoes a long single-stage combined procedure, which usually involves sacrifice of several segmental arteries, heavy blood loss, and hypotension. Any disruption of spinal cord perfusion after ligation of a major nutrient-feeding vessel will predispose the cord to ischemic injury and jeopardize its ability to withstand the stress associated with the application of strong multiplane corrective forces from rigid spinal instrumentation. For this same reason we advocate staged anterior and posterior spinal fusion to allow reestablishment of spinal cord homeostasis after anterior spinal release, especially for patients with severe kyphoscoliosis or difficulties maintaining a stable blood pressure. (**Caveat:** To avoid inadequate spinal cord perfusion resulting from hypotension, MAP should be kept

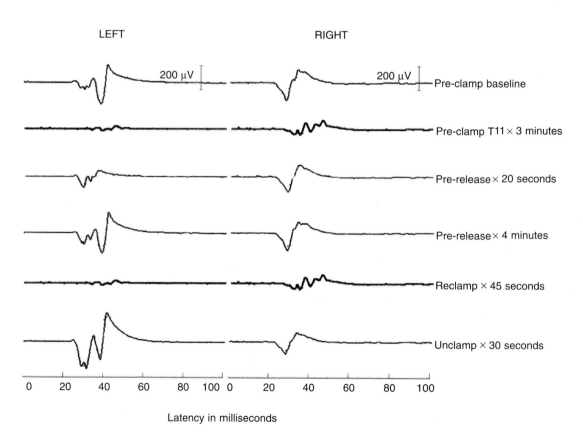

LEFT   RIGHT

200 µV

Pre-clamp baseline

Pre-clamp T11 × 3 minutes

Pre-release × 20 seconds

Pre-release × 4 minutes

Reclamp × 45 seconds

Unclamp × 30 seconds

0   20   40   60   80   100   0   20   40   60   80   100

Latency in milliseconds

Figure 8-1.   Neurophysiologic evidence of impending spinal cord ischemia secondary to temporary clipping of a nutrient-feeding segmental artery.

at 75 mm Hg for adults, above 65 mm Hg for children, and not below 80% of the baseline MAP for patients with preexisting hypertension.)

Posterior thoracic spine surgery often involves laminectomy and placement of various sublaminar and pedicle hooks, sublaminar wires/cables, and/or pedicle screws. The spinal cord is therefore at direct risk for contusion or stretch injury, which accounts for the majority of surgical alerts in these cases.

In cases of scoliosis or kyphosis, the deformity is usually corrected with three-dimensional derotation, distraction, and compression of the spinal column, which produce powerful stretching forces over the spinal cord and its vascular supplies. Lower extremity SSEPs should be monitored continuously to detect mechanical compression or vascular insufficiency, supplemented by TcMEPs recorded prior to and after every major maneuver.

If SSEP amplitude decreases greater than 50% in relation to a surgical manipulation, and/or TcMEPs show amplitude degradation of 75% or greater, the surgeon should be asked to pause temporarily from further surgical manipulation. (**Caveat:** Contrary to popular belief, we have not found latency to be of any significance in the interpretation of spinal cord monitoring data. We presume that the ubiquitous interpretation of 10% latency shift as the neurophysiologic signature of impending spinal cord injury leads to unnecessary false-positive alerts.)

The surgical maneuver thought to have provoked the event should be reversed, and the MAP should be raised to 90 mm Hg or greater to facilitate increased spinal cord perfusion. It is also good practice to initiate a spinal cord injury dose of steroids to minimize the adverse effects of intraoperative or postoperative edema. If TcMEPs recover to at least 50% of baseline amplitude over the next 10 to 20 minutes and SSEPs also start to recover, the surgery may resume with added caution. Otherwise, all instrumentation should be removed and surgery terminated to avoid further disturbance to the spinal cord. (See Schwartz[13] for a detailed decision matrix related to appropriate interventional strategies during thoracic spine surgery.)

RECOMMENDED INTERVENTION WHEN THERE IS SIGNIFICANT TcMEP OR SSEP AMPLITUDE CHANGE DURING CERVICAL OR THORACIC SPINE SURGERY

- Increase mean arterial pressure to 90 mm Hg.
- Initiate spinal cord injury steroid protocol.
- Adjust or remove interbody fusion graft.
- Adjust internal plate fixation.
- Remove sublaminar wire, laminar hook, thoracic pedicle screw, etc.
- Release distraction, derotation, or other corrective forces.
- Unclamp segmental vessel and consider sparing.
- Consider terminating surgery and removing all hardware if minimal or no amplitude recovery.

Special attention should be paid to sublaminar wires during and following passage because they may protrude into the spinal canal inadvertently, thereby causing spinal cord contusion. During tightening and application of powerful translational forces to the apex vertebrae and midline, there is heightened risk for spinal cord trauma as depicted in Figure 8-2. Observe the absence of any clinically significant changes in the SSEP and TcMEP responses up through the time that the wires were all passed. Upon tightening, however, there was a 50% decrease in the SSEP amplitude and, more importantly, complete loss of the TcMEPs recorded over anterior tibialis muscles. Consistent with our intervention protocol, surgery was temporarily halted, and the anesthesiologist was asked to raise the MAP from 68 to 95 mm Hg. Because TcMEPs were completely obliterated, the decision was made also to administer a spinal cord injury dose of methylprednisolone. Although the SSEP amplitude was noted to improve only 12 minutes following intervention, there was no change in the TcMEPs even after 15 to 20 minutes. Accordingly the surgeon was advised to remove the hardware and close. Ten minutes later the left TcMEP reemerged but at a reduced amplitude and distorted morphology, whereas the right leg response remained absent. The presence of improved posterior tibial nerve cortical SSEPs and unilateral reemergence of the TcMEP over the left anterior tibialis muscle led to the conclusion that the child would show postoperative left leg weakness and right leg paralysis. Upon anesthesia emergence these predictions were verified by physical examination. The timely identification of this neural injury in the making and immediate interventional steps to reverse the traumatic effects resulted in transient neurologic sequelae with complete return of bilateral function within 7 days.

INTRAOPERATIVE NEUROPHYSIOLOGIC MONITORING DURING LUMBOSACRAL SPINE SURGERY

An infrequent but possible complication of lumbosacral spine surgery and associated instrumentation is iatrogenic change in the functional status of lumbosacral spinal nerve roots, which result in sensory and/or motor deficits postoperatively. Consistent with the principals governing cervical and thoracic spine surgery, IONM during lumbar surgery provides the surgeon with essential timely information concerning altered neural function, thereby enabling reversal of potentially damaging surgical maneuvers, thus avoiding postoperative sequelae.

There is an increasing number of lumbosacral spine procedures, such as nonunions, spine instability, deformities, tumors, and trauma, during which intraoperative neuromonitoring is both applicable and helpful. Commonly monitored procedures include surgery for anterior interbody fusion (with either fusion cage or femoral ring), anterior vertebrectomy with strut graft and/or internal fixation device, and 360-degree fusions. A partial list of posterior surgeries monitored includes pedicle screw fixation and fusion, multilevel laminectomy for spinal stenosis, laminectomy with interbody

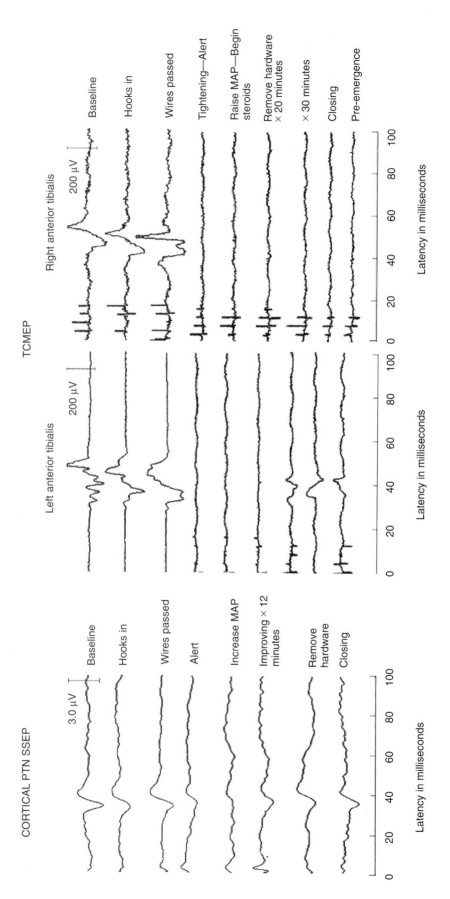

Figure 8-2. Neurophysiologic evidence of impending spinal cord shock following tightening of segmental wires and application of translational forces.

INTRAOPERATIVE NEUROPHYSIOLOGIC MONITORING (IONM) DURING LUMBAR SPINE SURGERY

AT OR ABOVE THE CONUS—NEED TO MONITOR SPINAL CORD AND NERVE ROOTS
- TcMEPs from lower extremity muscles
- PTN SSEPs
- spEMG from lower extremity and anal sphincter muscles to identify nerve root trauma during decompression, pedicle probing, pedicle marking, and pedicle screw placement
- stEMG for ensuring absence of cortical fracture following pedicle screw insertion

BELOW THE CONUS—NEED TO MONITOR NERVE ROOTS ONLY
- spEMG from lower extremity muscles to identify nerve root trauma during decompression, pedicle probing, pedicle marking, and pedicle screw placement
- stEMG for ensuring absence of cortical fracture following pedicle screw insertion
- spEMG from anal sphincter muscle if thecal sac is retracted for insertion of a fusion cage

---

fusion, cages, and laminectomy for excision of spinal nerve root tumors.

For spine cases corresponding to the level of the conus medullaris, such as an L1-L2 burst fracture, it is necessary to monitor both spinal cord and spinal nerve root function. The methods used to monitor both sensory and motor spinal cord function include SSEPs and TcMEPs that are identical to those reported previously for IONM during cervical and thoracic spine surgeries. Distal to L2 the neurophysiologist must make a paradigm shift and concentrate exclusively on monitoring spinal nerve roots.[19]

Early attempts at monitoring lumbosacral spinal nerve root function were based solely on unimodality SSEPs recorded either to femoral, peroneal, and/or posterior tibial nerve stimulation. This method is not suited for segmental nerve monitoring and is ineffectual due to the multiple nerve root entry of these mixed nerves. Because the mixed posterior tibial nerve has innervations from the L4 to S1 spinal nerve roots, it is entirely possible to miss a significant iatrogenic injury to an individual spinal nerve root due to the "masking effect" from contributions of the remaining intact spinal nerve roots as is illustrated in Figure 8-3. During the posterior portion of an anterior/posterior L2 corpectomy and subsequent fusion, the surgeon was retracting the thecal sac to gain access to an osteophytic deformity. Immediately upon retraction, there was significant high-amplitude, high-frequency spontaneous neurotonic electromyographic (spEMG) train activity from the left tibialis anterior muscle, thereby prompting immediate surgical alert. In response, the retraction was released, and the neurotonic activity subsided within 3 minutes. The surgery was completed, and the patient awoke

without any additional neurologic defects, consistent with the intraoperative neurophysiologic data. The salient feature of this example is not necessarily the spEMG activity, although this was pertinent to injury prevention, but rather the unchanged left posterior tibial nerve cortical SSEP during the intraoperative alert. Thus, mixed nerve SSEPs should not be used exclusively during monitoring of lumbosacral spinal nerve roots, but they should only be used as an adjunct to other modalities of neuromonitoring.

Other modalities of intraoperative monitoring that are more sensitive and specific to segmental spinal nerve root function or irritation include dEPs and electromyography, including both spEMG and stimulated EMG (stEMG). When dEPs are being used to monitor lower extremity spinal nerve root function, it is critical that the surgeon communicate to the neurophysiologist what level is being decompressed because only one stimulation site at a time can be utilized. Reliable communication is essential because it is impossible for the neurophysiologist to know at what level the surgeon is working. The merits and limitations of dEPs were covered earlier in the section on intraoperative cervical spine monitoring.

In addition to myelopathic signs precluding successful lower extremity dEPs, it is our experience that multilevel lumbosacral spinal stenosis or peripheral neuropathy secondary to systemic disease also precludes accurate monitoring of lower extremity dEPs. Evidence that lower extremity dermatomal areas overlap has been documented in the literature for several years. Kadish and Simmons[4] have shown a 14% incidence of nerve root anomalies, including anomalous levels of origin. Considering these confounding factors that complicate accurate intraoperative monitoring of spinal nerve root function by dEPs exclusively, it is important to rely on spEMG and stimulated EMG (stEMG) for monitoring the lumbosacral spine with occasional supplementary use of dEPs as needed.

Spontaneous EMG is used to minimize neural trauma to lumbosacral spinal nerve roots during decompression, hook or screw insertion, removal of bony fragments, tumor resection, distraction, or traction. EMG requires the absence of neuromuscular junction paralysis. Fortuitously, microtrauma to a spinal nerve root provokes ion depolarization, and the resultant muscle or motor unit potential can be recorded from a muscle innervated by that specific nerve root. Abrupt traction or mechanical contact with the spinal nerve root appears to be the most efficient stimulus for eliciting train or burst neurotonic activity, respectively. Gradual traction may elicit smaller or even no response. Thermal injury to a spinal nerve root can also evoke train potentials. Although bipolar cautery does restrict electrical current spread as compared with monopolar cautery, heat can still spread to adjacent neural tissue either by conduction or convection. An important concept to remember is that neuromonitoring is often precluded during electrocautery due to high-amplitude electrical artifact; therefore when bipolar cautery is necessary adjacent to neural tissue, it should be performed intermittently with

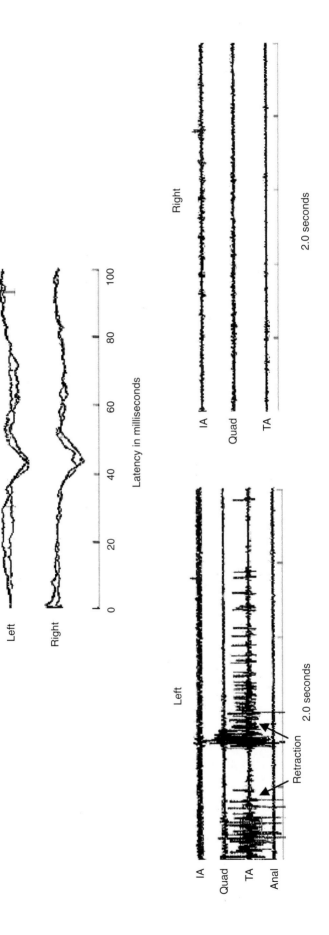

Figure 8-3. Absence of change in mixed posterior tibial nerve SSEPs with excessive surgical retraction of the thecal sac in the presence of significant neurotonic discharge evident on the spontaneous electromyographic (spEMG) recording.

brief periods to allow the neurophysiologist to assess neurologic function with artifact-free recordings.

Chronically compressed spinal nerve roots are often very sensitive and can exhibit train or burst activity to even mild surgical manipulation. Train potentials indicate some degree of spinal nerve root trauma and when present represent injury-related potentials that require immediate pause from surgical manipulation or release of traction until the activity subsides. In contrast, burst potentials resulting from mechanical contact with the spinal nerve root only rarely indicate microtrauma and surgical pause is therefore not indicated.

Spontaneous EMG neuromonitoring is also warranted whenever interbody fusion with cage instrumentation is utilized. Depending on the level of interbody cage placement, spEMG should be recorded from the following myotomes: L1—iliopsoas, L2—adductor, L3 to L4—vastus lateralis, L4 to L5—tibialis anterior, S1—gastrocnemius, and S2 to S5—external anal sphincter. During discectomy and subsequent placement of the interbody cage anteriorly and/or retraction of the thecal sac posteriorly, it is imperative to monitor not only the spinal nerves emerging through the intervertebral foramen between each of two adjacent vertebrae, but also all distal spinal nerve roots contained within the thecal sac. The distal spinal nerves within the thecal sac are subject to the distractive, concussive, and retraction forces used to impact and place an interbody cage. Figure 8-4 depicts an intraoperative surgical alert during

retraction of thecal sac prior to placement of a posterior L4 to L5 fusion cage. SpEMGs monitored from tibialis anterior and perianal muscles demonstrate significant neurotonic train activity from external anal sphincter muscles signifying excessive traction on the lower sacral roots, which subsided with immediate release of retraction. Clearly, inability to identify this precursor to serious sacral nerve root injury could have resulted in postoperative neurologic disaster.

Transpedicular screw fixation of the lumbosacral spine has become commonplace. Several studies have documented neurologic and/or mechanical complications as a result of improper screw trajectory resulting in a medial breech of the pedicle cortex and possible spinal nerve root injury.[1,6] Electrical impedance measurements reveal that the resistivity of cortical bone is 16,000 Ohms at low frequencies.[2] We know from basic research and from intraoperative monitoring data that an intact pedicle cortex will provide adequate impedance to current flow to prevent depolarization of a spinal nerve root at stimulus levels of at least 5.0 to 8.0 mA above the root's depolarization electrical threshold. If therefore one stimulates a spinal nerve root directly and it depolarizes with a stimulus intensity of 2.0 mA and then one stimulates the screw in the adjacent pedicle cortex at 10.0 mA with negative test results, (i.e., no compound muscle action potential [CMAP]), then there is strong rational evidence that the pedicle cortex is intact. These clinical findings have

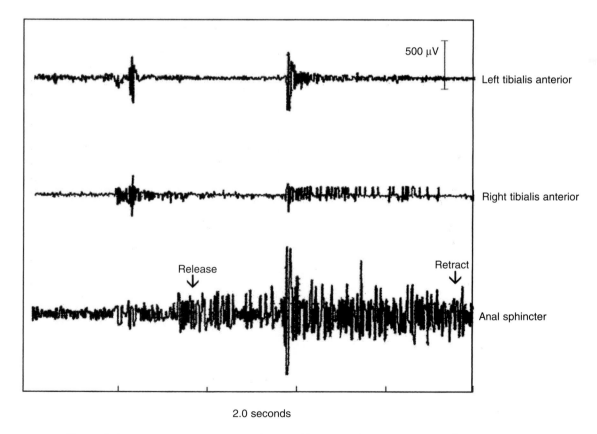

Figure 8-4. Spontaneous EMG evidence of low sacral nerve root injury following retraction of thecal sac prior to placement of posterior L4 to L5 BAK cage.

also been verified most recently by Toleikis et al.[23] Conversely, if the screw inadvertently perforated the pedicle, the resistance of the formerly intact cortical bone would be low, and because current follows the path of least resistance, it would flow through the medial breach to the nerve root. The current would provoke ion depolarization, and the subsequent CMAP can be recorded from a muscle innervated by that specific nerve root as illustrated in Figure 8-5. In this case, stimulation of the right S1 pedicle screw resulted in a large CMAP from the right gastrocnemius muscle, whereas that on the left side was expectedly silent. Accordingly the surgeon was asked to remove the screw and redirect such that the tip would be against intact bony cortex. Subsequent restimulation failed to produce a recordable CMAP.

Recently data were presented that reported higher electrical stimulation intensity is sometimes required to depolarize a chronically compressed or ischemic nerve root.[3] A chronically compressed and irritated nerve root might have thickened dura or fewer large-diameter functional fibers available for depolarization. Alternatively it can be demyelinated, have axonal degeneration, or can be ischemic as possible explanations accounting for its higher electrical threshold. This higher depolarization threshold could have a direct effect on the efficacy of stEMG for detection of cortical perforation. If upon direct stimulation a chronically compressed root was observed to depolarize at 6.0 mA rather than at the usual 1.0 to 2.0 mA, it is possible that the normal 10.0 mA screw-stimulation level would be too low and could fail to depolarize, thereby resulting in a false-negative test. To adapt to compressed spinal nerve roots that exhibit elevated electrical thresholds, we apply the following method: The surgeon is asked to stimulate the most pathologic root directly. If direct stimulation reveals a depolarization threshold of 5.0 mA, then instead of stimulating the screw at 10.0 mA we compensate for the elevated depolarization threshold and stimulate at 15 mA. If there is no CMAP recorded at this stimulus level, the pedicle cortex should be intact. If the most pathologic root fires at (X) mA, it would be justified to extrapolate that the rest of the spinal nerve roots would have similar or lower electrical thresholds.

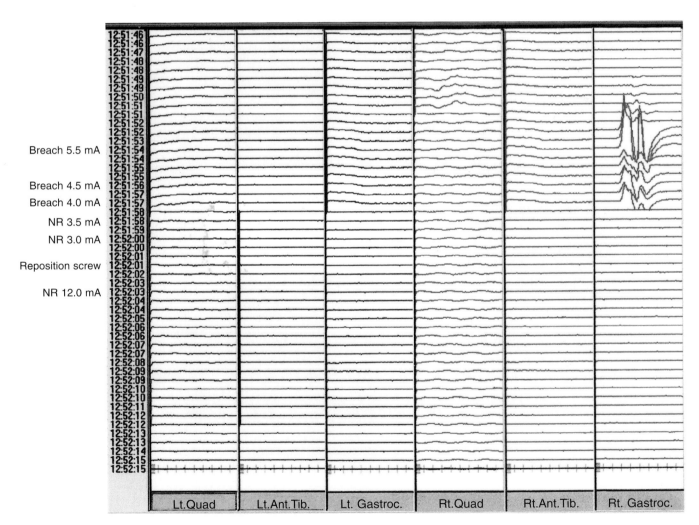

Figure 8-5. Stimulated EMG evidence of a significant breach of the right S1 pedicle cortex following bone screw insertion.

> ## SPINAL CORD AND NERVE ROOT MONITORING
>
> - Do not monitor spinal cord or nerve root integrity solely by SSEPs; use:
>   - TcMEPs
>   - Extensive clinical experience shows safety and efficacy
>   - Incorporate as direct intraoperative measure of efferent motor tracts
>   - Debatable: IONM for one- or two-level anterior cervical discectomies with or without interbody fusion; in favor of routine monitoring is identification of extensive neck extension, impending brachial plexopathy, C5 nerve root injury, or recurrent laryngeal nerve palsy

CONCLUSIONS

The scope of intraoperative neurophysiologic monitoring practice has broadened extensively in the past few years. No longer is it appropriate to rely on unimodality SSEPs to ensure spinal cord or nerve root integrity. The clinical safety and efficacy of TcMEPs have now been shown through extensive clinical experience. TcMEPs are so exquisitely sensitive to spinal cord injury that failure to incorporate this modality as a direct intraoperative measure of the efferent motor tracts will greatly impact the quality of patient care.

IONM during anterior cervical spine surgery, particularly single- or two-level discectomy with or without interbody fusion, continues to be a topic of debate. Opponents claim that the possibility of spinal cord injury is so remote that the cost of IONM is unjustified. Proponents, on the other hand, are able to attest not only to the direct benefits of identifying excessive neck extension with weight traction, vertebral body distraction, spinal cord concussion from an overimpacted fusion graft or ischemic injury, but also to tangential benefits such as identification of impending brachial plexus, C5 nerve root injury, or recurrent laryngeal nerve palsy. It would appear that the overall cost of IONM for a cervical discectomy, regardless of the presumed level of risk, pales in relation to that for iatrogenic injury to any associated neural element. It is not uncommon to have neurophysiologic alerts for impending brachial plexopathy from shoulder overtraction, C5 nerve root injury during anterior and/or posterior decompression, overextension of the neck due to excessive weight, and the like, which justify continuation of monitoring all cervical spine surgeries on a routine basis.

ACKNOWLEDGMENT

We wish to acknowledge the contributions of our colleagues at Surgical Monitoring Associates, who continuously strive to raise the threshold for excellence in IONM. Their support and dedication to the provision of superior quality of patient care is unmatched in this field.

SELECTED REFERENCES

Schwartz DM et al.: Neurophysiological monitoring during scoliosis surgery: a multimodality approach, *Semin Spine Surg* 9:97-111, 1997.

Schwartz DM et al.: Neurophysiological identification of iatrogenic neural injury during complex spine surgery, *Semin Spine Surg* 10:242-251, 1998.

Toleikis JR et al.: Spinally elicited peripheral nerve responses are sensory rather than motor, *Clin Neurophysiol* 111:736-742, 2000.

Toleikis JR et al.: The usefulness of electrical stimulation for assessing pedicle screw placement, *J Spinal Disord* 13:283-289, 2000.

REFERENCES

1. Esses SI, Sachs BL, Dreyzin V: Complications associated with the technique of pedicle screw fixation: a selected survey of ABS members, *Spine* 18:2231-2239, 1993.
2. Geddes LA, Baker LE: The specific resistance of biological material: a compendium of data for the biomedical engineer and physiologist, *Med Biol Eng* 5:271-293, 1967.
3. Holland NR et al.: Higher electrical stimulus intensities are required to activate chronically compressed nerve roots, *Spine* 23:224-227, 1998.
4. Kadish LJ, Simmons EH: Anomalies of the lumbosacral nerve roots: an anatomical investigation and myelographic study, *J Bone Joint Surg Br* 66(3):411-416, 1984.
5. Kostuik JP: Point of view, *Spine* 21:1223-1224, 1996.
6. Lubitz SE, Keith RW, Crawfor AH: Intraoperative experience with neuromotor evoked potentials, *Spine* 24:2030-2034, 1999.
7. Matsuzaki H et al.: Problems and solutions of pedicle screw plate fixation of lumbar spine, *Spine* 15:1159-1165, 1990.
8. Meylaerts SA et al.: Comparison of transcranial motor evoked potentials and somatosensory evoked potentials during thoracoabdominal aortic aneurysm repair, *Ann Surg* 230(6):742-749, 1999.
9. Owen JH: The application of intraoperative monitoring during surgery for spinal deformity, *Spine* 24:2649-2662, 1999.
10. Owen JH et al.: The clinical application of neurogenic motor evoked potentials to monitor spinal cord function during surgery, *Spine* 16(8 Suppl):S385-S390, 1991.
11. Péréon Y et al.: Successful monitoring of neurogenic mixed evoked potentials elicited by anterior spinal cord stimulation through thorocoscopy during spine surgery, *Spine* 24:2025-2029, 1999.
12. Rose RD: Sensory component of cervically elicited motor potentials, *Med Hypotheses* 46:577-579, 1996.
13. Schwartz DM: Intraoperative neurophysiological monitoring during cervical spine surgery, *Oper Tech Orthop* 6:6-12, 1996.
14. Schwartz DM, Drummond DS, Ecker ML: Influence of rigid spinal instrumentation on the neurogenic motor evoked potential, *J Spinal Disord* 9:439-445, 1996.
15. Schwartz DM et al.: Prevention of positional brachial plexopathy during surgical correction of scoliosis, *J Spinal Disord* 13:178-182, 2000.
16. Schwartz DM et al.: Neurophysiological monitoring during scoliosis surgery: a multimodality approach, *Semin Spine Surg* 9:97-111, 1997.
17. Schwartz DM et al: Influence of nitrous-oxide on posterior-tibial nerve cortical somatosensory evoked potentials, *J Spinal Disord* 10:80-86, 1997.
18. Schwartz DM et al.: Neurophysiological identification of iatrogenic neural injury during complex spine surgery, *Semin Spine Surg* 10:242-251, 1998.
19. Schwartz DM, Sestokas K, Wierzbowski LR: Intraoperative neurophysiological monitoring during surgery for spinal instability, *Semin Spine Surg* 8:318-331, 1996.
20. Su CF et al.: "Backfiring" in spinal cord monitoring: high thoracic spinal cord stimulation evoked sciatic response by antidromic sensory pathway conduction, not motor tract conduction, *Spine* 17:504-508, 1992.
21. Toleikis JR et al.: Spinally elicited neurogenic motor evoked potentials (NMEPs) assess sensory rather than motor function, *J Clin Neurophys* 16:169, 1999.
22. Toleikis JR et al.: Spinally elicited peripheral nerve responses are sensory rather than motor, *Clin Neurophysiol* 111:736-742, 2000.

23. Toleikis JR et al.: The usefulness of electrical stimulation for assessing pedicle screw placement, *J Spinal Disord* 13:283-289, 2000.
24. Wilson-Holden TJ et al.: Efficacy of intraoperative monitoring for pediatric patients with spinal cord pathology undergoing spinal deformity surgery, *Spine* 24:1685-1692, 1999.
25. Wilson-Holden TJ et al.: A prospective comparison of neurogenic mixed evoked potential stimulation methods: utility of epidural elicitation during posterior spinal surgery, *Spine* 25:2364-2371, 2000.
26. Winter RB et al.: Paraplegia resulting from vessel ligation, *Spine* 21:1232-1234, 1996.

Bone Graft and Fusion-Enhancing Substances: Practical Applications of Gene Therapy

K. Craig Boatright, Scott D. Boden

Despite many shortcomings, bone grafting is the current clinical method employed for biologic enhancement of spinal fusion. Understanding the events leading to fusion with bone graft helps direct research efforts to develop bone graft substitutes. Bone graft substitutes are being tested with success in multiple animal models, and recently the first successful human trials have occurred. Growth factors in combination with structural substances are the focus of this research to generate the ideal bone-forming environment. Future advances in biologic enhancement of bone formation will likely include gene therapy techniques, now in the early phases of investigation.

The first step in the systematic search for a superior bone generator is to gain a more complete understanding of the biology of spinal fusion. The well-studied set of events surrounding fracture healing of long bones and healing of segmental defects in long bones differs greatly from the incorporation of bone graft that occurs at the site of a spinal fusion mass. The biologic environment differs even between the various types of fusions found in the spine. The compressive environment of an interbody fusion is quite different from that found in posterolateral intertransverse process fusions,[60] the most common type of spinal arthrodesis performed in clinical practice.[52] Compressive forces play a much less significant role in intertransverse fusion since consolidation is necessary prior to any weight bearing by a newly formed posterolateral bone mass.[58]

The ideal bone generator for clinical use in spinal surgery will function to induce the migration of cells capable of becoming bone-forming cells and then activate the system of signals necessary to effect these cells to differentiate into osteoblasts. This bone generator must also supply the proper spatial environment for these bone-forming cells to function in; this requires that neovascularization occur in proximity to surface areas that provide physiologically resorbable scaffolding to act as a template for the various cells involved in bony remodeling. In this manner the grafted material can be replaced by functional bone that can be maintained physiologically over the patient's lifetime.

Interventions such as the implantation of hardware to better control the local biomechanical environment have improved the success rate of spinal arthrodesis. Still a nonunion rate of 10% to 15% exists.[88,90] Characterization of histologic and corresponding molecular events surrounding posterolateral fusion have led to exciting advances in our understanding of this process (Figures 9-1 to 9-4). This knowledge can be applied to the quest for a superior bone generator to replace autogenous bone graft, the present gold standard. As spinal surgery enters the new millennium, attention is focused on the biology of spine fusion to further enhance the rate of successful arthrodesis.[10]

CLASSIFYING BONE-GENERATING SUBSTANCES

A superior bone generator will need to meet many requirements. As an osteoconductive substance, it will provide the scaffolding that the cells of bone metabolism require. At least one component of the substance must

---

IDEAL BONE GENERATOR

PHYSICAL PROPERTIES
- Provides the proper spatial environment for neovascularization
- Provides a structural template for bone formation
- Is resorbable so new bone can form and provide lifelong physiologically maintainable structural support

BIOCHEMICAL PROPERTIES
- Induce the migration of progenitor cells able to become osteoblasts
- Effect differentiation of progenitor cells into osteoblasts

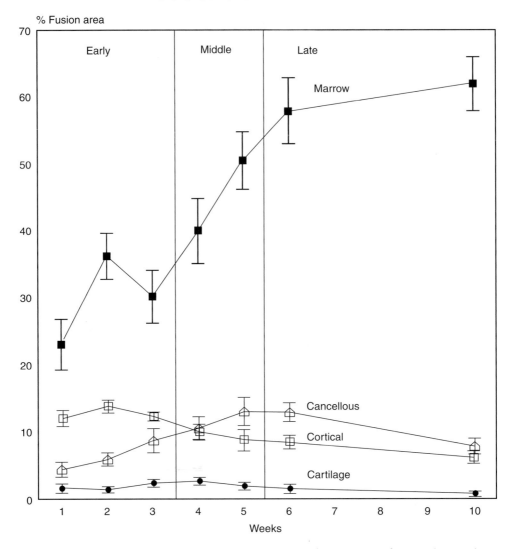

HISTOLOGY OF SPINAL FUSION

Figure 9-1.   Quantitative histologic healing sequence of rabbit spine fusions depicted graphically. Note the continuous increase in bone marrow content of the fusion mass beginning in the early phase and continuing through the late phase of healing. During the middle phase of healing a reversal of the cortical/cancellous bone ratio is seen as well as a small peak in the relative percentage of cartilage corresponding to the central region endochondral ossification. *(From Boden SD et al.: 1995 Volvo Award in Basic Sciences: the use of an osteoinductive growth factor for lumbar spinal fusion. I. The biology of spinal fusion, Spine 20:2626-2632, 1995.)*

provide osteoinduction. This is accomplished by inducing progenitor cells to differentiate into bone-forming cells. Growth factors such as bone morphogenetic proteins (BMPs) function to effect osteoinduction. Through osteoinduction the bone-forming environment becomes osteogenic.

Osteogenesis requires the presence of cells capable of forming bone. Autogenous bone graft is osteogenic under circumstances where osteoblasts remain viable after harvesting and implantation. Only autogenous bone graft and bone marrow contain bone-forming cells initially; all other substances must rely on osteoinduction to establish an osteogenic environment (Table 9-1).

PROPERTIES OF BONE FORMING SUBSTANCES

- *Osteoinduction*—induces differentiation of progenitor cells into bone forming cells
- *Osteoconduction*—provides a physical environment conducive to bone formation
- *Osteogenesis*—contains cells capable of generating bone

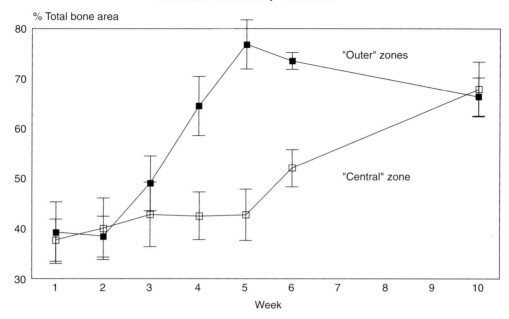

Cancellous Bone Area by Fusion Zone

Figure 9-2. Histologic fusion maturation depicted graphically with measurement of cancellous bone area (mean ± SEM). Note the temporally more advanced fusion maturation in the "outer" zones (near the transverse processes) as compared with the less mature fusion in the "central" zone. A similar temporal sequence of maturation occurred in the "central" zone, but it was delayed in time—"the lag effect." By 10 weeks, fusion maturation (as measured by cancellous bone area) was similar in both zones. *(From Boden SD et al.: 1995 Volvo Award in Basic Sciences: the use of an osteoinductive growth factor for lumbar spinal fusion. Part I: The biology of spinal fusion, Spine 20:2626-2632, 1995.)*

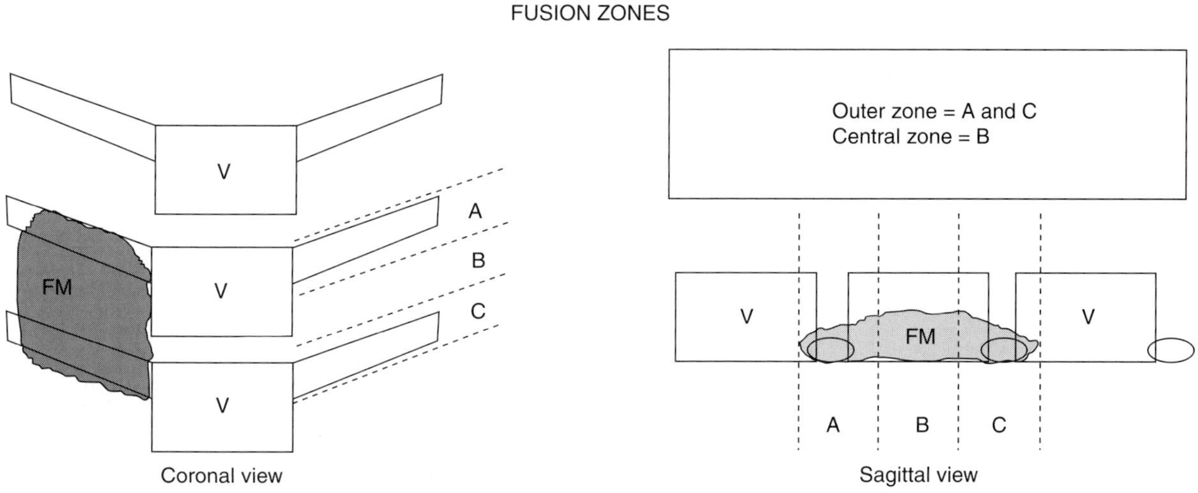

FUSION ZONES

Outer zone = A and C
Central zone = B

V

A
B
C

V

FM

V

Coronal view

V

FM

V

A   B   C

Sagittal view

Figure 9-3. Schematic diagram of lumbar spine fusion mass (*FM*) divided into thirds in the coronal and sagittal views and their relationship to the vertebral bodies (*V*). The two outer zones (*A* and *C*) are distinguished from the central zone (*B*). *(From Morone MA et al.: Gene expression during autograft lumbar spine fusion and the effect of bone morphogenetic protein-2, Clin Orthop 351:252-265, 1998.)*

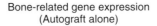

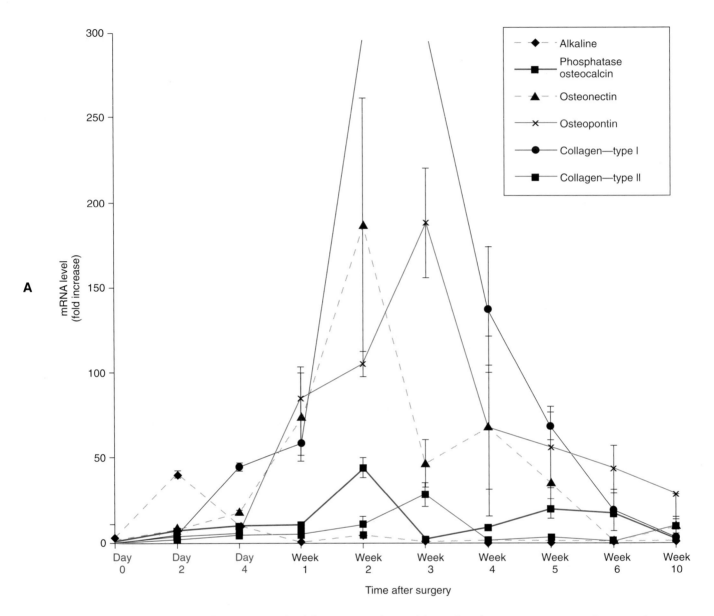

Figure 9-4.　**A,** Graph of the sequential osteoblast-related gene expression in the central zone of rabbit posterolateral spine fusion masses (n = 3 per time point) with autogenous bone graft. The values were determined by semiquantitative reverse transcriptase–polymerase chain reaction (RT-PCR) and expressed as fold increases over the level present in iliac crest bone (Day 0). A reproducible and orderly sequence of gene expression was seen that was paralleled in the central zone (not shown) but delayed by 1 to 3 weeks.

Continued

Available bone graft substitutes can be broadly classified under three major headings: bone graft extender, bone graft enhancer, or bone graft substitute. The terms *extender, enhancer,* and *substitute* all inherently reference the current gold standard, autogenous bone graft. One of the major shortcomings of autograft bone is the finite supply available in each patient. As the term implies, an extender is used to add to obtainable autograft in order to expand both volume and effect of the limited auto-

graft. By definition, rates of fusion are at best equal to that of autograft alone in a successful bone graft extender and autograft combination. In contrast, a bone graft enhancer is a substance that when used in conjunction with autograft will increase the successful rate of fusion above that reported for autograft alone (70% to 90% successful fusion rate) under the specific clinical circumstance. Finally, a bone graft substitute is unique in that it can replace autogenous bone graft by achieving equal

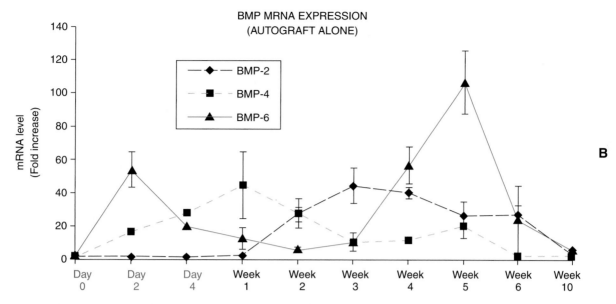

Figure 9-4, cont'd. **B,** BMP gene expression determined by RT-PCR in the outer zone of the spine fusion mass at specific times after surgery. The values of mRNA levels are given as fold increases over the level present in iliac crest bone (Day 0). A reproducible sequence of gene expression was seen with BMP-6 mRNA peaking earliest on Day 2, followed by BMP-4 mRNA, BMP-2 mRNA, and a second peak of BMP-6 mRNA. These results suggest different BMPs have unique temporal patterns of expression during the spine fusion healing process. *(From Morone MA, et al.: Gene expression during autograft lumbar spine fusion and the effect of bone morphogenetic protein-2, Clin Orthop 351:252-265, 1998.)*

Table 9-1	Bone Graft Material Characteristics		
Graft Material	**Osteoinductive**	**Osteoconductive**	**Osteogenic**
Autogenous bone	X	X	X
Allograft bone	X	X	
Bone marrow	?		X
Bone matrix (DBM)	X	X	
Collagen		X	
Ceramic		X	
Growth factors	X		

rates of fusion. A substitute obviates the need for autogenous bone graft harvest, thus avoiding its concomitant morbidity.

Clinical data exist to classify many of the available materials into one of these three categories for various grafting scenarios. Much of this chapter will concentrate on the performance results reported for spinal fusion with each substitute or combination of substitutes.

PRESENT OPTIONS FOR BIOLOGIC ENHANCEMENT OF SPINAL FUSION
Autogenous Bone Graft in Spinal Fusion

During the decade of the 1990s spinal fusion surgery became the most common reason for autologous bone grafting.[66] Despite the fact that autograft bone is osteoconductive, osteoinductive, and osteogenic, it has major

shortcomings as an ideal bone generator. The rate of nonunion after spinal arthrodesis is reported to range from 5% to 35%.[74] As noted earlier, the addition of internal fixation has lowered the nonunion rate, but pseudarthrosis can still be expected in 10% to 15% of instrumented cases when attempting posterolateral lumbar fusion.*

With the utilization of autogenous bone graft, a characteristic set of events must occur for a fusion mass to form.[14,19,58] First, osteoprogenitor cells must enter the fusion area via decortication; this allows cells to escape from the bone marrow into the fusion environment.[77] Differentiation of these cells must be effected in order for them to become osteoblasts. Osteoblasts can then deposit new bone matrix upon the structural component

---

*References 18, 37, 61, 76, 84, 88, 90.

AUTOGRAFT: THE CLINICAL GOLD STANDARD

- Osteoconductive, osteoinductive, and osteogenic
BUT
- Nonunion of 5% to 35%
- Complications in up to 25% of cases
  - Infection
  - Fracture of ileum
  - Abdominal herniations
  - Increased blood loss
  - Longer hospital stays
  - Increased postoperative pain
- Limited supply
  - Multilevel fusions
  - Previous graft harvests

CLINICALLY AVAILABLE BONE GRAFT SUBSTITUTES

- Allograft
- Osteoconductive substances
  - Calcium sulfate
  - Coralline substances
  - Ceramics
  - Collagen
- Osteoinductive substances
  - Demineralized bone matrix

---

of the transplanted bone graft. Finally, remodeling of the initial fusion mass occurs according to Wolff's law; this results in a mature fusion mass that is able to provide long-term, durable stability to the spine.[58]

Aside from the significant nonunion rate, bone graft harvest is associated with well-known complications in up to 25% of cases; these include infection, fracture of the ileum, abdominal herniations, increased blood loss, increased hospital stay, and increased postoperative pain.[2,35,87] In addition, autograft is available in a limited supply that can be inadequate for revisions or multilevel procedures. The clinical track record of autogenous bone graft makes it the present gold standard for spinal arthrodesis, but the motivation to find a superior alternative is obvious.

Allogenic Bone Graft in Spinal Fusion

Performance of allograft bone in spinal fusion varies greatly with each specific clinical scenario. With a few notable exceptions, it has functioned well for anterior structural grafts and poorly when used alone for posterior spinal fusion. It remains the most commonly used bone graft extender.[66]

Methods of sterilization and preservation kill the cells within allograft and damage other soft tissue components including proteins. For this reason, allograft does not function as an osteogenic substance and has only weak osteoinductive potential.[66] Cancellous allograft is the quintessential example of an osteoconductive material.[27,85]

Cortical allografts have been used with success in anterior cervical surgery as structural interbody implants. Fusion rates are reported to be equal to autograft for one-level anterior cervical discectomy and fusion (ACDF) with rates of 95% successful arthrodesis.[86,89] Use of allogenic strut grafts for anterior column support after complete or partial corpectomy is common throughout the spine. In this setting morselized autograft is placed at the site of the construct by most surgeons, and while the allograft strut may take up to a year to incorporate at both ends, clinical sequelae of pseudarthrosis are rare.[53]

With one notable exception, allograft bone as a bone graft substitute has functioned poorly in posterior spinal surgery.[1,51] The exception has been reported in adolescent idiopathic scoliosis where small amounts of local autogenous bone were mixed with allograft chips and found to have a fusion rate equal to iliac crest autograft and local autograft combination. Although this application does not represent use as a true stand-alone bone graft substitute (*local* autograft was added), secondary donor site morbidity was avoided and this was reflected in patient outcome.[31]

Allograft bone functions well for structural support of the anterior column and as a bone graft extender in cases where sufficient autograft is not available. At this time data do not support its use as a stand-alone bone graft substitute in posterior spinal surgery.

Osteoconductive Bone Graft Substitutes

The basic science of osteoconductive materials has centered on the analysis of the porous physical structure of compounds that have demonstrated efficacy as bone graft substitutes. Porosity allows vascularization and provides surface area for adherence of osteogenic cells, including osteoblasts and osteoclasts. The optimal pore size for bony ingrowth has been studied in detail and appears to be between 100 μm and 500 μm with a total porous volume of 75% to 80%.[27,85] The topographic structure of the channels appears to be most successful when it closely resembles that of natural bone. Also critical for the ultimate goal of bony union followed by physiologic remodeling is the ability of a material to be reabsorbed over a time course that encourages bony replacement.[20,46]

Calcium Sulfate

Reported in 1892 by Dresmann, plaster of Paris was the first substance used to fill bony defects in patients. He noted that bony voids filled with this calcium sulfate compound showed evidence of bone ingrowth.[65] Since that time multiple preparations of calcium-containing compounds have been used as bone graft extenders or substitutes with varying success.[75]

Calcium sulfate, the primary ingredient in plaster of Paris, continues to be available for clinical use albeit in a different form than that used by Dresmann in 1892. Compounds of calcium sulfate generate very little foreign body reaction,[65] and osteoclasts actively reabsorb calcium sulfate in a manner similar to physiologic bone remodeling.[73] Despite these desirable traits, previous heterogenous compounds were unreliable and dissolved quickly so that fibrous tissue formed instead of bone. Recently a more crystalline form of calcium sulfate that dissolves at a more predictable rate has become available. This substance is marketed as Osteoset (Wright Bio-Orthopaedics, Arlington, TN) and has shown promising results in several animal models, including a sheep posterolateral fusion model; there it performed as well as autograft.[29] It is marketed for clinical use as "bone void filler."

Coralline Substitutes

Similarity between the exoskeletons of certain naturally occurring marine corals and bone was first recognized by Chiroff[21] in the 1970s. This similarity has been exploited as naturally occurring corals have served as templates for the generation of various implants for bone grafting. The term *coralline* was coined to classify this subset of bone graft substitutes.

One of two general processes is used to prepare marine corals for implantation. The first uses the calcium carbonate exoskeleton directly after it has undergone a detergent-based process to remove the organic phase of the coral organism; this results in the product whose trade name is Biocoral (Inoteb, Saint-Gonnery, France). The second general process converts the calcium carbonate to hydroxyapatite via a hydrothermal exchange reaction known as replamineform. Products produced by this process are Prosteon and Interpore porous hydroxyapatite (Interpore Cross International, Inc, Irvine, CA).[72]

Multiple animal studies have demonstrated the biocompatibility as well as the bioactivity of coralline implants as osteoblasts and vascular tissues readily migrate into their matrix.[3,32,38] Remodeling also occurs as the implants are resorbed and replaced by host bone.[20,46] Remodeling of hydroxyapatite occurs slowly over years, although a newer formulation may resorb quicker. This process is described by Wolff's law and is accomplished via osteoclastic activity similar to physiologic bone remodeling.[20,47,72] Much of this data has been accumulated using long bone defect models, and, despite these encouraging results, these products have not proven to be stand-alone bone graft substitutes, especially in the challenging environment of posterolateral spinal fusion.[7,15]

Ceramics

Ceramic forms of calcium phosphates are formed by heating and pressurizing these nonmetallic materials. While the biocompatibility of these substances has been excellent as a group, bioresorbability has varied among the ceramics. In fact, several ceramic substances have been abandoned because the rate of resorption is too slow. The retained implant creates a stress riser within the fusion mass and thus compromises it mechanically.[48]

An example of poor resorbability is ceramic hydroxyapatite.[20,46,47] At the other extreme of resorbability are the calcium sulfate compounds mentioned earlier.[75] Intermediate are the tricalcium phosphate (TCP) implants that dissolve within 6 weeks, a time course that is still quite short for posterolateral fusion in primates.[41] One strategy used to deal with these shortcomings is to integrate two substances into one composite, thus providing a more favorable timeline of dissolution.[6,54]

Collagen

The use of collagen as a bone graft substitute was suggested by its role in normal bone physiology. Type I collagen functions to catalyze the events surrounding bone formation, acting in both a structural and biochemical manner.[64] The use of collagen as a stand-alone bone graft substitute has been unsuccessful, but it has been found to greatly potentiate the effects of other osteoinductive and osteoconductive substances, including bone marrow[83] and composites of hydroxyapatite and TCP.[50] While collagen has been a successful bone graft extender,[92] its primary future role will likely be as an ingredient in stand-alone bone graft substitute composites, since it appears to contribute to an ideal environment for new bone formation.[27]

Osteoinductive Bone Graft Substitutes: Demineralized Bone Matrix

Demineralized bone matrix (DBM) became available for clinical use in 1991. Since that time its use has grown, and it is estimated that in 1999 over 500,000 ml was implanted in the United States.[66] The seminal work of Urist,[79] first reported in 1965, proved the osteoinductive capacity of DBM, which is prepared from allograft by decalcification of cortical bone.[33,79] This process leaves the extracellular matrix, which contains type I collagen and nonstructural proteins including small amounts of growth factors. Among the growth factors are the bone morphogenic proteins that make up approximately 0.1% of the total weight of all proteins in bone and are responsible for the osteoinductive capacity of DBM.[62,66] Although DBM provides no structural integrity and is meant to be used in a stable environment, it still has variable osteoconductive potential due to the presence of collagen.[58]

Despite its widespread clinical use, prospective clinical data on DBM is very limited. Much of the data has been generated in small animal models where it has been shown to have variable osteoinductive potency depending on details of preparation, composite form, and healing environment being tested.[24,59] Data from animal studies are the greatest source of information on DBM in spinal fusion, where it has been tested as a bone graft substitute and as an autogenous bone graft extender. DBM consistently performs better than mineralized allograft bone but not as well as autogenous bone in small animal models.*

---

*References 24, 34, 39, 56, 62, 78.

Studies in human subjects are quite limited. Two retrospective evaluations have been reported. Sassard et al.[69] reported a retrospective comparison of patients undergoing instrumented posterolateral fusion with local autogenous bone graft and DBM (Grafton, Osteotech Inc, Eatontown, NJ) versus matched controls undergoing the same procedure using autograft alone. Radiographic comparisons were undertaken at 3-, 6-, 12-, and 24-month intervals postoperatively. Low fusion rates were reported for both groups, 60% and 56%, respectively; these rates represented no significant difference between the two groups. Lowery et al.[57] reported similar findings of equivalent results when comparing Grafton DBM and autograft composite with autograft alone in posterolateral fusion.

As the use of DBM has evolved, different variables have been studied in order to determine its optimum use. Morone and Boden,[62] using a validated rabbit model of lumbar posterolateral intertransverse process arthrodesis, have compared the fusion rates utilizing variable DBM gel to autograft ratios. Utilizing DBM as a bone graft extender, they showed that fusion rates with DBM gel/autograft ratios of 1:1 and 3:1 were both comparable to autograft alone. Further investigation in this same model compared the different composite forms of the DBM compound available for implantation. Interestingly, this comparison between Grafton DBM gel and newer putty and flex forms of Grafton DBM demonstrated function of both the putty and the flex composites as bone graft enhancers with rates of fusion of 100% when mixed in a 1:1 ratio with autograft. The flex formulation was also found to function in this rabbit model as a bone graft substitute with a stand-alone rate of fusion of 100%.[59]

As noted above, DBM has shown promising results as a bone graft extender in small-animal models. Care must be taken in extrapolating results from small-animal models to humans due to the increased difficulty of initiating osteoinduction in primates.[58] In evaluating the presently available DBM compounds, the prevailing clinical attitude is that DBM compounds function as bone graft extenders, not substitutes.

OPTIONS IN DEVELOPMENT FOR BIOLOGIC ENHANCEMENT OF SPINAL FUSION

Urist,[80,81] after initially identifying DBM and its osteoinductive ability, proceeded to fractionate the osteoinductive portion of the DBM. From this portion he eventually reported on a series of soluble, low molecular weight glycoproteins that were responsible for inducing bone formation. These became known as bone morphogenic proteins (BMPs) and are the most widely investigated group of growth factors that result in bone formation. By the early 1990s nine specific molecules, designated BMP 1 through 9, had been isolated and cloned using the molecular techniques of genetic engineering.[58] Through these processes recombinant human BMPs (rhBMPs) may be generated in standard potencies and unlimited quantities, making the study of these compounds easier. As a result these cloned growth factors are being applied to many models of bone healing with exciting results.

> ## OSTEOINDUCTIVE GROWTH FACTORS IN DEVELOPMENT
>
> **EXTRACTED**
> - Human or bovine
> - Mixture of factors
> - Various concentrations
>
> **RECOMBINANT**
> - In development: rhBMP-2 and rhOP-1 (rhBMP-7)
>   - Unlimited quantities

Extracted Bone Morphogenic Proteins: Bovine-Derived Bone Protein Extract

Bovine-derived bone protein extract, known as NeOsteo (NeOsteo; Intermedics Orthopaedics, Denver, CO) has been investigated by Boden et al.[15] in both rabbit and nonhuman primate models. This osteoinductive mixture is the product of improved techniques of extraction and purification and results in more concentrated bovine BMPs. Investigation in the previously discussed New Zealand rabbit model demonstrated a dose-dependent response to NeOsteo, suggesting a dosing threshold for bone formation exists when utilizing growth factors. Further investigation in adult rhesus macaque monkeys utilizing NeOsteo versus autograft again demonstrated successful arthrodesis but over a significantly longer time course of 18 to 24 weeks. Comparison of effect of NeOsteo delivered in several different carriers was undertaken, and results showed that NeOsteo functioned successfully for fusion when delivered in autograft, DBM, natural coral, or coralline hydroxyapatite.[6,7,15] Variables such as time to fusion, biomechanical properties, and histology of the resulting fusion masses were studied for each different combination.[12,13] Systematic investigation of this compound with various delivery systems in appropriate animal models demonstrated an effective methodology to investigate optimization of new growth factors.

Recombinant Bone Morphogenic Proteins
Recombinant Human Bone Morphogenic Protein-2 (rhBMP-2)

At this time recombinant human BMP-2 (Genetics Institute, Cambridge, MA) has been investigated longer than other BMPs. In 1990 this particular glycoprotein molecule was reported by Wang et al.[82] to induce ectopic bone formation in rats. Since that time it has been effective for bone generation in many spinal fusion models, including rabbits, dogs, sheep, and goats.* Recent results reported in nonhuman primates and in pilot human clinical trials have been very encouraging.[5,45]

To date, published primate research utilizing rhBMP-2 has focused on use in the interbody fusion environment. Hecht et al.[43] reported rhBMP-2–soaked collagen

---

*References 5, 36, 45, 63, 68, 71, 91.

sponges had superior results to autograft in a rhesus monkey anterior interbody fusion model comparing freeze-dried allograft bone dowels filled with either autograft or rhBMP-2–soaked collagen sponges. Specifically, the rhBMP-2/collagen sponge fusion sites demonstrated 100% fusion at 6 months and extensive replacement of allograft with new host bone. The autograft–filled dowel sites showed no similar remodeling of initial allograft dowels.[43] Boden et al.[5,9] reported similar successful results in adult rhesus monkeys also utilizing the lumbar interbody environment. In this experiment titanium cages were implanted with various doses of rhBMP-2–soaked collagen sponges in five animals; two control animals were implanted with cages containing collagen sponge without rhBMP-2. All animals receiving cages with rhBMP-2 showed solid fusion through the cages while neither of the controls fused.

These data set the stage for a recently published pilot study of single-level anterior lumbar interbody fusions in humans that has shown definitive evidence of osteoinduction by rhBMP-2 in humans. Fourteen patients with single-level lumbar degenerative disc disease were prospectively randomized to receive tapered cylindric threaded fusion cages filled with either rhBMP-2–soaked collagen sponges or autogenous iliac crest autograft. All 11 patients randomized to the rhBMP group were fused at 6 months postoperatively, while one of the three patients randomized to the control group receiving autograft in their cages was finally deemed a nonunion at 1 year.[16] These studies have provided data necessary to justify further human trials. Human trials investigating rhBMP in the human posterolateral intertransverse fusion environment are presently under way.

Recombinant Human Osteogenic Protein-1 (rhOP-1 or rhBMP-7)

Recombinant human osteogenic protein-1 (Stryker Biotech, Hopkinton, MA), also known as recombinant human bone morphogenic protein-7 (rhBMP-7), has been investigated in detail in long bone defect and fracture models.[22,23,26] In these environments it has functioned to promote filling of bone defects and speed healing. Results in spinal fusion have been reported for both an anterior thoracic interbody sheep model and a posterior laminar dog model. In both anterior interbody and posterior spinal fusion models it has been shown to act as a bone graft substitute achieving biomechanically stable fusions in much shorter times when compared with autograft under similar conditions.[25,28]

Human trials have been reported from northern Europe with mixed results. Successful long bone healing has been reported for high tibial osteotomy fibular defects when comparing rhOP-1 delivered on collagen sponge with controls of collagen sponge alone.[40] Injection of rhOP-1 into unstable single-level thoracolumbar fractures in five patients had disappointing results with failure of posterior fixation prior to healing of fractures in all five patients.[55] Use of rhOP-1 delivered on a collagen carrier for four attempted C1 to C2 fusions in rheumatoid patients resulted in three of four nonunions at 6 months.[49] Use of rhOP-1 for controlled human trials in posterolateral or anterior lumbar spinal fusion has not been reported.

MAXIMIZING BIOLOGIC ENHANCEMENT OF SPINAL FUSION

As the necessary ingredients for a bone generator are better understood, it becomes clearer why no *single* substitute has been able to supplant autograft. It is also easier to explain why even autograft is not uniformly successful, since at times it fails to provide a sufficient quantity of osteoinductive substances over an appropriate time course once it has been devitalized by the grafting process. Focus has now shifted to synthesis of a composite that maximizes the potential of each ingredient.

Growth factors, osteoconductive matrix, and an adequate supply of progenitor cells are the key to osteoinductivity. As discussed in the previous section, the glycoprotein molecules of the BMP family are effective bone-generating growth factors. The challenge now lies in delivering a potent growth factor over the appropriate time course for each specific clinical need. In nonhuman primate models the time course for spinal fusion protracted over several months, rather than weeks as seen in rodents. The normal physiologic half-life of glycoprotein molecules in the cellular environment is measured in hours and days, not the months that may be necessary for spinal fusion in primates.

In addition, it is necessary to find a "growth factor" that works early enough in the cascade of events leading to efficient bone formation such that all of the elements needed for bone formation will be in place at a clinical site with appropriate physiologic timing. The ideal factor will initiate bone formation by triggering the construction of the biochemical bone-forming environment, attracting and effecting differentiation of osteoprogenitor cells, and then potentiating the activity of those cells involved in physiologic bone formation and remodeling.

As more physiologic environments are characterized, the complexity of each has become increasingly evident. It is likely that bone generation requires a molecular milieu that is provided at specific phases of the wound-healing process. During each phase a different milieu of permissive factors is available. These factors are substances such as transforming growth factor-beta, fibroblast growth factor, glucocorticoids, and vitamin D. It is important that these permissive and/or potentiating factors be present within the bone-forming environment at the appropriate concentrations for factors such as the BMPs to be maximally effective.[8,17,42]

It is evident that each fusion environment, as characterized by the species of the animal, the location of the fusion within the animal, and the maturity of the animal, is unique. Much of this research centers on dosing of growth factor for each situation. Dosing thresholds for osteoinduction have been shown to differ by several orders of magnitude between successful cell response found in in vitro experiments and that necessary for in vivo bone induction.[42] Evidence suggests that fusion in primates is more difficult to achieve than in the rodents used for many fusion models. This difficulty has been directly related to dosing.[13,16]

Delivery of Growth Factors: The Dosing Dilemma

Current data on rhBMPs indicate that these substances can lead to bone formation within the spinal fusion environment. These growth factors must be delivered appropriately in both a spatial and temporal sense. Strategies for accomplishing this have included the utilization of different doses and/or carriers with different breakdown rates in the hope that some of the growth factor will be available at the appropriate times. Recent pilot studies have proven that it is possible for BMP to induce bone consistently in humans, but both NeOsteo and rhBMP-2 require higher dosing and take longer for osteoinduction in primates than in rodents.[16] These substances can be effective in primates, but the high doses necessary and the length of time to fusion demonstrate the need to refine these systems to make them more clinically practical.

Preformed Growth Factors Delivered on Carriers

One major strategy is to develop a better delivery system for growth factor. Multiple alternatives have been explored that utilize the various available osteoconductive substances soaked with growth factors. The administration of rhBMP-2 is being explored in detail in an attempt to generate the optimum regimen to achieve fusion with this growth factor.

Osteoconductive Carriers

The role of osteoconductive bone graft substitutes has changed considerably as more data have become available and bone-grafting strategies have evolved. At this time the use of osteoconductive implants has evolved away from use alone as bone graft substitutes. Despite this, interest in and development of these substances has intensified. The goal now is to integrate the use of an ideal osteoconductive substance with a potent osteoinductive substance to create a superior bone-generating composite.

Boden et al.[11] have explored various carrier/growth factor composites in an attempt to identify a mixture that provides the appropriate dose of growth factor, structural environment, and reabsorption kinetics for posterolateral fusions. Initial work utilized a previously validated New Zealand white rabbit model. Results were reported for natural particulate coral (Biocoral 1000: Inoteb, St. Gonnery, France) mixed with a 3% bovine type I collagen dispersion and various doses of bovine-derived osteoinductive bone protein extract (NeOsteo). Appropriate controls showed no fusion. Once the fusion threshold dose of NeOsteo was surpassed, fusion was 100% and a dose-dependent coral resorption rate and remodeling were seen.[15] In another study using this rabbit model a composite of coralline hydroxyapatite (Prosteon) and collagen

served as carrier for NeOsteo. Results for posterolateral fusion were compared with a Prosteon/autograft mix. Here the Prosteon/collagen/NeOsteo mix showed a 100% fusion rate versus only 50% in the Prosteon/autograft group.

These results demonstrate the efficacy of resorbable composites to serve as bone graft substitute in small-animal posterolateral spinal fusion models. Next Boden et al.[6] performed experiments in a nonhuman primate model utilizing a hydroxyapatite/TCP carrier with rhBMP-2. Dose-dependent new bone formation and a 100% fusion rate were demonstrated within the hydroxyapatite/TCP fusion blocks.

As noted above, collagen has been proven to contribute to a successful fusion environment; this is thought to be due to collagen's gradual release kinetics for growth factor.[42] Collagen and other substances such as polymers can be modified to offer a steady time release that provides an acceptable dosing profile.

Polymer Carriers

The excitement for polymer as a delivery substance is due to the ability to change release kinetics by altering the production procedure or component ratio of the polymer. These synthetic materials are not osteoinductive. Integrated with rhBMP, polymers have been explored in several posterolateral canine fusion models where rhBMP-2 in a biodegradable polymer was superior or equal to autogenous iliac crest bone graft for inducing transverse process arthrodesis and strength of fusion mass.[30,67,68] Sandhu et al.[68] found that rhBMP-2 in a polylactic acid carrier was superior to autogenous iliac crest bone graft for inducing transverse process arthrodesis. Also in a canine posterolateral spine fusion model, Muschler et al.[63] reported that rhBMP-2 in a similar biodegradable copolymer carrier of polylactic acid and glycolic acid had equivalent fusion rates and strength to autograft. Some polymers have been associated with a variable inflammatory response.

Under the paradigm of dosing via release kinetics, controlled release will certainly be necessary for the time course of spinal fusion in humans. New approaches such as gene therapy for de novo production of growth factor at the fusion site are presently being explored in an attempt to provide growth factor within the fusion environment at the ideal concentration and with the right timing.

Gene Therapy

Gene therapy is an alternative delivery system for growth factors. Utilizing various molecular strategies, genes encoding for factors of the bone formation cascade are inserted into the patient's own cells that exist at the site for fusion (in vivo) or that have been removed and will be reimplanted at the site of fusion (ex vivo).[70] Once these cells are in place, they will then produce a protein product from the transfected gene that leads to bone formation. In this manner the half-life of the cell or the gene within the cell and not the actual glycoprotein is the limiting temporal factor for presence of a specific growth factor at the fusion site.

A variant of this strategy has been used in a rat posterolateral spine fusion model with excellent results. A novel protein was recently reported that appears to function very early in the cascade of events leading to bone formation.[4] The protein is an intracellular signaling protein, named LIM mineralization protein-1 (LMP-1). It was isolated via molecular techniques, and its gene was identified. Utilizing an ex vivo methodology, this gene was transfected into harvested bone marrow cells of rats and then reimplanted at sites for posterolateral spine fusion. Sites implanted with cells containing the LMP-1 gene fused solidly, while control sites implanted with control cells had no fusion. This study validates the feasibility of local gene therapy to induce bone formation and spinal fusion in a mammal.

An in vivo strategy for gene therapy in a rodent model has also been reported. An adenovirus vector containing the growth factor rhBMP-9 was injected directly into the paraspinal musculature of rodents. These injections resulted in solid posterior arthrodesis at all experimental sites, thus demonstrating success in a rodent model with another strategy for gene therapy and a different growth factor.[44]

Optimizing gene therapy introduces even more challenges to the search for an ideal bone generator. Vectors for the delivery of genes into cells, the types of cells transfected, and the control of gene expression are all areas to be explored. As knowledge of each growth factor and its mechanism of action is elucidated, the most potent factor can be identified and exploited. As knowledge of spinal fusion expands on a molecular level, the search for a complete bone graft substitute will proceed in a more logical, systematic fashion and rely less on empirical trial and error.[17]

CONCLUSIONS

Previous goals for bone graft substitutes have been to match autologous bone-grafting techniques, the present gold standard, for fusion rates while avoiding the morbidity of bone graft harvest and extending the quantity of graft material available. As bone graft substitutes and growth factors become clinical realities, a new gold standard will be defined.

An ideal bone-generating *combination* is now the goal. It will integrate abundant osteoconductive matrix with growth factor delivery in a localized environment and over the appropriate time course attract and sustain osteoprogenitor cells as they differentiate into osteogenic cells. The osteoinductive growth factors may be delivered as proteins or be synthesized on site as the product of cells genetically engineered to produce these substances under specific conditions controlled by the physician. Finally, the ideal substitute will provide structural support as necessary, but as the graft site matures, the graft matrix will allow transition of functional weight bearing to the new host bone.

The next generation of stand-alone bone graft substitutes, likely made up of an optimum combination of the substances reviewed here, can realistically be expected to have an enhanced rate of fusion when compared with autograft.

SELECTED REFERENCES

Biology of Spine Fusion
Boden SD, Schimandle JH, Hutton WC: Lumbar intertransverse process spine arthrodesis using a bovine-derived osteoinductive bone protein, *J Bone Joint Surg* 77A:1404-1417, 1995.

Boden SD, Schimandle JH, Hutton WC: 1995 Volvo Award in Basic Sciences: the use of an osteoinductive growth factor for lumbar spinal fusion. II. Study of dose, carrier, and species, *Spine* 20:2633-2644, 1995.

Boden SD et al.: 1995 Volvo Award in Basic Sciences: the use of an osteoinductive growth factor for lumbar spinal fusion. I. The biology of spinal fusion, *Spine* 20:2626-2632, 1995.

Morone MA et al.: Gene expression during autograft lumbar spine fusion and the effect of bone morphogenetic protein-2, *Clin Orthop* 351:252-265, 1998.

Demineralized Bone Matrix
Cook SD et al.: In vivo evaluation of demineralized bone matrix as a bone graft substitute for posterior spinal fusion, *Spine* 20:877-886, 1995.

Morone MA, Boden SD: Demineralized bone matrix as a graft extender in posterolateral lumbar spine arthrodesis, *Spine* 23:159-167, 1998.

BMP-2
Boden SD et al.: The use of rhBMP-2 in interbody fusion cages: definitive evidence of osteoinduction in humans, *Spine* 25:376-381, 2000.

Hecht BP et al.: The use of recombinant human bone morphogenetic protein 2 (rhBMP-2) to promote spinal fusion in a nonhuman primate anterior interbody fusion model, *Spine* 24:629-636, 1999.

OP-1
Cook SD et al.: In vivo evaluation of recombinant human osteogenic protein (rhOP-1) implants as a bone graft substitute for spinal fusions, *Spine* 19:1655-1663, 1994.

Cunningham BW: Osteogenic protein versus autologous interbody arthrodesis in the sheep thoracic spine: a comparative endoscopic study using the Bagby and Kuslich interbody fusion device, *Spine*, 24:509-518, 1999.

Geesink RG, Hoefnagels NH, Bulstra SK: Osteogenic activity of OP-1 bone morphogenetic protein (BMP-7) in a human fibular defect, *J Bone Joint Surg Br* 81:710-718, 1999.

Gene Therapy
Boden SD et al.: 1998 Volvo Award in Basic Sciences: lumbar spine fusion by local gene therapy with a cDNA encoding a novel osteoinductive protein (LMP-1), *Spine* 23:2486-2492, 1998.

Helm G et al.: Use of bone morphogenetic protein-9 gene therapy to induce spinal arthrodesis in the rodent, *J Neurosurg* 92(2 Suppl):191-196, 2000.

Scaduto AA, Lieberman JR: Gene therapy for osteoinduction, *Orthop Clin North Am* 30:625-633, 1999.

REFERENCES

1. An HS et al.: Comparison between allograft plus demineralized bone matrix versus autograft in anterior cervical fusion: a prospective multicenter study, *Spine* 20:2211-2216, 1995.
2. Banwart JC, Asher MA, Hassanein RS: Iliac crest bone graft harvest donor site morbidity: a statistical evaluation, *Spine* 20:1055-1060, 1995.
3. Begley CT, Doherty MJ, Mollan RA: Comparative study of the osteoinductive properties of bioceramic, coral and processed bone graft substitute, *Biomaterials* 16:1181-1185, 1995.
4. Boden SD et al.: LMP-1, a LIM-domain protein, mediates BMP-6 effects on bone formation, *Endocrinology* 139:5125-5134, 1998.
5. Boden SD et al.: Laparoscopic anterior spinal arthrodesis with rhBMP-2 in a titanium interbody threaded cage, *J Spinal Disord* 11:95-101, 1998.
6. Boden SD et al.: Posterolateral lumbar intertransverse process spine arthrodesis with rhBMP-2/hydroxyapatite-tricalcium phosphate (HA-TCP) following laminectomy in the non-human primate, *Spine* 24:1179-1185, 1999.

7. Boden SD et al.: The use of coralline hydroxyapatite with bone marrow, autogenous bone graft, or osteoinductive bone protein extract for posterolateral lumbar spine fusion, *Spine* 24:320-327, 1999.

8. Boden SD et al.: Differential effects and glucocorticoid potentiation of bone morphogenetic protein action during rat osteoblast differentiation in vitro, *Endocrinology* 137:3401-3407, 1996.

9. Boden SD et al.: Video-assisted lateral intertransverse process arthrodesis: validation of a new minimally invasive lumbar spinal fusion technique in the rabbit and nonhuman primate (rhesus) models, *Spine* 21:2689-2697, 1996.

10. Boden SD, Schimandle JH: Biologic enhancement of spinal fusion, *Spine* 20:113S-123S, 1995.

11. Boden SD, Schimandle JH, Hutton WC: An experimental lumbar intertransverse process spinal fusion model: radiographic, histologic, and biomechanical healing characteristics, *Spine* 20:412-420, 1995.

12. Boden SD, Schimandle JH, Hutton WC: Lumbar intertransverse process spine arthrodesis using a bovine-derived osteoinductive bone protein, *J Bone Joint Surg* 77A:1404-1417, 1995.

13. Boden SD, Schimandle JH, Hutton WC: 1995 Volvo Award in Basic Sciences: the use of an osteoinductive growth factor for lumbar spinal fusion. II. Study of dose, carrier, and species, *Spine* 20:2633-2644, 1995.

14. Boden SD et al.: 1995 Volvo Award in Basic Sciences: the use of an osteoinductive growth factor for lumbar spinal fusion. I. The biology of spinal fusion, *Spine* 20:2626-2632, 1995.

15. Boden SD et al.: In vivo evaluation of a resorbable osteoinductive composite as a graft substitute for lumbar spinal fusion, *J Spinal Disord* 10:1-11, 1997.

16. Boden SD et al.: The use of rhBMP-2 in interbody fusion cages: definitive evidence of osteoinduction in humans, *Spine*. 25:376-381, 2000.

17. Bostrom M, Saleh K, and Einhorn T: Osteoinductive growth factors in preclinical fracture and long bone defects models, *Orthop Clin North Am* 30:647-658, 1999.

18. Bridwell KH et al.: The role of fusion and instrumentation in the treatment of degenerative spondylolisthesis with spinal stenosis, *J Spinal Disord* 6:461-472, 1993.

19. Burchardt H: Biology of bone transplantation, *Orthop Clin North Am* 18:187-196, 1987.

20. Chapman MW, Bucholz R, Cornell CN: Treatment of acute fractures with a collagen-calcium phosphate graft material: a randomized clinical trail, *J Bone Joint Surg Am* 18:495-502, 1997.

21. Chiroff RT et al.: Tissue ingrowth of replamineform implants, *J Biomed Res Symp* 6:29-45, 1975.

22. Cook S.: Preclinical and clinical evaluation of osteogenic protein-1 (BMP-7) in bony sites, *Orthopedics* 22:669-671, 1999.

23. Cook SD et al.: The effect of recombinant human osteogenic protein-1 on healing of large segmental bone defects, *J Bone Joint Surg Am* 6:827-838, 1994.

24. Cook SD et al.: In vivo evaluation of demineralized bone matrix as a bone graft substitute for posterior spinal fusion, *Spine* 20:877-886, 1995.

25. Cook SD et al.: In vivo evaluation of recombinant human osteogenic protein (rhOP-1) implants as a bone graft substitute for spinal fusions, *Spine* 19:1655-1663, 1994.

26. Cook SD et al.: Effect of recombinant human osteogenic protein-1 on healing of segmental defects in non-human primates, *J Bone Joint Surg* 77A:734-750, 1995.

27. Cornell CN: Osteoconductive materials as substitutes for autogenous bone grafts, *Orthop Clin North Am* 30:591-598, 1999.

28. Cunningham BW et al.: Osteogenic protein versus autologous interbody arthrodesis in the sheep thoracic spine: a comparative endoscopic study using the Bagby and Kuslich interbody fusion device, *Spine* 24:509-518, 1999.

29. Cunningham BW, Sefter JC, Buckley R: An investigational study of calcium sulfate for posterolateral spinal arthrodesis: an in vivo animal model. Presented at the 33rd annual meeting of the Scoliosis Research Society, New York, Sept 16-20, 1998.

30. David SM et al.: Lumbar spinal fusion using recombinant human bone morphogenetic protein-2 (rhBMP-2): a randomized, blinded and controlled study, *Spine* 22:14, 1995.

31. Dodd C et al.: Allograft versus autograft bone in scoliosis surgery, *J Bone Joint Surg Br* 70:431-434, 1988.

32. Doherty MJ, Schlag G, Schwartz N: Biocompatibility of xenographic bone, commercially available coral, a bioceramic and tissue sealant for human osteoblasts, *Biomaterials* 15:601-608, 1994.

33. Dubuc FL, Urist MR: The accessibility of the bone induction principle in surface-decalcified bone implants, *Clin Orthop* 55:217-223, 1967.

34. Feighan JE et al.: Induction of bone by a demineralized bone matrix gel: a study in a rat femoral defect model, *J Orthop Res* 13:881-891, 1995.

35. Fernyhough JC et al.: Chronic donor site pain complicating bone graft harvesting from the posterior iliac crest for spinal fusion, *Spine* 17:1474-1480, 1992.

36. Fischgrund JS et al.: Augmentation of autograft using rhBMP-2 and different carrier media in the canine spine fusion model, *J Spinal Disord* 10:467-472, 1997.

37. Fischgrund JS et al.: Degenerative lumbar spondylolisthesis with spinal stenosis: a prospective, randomized study comparing decompressive laminectomy and arthrodesis with and without spinal instrumentation, *Spine* 22:2807-2812, 1997.

38. Flatley TJ, Lynch KL, Benson M: Tissue response to implants of calcium phosphate ceramic in the rabbit spine, *Clin Orthop* 179:246-252, 1983.

39. Frenkel SR et al.: Demineralized bone matrix: enhancement of spinal fusion, *Spine* 18:1634-1639, 1993.

40. Geesink RG, Hoefnagels NH, Bulstra SK: Osteogenic activity of OP-1 bone morphogenic protein (BMP-7) in a human fibular defect, *J Bone Joint Surg Br* 81:710-718, 1999.

41. Goldberg VM, Stevenson S, Shaffer JW: Biology of autografts and allografts. In Friedlaender GE, Goldberg VM, eds: *Bone and cartilage allografts*, Park Ridge, Ill, 1991, American Academy of Orthopaedic Surgeons, pp. 3-12.

42. Groeneveld E, Burger E: Bone morphogenic proteins in human bone regeneration, *Eur J Endocrinol* 142:9-21, 2000.

43. Hecht BP et al.: The use of recombinant human bone morphogenic protein 2 (rhBMP-2) to promote spinal fusion in a nonhuman primate anterior interbody fusion model, *Spine* 24:629-636, 1999.

44. Helm G et al.: Use of bone morphogenic protein-9 gene therapy to induce spinal arthrodesis in the rodent, *J Neurosurg* 92(2 Suppl):191-196, 2000.

45. Holliger EH et al.: Morphology of the lumbar intertransverse process fusion mass in the rabbit model: a comparison between two bone graft materials—rhBMP-2 and autograft, *J Spinal Disord* 9:125-128, 1996.

46. Holmes R et al.: A coralline hydroxyapatite bone graft substitute, *Clin Orthop* 188:252-262, 1984.

47. Holmes RE, Bucholz RW, Mooney V: Porous hydroxyapatite as a bone graft substitute in metaphyseal defects, *J Bone Joint Surg Am* 68-A:904-911, 1986.

48. Jarcho M: Calcium phosphate ceramics as hard tissue prosthetics, *Clin Orthop* 157:259-278, 1981.

49. Jeppsson C et al.: OP-1 for cervical spine fusion: bridging bone in only 1 of 4 rheumatoid patients but prednisolone did not inhibit bone induction in rats, *Acta Orthop Scand* 70:559-563, 1999.

50. Johnson KD, Frierson K, Keller TS: Porous ceramics as bone graft substitutes in long bone defects: a biomechanical, histological, and radiographic analysis, *J Orthop Res* 14:351-369, 1996.

51. Jorgenson SS et al.: A prospective analysis of autograft versus allograft in posterolateral lumbar fusion in the same patient: a minimum of 1 year follow-up in 144 patients, *Spine* 19:2048-2053, 1994.

52. Katz JN: Lumbar spinal fusion, surgical rates, costs, and complications, *Spine* 20:78s-83s, 1995.

53. Kozak JA, Heilman AE, O'Brien JP: Anterior lumbar fusion operations: technique and graft materials, *Clin Orthop* 300:45-51, 1994.

54. Kurashina K, Kurita H, Hirano M: In vivo study of calcium phosphate cements: implantation of an alpha-tricalcium phosphate/dicalcium phosphate dibasic/tetracalcium phosphate monoxide cement paste, *Biomaterials* 18:539-543, 1997.

55. Laursen M et al.: Recombinant bone morphogenic protein-7 as an intracorporal bone growth stimulator in unstable thoracolumbar burst fractures in humans: preliminary results, *Eur Spine J* 8:485-490, 1999.

56. Lindholm TS, Ragni P, Lindholm TC: Response of bone marrow stroma cells to demineralized cortical bone matrix in experimental spinal fusion in rabbits, *Clin Orthop* 230:296-302, 1988.

57. Lowery GL et al.: Comparison of autograft and composite grafts of demineralized bone matrix and autologous bone in posterolateral fusions: an interim report, *Innov Tech Biol Med* 16:1-8, 1995.

58. Ludwig SC, Boden SD: Osteoinductive bone graft substitutes for spinal fusion, *Orthop Clin North Am* 30:635-645, 1999.

59. Martin G et al.: New formulations of demineralized bone matrix as a more effective graft alternative in experimental posterolateral lumbar spine arthrodesis, *Spine* 24:637-645, 1999.

60. McAfee PC et al.: The biomechanical and histomorphometric properties of anterior lumbar fusions: a canine model, *J Spinal Disord* 1:101-110, 1988.

61. McGuire RA, Amundson GM: The use of primary internal fixation in spondylolisthesis, *Spine* 18:1662-1672, 1993.

62. Morone MA, Boden SD: Demineralized bone matrix as a graft extender in posterolateral lumbar spine arthrodesis, *Spine* 23:159-167, 1998.

63. Muschler GF et al.: Evaluation of human bone morphogenetic protein 2 in a canine spinal fusion model, *Clin Orthop* 308:229-240, 1994.

64. Muschler GF, Lane JM, Dawson EG: The biology of spinal fusion. In Cotler J, Cotler H, eds: *Spinal fusion*, New York, 1991, Springer-Verlag, pp. 9-21.

65. Peltier L: The use of plaster of paris to fill large defects in bone, *Am J Surg* 97:311-315, 1959.

66. Sandhu HS, Grewal HS, Parvataneni H: Bone grafting for spinal fusion, *Orthop Clin North Am* 30:685-698, 1999.

67. Sandhu HS et al.: Effective doses of recombinant bone morphogenetic protein-2 in experimental spinal fusion, *Spine* 21:2115-2122, 1996.

68. Sandhu HS et al.: Evaluation of rhBMP-2 with an OPLA carrier in a canine posterolateral (transverse process) spinal fusion model, *Spine* 20:2669-2682, 1995.

69. Sassard WR, Eidman DK, Gray PM: Analysis of spine fusion utilizing demineralized bone matrix, *Orthop Trans* 18:886-887, 1994.

70. Scaduto AA, Lieberman JR: Gene therapy for osteoinduction, *Orthop Clin North Am* 30:625-633, 1999.

71. Schimandle JH, Boden SD: The use of animal models to study spinal fusion, *Spine* 19:1998-2006, 1994.

72. Shors EC: Coralline bone graft substitutes, *Orthop Clin North Am* 30:599-613, 1999.

73. Sidqui M, Collin P, Vitte C: Osteoblast adherence and resorption activity of isolated osteoclasts on calcium sulfate hemihydrate, *Biomaterials.* 16:1327-1331, 1995.

74. Steinmann JC, Herkowitz, HN: Pseudarthrosis of the spine, *Clin Orthop* 284:80-90, 1992.

75. Tay B, Patel V, Bradford D: Calcium sulfate and calcium phosphate based bone substitutes, *Orthop Clin North Am* 30:615-623, 1999.

76. Thomsen K et al.: The effect of pedicle screw instrumentation on functional outcome and fusion rates in posterolateral lumbar spinal fusion: a prospective, randomized clinical study, *Spine* 22:2813-2822, 1997.

77. Toribatake Y et al.: Revascularization of the fusion mass in a posterolateral intertransverse process fusion, *Spine* 23:1149-1154, 1998.

78. Turner CH et al.: A noninvasive, in vivo model for studying strain adaptive bone modeling, *Bone* 12:73-79, 1991.

79. Urist MR: Bone: formation by autoinduction, *Science* 150:893-899, 1965.

80. Urist MR et al.: Inductive substrates for bone formation, *Clin Orthop* 59:59-96, 1968.

81. Urist MR, Mikulski A, Lietze A: Solubilized and insolubilized bone morphogenetic protein, *Proc Natl Acad Sci* 76:1828-1832, 1979.

82. Wang EA et al.: Recombinant human bone morphogenetic protein induces bone formation, *Proc Natl Acad Sci USA* 87:2220-2224, 1990.

83. Werntz J et al.: The repair of segmental bone defects with collagen and marrow, *Trans Orthop Res Soc* 32, 108, 1986 (abstract).

84. West JL III, Bradford DS, Ogilvie JW: Results of spinal arthrodesis with pedicle screw plate fixation, *J Bone Joint Surg Am* 73:1179-1184, 1991.

85. White E, Shors EC: Biomaterial aspects of interpore-200 porous hydroxyapatite, *Dent Clin North Am* 30:250-256, 1986.

86. Young W, Rosenwasser R: An early comparative analysis of the use of fibular allograft versus autologous iliac crest graft for interbody fusion after anterior cervical discectomy, *Spine* 18:1123-1124, 1993.

87. Younger EM, Chapman MW: Morbidity at bone graft donor sites, *J Orthop Trauma* 3:192-195, 1989.

88. Yuan HA, Garfin S, Dickman C: A historical cohort study of pedicle screw fixation in thoracic, lumbar and sacral spinal fusions, *Spine* 19(Suppl 20):2279s-2296s, 1994.

89. Zdeblick T, Ducker T: The use of freeze-dried allograft bone for anterior cervical fusions, *Spine* 16:729, 1991.

90. Zdeblick TA: A prospective, randomized study of lumbar fusion: preliminary results, *Spine* 18:983-991, 1993.

91. Zdeblick TA et al.: Cervical interbody fusion cages: an animal model with and without bone morphogenetic protein, *Spine* 23:758-766, 1998.

92. Zerwekh JE et al.: Fibrillar collagen-biphasic calcium phosphate composite as a bone graft substitute for spinal fusion, *J Orthop Res* 10:562-572, 1992.

Metabolic Bone Disease

II

Treatment of Spinal Deformities in the Setting of Osteoporosis

John P. Kostuik

Osteoporosis is a major public health concern in the industrialized world. It is estimated that 25 million women in the United States have osteopenia or osteoporosis. The lifetime risk of death as a result of fractures is equal to that of breast cancer.

Osteoporosis should be considered as a preventable disorder and not a disease. The course of bone loss and fracture can be altered through various therapies.

The impact of osteoporosis is significant for families and patients as a result of pain, deformity, dependency, depression, fear of falling, and premature death.

Considerable demographic trends in the aging of America are occurring. Baby boomers are not aging gracefully. The elderly, over age 65 years, and the very old, over age 80 years, are the fastest-growing portions of our population. It is estimated that by the year 2020 more than 30% of the U.S. population will be over age 65 years. The median age of the U.S. population will increase from the mid-20s in 1970 toward approximately 40 years by 2025.

Osteoporosis is a disease of aging. At age 50 years at least 10% of people have osteoporosis; by age 65 years this rises to between 20% and 25%; and by age 75 years to 40%. Greater than 50% of patients with osteoporosis will sustain some form of fracture, of which vertebral compression fractures are the most common. Among the common diseases of aging, osteoporosis ranked third in prevalence behind heart disease and arthritis but ahead of such disorders as depression, diabetes, cancer, Alzheimer's disease, and Parkinson's disease.

In 1984 an estimated 0.6 million people were at risk of spinal fractures from osteoporosis with a cost of approximately 6 billion dollars. By 1997 this had risen to an estimated 13 billion dollars; by 2050 the cost of care for osteoporotic spinal fracture is estimated to be as high as 240 billion dollars.

Osteopenia is a radiologic descriptive term meaning "reduced radiodensity" and indicates a reduction in total bone mass of at least 30%. The major implication is decreased vertebral body strength. Osteoporosis is a syndrome characterized by decreased amounts of normal bone, leading to increased susceptibility to fracture. Peak bone mass is reached somewhere shortly before age 30 years, and thereafter bone decreases in both males and females. Because of bone voids, the osteoporotic spine may develop kyphosis, vertebral wedging, concave fractures, and scalloped end plates. The cortical shell is responsible for 10% of vertebral body compressive strength.

Osteoporosis is of two types: primary osteoporosis type I, which is a postmenopausal osteoporosis that starts 3 to 8 years after menopause as a result of estrogen deficiency, and primary osteoporosis type II, or senile osteoporosis, which is seen in men and women over age 70 years. Type II is related to aging and may be related to long-term calcium deficiency. Currently an estimated 30 to 35 million people are at risk for osteoporosis, of which 700,000 will sustain vertebral fractures, more than 200,000 will require narcotics, and 150,000 will require hospitalization.

Various myths and legends challenge reality about osteoporosis and spinal fractures. The reality is that most of these fractures are painful. Sixty percent of people get better within 3 months. Bed rest as a treatment is contraindicated, since 10% of bone mass loss may occur within 2 weeks.

OSTEOPOROSIS AND OSTEOPENIA: EPIDEMIOLOGY AND DEFINITIONS

- Estimated 25 million women in the United States have osteopenia or osteoporosis, with lifetime risk of death resulting from fractures equal to that of breast cancer
  - Most common: Vertebral compression fractures
- By 2020, more than 30% of U.S. population will be over age 65
  - By age 50: At least 10% of people have osteoporosis
  - By age 65: 20% to 25% of people have osteoporosis
  - By age 75: Up to 40% of people have osteoporosis
- Two types of osteoporosis
  - Primary osteoporosis or type I: 3 to 8 years after menopause as result of estrogen deficiency
  - Primary osteoporosis type II: Senile osteoporosis seen in men and women over age 70; may be related to long-term calcium deficiency

The natural history is not clearly understood. In a recent study of osteoporotic fractures in 9000 women over age 65 years followed up for more than 8 years, there were 1915 with fractures at baseline. The study was adjusted for age, comorbidities, and smoking. If a woman had one fracture, the average increase in kyphosis was 12 degrees, vital capacity decreased approximately 90%, and the risk of further fractures increased more than 500%. Any fracture resulted in a 23% increase in mortality; a severe fracture was associated with a 37% increase in mortality and increased risk of pulmonary death of at least 300%. The myths to be dispelled are that these fractures do not disable people and do not hurt much. Another myth is that of letting the person rest until healing occurs. Finally, there is the myth that there are no long-term problems.

Anterior, posterior, and lateral x-rays of the thoracic and lumbar spine may be all that is necessary to diagnose osteopenia, and these may help to establish baseline bone density. In addition, plain x-rays may help to classify fracture types. Magnetic resonance imaging (MRI) of course is the most helpful study and may show a decrease in marrow fat signal. It can assess canal compromise and show evidence of osteonecrosis. To assess whether a fracture is new or old, a bone scan may be of value.

PREVENTION AND MEDICAL TREATMENT

Current treatment consists of a careful assessment of the patient, including neurologic examination, deformity evaluation, osteoporotic risks, radiographs, and consideration of other studies such as a computed tomography (CT) scan, MRI, and bone scanning as indicated.

The current treatment options for symptomatic spinal osteoporotic fractures include prevention, medical management (including analgesics), bracing, and surgical intervention, particularly for chronic pain and neurologic problems. The problem with all these current treatments is that prevention does not reverse severe cases. With symptomatic control, deformity remains, often with chronic pain. Surgical intervention is invasive and often subject to fixation failure. The main means of prevention is exercise. Building bone mass when young with adequate calcium and vitamin D intake and weight-bearing exercises can lead to prevention provided postmenopausal care is used, including estrogen and calcium replacement. If a female engages in a weight-bearing exercise for 20 minutes, four times a week, 10 years prior to menopause, she will not develop primary osteoporosis. These exercises can include spinal exercises, walking, isometric and abdominal exercises, water exercises, being on one's feet 4 to 6 hours a day, light free weights, or proprioceptive skills.

Other preventive measures for postmenopausal women include hormone replacement with estrogens. Estrogen therapy unequivocally reduces fractures, and if there are no contraindications, all women at risk should be considered for estrogen therapy. Estrogen therapy prevents rapid postmenopausal bone loss but does not increase bone density. This is recommended as a primary treatment and may be combined with progesterone. Controversy continues concerning its contraindications with the history of cancer. Estrogen use in postmenopausal osteoporotic women with at least one vertebral fracture has been shown to decrease subsequent fracture risk by 125%.

Intranasal calcitonin is indicated for elderly patients with low bone mass who cannot or refuse to take estrogens. This may result in an increased bone density, particularly in the spine, with a plateau effect at about 18 months. Calcitonin is also available in the injectable form, and it requires subcutaneous injections every 2 weeks. It has been shown to increase bone mass. In addition, intranasal calcitonin may have an analgesic effect.

Antiosteoclastic drugs such as alendronate or biphosphonate therapy are available. The effect on fracture incidence reduction is not yet clear with the use of biphosphonates, and alendronate does have few side effects. Oral alendronate (Fosamax) decreases fracture risk about 35% and has analgesic effect in fresh fractures. It does, however, have a high rate of gastrointestinal effects and must be taken very specifically. It is contraindicated if there is reflux.

Intravenous pamidronate increases bone mass as well, and it requires infusions every 2 to 3 months.

Selective estrogen receptor modulators are the newest drug class in prevention.

Calcium supplements should be between 1200 and 1500 mg per day. Radiographs should be used for follow-up and for progression.

FRACTURES: EPIDEMIOLOGY AND APPROACHES

- Most fractures due to axial compression failure (most commonly in upper thoracic spine)
  - Wedged with anterior column collapse
  - May retain relative square-to-trapezoidal shape with associated biconcave end plate failure
  - May be crushed with anterior and middle column failure, so-called burst fractures
    - Potential for instability and neurologic compromise
- 50% asymptomatic
- Progressive collapse may ensue secondary to avascular necrosis
- Bracing: Often poorly tolerated in elderly, women in particular, as many are thin and intolerant of skin irritation of appropriate bracing
- Analgesics: Mainstay of symptomatic control
- Nutrition
  - Assess to rule out osteomalacia and for prevention
  - Assess serum albumin level, total lymphocyte count, calorie count, and serum transferrin level

---

SURGICAL INDICATIONS AND APPROACHES

- Indications
  - Progressive deformity with intractable pain
  - Burst fractures with neurologic deficit, which are rare
  - Progressive deformity with spinal stenosis
  - Instability associated with symptoms of spinal stenosis
- Greatly decreased mechanical strength of bone in osteoporosis
  - Pedicle
    - Strongest point for fixation
    - Maximal diameter of pedicle screw used because of thin pedicle cortex that exists in osteoporotic spine
  - Anterior cortex fixation: Important in sacrum
  - Far cortex fixation: Important for anterior screw fixation in vertebral bodies proximal to sacrum
  - Hooks: Increase risk of laminar fracture and pullout
  - Pullout less with screws
- Burst fractures with neurologic problems: Anterior approach is preferred but may be contraindicated in severe respiratory depression
- Other approaches: Posterior approaches, posterolateral decompression, eggshell procedure (decancelization), combined approaches

---

A study evaluating the efficacy of calcium and vitamin D in 1255 postmenopausal women with osteoporosis was undertaken. At inception 265 had no prevalent fractures, 926 had one to five prevalent fractures, and 64 had greater than five prevalent fractures. All patients received 1000 mg of calcium and 400 IU of vitamin D per day and were followed annually for 5 years. At follow-up, a significant reduction of fractures occurred in patients receiving 200 IU of calcitonin.

FRACTURE TYPE

The majority of fractures are due to axial compression failure. They may be wedged with anterior column collapse; they may retain their relative square-to-trapezoidal shape with associated biconcave end plate failure; or they may be crushed with anterior and middle column failure, the so-called burst fractures. The implications for the latter are the potential for instability and neurologic compromise.

The upper thoracic spine is most commonly affected, with 50% asymptomatic. The pain is more prevalent with fractures in the lumbar spine. Progressive collapse may ensue secondary to avascular necrosis. Patients with thoracic fractures may experience radicular pain, which always precedes any motor deficit secondary to cord compression. A neurologic deficit or radicular symptoms may develop weeks or months after the initial fracture. Delayed collapse may be insidious and progressive. The posterior cortex of the vertebral body is more involved than it was previously felt, resulting in the so-called burst fracture. As a result, all osteoporotic fractures should be followed for a minimum of 1 year. It is important to rule out osteomalacia, particularly in the elderly living in inner cities or where access to regular sunlight may be difficult.

BRACING

Bracing is often poorly tolerated in the elderly, women in particular, as many of them are thin and do not tolerate the skin irritation that accompanies appropriate bracing. Corset-type bracing may be valuable in the lumbar spine, but more rigid bracing is necessary in the thoracolumbar area. Because of rib support and inadequacy of bracing, upper thoracic fractures generally are not helped by bracing.

ANALGESICS

Analgesics are the mainstay of symptomatic control. Strong narcotics or long-standing narcotics should be avoided in the elderly as these often produce confusion. In addition, preventive measures, noted previously, should be administered.

NUTRITION

Nutrition should be assessed to rule out osteomalacia and to assess adequate nutrition for prevention. This is particularly important preoperatively. Serum albumin level, total lymphocyte count, calorie count, and serum transferrin level should all be assessed.

SURGICAL INDICATIONS

Indications for surgery include progressive deformity with intractable pain, burst fractures with neurologic deficit, which are rare, progressive deformity with spinal stenosis, and instability associated with symptoms of spinal stenosis.

Although surgery is not commonly indicated, at the present time the indications and numbers are rapidly increasing because of the changing aging demographics of our population, as pointed out earlier in this chapter.

Critical surgical concepts include the greatly decreased mechanical strength of bone in an osteoporotic individual. The pedicle is the strongest point for fixation. Anterior cortex fixation is important in the sacrum, and far cortex fixation is important for anterior screw fixation in vertebral bodies proximal to the sacrum. In anterior approaches, the sacral promontory is a better point of fixation than the ala. Methyl methacrylate supplementation of vertebral body may be important as well, and it will be discussed later.

Surgery should be individualized to the patient and his/her comorbidities. Ideally for burst fractures with neurologic problems the anterior approach is preferred, but it may be contraindicated in severe respiratory depression. Other approaches may include posterior approaches, posterolateral decompression, an eggshell procedure (decancelization), or combined approaches.

Technical considerations in spinal fixation must be considered. Osteoporosis does affect fixation. There is an increased risk of laminar fracture and pullout when hooks are used. Pullout is less with screws. A maximal diameter of pedicle screw should be used because of the thin pedicle cortex that exists in the osteoporotic spine.

Continued low back and pelvic pain should include ruling out the possibility of occult sacral fractures and pelvic fractures.

VERTEBRAL BODY AUGMENTATION

Intravertebral injections were initially done for sclerosis of vascular lesions preoperatively in the early 1980s and were found to be therapeutic for tumor pain. In 1984 polymethyl methacrylate was injected into the vertebral bodies for the treatment of aggressive angioma, resulting in pain relief and stability. The use of polymethyl methacrylate for vertebral compression fractures was reported by the French in 1991, with about 75% to 80% satisfactory results for relief of pain. A series in 1996 was reported in 22 patients. Injections were not without risk, with 2 of 22 patients developing neurologic problems. At this time it was recognized that the posterior cortex must be intact prior to vertebral body injection. In a more recent study in the French literature, 36 of 37 patients had good, lasting pain relief with no neurologic problems. There was evidence on CT scanning of some extraosseous polymethyl methacrylate in 20% of the patients. There have been no long-term reports on the effect of polymethyl methacrylate injections for osteoporotic compression injuries. Anecdotally, this has been used for vertebral screw fixation anteriorly for more than 25 years by the author with no evidence of any untoward problems reported. In a review of the first 20 patients with compression fracture at Johns Hopkins treated transpedicularly in 1997 and 1998, 25 of 27 treated levels had good pain relief with no neurologic problems. Two patients did develop fractures at other levels at a later time. More recently another 300 patients have been treated.

INTRAVERTEBRAL INJECTIONS

- 1980s
  - Initially done for sclerosis of vascular lesions preoperatively and found to be therapeutic for tumor pain
  - Polymethyl methacrylate injected into the vertebral bodies for the treatment of aggressive angioma, resulting in pain relief and stability
- 1990s
  - Polymethyl methacrylate for vertebral compression fractures with about 75% to 80% satisfactory results for relief of pain
  - Posterior cortex must be intact prior to vertebral body injection to minimize risk of developing neurologic problems
  - Traditional augmentation of vertebral body via pedicle, but posterolateral approach is safer, more rapid, and equally as effective
- Intraoperatively polymethyl methacrylate introduced into vertebral body via 14-gauge catheter injecting 2 ml to 4 ml
- Injection very slow since is quite liquid and subject to flow outside of intended point
- Cement not injected directly into pedicle as studies show variety of incidences of pedicle hole perforation as high as 20% during screw hole preparation

---

AUGMENTATION CHOICES

- Ideal vertebral body for augmentation
  - Has collapsed less than 50%
  - Significant collapse beyond 50% or avascular collapse not amenable to augmentation therapy
- Augmentation of vertebral body may help alleviate pain but does not correct deformity
- Reduction of deformity and restoration of vertebral body height achieved by balloon expansion of compressed vertebral body
  - Pedicle approach followed by augmentation of void created by balloon with polymethyl methacrylate
  - Currently advocated for compression fractures with 50% loss of height or less, within first 4 to 6 weeks of fracture (extended up to 6 months in some cases, particularly steroid induced)
  - Clinical trials on balloon expansion of compression fractures with above indications under way

---

Studies in 1991 in our laboratory looked at stiffness related to osteoporotic controls using 3 ml, 6 ml, and 9 ml of polymethyl methacrylate augmentation of the vertebral body. Vertebral stiffness increased 40%, 45%, and 60%, respectively. Energy to fracture increased 2.5 times with 3-ml augmentation and 3 times for 6 ml of augmentation. Compressive strength improved between 33% and 100%. Further studies of energy to fracture using a unilateral pedicle injection with 3 ml indicated improvement of 40%, and with 6 ml a 150% improvement was noted. A bilateral injection with 5 ml was equivalent to or slightly greater than unilateral 6-ml injection. Further studies were done on pedicle screw augmentation experimentally. These were randomized by pedicle to a control group with no polymethyl methacrylate injection and a direct injection of 1 ml of polymethyl methacrylate into the vertebral body via the pedicle. The screw diameters of 5 mm, 6 mm, and 7 mm were assessed. Augmentation of 1 ml increased the pullout strength by 100%, 2 ml by 400%, and 3 ml by 1000%.

The traditional augmentation of the vertebral body has been via the pedicle. More recently Bhatnagar has advocated a posterolateral approach, which is safer, more rapid, and equally as effective.

Intraoperatively polymethyl methacrylate can be introduced into the vertebral body via a 14-gauge catheter injecting 2 ml to 4 ml of polymethyl methacrylate. A variety of polymethyl methacrylates can be used, including the standard materials used for joint replacement, which, if left in the refrigerator for an hour prior to injection, become more liquid and slower to set. Cranioplasty has been advocated as used primarily by neuroradiologists. Injection must be very slow since this is quite liquid and subject to flow outside of its intended point. Cement should not be injected directly into the pedicle as studies have shown a variety of incidences of pedicle hole perforation as high as 20% during screw hole preparation.

AUGMENTATION FOR VERTEBRAL BODY OSTEOPOROTIC FRACTURES

The ideal vertebral body for augmentation is one that has collapsed less than 50%. Avascular collapse or significant collapse beyond this is not amenable to augmentation therapy. The main problem is the natural history since at least 60% of fractures are asymptomatic within a few months of their onset. It is also important to follow these fractures closely following their presentation to make sure that further collapse is not happening in the first few months.

OTHER INDICATIONS FOR VERTEBRAL BODY AUGMENTATION

In addition to the treatment of osteoporotic vertebral body fractures as indicated, other uses include augmentation of vertebral bodies for pedicle screw fixation and prevention of the topping-off syndrome.

KYPHOPLASTY

Although augmentation of vertebral body may help alleviate pain, deformity is not corrected. Recently a technique using balloon expansion of the compressed vertebral body via a pedicle approach has been advocated for reduction of the deformity and restoration of vertebral body height followed by augmentation of the void created by the balloon with polymethyl methacrylate.

Indications remain unclear, and currently it is advocated for compression fractures with 50% loss of height or less, within the first 4 to 6 weeks of fracture. In some cases, particularly steroid induced, the time has been extended up to 6 months from the time of fracture.

Although the initial results seem promising, the real question remains, what is the natural history of such a fracture? It is recognized that the vast majority of the osteoporotic compression fractures will be pain free without major sequelae, which brings to question the timing of such intervention. Currently clinical trials on balloon expansion of compression fractures with the above indications are under way, and hopefully answers will be provided.

SELECTED REFERENCES

Barr J et al.: Percutaneous vertebroplasty for pain relief and spinal stabilization, *Spine* 25:923-928, 2000.

Chiras J et al.: Percutaneous vertebroplasties: technique and indications, *J Neuroradiol* 24:45-59, 1977.

Dunnagan S, Knox M, Deaton S: Osteoporotic compression fracture with persistent pain: treatment with percutaneous vertebroplasty, *J Ark Med Soc* 96:258-259, 1999.

Einhorn T: Vertebroplasty: an opportunity to do something really good for patients, *Spine* 25(9):1051-1052, 2000.

Grados F et al.: Treatment of vertebral compression fractures by vertebroplasty, *Rev Rheum Engl Educ* 64:38, 1997 (abstract).

Jensen M et al.: Percutaneous polymethylmethacrylate vertebroplasty in the treatment of osteoporotic vertebral body compression fractures: technical aspects, *Am J Neuroradiol* 18:1987-1984, 1997.

Tohmeh A et al.: Biomechanical efficacy of unipedicular versus bipedicular vertebroplasty for the management of osteoporotic compression fractures, *Spine* 24:1772-1766, 1999.

Wasnich U: Vertebral fracture epidemiology, *Bone* 18:1795-1835, 1996.

Wilson D et al.: Effect of augmentation on the mechanics of vertebral wedge fractures, *Spine* 25:158-165, 2000.

REFERENCES

1. Al-Assair I et al.: Percutaneous vertebroplasty: a special syringe for cement injection, *Bone* 25(2 Suppl):11S-15S, 1999.
2. Arden N, Cooper C: Present and future of osteoporosis: epidemiology. In Meunier PJ: *Osteoporosis: diagnosis and management*, St. Louis, 1997, Mosby.
3. Bai B et al.: The use of an injectable, biodegradable calcium phosphate bone substitute for the prophylactic augmentation of osteoporotic vertebrae and the management of vertebral compression fractures, *Spine* 24(15)1521-1526, 1999.
4. Barr J et al.: Percutaneous vertebroplasty for pain relief and spinal stabilization on spine, *Spine* 25:923-928, 2000.
5. Beckenbaugh R, Tressler H, Johnson E: Results of hemiarthroplasty of the hip using a cemented femoral prosthesis: a review of 109 cases with an average follow up of 36 months, *Mayo Clin Proc* 52:349-353, 1977.
6. Belkoff S, Fenton F, Mathis J: Biomechanical comparison of two bone cements for use in vertebroplasty. Presented at the 45th annual meeting of the Orthopaedic Research Society, Anaheim, Feb 1-4, 1999.
7. Belkoff S et al.: An in vitro biomechanical evaluation of bone cements used in percutaneous vertebroplasty, *Bone* 25(2 Suppl):23S-26S, 1999.
8. Belkoff S et al.: Biomechanical evaluation of a new bone cement for use in vertebroplasty, *Spine* 25(9):1061-1064, 2000.
9. Bhatnagar M, Mathur S, Mess C: Case report: fatal pulmonary embolism caused by acrylic cement: an unseen complication in vertebroplasty (to be submitted).
10. Chiras J et al.: Percutaneous vertebroplasties: technique and indications, *J Neuroradiol* 24:45-59, 1977.
11. Convery F et al.: The relative safety of PMMA, *J Bone Joint Surg Am* 57A:57-64, 1975.

12. Cooper C et al.: Population study of survival following osteoporotic fractures, *Am J Epidemiol* 137:1001-1005, 1993.

13. Cortet B et al.: Percutaneous vertebroplasty in patients with osteolytic metastases or multiple myeloma, *Rev Rheum Engl Educ* March 1997, pp. 177-183.

14. Cotton A et al.: Percutaneous vertebroplasty for osteolytic metastases and myeloma: effect of the percentage of lesion filling and the leakage of methyl methacrylate at clinical follow up, *Radiology* 200:525-530, 1996.

15. Cunin G et al.: Experimental vertebroplasty using osteoconductive granular material, *Spine* 25(9):1070-1076, 2000.

16. Cyteval C et al.: Acute osteoporotic vertebral collapse: open study on percutaneous injection of acrylic surgical cement in 20 patients, *Am J Roentgenol* 173:1685-1690, 1999.

17. DePriester C et al.: Percutaneous vertebroplasty: indications, technique and complications.

18. Deramond H, Wright N, Belkol TS: Temperature elevation caused by bone cement polymerization during vertebroplasty, *Bone* 25(2 Suppl):17S-21S, 1999.

19. Duncan J: Intraoperative collapses or death related to the use of acrylic cement in hip surgery, *Anesthesia* 44:149-153, 1989.

20. Dunnagan S, Knox M, Deaton S: Osteoporotic compression fracture with persistent pain: treatment with percutaneous vertebroplasty, *The Journal* 96:258-259, 1999.

21. Einhorn T: Vertebroplasty: an opportunity to do something really good for patients, *Spine* 25(9):1051-1052, 2000.

22. Feydy A et al.: Acrylic vertebroplasty in symptomatic cervical hemangiomas: report of 2 cases, *Neuroradiology* 38:389-391, 1996.

23. Gangi A, Kastler B, Dietermann J: Percutaneous vertebroplasty guided by a combination of CT and fluoroscopy, *Am J Neuroradiol* 15:83-86, 1994.

24. Garfin S et al.: Challenges of spine fixation in the adult. Presented at the NASS Annual Meeting, San Francisco, Oct 31,1998.

25. Grados F et al.: Treatment of vertebral compression fractures by vertebroplasty, *Rev Rheum Engl Educ* 64:38, 1997 (abstract).

26. Ide C et al.: Vertebral hemangiomas with spinal cord compression: the place of preoperative percutaneous vertebroplasty with methyl methacrylate, *Neuroradiology* 38:585-589, 1996.

27. Jensen M et al.: Percutaneous polymethylmethacrylate vertebroplasty in the treatment of osteoporotic vertebral body compression fractures: technical aspects, *Am J Neuroradiol* 18:1987-1984, 1997.

28. Kostuik J: *The adult spine: principles and practice*, Vol 1, Philadelphia, 1998, Lippincott, pp. 661-677.

29. Martin J, Sugiu J, Ruiz D: Vertebroplasty: clinical experience and follow up results, *Bone* 25(2 Suppl):11S-15S, 1999.

30. McLaughlin R et al.: Blood clearance and acute pulmonary toxicity of methylmethacrylate in dogs after simulated arthroplasty and intravenous injection, *J Bone Joint Surg Am* 55A:1621-1628, 1973.

31. Padovani B et al.: Pulmonary embolism caused by acrylic cement: a rare complication of percutaneous vertebroplasty, *Am J Neuroradiol* 20:375-377, 1999.

32. Philips H, Cole P, Letton A: Cardiovascular effects of implanted acrylic bone cement, *Br Med J* 3:460-461, 1971.

33. Taurel P et al.: Acute osteoporotic vertebral collapse: open study of percutaneous injection of acrylic surgical cement in 20 patients, *Am J Roentgenol* 173:1685-1690, 1999.

34. Tohmeh A et al.: Biomechanical efficacy of unipedicular versus bipedicular vertebroplasty for the management of osteoporotic compression fractures, *Spine* 24:1772-1776, 1999.

35. Wasnich U: Vertebral fracture epidemiology, *Bone* 18:1795-1835, 1996.

36. Weill A et al.: Spinal metastases: indications for and results of percutaneous injection of acrylic surgical cement, *Radiology* 199:241-247, 1996.

37. Wijn de J, Slooff T, Driessens F: Characterization of bone cements, *Acta Orthop Scand* 46:38-51, 1975.

38. Wilson D et al.: Effect of augmentation on the mechanics of vertebral wedge fractures, *Spine* 25:158-165, 2000.

39. Wolff A, Dixon A: Fractures in osteoporosis. In *Osteoporosis: a clinical guide*, ed 2, St. Louis, 1998, Mosby, pp. 153-176.

The Nonoperative and Operative Management of Spinal Pathology in the Setting of Paget's Disease

Ashwini D. Sharan, Gregory J. Przybylski

Paget's disease was originally termed *osteitis deformans* in 1877 by Sir James Paget, who described five patients with skeletal abnormalities.[22] Although only two of these patients had spinal manifestations, subsequent observers have identified frequent spinal involvement, typically causing spinal pain. Consequently, it is important for the spinal surgeon to be able to identify the varied presentations of Paget's disease and be familiar with various therapies for symptomatic disease.

EPIDEMIOLOGY

Paget's disease is observed more frequently with increasing age, affecting approximately 3% of the population over 40 years of age[11] and 10% of those beyond 80 years old.[11] The disease occurs more commonly in men, and Paget's may be more prevalent in England and northern Europe.[3] Interestingly, most patients are asymptomatic.

Although Paget's disease may affect any bone in the body, the spine is most frequently involved (in 75% of patients), followed by the skull (in 65%). The pelvis and long bones are less commonly involved (in 40% and 35%, respectively).[11] The distribution among spinal regions favors the lumbar spine, followed by thoracic spine and sacrum. However, cervical involvement is uncommon.[18] Paget's disease may involve single or multiple vertebrae. However, additional vertebrae usually become involved later in the course of the disease. Other manifestations have been demonstrated in the intervertebral disc and other extradural tissues of the spine.[4,9,16] Finally, 14% to 30% of patients with Paget's disease will also have Forestier disease (disseminated idiopathic skeletal hyperostosis) with additional bony lesions.[1,8,13]

PATHOLOGY

Although Paget's disease is a chronic, focal process, it can affect multiple bones. Although the cause of this disease is uncertain, several possible causes have been considered. For example, Paget originally suggested an inflammatory pathogenesis.[22] Moreover, investigations of families with Paget's disease have identified an association with the HLA-B27 antigen. However, others have suggested that Paget's disease results from a slow virus infection.[19]

Histopathologic examination of the bone involved with Paget's disease shows hyperactive osteoclastic activity with abnormal and disorganized bone reformation. The newly formed bone has weaker structural properties compared with normal bone.[11] This process evolves over three phases, during which normal bone is gradually replaced. Initially, increased osteoclastic activity causes marrow replacement by vascular ingrowth. Subsequently, disorganized bone formation occurs. Finally, the abnormal bone is replaced by lamellar bone in a chaotic, "mosaic" pattern. Different stages of osteolysis and bony sclerosis will be observed in the various bony lesions. Moreover, proliferation of arterioles in the affected bone has been observed.

EPIDEMIOLOGY

- 3% incidence over age 40 years
- 10% incidence over age 80 years
- More common in men
- Spine affected in 75% of patients
- Associated with Forestier disease

PATHOGENESIS

- Staged, inflammatory process
- Osteoclastic activity followed by disorganized hyperostotic bone reformation
- Arteriolar infiltration

CLINICAL MANIFESTATIONS IN THE SPINE

Because the vast majority of patients with Paget's disease are asymptomatic, the disease is usually discovered incidentally on plain radiographs obtained for unrelated reasons. Symptomatic patients typically complain of pain with weight bearing and activity. This pain is typically relieved with nonsteroidal antiinflammatory medications as well as drugs specifically targeting the abnormal bone behavior.[11] Although back pain is the most common complaint, occurring in 11% to 43% of patients, Paget's disease is rarely the only cause of this pain.[8,18]

The symptoms of Paget's disease may be related to several causes, including altered bone formation, vascular infiltration, and neoplasia. For example, because the hyperostotic bone predisposes the patient to spinal canal and foraminal stenosis, additional symptoms may result from neural compression, including radiculopathy, cauda equina syndrome, and myelopathy.[6,12,29] In addition, the replacement of the normal vertebral ultrastructure with mechanically impaired, disorganized bone predisposes patients to the development of multiple bony fractures.* In fact, Paget's disease may lead to vertebral collapse and kyphosis (Figure 11-1). Therefore, symptoms may result from progressive spinal deformity. Moreover, basilar impression (platysbasia) may occur, causing compression of the cervicomedullary junction, resulting in symptoms of sleep apnea, nystagmus, or quadraparesis.

In addition to symptoms related to altered bone function, vascular complications have also been associated with Paget's disease. The proliferation of arterioles in bone affected by Paget's disease results in greater blood flow traversing the vertebra. This may be related to the infrequent but reported occurrence of spontaneous hemorrhage.

Lee et al. first described a spontaneous epidural hematoma that occurred in a 74-year-old man treated with etidronate for Paget's disease who developed weakness in the right leg without trauma and was found to have epidural hematoma needing surgical evacuation.[10,17] Perhaps small fractures in the setting of increased vascularity can cause a sudden epidural hematoma without trauma. In some patients, cardiac output may increase as a consequence of the increased vascularity, causing congestive heart failure. Finally, symptoms may result from an arterial steal phenome-

non. Despite an absence of compression, some patients with Paget's disease will experience progressive neurologic dysfunction. Shunting of blood from the anterior spinal artery at the level of the involved vertebra into the hypervascular bone may cause spinal cord ischemia.[8,14]

Finally, several neoplastic processes have been associated with Paget's disease. For example, benign giant cell tumors of the face or skull bones as well as parathyroid adenomas have been reported.[24] Moreover, neoplastic transformation of the bone involved with Paget's disease may occur. This sarcomatous change may be heralded by severe spinal pain, a change in symptom severity, or a rapidly deteriorating course. Limited survival of 5 months after diagnosis of an associated sarcoma has been reported.[15,25]

DIAGNOSIS

The initial diagnosis of Paget's disease is achieved with blood tests to identify markers of osteoblastic and osteoclastic activity. Although serum alkaline phosphatase is a marker for bone formation, its serum level may be affected by extraskeletal sources of the enzyme. Alternatively, greater specificity can be achieved with bone-specific serum alkaline phosphatase. In contrast, elevated urine hydroxyproline levels reflect the bone resorption seen. These serum markers can serve to evaluate patients for their response to treatment. Interestingly, although serum calcium levels may be elevated, levels are typically normal because the rates of bone reformation and resorption are usually matched.

SIGNS AND SYMPTOMS

- Most patients asymptomatic
- Most common symptom: Pain
- Neurologic symptoms from central and foraminal stenosis
- Central and foraminal stenosis, less common, spontaneous bleeding or neoplastic changes, deformity: Vertebral collapse, kyphosis, or basilar impression.

---

*References 2, 5, 7, 21, 23, 27.

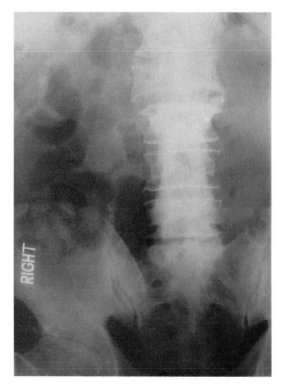

Figure 11-1. Anteroposterior lumbar radiograph demonstrates vertebral collapse from Paget's disease involving the L2 vertebral body.

Radiographic studies are typically sufficient to diagnose Paget's disease. One can identify vertebrae with osteolytic and osteoblastic lesions that are irregularly dispersed. In addition, there may be evidence of recent fracture or subsequent healing. Initially, Paget's disease causes osteolysis, resulting in radiolucent areas on radiographs. Subsequent stages of bone reformation appear as thickened and coarse trabecular

bone expanding beyond their normal boundaries, resulting in greater anteroposterior diameter of the vertebral body with decreased body height (Figure 11-2). Alternatively, dense condensation of the endplates with a flaky appearance of the cortex and a lucent central portion may appear like a "picture frame."[11] Less commonly, massive and homogenous condensation of the vertebral body may result in an "ivory" vertebra.[8]

Computed tomography (CT) may provide additional detail of the bony involvement in Paget's disease (Figure 11-3, *A*). In a study by Zlatkin and colleagues, facet arthropathy, defined as articular cartilage loss from the facet, was observed in more than 75% of patients with the disease.[30] CT also showed expansile remodeling of both the vertebral body and the neural arch in 53 out of 65 vertebra (Figure 11-3, *B*). Finally, moderate to severe spinal stenosis was identified in more than half of the patients.[30]

DIAGNOSIS

LABORATORY TESTS
- Serum alkaline phosphatase elevated
- Urine hydroxyproline elevated
- Calcium levels may be normal

PLAIN RADIOGRAPHS
- Vertebrae with mixed osteolytic and osteoblastic lesions
- "Picture frame" appearance of dense end plates, flaky cortex, lucent center

COMPUTED TOMOGRAPHY
- Expansile remodeling of vertebral body and neural arch
- Spinal stenosis

RADIOISOTOPE BONE SCANNING
- Demonstrates extent of disease
- Identifies areas of arteriolar proliferation

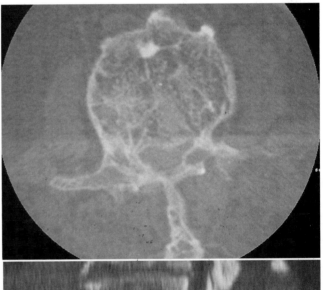

A

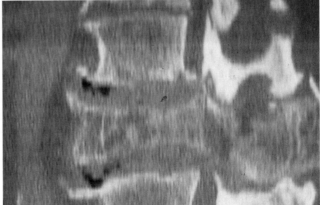

B

Figure 11-3. **A,** Axial CT demonstrates irregularly dispersed osteolytic and osteoblastic lesions. This has been accompanied by bone reformation with expansion beyond the normal boundaries, resulting in severe spinal stenosis. **B,** Sagittal CT reconstruction demonstrates expansile remodeling of both the vertebral body and the neural arch.

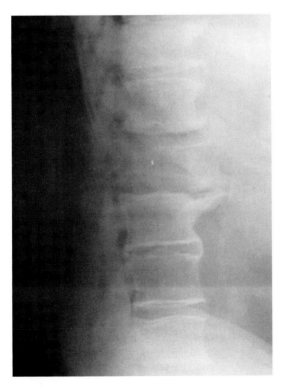

Figure 11-2. Lateral lumbar radiograph demonstrates osteolytic and osteoblastic changes with expansion of the anteroposterior diameter and vertebral body collapse.

However, the most sensitive method for identifying Paget's disease uses radioisotope bone scanning.[26] Bony areas containing arteriolar proliferation are typically identified with these images. Although this facilitates determination of the extent of the disease, it should not replace plain radiographs of each involved region. Repeat scanning or imaging may be warranted when symptoms change significantly.

TREATMENT

Paget's disease is a chronic illness that requires prolonged therapy. The primary treatment of Paget's disease includes medications that inhibit osteoclastic-mediated bone resorption, not only to control progression but also to induce disease remission. For example, calcitonin inhibits the activity of both normal osteoclasts and those in Paget's disease. As a result, calcitonin relieves bone pain after 2 to 3 weeks of treatment in the majority of patients. However, medications should not be the sole treatment if the patient is neurologically deteriorating.[28] With calcitonin treatment, urine hydroxyproline excretion falls immediately. However, bone scan images fail to show improvement for 1 to 3 years.[28] Furthermore, there is a rapid loss of therapeutic effect after stopping treatment with calcitonin.[26] Patients commonly experience problems with flushing and nausea after subcutaneous injection of calcitonin. Small incremental dosing of the medication may reduce this side effect.

In contrast, bisphosphonates, such as etidronate, pamidronate, alendronate, and tiludronate, represent newer and more advanced therapy for Paget's disease. These compounds contain two carbon-phosphorus bonds that inhibit normal calcification by interfering with the calcium phosphate crystal growth. At a cellular level, they may also alter bone resorption. More importantly, the bisphosphonates have the ability to induce prolonged remissions. Altman, Brown, and Gargano identified a dose-response relationship in a double-blind controlled study examining the influence of etidronate on pain.[1] Moreover, Nicholas and colleagues demonstrated radiographic improvement following etidronate administration.[20] However, no greater efficacy of one bisphosphonate over another has been demonstrated. In addition, one should be aware that etidronate can induce mineralization defects, which may lead to pathologic fractures in patients with preexisting osteomalacia.

Although calcitonin and bisphosphonates can help symptomatic patients, medical therapy for Paget's disease may also be useful in asymptomatic patients with elevated biologic markers for the disease whose bony involvement has occurred at sites where complications can result in serious morbidity. Medical therapy may also help reduce the effects of vascular steal syndrome among patients in whom mechanical compression cannot be demonstrated. Finally, medications may prevent local progression of the disease or facilitate surgical treatment when medical therapy is inadequate. For example, Walpin and Singer observed reduced bony bleeding when patients were pretreated with calcitonin.[28]

Although spinal surgery is used primarily for decompression in the setting of failed medical therapy or rapidly progressive neurologic deterioration, the spine surgeon must consider the vascular nature of the disease. In fact, surgical hemostasis is imperative, requiring frequent use of bone wax. One should also consider blood salvage with cell saver and pretreatment with medications to reduce operative blood loss. Finally, high-speed drilling may facilitate decompression while reducing bleeding volume. Surgery should be followed by suppressive therapy because previous reports have described disease recurrence at other spinal levels years after initial surgical intervention.[28]

CONCLUSIONS

Paget's disease is a pathologic process resulting in abnormal bone remodeling. The pathogenesis is unknown, but it may represent an inflammatory process. Although most patients are asymptomatic, the progressive hyperostosis and weakening of vertebra can lead to symptomatic stenosis or fractures. In addition, the hypervascularity of involved vertebrae can result in spontaneous hemorrhage or spinal cord ischemia. Medical therapy with calcitonin or bisphosphonates is successful in managing most symptomatic patients and may even result in remission of the disease.

SELECTED REFERENCES

Hadjipavlou A, Lander P: Paget disease of the spine, *J Bone Joint Surg Am* 73:1376-1381, 1991.
Marcelli C et al.: Pagetic vertebral ankylosis and diffuse idiopathic skeletal hyperostosis, *Spine* 20:454-459, 1995.
Poncelet A: The neurologic complications of Paget's disease, *J Bone Miner Res* 14:88-91, 1999.
Ryan MD, Taylor TKF: Spinal manifestations of Paget's disease, *Aust N Z J Surg* 62:33, 1992.
Tiegs RD: Paget's disease of bone: indications for treatment and goals of therapy, *Clin Ther* 19:1309-1329, 1997.

REFERENCES

1. Altman RD, Brown M, Gargano F: Low back pain in Paget's disease of bone, *Clin Orthop* 217:152-161, 1987.
2. Bidner S, Finnegan M: Femoral fractures in Paget's disease, *J Orthop Trauma* 3:317-322, 1989.

TREATMENT

MEDICAL TREATMENT
- Calcitonin: Inhibits osteoclastic activity
- Bisphosphonates: Cause remission by altering bone resorption and calcification

SURGICAL TREATMENT
- Decompression: In the setting of progressive neurologic deficit
- Subsequent suppressive medical therapy: May reduce recurrence
- Must be prepared for substantial bleeding

3. Bone HG, Kleerekoper M: Paget's disease of bone, *J Clin Endocrinol Metab* 75:1179, 1992.

4. Clarke PR, Williams HI: Ossification in extradural fat in Paget's disease of spine, *Br J Surg* 62:571-572, 1975.

5. Davis DP, Bruffey JD, Rosen P: Coccygeal fracture and Paget's disease presenting as acute cauda equina syndrome, *J Emerg Med* 17:251-254, 1999.

6. Dinneen SF, Buckley TF: Spinal nerve root compression due to monostotic Paget's disease of a lumbar vertebra, *Spine* 12:948-950, 1987.

7. Gigliotti S, Giuzio E, De Durante C: Fractures in Paget's disease, *Chir Organ Mov* 75:331-336, 1990.

8. Hadjipavlou A, Lander P: Paget disease of the spine, *J Bone Joint Surg Am* 73:1376-1381, 1991.

9. Hadjipavlou A et al.: Pagetic spinal stenosis with extradural pagetoid ossification, *Spine* 13:128-130, 1988.

10. Hanna JW et al.: Spontaneous spinal epidural hematoma complicating Paget's disease of the spine: case report, *Spine* 14:900-902, 1989.

11. Harkey HL: Osteoporosis, osteomalacia, and Paget's disease. In Menezes AH, Sonntag VK, eds: *Principles of spinal surgery*, New York, 1996, McGraw-Hill, pp. 493-504.

12. Hartman JT, Dohn DF: Paget's disease of the spine with cord or nerve-root compression, *J Bone Joint Surg Am* 48:1079-1084, 1966.

13. Hepgul K, Nicoll JA, Coakham HB: Spinal cord compression due to Pagetic spinal stenosis with involvement of extradural soft tissues: a case report, *Surg Neurol* 35:143-146, 1991.

14. Herzberg L, Bayliss E: Spinal-cord syndrome due to non-compressive Paget's disease of bone: a spinal-artery steal phenomenon reversible with calcitonin, *Lancet* 2:13-15, 1980.

15. Huang TL et al.: Osteosarcoma complicating Paget's disease of the spine with neurologic complications, *Clin Orthop* 141:260-265, 1979.

16. Lander P, Hadjipavlou A: Intradiscal invasion of Paget's disease of the spine, *Spine* 16:46-51, 1991.

17. Lee KS, McWhorter JM, Angelo JN: Spinal epidural hematoma associated with Paget's disease, *Surg Neurol* 30:131-134, 1988.

18. Marcelli C et al.: Pagetic vertebral ankylosis and diffuse idiopathic skeletal hyperostosis, *Spine* 20:454-459, 1995.

19. Mirra JM: Pathogenesis of Paget's disease based on viral etiology, *Clin Orthop* 217:162-170, 1987.

20. Nicholas JJ et al.: Clinical and radiographic improvement of bone of the second lumbar vertebra in Paget's disease following therapy with etidronate disodium: a case report, *Arthritis Rheum* 32:776-779, 1989.

21. Ogilvie-Harris DJ, Fornasier VL: Pathologic fractures of the hand in Paget's disease, *Clin Orthop* 143:168-170, 1979.

22. Paget J: On a form of chronic inflammation of bones (osteitis deformans), *Med Chir Tr* 60:37-63, 1877.

23. Poncelet A: The neurologic complications of Paget's disease, *J Bone Miner Res* 14:88-91, 1999.

24. Posen S, Clifton-Bligh P, Wilkinson M: Paget's disease of bone and hyperparathyroidism: coincidence or causal relationship? *Calcif Tissue Res* 26:107, 1978.

25. Ryan MD, Taylor TKF: Spinal manifestations of Paget's disease, *Aust N Z J Surg* 62:33, 1992.

26. Tiegs RD: Paget's disease of bone: indications for treatment and goals of therapy, *Clin Ther* 19:1309-1329, 1997.

27. Verinder DG, Burke J: The management of fractures in Paget's disease of bone, *Injury* 10:276-280, 1979.

28. Walpin LA, Singer FR: Paget's disease: reversal of severe paraparesis using calcitonin, *Spine* 4:213-219, 1979.

29. Wyllie WG: The occurrence in osteitis deformans of lesions of the central nervous system with a report of four cases, *Brain* 46:336-351, 1923.

30. Zlatkin MB et al.: Paget disease of the spine: CT with clinical correlation, *Radiology* 160:155-159, 1986.

Natural History and Surgical Treatment for Ossification of the Posterior Longitudinal Ligament

Kiyoshi Hirabayashi, Kazuhiro Chiba, Kazuhiko Satomi

The pathogenesis of ossification of the posterior longitudinal ligament (OPLL) has not yet been clarified, but it is considered a part of the spectrum of conditions involving ossification of the various ligaments, such as diffuse idiopathic skeletal hyperostosis (DISH).

Severe myelopathy may be caused by OPLL, which is much more common in Japanese and other Asian individuals than in white persons. In the natural course of cervical myelopathy caused by OPLL, myelopathy worsened over 10 years in 40% of patients who already had myelopathy at the initial examination, and it appeared in 20% of patients who were nonmyelopathic at their initial examination.

Surgery is indicated in patients with cervical OPLL whose Japan Orthopaedic Association (JOA) scores are less than 12 points and who do not obtain sufficient improvement by conservative treatments. Even if their myelopathy is not severe, surgery may be indicated when patients are relatively young and have severe spinal stenosis.

Anterior decompressive surgery is performed in patients with mixed and localized types of OPLL when fewer than three disc levels are affected.

In continuous and mixed types of OPLL with kyphotic deformity, we advocate combined posterior and anterior decompressive surgeries because sufficient decompression cannot be achieved by posterior decompression alone. In these cases anterior decompression with fusion is applied only at the most prominent portion of the OPLL after posterior decompressive surgery.

As a posterior decompressive procedure, expansive open-door laminoplasty is considered a safer and easier procedure for the severely deteriorated spinal cord compared with anterior decompressive surgery. In posterior decompressive surgery the postoperative lordotic curvature of the cervical spine allows a posterior shift of the compressed spinal cord; therefore it is important to maintain this lordotic curvature.

In OPLL patients the degree of decompression may need to be extended more than in a spondylotic myelopathic patient due to the potential for postoperative progression of OPLL as a result of biologic stimulation.

The first report on cervical compressive myelopathy caused by ossification of the longitudinal ligament (OPLL) was made by Key in 1938.[10] Tsukimoto was the first Japanese author to describe OPLL in 1960 using autopsy findings.[24] Since then, numerous reports on this disease have been published in Japan.[16,18]

The pathogenesis of OPLL has not yet been clarified, but severe myelopathy or radiculopathy may be caused by OPLL, which is much more common in Japanese and other Asian persons than among white persons.[11,25] In eastern Asian countries, including Japan, OPLL is observed in approximately 2% to 3% of the cervical radiographs obtained from outpatients, compared with 0.2% of those at the Mayo Clinic and 0.6% of those in Hawaii.[26] The incidence of a symptomatic ossification showed a roughly linear increase with advancing age: 11% of healthy individuals in their sixth decade of life had radiographic changes suggestive of ossification. The male/female ratio is 2:1 in cervical OPLL, but thoracic OPLL is more frequent in female than in male patients.

PATHOGENESIS

- Not yet clarified but, in part, hereditary
- Related to DISH (diffuse idiopathic skeletal hyperostosis)
- More common in Japanese and Asian persons
- Linear progression with advancing age

OPLL was once called a Japanese disease; however, the relation of DISH and OPLL, reported by Resnick et al., has recently attracted attention.[17]

NATURAL HISTORY OF MYELOPATHY CAUSED BY OPLL

It is widely recognized that most patients with OPLL do not have disturbances in the activities of daily living but have only mild subjective complaints, such as neck pain and numbness in their hands (Table 12-1). Spastic gait disturbance and clumsiness of the fingers are recognized objectively in 15% and 10% of patients with these symptoms, respectively. The average age at onset of initial symptoms is 51.2 years in men and 48.9 years in women. Acute spinal cord injury, including central cord injury (Schneider)[22] or aggravation of tetraparesis after a minor neck trauma, such as falling down, has been reported in 20.6% of myelopathic cases.

After more than 5 years of follow-up of patients with OPLL who were treated conservatively for mild disturbances in their activities of daily life due to myelo-radiculopathy, 54.8% showed no change in symptoms, 26.7% showed improvement, and 18.5% showed aggravation of symptoms (according to the Japanese Ministry of Public Health and Welfare Investigation Committee reports, 1986).[15] Matsunaga et al. found that myelopathic symptoms were already present in 18% of patients at the initial examination and that clinical symptoms were unchanged thereafter in 66% of patients over 10 years.[13] Symptoms of myelopathy, however, appeared in 20% of patients who were not myelopathic at the initial examination.

A radiologic study of OPLL patients at least 50 years old revealed that 52% of them had the segmental type, 33% had the continuous type, and 15% had the mixed type of OPLL. The Japanese Ministry of Public Health and Welfare Investigation Committee accumulated information on 633 cases consisting of 338 nonoperative cases and 295 operative cases that were followed for at least 5 years. From the analysis of these individuals' information, it was clear that the prevalence of progression of OPLL was higher in postoperative cases than in nonoperative cases. Radiographic evidence of OPLL increased in the axial direction in 62% of nonoperative patients and 74% in operative cases. It progressed in the transverse direction in 58% of the nonoperatively treated patients and 74% of operatively managed cases. During this period, 16.7% of those with the segmental type transformed to the mixed type and 7.6% into the continuous type, and 17.4% of those with the mixed type transformed into the continuous type (Figure 12-1).

TYPE OF OPLL

- Segmental type: 52%
- Continuous type: 33%
- Mixed type: 15%

PROGRESSION OF OPLL OVER 5-YEAR PERIOD

- Higher in postoperative than nonoperative cases
- Transformation from segmental type to mixed: 17%
- Transformation from segmental type to continuous: 8%
- Transformation from mixed type to continuous: 17%

NATURAL COURSE

- At initial examination
  - 20% myelopathy vs. 80% pain or dysesthesia only
- During 10-year follow-up
  - Myelopathy appears in 20% of initially nonmyelopathic patients
  - Myelopathy worsens in 40% of patients

Table 12-1	Initial Symptoms of OPLL
Symptoms	Frequency (%)
Pain or dysesthesia in upper extremities	47.7
Neck pain	41.9
Dysesthesia in lower extremities	19.0
Motor dysfunction in lower extremities	15.4
Motor dysfunction in upper extremities	10.4
Sensory disturbance in upper extremities	7.4
Sensory disturbance in lower extremities	5.0
Bladder disturbance	1.0
Total number of patients: 2162	

Modified from: Tsuyama N et al.: The ossification of the posterior longitudinal ligament of the spine (OPLL), *J Jpn Orthop Assoc* 55(14):83, 1981.

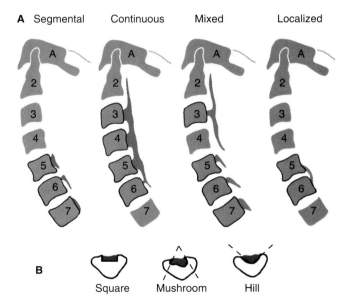

Figure 12-1. Schematic presentation of each type of ossification of the posterior longitudinal ligament (OPLL) on lateral roentgenogram (A) and shapes of OPLL on computed tomography (B).

OPLL may be classified into two patterns, hyperostotic and nonhyperostotic. The former pattern implies the multisegmental, continuous, and mixed type OPLL, which has a high potential for progression, whereas the latter refers to the less-involved segmental type, which has a low potential of progression. These observations may affect the degree or extent of surgical decompression as a result of the potential for progression of the OPLL, whether in axial or transverse direction.

Hirai et al. reported that patients with an area of low or iso signal intensity in the ossification on MRI (which may correspond to proliferation of small vessels in the hyperplastic ligament) showed axial progression in 46% and transverse progression in 72% of the continuous type, and 52% axial and 52% transverse progression in the mixed type OPLL.[9] Patients with no such signal (corresponds to either compact bone with a lamellar structure or massive calcification in the ligament) or with high signal intensity area (corresponds to bone marrow including fat in the center of the ossified mass) showed little progression in either type.[9]

With regard to the relation between progression of myelopathy and OPLL, myelopathy appeared or was worsened in 32% of patients with thickening of the ossification, but in 17% it occurred without thickening. Progression in the thickness of ossification is an important factor in the onset and worsening of myelopathic symptoms.

With regard to the relation between myelopathy and range of motion (ROM) of the cervical spine, myelopathy is less likely to appear despite the presence of severe spinal stenosis when ROM is severely limited. This means that dynamic factors are important in the development of myelopathy in addition to static compression caused by OPLL.

SURGICAL TREATMENT
Indications

Conservative treatment for OPLL patients with mild myelopathy of more than 14 points (JOA score) consists of continuous skull traction using a halo brace, bed rest with a halter traction, and application of a neck brace. Such conservative treatment eliminates dynamic irritating factors; however, very few patients with severe myelopathy improve sufficiently by conservative therapy. After more than 5 years of follow-up of nonoperated and operated cases, clinical evaluation by JOA score was not changed significantly in the nonoperated cases, but the condition was remarkably improved in the operated cases.[14]

Anterior Decompressive Surgery
Indications

In the anterior approach, the ossified ligaments compressing the spinal cord are removed to allow direct decompression of the thecal sac.[3] In OPLL below the C3 to C4 level, an anterior decompression followed by fusion is often selected when fewer than three disc levels are affected.[8]

In cases of mixed type OPLL, which has locally prominent ossified masses, a two-stage combined operation is occasionally applied. The first operation, a posterior decompression, is performed to provide space for the compressed spinal cord to shift in a posterior direction. An anterior decompression is performed 3 to 6 weeks later (Figure 12-2). This combined posteroanterior operation is probably safer than the combined surgery in the reverse order.[20]

In 1975 Yamamura et al. devised an anterior floating method as an anterior decompressive method for OPLL.[12] It provides anterior decompression of the compressed spinal cord by anterior shift (floating) of OPLL without complete removal to avoid leakage of cerebrospinal fluid (CSF) as a result of the OPLL tightly adhering to the dura. This operation is routinely used in the hyperostotic type of OPLL, in which the ligament is greater than 6 mm thick. Elderly patients or patients at high medical risk with spinal canal stenosis are not considered candidates for an anterior operation.

Operative Technique

It is important to expose widely both uncinate processes to confirm localization of OPLL in relationship to the vertebral body. The width of the vertebral bodies to be resected is determined, which is usually around 1.5 cm, judging from the extent of the OPLL on computed tomography (CT).

MECHANISM OF DEVELOPMENT OF MYELOPATHY

- Static factor = thickness of OPLL
- Dynamic factor = neck motion, unstable spine

INDICATION FOR INDIVIDUAL OPERATIVE METHODS

- Anterior decompression and fusion
  - Segmental type, fewer than two intervertebral levels
  - Localized type
  - Associated with disc herniation
- Posterior decompression (expansive open-door laminoplasty)
  - Widely extensive continuous or mixed type
  - Multisegmental type, more than three intervertebral levels
  - Associated with spinal canal stenosis
  - Aged patients
- Scheduled two-stage combined operation
  - Favorable indication: Multisegmental type with more than three intervertebral levels, combined with spinal canal stenosis, and locally kyphotic deformity
  - Relative indication: Widely extensive ossification and locally prominent ossification

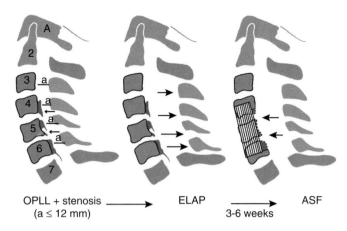

OPLL + stenosis ⟶ ELAP ⟶ ASF
(a ≤ 12 mm)   3-6 weeks

Figure 12-2. Anterior spinal fusion (ASF) is a scheduled two-stage combination operation (posterior to anterior) for patients with ossification of the posterior longitudinal ligament. ASF is performed 3 to 6 weeks after expansive laminoplasty (ELAP).

OPLL: ANTERIOR DECOMPRESSIVE APPROACH

- Expose widely both uncinate processes to expose boundaries of OPLL
- Width of vertebral body resected is around 1.5 cm
- Utilize anterior floating method if risk of dural or neurologic injury is high
- Alternately separate posterior longitudinal ligament at lateral gutters where compression is often minimal
- Microfibrillar collagen held with gentle pressure assists in blood coagulation

---

When it is too risky to remove the ossified mass en bloc because of significant epidural bleeding or CSF leakage due to adhesion of the ossified ligament to the dura, removal of the ossified mass is unnecessary and the anterior floating method of decompression may be chosen. Alternatively, the ossified mass can be removed without much difficulty or risk if the posterior longitudinal ligament is separated from the dura at the lateral gutter, where compression of the spinal cord is relatively mild.

When epidural bleeding cannot be coagulated with bipolar forceps, microfibrillar collagen (Avitena) held in place with meticulous soft pressure is usually effective. When the floating method of resection is chosen, the OPLL mass, which is adherent to the dura, must be managed gently because over-manipulation may compromise cord function.

Operative Results

Kurosa et al. reported that the average preoperative JOA score of 8.0 increased to 14.2 (recovery rate, 71%) at the final follow-up in 100 patients operated on by the anterior floating method.[12] However, six patients had remaining canal stenosis as a result of insufficient floating of the ossified ligament, and three individuals

---

MECHANISM OF POSTERIOR DECOMPRESSION OF THE COMPRESSED SPINAL CORD

- Local dorsal decompression
- Diffuse ventral decompression by dorsal shifting of the spinal cord in lordotic curvature

---

had residual lateral compression by the ossified mass.[12] Five patients showed worsening of postoperative outcome over the long term.

Radiographically, the floating ossified mass forms the anterior wall of the spinal canal and has the appearance of mature bone. The progression of OPLL is halted completely. The floating ossified mass eventually forms a gentle slope by fusing to the remaining OPLL at the cranial and caudal boundaries of the decompression. Postoperative growth of OPLL in the region rarely occurs; however, three patients did have growth of at least 1 mm thick.

Complications

Notable complications of this procedure include C5 paresis and spinal cord injury due to unstable movement of the ossified mass during the operative procedure. Including CSF leakage and dislodgment or nonhealing of the fusion graft, the overall complication rate is approximately 24%, and the rate of reoperation approximately 12.5%.[23]

Posterior Decompressive Surgery
Indications

In addition to creating a local decompressing effect, posterior surgery, including expansive laminoplasty and laminectomy, allows a global decompression of the spinal cord resulting from the posterior shift of the spinal cord, if the patient's cervical alignment is maintained in lordosis (Figure 12-3). Because this total decompressing effect may not work in patients with cervical kyphosis, expansive laminoplasty has a certain biomechanical advantage over laminectomy, in which postoperative severe kyphosis may occasionally occur. In fact, kyphotic deformity or instability after laminoplasty requiring corrective anterior spinal fusion has never been experienced in our clinic.[21]

If the OPLL is continuous and involves more than three levels, extensive laminectomy or expansive laminoplasty (ELAP) for posterior decompression is recommended.[7,8,27] Posterior decompression is routinely performed one level below and above the stenotic site. Although posterior surgery is not a radical decompressive surgery for the spinal cord anteriorly compressed by OPLL, it is considered a much safer and easier procedure for a severely deteriorated spinal cord compared with anterior surgery.[1,2]

After a posterior decompressive surgery, the OPLL is still present, with the possibility of postoperative

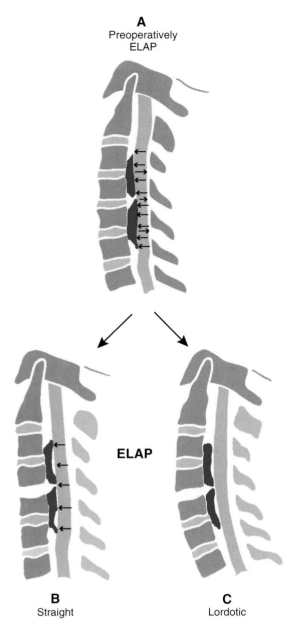

A
Preoperatively
ELAP

ELAP

B
Straight

C
Lordotic

Figure 12-3. Effect of dorsal shift of the spinal cord in lordotic curvature in the cervical spine. **A,** Preoperatively, the spinal cord is compressed ventrally due to ossification of posterior longitudinal ligament and pushed toward the posterior wall of the spinal canal. **B,** Postoperatively, ventral compression to the spinal cord remains in straight or kyphotic curvature. **C,** Postoperatively, ventral compression is also relieved due to dorsal shift of the spinal cord in lordotic curvature.

PRINCIPLE OF ELAP FOR OPLL

- Make expansion one level above and one below stenotic levels.
- Open the laminae widely to obtain the maximum cross-sectional area of the spinal canal.

---

progression of the ossification.[5] Accordingly, in expansive open-door laminoplasty for OPLL, it is necessary to sufficiently widen the sagittal spinal canal.

Operative Technique

As a posterior decompressive operation, ELAP was developed by Dr. Hirabayashi in 1977.[5,6] Since then, the authors have improved this procedure in the following four ways.[4] The first improvement is the placement of retention sutures between the facet joint capsule and the base of the spinous process to prevent reclosure of the opened laminae. This was thought of as a result of our experience with our first two cases of reoperation due to reclosure of the laminae in the postoperative period (Figure 12-4).

The second improvement is to make sure that all surgical steps are completed before the hinge is made. This was developed due to the occurrence of hinge breakage when work was being performed on the open side.

The third improvement involves preserving the supraspinous and interspinous ligaments together with the spinous processes (see Figure 12-4). This technique was devised in an attempt to maintain cervical lordosis, which plays an important role in allowing dorsal shift of the spinal cord to provide effective decompression and potentially correct a mild preoperative kyphotic curvature in some cases to a lordotic posture. When the lamina is opened, the attachment of the aforementioned ligaments to the noninvolved lamina and spinous processes become tight, making it difficult to expand the degree of decompression. To avoid this situation, an osteotomy is carried out at the base of inferior spinous process adjacent to the decompressed posterior elements, which is then bent toward the hinge side.

The fourth improvement is also designed to maintain and secure cervical lordosis. Just before opening the laminae, the patient's neck position is changed from a flexed position to a neutral position followed by the opening procedure. There are some merits to this technique; for example, the degree of lordosis in the neutral position can be confirmed via direct visualization and reconstruction of the muscular layers is easier as the tension of the neck muscles is relieved. The correction of a preoperatively established kyphotic deformity seems to be difficult, but that of a straight deformity may be possible and, moreover, maintenance of a preoperative lordotic position is the most important point of this technique (Figure 12-5).

Compared with other techniques of expansive laminoplasty, the ELAP method involves minimal technical maneuvers and appears to be the simplest and safest of all laminoplasty procedures.

The greatest concern is the reclosure of the opened laminae. This is addressed by other methods, which use implantation of bone grafts or spacers on the open side in an attempt to prevent this problem.[19] This concern can be lessened by the following precautions: Do not make the hinge trough too thick; make the expansion canal a bit larger, especially in the case of OPLL; and make the retention sutures go around and firmly hold the joint capsules.

1 Laminectomy (lam)

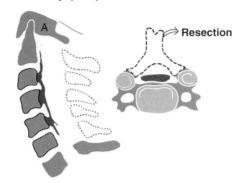

2 Expansive laminoplasty (ELAP)

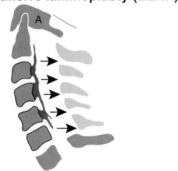

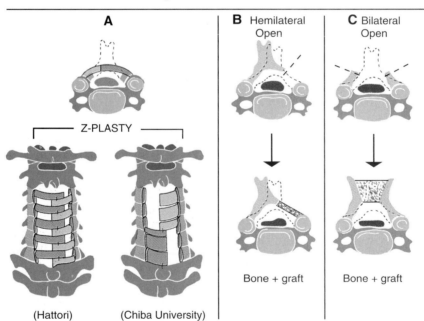

Figure 12-4. Schematic presentation of posterior decompressive procedures as shown in laminectomy *(1)* and expansive laminoplasty (ELAP) *(2)*, and various modifications of expansive laminoplasties as shown in Z-plasty type **(A),** hemilateral open type **(B),** and bilateral open type **(C).**

Operative Results

The results of 87 patients who were operated on by ELAP were reviewed. Their preoperative JOA scores averaged 8.7 and had increased to an average of 11.9 (recovery rate, 38%) at discharge, 13.0 (48%) at 1-year follow-up, 13.4 (55%) at 3 years,[9,13] 13.7 (57%) at 5 years, and 14.0 (59%) at 7 years,[21] which suggests that improvement in

their clinical condition was well maintained for a long period of time.

Loss of widening of the spinal canal was observed in seven patients, among whom four patients maintained their clinical recovery; however, the other three showed worsening due to postoperative progression of OPLL. The range of cervical spine motion, between C3 and C7

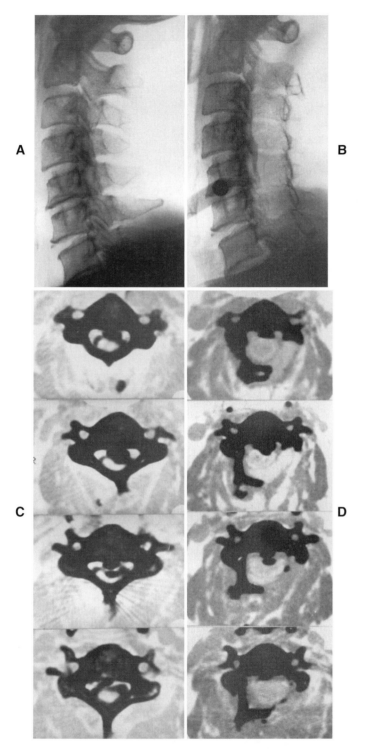

Figure 12-5. **A,** Preoperative lateral x-ray view. **B,** Postoperative lateral x-ray view. **C,** On preoperative computed tomography (CT)-myelogram, metrizamide ring is compressed dorsally. **D,** On plain CT 1 year after operation, decompression of the dural tube and the spinal cord is obvious.

on flexion-extension films, decreased at each follow-up point after operation as follows: on average, the range decreased from 29.9 to 13.6 degrees at 1 year and to 9.3 degrees at 5 years. Severe kyphotic deformity was not observed in any case after operation.

> ## OPLL: POSTERIOR DECOMPRESSIVE SURGERY—EXPANSIVE OPEN-DOOR LAMINOPLASTY (ELAP)
>
> - ELAP is routinely performed one level above and below the stenotic levels.
> - To prevent closure of door, place retention sutures between facet capsule and base of spinous process.
> - Complete the hinge trough last.
> - Preserve the attachment of the supra and interspinous ligaments with the spinous processes of the nondecompressed levels.
> - Osteotomize the base of the subadjacent spinous process to facilitate laminae door opening.
> - Before opening laminae, change neck position from a flexed to neutral position to improve sagittal alignment.

The maximal thickness of the ossified mass increased from 6.3 mm to 7.5 mm on average at the final follow-up. Among patients with 5-year follow-up, postoperative thickness growth of ossification of more than 2 mm or longitudinal extension over one vertebral body length was observed in 40% of patients. Those with larger enlargement of their spinal canal had significantly better results ($p < 0.05$). It is important when performing an ELAP to gain and maintain a sufficient enlargement of the spinal canal in OPLL patients.

Complications

Closure of the opened laminae is a major complication of open-door laminoplasty. However, closure has not occurred since the opened laminae were secured with stay sutures or lamina spacers.[6,19]

Other complications are transient muscle paraparesis of the shoulder girdle and severe neck pain, resulting from disjointing of the hinge, traumatic tissue damage during the operation, or tethering of the nerve roots of C5 or C6. To prevent disjointing of the hinge, it is important that the hinge side of the bony gutter be drilled after completing the bony gutter on the open side. Hinge stability should be checked frequently by pushing the spinous processes while making the gutter. Although there is no way to prevent neurologic complications resulting from the tethering of the nerve roots, fortunately, spontaneous recovery can be expected in most cases within 2 years after the operation.[21]

Factors Influencing Outcome

Operative results of surgery for OPLL are influenced by various preoperative and postoperative factors. Operative results tend to be worse in patients older than 65 years of age, those with severe clinical symptoms (less than 7 points in the JOA scoring system), those with myelopathy for more than 2 years preoperatively, those with a traumatic onset, those with severe stenosis of the spinal canal (more than 60% stenosis), those with a kyphotic curvature, and those with progression of thoracic OPLL.[19]

Postoperatively, OPLL sometimes grows in either a longitudinal or a transverse direction. Growth in the continuous and mixed types is more frequent than in the segmental type. This also influences the long-term outcome. In our series, the incidence of postoperative growth of the continuous and mixed types of OPLL was 89% in the laminectomy group, 34% in the laminoplasty group, and 20% in the anterior spinal fusion group. A comparison of the laminectomy and laminoplasty groups revealed a significant difference in transverse growth but not in longitudinal growth. The structural weakness caused by laminectomy may evoke postoperative growth of OPLL as a compensatory stabilizing process. The postoperative results in patients with no progression of ossification were significantly better ($p < 0.15$), which resulted in the suggestion of expanding initially the degree of longitudinal and transverse decompression during the ELAP procedure for OPLL.

CONCLUSIONS

Conservative treatments are acceptable in patients with mild myelopathy and in relatively elderly patients with chronic moderate myelopathy, as long as neck trauma, which is likely to evoke spinal cord injury, can be avoided throughout their lives.

Consequently, it is our principle to recommend early surgical decompression, especially in relatively young patients with a narrow spinal canal who show mild to moderate myelopathic symptoms, so as to obtain better outcomes from decompressive surgery before the spinal cord irreversibly deteriorates.

Expansive laminoplasty is the treatment of choice for almost all patients with multilevel myelopathy caused by OPLL. The exceptions are patients with a preoperatively established kyphotic deformity, because they are good candidates for anterior spinal decompression.

SELECTED REFERENCES

Matsunaga S et al.: The natural course of myelopathy caused by ossification of the posterior longitudinal ligament in the cervical spine, *Clin Orthop* 305:168-177, 1994.

Resnick D et al.: Association of diffuse idiopathic skeletal hyperostosis (DISH) and calcification and ossification of the posterior longitudinal ligament, *Am J Roentgenol* 131:1049-1053, 1978.

Sakou T, Matsunaga S, Koga H: Recent progress in the study of pathogenesis of ossification of the posterior longitudinal ligament, *J Orthop Sci* 5:310-315, 2000.

Satomi K et al.: Long term follow-up studies of open-door expansive laminoplasty for cervical stenotic myelopathy, *Spine* 19:507-510, 1994.

Tsuyama N: Ossification of the posterior longitudinal ligament of the spine, *Clin Orthop* 184:71-84, 1984.

REFERENCES

1. Baba H et al.: Osteoplastic laminoplasty for cervical myeloradiculopathy secondary to ossification of the posterior longitudinal ligament, *Int Orthop* 19:40-45, 1995.
2. Cheng WC et al.: Surgical treatment for ossification of the posterior longitudinal ligament of the cervical spine, *Surg Neurol* 41:90-97, 1994.
3. Epstein N: The surgical management of ossification of the posterior longitudinal ligament in 51 patients, *J Spinal Disord* 6:432-455, 1993.
4. Hirabayashi K: Expansive open-door laminoplasty. In Sherk HH et al, eds: *The cervical spine: an atlas of surgical procedures*, Philadelphia, 1994, Lippincott, pp. 233-250.
5. Hirabayashi K et al.: Operative results and postoperative progression of ossification among patients with ossification of cervical posterior longitudinal ligament, *Spine* 6:354-364, 1981.
6. Hirabayashi K, Satomi K: Operative procedure and results of expansive open-door laminoplasty, *Spine* 13:870-876, 1988.
7. Hirabayashi K, Satomi K, Toyama Y: *Surgical management of OPLL: anterior versus posterior approach. II. The cervical spine*, ed 3, Philadelphia, 1999, Lippincott, pp. 876-887.
8. Hirabayashi K, Toyama Y: *Choice of surgical procedure for cervical ossification of the posterior longitudinal ligament: the OPLL*, Tokyo, 1997, Springer Verlag, pp. 135-142.
9. Hirai N et al.: The progression of OPLL in the cervical spine, the relationship with MRI of the ossified area (in Japanese), *Seikeigba* 44:1139-1146, 1993.
10. Key CA: Paraplegia depending on disease of the ligaments of the spine, *Guy's Hosp Rep* 3:17-34, 1938.
11. Klara M, McDonnell DE: Ossification of the posterior longitudinal ligament in Caucasians: diagnosis and surgical intervention, *Neurosurgery* 19:212-217, 1986.
12. Kurosa Y et al.: Long term results of the anterior floating method for OPLL myelopathy (in Japanese), *Seikeigba* 44:1225-1232, 1993.
13. Matsunaga S et al.: The natural course of myelopathy caused by ossification of the posterior longitudinal ligament in the cervical spine, *Clin Orthop* 305:168-177, 1994.
14. Ohtsuka K et al.: Over five years follow-up studies on ossification of the posterior longitudinal ligament of cervical spine. Annual report of the Investigation Committee on Ossification of the Spinal Ligament, Japanese Ministry of Public Health and Welfare Investigation Committee, 1987, pp. 20-21.
15. Ohtsuka K et al.: A radiological population study on the ossification of the posterior longitudinal ligament in the spine, *Arch Orthop Trauma Surg* 106:89-93, 1987.
16. Okamoto Y, Yasuma T: Ossification of the posterior longitudinal ligament of cervical spine with or without myelopathy, *J Jpn Orthop Assoc* 40:1349-1360, 1967.
17. Resnick D et al.: Association of diffuse idiopathic skeletal hyperostosis (DISH) and calcification and ossification of the posterior longitudinal ligament, *Am J Roentgenol* 131:1049-1053, 1978.
18. Sakou T, Matsunaga S, Koga H: Recent progress in the study of pathogenesis of ossification of the posterior longitudinal ligament, *J Orthop Sci* 5:310-315, 2000.
19. Satomi K, Hirabayashi K: *Ossification of the posterior longitudinal ligament: the Spine*, ed 4, Philadelphia, 1999, WB Saunders, pp. 565-579.
20. Satomi K et al.: Staged posterior and anterior decompressive surgery for cervical spondylotic myelopathy with narrow spinal canal (in Japanese), *Seikeigeba* 28:1618-1626, 1977.
21. Satomi K et al.: Long term follow-up studies of open-door expansive laminoplasty for cervical stenotic myelopathy, *Spine* 19:507-510, 1994.
22. Schneider RC: The syndrome of acute central cervical spinal cord injury, *J Neurol Neurosurg Psychiatry* 21:216-227, 1958.
23. Shinomiya K et al.: An analysis of failures in primary cervical anterior spinal cord decompression and fusion, *J Spinal Disord* 6:277-288, 1993.
24. Tsukimoto H: A case report: autopsy of syndrome of compression of spinal cord owing to ossification within spinal canal of cervical spine (in Japanese), *Nippon Geka Hokan* 29:1003-1007, 1960.
25. Tsuyama N: Ossification of the posterior longitudinal ligament of the spine, *Clin Orthop* 184:71-84, 1984.
26. Tsuyama N et al. The ossification of the posterior longitudinal ligament of the spine (OPLL), *J Jpn Orthop Assoc* 55:425-440, 1981.
27. Yonenobu K: Laminoplasty versus subtotal corpectomy: a comparative study of results in multisegmental cervical spondylotic myelopathy, *Spine* 17:1281-1284, 1992.

III

Tumor/Infection

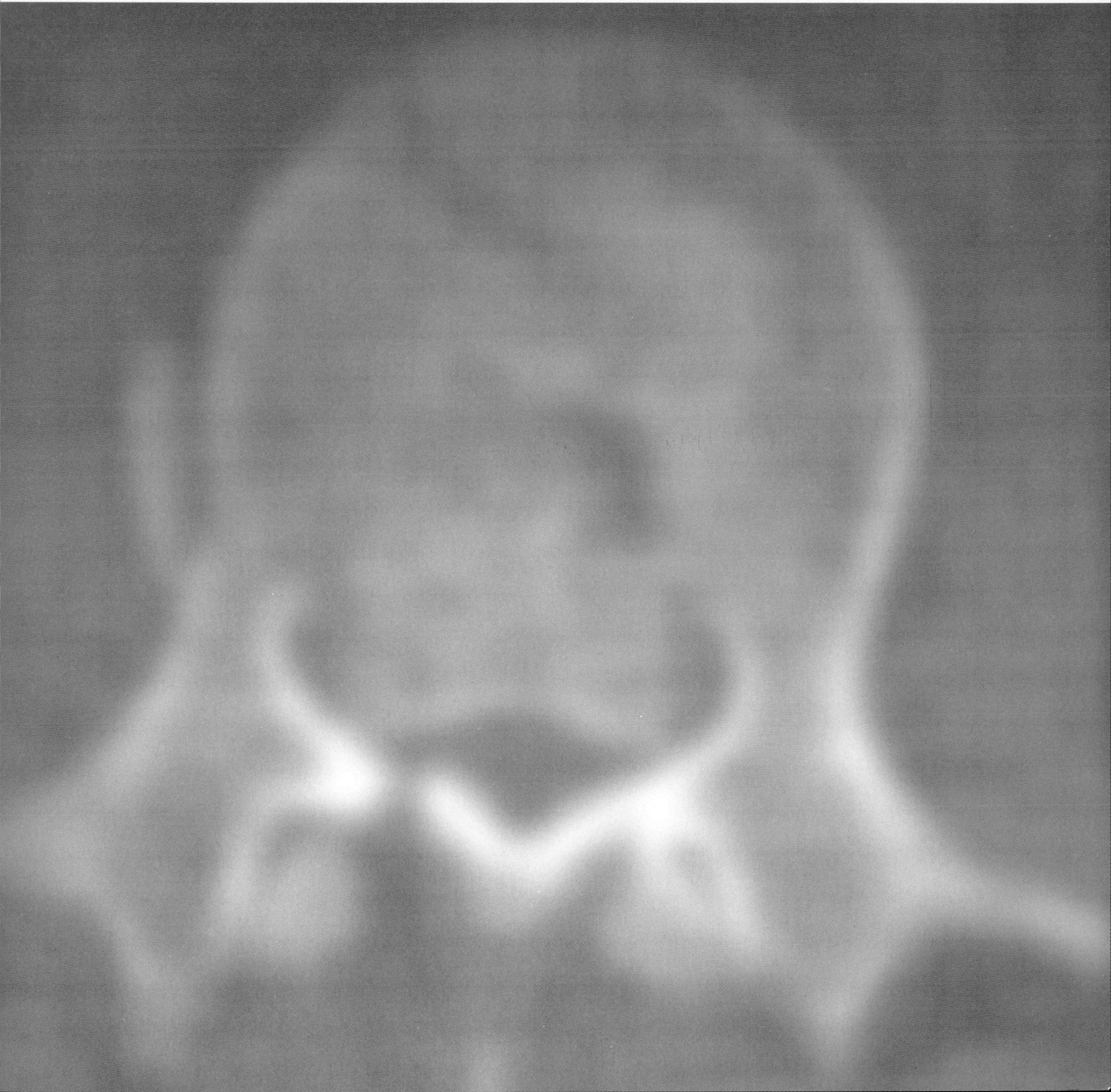

Spinal Infections, Pyogenic Osteomyelitis, and Epidural Abscess

Alexander R. Vaccaro, Basil M. Harris, Luke Madigan

Vertebral osteomyelitis and discitis remain relatively rare diseases. A rise in the number of immunocompromised patients, the aging of the population, and an increase in spinal procedures, however, have precipitated a rise in the incidence of spinal infections, including the resurgence of *Mycobacterium tuberculosis* infections. Timely identification and treatment of vertebral osteomyelitis and discitis are essential to limiting the complications of epidural abscess, osteomyelitis, sepsis, paralysis, and even death. Management schemes, except in rare cases, include a trial of nonsurgical therapy with antibiotics and spinal immobilization. Failure of conservative therapy warrants surgical intervention. The mainstay of surgical therapy is adequate debridement and, when necessary, spinal reconstruction.

PATIENTS

The clinical presentation and demographic features of patients with vertebral discitis and osteomyelitis have gradually changed over the last several decades with advances in medical care and the aging of the population. In North America clinically challenging spinal infections are often encountered in elderly immunocompromised patients and in long-term abusers of illicit intravenous (IV) drugs. Often the management of vertebral osteomyelitis and discitis is addressed in general terms without regard to patient age.

EPIDEMIOLOGY

Vertebral osteomyelitis comprises approximately 2% to 7% of all cases of osteomyelitis in developed countries, ranking third in incidence after infections of the femur and tibia. The relative rarity of vertebral osteomyelitis combined with a nonspecific presentation may hinder a timely diagnosis, leading to a delay in appropriate treatment. Made more difficult by the patient's delay in seeking immediate medical attention for neck or back pain, the diagnosis may not be achieved for several weeks to many months.[3,8,37] Minimizing delays in diagnosis through increased clinician awareness and the use of advanced imaging modalities may limit or prevent the complications associated with a progressive spinal infection, such as invasion into the epidural space, structural deformities, chronic osteomyelitis, sepsis, paralysis, and even death.

Although pyogenic vertebral osteomyelitis remains uncommon, the incidence is unfortunately on the rise. This increase stems from a growing population of aged and immunocompromised persons, a rise in intravenous drug abuse, and an increase in invasive diagnostic and therapeutic medical procedures—particularly urologic interventions. Infections of the genitourinary tract, skin, or respiratory tract are common primary sources of spinal infections, encountered in roughly 40% of patients who develop vertebral osteomyelitis.[26] Risk factors for pyogenic vertebral osteomyelitis cited in three current studies are summarized in Table 13-1; they include intravenous drug use (37% to 42%), diabetes mellitus (10% to 29%), multiple medical illnesses (21% to 23%), penetrating trauma (4% to 17%), recent genitourinary procedure (33%), urinary tract infection (12%), prior spinal surgery (15%), alcohol abuse (14%), morbid obesity (9%), spinal nerve block (7%), human immunodeficiency virus infection/acquired immune deficiency syndrome (HIV/AIDS) (9% to 18%), end-stage renal disease (3% to 8%), malignancy (8% to 10%), rheumatoid arthritis (8%), and male sex (60% to 82%).[8,37,40] Other risk factors may include endocarditis, hemoglobinopathy, and advanced age.[15,23]

The exact cause of vertebral osteomyelitis and discitis remains to be elucidated. There is ongoing debate, particularly as to the precise route of infection spread. Most evidence suggests that an isolated discitis primarily occurs in children and young adults, whereas primary involvement of the vertebra is more common in adulthood.[3,7] The intervertebral disc is

Table 13-1	Risk Factors for Pyogenic Vertebral Osteomyelitis		
Risk Factors	Study 1 (57 Patients)[37] (%)	Study 2 (111 Patients)[8] (%)	Study 3 (75 Patients)[40] (%)
Intravenous drug abuse	42	NR	37
Diabetes mellitus	10	25	29
Multiple medical illnesses	NR	21	23
Trauma (penetrating)	4	NR	17
Recent genitourinary procedure	NR	33	NR
Urinary tract infection	NR	12	NR
Prior spinal procedure	NR	NR	15
Alcohol abuse	14	NR	NR
Morbid obesity	NR	NR	9
Spinal nerve block	NR	NR	7
HIV/AIDS	18	NR	9
End-stage renal disease	8	3	8
Malignancy	8	10	NR
Rheumatoid arthritis		8	NR
Male sex	82	60	64

NR, Factor was not reported in study.

EPIDEMIOLOGY

VERTEBRAL OSTEOMYELITIS
- Rare: 1:250,000 cases per year
- Comprises only 2% to 7% of all cases of pyogenic osteomyelitis
- Incidence rising with increased size of immunocompromised population and increases in number of spinal operative procedures

ETIOLOGY OF DISCITIS AND VERTEBRAL OSTEOMYELITIS
- Children: Vascularity extends into nucleus pulposus, allowing direct deposition of bacterial emboli into nucleus of the intervertebral disc
- Adults: Vascularity extends only to annulus fibrosis, limiting deposition of bacterial emboli in vertebral body metaphysis; result: bony ischemia, infarct, eventual contiguous spread into disc space

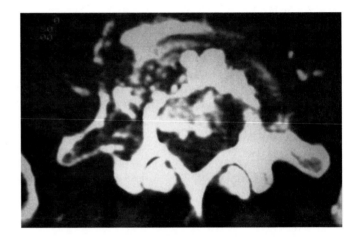

Figure 13-1. A 45-year-old female with biopsy-proven *S. aureus* osteomyelitis of the L4 and L5 vertebral bodies with destruction of the L4 to L5 intervertebral disc.

highly vascularized in children, with direct vascular perfusion of the nucleus pulposus. In adults, however, the blood supply to the disc is limited to the annulus fibrosis. Therefore, in adults, the initial route of inoculum may be the metaphysis of a vertebral body at the end sinusoids, and spread to the disc may be a secondary phenomenon.

CAUSATIVE ORGANISMS

Staphylococcus aureus is the most common infecting organism of the spine and is found in 50% to 65% of the cases of vertebral osteomyelitis (Figure 13-1). *S. aureus* was responsible for virtually all cases in the era before antibiotics.[11,23,40] Other organisms associated with spinal infections include *Escherichia coli* and other enteric bacteria (20%), methicillin-resistant staphylococci (15%), *Streptococcus* species (8%), *Staphylococcus epidermidis* (5%), *Pseudomonas* species (4%), *M. tuberculosis*, *Acinetobacter* species, and others.[5,23,24,37]

SIGNS AND SYMPTOMS

The diagnosis of vertebral osteomyelitis is often delayed in the patient with subtle or nonspecific complaints of neck or back pain without neurologic abnormalities. The difficulty of diagnosis is compounded by the rarity of the disease, leading to diagnostic delays of weeks to months. Back pain is the most common complaint and may be the only presenting symptom.[8,16,29,33] Patients with vertebral osteomyelitis may present with back pain (60% to 95%), muscle weakness (33% to 68%), gait difficulties (55%), sensory complaints (49%), fever (16% to 46%), or sphincter disturbance (25%).[8,35,37] Severe paraspinal muscle spasm with spinal tenderness and a decreased range of motion may be found on physical examination.[3] Pyogenic vertebral osteomyelitis should be considered in patients presenting with a pleural effusion of undetermined cause, especially if accompanied by back pain.[2]

CAUSATIVE FACTORS

- Risk factors for pyogenic spinal infection
  - Systemic: Immunodeficiency, diabetes, advanced age
  - Traumatic: Penetrating trauma
  - Infectious: Urinary tract infection
  - Iatrogenic: Recent genitourinary procedure, deep wound infection
  - History: Smoking, obesity, malnutrition, diabetes, steroids, prolonged hospitalization, radiation, malignancy
- Causative organisms
  - *S. aureus*: 60%
  - *S. epidermidis*: 15%
  - *Streptococcus hemolyticus*: 5%
  - *Streptococcus viridans*: 5%
  - *Peptococcus*: 5%
  - *Escherichia coli*: 5%
- Location of vertebral osteomyelitis
  - Lumbar (50%) > thoracic > cervical
  - Tuberculosis: Thoracolumbar spine
  - IV drug users: Cervical spine

CLINICAL AND LABORATORY DATA

- Signs and symptoms
  - Focal back pain: 97% pyogenic, 90% tuberculous
  - Fever
  - Radicular pain
  - Myelopathy
  - Neurologic deficit: 3% to 4% of cases
  - Paralysis: Incidence decreasing; associated with advanced age, rheumatoid arthritis, diabetes, systemic steroids, and infection with *S. aureus*
- Laboratory findings
  - Early diagnostic tests: Increased white blood cells, ESR, and C-reactive protein
  - Blood cultures: Slow and positive in only 50% of cases
  - PCR: Rapid diagnosis but still problems with cross-contamination

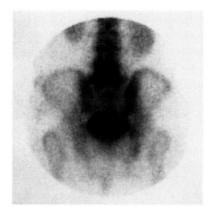

Figure 13-2. A bone scan reveals increased uptake of tracer involving the L4, L5 vertebral bodies as well as the L4 to L5 intervertebral disc.

LABORATORY FINDINGS

As with the physical findings, the laboratory results may provide only nonspecific data. Nevertheless, an abnormal elevation in the markers of inflammation should alert the physician to the possibility of a spinal infection. An elevated leukocyte count is found in about one third of the cases, an elevated erythrocyte sedimentation rate (ESR)—greater than 20 mm/h—is found in over 95% of the cases, and an elevated C-reactive protein level may be found in virtually all cases.[8,35,37] Following an invasive procedure without any postoperative infectious complications, the ESR or C-reactive protein level may be significantly elevated, even in the absence of infection. The ESR will peak between the fourth and the sixth postoperative day and will typically normalize within 2 weeks. The C-reactive protein will normalize by the sixth postoperative day.[23]

Blood cultures are positive in 50% to 75% of all cases of vertebral osteomyelitis and should be drawn to attempt to identify the infective organism.[35,37,46] Many organisms are difficult to culture, and a more rapid diagnosis may be obtained by DNA amplification techniques using the polymerase chain reaction (PCR), thereby allowing an early initiation of focused antibiotic therapy.[23] A tentative diagnosis of vertebral osteomyelitis may be based on the clinical examination and imaging studies alone; however, the suspicion should be corroborated by additional studies (including blood cultures, PCR data, or vertebral biopsy). A positive urine culture may indicate this as the source of spinal infection; however, other causes should be sought because nonsimilar organisms may be identified at the time of vertebral biopsy.[3,11]

SPINAL IMAGING

Plain radiographic changes as a result of a vertebral body or disc infection are usually apparent by the second to the fourth week, but they may not become evident until the eighth week.[4,38] Disc-space narrowing with the end plate blurring and soft-tissue swelling are usually the earliest radiographic signs of vertebral osteomyelitis. Osteosclerosis may be visible by weeks 8 to 12.[38] Radionuclide bone scans with technetium-99m methylene diphosphonate (MDP) are more sensitive, but they highlight any bone-forming process and thus are not specific for inflammatory disorders.[4,38] Bone scans with gallium-67–labeled or indium-111–labeled leukocytes are more specific for inflammatory processes (Figure 13-2), and the combination of gallium and technetium has increased sensitivity and specificity above either alone.[4] Computed tomography (CT) may indicate infection as small areas of hypodensity in the disc and end plate destruction earlier than would be possible with plain radiographs (Figure 13-3).[4,30,38] Magnetic resonance imaging (MRI) is the imaging method of choice for detection of vertebral osteomyelitis, with a sensitivity greater than 82% and a specificity between 53% and 94%.[4,9,25,38] The high sensitivity of MRI in the early detection of

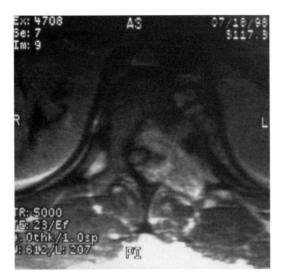

Figure 13-3. A CT scan at the level of the L5 vertebral pedicles reveals marked destruction/erosion of the superior L5 vertebral body.

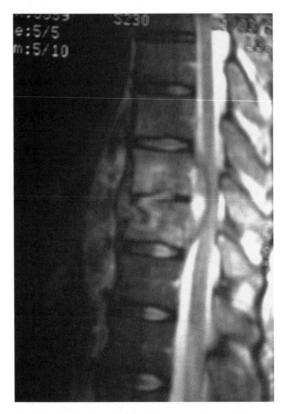

Figure 13-4. A sagittal MRI of the thoracolumbar spine revealing evidence of an epidural abscess of the T12 to L1 level with osteomyelitic involvement of the T12 to L1 vertebral bodies and destruction of the intervening disc space.

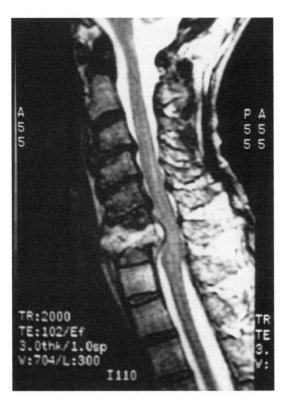

Figure 13-5. A sagittal MRI revealing severe destruction of the C6 to C7 intervertebral disc space and adjacent vertebral bodies as a result of discitis/osteomyelitis and associated anterior epidural abscess.

IMAGING

- Plain films
  - Changes not evident until 2 to 4 weeks after onset of infection
  - Changes include disc space narrowing and endplate blurring
- CT
  - Reveal areas of hypodensity
  - Trabecular, cortical, and endplate destruction
- Technetium bone scan
  - Very sensitive but not specific
- Gallium scan
  - Less sensitive but more specific for inflammatory processes
- MRI
  - Most sensitive (93% to 96%) and specific (92% to 97%)
  - T1: Decreased enhancement of vertebral marrow/disc
  - T2: Increased intensity of vertebral marrow/disc
  - Increased enhancement of marrow with gadolinium administration
  - Following discectomy posterior annulus change is normal but change in vertebral marrow/nucleus pulposus is abnormal

---

vertebral osteomyelitis is attributed to the characteristic changes of the bone marrow during inflammation; the infected regions appear with decreased intensity on T1 weighted images and increased intensity on T2 weighted images (Figures 13-4 and 13-5).[4]

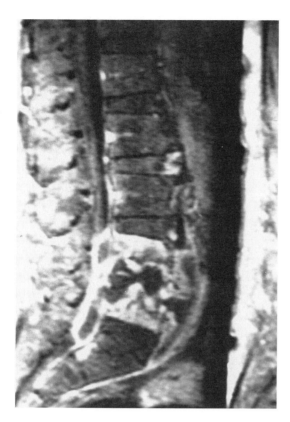

Figure 13-6. A sagittal MRI with gadolinium reveals significant enhancement of the involved L4 and L5 vertebral bodies and intervening disc space.

Gadolinium administration increases the signal intensity of infection on T1 weighted images (Figure 13-6).[4,30,38] Postoperative MRI imaging changes may be normal (e.g., as those exclusively involving the posterior annulus), or imaging changes may be indicative of infection if changes in the posterior annulus are accompanied by changes involving the nucleus pulposus and the adjoining vertebral marrow or any changes to the disc space itself in cases not involving disc removal.

EPIDURAL ABSCESS

A serious complication of vertebral osteomyelitis and discitis is the development of a spinal epidural abscess.[12,20] Rarely is a purulent epidural collection present without involvement of the vertebral body or the disc space. In general, the majority of collections are anterior, originating from the posterior aspect of the vertebral body and disc space. An epidural abscess originating from hematogenous sources is usually associated with a posterior soft tissue abscess, and often patients with such abscesses have positive blood cultures. Common sources of hematogenous seeding include skin or soft tissue infections, infected vascular access sites, or invasive spinal procedures. MRI is extremely sensitive in the visualization of an epidural collection except in the presence of meningitis.[34] The management of spinal epidural abscess is generally surgical, except occasionally in the lumbar region in the

EPIDURAL ABSCESS

- Rare in absence of disc/vertebral body infection
- Most collections anterior, except with hematogenous seeding
- MRI sensitive, except with coexisting meningitis
- Timely surgical treatment needed, except in lumbar abscess without a neurologic deficit

absence of a neurologic deficit. Due to the potential for rapid progression of neurologic dysfunction, nonoperative management in the cervical and thoracic spine has been discouraged. Mechanical compression alone often does not account for the degree of neurologic loss present, suggesting a role for vascular dysfunction, especially venous congestion.[13]

NONOPERATIVE TREATMENT

Management of vertebral osteomyelitis typically includes a trial of nonsurgical therapy with spinal immobilization, early ambulation, and antibiotics (intravenous followed by oral antibiotics). As many as three quarters of all patient will experience the resolution of spine pain and often fuse spontaneously. In general, patients younger than 60 years of age with normal immune function and a decreasing sedimentation rate do well with nonsurgical therapy.[8,10,23,43] Failure of the conservative therapy warrants surgical intervention, including adequate debridement and spinal reconstruction, if necessary.

The outcomes of adult patients with vertebral osteomyelitis and discitis have dramatically improved with antibiotics. A 4- to 6-week regimen of high-dose parenteral antibiotics with spinal immobilization, followed by oral antibiotic treatment, may be sufficient in the clinically stable patient. The duration of the antibiotic treatment may be curtailed if the ESR has resolved to one half of the pretreatment value.

In staphylococcal infections, high-dose penicillins (e.g., nafcillin, 2 g intravenously every 6 hours) are usually recommended. Patients allergic to penicillins may be given first- or second-generation cephalosporins (e.g., cefazolin, 1 g intravenously every 8 hours), and for methicillin-resistant *S. aureus*, vancomycin is the agent of choice.[41,42] For pseudomonal infections, two-drug regimens are recommended (e.g., ceftazidime plus tobramycin or gentamycin may be used, depending on specific strain susceptibilities).[42]

Carragee reported on 111 patients with vertebral osteomyelitis, of whom 72 were initially treated nonoperatively with antibiotics.[8] Over one third of patients failed conservative therapy, with the final outcome related to age and the patient's immune status.[8]

OPERATIVE TREATMENT

Indications for surgical therapy may include static or progressive neurologic impairment, the presence of a

> ## NONSURGICAL OPTIONS
>
> ### NONOPERATIVE TREATMENT
> - Spinal immobilization: Cast or bracing
> - IV followed by oral antibiotics
> - Early ambulation
> - Three fourths of patients respond with resolution of pain and often spontaneous fusion
> - Severely immunocompromised patients tend to fail conservative therapy
> - Markers of favorable outcome
>   - Age <60 years, decreasing ESR
>   - Nonstaphylococcal infection
>
> ### ANTIBIOTIC THERAPY
> - Immobilization and appropriate IV antibiotics
> - Discontinued when purulent abscess is absent, patient is stable, ESR is resolved to half its original value
> - Choice of antibiotic depends on the following:
>   - Isolation of organism
>   - Identification of sensitivities

> ## SURGICAL THERAPY
>
> - Indications
>   - Organism identification: Open biopsy
>   - Failure of conservative therapy
>   - Symptomatic neural compression
>   - Deformity: Potential or progressive
>   - Persistent, severe pain
> - Surgical principles
>   - Thorough debridement
>   - Provision of adequate blood flow
>   - Restoration/maintenance of spinal stability

> ## POSTERIOR DECOMPRESSION
>
> - Without fusion
>   - Potentially leads to progression of deformity, instability, and neurologic deterioration
>   - Reserved for rare cases of isolated posterior epidural abscess without anterior vertebral involvement
> - With fusion and instrumentation
>   - Rarely indicated, often on delayed basis
>   - Cases of posterolateral decompression of primary anterior focus of infection

spinal abscess, sepsis, severe pain in the presence of external immobilization, a progressive spinal deformity, gross instability, the need for organism identification (open biopsy), and the failure of nonoperative treatment.[23,32] Common to all surgical approaches are three main principles: thorough debridement of all necrotic and infected tissues, the deliverance of adequate blood flow through debridement or vascularized soft-tissue transfer, and the maintenance or creation of adequate spinal stability.

Posterior Decompression Without Fusion

An isolated posterior decompression (i.e., a laminectomy without accompanying fusion) is indicated only in the rare event of a posterior epidural infection sparing involvement of any anterior vertebral elements. Otherwise, a posterior laminectomy often results in an unfavorable clinical outcome, including progressive deformity, increasing instability, and worsening neurologic impairment. In a retrospective view of 61 patients with vertebral osteomyelitis, Eismont et al. described seven patients surgically treated by laminectomy, three of whom worsened neurologically and four of whom remained unchanged postoperatively.[13] Generally, the anterior view elements are seldom spared involvement, whereas the posterior elements are typically uninvolved. The poor clinical outcomes of patients following a posterior decompression without fusion stems from the failure to directly address the primary pathology (anterior involved spinal elements) compounded with the disruption of the stabilizing posterior spinal elements.[13,23]

Posterior Decompression With Fusion and Instrumentation

The posterior debridement of an epidural abscess originating from the anterior spinal elements (posterolateral or extracavitary approach) risks the potential for anterior vertebral column collapse and progressive deformity whether or not the anterior column is reconstructed with a structural autologous bone graft. A two-stage procedure following soft-tissue healing using posterior instrumentation is often useful, because placement of instrumentation at the time of initial debridement is not desirable.[40] In a retrospective review of 32 surgically managed patients with pyogenic vertebral osteomyelitis, McGuire and Eismont described five patients successfully managed with such a two-stage debridement and reconstructive procedure.[31]

Variations of the extracavitary or costotransversectomy approaches afford posterior access to the anterior vertebral elements for debridement or placement of a structural bone graft. However, this approach provides only a limited exposure of the anterior thecal sac and is technically more difficult to use when attempting to place an anteriorly situated structural graft. Some surgeons have advocated primary placement of posterior instrumentation at the time of debridement if the posterior soft tissues, epidural space, or bony elements are not involved. Rath et al. reported on 43 surgically managed patients with vertebral osteomyelitis, including 18 patients who underwent a single-stage posterior debridement and autologous bone grafting with instrumentation.[35] Of these 18 patients, 17 (94%) achieved a successful fusion.[35]

Anterior Decompression With and Without Autologous Bone Graft

Aggressive debridement without reconstruction has been used with moderate success in the surgical management of tuberculous infections of the spine. Follow-up series have highlighted the benefits of autologous bone reconstruction or grafting of bony voids following debridement in this setting.[1] Rarely is debridement alone, without autologous grafting, performed in the treatment of progressive vertebral osteomyelitis. Cahill et al. reported on 10 patients with vertebral pyogenic osteomyelitis with severe vertebral segment destruction and instability.[6] All 10 patients underwent anterior debridement and fusion without instrumentation and subsequent immobilization with casting or bracing for 3 months. Although the patients were successfully treated, the authors suggested that instrumentation may have decreased the need for prolonged external immobilization.[6] Fang et al. reported on 43 patients with pyogenic vertebral osteomyelitis, of whom 39 were treated with anterior debridement and fusion without instrumentation.[14] At 5-year follow-up of 30 patients, 29 were improved clinically without evidence of recurrence.[14] Lifeso also reported on 20 patients with vertebral osteomyelitis and discitis.[28] All patients were successfully treated surgically, with 11 receiving anterior decompression and fusion and 9 receiving anterior debridement alone.[28]

Autologous bone grafting is a useful method to promote local bone healing and prevent late deformity by accelerating the attainment of spinal stability. The addition of posterior instrumentation in a noncontaminated field may be the optimal treatment method to avoid graft displacement or collapse, while providing enough stability to allow early rehabilitation and improved functional outcome.[6,14,23,31]

Anterior Decompression and Fusion With Posterior Instrumentation Stabilization

Posterior instrumentation stabilization following aggressive anterior debridement with bone grafting allows early patient mobilization, thereby lessening the morbidity associated with prolonged recumbency. Early ambulation and return to activities of daily living often result in improved patient satisfaction and functional outcome (Figures 13-7 and 13-8).[22,23,36,39]

Krödel et al. reported on 41 patients with vertebral osteomyelitis surgically managed with anterior debridement and interbody fusion followed by posterior instrumentation.[24] All patients were mobile without external support after about 4 days of bed rest. Thirty-three patients were followed-up at 1 year, with a documented fusion success of 100%, with two patients experiencing reinfection and two requiring reoperation as a result of instrumentation failure.[24] Liebergall et al. reported on 14 patients with symptomatic vertebral osteomyelitis and discitis managed surgically with anterior debridement and fusion.[27] Only two of the patients underwent an additional posterior stabilization procedure with instrumentation, allowing them to avoid the 3- to 6-month period of external mobilization required of the remain-

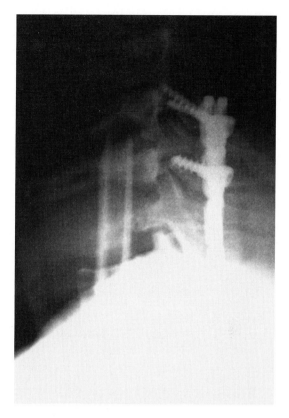

Figure 13-7. A lateral x-ray following an anterior cervical debridement and fusion with autologous fibular graft, followed by posterior cervical stabilization with lateral mass plates and screws.

ing 12 patients.[27] Redfern et al. also reported on the successful surgical management of six patients with spinal infections.[36] All patients underwent an anterior debridement and fusion followed by posterior instrumentation stabilization and early postoperative mobilization.

Anterior Decompression and Fusion With Anterior Instrumentation

Placing instrumentation in the same surgical field during the initial debridement of pyogenic vertebral osteomyelitis is generally avoided, considering the risk of hardware contamination and subsequent clinical reinfection of the surgical site.[27] However, some have argued that in the cervical spine, anterior cervical plating immediately after debridement and grafting offers immediate stabilization and prevents graft dislodgment while possibly avoiding an additional posterior surgical procedure. Hughes et al. reported successful management of 12 patients after applying anterior instrumentation following an anterior debridement and fusion for cervical osteomyelitis and discitis.[21] Woo et al. reported on 12 patients with anterior cervical osteomyelitis and discitis treated with anterior instrumentation following debridement and fusion.[44] Seven of the patients had no further operations, four patients had a supplemental posterior stabilization procedure, and one patient experienced graft displacement and increased cervical deformity in the face of continued

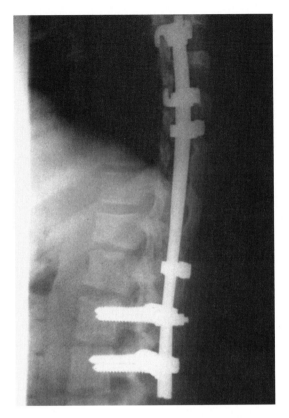

Figure 13-8. A 19-year-old female with biopsy-proven tuberculosis involving the left-sided posterior elements (lamina, pedicle) with extension into the paraspinal soft tissues. An open left-sided posterolateral debridement was performed involving two contiguous vertebral levels and paraspinal soft tissues. Because of the potential of instability, a posterior stabilization procedure using rods, screws, hooks, and autologous bone graft was performed (lateral plain x-ray).

ANTERIOR DECOMPRESSION

- Anterior decompression plus autograft fusion
  - Anterior debridement followed by autograft placement: Autograft promotes local bone healing, adds stability, and prevents late deformity
  - In situ fusion without instrumentation effective in treatment of tuberculosis
- Anterior decompression plus fusion with posterior stabilization
  - Majority of pyogenic osteomyelitis
  - Anterior graft promotes healing and vascular return
  - Posterior stabilization results
  - Increased circumferential stability
  - Improvement in functional outcome
  - Decrease in pain
  - Overall increase in patient satisfaction
- Anterior decompression plus fusion with anterior stabilization
  - Pyogenic vertebral osteomyelitis/discitis (reports limited to cervical spine)
  - Viable approach in tuberculosis

---

intravenous drug abuse. The measured sagittal plane alignment improved 21 degrees on average following graft placement with instrumentation.[44] Heary et al. reported the successful use of anterior instrumentation in one patient with vertebral osteomyelitis.[18]

Vascularized Bone Graft

In selected cases of osteomyelitis, the use of vascularized tissue grafts during revision procedures affords immediate continuous blood supply to the donor graft, protects against late weakening and fatigue failure of the grafting substance, and substantially increases the rate and success of graft incorporation.[17,45] The internal oblique muscle provides a versatile source of vascularization for iliac crest grafts used from approximately T8 to the sacrum. The flap draws its supply from anastomosis of the deep circumflex iliac artery by way of the first and second lumbar arteries. Alternatively, a less versatile source is the internal oblique muscle–iliac crest myocutaneous flap supplied by the deep circumflex iliac artery. The rib and the fibula provide other vascularized graft options. Hayashi et al. reported successful fusion in six patients with pyogenic or tubercular infection treated with a vascularized graft source.[17] With the exception of vessel occlusion, most complications related to the use of vascularized grafts are caused by graft harvesting and include femoral nerve palsies, donor-site hematomas, and hernia formation.[23]

Antibiotic Beads

In highly contaminated surgical fields, especially if the use of instrumentation is necessary, the temporary placement of antibiotic-impregnated cement beads may be useful to locally deliver antibiotics to the surrounding soft tissues and bone and to provide effective dead-space management and expansion of contracted tissues. Persistent bead contamination, infection, and possible inhibition of normal leukocyte function have been associated with the use of methylmethacrylate chains.[18,19]

Percutaneous Techniques

Percutaneous techniques for the treatment of vertebral osteomyelitis described by Jeanneret and Magerl include the percutaneous drainage of paraspinal abscesses, the percutaneous suction/irrigation of disc-space infections, and the percutaneous placement of external spinal fixation for stabilization.[22] Percutaneous external fixation is an alternative to open debridement and internal fixation in selected patients with vertebral osteomyelitis and bony destruction who are unable to be supported by an external orthotic device alone or are medically unfit for an open anterior debridement.[22] Jeanneret and Magerl reported on 23 patients with vertebral osteomyelitis managed surgically either with percutaneous techniques or in concert with a planned secondary anterior debridement. All of the patients received posterior external spinal fixation. Twelve were managed successfully with this treatment and required

VASCULARIZED BONE GRAFT, ANTIBIOTIC BEADS, AND PERCUTANEOUS TECHNIQUES

VASCULARIZED BONE GRAFT
- Advantages: Decreased graft resorption, superior strength, accelerated union
- Complications (from harvesting): Femoral nerve palsies, donor site hematomas, hernia formations
- Many vascularized bone graft options include internal oblique muscle flap, IOM-iliac crest myocutaneous flap, vascularized fibula, vascularized rib

ANTIBIOTIC BEADS
- Indications for temporary placement: Dead space management, expansion of contracted tissues, local antibiotic delivery
- Can become contaminated and lead to reinfection
- May inhibit leukocyte function

PERCUTANEOUS TECHNIQUES
- Percutaneous suction/irrigation for biopsy or debridement
- Percutaneous external spinal fixator (PESF)
  - Possible between T3 and S1
  - Option when external orthotic device is inadequate and open instrumentation is contraindicated

SUMMARY

- Diagnosis of vertebral osteomyelitis and discitis is based on clinical suspicion and imaging confirmation (MRI).
- Timely diagnosis and management limit serious complications.
- Organism identification, IV antibiotics, and spinal bracing are usually sufficient.
- With surgical therapy, autologous bone sources are preferable.
- Avoid instrumentation at the site of infection.
- Consider circumferential stability.

no further intervention. Two patients with progressive bony destruction required an unplanned anterior debridement and bone grafting.

CONCLUSIONS

Fortunately, vertebral osteomyelitis is uncommon; however, its relative rarity combined with a nonspecific presentation may hinder timely diagnosis, leading to delay in appropriate treatment. Spinal infection should be suspected in a patient with significant back pain, fever, and laboratory evidence of an acute inflammatory process. Minimizing delays in diagnosis through increased clinician awareness and the use of advanced imaging modalities may limit or prevent the complications associated with a progressive spinal infection, such as invasion into the epidural space, structural deformities, chronic osteomyelitis, sepsis, paralysis, and even death. MRI is the most sensitive and specific imaging tool for a suspected diagnosis of vertebral osteomyelitis. It allows early detection of the subtle pathologic changes of inflammation before abscess formation or vertebral destruction. Identification of the offending pathogen should be sought through blood cultures or vertebral biopsy using, if available, advanced microbiologic techniques for rapid organism identification (e.g., PCR DNA amplification of difficult-to-culture organisms).

Nonoperative therapy is effective in as many as three quarters of all patients and includes parenteral antibiotic administration, spinal immobilization, and early ambulation. Surgical therapy is indicated in patients with neurologic impairment (static or progressive), the presence of a spinal abscess, sepsis, severe pain in the presence of external immobilization, a progressive spinal deformity, or gross instability; in those with the need for organism identification (open biopsy); and in those who have experienced failure of nonoperative treatment. The most widely accepted approach for surgical management of vertebral osteomyelitis combines an anterior debridement and autologous bone grafting with posterior instrumentation stabilization performed in a single- or two-stage procedure. The addition of instrumentation stabilization anteriorly immediately following an anterior debridement is advocated by some, but it remains to be investigated with long-term patient follow-up.

SELECTED REFERENCES

Cahill DW, Love LC, Rechtine GR: Pyogenic osteomyelitis of the spine in the elderly, *J Neurosurg* 74:878-886, 1991.
Eismont FJ et al.: Pyogenic and fungal vertebral osteomyelitis with paralysis, *J Bone Joint Surg Am* 65:19-29, 1983.
Fang D et al.: Pyogenic vertebral osteomyelitis: treatment by anterior debridement and fusion, *J Spinal Disord* 7:173-180, 1994.
Hayashi A et al.: Vascularized iliac bone graft based on a pedicle of upper lumbar vessels for anterior fusion of the thoracolumbar spine, *Br J Plast Surg* 41:425-430, 1994.
Heary R, Hunt C, Wolansky LJ: Rapid bony destruction with pyogenic vertebral osteomyelitis, *Surg Neurol* 41:34-39, 1994.
Heggeness MH et al.: Late infection of spinal instrumentation by hematogenous seeding, *Spine* 18:492-496, 1993.
Hughes J, DiGiacinto G, Sundaresan N: *Anterior instrumentation in cervical osteomyelitis*, Cervical Spine Research Society, Rancho Mirage, Calif, Dec. 1997.
Jeanneret B, Magerl F: Treatment of osteomyelitis of the spine using percutaneous suction/irrigation and percutaneous external spinal fixation, *J Spinal Disord* 7:185-205, 1994.
Lifeso RM: Pyogenic spinal sepsis in adults, *Spine* 15:1265-1271, 1990.
Medical Research Council Working Party on Tuberculosis of the Spine, Griffiths DLL, Seddon H, Ball J: A 15-year assessment of controlled trials of the management of tuberculosis of the spine in Korea and Hong Kong, *J Bone Joint Surg Br* 80:456-462, 1998.
Medical Research Council Working Party on Tuberculosis of the Spine, Griffiths DLL, Seddon H, Ball J: A 10-year assessment of a controlled trial comparing debridement and anterior spinal fusion in the management of tuberculosis of the spine in patients on standard chemotherapy in Hong Kong. Thirteenth Report of the Medical Research Council Working Party on Tuberculosis of the Spine. *J Bone Joint Surg Br* 64:393-398, 1982.
Sapico FL: Microbiology and antimicrobial therapy of spinal infections, *Orthop Clin North Am* 27:9-13, 1996.
Spies EH, Stücker R, Reichelt A: Conservative management of pyogenic osteomyelitis of the occipitocervical junction, *Spine* 24:818-822, 1999.

Wiedau-Pazos M, Curio G, Grüsser C: Epidural abscess of the cervical spine with osteomyelitis of the odontoid process, *Spine* 24:133-136, 1999.

Woo H, Rezai A, Cooper P: *Modern management of cervical osteomyelitis*, Cervical Spine Research Society, Rancho Mirage, Calif, December 1997.

REFERENCES

1. Medical Research Council Working Party on Tuberculosis of the Spine: A 15-year assessment of controlled trials of the management of tuberculosis of the spine in Korea and Hong Kong, Thirteenth Report of the Medical Research Council Working Party on Tuberculosis of the Spine, *J Bone Joint Surg Br* 80(3):456-462, 1998.

2. Bass SN et al.: Pyogenic vertebral osteomyelitis presenting as exudative pleural effusion: a series of five cases, *Chest* 114(2):642-647, 1998.

3. Blumberg KD, Silveri CP, Balderston RA: Presentation and treatment of pyogenic vertebral osteomyelitis, *Semin Spine Surg* 8(2):115-125, 1996.

4. Boutin RD et al.: Musculoskeletal imaging update, part II: update on imaging orthopedic infections, *Orthopc Clin North Am* 29(1):41-66, 1998.

5. Broner FA, Garland DE, Zigler JE: Spinal infections in the immunocompromised host, *Orthop Clin North Am* 27(1):37-46, 1996.

6. Cahill DW, Love LC, Rechtine GR: Pyogenic osteomyelitis of the spine in the elderly, *J Neurosurg* 74:878-886, 1991.

7. Calderone RR, Larsen JM: Overview and classification of spinal infections, *Orthop Clin North Am* 27(1):1-8, 1996.

8. Carragee EJ: Pyogenic vertebral osteomyelitis, *J Bone Joint Surg Am* 79(6):874-880, 1997.

9. Carragee EJ: The clinical use of magnetic resonance imaging in pyogenic vertebral osteomyelitis, *Spine* 22(7):780-785, 1997.

10. Carragee EJ et al.: The clinical use of erythrocyte sedimentation rate in pyogenic vertebral osteomyelitis, *Spine* 22(18):2089-2093, 1997.

11. Currier BL: Spinal infections: principles and techniques of spine surgery. In An HS, ed: 1996, pp. 567-603, Philadelphia, Lippincott Williams & Wilkins.

12. Del Curling OJ, Gower D, McWhorter J: Changing concepts in spinal epidural abscess: a report of 29 cases, *Neurosurgery* 27:185-192, 1990.

13. Eismont FJ et al.: Pyogenic and fungal vertebral osteomyelitis with paralysis, *J Bone Joint Surg Am* 65(1):19-29, 1983.

14. Fang D et al.: Pyogenic vertebral osteomyelitis: treatment by anterior debridement and fusion, *J Spinal Disord* 7(2):173-180, 1994.

15. Frank CJ, Hanley EN Jr: Profiles of patients with spine infections and infections that have a predilection for the spine, *Semin Spine Surg* 8(2):95-104, 1996.

16. Ghanayen AJ, Zdeblick TA: Cervical spine infections, *Orthop Clin North Am* 27(1):53-67, 1996.

17. Hayashi A et al.: Vascularized iliac bone graft based on a pedicle of upper lumbar vessels for anterior fusion of the thoracolumbar spine, *Br J Plast Surg* 47:425-430, 1994.

18. Heary RF, Hunt CD, Wolanski LJ: Rapid bony deconstruction with pyogenic vertebral osteomyelitis, *Surg Neurol* 41:34-39, 1994.

19. Heggeness MH et al.: Late infection of spinal instrumentation by hematogenous seeding, *Spine* 18(4):492-496, 1993.

20. Hlavin M et al.: Spinal epidural abscess: a ten year perspective, *Neurosurgery* 27:177-184, 1990.

21. Hughes J, DiGiancinto G, Sundaresan N: Anterior instrumentation in cervical osteomyelitis. Presented at the 25th Annual Meeting of the Cervical Spine Research Society, Rancho Mirage, Calif, Dec. 1997.

22. Jeanneret B, Magerl F: Treatment of osteomyelitis of the spine using percutaneous suction/irrigation and percutaneous external spine fixation, *J Spinal Disord* 7(3):185-205, 1994.

23. Khan IA, Vaccaro AR, Zlotolow DA: Management of vertebral diskitis and osteomyelitis, *Orthopedics* 22(8):758-765, 1999.

24. Krödel A et al.: Anterior debridement, fusion and extrafocal stabilization in the treatment of osteomyelitis of the spine, *J Spinal Disord* 12(1):17-26, 1999.

25. Küker W et al.: Epidural spine infection: variability of clinical and magnetic resonance imaging findings, *Spine* 22(5):544-550, 1997.

26. Lestini WF, Bell GR: Spinal infection: patient evaluation, *Semin Spine Surg* 8(2):81-94, 1996.

27. Liebergall M et al.: Pyogenic vertebral osteomyelitis with paralysis prognosis and treatment, *Clin Orthop* 269:142-150, 1991.

28. Lifeso RM: Pyogenic spinal sepsis in adults, *Spine* 15(12):1265-1271, 1990.

29. Mackenzie AR et al.: Spinal epidural abscess: the importance of early diagnosis and treatment, *J Neurol Neurosurg Psychiatry* 65(2):209-212, 1998.

30. Maiuri F et al.: Spondylodiskitis: clinical and magnetic imaging diagnosis, *Spine* 22(15):1741-1746, 1997.

31. McGuire RA, Eismont FJ: The fate of autogenous bone graft in surgically treated pyogenic vertebral osteomyelitis, *J Spinal Disord* 7:206-215, 1994.

32. Ozuna RM, Delamarter RB: Pyogenic vertebral osteomyelitis and postsurgical disk space infections, *Orthop Clin North Am* 27(1):87-94, 1996.

33. Perronne C et al.: Pyogenic and tuberculous spondylodiskitis (vertebral osteomyelitis) in 80 adult patients, *Clin Infect Dis* 19(4):746-750, 1994.

34. Post M et al.: Spinal infection: evaluation with MR imaging and intraoperative US, *Radiology* 169:765-771, 1998.

35. Rath SA et al.: Neurosurgical management of thoracic and lumbar vertebral osteomyelitis and discitis in adults: a review of 43 consecutive surgically treated patients, *Neurosurgery* 38(5):926-933, 1996.

36. Redfern RM et al.: Stabilization of the infected spine, *J Neurol Neurosurg Psychiatry* 5: 803-807, 1988.

37. Rezai AR et al.: Contemporary management of spinal osteomyelitis, *Neurosurgery* 44(5):1018-1025, 1999.

38. Rothman, SLG: The diagnosis of infections of the spine modern imaging techniques, *Orthop Clin North Am* 27(1):37-46, 1996.

39. Safran O et al.: Sequential or simultaneous, same-day anterior decompression and posterior stabilization in the management of vertebral osteomyelitis of the lumbar spine, *Spine* 23(7):1885-1890, 1998.

40. Sampath P, Rigamonti D: Spinal epidural abscess: a review of epidemiology, diagnosis, and treatment, *J Spinal Disord* 12(2):89-93, 1999.

41. Sapico FL: Microbiology and antimicrobial therapy of spinal infections, *Orthop Clin North Am* 27(1):9-13, 1996.

42. Savoia M: An overview of antibiotics in the treatment of bacterial, mycobacterial, and fungal osteomyelitis, *Semin Spine Surg* 8(2):105-114, 1996.

43. Spies EH, Stücker R, Reichelt A: Conservative management of pyogenic osteomyelitis of the occipitocervical junction, *Spine* 24(8):818-822, 1999.

44. Woo H, Rezai A, Cooper P: Modern management of cervical osteomyelitis. Presented at the 25th annual meeting of the Cervical Spine Research Society, Rancho Mirage, Calif, Dec. 1997.

45. Yelizarov VG et al.: Vascularized bone flaps for thoracolumbar spinal fusion, *Ann Plast Surg* 31:532-558, 1993.

46. Zeidman SM, Ducker TB: Infectious complications of spine surgery: spine surgery techniques complication avoidance, and management. In Benzel EC, ed. New York, 1999, Churchill Livingstone.

{AU: Please supply original halftones for Figures 13-1 through 13-8—cannot scan from this sort of paper}

Tuberculous Infections of the Spine

Seth K. Williams, Christopher P. Kauffman, Liz Stimson, Steven R. Garfin

Within the past decade granulomatous diseases of the spine have reemerged as a condition of sufficient prevalence to warrant awareness by spine surgeons both abroad and in the United States. Granulomatous disease of the spine may be caused by a wide variety of organisms, including fungi, spirochetes, and mycobacterium. *Mycobacterium tuberculosis* is the most common and extensively studied. Granulomatous infections of the spine are characterized by their insidious onset, and diagnosis is often delayed. Neurologic compromise is common. Effective medical treatment of these problems requires a multiple-drug regimen and spinal immobilization for many months. Surgical treatment must include radical debridement, followed by reconstruction and maintenance of spinal stability, as well as appropriate antibiotic coverage.

Tuberculosis is one of the most common human pathogens in the world today. Although thought of as a disease of the past in North America, tuberculosis has reemerged as a common source of morbidity and mortality. It is difficult to treat. Resurgence of tuberculosis can be linked to several factors. The first is noncompliance with the long-term therapy required for eradication of the organism. The second is the rising population of immunocompromised hosts. These factors have also led to the emergence of multidrug-resistant strains. Antimicrobial resistance, human immunodeficiency virus (HIV) infection, and therapeutic immunosuppression (organ transplants) have all contributed to the rising incidence of tuberculosis infecton.[15-23] The foundation of treatment is early management with appropriate antibiotics and surgical intervention when indicated for preservation of spinal stability and neurologic function.

EPIDEMIOLOGY

One third of the world's population is infected by tuberculosis, 3 million of whom succumb each year.[10,62] Most infections are controlled in the primary phase, but 5% of infections progress to secondary disseminated tuberculosis. Of these, 50% result in a fatal outcome. Tuberculosis is endemic in developing countries, where

---

EPIDEMIOLOGY OF TUBERCULOSIS

- Infects one third of the world's population
- 50% of those infected have spinal involvement
- Incidence rising with increased numbers of immunocompromised hosts
- Risk factors
  - HIV
  - Immunosuppression (e.g., transplant)
  - Alcoholism and drug abuse
- Most common cause of nontraumatic paraplegia in developing countries

---

pediatric involvement predominates. Adult infection is more common in North America, Europe, and the Middle East, where the incidence of disease is lower.[2,40,54,56,57] Within developed nations the highest risk groups are recent immigrants, the homeless, alcoholics and drug abusers, and patients with acquired immunodeficiency syndrome (AIDS).[18,21]

Approximately 10% of patients with active tuberculosis have skeletal involvement, 50% of whom have involvement of the spine.[67] Of these, 10% to 45% will have a corresponding neurologic deficit.[39] In developing countries tuberculous spondylitis is the most common cause of nontraumatic paraplegia.[69]

MICROBIOLOGY: CAUSATIVE ORGANISMS

Mycobacteria are aerobic bacilli with a capsule that retains red stain upon treatment with acid, hence the term *acid-fast bacillus*.[17] Two organisms cause tuberculosis: *M. tuberculosis* and *Mycobacterium avium-intracellulare*. *M. tuberculosis* is spread by inhalation of aerosolized tubercle bacilli. *M. avium-intracellulare* is contracted by drinking contaminated milk in developing countries. A delayed-type hypersensitivity reaction usually eradicates the organism, leaving as evidence calcified scar in the lung parenchyma and hilar lymph nodes, which together constitute the Ghon complex.[21]

CAUSATIVE ORGANISMS

- *Mycobacterium tuberculosis*
- *Mycobacterium avium-intracellulare*
- *Actinomyces israelii*
- *Nocardia asteroides*
- *Brucella*
- *Coccidioides immitis*
- *Blastomyces dermatitidis*
- *Cryptococcus neoformans*
- *Candida*
- *Aspergillus*
- *Treponema pallidum*

GRANULOMATOUS INFLAMMATION

- Human immune response causes the pathology
- Chronic in nature
- T-cell immunity—delayed-type hypersensitivity reaction
- Granuloma formation
- Tubercle—granuloma with central caseating necrosis (see Figure 14-1)

PATHOLOGY

The spectrum of inflammatory responses to infection of human tissue depends on the condition of the host and the offending organism. Suppurative inflammation is the hallmark of infection with gram-positive cocci and gram-negative rods. These organisms cause increased vascular permeability and release chemoattractants that result in massive tissue infiltration by polymorphonuclear neutrophils.[76] Pus is simply a collection of these neutrophils. Suppurative inflammation differs from granulomatous inflammation in etiology, pathophysiology, natural course, and treatment.

Granulomatous inflammation is a reaction to foreign bodies or persistent organism particles. Associated disease states are chronic in nature, and the response strongly linked to T-cell immunity. Focal areas of granulomatous inflammation are marked by granulomas, which are identified by their distinct inflammatory cell morphology. Such a microscopic finding narrows the differential diagnosis to a subset of infectious and immune-linked diseases. Tuberculosis, fungal infection (e.g., coccidioidomycosis, histoplasmosis), leprosy, syphilis, sarcoidosis, schistosomiasis, Crohn's disease, cat-scratch disease, and presence of foreign bodies result in a granulomatous response. Tuberculosis is the archetype and is distinguished by demonstration of granulomas with central caseating necrosis (Figure 14-1). This type of granuloma, though not quite pathognomonic of tuberculosis, is referred to as a tubercle.[21]

Involvement of the spine is usually secondary to seeding from a remote source, typically the lungs and less frequently the genitourinary system.[11] Direct extension from a paraspinal site occurs rarely.[11,20,32]

Involvement of the spine may be classified as peridiscal, anterior, or central.[29] Posterior arch involvement and infection of the cord alone are atypical of tuberculous infection.[4,74] Over one half of adult cases are peridiscal.[11]

With peridiscal involvement the infection begins within the metaphysis. Spread to adjacent vertebral bodies occurs underneath the anterior longitudinal ligament. Sparing of the disc is characteristic, as opposed to pyogenic infection (Figures 14-2 and 14-3). However, disc space narrowing does occur, as does infection of the disc itself.[11,20] Anterior involvement includes spread beneath the anterior longitudinal ligament, with erosion of the anterior segment of vertebral bodies over several segments. Central lesions begin within the middle of the vertebral body and tend to remain restricted to one segment (Figures 14-4 and 14-5). Collapse is typical, often causing spinal deformity.[11,29]

Secondary tuberculosis implies disseminated disease. This occurs by reactivation of dormant disease, direct progression from primary stage, reinfection, or inadequately treated cases. Granulomas then appear in the apex of the lung and any other organ system. Differing presentations may imitate a multitude of diseases.[21]

Other infectious organisms cause granulomatous reactions as well and may involve the spine. *Actinomyces israelii* is an anaerobic gram-positive bacterium known for its propensity to form draining sinuses. The organisms require trauma, surgery, or other infection to penetrate the mucosa. *Nocardia asteroides* is an aerobic bacterium that causes respiratory tract infection and pulmonary granulomas primarily in immunocompromised hosts. *Nocardia* disseminates to the brain, meninges, and spinal cord in 23% of cases, but vertebral involvement is rare. *Brucella* is an aerobic gram-negative organism contracted from direct contact with domestic animals or contaminated products. Fungal infections such as coccidioidomycosis, histoplasmosis, blastomycosis, cryptococcosis, and aspergillosis are being seen in increasing frequency in immunocompromised hosts.

Treponema pallidum, more commonly known as syphilis, has been called the "great imitator" and causes two types of lesions in the spine. Charcot's spine is the most common. Bony erosion, compiled with excessive reactive bone development, typically occurs related to insensitivity. It is caused by involvement of the posterior columns of the spinal cord, not a primary lesion in the bone. This is tabes dorsalis and is manifested as postural instability with paroxysmal radiating pain and paresthesias to the lower extremities. The second type of lesion is gummatous lesions of the spine itself. The treatment of choice for syphilis remains penicillin.

The treatment of these organisms varies pharmacologically, but the surgical principles remain the same. Biopsy is necessary for definitive diagnosis and to guide appropriate antibiotic therapy. The pharmacologic treatment of fungal infections is difficult, often necessitating long-term and sometimes lifetime antifungal chemotherapy. The surgical options are the same as for tuberculosis and are guided by the same algorithm.

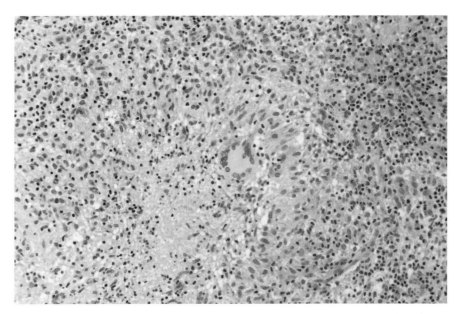

Figure 14-1. Granuloma with caseating necrosis. *(From Kauffman CP et al.: Spinal granulomatous infection, Semin Spine Surg 12[4]:191-201, 2000.)*

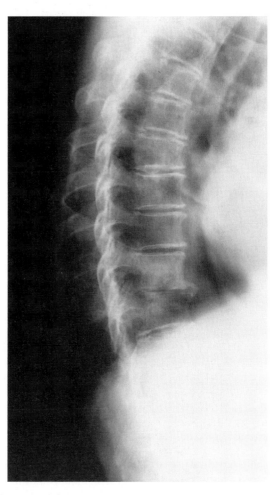

Figure 14-2. Tuberculosis T9 to T10. *(From Kauffman CP et al.: Spinal granulomatous infection, Semin Spine Surg 12[4]:191-201, 2000.)*

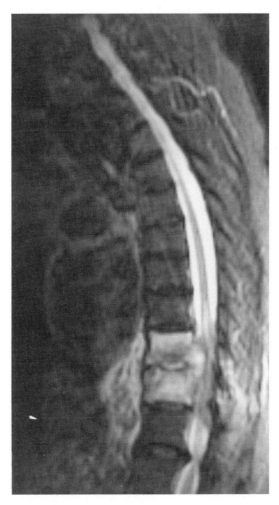

Figure 14-3. MRI findings—patient in Figure 14-2. Note sparing of disc space. *(From Kauffman CP et al.: Spinal granulomatous infection, Semin Spine Surg 12[4]:191-201, 2000.)*

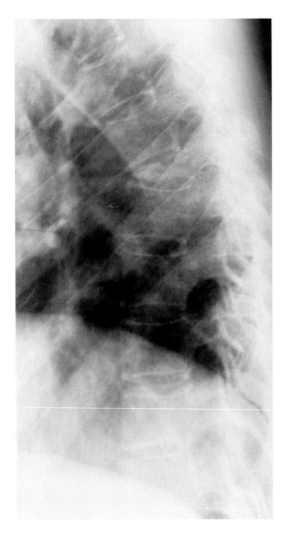

Figure 14-4. Tuberculosis of T6 with collapse/kyphosis. *(From Kauffman CP et al.: Spinal granulomatous infection, Semin Spine Surg 12[4]:191-201, 2000.)*

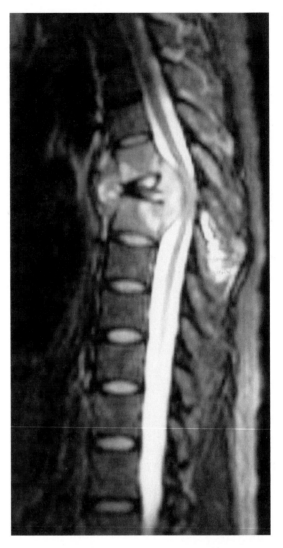

Figure 14-5. Same patient as Figure 14-4. MRI shows involvement of adjacent bodies, also large epidural granuloma. *(From Kauffman CP et al.: Spinal granulomatous infection, Semin Spine Surg 12[4]:191-201, 2000.)*

SPINAL INVOLVEMENT

- Usually secondary from lungs or genitourinary tract
- Three common types
  - Peridiscal (50%)
    - Starts in metaphysis
    - Spreads under anterior longitudinal ligament
    - Commonly spares disc spaces (see Figures 14-2 and 14-3)
  - Anterior
    - Spreads under anterior longitudinal ligament
    - Erosions of anterior columns of several adjacent vertebrae
  - Central
    - Usually restricted to one segment (see Figures 14-4 and 14-5)
- Posterior involvement rare
- Secondary pyogenic infection possible

Neurologic involvement may occur during the course of active disease or after resolution. During active disease, neurologic involvement is secondary to external pressure, invasion of the dura, kyphotic deformity, subluxation, or dislocation. After resolution, fibrosis, persistent granulomas, or progressive deformity due to instability may cause neurologic symptoms. Most lesions are anterior, but involvement of the arches with posterior compression does occur. Rarely, direct involvement of the spinal cord or nerve roots is responsible for the neurologic deficit.[31,45,54,64]

Secondary pyogenic infection may complicate tuberculous spondylitis. Inoculation occurs via draining sinus tracts from paraspinal abscesses or after debridement.[20]

NEUROLOGIC INVOLVEMENT

- Active infection
  - External pressure
  - Kyphotic deformity
  - Invasion of the dura
  - Subluxation
  - Dislocation
- Chronic infection
  - Persistent granulomas—direct pressure
  - Fibrosis
  - Progressive deformity
- Direct cord or meningeal involvement rare

CLINICAL PRESENTATION

- Back pain
- Draining sinuses
- Deformity
- Neurologic involvement
- Paraplegia
  - Cervical
  - Thoracic
  - More likely in adults, although disease more extensive in children

---

PATHOPHYSIOLOGY

Virulence is linked to the ability of the tubercle bacillus to escape immune mechanisms and induce a delayed-type hypersensitivity reaction. *M. tuberculosis* has no known exotoxins, endotoxins, or histolytic enzymes. Its destructiveness in tissues is believed to be a result of continued immune function as a response to persistence of the organism.[18,25] The human immune response causes the pathology. Because granulomatous infection tends to run a chronic, indolent course, early diagnosis is typically not vital, as it may be in a case of acute pyogenic infection.

HISTORIC PERSPECTIVE

Spinal tuberculosis was first described by Sir Percival Pott in 1779 and came to be referred to as Pott's disease. Nonsurgical treatment was typically limited to fresh air, sunlight, bed rest, and nutrition.[11] Pott was the first to advocate drainage of a tubercle abscess in the face of paraplegia.[65] This was the first form of surgical debridement for tuberculosis of the spine and led others to more radical debridement.

The advent of pharmacotherapeutic measures revolutionized the approach to treatment and remains the cornerstone of cure.[54] Surgical intervention has evolved into an important adjunct to pharmacotherapy. In many cases cure cannot be expected without operative treatment (debridement and fusion).[56]

Albee originally described spinal instrumentation for the treatment of spinal tuberculosis in 1911.[3] Instrumentation of the spine allowed for more radical debridement while maintaining stability and protection of the spinal cord. Stabilization with instrumentation also provided higher fusion rates. It was the combination of Sir Percival Pott's ideas for debridement and Albee's instrumented fusion that has evolved into the current surgical treatment for spinal infection.

CLINICAL PRESENTATION

Clinical presentation is extremely variable and depends upon the site of involvement, severity of disease, and duration of infection. Classically the patient has sys-temic manifestations such as weight loss, fever, fatigue, and malaise, as well as complaints of back pain. The pain corresponds to the site of involvement. It is most common in the thoracic spine, less common in the lumbar spine, and rare in the cervical spine, sacrum, and coccyx. Abscesses, with or without draining sinus tracts, may occur at any site.[43,58,59]

Neurologic deficit and deformity are variably present. Paraplegia is the most common neurologic deficit and is seen mainly with cervical and thoracic spine lesions. With respect to cervical involvement, adults are much more likely to suffer from paraplegia than children, even though children often have more extensive involvement.[1,5,13,60,61]

DIAGNOSIS

Tuberculous spondylitis is suggested when characteristic symptoms and imaging studies are present and the tubercle bacillus is identified in a sputum sample, urine sample, or aspirated abscess. In order to make the diagnosis, organisms must be isolated from the spine lesion.[51] If surgery is indicated based on clinical presentation and imaging studies, samples can be taken intraoperatively and cultures and sensitivities obtained to guide chemotherapy. If surgery is not clearly indicated, a percutaneous biopsy may be obtained in order to culture the organism, establish a diagnosis, and guide chemotherapy.

Laboratory Findings

Diagnosis is made by the demonstration of acid-fast organisms in an appropriate clinical specimen and is confirmed with cultures. Characteristic radiographic findings are supportive of diagnosis. Because the tubercle bacillus grows slowly in culture, final confirmation is not available 6 to 8 weeks.[7,53] More rapid confirmation may be made by biochemical techniques, such as polymerase chain reaction (PCR). These rapid techniques may be limited by their exquisite specificity. The tests typically detect sequences specific to one species of mycobacterium, thereby potentially returning a negative result in the event of infection with an unexpected species.[8,16,22,24]

Evidence of prior exposure is elicited by placing purified protein derivative (PPD) under the skin, which

DIAGNOSIS

- Organisms isolated from spinal lesion
- Acid-fast staining
- Growth in culture—requires 6 to 8 weeks
- Polymerase chain reaction (PCR)
  - Rapid
  - Most specific test will only identify **exact** organism tested
    - Must order PCR for each organism suspected
    - Not available for all organisms or species
- Purified protein derivative (PPD) test
  - Best as screening tool
  - Only indicates prior exposure
  - Not indicative of active disease or infectiousness
- White blood cell count (WBC) not usually helpful
- Erythrocyte sedimentation rate (ESR) elevated but nonspecific

DIAGNOSTIC IMAGING

PLAIN RADIOGRAPHS
- Early findings
  - Often negative
  - Bone rarefaction
- Late findings
  - Peridiscal
    - Disc space narrowing
    - See Figures 14-6 and 14-7—tuberculosis of L2 to L3
  - Anterior
    - Characteristic scalloped appearance over several adjacent levels
  - Central
    - Rarefaction in body often confused with metastatic cancer
- Note: By time of presentation often see advanced kyphotic deformity/collapse

MAGNETIC RESONANCE IMAGING (MRI)
- Diagnostic imaging modality of choice
- Often distinguishes between pyogenic infection, granulomatous infection, and tumor
- Relative sparing of disc spaces (also seen in neoplastic processes)
- Large paraspinal masses (see Figures 14-3 and 14-5)
- Gadolinium-enhanced MRI
  - Granulomas enhance throughout
  - Pyogenic abscesses enhance on periphery only
- Combination of disc space sparing and enhancing granulation tissue—highly suggestive but not pathognomic
  CAUTION (Figures 14-8 and 14-9)

COMPUTED TOMOGRAPHY (CT)
- Useful for minimally invasive biopsy
- Extent of bony destruction
- Extent of soft tissue changes

RADIONUCLIDE SCANNING
- No real role in evaluation of granulomatous infection

elicits a delayed-type hypersensitivity response. This response is dependent upon presence of memory T cells and becomes positive 1 to 3 weeks after exposure. The PPD is not indicative of active disease or degree of infectiousness. This technique is best utilized as a screening tool.[7,21] All patients with suspected tuberculosis require a PPD test and anergy panel as part of the diagnostic work-up.

White blood cell counts (WBCs) may be helpful in distinguishing pyogenic from granulomatous infections, but in the WBC may be normal or only slightly elevated. The erythrocyte sedimentation rate (ESR) is often increased but is also nonspecific.[54]

Diagnostic Imaging

Imaging studies begin with plain anteroposterior (AP) and lateral radiographs of the spine (Figures 14-6 and 14-7). Findings depend upon the type, extent, and chronicity of infection. Tuberculous infection of the spine is typically indolent, as compared with an acute pyogenic infection. Initial radiographs may be negative in both diseases, although with the typically late presentation of patients with Pott's disease, the radiographic demonstration of bony changes and collapse are often advanced. Bone rarefaction is a common early finding. With peridiscal infection, disc space narrowing precedes bone destruction. Anterior involvement over several segments produces a characteristic "scalloped" appearance. Central body involvement is often mistaken for a tumor, with central rarefaction progressing to collapse.[19,29,44,68] Chest films should be obtained to evaluate for pulmonary involvement and for paraspinal soft tissue masses.

Magnetic resonance imaging (MRI) is the imaging study of choice to obtain when tuberculous spondylitis is suspected. MRI findings in Pott's disease show differences from both pyogenic infection and tumor. There is a relative sparing of the disc spaces, which is similar to, but usually distinguishable from, findings in metastatic cancer (Figure 14-8). The sparing of the disc space reflects disc resistance to tuberculous infection. An anterior lesion spreading over several segments or isolated posterior involvement raises the likelihood of tuberculous spondylitis. Paraspinal masses are usually larger in granulomatous infection and in pyogenic infection and can be differentiated with the use of contrast. On gadolinium-enhanced scans granulation tissue enhances throughout, whereas an abscess tends to enhance only at the periphery. The combination of disc space sparing and enhancing granulation tissue is highly suggestive of tuberculosis.[27,36,50,70,71] Because granulomatous and pyogenic processes may present similarly and no MRI finding is pathognomonic, biopsy must be obtained to establish the diagnosis.

Other imaging may aid in the diagnosis. Plain films of the chest may show characteristic apical lesions or the Ghon complex. Bone scans may help demonstrate extent of involvement but are nonspecific. Computed tomography (CT) scans may be useful in evaluating perispinal soft tissue changes and in determining the

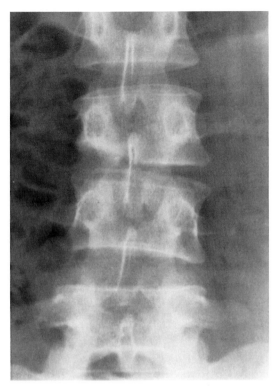

Figure 14-6. Tuberculosis of L2 to L3, AP view. *(From Kauffman CP et al.: Spinal granulomatous infection, Semin Spine Surg 12[4]:191-201, 2000.)*

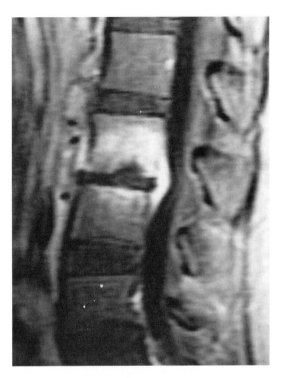

Figure 14-8. Same patient as in Figures 14-6 and 14-7. MRI: tuberculosis of L2 to L3. *(From Kauffman CP et al.: Spinal granulomatous infection, Semin Spine Surg 12[4]:191-201, 2000.)*

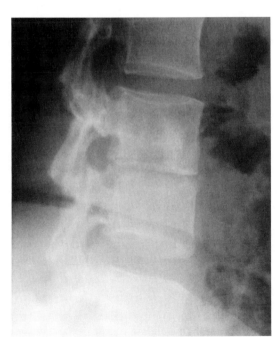

Figure 14-7. Same patient as in Figure 14-6. Tuberculosis of L2 to L3, lateral view. *(From Kauffman CP et al.: Spinal granulomatous infection, Semin Spine Surg 12[4]:191-201, 2000.)*

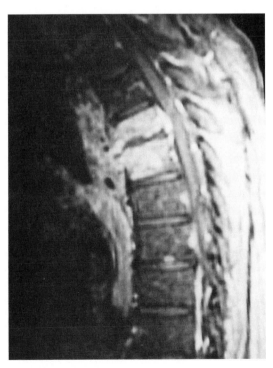

Figure 14-9. MRI: patient with *Staphylococcus aureus* infection. MRI highly suggestive of tuberculosis, sparing of disc spaces, large enhancing anterior soft tissue mass. This patient turned out to have *S. aureus* infection. *(From Kauffman CP et al.: Spinal granulomatous infection, Semin Spine Surg 12[4]:191-201, 2000.)*

extent of bony involvement.[48] CT can also be used to obtain needle biopsy when radical debridement is not indicated. One problem with needle biopsy remains the amount of tissue obtainable and a higher false-negative biopsy rate. In the event acid-fast bacilli are not seen on staining, a delay in diagnosis occurs because cultures take up to 8 weeks for final results.

TREATMENT

The treatment of patients with established tuberculosis depends on their neurologic status at the time of presentation. The goal of treatment is prevention or improvement of neurologic deficit and spinal deformity. Patients without neurologic deficit or significant kyphosis should be treated with a multidrug regimen for 9 months. Management initially includes a biopsy to establish the diagnosis and allow for cultures to guide pharmacotherapy. The first biopsy can be done by interventional radiology techniques, but an open biopsy may be necessary if insufficient tissue is obtained by percutaneous methods. When open biopsy is necessary, posterior approaches, either transpedicular or costotransversectomy, are appropriate. If it is necessary to use an anterior approach for biopsy, then radical debridement and fusion should be considered at the time of biopsy.

Pharmacotherapy

Pharmacotherapy directed against the tubercle bacillus began with the discovery of streptomycin by Waksman in 1943, followed by the fortuitous discovery of isoniazid by Chorine in 1945.[38,39] The earliest studies were performed on streptomycin.[12] Five years after its introduction the mortality rate at Sea View Hospital in New York decreased by 72.5%.[14] Isoniazid came to be recognized as a more effective agent, and to this day isoniazid remains the most important antituberculous agent worldwide.[26,34] As resistance emerged, however, treatment with isoniazid alone became ineffective. Pyridoxine (vitamin B₆) should be given concurrently, because it prevents the side effect of peripheral neuritis, which occurs in 2% of patients taking isoniazid.[72]

Rifampin is an important adjunct to isoniazid. Given alone, resistance to rifampin develops quickly. However, the combination of rifampin and isoniazid is more effective than either one alone and is sufficient in areas where primary resistance to isoniazid is rare. Primary resistance to isoniazid occurs in approximately 10% of all isolates. In areas of the United States where resistance occurs most frequently, such as large cities, borders with Mexico, and sites of immigration, empiric therapy is often initiated with four agents. Cultures are not mature for 6 to 8 weeks, and all agents must be continued until susceptibility results are available. When definitive sensitivities are established, some of the drugs may be discontinued.[6,9]

Multidrug treatment is now standard due to increasing resistance to single agents and even combination of agents. Selection of drug combinations is based on regional patterns of sensitivity, side-effect profiles, and

> ## PHARMACOTHERAPY
>
> - Key: Long-term, multidrug treatment regimen
> - Patient compliance issues
> - Based on tuberculous organisms both intracellularly and extracellularly
> - Isoniazid (INH)
>   - Remains primary drug of choice
>   - Acts intracellularly/extracellularly
>   - Pyridoxine (vitamin B₆) given to prevent peripheral neuritis
> - Rifampin
>   - Always added because resistance to isoniazid develops quickly
>   - Acts intracellularly/extracellularly
> - Pyrazinamide (PZA)
> - Acts intracellularly
> - Streptomycin
> - Acts extracellularly
> - Ethambutol
> - Endemic areas and high-risk groups require four-drug regimens

mechanisms of action. Tuberculous organisms may exist in the intracellular and extracellular spaces. Isoniazid and rifampin are bactericidal against both forms. Streptomycin is active extracellularly and therefore is often used to complement the intracellular action of pyrazinamide.[9,34,47,66,73]

First-line agents are isoniazid, rifampin, pyrazinamide, and streptomycin (or ethambutol). Second-line agents may be used in some cases where multidrug-resistant strains are isolated, in complicated patients such as those who are immunosuppressed, or in those with intolerance to first-line agents. Total duration of medical treatment typically comprises a 6- to 9-month period.[26,34,66]

Tubercle bacillus isolates demonstrate increasing tendency towards resistance. Multidrug-resistant strains are a result of selective pressure in those patients who are noncompliant or partially compliant with therapy. These strains pose significant treatment challenges, to the extent that the trend towards decreased incidence of tuberculoses infection has reversed.[28,33]

Operative Management

The surgical indications for treatment of tuberculosis are neurologic deficit, failure of response after 3 to 6 months of nonoperative treatment, uncertain diagnosis, instability, progressive kyphotic deformity, or recurrence of disease. The surgical options include anterior debridement and strut graft, with or without posterior instrumentation and fusion. Posterior surgery without anterior debridement is reserved for patients with disease of the posterior elements causing neurologic sequelae.

Neurologic Involvement

The treatment of neurologic deficit deserves special consideration. As early as 1779 Pott found that patients

SURGICAL MANAGEMENT

SURGICAL INDICATIONS
- Neurologic deficit
- Failure of response after 3 to 6 months of nonoperative treatment
- Uncertain diagnosis
- Instability
- Progressive kyphotic deformity
- Recurrence of disease

OPERATIVE OPTIONS
- Anterior debridement and strut graft done alone or with posterior instrumentation and fusion
- Posterior surgery without anterior debridement
  - Only for isolated posterior disease
  - When done for anterior disease leads to
    - Relentless progression deformity
    - Increase in neurologic deficit

NEUROLOGIC INVOLVEMENT

- Improves with drainage
- Pharmacologic treatment alone yields inferior results; only 38% of patients with paraplegia, quadriplegia improve with drug therapy alone
- Direct correlation between duration of preoperative symptoms and neurologic recovery
- Earlier debridement leads to faster and better neurologic recovery
- Early surgery
  - Easier because planes well defined
  - Response to drug therapy faster
  - Overall surgical mortality rate is 3%

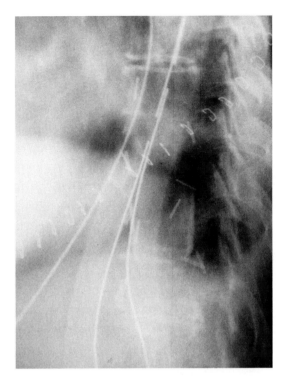

Figure 14-10. Radical debridement T5, T6, and T7 allograft strut. (*From Kauffman CP et al.: Spinal granulomatous infection,* Semin Spine Surg *12[4]:191-201, 2000.*)

demonstrated recovery of their lower extremity function following drainage of a tuberculous abscess in the spine.[65] Since that time debridement of the spine has been the accepted treatment for any patient with neurologic compromise. The approach to intervention has varied from simple debridement to anterior and posterior reconstruction of the spine. There have been attempts to treat neurologically compromised patients with pharmacotherapy alone, but the results have proven inferior to surgical decompression.

Tuli presented what he termed a "middle-path" to the treatment of spinal tuberculosis. He treated all patients, including those with neurologic deficit, initially with chemotherapy alone. Surgery was later performed on those patients who failed chemotherapy regimens. Examination of his results reveals that only 38% of patients having paraparesis, paraplegia, tetraparesis, or tetraplegia improved with drug regimens alone. Of the patients failing medical treatment, only 69% recovered with surgery.[75]

Hodgson and Stock have shown a direct correlation between duration of neurologic symptoms prior to surgery and neurologic recovery afterward.[41] Others have

documented that recovery is faster, better, and safer in patients having surgery with active disease rather than with resolved disease. The difference in recovery is thought to be due to compression of the cord by granuloma in early disease versus hard osteophytes in resolved disease, the latter suggesting longer-term compression and permanent damage.[45]

When surgery is indicated, it is best performed earlier in the treatment course, because abscesses tend to dissect along tissue planes, making the surgical dissection less demanding. When surgery is delayed, fibrosis results in scarring and subsequent loss of the planes between structures. Surgery on active disease has been shown to be safer and the response to treatment faster.[45]

Anterior Debridement

Some authors have advocated anterior debridement alone, without fusion of the spine, but the results have not proven to be as consistent as with debridement and reconstruction. The spontaneous fusion rate is lower than with the addition of strut graft (Figure 14-10).[61] Authors have also reported problems with progression of kyphotic deformity, with 18% progressing 30 degrees or more.[52] Currently anterior debridement alone is not recommended.

Posterior Decompression

Posterior decompression alone is only used for decompression of neurologic compromise from isolated

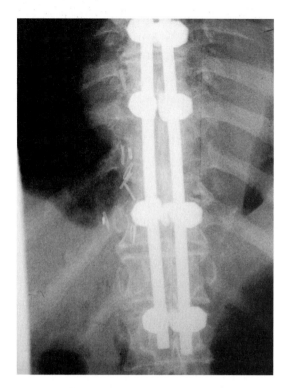

Figure 14-11. Anterior debridement/strut. Graft posterior instrumentation and fusion. *(From Kauffman CP et al.: Spinal granulomatous infection, Semin Spine Surg 12[4]:191-201, 2000.)*

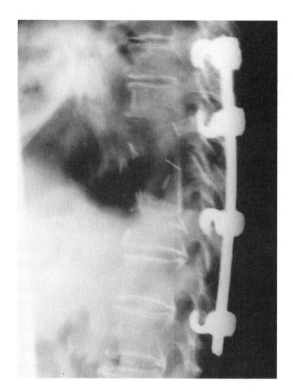

Figure 14-12. Anterior debridement/strut graft. Posterior instrumented fusion. *(From Kauffman CP et al.: Spinal granulomatous infection, Semin Spine Surg 12[4]:191-201, 2000.)*

POSTERIOR APPROACHES

POSTERIOR FUSION
- Part of staged procedure
- Alone does not control progressive kyphosis—radical debridement of disease essential
- With or without instrumentation
- Instrumentation does NOT affect ability to eradicate disease (Figures 14-11 and 14-12)

POSTERIOR DECOMPRESSION
- Only for isolated posterior disease

---

atypical posterior disease. When laminectomy is performed in the presence of anterior disease, there may be initial neurologic improvement, followed by the inevitable development of progressive kyphosis and paraplegia.[12]

Posterior Fusion

The current role of posterior fusion is in staged procedures with posterior instrumented spinal fusion following anterior debridement and grafting. Posterior fusion alone does not control the progression of kyphosis.[37] Moon and colleagues have reported their results using staged anterior and posterior procedures. They reported

cure of infection in all cases, and the loss of correction did not exceed 3 degrees at follow-up.[63] Moon has advocated the addition of posterior fusion in the skeletally immature because there is a risk of progressive deformity with growth.[42] Spinal instrumentation may be used with active tuberculous infection, because it does not affect ability to eradicate the disease. Surgical treatment, however, cannot stand alone. Appropriate antibiotic therapy must also be given.

Graft Choice

The choice of graft material depends on the anatomic location of surgery and the availability of bone graft. Most studies have used either iliac crest graft or rib graft. The use of rib graft is not recommended in adults, because there is a 32% incidence of graft fracture and average increase of 20 degrees of kyphosis.[49] The use of fibular graft has been studied. The major concern is the grafts are markedly weakened between 6 weeks and 6 months. The strength is almost normal at 1 year.[30] Vascularized rib grafts have been used successfully for spinal tuberculosis.[55] Fresh-frozen cortical allograft humeral segments have also been used successfully in the anterior debridement and grafting procedures.[35] Among the types of graft used successfully, choice of materials depends upon surgeon preference and availability of an allograft or sufficient quantity of autografts.

> ## GRAFT CHOICE
>
> NOTE: All are acceptable and depend on surgeon preference, size of defect, and availability
> - Autograft
>   - Iliac crest
>   - Rib—not recommended in adults
> - Allograft
> - Vascularized fibula

Complications

The complications associated with surgical treatment of tuberculosis are the same as those associated with the approach used for the surgery. Complications are frequent, and overall mortality rate is about 3%.[42] The relapse rate with current regimens is close to zero.

CERVICAL DISEASE

Tuberculosis of the cervical spine is especially concerning because there is a 40% incidence of cord compression. Lesions in this area deserve aggressive treatment, including surgical debridement and strut grafting.[46] The surgical approach is the standard anterior cervical approach used for corpectomy. Anterior debridement and strut grafting may need to be staged with a posterior instrumented fusion. Laminectomy is contraindicated in the cervical spine.

CONCLUSIONS

Tuberculosis is the most common cause of nontraumatic paraplegia and quadriplegia throughout the world in developing countries. It is estimated that one third of the world's population has been infected with tuberculosis. There is a resurgence of tuberculosis in North America that can be attributed to a rising population of immunocompromised hosts, including patients with disease and those undergoing therapeutic treatment. It is necessary for physicians treating spinal disorders to be familiar with the presentation, diagnosis, and treatment of granulomatous infection.

The treatment of granulomatous infections of the spine differs from pyogenic infections because of the slow, insidious nature of the disease. The role of the spine surgeon is in both the diagnosis and treatment of the disease. There are several key points to consider when taking care of these patients. Definitive diagnosis is necessary prior to treatment because different granulomatous infections not only require different pharmacologic treatment regimens but also may radiographically mimic tumor. Patients with neurologic deficit require early evaluation for decompressable lesions, and initiation of treatment should be considered early in the treatment course. This is especially true in cervical disease. Anterior debridement and reconstruction at the site of pathology has shown the best long-term neurologic and structural results with a very high successful clinical outcome. Treatment is best performed using a team approach among spine surgeons and medical and infectious disease specialists.

SELECTED REFERENCES

Bloch AB et al.: Nationwide survey of drug-resistant tuberculosis in the United States, *JAMA* 271:665-671, 1994.

Desai SS: Early diagnosis of spinal tuberculosis by MRI, *J Bone Joint Surg Br* 76:863-869, 1994.

Medical Research Council Working Party on Tuberculosis of the Spine: A 15-year assessment of controlled trials of the management of tuberculosis of the spine in Korea and Hong Kong, *J Bone Joint Surg Br* 80:456-462, 1998.

Naim-Ur-Rahman, Al-Arabi KM, Khan FA: Atypical forms of spinal tuberculosis, *Acta Neurochir (Wien)* 88:26-33, 1987.

REFERENCES

1. Adams ZB: Tuberculosis of the spine in children: a review of sixty-three cases from the Lakeville State Sanitorium, *J Bone Joint Surg* 22:860-861, 1940.
2. Adendorff JJ, Boeke EJ, Lazarus C: Tuberculosis of the spine: results of management of 300 patients, *J R Coll Surg Edinb* 32:152-155, 1987.
3. Albee FH: Transplantation of a portion of the tibia into the spine for Pott's disease: a preliminary report, *JAMA* 57:885-886, 1911.
4. Babhulkar SS, Tayade WB, Babhulkar SK: Atypical spinal tuberculosis, *J Bone Joint Surg Br* 66:239-242, 1984.
5. Bailey HL et al.: Tuberculosis of the spine in children, *J Bone Joint Surg Am* 54:1633-1657, 1972.
6. Bass JB Jr et al.: Treatment of tuberculosis and tuberculosis infection in adults and children, *Am J Respir Crit Care Med* 149:1359-1374, 1994.
7. Bates JH: Diagnosis of tuberculosis, *Chest* 76:757-763, 1979.
8. Berk RH et al.: Detection of *Mycobacterium tuberculosis* in formaldehyde solution-fixed, parafin-embedded tissue by polymerase chain reaction in Pott's disease, *Spine* 21:1991-1995, 1996.
9. Bloch AB et al.: Nationwide survey of drug-resistant tuberculosis in the United States, *JAMA* 271:665-671, 1994.
10. Bloom BR, Murray CJ: Tuberculosis: commentary on a reemergent killer, *Science* 257:1055-1064, 1992.
11. Boachie-Adjei O, Squillante RG: Tuberculosis of the spine, *Orthop Clin North Am* 27:95-103, 1996.
12. Bosworth DM, Pietra AD, Farrell RF: Streptomycin in tuberculous bone and joint lesions with mixed infection sinuses, *J Bone Joint Surg Am* 32:103-108, 1950.
13. Bosworth DM, Pietra AD, Rahilly G: Paraplegia resulting from tuberculosis of the spine, *J Bone Joint Surg Am* 35:735-740, 1953.
14. Bouchez B, Arnott G, Delfosse JM: Acute spinal epidural abscess, *J Neurol* 231:343-344, 1985.
15. Bradford WZ, Daley CL: Multiple drug-resistant tuberculosis, *Infect Dis Clin North Am* 12:157-172, 1998.
16. Brisson-Noel A et al.: Rapid diagnosis of tuberculosis by amplification of mycobacterial DNA in clinical samples, *Lancet* 2:1069-1071, 1989.
17. Burdash NM et al.: Evaluation of the acid-fast smear, *J Clin Microbiol* 4:190-191, 1976.
18. Cantwel MF et al.: Epidemiology of tuberculosis in the United States, 1985 through 1992, *JAMA* 272:535-539, 1994.
19. Chapman M, Murray RO, Stoker DJ: Tuberculosis of bones and joints, *Semin Roentgenol* 14:266-282, 1979.
20. Compere EL, Garrison M: Correlation of pathologic and roentgenologic findings in tuberculosis and pyogenic infections of the vertebra: the fate of the intervertebral disk, *Ann Surg* 104:1038-1067, 1936.
21. Cotran RS, Kumar V, Robbins SL: *Robins pathologic basis of disease*, ed 5, Philadelphia, 1994, WB Saunders.
22. Cousins DV et al.: Use of polymerase chain reaction for rapid diagnosis of tuberculosis, *J Clin Microbiol* 30:255-258, 1992.
23. Daley CL, Small PM, Schecter GF: An outbreak of tuberculosis with accelerated progression among persons infected with the human immunodeficiency virus, *N Engl J Med* 326:231-235, 1992.

24. Daniel TM: The rapid diagnosis of tuberculosis: a selective review, *J Lab Clin Med* 116:277-282, 1990.
25. Dannenberg AM Jr: Delayed-type hypersensitivity and cell-mediated immunity in the pathogenesis of tuberculosis, *Immunol Today* 12:228-233, 1991.
26. Davidson PT: Treating tuberculosis: what drugs, for how long? *Ann Intern Med* 112:393-395, 1990.
27. Desai SS: Early diagnosis of spinal tuberculosis by MRI, *J Bone Joint Surg Br* 76:863-869, 1994.
28. Dooley SW et al.: Multidrug-resistant tuberculosis, *Ann Intern Med* 117:257-259, 1992.
29. Doub HP, Badgley CE: The roentgen signs of tuberculosis of the vertebral body, *Am J Roentgenol* 27:827-837, 1932.
30. Enneking WF et al.: Physical and biological aspects of repair in dog corticol bone transplants, *J Bone Joint Surg Am* 57:237-252, 1975.
31. Freilich D, Swash M: Diagnosis and management of tuberculous paraplegia with special reference to tuberculous radiculomyelitis, *J Neurol Neurosurg Psychiatry* 42:12-18, 1979.
32. Friedman B: Chemotherapy of tuberculosis of the spine, *J Bone Joint Surg Am* 48:451-474, 1966.
33. Goble M et al.: Treatment of 171 patients with pulmonary tuberculosis resistant to isoniazid and rifampin, *N Engl J Med* 328:527-532, 1993.
34. Goldman AL, Braman SS: Isoniazid: a review with emphasis on adverse effects, *Chest* 62:71-77, 1972.
35. Govender S, Parbhoo AH: Support of the anterior column with allografts in tuberculosis of the spine, *J Bone Joint Surg Br* 81:106-109, 1999.
36. Gundry CR, Fritts HM: Magnetic resonance imaging of the musculoskeletal system: the spine, *Clin Orthop* 346:262-278, 1998.
37. Halpern AA et al.: Coccidiomycosis of the spine: unusual roentgenographic presentations, *Clin Orthop* 140:78-79, 1979.
38. Hardman JG et al.: Antimicrobial agents: drugs used in the treatment of tuberculosis and leprosy. In *Goodman and Gilman's the pharmacological basis of therapeutics*, ed 9, New York, 1996, McGraw-Hill, pp. 1155-1174.
39. Herkowitz HN et al.: Infections of the spine. In Herkowitz HN et al.: *Rothman-Simeone the spine*, ed 4, Philadelphia, 1999, WB Saunders, pp. 1207-1258.
40. Hodgson AR: Report of the findings and results in 300 cases of Pott's disease treated by anterior fusion of the spine, *J West Pacitc Orthop Assoc* 1:3, 1964.
41. Hodgson AR, Stock FE: Anterior spinal fusion for the treatment of tuberculosis of the spine: the operative findings and results of treatment in the first one hundred cases, *J Bone Joint Surg Am* 42A:295-310, 1960.
42. Hodgson AR, Stock FE, Fang HSY: Anterior spinal fusion: the operative approach and pathologic findings in 412 patients with Pott's disease of the spine, *Br J Surg* 48:172-178, 1960.
43. Hodgson AR et al.: A clinical study of one hundred consecutive cases of Pott's paraplegia, *Clin Orthop* 36:128-150, 1964.
44. Hopewell PC: A clinical view of tuberculosis, *Radiol Clin North Am* 33:641-653, 1995.
45. Hsu LCS, Cheng CL, Leong JCY: Pott's paraplegia of late onset: the cause of compression and results after anterior decompression, *J Bone Joint Surg Br* 70:534-538, 1988.
46. Hsu LCS, Leong JCY: Tuberculosis of the lower cervical spine (C2-C7): a report on 40 cases, *J Bone Joint Surg Br* 66:1-5, 1984.
47. Iseman MD: Treatment of multidrug-resistant tuberculosis, *N Engl J Med* 329:784-791, 1993.
48. Jain R, Sawhney S, Berry M: Computed tomography of vertebral tuberculosis: patterns of bone destruction, *Clin Radiol* 47:196-199, 1993.
49. Kemp HBS et al.: Anterior fusion of the spine for infective lesions in adults, *J Bone Joint Surg Br* 55:715-734, 1973.
50. Kim NH, Lee HM, Suh JS: Magnetic resonance imaging for the diagnosis of tuberculous spondylitis, *Spine* 19:2451-2455, 1994.
51. Kirkaldy-Willis WH, Thomas TG: Anterior approaches in the diagnosis and treatment of infections of the vertebral bodies, *J Bone Joint Surg Am* 47:87-110, 1965.

52. Konstam PG, Besovsky A: The ambulatory treatment of spinal tuberculosis, *Br J Surg* 50:26-38, 1962.
53. Levy H et al.: A reevaluation of sputum microscopy and culture in the diagnosis of pulmonary tuberculosis, *Chest* 95:1193-1197, 1989.
54. Lifeso RM, Weaver P, Harder EH: Tuberculous spondylitis in adults, *J Bone Joint Surg Am* 67:1405-1413, 1985.
55. Louw JA: Spinal tuberculosis with neurologic deficit: treatment with anterior vascularized rib grafts, posterior osteotomies and fusion, *J Bone Joint Surg Br* 72:686-693, 1990.
56. Martin NS: Tuberculosis of the spine: a study of the results of treatment during the last twenty-five years, *J Bone Joint Surg Br* 52:613-628, 1970.
57. Medical Research Council Working Party on Tuberculosis of the Spine: a controlled trial of ambulant out-patient treatment and in-patient rest in bed in the management of tuberculosis of the spine in young Korean patients on standard chemotherapy, *J Bone Joint Surg Br* 55:678-697, 1973.
58. Medical Research Council Working Party on Tuberculosis of the Spine: A controlled trial of debridement and ambulatory treatment in the management of tuberculosis of the spine in patients on standard chemotherapy: a study in Bulawayo, *Rhodesia. J Trop Med Hyg* 77:72-92, 1974.
59. Medical Research Council Working Party on Tuberculosis of the spine: Five-year assessment of controlled trials of ambulatory treatment, debridement and anterior spinal fusion in the management of tuberculosis of the spine, *J Bone Joint Surg Br* 60:163-177, 1978.
60. Medical Research Council Working Party on Tuberculosis of the Spine: A 10-year assessment of a controlled trial comparing debridement and anterior spinal fusion in the management of tuberculosis of the spine in patients on standard chemotherapy in Hong Kong, *J Bone Joint Surg Br* 64:393-398, 1982.
61. Medical Research Council Working Party on Tuberculosis of the Spine: A 15-year assessment of controlled trials of the management of tuberculosis of the spine in Korea and Hong Kong, *J Bone Joint Surg Br* 80:456-462, 1998.
62. Moon MS: Tuberculosis of the spine: controversies and a new challenge, *Spine* 22:1791-1797, 1997.
63. Moon MS et al.: Posterior instrumentation and anterior interbody fusion for tuberculous kyphosis of dorsal and lumbar spines, *Spine* 20:1910-1916, 1995.
64. Naim-Ur-Rahman, Al-Arabi KM, Khan FA: Atypical forms of spinal tuberculosis, *Acta Neurochir (Wien)* 88:26-33, 1987.
65. Pott P: *Remarks on that kind of palsy of the lower limbs which is frequently found to accompany a curvature of the spine and is supposed to be caused by it: together with its method of cure*, London, 1779, J Johnson, pp. 1-84.
66. Radner DB: Toxicologic and pharmacologic aspects of rifampin, *Chest* 64:213–216, 1973.
67. Rajasekaran S et al.: Tuberculous lesions of the lumboscaral region: a 15-year follow-up of patients treated by ambulant chemotherapy, *Spine* 23:1163-1167, 1998.
68. Ridley N et al.: Radiology of skeletal tuberculosis, *Orthopedics* 21:1213-1220, 1998.
69. Scrimgeour EM, Kaven J, Gajdusek DC: Spinal tuberculosis: the commonest cause of non-traumatic paraplegia in Papua New Guinea, *Trop Georgr Med* 39:218-221, 1987.
70. Sharif HS et al.: Granulomatous spinal infections: MR imaging, *Radiology* 177:101-107, 1990.
71. Smith AS et al.: MR imaging characteristics of tuberculous spondylitis vs vertebral osteomyelitis, *Am J Roentgenol* 153:399-405, 1989.
72. Snider DE Jr: Pyridoxine supplementation during isoniazid therapy, *Tubercle* 61:191-196, 1980.
73. Snider DE Jr, Roper WL: The new tuberculosis, *N Engl J Med* 326:703-705, 1992.
74. Travlos J, Du Tott G: Spinal tuberculosis: beware the posterior elements, *J Bone Joint Surg Br* 72:722-723, 1990.
75. Tuli SM: Results of treatment of spinal tuberculosis by "middle-path" regime, *J Bone Joint Surg Br* 57:13-23, 1975.
76. Woods GL, Guttierez Y: *Diagnostic pathology of infectious diseases*, Philadelphia, 1993, Lea and Febiger.

Primary Spinal Tumors

Bobby K.-B. Tay, Frank J. Eismont

Neoplasms of the spine can be broadly divided into primary and metastatic tumors. These in turn are subdivided into intradural and extradural lesions. This chapter focuses on the evaluation and treatment of primary extradural neoplasms of the spinal column. The evaluation and treatment of primary tumors of the spinal column have remained extremely challenging. General indications for surgery are to prevent or address spinal instability and to decompress neural elements in the face of neurologic deficit. The operative plan for each patient with a spinal neoplasm must be customized to the type, grade, and stage of the tumor, as well as to the patient's individual circumstances.

Primary spinal tumors comprise about 0.04% of all tumors and about 10% of all bony tumors. Because of their rarity, the community orthopedist or spinal surgeon is unlikely to encounter a sufficient number of these tumors to develop any significant expertise in their treatment. However, an understanding of these tumors will allow the physician to initiate the work-up to accurately evaluate and treat these patients.

The management of patients presenting with a specific neoplasm of the vertebral column depends on multiple factors including the age of the patient; his or her associated medical conditions; the type, grade, and stage of the tumor; the extent of bony involvement; spinal column stability; and the presence or absence of a neurologic deficit. Clearly, the treatment must be individualized to each patient and his or her unique circumstances. In an optimal setting, the care of the patient should be multidisciplinary, involving the concerted efforts of the spinal surgeon and the oncologist.

GENERAL OVERVIEW

Some generalizations can be made to provide a structure by which the individual tumor can be understood more easily. The age of the patient at presentation is highly correlated with the presence of a benign or malignant lesion. Benign tumors typically occur in the younger age-group (under 21 years), whereas up to 70% of malignant tumors are found in patients over 21 years of age.[108] The location of the tumor may also suggest a benign or malignant process. The majority of malignant

---

GENERALIZATIONS

- Benign tumors usually occur in patients under 21 years of age. Malignant tumors occur in patients over 21 years of age.
- Most common symptom: Pain, especially night pain.
- Neurologic deficit is rarely the first sign, but up to 70% of patients manifest weakness by diagnosis.
- Twenty percent of patients have signs or symptoms of spinal cord compression.

---

tumors originate anteriorly in the vertebral body, whereas benign tumors tend to occur in the posterior elements.

Although patients with spinal tumors can present with a variety of symptoms, the most common symptom is pain. Classically, pain that wakes a patient up at night is highly suggestive of an underlying neoplastic process. Some patients may present with both pain and deformity caused by mechanical instability or paraspinous muscle spasm. Other patients may present initially with bowel and bladder dysfunction or paraparesis or tetraparesis from spinal cord compression.

Neurologic deficit is rarely the patient's presenting complaint in neoplastic conditions of the spinal column. However, as many as 70% of patients will manifest weakness by the time that the correct diagnosis is made.[61,93] Nearly 20% of patients with spinal tumors develop symptoms of spinal cord compression such as weakness, long tract signs, and bowel and bladder dysfunction.[95] Rapidly progressive neurologic deficit is most commonly associated with malignant tumors. Before the time of magnetic resonance imaging (MRI), there were case reports in which spinal tumors masqueraded as lumbar disc herniations.[96]

PHYSICAL EXAMINATION AND IMAGING

After a careful and complete history and physical examination (including a detailed neurologic examination), appropriate imaging studies are invaluable in obtaining a diagnosis and in differentiating lesions that will require further work-up from those that can be followed without treatment. Plain radiographs were and still are the first imaging modality used in the work-up of a spinal lesion. The subtle "winking pedicle" sign may or may not be seen. This classic sign results from destruction of the pedicle secondary to tumor infiltration. The vertebral body may show signs of collapse from bony erosion of the supporting columns leading to pathologic fracture. The major disadvantage of plain radiographs is the lack of sensitivity in detecting small tumors. Radiographic evidence of bony destruction is not seen until 30% to 50% of the trabecular bone has been lost.[23]

Despite their lack of sensitivity, plain x-rays can give important clues about the nature of the tumor. In addition, flexion and extension lateral x-rays allow an assessment of spinal stability. The pattern of bony destruction provides an estimation of the malignant potential of the lesion. Geographic lesions with well-circumscribed margins suggest a more benign process. In contrast, a permeative lesion suggests the presence of a malignant neoplasm. Early on, it is often difficult to distinguish a neoplastic process from an infectious one. Indeed, cases exist in which spinal infections have been mistakenly irradiated because they were initially diagnosed as tumors. Cases also exist where infection and neoplasm co-exist.[24]

Computed tomography (CT) is more reliable and significantly more sensitive than plain radiographs. It allows an accurate estimation of the degree of bony destruction and can play an essential role in the preoperative planning for surgical stabilization or reconstruction. The main limitation of CT is its impracticality for use as a screening tool. The lesion must be localized to a specific area using a bone scan, screening radiographs, or an MRI.

The bone scan was, in the past, the most sensitive test to localize the majority of neoplastic lesions of the spine. It is highly sensitive to areas of increased osteoid formation. Its utility is most notable in the evaluation of metastatic disease. When used in combination with gallium scanning, Tc-99 bone scans can help differentiate between tumors and infections. Today, to detect and evaluate primary tumors of the spine, bone scans have been largely supplanted by MRI.

MRI is the study of choice in the diagnosis and evaluation of primary neoplasms of the spine. Its advantages include superior soft tissue visualization, the availability of multiplanar images, and its ability to evaluate the extent of neural compression or infiltration.

In most cases the imaging studies alone will allow the tumor to be staged. The best staging system for spinal tumors was recently described by Boriani in 1997 (Figure 15-1). This system (named the Weinstein-Boriani-Biagini system) is a modification of the classic Enneking staging system and also takes into account the precise location of the tumor in the vertebral column (Figure 15-2).[8] If the imaging studies fail to provide a definitive diagnosis, a biopsy is then required. Three forms of biopsy exist: needle biopsy, incisional biopsy, and excisional biopsy. Needle biopsy is the least invasive, and sufficient tissue can be obtained to make a diagnosis in most cases. Both incisional and excisional biopsy will provide a definitive

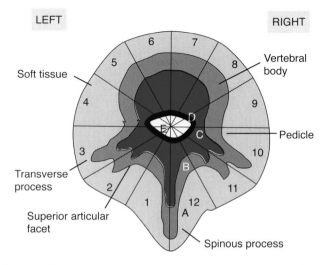

Figure 15-1. Weinstein-Boriani-Biagini Staging System for spinal tumors. *A,* Extraosseous soft tissue. *B,* Superficial intraosseous. *C,* Deep intraosseous. *D,* Extraosseous extradural. *E,* Extraosseous intradural. *(Modified from Hart R et al.: A system for surgical staging and management of spine tumors, Spine 22(15):1773-1783, 1997.)*

DIAGNOSTIC TIPS

- Requires a complete history and physical examination with detailed neurologic examination
- Plain radiographs not very sensitive for small lesions—30% to 50% trabecular bone loss for radiographic evidence of bone destruction
- Geographic lesions suggest benign process; permeative lesions suggest malignant process
- CT more sensitive than plain radiographs but lesion localized by another study first
- Bone scan combined with gallium scan differentiates tumors from infections
- MRI the most sensitive and specific test; shows relationship of tumor to neural elements
- Biopsy required when imaging studies cannot delineate lesion

---

pathologic diagnosis, but they are more invasive and require a significant amount of preoperative planning to determine the optimal approach and reconstruction (if necessary).

If removal of the tumor is necessary, the surgeon must determine the best approach for excision. Tumor excision can be broadly categorized into intralesional and en bloc excision. Curettage describes the piecemeal removal of the tumor and is always considered to be intralesional. En bloc excision is an attempt to remove the entire tumor in one piece, which on pathologic examination can be either intralesional, marginal, or wide. If the surgeon has cut into the tumor mass, the excision is intralesional. Marginal excision occurs when the tumor has been removed by dissection along its pseudocapsule. Wide excision is accomplished if the

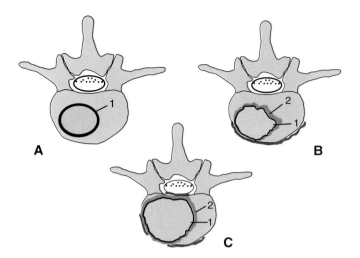

Figure 15-2. Enneking Staging System for spinal tumors. **A,** Stage 1 lesion with complete containment of the tumor within a capsule *(1)* with no reactive zone. **B,** Stage 2 lesion with active, growing tumor with a thin capsule *(1)* and a surrounding reactive zone *(2)*. **C,** Stage 3 lesion with a thin discontinuous capsule *(1)* and a wide reactive zone *(2)*. *(Modified from Hart R et al.: A system for surgical staging and management of spine tumors, Spine 22(15):1773-1783, 1997.)*

tumor is removed along with a continuous shell of normal tissue.

BENIGN TUMORS OF THE SPINE

Benign spinal tumors are usually slow-growing, well-circumscribed lesions that generally occur in the younger age-group (under 21 years). These include osteochondromas, osteoid osteomas, osteoblastomas, aneurysmal bone cysts, giant cell tumors, and eosinophilic granulomas. Benign tumors of the spinal column should be differentiated from similar tumors that occur in a peripheral location. The adjective *benign* can be a misnomer, because a benign lesion in a critical location in the spine may cause significant morbidity or mortality and may preclude complete tumor excision.

Osteochondroma

Isolated osteochondromas are one of the most common benign lesions of bone. These tumors tend to occur in the younger age-group. Multiple osteochondromatosis is the most common of all skeletal dysplasias, and about 7% of patients with multiple osteochondromatosis have vertebral involvement[57] (Figure 15-3). Treatment of

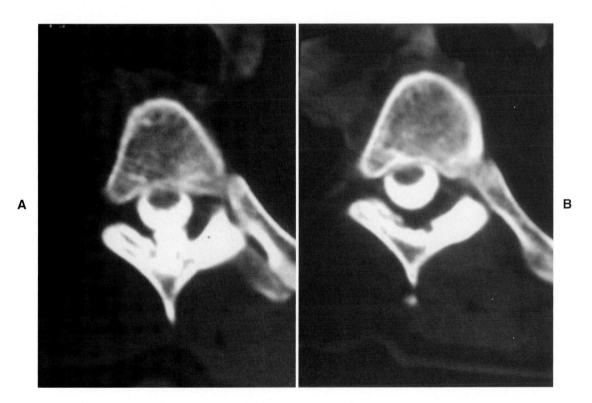

Figure 15-3. Osteochondroma. This 45-year-old woman had severe midthoracic spine pain that did not respond to any type of conservative treatment. She had no history of other osteochondromas in other areas. **A,** A postmyelogram CT scan was performed and the only abnormality was at the T7 level, where she had a protrusion into the spinal canal from her lamina, which was in contact with her dura. **B,** A simple laminectomy was performed at this one level, removing this abnormality. Pathologic examination showed this to be a simple osteochondroma. The patient's symptoms completely resolved following this surgical excision.

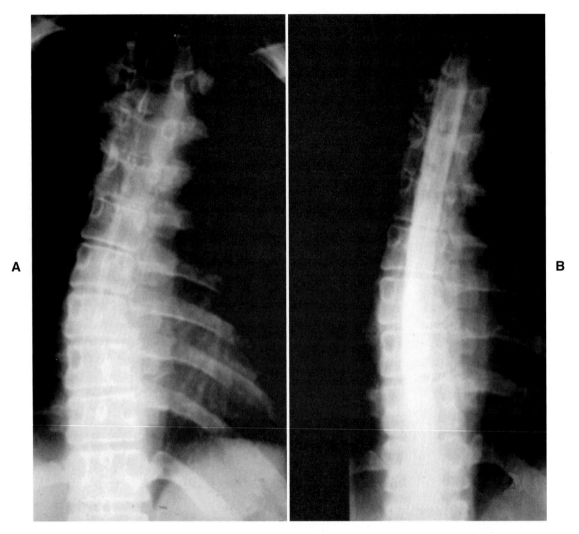

A

B

Figure 15-4.   Osteoid osteoma. This 16-year-old boy presented with a painful scoliosis. Because of the associated pain a myelogram followed by a CT scan was performed. **A,** This AP view of the thoracic spine shows the original scoliosis curvature. **B,** No significant compression of the myelogram dye can be seen.

OSTEOCHONDROMAS

- The most common benign lesions of bone
- 7% have spinal involvement

spinal osteochondromas consists of excision if neurologic deficit is present.

Osteoid Osteoma and Osteoblastoma

Osteoid osteoma and osteoblastoma are osteoblastic lesions that are differentiated from each other by size. Lesions smaller than 2 cm are arbitrarily named osteoid osteomas, whereas tumors larger than 2 cm are called osteoblastomas. These tumors tend to occur in the second and third decades of life. They occur twice as often in men than in women. These tumors are usually found in the posterior elements of the spinal column. The most common symptom is back pain that wakes the patient up at night. This is the case for osteoid osteomas. In contrast, night pain is not as frequent in osteoblastomas. Classically, the pain is relieved by salicylates and nonsteroidal antiinflammatory drugs (NSAIDs). Lesions in the thoracic spine can produce various degrees of neurologic defect ranging from radiculopathy to frank paraparesis.[7]

Osteoid osteomas appear radiographically as a nidus surrounded by densely sclerotic bone. Tumors that grow close to the periosteum may cause a fusiform thickening of the overlying cortex secondary to hyperemia. Both the nidus and periosteal reaction can sometimes be seen on plain radiographs but are most easily delineated on the axial cuts of a CT scan (Figures 15-4 to 15-6). Bone scan and MRI are also effective in localizing the tumor. MRI will overestimate the size of the tumor because of the surrounding hyperemia. Grossly, the tumor is composed of a firm red-gray tissue. On microscopic examination

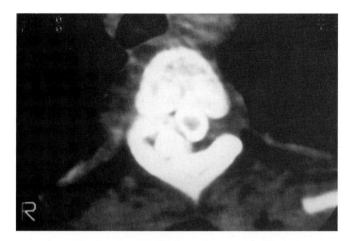

Figure 15-5. Osteoid osteoma. This postmyelogram CT scan shows a right-sided bone tumor arising from the posterolateral elements of the vertebra. This is consistent with an osteoid osteoma. The patient was treated with surgical excision and local fusion.

OSTEOID OSTEOMAS

- Smaller than 2 cm; occurs in second and third decades, usually in males
- Night pain common, relieved by salicylates
- Radiographs show nidus but lesion most easily seen on CT
- MRI overestimates tumor size because of surrounding hyperemia

OSTEOBLASTOMAS

- Larger than 2 cm
- Primary presenting symptom is pain, but night pain not frequent as in osteoid osteomas
- Radiolucent lesions with a ground-glass appearance; expansion of surrounding bone
- 41% to 46% in spine, over half in lumbar spine
- Can cause scoliosis

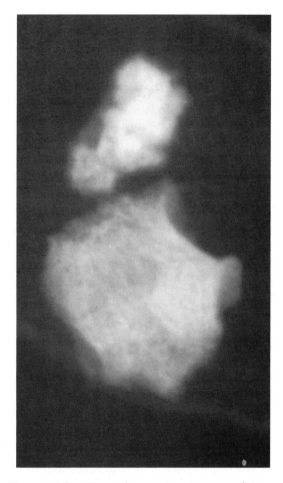

Figure 15-6. Osteoid osteoma. An x-ray of the excised tumor confirms the presence of the nidus, as well as the adjacent sclerotic bone. Following excision of this tumor, the patient's symptoms completely resolved. He was treated in a thoracolumbar sacral orthosis (TLSO) brace for 3 months until the fusion was solid.

delicate trabeculae of osteoid are rimmed with numerous osteoblasts enclosed in a vascularized spindle cell stroma. As the lesion matures, the tangled islands of partially mineralized osteoid and bony trabeculae become more prominent in the fibrous stroma.

When these benign tumors grow larger than 2 cm, they are called osteoblastomas. Because of this almost-arbitrary determination, osteoblastomas were sometimes called giant osteoid osteomas. Osteoblastomas occur less frequently than aneurysmal bone cysts, solitary plasmacytomas, and osteoid osteomas. Pain is the primary presenting symptom, but night pain is not as frequent as in patients with osteoid osteomas. In contrast to their smaller counterparts, osteoblastomas are more easily detected on plain radiographs (Figures 15-7 and 15-8). They are radiolucent lesions with a ground-glass appearance, are generally poorly marginated, and cause expansion of the surrounding bone. On CT evaluation there may be marginal sclerosis and matrix calcification (Figures 15-9 and 15-10). Like osteoid osteomas, osteoblastomas have a propensity to occur in the pedicle and posterior elements.[64] In Marsh review of 197 osteoblastomas, 41% were located in the spine, and all were localized to the posterior elements.[64] In Boriani's series of 65 patients with osteoblastomas, 46% of the tumors were of spinal origin. Fifty-three percent of the spinal osteoblastomas were found in the lumbar spine, and the rest were equally distributed in the thoracic and cervical spine.[7] Vertebral involvement almost always occurs due to secondary expansion from the pedicle, and there may be an associated soft tissue mass.

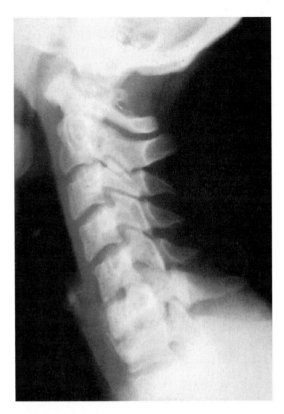

Figure 15-7. Osteoblastoma. This 19-year-old woman presented with severe unremitting neck pain. The patient had some improvement of her symptoms with nonsteroidal antiinflammatory drugs, but the pain was still presistent and disabling. This lateral x-ray of the cervical spine shows abnormalities involving the C6 vertebral body predominantly, but there are some abnormalities also in the superior portion of C7 vertebra.

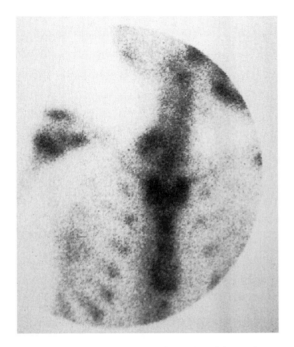

Figure 15-8. Osteoblastoma. This oblique bone scan of the 19-year-old woman (see Figure 15-7) shows marked uptake on the right side of her spine at the level of C6 and C7.

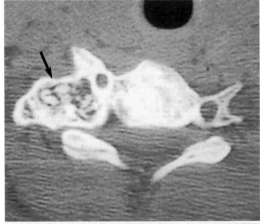

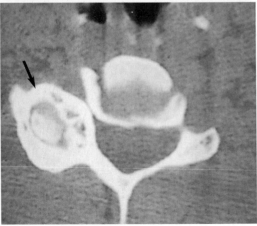

Figure 15-9. Osteoblastoma. The CT images show marked sclerotic changes in the right lateral mass of C6. A nidus can also be seen. Because of its size, this would be considered an osteoblastoma.

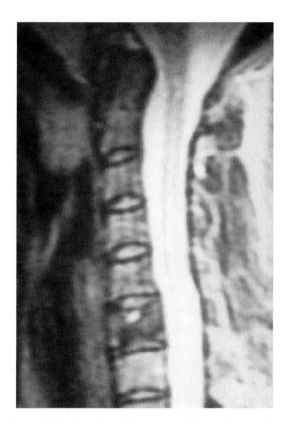

Figure 15-10. Osteoblastoma. This midsagittal MRI scan shows that the C6 vertebral body has signal changes within the body even though the tumor involves predominantly the lateral mass of C6. It is very common to see this type of hyperemic change in the adjacent bone.

Both osteoid osteomas and osteoblastomas are spinal tumors known to cause scoliosis (see Figure 15-4). Marsh noted that 50% of his patients with tumors localized to the thoracolumbar spine or from the ribs also had a spinal curvature.[64] Pettine and Klassen reported a 63% incidence of scoliosis in 41 patients with these benign tumors.[76] The lesion is typically located on the concavity of the curvature, and unilateral paravertebral spasm is thought to be the cause of the scoliosis. Over time, however, the curvature becomes structural (typically 15 months to 2 years). If the curvature is flexible, the scoliosis typically resolves after the removal of the tumor.[76,81]

Curettage can offer a high rate of disease remission when the lesions are well contained within the vertebral bone.[7] Wide excision of the lesion is always curative and may also provide reliable pain relief and resolution of the spinal deformity. However, marginal excision is safer and also provides an excellent cure rate. Thus marginal excision is the treatment of choice for these tumors (Figure 15-11). Even partial excision may offer symptom resolution if the nidus is removed. This can be aided by the use of adjuvant radiotherapy.[31] The local recurrence rate can be up to 10% for some osteoblastomas, but malignant degeneration is a rare occurrence.

ANEURYSMAL BONE CYSTS

- Rare lesions
- 80% of patients are 20 years of age
- Most common symptom: Pain
- Radiographs: Eccentric, lytic lesion with ballooning of host bone
- CT and MRI: Fluid-fluid levels
- Intralesional excision provides 87% cure rate
- Possibility of coexisting neoplasm

Aneurysmal Bone Cysts

Aneurysmal bone cysts (ABCs) are very rare lesions. Approximately 80% of patients are under 20 years of age. From 12% to 30% of these neoplasms occur in the spine, especially the lumbar areas. The tumor involves the posterior elements 60% of the time. In addition, ABCs are among the few benign lesions that tend to affect adjacent vertebrae. Pain is the most common symptom.

Plain radiographs will typically show an expansile osteolytic cavity with a bubbly appearance. Sometimes ABCs can cause significant vertebral collapse and can be misdiagnosed as the "vertebra-plana" of eosinophilic granuloma[74] (Figure 15-12). Radiographs show an eccentric, lytic lesion with expansion or "ballooning" of the host bone. On CT scans an extremely thin but continuous outer rim of bone can be seen surrounding the tumor (Figure 15-13). Fluid-fluid levels may be seen on both CT and MRI imaging.

Papagelopoulos et al. reported a 90% cure rate after an average 10 years of follow-up in 40 patients treated with intralesional excision[75] (Figure 15-14). Radical resection allows good local control[106] (Figure 15-15). Recurrences can be successfully managed by reexcision.[36] Appropriate treatment of aneurysmal bone cysts requires an understanding that it may arise from or coexist with a preexisting neoplasm.[49,67] Clearly, the treatment plan must address the secondary lesion to ensure an optimal outcome.

Hemangiomas

In contrast to aneurysmal bone cysts, hemangiomas are much more common in the spine. They comprise about 7% of all benign tumors. Hemangiomas are rarely symptomatic. However, of the five patients with spinal hemangiomas treated by the senior author, all five developed significant neurologic deficit secondary to pathologic fracture. Radiographically, individuals with spinal hemangiomas present with classic vertebral striations resulting from the abnormally thickened bony trabeculae. CT scans easily delineate the lesion, and MRI shows high signal intensity on T2 weighted images and low signal intensity on T1 weighted images (Figure 15-16).

If the tumor becomes symptomatic, radiotherapy is an effective treatment. If surgical excison is considered, preoperative angiography and embolization of the

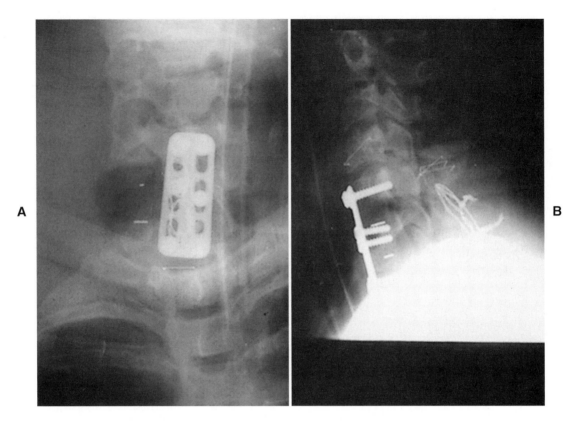

Figure 15-11. Osteoblastoma. **A,** An anterior approach was performed to remove the vertebral body of C6 up to the pedicle of C6. The vertebral artery at the C6 level was isolated and dissected free from the bone at the C6 level, up toward the C5, and down toward the C7 levels. **B,** A posterior approach was then used to perform a hemilaminectomy combined with an excision of the lateral mass of C6. This reconstruction allowed the patient to be mobilized in a rigid cervical collar. Immediately postoperatively it was apparent to the patient that her previous pain was completely resolved. She has had no recurrence of her pain.

HEMANGIOMAS

- Comprise 7% of all benign tumors
- Rarely symptomatic
- Classic vertebral striations on radiographs
- MRI: High signal on T2 and low signal on T1
- Radiotherapy effective
- Preoperative angiography and embolization useful if surgical resection is needed for neurologic deficit

---

feeder vessel with polyvinyl alcohol particles or metallic coils may make surgical resection easier and safer.[11,91]

Percutaneous vertebroplasty can also be an effective treatment option.[14,19,21] In addition, the surgeon must be aware of and prepared for the development of consumptive coagulopathy that can cause significant blood loss at the time of excision.[58]

Giant Cell Tumors

Giant cell tumors comprise about 10% of all primary bone tumors. These tumors occur in people between the ages of 20 and 40 years with a slight female predominance (70.8%).[85,86] Spinal involvement is seen in patients in the third and fourth decades of life. Savini et al. reported a 3.2% incidence of spinal involvement in his series of nine patients.[86] In the Mayo clinic series, giant cell tumors of the spine constituted 6.5% of all of the giant cell tumors seen.[85] In this series the tumors were equally distributed among the cervical, thoracic, and lumbar spine. The vast majority of giant cell tumors are slow-growing, locally aggressive neoplasms that do not metastasize.

Pain is typically the presenting symptom, and up to one third of patients with giant cell tumors will have a neurologic deficit.[85] The majority of these tumors are found in the vertebral body and often expand into and destroy the surrounding cortical bone[85] (Figures 15-17 to 15-19). Plain radiographs will show a lytic lesion with matrix calcification and sclerosis. Large tumors may cause pathologic fractures and may have an associated soft tissue component. Grossly, the tumor is solid with scattered zones of hemorrhagic necrosis. Histologically, the giant cell tumor is composed of normochromatic, ovoid stromal cells with a variable number of multinucleated giant cells.

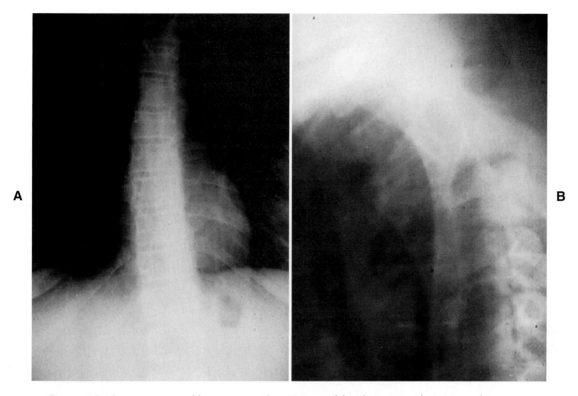

Figure 15-12. Aneurysmal bone cyst. This 16-year-old girl presented to our scoliosis clinic complaining of pain in her upper thoracic spine. The pain had been present for approximately 1 year and was gradually worsening. Her pain was present at night, as well as during the day. Standard AP (**A**) and lateral (**B**) x-rays revealed some anterior bony destruction and collapse in the upper thoracic spine and a very mild secondary scoliosis.

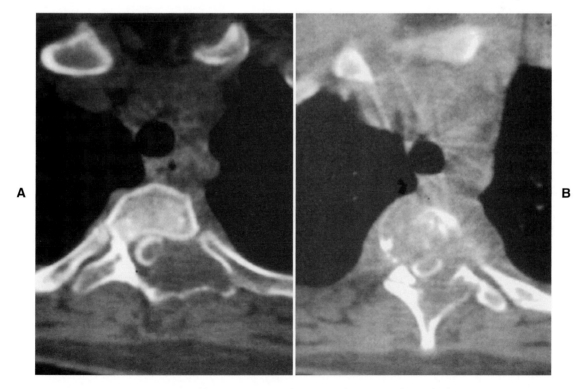

Figure 15-13. Aneurysmal bone cyst. Myelo-CT axial sections through the tumor (**A** and **B**) show spinal cord compression and a significant soft tissue component to the tumor. The posterior spine has an extremely thin cortical rim.

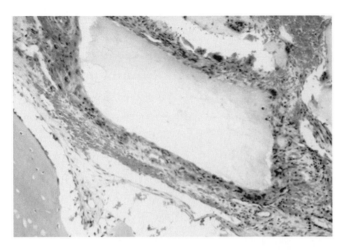

Figure 15-14.   Aneurysmal bone cyst. A large bone biopsy revealed this to be a giant cell tumor of bone. The tumor was treated with a combined anterior and posterior approach to perform a very thorough intralesional excision.

GIANT CELL TUMORS

- 10% of all bone tumors
- Spinal involvement in 3.2% to 6.5%
- Slow growing, locally aggressive
- Presenting symptom: Pain
- Neurologic deficit in 33%
- Imaging studies: Lytic lesion with matrix calcification and sclerosis
- Marginal resection necessary for cure
- Curettage alone has a high recurrence rate, improved with cryotherapy or packing methylmethacrylate (PMMA)
- 10% incidence of sarcomatous change with irradiation therapy

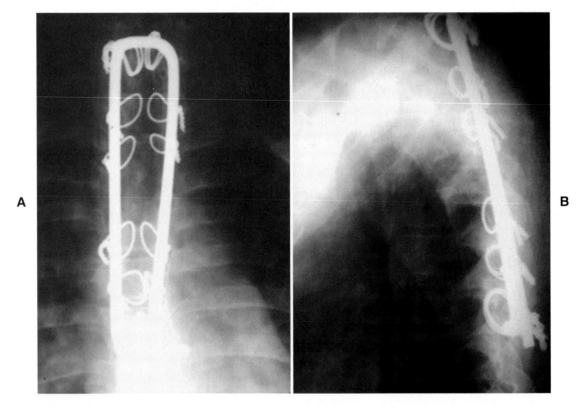

Figure 15-15.   Aneurysmal bone cyst. AP **(A)** and lateral **(B)** views of the spine following reconstruction with anterior structural bone graft, as well as posterior segmental fixation and fusion. There has been no evidence of this tumor recurrence.

Treatment of giant cell tumors of the spine requires marginal resection (usually by vertebrectomy) for cure (Figure 15-20). Shikata, Stener, and Stener and Johnsen have reported disease-free intervals of up to 6 years with marginal resection and reconstruction.[92,97,99] Wide resection via en bloc spondylectomy is also curative and may be possible in the thoracic and lumbar spine but is impossible in the cervical spine. In these cases the risk:benefit ratio must be considered. For giant cell tumors of the extremities, marginal excison has been replaced by intralesional curettage and cementation. Intralesional curettage alone leads to a high local recurrence rate (25% to 50%). However, in extremity and sacral lesions, curettage in combination with an adjunc-

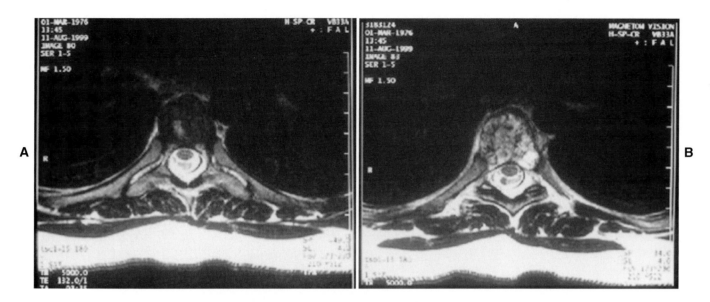

Figure 15-16. Hemangioma. This patient presented with upper thoracic spine pain after a minor fall with a high thoracic compression fracture. **A** and **B** show sequential axial T2 weighted MRI images consistent with a hemangioma of the vertebra at this level.

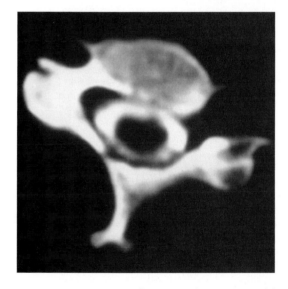

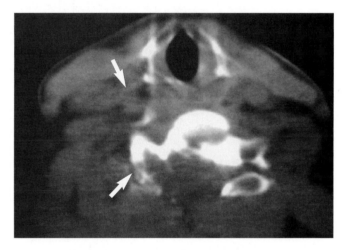

Figure 15-18. Giant cell tumor. Taken at the same time as the image in Figure 15-17, this CT scan at the C7 level showed no myelogram dye despite the fact that a laminectomy had been performed at this level. The tumor can also be seen involving the lateral mass on the right side (*top arrow*). There is also soft tissue extension into the paraspinous muscles and into the longus colli muscles anteriorly on the right side (*bottom arrow*).

Figure 15-17. Giant cell tumor. This 22-year-old woman was referred to our institution with severe weakness of her upper extremity, with the hands being most severely involved and some diffuse weakness of both legs. A three-level posterior cervical laminectomy had been performed elsewhere, and a giant cell tumor was encountered and debrided at that time. She was then sent to our institution for further treatment. A myelogram and postmyelo-CT scan were performed. This CT scan at the C3 level shows a normal spinal canal and normal bone.

tive procedure such as liquid nitrogen treatment of the margin or packing the cavity with methylmethacrylate significantly reduces the local recurrence rate.[18,63] The use of irradiation therapy for incompletely resected lesions remains controversial, because there is a 10% reported risk of sarcomatous change.[12,85,86] Follow-up examination should include routine CT scanning to look for recurrent tumor. Hart et al. reported a 24% recurrence rate when the tumor involved both anterior and posterior elements compared with no recurrences when the tumor involved only the vertebral body.[35] In addition, if there was extraosseous extension into both the canal and the paraspinous musculature, the recurrence rate was 21% compared with 10% if either one was affected alone.[35] Isolated lung metastasis is easily

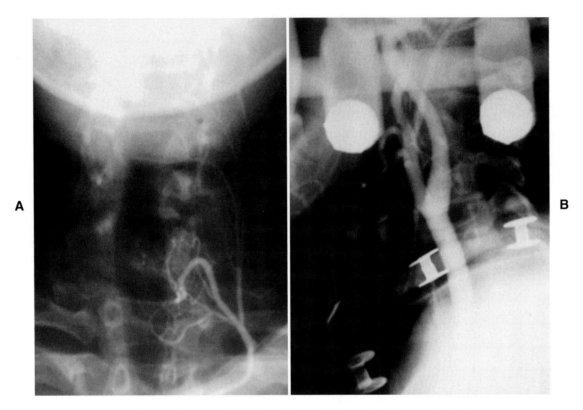

Figure 15-19. Giant cell tumor. AP **(A)** and lateral **(B)** views of the cervical spine. An arteriogram has been performed to verify that both vertebral arteries and both carotid arteries were completely patent. At the time of surgery, the patient's right vertebral artery was explored and cleared of tumor.

managed by resection and is not a sign of malignant disease.

Eosinophilic Granuloma

Eosinophilic granuloma is a variant of Langerhans' cell histiocytosis, a disease entity that includes Hand-Schüller-Christian disease and Letterer-Siwe disease. The tumor was first described in 1925 by Calve, who thought that it was a form of osteochondrosis. Eosinophilic granuloma is a proliferative disorder of the Langerhans' cells that is commonly seen in young children under 10 years of age and rarely in adults. The disease has a male preponderance. Vertebral involvement is seen in 7% to 15% of cases and typically presents with the sudden onset of neck pain and torticollis.[90] Spinal cord compression is a rare but reported event.[1,50,60,87]

Eosinophilic granuloma can present with a spectrum of radiographic manifestations, depending on the stage of the tumor. Early on, the tumor presents as a central, lytic lesion with poorly defined margins. Plain radiographs show permeative bony destruction with a marked periosteal reaction. At this stage the tumor is difficult to distinguish from a high-grade sarcoma such as Ewing's sarcoma. Later in the evolution of the tumor, there is vertebral body collapse leading to a flattening of the vertebral bone between the adjacent intact discs.

> ### EOSINOPHILIC GRANULOMA
>
> - A proliferative disorder of Langerhans' cells
> - Commonly seen in young children
> - Vertebral involvement in 7% to 15% of cases
> - Spectrum of radiographic presentations—classic vertebra plana
> - Must distinguish isolated lesion from systemic disease
> - Symptomatic lesions treated with immobilization and radiotherapy

This phenomenon results in the classic "coin on end" appearance and "vertebra plana"[17,90] (Figures 15-21 to 15-23).

Clinically it is important to distinguish an isolated lesion from systemic disease because the prognosis is significantly altered by the presence of systemic manifestations. Treatment for symptomatic lesions consists of radiation therapy (500 to 1000 rads) and immobilization. Excision of the tumor is rarely required.[30] However, surgery should be reserved for patients exhibiting a neurologic deficit. In a growing child, the vertebral collapse will remodel and reconstitute over time with immobilization.[62,80]

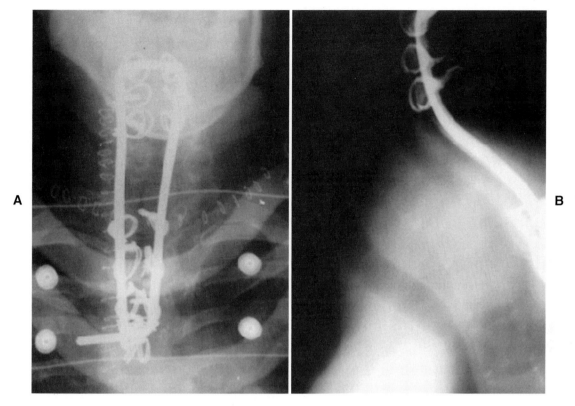

Figure 15-20. Giant cell tumor. AP **(A)** and lateral **(B)** radiographs of the cervical spine and upper thoracic spine. We performed revision posterior surgery with removal of all visible tumor and bone that was abnormal on the patient's CT scan. This also included anterior fusion and a posterior fusion with segmental instrumentation. The patient was also placed in a halo vest at that same time. Her lower extremity function returned to normal, and her upper extremity function of C5 and C6 remained normal. The C7, C8, and T1 nerve roots have remained weak in the range of ⅕ to ⅗. At 16 years after our surgery she has had two smaller operations for limited recurrence. At the time of her second operation, 5 years after our index procedure, she was also treated with radiation. She is followed yearly for evidence of significant recurrence.

MALIGNANT TUMORS OF THE SPINE

Malignant tumors of the spine are generally fast growing and permeative. They include multiple myeloma, solitary plasmacytoma, osteosarcoma, chondrosarcoma, Ewing's sarcoma, chordoma, and lymphoma.

Multiple Myeloma and Solitary Plasmacytoma

Multiple myeloma and solitary plasmacytoma are B-cell lymphoproliferative diseases composed of abnormal aggregates of plasma cells. The neoplasm has a peak occurrence between the ages of 50 and 60 years, with an equal distribution between the sexes. Multiple myeloma is a multifocal plasma cell cancer of the osseous system whose neoplastic cells produce complete or incomplete immunoglobulins. The annual incidence of myeloma is about 2 to 3 per 100,000 among the general population. Genetic analysis of the tumor cells have demonstrated abnormalities in band q32 of chromosome 14. The diagnosis is made on serum and urine evaluation for abnormal immunoglobulin levels. Serum protein electrophoresis will show increases in the levels of one of the immunoglobulin classes. The M-component is IgG in 55% of cases, IgA in 25% of cases, and rarely IgE, IgD, or IgM. Urine protein electrophoresis may detect the presence of immunoglobulin light chains called Bence Jones proteins in up to 99% of patients. In 60% of patients afflicted with multiple myeloma, both Bence Jones proteins and abnormal serum immunoglobulin levels will be detected.

On plain radiographs, myeloma appears as "punched-out" lytic lesions. The vertebral column is the most common site of skeletal involvement, followed by the ribs, skull, pelvis, clavicle, and scapula. Compression fractures from vertebral column lesions have the same distribution as osteoporotic compression fractures.[53,54] Unlike the majority of spinal neoplasms, the lesions frequently show no uptake on Tc-99 bone scan. MRI has an 86% sensitivity in the detection of multiple myeloma. This study will demonstrate diffuse signal abnormalities in the vertebral body bone (Figures 15-24, *A* and *B*). MRI also has the ability to distinguish multiple myeloma

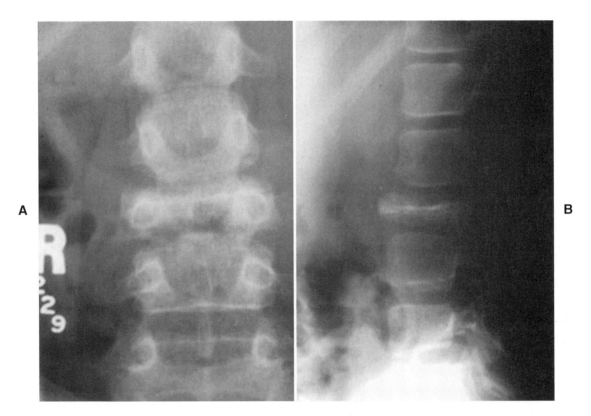

Figure 15-21. Eosinophilic granuloma. This 5-year-old girl presented to the spine clinic with a 2- to 3-month history of lumbar spine pain. AP **(A)** and lateral **(B)** radiographs of the lumbar spine show an L3 vertebra plana.

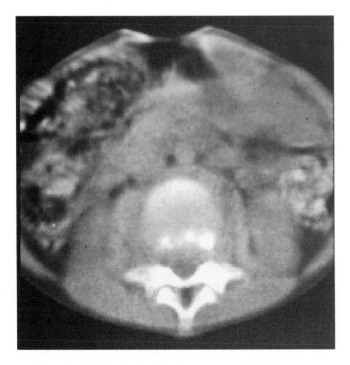

Figure 15-22. Eosinophilic granuloma. This transverse CT image shows considerable soft tissue extension laterally from the spine.

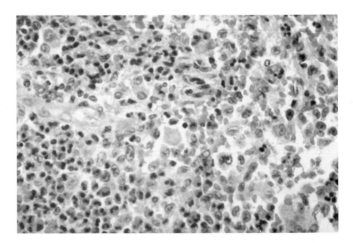

Figure 15-23. Eosinophilic granuloma. A biopsy of the spine revealed pathology typical for an eosinophilic granuloma. The patient was treated with low-dose radiation (500 to 1000 rads is effective), and she was immobilized in a thoracolumbar sacral orthosis (TLSO) brace. Her symptoms resolved over a period of 4 to 6 weeks.

from other monoclonal gammopathies. The bony destruction is caused by osteoclasts, which are activated by humoral factors released from the myeloma cells. These factors include interleukin-1 (IL-1), tumor necrosis factor (TNF), and lymphotoxin.[27] Grossly, the tumors are red, soft, and gelatinous. Microscopically, the myeloma is composed of abnormal aggregates of plasma cells containing acidophilic inclusions called Russell bodies.

Despite the fact that the vertebral column is a common site of involvement for multiple myeloma, it is important to recognize that the neoplasm is a systemic illness. Renal involvement can result in "myeloma nephrosis" that can lead to renal failure. The myeloma cells can directly infiltrate into nerves or can secrete factors that result in a nonspecific carcinomatous polyneuropathy. Hypercalcemia of malignancy can cause confusion, lethargy, weakness, constipation, and polyuria. The immunosuppressive effect of bone marrow replacement by tumor cells and the production of defective immunoglobulins can predispose the patient to recurrent infections by encapsulated bacteria. The myeloma cells can also produce antibodies to red blood cells, causing hemolytic anemia and coagulation defects.[25] Spontaneous epidural hematomas can occur from injury to inflamed epidural vessels over the area of

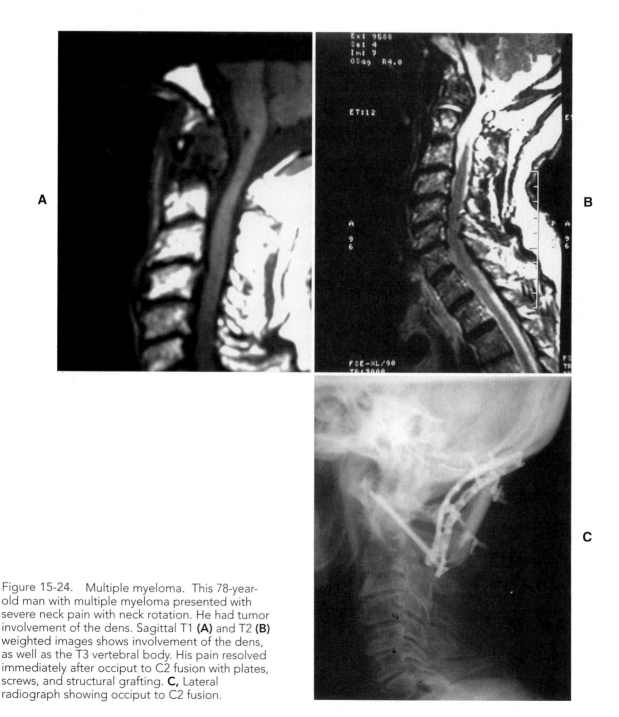

Figure 15-24. Multiple myeloma. This 78-year-old man with multiple myeloma presented with severe neck pain with neck rotation. He had tumor involvement of the dens. Sagittal T1 (**A**) and T2 (**B**) weighted images shows involvement of the dens, as well as the T3 vertebral body. His pain resolved immediately after occiput to C2 fusion with plates, screws, and structural grafting. **C,** Lateral radiograph showing occiput to C2 fusion.

MULTIPLE MYELOMA

- Composed of abnormal aggregates of plasma cells
- Peak occurrence between ages 50 and 60 years
- Diagnosis based on serum and urine protein electrophoresis
- Radiographs show "punched-out" lesions
- No uptake on bone scan, but MRI has 86% sensitivity in diagnosis
- Primary causes of death: Renal failure and infections
- Treated with combination chemotherapy and local irradiation
- Surgery reserved for neurologic deficit and spinal instability
- 18% 5-year survival and median survival of 24 months

PRIMARY OSTEOSARCOMA

- Usually affects patients under age 20 years with a slight male preponderance
- 1% to 2% arise primarily in spine
- Radiographs: mixed lytic and sclerotic lesion with soft tissue calcification
- Treatment with wide resection, combination chemotherapy, and local radiotherapy
- Main cause of treatment failure: Failure to obtain local control
- Median survival: 6 to 10 months

---

tumor infiltration.[37] The primary causes of death in this population are renal failure and infection. Clearly, an awareness of the systemic manifestations of the disease is vital to determine the appropriate treatment for each patient.

The initial treatment of myeloma consists of chemotherapy and irradiation. Chemotherapy is an effective means of controlling the advancement of the disease process but may increase the risk of secondary leukemia.[6] The commonly employed agents include melphalan and prednisone. Newer agents such as gallium nitrate may attenuate the rate of skeletal bone loss from the disease and from steroid treatment. Radiation to affected osseous sites may reduce pain and prevent vertebral collapse, deformity, and neural compression.[52] However, despite the advances in both radiation therapy and chemotherapy, the survival rate for patients with multiple myeloma remains dismal. The disease is rapidly progressive and may be fatal within 2 to 3 years from the time of diagnosis. The estimated 5-year survival is 18%, and the median survival is 24 months. Patients with cancer that produces only gamma light chains may have a shorter survival than their cohorts. Surgery is reserved for the treatment of vertebral instability and neural compression with a neurologic deficit that fails to respond to radiation therapy and to chemotherapy (see Figure 15-24, C). Before surgical treatment is attempted, the surgeon must be certain that the adjacent vertebral bodies have sufficient bone stock to support spinal reconstruction. Improvement in neurologic status after decompression may be hampered by the coexistence of carcinomatous polyneuropathy.

In contrast to the dismal prognosis for multiple myeloma, patients with solitary plasmacytoma tend to have a prolonged survival despite eventual progression. Solitary plasmacytomas comprise 3% to 5% of all plasma cell neoplasms.[20] Solitary plasmacytoma appears as an isolated lesion with the same "punched out" appearance on radiographs as a myeloma. Elevated M-proteins and Bence Jones proteinuria are found in only 25% of cases.[51] As its name implies, systemic disease is not a hallmark of solitary plasmacytoma. This characteristic is the primary reason that these patients have a significantly longer median survival (86 months). Treatment with

4000 to 5000 rads gives dependable local control.[20] The disappearance of myeloma protein on serum protein electrophoresis following irradiation is highly correlated with the likelihood of cure.[55] The serum analysis also provides a means to monitor the patient for recurrent disease. Surgical resection is often curative if radiation therapy fails to alleviate the symptoms.

Primary Osteosarcoma

Primary osteosarcoma is a malignant tumor of mesenchymal cells characterized by the direct formation of osteoid or bone by the tumor cells. It is the second most common primary neoplasm of bone behind myeloma. Most appear in persons under 20 years of age before epiphyseal closure. There is a slight male preponderance. In a series of patients with osteosarcoma, Barwick et al. noted that 1% to 2% arose initially in the spine.[4] Primary osteosarcomas can arise de novo in the absence of underlying carcinogenic influences. Genetic influences certainly play a role in the development of the neoplasm. Patients with retinoblastoma (caused by a hereditary mutation in the q14 band of chromosome 13, which codes for a tumor suppressor gene) have a 500-fold greater risk of developing osteosarcoma. The overall consensus is that these tumors have a multifactorial origin involving genetic, constitutional, and environmental influences.

Radiographically, osteosarcomas present as mixed lytic and sclerotic lesions that cause cortical destruction and soft tissue calcification. In advanced stages vertebral collapse occurs from replacement of the structural elements of the spine with tumor. On pathologic section the tumors appear as gray-white heterogeneous masses with areas of hemorrhage and cystic softening. Their consistency varies depending on the relative proportions of fibrous tissue, chondroid tissue, necrotic tissue, and osteoid. Osteosarcomas tend to be aggressive neoplasms that have the propensity to metastasize widely via the hematogenous route, causing pulmonary, bony, and pleural metastasis.[4]

The treatment of spinal osteosarcomas is difficult, and the overall outcomes are poor. Although en bloc spondylectomy has been shown to be curative, most of these tumors are not amenable to this type of approach because of loss of containment. In addition, the proxim-

---

SECONDARY OSTEOSARCOMA

- Arises from dysplastic or previously irradiated bone
- Accounts for up to 30% of osteosarcomas of the spine
- Paget's sarcoma in patients in sixth decade
- Postirradiation osteosarcoma in patients in their forties and fifties with a long latency period between irradiation treatment (usually >5000 rads) and tumor development
- Paget's sarcoma: Less than 5% long-term survival rate
- Postirradiation osteosarcoma: 7.5% to 17% 5-year survival rate

---

CHONDROSARCOMA

- Occurs in middle to later years of life with a male preponderance
- Primary or secondary incidence of malignant change is 20%
- 6% to 10% of all chondrosarcomas arise from spine
- Symptoms: Pain (most common), neurologic deficit (4.5%)
- Radioresistant—mainstay of treatment is wide surgical excision
- Five-year survival rate 21% to 55%, with a median survival of 6 years

---

ity of the spinal cord and major vessels to the tumor mass makes wide excision extremely hazardous.[45] Traditional therapy has involved limited tumor resection and radiotherapy. A more aggressive approach with wide resection, combination chemotherapy, and local radiotherapy, as described by Sundaresan et al. and Weinstein and McLain, demonstrated promising early results.[104,108] In their series and in others, failure to obtain local control was the main cause of treatment failure.[42,104] The prognosis for patients with spinal osteosarcomas is dismal. Barwick reported a median survival of 6 months for his 10 patients.[4] Shives reported a similar median survival of 10 months in his series of 27 patients.[93]

Secondary Osteosarcoma

Secondary osteosarcoma, as its name implies, arises from dysplastic or previously irradiated bone. It may occur in the setting of Paget's disease, multiple enchondromatosis, multiple osteochondromatosis, chronic osteomyelitis, or fibrous dysplasia.[66] Secondary osteosarcomas account for 3.6% to 5.5% of all intramedullary osteosarcomas and up to 30% of all osteosarcomas of the spine.[4,40,93] Paget's sarcoma presents in the sixth decade in patients with polyostotic disease. This form of osteosarcoma is locally aggressive and metastasizes early. Postirradiation osteosarcoma is typically present in patients in their fourth or fifth decades. Most of these patients have received >5000 rads in the treatment of nonosseous disease or for the treatment of giant cell tumor or Ewing's sarcoma. There is usually a long latency period between the irradiation and the presentation of the tumor. However, once the tumor has advanced enough to be detected or to cause symptoms, rapid progression is the rule.[102,103] Patients with Paget's sarcoma have less than a 5% long-term survival rate.[78] Postirradiation osteosarcoma carries a median survival rate of 1 year and a 5-year survival of 7.5% to 17%.[12,40,41]

Chondrosarcoma

Chondrosarcoma is the third most common primary bone tumor behind myeloma and osteosarcoma. Primary chondrosarcomas occur in the middle to later years of life and have a slight male preponderance. Like osteosarcomas, chondrosarcomas can be primary or secondary. Primary lesions arise de novo, and secondary lesions arise in the context of dysplastic bone or a pre-existing bony neoplasm such as multiple enchondromatosis or multiple hereditary exostosis.[112,113] In this setting, the incidence of malignant change is 20%.[13] Typically the neoplasm affects the bones of the shoulder and pelvic girdle, the long tubular bones, and the ribs. Of all chondrosarcomas, 6% to 10% arise in the spine.[22,105] The clinical behavior of the tumor depends on the degree of cellular anaplasia, but most are slow growing and metastasize late.

Pain in the area of involvement is the first symptom. Fifty percent of patients will have a palpable mass before being diagnosed. About 4.5% will have some form of neurologic deficit varying from sensory deficits to frank paraplegia.

Plain radiographs will demonstrate a large area of bony destruction and a soft tissue mass with matrix calcification (Figures 15-25 and 15-26). MRI will help to delineate the extent of soft tissue and bony involvement. Grossly the tumor is composed of gray-white translucent tissue with a variable amount of central necrosis. Histologically, anaplasia of the lacunar cells will differentiate it from the more benign chondroma.

Chondrosarcomas are radio-resistant. Thus the mainstay of treatment is wide excision (Figure 15-27). Survival is closely related to obtaining a clear surgical margin at the time of surgical excision.[94] In the Mayo Clinic series, 15 (75%) of 20 patients with chondrosarcoma died of local progression. Their 5-year survival rate was 21% to 55%, with a median survival of 6 years.[13,94] High-dose irradiation therapy may have limited benefit for inoperable lesions.[47]

Ewing's Sarcoma

Ewing's sarcoma is a malignant round cell tumor with a peak incidence in the second decade of life. The sarcoma was first described in 1921 by James Ewing, who called it an endothelial myeloma. The neoplasm occurs twice as often in men than in women.[111] Spinal involvement is seen in 3.5% of all Ewing's sarcomas, and a large proportion of these arise in the sacrum.[110] If the sacrum is excluded, only 0.9% of these tumors occur

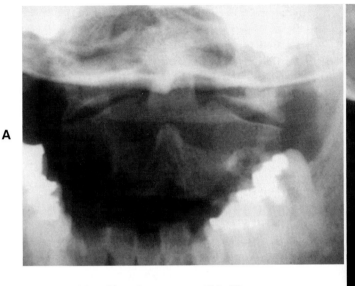

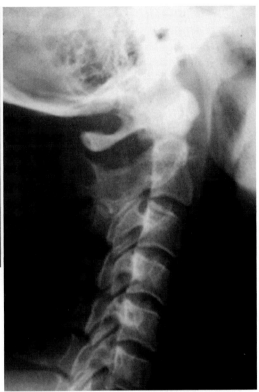

Figure 15-25. Chondrosarcoma. This 32-year-old woman had a 2-year history of severe and unremitting pain in her upper cervical spine. The pain increased over time and did not improve with any conservative measures. Open mouth view **(A)** and lateral view **(B)** of her cervical spine show decreased density in the right lateral mass and pedicle of C2.

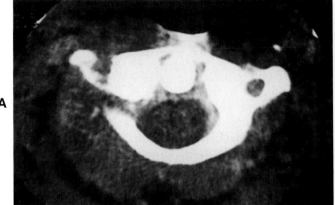

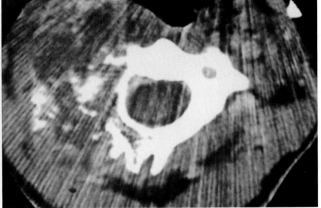

Figure 15-26. Chondrosarcoma. **A,** CT transverse image at C2 shows complete destruction of the right pedicle, right lamina, and right lateral mass of C2 with large soft tissue extension. **B,** Soft tissue windows show destruction of the right side of C1 with soft tissue extension laterally at the C1 level as well. It was suspected from the radiographic appearance that this was a chondrosarcoma.

in the remainder of the vertebral column. The main symptom is pain. In addition, Grubb et al. and Pilepich et al. noted that 50% to 58% of patients with spinal Ewing's had neurologic deficit.[32,77]

On MRI examination, the tumor is hypo-intense on T1 weighted images. Radionuclide imaging and chest CT scanning are essential in the evaluation of disseminated disease.

Grossly the tumor is gray-white and soft, and it causes an expansion of the surrounding bone. Microscopically the neoplasm is composed of sheets of small round cells resembling lymphocytes that occasionally surround a central clearing, forming the classic "pseudo-rosette" pattern. The cells stain with periodic acid-Schiff (PAS+) because they contain glycogen. Genetic analysis of the tumor cells suggests a possible

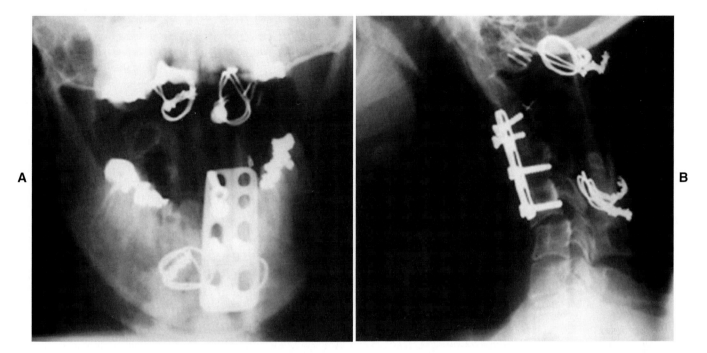

Figure 15-27. Chondrosarcoma. Postoperative AP **(A)** and lateral **(B)** radiographs of the cervical spine. The chondrosarcoma was treated with an en bloc excision of C1, C2, and C3, removing the entire right side along with the right vertebral artery and adjacent soft tissue in one specimen. This was achieved with a combination of a right lateral approach, a right anterior approach, and a midline occipitocervical approach. Following excision the tumor margins appeared to be free of tumor by gross and microscopic analysis. The patient was neurologically normal preoperatively, as well as postoperatively. On her right side the C1, C2, and C3 nerve roots were sectioned and sent with the tumor. The patient's diaphragm and arm function remain normal. Four years after excision the patient presented with a cervical myelopathy and recurrence of the tumor within her spinal canal. She was treated with repeat excision locally, combined with radiation therapy. Eight years after the original surgery she again was treated for a limited recurrence. Twelve years after surgical excision she was found to have extension into her cranium, which was treated through a transoral approach with excision.

EWING'S SARCOMA

- Malignant round cell tumor
- Peak incidence: Second decade of life
- Spinal involvement: 3.5% of Ewing's sarcomas—most in sacrum
- Main symptoms: Pain, neurologic deficit in up to 58%
- Cell stain PAS+ due to glycogen stores
- Treatment: Combination chemotherapy and high-dose radiation
- Surgery: Reserved for spinal instability and neurologic deficit
- Five-year survival of 32%-43%: mean survival of 2.9 years with 31% recurrence rate

The treatment of Ewing's sarcoma of the spine consists of combination chemotherapy and high-dose radiation therapy.[3,83,88] The most common chemotherapeutic regimen includes vincristine, actinomycin, and cyclophosphamide, with or without Adriamycin.[88] Surgical treatment is indicated in the presence of spinal instability and neurologic deficit. The prognosis for patients with spinal involvement is poorer than for patients with extremity lesions. With radiation and chemotherapy alone, the 5-year survival rate is reported to be 32% to 43.5%, with a 31% local recurrence rate.[3,32] Grubb reported a mean survival of 2.9 years from the time of diagnosis.[32] Death is usually the result of widespread hematogenous dissemination.

Chordoma

Chordoma arises from tests of primitive notochord cells in the spine. Physaliphorous cells, containing abundant vacuoles filled with glycogen and oxidative enzymes, are the distinctive cells of this neoplasm. Molecular analysis has shown that chordoma cells express galectin-3, a carbohydrate-binding protein that plays a role in cell

neuroectodermal origin with a characteristic reciprocal translocation of the long arms of chromosomes 11 and 22.[109] Sharma, Khosla, and Banerjee noted that metastasis can arise from the epidural space without bony involvement.[89]

differentiation, morphogenesis, and cancer biology.[29] The neoplasm usually occurs in the fifth and sixth decades of life and afflicts men twice as often as women. The majority of the tumors appear in the sacrococcygeal area (50%) followed by the basioccipital area (35%). The remainder are distributed over the rest of the spine. The symptoms are vague and usually occur as a result of local compression once the tumor has grown to a signi-

ficant size. This fact contributes to the generally late diagnosis of the tumor. By the time of diagnosis, sacral chordomas are usually staged 1B. Symptoms may include constipation, frequent urination, and radiculopathy. Patients with cervicothoracic tumors can present with progressive dyspnea.[38] A firm, fixed presacral mass may be found on rectal examination.

Radiographs usually show destruction of several segments of the sacrum. The tumor is centrally placed and associated with an anterior soft tissue mass. A bone scan, although unnecessary for diagnosis, will show no uptake for both Tc-99 and gallium tracers.[101] CT scan will show the extent of bony destruction and may help plan the reconstruction. MRI is the study of choice to diagnose and stage these lesions. Chordomas will stand out in high contrast to the adjacent soft tissues on T2 weighted images (Figures 15-28 to 15-30).

Wide excision of the tumor offers the only chance for a cure. En bloc excision or high sacral amputation through a posterior approach or a combined approach is the preferred procedure for tumors of the mobile spine and sacral-based tumors, respectively[26,28,98] (Figures 15-31 and 15-32). During high sacral amputation, sparing of the S3 roots will permit maintenance of normal bowel and bladder function.[16] Saving the S2 nerve roots will allow the patient to retain some bowel and bladder function. Great care must be taken to prevent tumor spillage during

---

CHORDOMA

- From notochordal tests in spine: Typical cell type called physaliphorous cells
- Occurs in fifth and sixth decades and twice as often in men as in women
- Most in sacrum (50%) and basioccipital area (35%)
- Symptoms: Vague; occur due to local compression of viscera and nerves
- MRI: study of choice—high intensity on T2 images
- Wide resection only chance for a cure
- S2 roots to retain some bowel/bladder function
- Adjuvant irradiation indicated for intraoperative tumor spillage or incomplete excision
- 29% to 52% 10-year survival, 64% local recurrence with tumor spillage

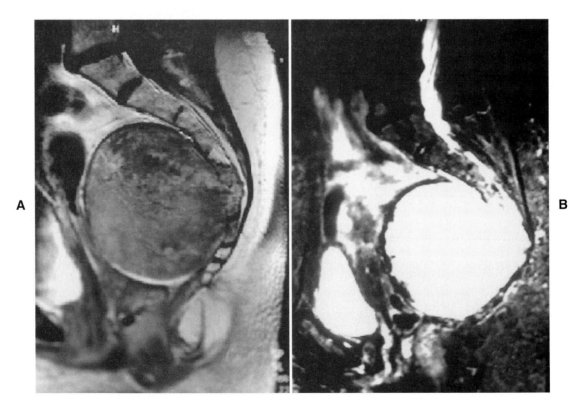

A **B**

Figure 15-28. Chordoma. This 70-year-old woman had a 6-month history of severe coccygeal pain. It was impossible for her to sit without aggravating her pain. The pain was even present when she was lying on her side. A biopsy of this tumor had been performed at another institution through the rectum. The biopsy showed that this tumor was a chordoma. These sagittal T1 **(A)** and T2 **(B)** MRI images show that the tumor is arising from the lower sacrum at approximately the S3 level.

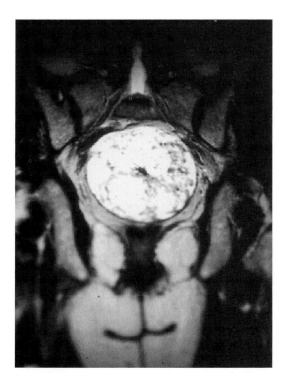

Figure 15-29. Chordoma. This coronal image shows the width of the tumor.

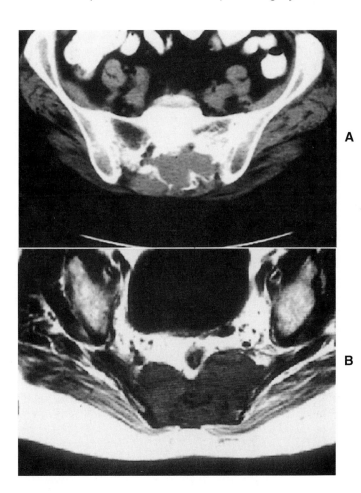

Figure 15-30. Chordoma. This transverse CT image (**A**) and transverse MRI image (**B**) show that the tumor posteriorly extends up to the S2 level. The lateral margin of the tumor, especially on the right side, extends to the sciatic notch.

resection because spillage can increase the local recurrence rate from 28% to 64%.[44,114] Adjuvant radiation therapy is indicated when complete resection is impossible or when tumor spillage occurs at the time of resection. Radiation therapy may allow an increased continuous disease-free survival.[16,115] Preoperative irradiation of 50 Gy may also be useful if contamination is expected at the time of wide excision.[15] Soft tissue and skin defects after wide resection are well addressed using a local rotational flap or a transpelvic transverse rectus myocutaneous flap.[65] Fast-neutron or proton beam radiation therapy for inoperable tumors has a 61% 4-year survival rate and a 54% to 65% 10-year survival rate in some small series.[9,68,84]

Cheng et al. reported an 86% overall 5-year survival, a continuous disease-free survival rate of 58%, and a local recurrence–free survival of 60%.[16] Other surgeons report similar results, with a 71% to 76% 5-year survival for patients who had complete surgical resection.[84] Ten-year survival for patients treated with surgical resection is between 29% and 52%.[46,114] Local recurrence is a poor prognostic sign.

Lymphoma

When lymphoma occurs as an isolated bony lesion, it is called a reticulum cell sarcoma. In Ostrowsky, Krishnan, and Banks's series of 422 patients, 12% had spinal involvement and 5% had primary lesions in the spine.[73]

A well-localized lesion can be successfully treated by radiotherapy (40 Gy to the tumor and 10 Gy to the sur-

---

LYMPHOMA

- Isolated lesions called reticulum cell sarcomas
- Well-localized lesions successfully treated with irradiation
- 58% 5-year and 53% 10-year survival rate for isolated lesions

---

rounding lymph nodes).[2] Diffuse histiocytic lymphoma is best treated with adjuvant chemotherapy, which offers a 41% complete remission rate and a 9% recurrence rate. The stage of the disease is the most important factor influencing a patient's prognosis. An isolated bony lesion carries a 58% 5-year and 53% 10-year survival rate. Multifocal osseous lesions have a 42% 5-year and a 35% 10-year survival rate. The presence of both bony and soft tissue involvement carries a poorer prognosis, with a 22% 5-year and a 12.5% 10-year survival rate.[73]

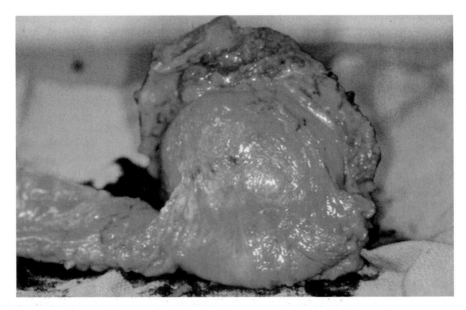

Figure 15-31.   Chordoma. This tumor specimen after excision shows that a colostomy was necessary. The fact that the original biopsy had been done through the rectum necessitates this more radical treatment.

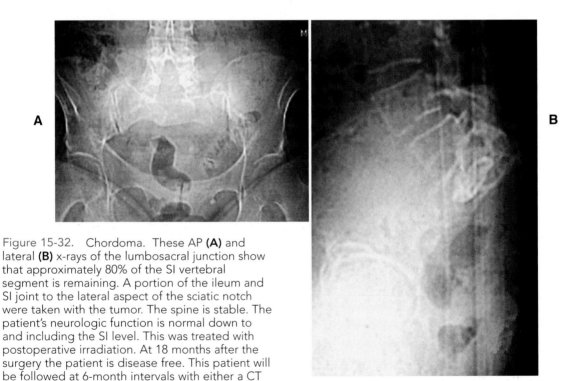

Figure 15-32.   Chordoma. These AP (**A**) and lateral (**B**) x-rays of the lumbosacral junction show that approximately 80% of the SI vertebral segment is remaining. A portion of the ileum and SI joint to the lateral aspect of the sciatic notch were taken with the tumor. The spine is stable. The patient's neurologic function is normal down to and including the SI level. This was treated with postoperative irradiation. At 18 months after the surgery the patient is disease free. This patient will be followed at 6-month intervals with either a CT scan or an MRI scan at each visit in order to detect any recurrence at the earliest possible date.

MISCELLANEOUS TUMORS OF THE SPINE
Paragangliomas

Paragangliomas are benign, slow-growing tumors of neural crest origin that arise from the paraganglia of the autonomic nervous system. They have also been called glomus tumors, chemodectomas, and chromaffin and nonchromaffin paragangliomas. The majority of these tumors arise in the carotid bodies and the glomus jugulare in the neck.[39,82] Spinal involvement is rare and is usually intradural at the level of the cauda equina.[10,71,82] These tumors are classified by the location of the primary tumor and on the endocrine status of the tumor.

Most patients will present with pain and signs of neural compression. Plain radiographs, MRI with gadolinium, and CT scans are useful to plan out the degree of soft tissue and bony involvement to plan the optimal approach for resection and reconstruction (if necessary). Serum and urine catecholamine assays, if positive, help to define the nature of the tumor and may provide a way to monitor for recurrence. Histologically, paragangliomas are composed of clusters of chief cells (Zellballen) with a highly vascular stroma. These cells contain multiple secretory granules. On a molecular level, the tumors express angiogenic growth factors including vascular endothelial growth factor and platelet-derived endothelial cell growth factor.[43]

Surgical resection is the mainstay of treatment of paragangliomas. The surgical approach should be tailored to the location, size, and extension of the tumor. Radiation is useful for adjunctive treatment.[10,82] Progress of patients with paragangliomas should be followed carefully because metastatic lesion can occur many years after the initial diagnosis and treatment of the tumor.

Hemangiopericytomas

Hemangiopericytomas are rare tumors derived from pericytes. Spinal involvement is uncommon. As of 1996 only 53 cases of spinal hemangiopericytomas had been reported in the literature. Nine involved the vertebral bone, and the remaining forty-four had meningeal involvement.[56] These tumors have a propensity for metastasis via hematogenous dissemination. The rate of metastatic spread has been reported to range from 15% to 56.5%.[69] Thus, a detailed work-up including radiographs, CT, MRI, and spinal angiography should be obtained prior to planning definitive treatment.[69] MRI will demonstrate a hypodense lesion with moderate enhancement on T1 and T2 weighted images.[56] On routine histology, hemangiopericytomas are composed of sheets of spindle-shaped tumor cells with prominent capillaries separated from neoplastic cells by an intact basement membrane.[34]

Treatment of hemangiopericytomas consists of surgical resection. Preoperative embolization may be helpful to reduce intraoperative blood loss and may allow complete tumor excision.[69] Postoperative irradiation therapy is also recommended.[100] These tumors have a high risk for recurrence, and patient follow-up should include repeated bone scans.[70] Advanced inoperable hemangiopericytomas can be treated by palliative radiation therapy and combination chemotherapy consisting of doxorubicin (Adriamycin) and dacarbazine (DTIC).[5]

Angiolipomas

Angiolipomas are benign tumors accounting for approximately 0.14% of all spinal tumors.[72] These tumors consist of both lipomatous and vascular components and are predominantly neoplasms of adulthood. They can be found in both the anterior and the posterior elements of the vertebral column. However, the majority (>90%) are found in the epidural space, where they

cause neural compression.[48,107] Two forms of this tumor exist: the more common infiltrating form and the noninfiltrating form.

The patients will present with symptoms of neural compression. There is typically a slow onset of symptoms that may progress over 1 to 2 years or more.[33,72] There are some reports of rapid symptom progression after the use of vasodilators, presumably from enlargement of the tumor through vascular engorgement.[72] Radiographically, the infiltrating form will show evidence of bony erosions, and the noninfiltrating form will show no bony destruction. CT will demonstrate a hypodense lesion in 80% of cases and an isodense lesion in the remaining 20%.[107] MRI will show a lipomatous mass containing signal voids, suggesting a vascular component. On T1 these vascular regions will be hypointense. The addition of gadolinium will help to assess the degree of vascularity of the tumor.[72,79,107]

Angiolipomas are best treated with surgical resection. Complete resection is often curative and leads to neurologic recovery.[33,59,72]

CONCLUSIONS

The evaluation and treatment of primary tumors of the spinal column have remained extremely challenging. With the advent of newer and more effective chemotherapeutic agents and improved technologies in radiation oncology, the possibility of increasing survival rates remains optimistic. Advances in molecular biology and genetics have added significantly to our understanding of these tumors and offers the promise of new treatments directed to the specific type of tumor cell. In addition, significant improvements in spinal fixation systems over the last 10 years have allowed improved methods of spinal stabilization and reconstruction. General indications for surgery are to prevent or address spinal instability and to decompress neural elements in the face of neurologic deficit. In addition, surgical excision offers a chance for cure if the neoplasm is isolated and if a good margin is obtainable at the time of resection. In most instances, however, surgery is an adjunct to maximal medical treatment. The operative plan for each patient with a spinal neoplasm must be customized to the type, grade, and stage of the tumor, as well as to the patient's individual circumstances. Clearly, a multidisciplinary approach is crucial to optimize the outcome.

SELECTED REFERENCES

Boriani S et al.: Osteoblastoma of the spine, *Clin Orthop* 1992, pp. 37-45.

Boriani S, Weinstein JN, Biagini R: Primary bone tumors of the spine: terminology and surgical staging, *Spine* 22:1036-1044, 1997.

Lecouvet FE et al.: Vertebral compression fractures in multiple myeloma. I. Distribution and appearance at MR imaging, *Radiology* 204:195-199, 1997 (see comments).

Lecouvet FE et al.: Vertebral compression fractures in multiple myeloma. II. Assessment of fracture risk with MR imaging of spinal bone marrow, *Radiology* 204:201-205, 1997 (see comments).

Sharafuddin MJ et al.: Treatment options in primary Ewing's sarcoma of the spine: report of seven cases and review of the literature, *Neurosurgery* 30:610-618, discussion 618-619, 1992.

REFERENCES

1. Acciarri N et al.: Langerhans cell histiocytosis of the spine causing cord compression: case report, *Neurosurgery* 31:965-968, 1992.
2. Bacci G et al.: Therapy for primary non-Hodgkin's lymphoma of bone and a comparison of results with Ewing's sarcoma: ten years' experience at the Istituto Ortopedico Rizzoli, *Cancer* 57:1468-1472, 1986.
3. Barbieri E et al.: Radiotherapy in vertebral tumors. Indications and limits: a report on 28 cases of Ewing's sarcoma of the spine, *Chir Organi Mov* 83:105-111, 1998.
4. Barwick KW, Huvos AG, Smith J: Primary osteogenic sarcoma of the vertebral column: a clinicopathologic correlation of ten patients, *Cancer* 46:595-604, 1980.
5. Beadle GF, Hillcoat BL: Treatment of advanced malignant hemangiopericytoma with combination Adriamycin and DTIC: a report of four cases, *J Surg Oncol* 22:167-170, 1983.
6. Bergsagel DE et al.: The chemotherapy on plasma-cell myeloma and the incidence of acute leukemia, *N Engl J Med* 301:743-748, 1979.
7. Boriani S et al.: Osteoblastoma of the spine, *Clin Orthop* 37-45, 1992.
8. Boriani S, Weinstein JN, Biagini R: Primary bone tumors of the spine: terminology and surgical staging, *Spine* 22:1036-1044, 1997.
9. Breteau N et al.: Fast neutron therapy for inoperable or recurrent sacrococcygeal chordomas, *Bull Cancer Radiother* 83:142s-145s, 1996.
10. Brodkey JA, Brodkey JS, Watridge CB: Metastatic paraganglioma causing spinal cord compression, *Spine* 20:367-372, 1995.
11. Bucknill T et al.: Haemangioma of a vertebral body treated by ligation of the segmental arteries: report of a case, *J Bone Joint Surg Br* 55:534-539, 1973.
12. Cahan WG, Woodward HQ, Higinbotham NL: Sarcoma arising in irradiated bone, *Cancer* 1:3-29, 1948.
13. Camins MB et al.: Chondrosarcoma of the spine, *Spine* 3:202-209, 1978.
14. Cardon T et al.: Percutaneous vertebroplasty with acrylic cement in the treatment of a Langerhans cell vertebral histiocytosis, *Clin Rheumatol* 13:518-521, 1994.
15. Catton C et al.: Chordoma: long-term follow-up after radical photon irradiation, *Radiother Oncol* 41:67-72, 1996.
16. Cheng EY et al.: Lumbosacral chordoma. Prognostic factors and treatment, *Spine* 24:1639-1645, 1999.
17. Compere EL, Johnson WE, Coventry MB: Vertebra plana (Clave's disease) due to eosinophilic granuloma, *J Bone Joint Surg Am* 36:969-980, 1954.
18. Conrad EV, Springfield DS: Giant-cell tumor treated with curettage and cementation. In *Limb salvage in musculoskeletal oncology*, New York, 1987, Churchill Livingstone, pp. 516-519.
19. Cortet B et al.: Percutaneous vertebroplasty in patients with osteolytic metastases or multiple myeloma, *Rev Rheum Engl Educ* 64:177-183, 1997 (see comments).
20. Corwin J, Lindberg RD: Solitary plasmacytoma of bone vs. extramedullary plasmacytoma and their relationship to multiple myeloma, *Cancer* 43:1007-1013, 1979.
21. Cotten A et al.: Preoperative percutaneous injection of methyl methacrylate and N-butyl cyanoacrylate in vertebral hemangiomas, *Am J Neuroradiol* 17:137-142, 1996.
22. Dahlin DC: *Bone tumors: general aspects and data on 6221 cases*, ed 3, Springfield, Ill, 1978, Thomas.
23. Edelstyn GA, Gillespie PJ, Grebbell FS: The radiological demonstration of osseous metastases: experimental observations, *Clin Radiol* 18:158-162, 1967.
24. Eismont FJ et al.: Coexistent infection and tumor of the spine: a report of three cases, *J Bone Joint Surg Am* 69:452-458, 1987.
25. Farhangi M, Merlini G: The clinical implications of monoclonal immunoglobulins, *Semin Oncol* 13:366-379, 1986.
26. Fujita T et al.: Chordoma in the cervical spine managed with en bloc excision, *Spine* 24:1848-1851, 1999.
27. Garrett IR et al.: Production of lymphotoxin, a bone-resorbing cytokine, by cultured human myeloma cells, *N Engl J Med* 317:526-532, 1987.
28. Gennari L, Azzarelli A, Quagliuolo V: A posterior approach for the excision of sacral chordoma, *J Bone Joint Surg Br* 69:565-568, 1987.
29. Gotz W et al.: Detection and distribution of the carbohydrate binding protein galectin-3 in human notochord, intervertebral disc and chordoma, *Differentiation* 62:149-157, 1997.
30. Green NE, Robertson WW Jr, Kilroy AW: Eosinophilic granuloma of the spine with associated neural deficit: report of three cases, *J Bone Joint Surg Am* 62:1198-1202, 1980.
31. Griffin JB: Benign osteoblastoma of the thoracic spine: case report with fifteen-year follow-up, *J Bone Joint Surg Am* 60:833-835, 1978.
32. Grubb MR et al.: Primary Ewing's sarcoma of the spine, *Spine* 19:309-313, 1994.
33. Haddad FS, Abla A, Allam CK: Extradural spinal angiolipoma, *Surg Neurol* 26:473-486, 1986.
34. Harris DJ, Fornasier VL, Livingston KE: Hemangiopericytoma of the spinal canal: report of three cases, *J Neurosurg* 49:914-920, 1978.
35. Hart RA et al.: A system for surgical staging and management of spine tumors: a clinical outcome study of giant cell tumors of the spine, *Spine* 22:1773-1782, discussion 1783, 1997.
36. Hay MC, Paterson D, Taylor TK: Aneurysmal bone cysts of the spine, *J Bone Joint Surg Br* 60:406-411, 1978.
37. Hayem G et al.: Spontaneous spinal epidural hematoma with spinal cord compression complicating plasma cell myeloma: a case report, *Spine* 23:2432-2435, 1998.
38. Hester TO et al.: Cervicothoracic chordoma presenting as progressive dyspnea and dysphagia, *Otolaryngol Head Neck Surg* 120:97-100, 1999.
39. Hoffmann J et al.: Polytopic manifestations of paragangliomas: diagnosis, differential diagnosis and indications for therapy, *Mund Kiefer Gesichtschir* 4:53-56, 2000.
40. Huvos AG: Osteogenic sarcoma of bones and soft tissues in older persons: a clinicopathologic analysis of 117 patients older than 60 years, *Cancer* 57:1442-1449, 1986.
41. Huvos AG et al.: Postradiation osteogenic sarcoma of bone and soft tissues: a clinicopathologic study of 66 patients, *Cancer* 55:1244-1255, 1985.
42. Jaffray D, Hoyle M, O'Brien JP: Anterior decompression of vertebral osteosarcomas to relieve paraparesis: report of two cases, *Clin Orthop* 210-216, 1987.
43. Jyung RW et al.: Expression of angiogenic growth factors in paragangliomas, *Laryngoscope* 110:161-167, 2000.
44. Kaiser TE, Pritchard DJ, Unni KK: Clinicopathologic study of sacrococcygeal chordoma, *Cancer* 53:2574-2578, 1984.
45. Kawahara N et al.: Osteosarcoma of the thoracolumbar spine: total en bloc spondylectomy: a case report, *J Bone Joint Surg Am* 79:453-458, 1997.
46. Keisch ME, Garcia DM, Shibuya RB: Retrospective long-term follow-up analysis in 21 patients with chordomas of various sites treated at a single institution, *J Neurosurg* 75:374-377, 1991.
47. Kim RY, Salter MM, Brascho DJ: High-energy irradiation in the management of chondrosarcoma, *South Med J* 76:729-731, 735, 1983.
48. Klisch J et al.: Radiological and histological findings in spinal intramedullary angiolipoma, *Neuroradiology* 41:584-587, 1999.
49. Kransdorf MJ, Sweet DE: Aneurysmal bone cyst: concept, controversy, clinical presentation, and imaging, *Am J Roentgenol* 164:573-580, 1995.
50. Kruger L, Schmitt E: Solitary involvement of the fourth thoracic vertebral body with eosinophilic granuloma and development of incomplete paraparesis, *Eur Spine J* 4:313-316, 1995.
51. Kyle RA: Diagnosis and management of multiple myeloma and related disorders, *Prog Hematol* 14:257-282, 1986.
52. Lecouvet FF et al.: Long-term effects of localized spinal radiation therapy on vertebral fractures and focal lesions appearance in patients with multiple myeloma, *Br J Haematol* 96:743-745, 1997.
53. Lecouvet FE et al.: Vertebral compression fractures in multiple myeloma. II. Assessment of fracture risk with MR imaging of spinal bone marrow, *Radiology* 204:201-205, 1997 (see comments).
54. Lecouvet FE et al.: Vertebral compression fractures in multiple myeloma. I. Distribution and appearance at MR imaging, *Radiology* 204:195-199, 1997 (see comments).
55. Liebross RH et al.: Solitary bone plasmacytoma: outcome and prognostic factors following radiotherapy, *Int J Radiat Oncol Biol Phys* 41:1063-1067, 1998.
56. Lin YJ et al.: Primary hemangiopericytoma in the axis bone: case report and review of literature, *Neurosurgery* 39:397-399, discussion 399-400, 1996.

57. Loftus CM et al.: Solitary osteochondroma of T4 with thoracic cord compression, *Surg Neurol* 13:355-357, 1980.
58. Lozman J, Holmblad J: Cavernous hemangiomas associated with scoliosis and a localized consumptive coagulopathy: a case report, *J Bone Joint Surg Am* 58:1021-1024, 1976.
59. Maggi G et al.: Spinal intramedullary angiolipoma, *Childs Nerv Syst* 12:346-349, 1996.
60. Maggi G et al.: Eosinophilic granuloma of C4 causing spinal cord compression, *Childs Nerv Syst* 12:630-632, 1996.
61. Malat J, Virapongse C, Levine A: Solitary osteochondroma of the spine, *Spine* 11:625-628, 1986.
62. Mammano S, Candiotto S, Balsano M: Cast and brace treatment of eosinophilic granuloma of the spine: long-term follow-up, *J Pediatr Orthop* 17:821-827, 1997.
63. Marcove RC et al.: Conservative surgery for giant cell tumors of the sacrum: the role of cryosurgery as a supplement to curettage and partial excision, *Cancer* 74:1253-1260, 1994.
64. Marsh BW et al.: Benign osteoblastoma: range of manifestations, *J Bone Joint Surg Am* 57:1-9, 1975.
65. McAllister E et al.: Perineal reconstruction after surgical extirpation of pelvic malignancies using the transpelvic transverse rectus abdominal myocutaneous flap, *Ann Surg Oncol* 1:164-168, 1994.
66. Mischis-Troussard C et al.: Osteosarcoma of the sacrum complicating Paget's disease of bone, *Rev Rheum Engl Educ.* 65:361-362, 1998 (letter).
67. Morton KS: Aneurysmal bone cyst: a review of 26 cases, *Can J Surg* 29:110-115, 1986.
68. Munzenrider JE, Liebsch NJ: Proton therapy for tumors of the skull base, *Strahlenther Onkol* 175(Suppl 2):57-63, 1999.
69. Muraszko KM et al.: Hemangiopericytomas of the spine, *Neurosurgery* 10:473-479, 1982.
70. Nonaka M et al.: Metastatic meningeal hemangiopericytoma of thoracic spine, *Clin Neurol Neurosurg* 100:228-230, 1998.
71. North CA et al.: Multiple spinal metastases from paraganglioma, *Cancer* 66:2224-2228, 1990.
72. Oge HK et al.: Spinal angiolipoma: case report and review of literature, *J Spinal Disord* 12:353-356, 1999.
73. Ostrowsky ML, Krishnan KU, Banks PM: Malignant lymphoma of bone, *Cancer* 58:2646-2655, 1986.
74. Papagelopoulos PJ et al.: Vertebra plana of the lumbar spine caused by an aneurysmal bone cyst: a case report, *Am J Orthop* 28:119-124, 1999.
75. Papagelopoulos PJ et al.: Aneurysmal bone cyst of the spine: management and outcome, *Spine* 23:621-628, 1998.
76. Pettine KA, Klassen RA: Osteoid-osteoma and osteoblastoma of the spine, *J Bone Joint Surg Am* 68:354-361, 1986.
77. Pilepich MV et al.: Ewing's sarcoma of the vertebral column, *Int J Radiat Oncol Biol Phys* 7:27-31, 1981.
78. Price CHG, Goldie W: Paget's sarcoma of bone: a study of 80 cases, *J Bone Joint Surg Br* 51:205-224, 1969.
79. Provenzale JM, McLendon RE: Spinal angiolipomas: MR features, *Am J Neuroradiol* 17:713-719, 1996.
80. Raab P et al.: Vertebral remodeling in eosinophilic granuloma of the spine: a long-term follow-up, *Spine* 23:1351-1354, 1998.
81. Ransford AO et al.: The behaviour pattern of the scoliosis associated with osteoid osteoma or osteoblastoma of the spine, *J Bone Joint Surg Br* 66:16-20, 1984.
82. Razakaboay M et al.: Bone metastases from a paraganglioma: a review of five cases, *Rev Rheum Engl Educ* 66:86-91, 1999.
83. Rosen G et al.: Ewing's sarcoma: ten-year experience with adjuvant chemotherapy, *Cancer* 47:2204-2213, 1981.
84. Samson IR et al.: Operative treatment of sacrococcygeal chordoma: a review of twenty-one cases, *J Bone Joint Surg Am* 75:1476-1484, 1993.
85. Sanjay BK et al.: Giant-cell tumours of the spine, *J Bone Joint Surg Br* 75:148-154, 1993.
86. Savini R et al.: Surgical treatment of giant-cell tumor of the spine: the experience at the Istituto Ortopedico Rizzoli, *J Bone Joint Surg Am* 65:1283-1289, 1983.
87. Scarpinati M, Artico M, Artizzu S: Spinal cord compression by eosinophilic granuloma of the cervical spine: case report and review of the literature, *Neurosurg Rev* 18:209-212, 1995.
88. Sharafuddin MJ et al.: Treatment options in primary Ewing's sarcoma of the spine: report of seven cases and review of the literature, *Neurosurgery* 30:610-618, discussion 618-619, 1992.
89. Sharma BS, Khosla VK, Banerjee AK: Primary spinal epidural Ewing's sarcoma, *Clin Neurol Neurosurg* 88:299-302, 1986.
90. Sherk HH, Nicholson JT, Nixon JE: Vertebra plana and eosinophilic granuloma of the cervical spine in children, *Spine* 3:116-121, 1978.
91. Shi HB et al.: Preoperative transarterial embolization of spinal tumor: embolization techniques and results, *Am J Neuroradiol* 20(10):2009-2015, 1999.
92. Shikata J et al.: Surgical treatment of giant-cell tumors of the spine, *Clin Orthop*, 1992, pp. 29-36.
93. Shives TC et al.: Osteosarcoma of the spine, *J Bone Joint Surg Am* 68:660-668, 1986.
94. Shives TC et al.: Chondrosarcoma of the spine, *J Bone Joint Surg Am* 71:1158-1165, 1989.
95. Siegal T: Current considerations in the management of neoplastic spinal cord compression, *Spine* 14:223-228, 1985.
96. Sim FH et al.: Primary bone tumors simulating lumbar disc syndrome, *Spine* 2:65-74, 1977.
97. Stener B: Complete removal of vertebrae for extirpation of tumors: a 20-year experience, *Clin Orthop*, 1989, pp. 72-82.
98. Stener B, Gunterberg B: High amputation of the sacrum for extirpation of tumors: principles and technique, *Spine* 3:351-366, 1978 (published erratum appears in *Rev Chir Orthop* 73[3]:following 217, 1987).
99. Stener B, Johnsen OE: Complete removal of three vertebrae for giant-cell tumour, *J Bone Joint Surg Br* 53:278-287, 1971.
100. Stern MB, Grode ML, Goodman MD: Hemangiopericytoma of the cervical spine: report of an unusual case, *Clin Orthop*, 1980, pp. 201-204.
101. Suga K et al.: Bone and gallium scintigraphy in sacral chordoma: report of four cases, *Clin Nucl Med* 17:206-212, 1992.
102. Sundaresan N et al.: Postradiation sarcoma involving the spine, *Neurosurgery.* 18:721-724, 1986.
103. Sundaresan N et al.: Postradiation osteosarcoma of the spine following treatment of Hodgkin's disease, *Spine* 11:90-92, 1986.
104. Sundaresan N et al.: Combined treatment of osteosarcoma of the spine, *Neurosurgery* 23:714-719, 1988.
105. Thomsen K, Bunger CE: Chordoma localized in the spine, *Ugeskr Laeger* 155:2480, 1993 (letter; comment).
106. Turker RJ, Mardjetko S, Lubicky J: Aneurysmal bone cysts of the spine: excision and stabilizations, *J Pediatr Orthop* 18:209-213, 1998.
107. Weill A et al.: Spinal angiolipomas: CT and MR aspects, *J Comput Assist Tomogr* 15:83-85, 1991.
108. Weinstein JN, McLain RF: Primary tumors of the spine, *Spine* 12:843-851, 1987.
109. Whang-Peng J et al.: Cytogenetic characterization of selected small round cell tumors of childhood, *Cancer Genet Cytogenet* 21:185-208, 1986.
110. Whitehouse GH, Griffiths GJ: Roentgenologic aspects of spinal involvement by primary and metastatic Ewing's tumor, *J Can Assoc Radiol* 27:290-297, 1976.
111. Wilkins RM et al.: Ewing's sarcoma of bone: experience with 140 patients, *Cancer* 58:2551-2555, 1986.
112. Wuisman PI, Jutte PC, Ozaki T: Secondary chondrosarcoma in osteochondromas: medullary extension in 15 of 45 cases, *Acta Orthop Scand* 68:396-400, 1997.
113. Wuisman PI, Noorda RJ, Jutte PC: Chondrosarcoma secondary to synovial chondromatosis: report of two cases and a review of the literature, *Arch Orthop Trauma Surg* 116:307-311, 1997.
114. Yonemoto T et al.: The surgical management of sacrococcygeal chordoma, *Cancer* 85:878-883, 1999.
115. York JE et al.: Sacral chordoma: 40-year experience at a major cancer center, *Neurosurgery* 44:74-79, discussion 79-80, 1999.

Metastatic Tumors of the Spine

Alexander J. Ghanayem

Metastasic lesions to the spine represent a continuum of the disease process that affects patients with cancer. More than any other disease process, spine metastasis truly requires the coordinated effort of multiple health care providers, including the spine surgeon, radiation oncologist, medical oncologist, orthotist, and other oncologic health care providers. Treatment outcomes are difficult to measure when one is faced with making clinical decisions in the context of "quality of remaining life." Most metastatic lesions to the vertebral column can be treated by nonoperative means. A treatment algorithm is outlined that provides a framework to identify surgical, nonsurgical, and combined treatment plans. For the spine surgeon to navigate this algorithm, one must understand the disease process, including the pathophysiology of the disease process, patient presentation, diagnostic workup, and natural history, and one must have a clear understanding of the goals of treatment for each patient. The patient's overall medical condition, nutritional status, and life expectancy must all be considered. Communication among all of the health care providers involved with care of the patient with cancer, along with the patient and the patient's family, allows the spine surgeon to be effective in his or her treatment plan.

The medical treatment of patients with cancer has made great advances since the 1980s. As a result, patients are surviving longer and more are requiring treatment for involvement of the spine. Surgical treatment for tumors of the spine has also evolved significantly during this time period. With the development of new approaches and fixation techniques, outcomes have improved dramatically and diminished many of the postoperative complications reported by earlier investigators. Because of these advances, surgical indications have expanded and procedures that were once considered radical are now seen as commonplace.

Breast, lung, and prostate tumors account for the majority of spinal metastases.[26] Tumors of the kidney, thyroid, and gastrointestinal tract account for the majority of the remaining spinal metastases. Breast cancer is the most common source of bony metastasis, with the development of skeletal disease in up to 85% of women with breast cancer before death. Lung and prostate carcinomas are the most common source of metastasis in men. Lymphoreticular malignancies, including lymphoma and myeloma, are common sources of spinal involvement; however, they are systemic diseases, do not represent true metastasis, and are not included in many clinical series. The true incidence of spinal metastases varies from series to series and depends on the type of series reviewed (i.e., autopsy studies or clinical studies).[5,26] Patients with either breast or prostate cancer who survive for long periods of time are more likely to require treatment for their spinal disease. Conversely, patients with lung cancer, whose survival is much more limited, often do not require more than supportive treatment for their spinal lesion.

Because of improved patient survival and the dramatic impact that appropriate surgical treatment can have, it is important for treating physicians to develop a logical approach when evaluating patients suspected of having a metastatic spine tumor. Unfortunately, there is no uniform approach to the evaluation and treatment of patients with metastatic spine tumors. The goals of treatment are to preserve neurologic function, promote pain relief, and provide functional improvement. This chapter outlines the principles in the evaluation and management of patients with metastatic tumors to the spine.

PATHOPHYSIOLOGY

Metastatic tumors that involve the spine metastasize to the spine via either the bloodstream or the lymphatics.[3,7] This explains the predilection of malignancies for various parts of the spine. Breast tumors drain through the azygous venous system and commonly spread to the thoracic spine. The prostate drains via the pelvic venous plexus, and thus these tumors are more common in the lumbar spine. Tumors of the lung most commonly occur in the thoracic spine and may seed the thoracic spinal column directly through segmental arteries.

Batson first described the importance of the paravertebral venous plexus in the pathophysiology of spinal metastases.[3] This plexus consists of small, thin-walled valveless vessels in the sinuses with a low intraluminal pressure. Tumor cells may become implanted in the vertebral column via retrograde flow through Batson's plexus. Batson's plexus is most significant in tumors of the breast, lung, and prostate.

Tumor cells lack normal cellular control mechanisms, making it difficult for the body to eradicate them. These cells lack the normal contact inhibition and cell cohesiveness demonstrated by normal cells; this allows unimpeded overgrowth of tumor cells. Tumor cells also secrete degradative enzymes (proteases and hydrolases), which provide another mechanism for invasion into surrounding tissues. Additional attributes of tumor cells, which enhance their survival, include the production of a fibrin-platelet coat that protects them from the host's immunologic response (macrophage system). Despite these mechanisms, it is estimated that less than 0.1% of the circulating tumor cells survive transport from the primary tumor site.

For a metastatic tumor to proliferate, a blood supply must be established. Metastatic tumor cells can remain in a dormant state until their blood supply is established. Thus, late metastasis may occur when tumor cells, which were previously dormant due to lack of blood supply, acquire sufficient vascularity. Tumors secrete an angiogenic factor that allows the establishment of a blood supply. The vertebral body maintains an active red marrow and capillary network throughout life, thus allowing tumor cells easy access and a suitable biochemical environment for survival.

PATIENT PRESENTATION

Pain is the most common initial complaint of patients presenting with a suspected metastatic lesion (Table 16-1).[18] The history and physical examination should narrow the differential diagnosis, help exclude nontumor sources of back pain, and identify any neurologic deficit. Patients with spine metastasis develop symptoms for one of the following reasons: (1) expansion of the cortex of the vertebral body, (2) pathologic fracture, (3) spinal instability, or (4) compression of nerve roots or spinal cord.[10]

The nature of the back pain can help differentiate between mechanical and nonmechanical pain. Mechan-

ical back pain is usually activity related and is relieved with rest. In contrast, back pain secondary to a tumor is usually not relieved by rest and is often unrelenting and intensifies at night. The majority of patients with a spinal metastasis present with back pain that is usually subacute and progressive over several weeks to months. Pain may precede neurologic symptoms by a variable length of time depending on the growth rate of the tumor. In patients with breast or prostate cancer, this may be as long as 12 months. Aggressive renal or lung tumors can progress from pain to neurologic involvement in less than 2 months. In descending order of frequency, the most prominent symptoms at presentation are back pain, radicular pain, weakness in the lower extremities, sensory loss, and loss of sphincter control.

Even though the lumbar vertebrae are most commonly affected by tumor metastases, it is in the thoracic spine that spinal cord compression most often occurs. The spinal cord at the thoracic level is the largest relative to the space available for the cord and thus is most susceptible at this level to compression by tumor cells. In Gilbert et al's series, 68% of patients had spinal cord compression from tumor involvement in the thoracic spine, 16% (thecal sac) from involvement in the lumbar spine, and 15% from involvement in the cervical spine.[9] When evaluating patients with spinal cord compression, it is important to be vigilant for noncontiguous areas of compression. Spinal cord compression usually occurs as a result of one of the following mechanisms: (1) compression by bone or a tumor mass after a pathologic fracture, (2) direct pressure from tumor extension into the epidural space, (3) kyphosis after vertebral collapse, or (4) pressure from intradural metastasis.[9]

The pain of epidural spinal cord compression may be accompanied by motor, sensory, and autonomic dysfunction. Because the compression usually occurs anteriorly from the vertebral body, the motor functions of the anterior part of the spinal cord are usually compromised first. Sensory disturbance occurs less frequently, and the level of sensory loss is not a reliable indicator of compression of the spinal cord. It is very unusual for patients with cord compression to present without pain; however, patients with lung or renal metastases or with lymphoma may present with a neurologic deficit in the absence of pain.

Timely diagnosis is extremely important because the neurologic status at the time of diagnosis is one of the most important prognostic factors that affects outcome. Of those patients who have the ability to walk at the time diagnosis is made, up to 90% retain that ability after treatment. Patients who have significant weakness are much less likely to continue to ambulate after treatment, and only 30% of patients who are paraplegic regain the ability to ambulate.[10,12] Prognostically, the ability to walk and the absence of myelopathy are correlated with the preservation of the ability of the patient to ambulate after treatment. Other factors affecting prognosis include the rapidity of onset. Patients who experience major neurologic deficit within 24 hours have a much poorer prognosis than do those who have their deficit occur over a longer period of time.[11]

Table 16-1	Presenting Symptoms in Patients With Spine Tumors
Presenting Symptoms	**Patients (%)**
Pain	**84**
Back pain	30
Radicular pain	10
Pain and weakness	28
Pain and mass	11
Weakness	**42**
Weakness alone	9
Weakness and pain	28
Mass	**16**
Mass alone	5
Mass and pain	11
Asymptomatic	**3**

From Weinsten JN, McLain RF: Primary tumors of the spine, *Spine Surg* 12:843-851, 1987.

PHYSICAL EXAMINATION

Physical examination must include an assessment of local tenderness, deformity, range of motion, and neurologic evaluation. Pain on palpation of the spine may be the earliest finding in patients with tumors in the posterior elements. The presence of kyphosis or a gibbous deformity may indicate a pathologic fracture.

The neurologic examination is the most important part of the physical examination. The neurologic assessment should include testing of muscle function in the upper and lower extremities. Sensory examination should include testing pin prick and light touch, particularly in the sacral dermatomes, as well as proprioception. Deep tendon reflexes should be tested and any hyperreflexia or asymmetry noted. Pathologic reflexes, including Babinski, Hoffman, and clonus, must be documented. Rectal examination may disclose a presacral mass indicative of a chordoma or show a mass or enlarged prostate. Neurologic deficits occur both with rapidly expanding malignant lesions and with slowly progressive expansile lesions.

IMAGING TECHNIQUES
Plain Radiographs

Plain radiographs of the spine are the initial imaging studies obtained in the workup of a patient with a spine lesion. Plain radiographs aid in the differential diagnosis of spine lesions, both by the radiographic appearance of the lesion and by the location in the vertebrae. Primary tumors of the spine are usually localized to single vertebra. Metastatic lesions of the spine may involve multiple adjacent vertebrae.

Plain radiographs of the spine have been reported to identify 30% to 70% of spine tumors at the time patients begin to experience back pain. Early lesions are difficult to detect because 30% to 50% of the trabecular bone must be destroyed before they are able to be detected on plain radiographs. Because so much of the cancellous bone in the vertebral body must be destroyed before it is detected on plain radiographs, the earliest radiographic sign of vertebral involvement is often the absence of the pedicle when seen on an anteroposterior view. The destruction of the cortical bone of the pedicle is much easier to detect than subtle loss of the cancellous bone of the vertebral body.

It is difficult to distinguish between a destructive lesion caused by tumor and one caused by infection. In general, the intervertebral disc space is preserved in patients with tumors.[4] Destruction of the intervertebral disc and adjacent end plates is suggestive of an infection. The intervertebral disc is very resistant to tumor invasion and usually maintains its height even in the face of extensive destruction of the vertebral body by tumor.

Bone Scan

A bone scan is a sensitive but nonspecific test that is used in the evaluation of spinal metastasis. The bone scan is a reflection of the concentration of newly formed osteoid. Bone scans are able to detect lesions as small as 2 mm, whether in trabecular or cortical bone, and may pick up lesions 3 to 18 months before their appearance on plain radiographs. A bone scan has a broad differential diagnosis when positive, including trauma, tumor, infection, inflammation, and degenerative conditions. Because of this high sensitivity and low specificity, bone scans are useful as a screening test but are not as helpful in making a specific diagnosis. They are, however, useful for determining the extent of metastasis throughout the skeleton.

False-negative bone scan results can occur in lesions that are rapidly destructive and lack significant bone formation or vascular response. Bone scans are negative in as many as 60% of patients with multiple myeloma. Patients receiving chemotherapy may also have a false-negative bone scan result.

Computed Tomography–Myelography

Computed tomography (CT)–myelography historically has been considered the gold standard for evaluating spinal cord compression, but it has been replaced by magnetic resonance imaging (MRI). There are significant drawbacks to the use of myelography in cases of suspected complete myelographic block. Up to 25% of patients with complete myelographic block demonstrate a significant, rapid deterioration neurologically after lumbar punctures due to cerebrospinal fluid pressure shifts. Also, in cases with complete myelographic block, in addition to a lumbar puncture, a C1 to C2 puncture must be performed to rule out multiple levels of compression and to fully evaluate the extent of the myelographic block. Current indications for CT-myelography include patients who experience recurrence of symptoms after surgery with instrumentation that would significantly degrade an MRI.

Plain CT is a very sensitive test to detect even very small areas of vertebral destruction and is a useful adjuvant neurodiagnostic imaging study. CT scans provide excellent images of the cross-sectional bony anatomy of the spine, allowing full delineation of the extent of bony destruction. CT scanning currently offers better definition of bony architecture than MRI and therefore more precise definition of the remaining bone and feasibility of fixation. It is less effective than MRI in showing the soft tissue anatomy and tumor extension.

Magnetic Resonance Imaging

MRI has become the imaging modality of choice in evaluating metastatic lesions of the spine.[2,6,19] MRI characterizes the lesion not only on the basis of morphology and location but also according to signal intensity characteristics. Before the development of MRI, bone scans were considered the most sensitive means of detecting suspected tumors of the vertebral body. MRI has been shown to be more sensitive to marrow abnormalities. In addition, MRI is able to detect lesions that frequently have false-negative results on a bone scan, such as multiple myeloma and lymphoma.

BENIGN VERSUS MALIGNANT COMPRESSION FRACTURES

Compression fractures secondary to osteopenia usually occur in the elderly patient with minimal trauma. Cancer with metastasis to the spine also usually occurs in the elderly population. It can be very difficult to differentiate a benign compression fracture secondary to osteoporosis from a pathologic fracture, especially if the patient has a history of a primary neoplasm. It has been estimated that up to one third of vertebral compression fractures in elderly patients with malignancies are benign. It is important to differentiate between benign and malignant compression fractures because the treatment and prognosis are very different for each process.

Studies looking at the reliability of differentiating benign from malignant compression fractures have shown mixed results. Some suggest that MRI can be useful in patients with compression fractures of the vertebral bodies to differentiate between benign osteoporotic collapse and neoplastic replacement.[19,31] Yuh et al. showed that 88% of metastatic fractures demonstrated complete bone marrow replacement on T1 images, whereas in 77% of benign fractures, there was some preservation of normal marrow elements.[31] They also noted that malignant processes resulted in an ill-defined and irregular pattern of bone marrow replacement, whereas benign compression fractures with partial preservation of marrow had smooth margins. MRI findings that were more common in fractures secondary to malignant lesions include homogeneous replacement of marrow with a decreased signal intensity on T1 and a high signal intensity on T2, diffuse and irregular borders of marrow involvement, other sites of metastasis, pedicle or posterior element involvement, paraspinal mass, and the return of signal intensity to normal in benign lesions during a 3-month time period (Table 16-2).[1]

Other studies have shown a high false-positive rate when using MRI to detect malignant compression fractures, especially acutely, because both malignant and benign compression fractures show a low signal on T1 images. The early healing process of benign compression fractures may mimic the findings of compression fractures secondary to metastatic lesions. The use of gadolinium-enhanced MRI improves the sensitivity in detecting pathologic fractures secondary to malignancy. A benign lesion would show diminished contrast enhancement at 1 to 2 months after the onset of symptoms, whereas a metastatic lesion would show progression of tumor involvement of the spine. Therefore, it may not be possible to determine in the acute stages whether a compression fracture is a benign osteopenic lesion or a pathologic fracture. A reasonable treatment approach to patients who present with an acute compression fracture, who are neurologically intact, is to treat them with an appropriate brace and to follow them radiographically and clinically, including a workup for a primary tumor.

METASTASIS: SPECIFIC TUMOR TYPES
Lung

Lung carcinoma commonly metastasizes to the liver, skeleton, bone marrow, and brain. There are four histologic types of lung cancer: epidermoid, adenocarcinoma, and small cell and large cell carcinoma. Small cell carcinoma has the best overall prognosis and longer survival rate, and thus patients with this type of lung cancer have the highest likelihood of the development of skeletal metastases. The treatment of lung carcinoma is dependent on the type of tumor. Small cell lung carcinoma is more responsive to chemotherapy and radiation therapy. Given the limited survival in patients with lung cancer at the time of diagnosis, they often are not candidates for surgical treatment (Table 16-3).

Breast

Because the survival time after the diagnosis of breast cancer is relatively long, the incidence of patients who are diagnosed with skeletal metastasis is high. In addition, venous drainage from the breast via the azygous veins and their communication to the paravertebral venous plexus accounts for the high percentage of thoracic spine metastases in patients with breast cancer. The incidence of women with breast cancer who develop skeletal metastasis has been estimated as high as 74%.

Table 16-2	Distinguishing Magnetic Resonance Imaging Characteristics Between Benign and Malignant Compression Fractures
Benign	**Malignant**
Preservation of some normal marrow elements on T1	Complete marrow replacement on T1
Smooth, linear margin	Irregular, ill-defined pattern
No associated soft tissue mass	Paraspinal or epidural mass
Anterior and middle column involvement only	Posterior element involvement
Usually isolated	Associated with multifocal or metastatic disease
Signal reverts to normal in 2 to 3 months	Increase in abnormal marrow signal with time

Table 16-3	Primary Site of Neoplasm in Patients With Spinal Metastasis in 1432 Patients	
Primary Site		**Patients (%)**
Breast		21
Lung		19
Unknown		10
Prostate		10
Lymphoma		8
Kidney		6
Myeloma		5
Gastrointestinal		4

From Grant R, Papadopoulos SM, Greenberg HS: Metastatic epidural spinal cord compression, *Neurol Clin* 825-841, 1991.

The metastatic lesions are most commonly osteolytic; however, in 10% to 15% of metastases, the lesions are purely blastic. Metastatic breast cancer often remains confined to the skeleton for a prolonged period of time. Patients who initially had metastasis of their primary breast tumor to the skeleton had a longer survival compared with those with extraskeletal metastasis. Breast tumors that metastasize to bone have been shown to be more frequently estrogen receptor positive and better differentiated than breast tumors that have metastasized to the lungs or liver.

Prostate

Metastases to the spine are common in prostate cancer. The most common radiographic appearance of prostate lesions is osteoblastic (80%); 12% present a mixed lytic and blastic appearance, and 4% appear to be purely lytic. Because these metastatic lesions are usually blastic, pathologic fractures are relatively rare in prostate carcinoma. Likewise, neurologic involvement is uncommon in blastic lesions. However, lytic lesions in the spine, although rare, can cause neurologic involvement. Treatment for prostate cancer can involve different modalities such as hormonal manipulation, radiation, chemotherapy, and surgery.

Renal

Patients with renal carcinoma have metastases to bone in 50% of cases. By the time the primary tumor is diagnosed, it has often reached an advanced stage. Renal cell carcinoma represents less than 10% of all cases of metastatic carcinoma to the spine but is the fourth most common primary tumor seen. Renal cell carcinoma is commonly hypervascular and enlarges rapidly. Radiographically, these tumors appear as lytic lesions with indistinct margins and expansion into the surrounding soft tissues. Pathologic fractures are common.

Chemotherapy and hormonal therapy have been shown to be ineffective. Although radiation treatment is often used, the tumor is relatively radioresistant. Therefore, failure to respond to radiation therapy or relapse after radiotherapy is not uncommon. Despite this, the role of surgery in the treatment of renal cell metastases to the spine is controversial. The surgical management of renal cell metastases to the spine is indicated in patients with intractable pain or with a neurologic deficit that has not responded to radiotherapy or has relapsed after radiotherapy. Patients with extensive bone destruction of the spinal column due to tumor often do not improve with radiation therapy alone. Instability should be treated with surgical decompression and stabilization followed by postoperative radiation. Preoperative arteriograms have been recommended to assess the vascularity of the tumor and preoperatively embolize its arterial blood supply. Accurate identification of the spinal cord blood supply is necessary to prevent its inadvertent embolization.

Survival in patients with metastatic renal cell carcinoma is most dependent on the pathologic characterization of the primary tumor. Survival has also been correlated with the severity of the neurologic deficit, as well as the presence of other metastases.

Thyroid

Thirty percent of patients with thyroid carcinoma have bone metastases at presentation. The actual prevalence of metastases to the spine from thyroid carcinoma is low because thyroid carcinoma is a rare disease. The risk of the development of bone metastases is highest with the follicular type of thyroid carcinoma and lowest in the medullary and papillary forms. Bone metastases are most common in patients older than 50 and with tumors larger than 4 cm. As with renal cell carcinoma, these tumors may be highly vascular and are usually lytic. The margins are usually poorly defined, and it is unusual for these lesions to demonstrate a periosteal reaction. Metastatic lesions usually show increased uptake of nucleotide on a bone scan. False-negative bone scans have been reported due to a low rate of osteoblastic activity.

Multiple Myeloma

Multiple myeloma is most common in patients older than 40. Multiple melanoma and solitary plasmacytoma are considered manifestations of the same lymphoproliferative disease, although the prognosis of plasmacytoma is considerably better. The majority of myeloma lesions in the skeleton are lytic. Bone scans may be negative in a significant number of cases with skeleton involvement. The prognosis for solitary plasmacytoma versus multiple myeloma is dramatically different. The course of multiple myeloma is usually rapidly progressive. By definition, solitary plasmacytoma is an isolated lesion, and the treatment of this lesion may provide long-term disease-free survival or cure. The spinal lesion in multiple myeloma represents a metastasis in a progressive, systemic disease with a survival of usually less than 2 years despite systemic and local treatment. The 5-year survival rate for patients with disseminated multiple myeloma is 18%, with a median survival of 28 months. With cases involving the spine, the outcome is worse: 76% of patients die within 1 year. The 5-year disease-free survival rate for patients with solitary plasmacytoma was 60% with a median survival of 92 months.

The treatment for both solitary plasmacytoma and multiple myeloma includes radiation. The main surgical indication is spinal instability or the onset of neurologic deficits.

Lymphoma

Lymphomas are a group of malignant diseases of the lymphoreticular system that account for a large number of spinal neoplasms. Patients with spinal involvement most commonly present with back pain. Lymphoma can also cause epidural spinal cord compression without significant bony destruction. In patients with epidural spinal cord compression due to lymphoma, some recommend a combination of surgical decompression followed by irradiation. Others advocate radiation treatment alone.

TREATMENT: DECISION MAKING

The historic treatment of vertebral column metastatic disease has included radiation therapy alone or in combination with laminectomy.* In patients with pathologic fractures secondary to anterior metastatic disease, the results were less than satisfactory. In patients with circumferential spinal canal compression, Hall and MacKay reported a 39% success rate in treating neurologic deficits by laminectomy.[10] However, in patients with anterior compression alone, there was only a 9% success rate. The use of laminectomy alone has resulted in an unsatisfactory outcome, approaching 65% with a 10% to 20% rate of acute neurologic deterioration after laminectomy. Finally, Gilbert et al. compared nonsurgical treatment of vertebral column metastasis with combined laminectomy and radiation therapy and found an equally satisfactory outcome in the two groups.[9]

In response to the less-than-satisfactory results of laminectomy for vertebral metastasis with pathologic fracture, Harrington began to treat these patients with anterior procedures.[11] His work was expanded on by Kostuik,[13] Kostuik et al.,[14] Siegal,[24,25] and Sundaresan et al.[27] Throughout the 1980s, the indication for anterior decompression and stabilization, with or without supplemental posterior stabilization, was developed and subsequently modified with the advent of anterior and posterior segmental spine stabilization systems.[13,14,17] With the development of these systems and the success of multiple surgeons, an algorithm for the treatment of patients with vertebral metastasis was developed (Figure 16-1). This algorithm assumes that the primary tumor is known and that the apparent metastatic lesion is from that primary tumor.

The first decision point in this algorithm is the presence or absence of a neurologic deficit. In patients without deficits, the next question to be answered is whether there is the presence of a spinal deformity or the potential for deformity. In patients without deformity or the potential for spinal deformity, radiation treatment is successful. An example of this is a patient with a metastatic lesion of the lamina or spinous process without involvement of the facet joints, pedicle, or vertebral body. If there is no neurologic deficit but there exists a potential for spinal deformity or there is the presence of a minimal spinal deformity, treatment should then include radiation therapy and protective bracing (Figure 16-2). The rationale for brace treatment is to prevent further deformity from occurring while the metastatic tumor undergoes necrosis from the radiation. While the tumor undergoes necrosis, and for a period of time after radiation therapy, the weight-bearing anterior and middle columns of the vertebral body are weakened and require 6 to 12 weeks to allow fibrous ingrowth into the defect once occupied by the tumor. Once this has occurred, the structural integrity of the vertebral column may be maintained and use of the brace discontinued. Another example of this is a patient with metastatic

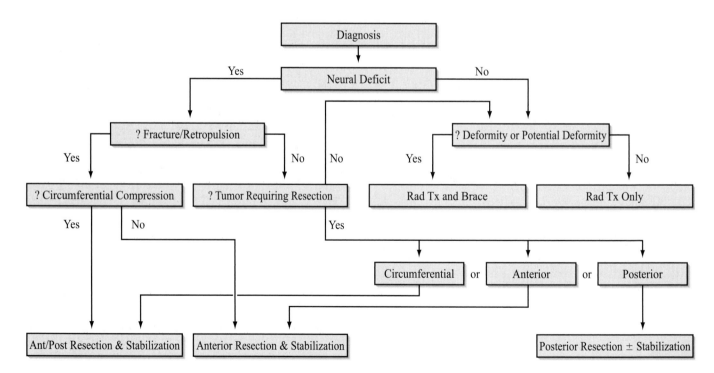

Figure 16-1. Treatment algorithm for patients with metastatic lesions to the spine.

*References 4, 8, 15, 20, 22, 28, 30.

prostate carcinoma to the L1 vertebral body with a pathologic compression fracture and minimal kyphosis. During radiation therapy, the goal of bracing would be to prevent subsequent increase in fracture severity and progressive deformity.

Radiation therapy is one of the primary treatment modalities for metastatic lesions to the spine. The administration of small daily radiation doses, as opposed to one or a few relatively large doses, has been shown to maximize radiation damage to tumors, while at the same time reducing complications from radiation damage to normal tissue. It is recommended that the total dose not exceed 5000 cGy to a large segment of the cord. This is usually administered in fractions of 180 to 200 cGy. The patient's functional status posttreatment is most dependent on pretreatment neurologic status. From 80% to 90% of patients with minimal weakness and the ability to bear weight will retain that ability. Only 30% of nonambulatory patients will regain sufficient ability to walk, regardless of other treatment options, including surgery.

If there is a neurologic deficit, the treating physician must ascertain whether there is a pathologic fracture. If there is no pathologic fracture, then the deficit must be caused by either an epidural-intradural metastasis or bony metastasis with direct extension into the spinal canal. Epidural-intradural metastatic lesions without bony involvement usually require radiation treatment only. For example, metastatic seminoma can present with an epidural lesion and acute neurologic deficit that responds rapidly to radiation therapy. The presence of a bony lesion with extension into the spinal canal must be evaluated for the potential for subsequent spinal deformity. If this is a potential, brace treatment may be instituted at the time of radiotherapy. If surgical decompression is planned along with adjuvant radiotherapy, the lesion should be treated as if it were a pathologic fracture (Figure 16-3).

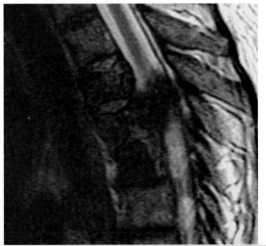

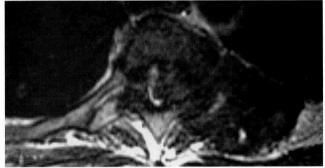

Figure 16-3. Axial and sagittal magnetic resonance image of a patient with metastatic prostate cancer. He presented with an acute inability to walk. Radiographs revealed no pathologic fracture in the thoracic spine. Magnetic resonance image reveals tumor involvement including the posterior chest wall, T3 to T6 vertebral bodies, and predominately lateral and posterior compression of the spinal cord at the T4 level. This patient underwent emergent laminectomy with debulking of the tumor followed by postsurgical irradiation and bracing. Although he did regain neurologic function in the lower extremities and was able to preserve complete bowel and bladder function, he never regained the ability to ambulate.

Figure 16-2. Sagittal magnetic resonance image of a patient with metastatic breast cancer in the cervical spine. The relative lordosis of the cervical spine is maintained, and there is no pathologic fracture. This patient responded to radiation therapy and 2 months of protective bracing after the last radiation treatment.

If there is a pathologic fracture with canal compromise or significant spinal deformity, with or without a neurologic deficit, the treating physician must determine the location of canal occlusion (i.e., anterior only or circumferential canal compromise) from the metastatic lesion. If canal compromise is circumferential, then the patient may benefit from an anterior and posterior resection and stabilization procedure. If compression is related to retropulsed bony fragments from the middle column, direct tumor extension into the anterior portion of the spinal canal, or significant kyphotic deformity secondary to a pathologic fracture, the treatment of choice would be anterior decompression with reconstruction of the anterior defect and stabilization (Figure 16-4). Postoperative radiation therapy is also indicated but should be delayed to allow wound and fusion healing.

There are many goals that should be met when performing an anterior stabilization procedure. Reconstruction of the anterior and middle column should be performed with a load-sharing strut graft. Strut graft migration should be prevented while restoring spinal stability. Internal fixation should be performed with MRI-compatible titanium implants to follow patients for recurrent disease. Because many patients with metastatic disease are of an advanced age, the reconstruction construct should allow immediate mobilization of the patient and keep external immobilization requirements feasible and easy to comply with.

Patients with metastatic disease may have significant life expectancies, especially those with prostate cancer (Table 16-4). Therefore, the material used to reconstruct the anterior and middle columns after an anterior pro-

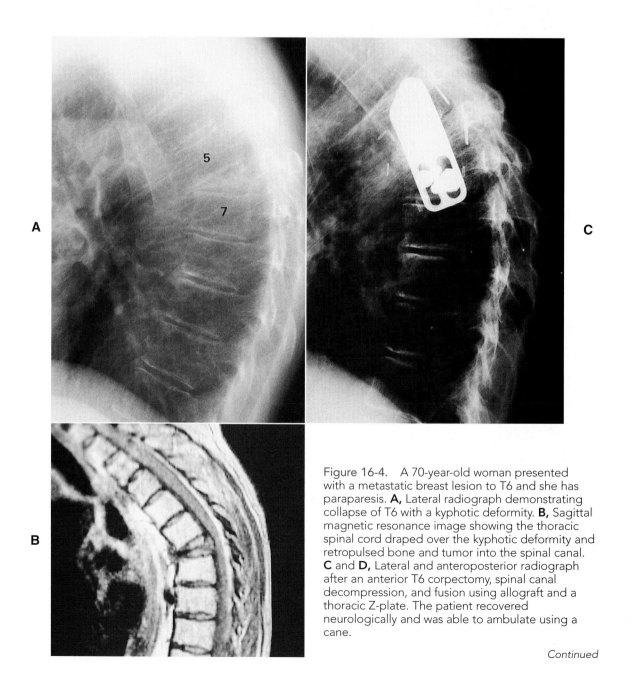

Figure 16-4. A 70-year-old woman presented with a metastatic breast lesion to T6 and she has paraparesis. **A,** Lateral radiograph demonstrating collapse of T6 with a kyphotic deformity. **B,** Sagittal magnetic resonance image showing the thoracic spinal cord draped over the kyphotic deformity and retropulsed bone and tumor into the spinal canal. **C** and **D,** Lateral and anteroposterior radiograph after an anterior T6 corpectomy, spinal canal decompression, and fusion using allograft and a thoracic Z-plate. The patient recovered neurologically and was able to ambulate using a cane.

Continued

cedure should allow for biologic incorporation. The use of methylmethacrylate cement spacers without simultaneous internal fixation results initially in a more stable construct than rib or iliac crest grafts without internal fixation. Whitehill et al. demonstrated that methylmethacrylate used in posterior constructs can restore immediate stability, but in patients who live longer than 3 months, the constructs fail.[29] McAfee et al. have also shown that cement constructs have a high incidence of failure with longer patient survival[16]; they reported that the mean time to failure of methylmethacrylate in their retrospective series of 24 patients was 200 days. Panjabi

et al. demonstrated that a wire-methylmethacrylate construct in the cervical spine fails at physiologic loads with flexion of the neck and that the initial rigidity of cement constructs decreases with time.[21] Methylmethacrylate used posteriorly has also been shown to increase the incidence of wound complications, including dehiscence and wound breakdown. Methylmethacrylate does not have the potential for biologic incorporation. The use of autogenous bone grafts with supplemental internal fixation can provide highly stable constructs and allow early patient mobilization. If sufficient autogenous graft material is not available, the use of bulk allografts (tibia, femur, or humerus) can be used to reconstruct the anterior and middle column defects. Although the incorporation of bulk allografts is slow, they do possess the potential to form a biologic arthrodesis that is not possible with methylmethacrylate. Bone-filled titanium composite spacers have also been used with clinical success.

This treatment algorithm is by no means comprehensive. There are many cases that cannot be addressed by this algorithm. Anterior lesions of the upper cervical spine are not amenable to anterior-only decompression and stabilization procedures. Access to the cervicothoracic junction and lumbosacral junction is limited by the regional anatomy and is not readily amenable to anterior stabilization procedures as well. Patients with multiple levels of involvement in the upper and lower thoracic

Table 16-4	Mean Survival Times From Time of Diagnosis in Patients With Spine Tumors	
Site		**Survival (Mo)**
Breast		14
Prostate		12
Lymphoma/myeloma		9
Kidney		9
All		8

From Sorensen PS, Borgesen SE, Rhode K: Metastatic epidural spinal cord compression: results of treatment and survival, *Cancer* 65:1502, 1990.

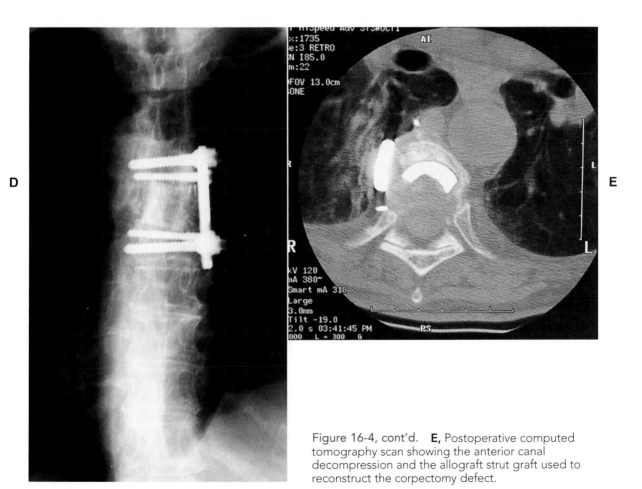

Figure 16-4, cont'd. **E,** Postoperative computed tomography scan showing the anterior canal decompression and the allograft strut graft used to reconstruct the corpectomy defect.

spine may benefit from multilevel posterolateral decompression via a costotransversectomy followed by posterior stabilization.[23] Finally, patients with recurrent disease require an individualized approach to their disease.

Contraindications to surgery include a limited life expectancy and the inability to tolerate surgery medically.[17] It is often difficult to project a particular patient's life expectancy, and the definition of what is an acceptable duration of remaining life is debatable. Sundaresan et al. excluded patients whose life expectancies were less than 3 months or in patients with significant concomitant comorbidities that would preclude surgery.[27] They also excluded patients who were completely paraplegic. McLain and Weinstein[18] believed that any patient with a life expectancy of greater than 6 weeks who was not bedridden should be given consideration for surgery.

CONCLUSIONS

The great majority of metastatic lesions to the vertebral column can be treated by nonoperative means. This requires a coordinated effort among the spine surgeon, radiation oncologist, medical oncologist, and orthotist. The treatment algorithm outlined is useful in that it provides a framework to identify areas of pathology and approaches to address them. This algorithm must not be used as the sole method in rendering care with metastatic lesions of the vertebral column. The patient's overall medical condition, nutritional status, life expectancy, and expectations must all be considered. These issues can be addressed successfully with a team approach to the patient with metastatic disease of the vertebral column.

SELECTED REFERENCES

An HS et al.: Can we distinguish between benign vs. malignant compression fractures of the spine by magnetic resonance imaging? *Spine* 20:1776, 1995.

Harrington KD: Current concepts review: metastatic disease of the spine, *J Bone Joint Surg* 68A:1110-1115, 1986.

McAfee PC, Zdeblick TA: Tumors of the thoracic and lumbar spine: surgical treatment via the anterior approach, *J Spinal Disord* 2:145-154, 1989.

McLain RF, Weinstein JN: Tumors of the spine, *Semin Spine Surg* 2:157-180, 1990.

Shimizu K et al.: Posterior decompression and stabilization for multiple metastatic tumors of the spine, *Spine* 17:1400, 1992.

REFERENCES

1. An HS et al.: Can we distinguish between benign vs. malignant compression fractures of the spine by magnetic resonance imaging? *Spine* 20:1776, 1995.
2. Avrahami E et al.: Early MR demonstration of spinal metastases in patients with normal radiographs and CT and radionuclide bone scans, *J Comput Assist Tomogr* 13:598, 1989.
3. Batson OV: The function of the vertebral veins and their role in the spread of metastases, *Ann Surg* 112:138-139, 1940.
4. Black P: Spinal metastasis: current status and recommended guidelines for management, *Neurosurgery* 5:726-746, 1979.
5. Boland PJ, Lane JM, Sundaresan N: Metastatic disease of the spine, *Clin Orthop* 169:95, 1982.
6. Carmody R et al.: Spinal cord compression due to metastatic disease: diagnosis with MR imaging vs. myelography, *Radiology* 173:225, 1989.
7. Comar, DR, DeLong, RP: The role of the vertebral venous system in the metastasis of cancer to the spinal column: experiments with tumor-cell suspensions in rats and rabbits, *Cancer* 4:610, 1951.
8. Constans JP et al.: Spinal metastases with neurological manifestations: review of 600 cases, *J Neurosurg* 59:111, 1983.
9. Gilbert RW, Kim JH, Posner JB: Epidural spinal cord compression from metastatic tumor: diagnosis and treatment, *Ann Neurol* 3:40-51, 1978.
10. Hall AJ, MacKay NNS: The results of laminectomy for compression of the cord or cauda equina by extradural malignant tumor, *J Bone Joint Surg* 55B:497-505, 1973.
11. Harrington KD: Current concepts review: metastatic disease of the spine, *J Bone Joint Surg* 68A:1110-1115, 1986.
12. Harrington KD: Anterior decompression and stabilization of the spine as a treatment for vertebral collapse and spinal cord compression from metastatic malignancy, *Clin Orthop* 233:177-197, 1988.
13. Kostuik JP: Anterior spinal cord decompression for lesions of the thoracic and lumbar spine: techniques, new methods of internal fixation, results, *Spine* 8:512-531, 1983.
14. Kostuik JP et al.: Spinal stabilization of vertebral column tumors, *Spine* 13:250, 1988.
15. Lord CF, Herndon, JH: Spinal cord compression secondary to kyphosis associated with radiation therapy for metastatic disease, *Clin Orthop* 210:120, 1986.
16. McAfee PC et al.: Failure of stabilization of the spine with methylmethacrylate, *J Bone Joint Surg* 68A:1145-1157, 1986.
17. McAfee PC, Zdeblick TA: Tumors of the thoracic and lumbar spine: surgical treatment via the anterior approach, *J Spinal Disord* 2:145-154, 1989.
18. McLain RF, Weinstein JN: Tumors of the spine, *Semin Spine Surg* 2:157-180, 1990.
19. Modic MT, Masyrek T, Paushter DM: Magnetic resonance imaging of the spine, *Radiol Clin North Am* 24:229, 1986.
20. Nather A, Bose K: The results of decompression of cord or cauda equina compression from metastatic extradural tumors, *Clin Orthop* 169:103-108, 1982.
21. Panjabi MM et al.: Biomechanical study of cervical spine stabilization with methylmethacrylate, *Spine* 10:198, 1985.
22. Schocker JD, Brady LW: Radiation therapy for bone metastasis, *Clin Orthop* 169:38, 1982.
23. Shimizu K et al.: Posterior decompression and stabilization for multiple metastatic tumors of the spine, *Spine* 17:1400, 1992.
24. Siegal T: Surgical decompression of anterior and posterior malignant epidural tumors compressing the spinal cord: a prospective study, *Neurosurgery* 17:424-432, 1985.
25. Siegal T: Current considerations in the management of neoplastic spinal cord compression, *Spine* 14:223-228, 1988.
26. Silverberg E, Lubera JA: Cancer statistics, *Cancer* 38:5, 1988.
27. Sundaresan N et al.: Treatment of neoplastic epidural cord compression by vertebral body resection and stabilization, *J Neurosurg* 63:676-684, 1985.
28. White WA, Patterson RH, Bergland RM: Role of surgery in the treatment of spinal cord compression by metastatic neoplasm, *Cancer* 27:558-561, 1971.
29. Whitehill R et al.: Posterior cervical fusions using cerclage wires, methylmethacrylate and autogenous bone graft, *Spine* 12:12, 1987.
30. Young RF, Post EM, King GA: Treatment of spinal epidural metastases: randomized prospective of comparison of laminectomy and radiotherapy, *J Neurosurg* 53:741-748, 1980.
31. Yuh WT, Zachar C, Barloon T: Vertebral compression fractures: distinction between benign and malignant causes with MR imaging, *Radiology* 172:215, 1989.

Intradural Intramedullary and Extramedullary Tumors

Seth M. Zeidman

Tumors involving the spinal cord or nerve roots have similarities to intracranial tumors in cellular type. Spinal cord tumors account for about 15% of central nervous system (CNS) neoplasms. They may arise from the spinal cord parenchyma, nerve roots, meningeal coverings, intraspinal vascular network, sympathetic chain, or vertebral column. In addition, they can metastasize from elsewhere in the CNS or from any site within the body. However, metastatic involvement of the spinal intradural compartment as a mass lesion occurs rarely. Intradural spinal cord tumors are broadly categorized according to their relationship to the spinal cord.

The patient's signs and symptoms, the radiologic features of a spinal cord tumor, and the surgical approach to the tumor are more a function of the involved anatomic compartment than the distinct tumor histology. The majority of these intradural tumors arise from the cellular constituents of the spinal cord and filum terminale, nerve roots, or meninges. Intradural tumors have been classically divided into extramedullary and intramedullary lesions. Intramedullary tumors arise within the substance of the spinal cord, whereas extramedullary tumors are extrinsic to the cord.

Discussion of spinal cord tumors is usually organized according to location in the spinal canal: (1) extradural, (2) intradural-extramedullary, or (3) intradural-intramedullary.

1. Extradural (ED) tumors (55%): These lesions are the most common spine tumors, and they arise outside the dura in vertebral bodies or epidural tissues. Metastatic lesions constitute the majority of ED tumors.
2. Intradural-extramedullary tumors (ID-EM) (40%): These lesions arise in the leptomeninges or roots. Only 4% of metastases occur here.
3. Intramedullary spinal cord tumors (IMSCT) (5%): These lesions arise within the substance of the spinal cord and displace or invade white matter tracts and neuron bodies. Only 2% of metastases occur in this compartment.

INTRADURAL-EXTRAMEDULLARY TUMORS

Included within this group are meningiomas, nerve sheath tumors, and filum terminale ependymomas, which constitute approximately 85% of all ID-EM tumors. Sarcoma and lipoma account for an additional 10%. Less common entities include dermoid, epidermoid, angioma, and lymphoma tumor cell types.

Meningiomas

Meningiomas arise from arachnoid villi cells embedded in the dura at the nerve root sleeve, thus explaining their propensity for lateral or ventrolateral locations (Figure 17-1). They can usually be separated from the nerve roots. About 80% occur in the thoracic spine. Thoracic meningiomas are generally posterolateral, whereas upper cervical tumors are more commonly found in the anterolateral canal. Lower cervical and lumbar meningiomas are unusual.

SPINAL CORD TUMOR LOCATIONS

EXTRADURAL (ED) TUMORS (55%)
- Most common spine tumors
- Arise outside the dura in vertebral bodies or epidural tissues

INTRADURAL-EXTRAMEDULLARY TUMORS (ID-EM) (40%)
- Arise in leptomeninges or roots

INTRAMEDULLARY SPINAL CORD TUMORS (IMSCT) (5%)
- Arise within substance of spinal cord

SPINAL MENINGIOMA

- Typical patient
  - Female
  - Older
  - Solitary
- Typical lesion
  - Entirely intradural

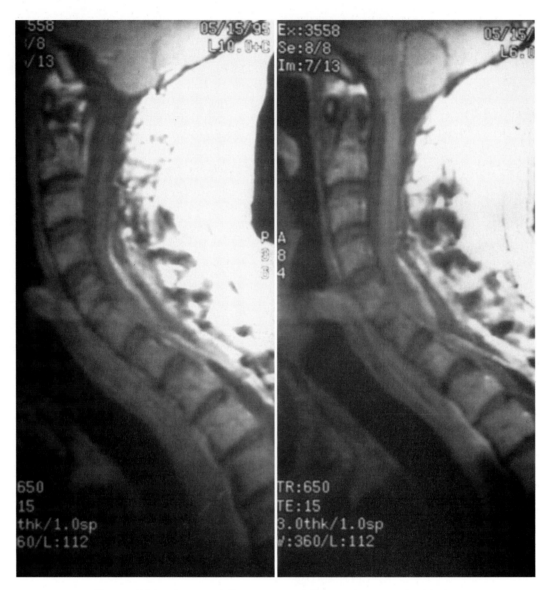

Figure 17-1. Intramedullary-extramedullary tumor—meningioma.

The typical patient with a spinal meningioma is female (female/male ratio is 10:1), older (majority in the fifth and seventh decade), with a solitary lesion (multiple tumors occur only 2% of the time) that is entirely intradural (10% of lesions involve both intradural and extradural compartments).

Nerve Sheath Tumors

The classification of nerve sheath tumors is complicated by the use of the terms *neurofibroma* and *schwannoma*, and the persistence of the inaccurate terms *neuroma*, *neurinoma*, and *neurolemmoma*. In patients with neurofibromatosis (NF-1), nerve sheath tumors are usually asymptomatic and multiple with histology consistent with neurofibromas. In patients with neurofibromatosis, these tumors are multiple and occur at numerous levels of the spinal canal. In the absence of neurofibromatosis, the tumors are almost always schwannomas.

Table 17-1	Neurofibroma vs Schwannoma	
	Neurofibroma	Schwannoma
Origin	Uncertain	Schwann cell
Neurofibromatosis	Present	Absent
Separable from root	Rarely	Often

Nerve sheath tumors typically arise from the dorsal roots. These tumors are relatively avascular, globoid, and without calcification. The dorsal root is intimately involved in the tumor and can rarely be preserved during surgical resection.

Schwannomas originate from Schwann cells, but the origin of neurofibromas is uncertain (Table 17-1). It has been postulated that neurofibromas arise from mesenchymal cells (fibroblasts). Neurofibromas produce a fusiform dilation of the involved sensory nerve root, with

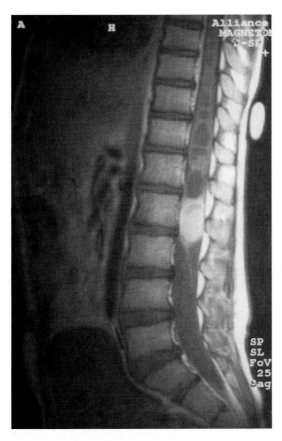

Figure 17-2. Intramedullary-extramedullary tumor—neurofibroma.

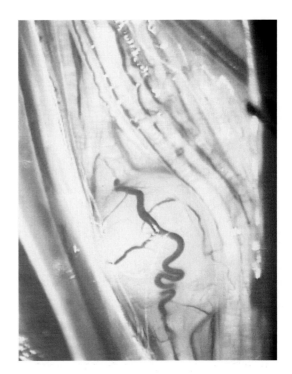

Figure 17-3. Intramedullary-extramedullary tumor—schwannoma.

no apparent plane between nerve and tumor (Figure 17-2). Occasionally they straddle the neural foramen and enlarge in the paraspinal tissues, resulting in a so-called dumbbell tumor with the narrowest portion in the foramen. When these tumors have a dumbbell configuration, the size of the extradural component may exceed the intradural component. Multiple neurofibromas contribute to establishing the diagnosis of neurofibromatosus (NF), but the entity should be considered in any patient with even a solitary tumor.

The overwhelming majority of intraspinal nerve sheath tumors are schwannomas. They occur with approximately the same frequency as meningiomas but in a more even distribution along the spine. They are slightly more common in men, with a peak incidence in the third and fifth decade. Like neurofibromas, schwannomas originate from sensory roots. In contrast with neurofibromas, schwannomas can often be separated from the nerve root. They are generally connected to a few fascicles without fusiform root enlargement (Figure 17-3).

Filum Ependymomas

Ependymomas account for only about 5% of intracranial tumors but about 30% of intraspinal tumors. Approximately half of spinal ependymomas occur at the filum terminale, reflecting the ependyma native to this region. Pathologists classify all spinal ependymomas as intramedullary due to their neuroectodermal origin, but from a clinical and surgical viewpoint the filum ependymoma is an extramedullary lesion. Filum ependymomas occur at any age but are most common between the third and fifth decades. These patients present earlier than those with intramedullary ependymomas.

Although unencapsulated, filum ependymomas are typically well circumscribed and seldom infiltrate the thecal sac; they can often be totally resected if detected early. Unfortunately, their slow growth, pliable texture, and location in the relatively spacious region near the cauda often contribute to a delayed diagnosis with consequent subtotal resection.

Clinical Features

The clinical manifestations of extramedullary intradural tumors are neither unique nor distinct. Classically these tumors present with radicular symptoms that evolve into myelopathy as the tumor enlarges and compresses the spinal cord. Preoperative symptom duration is variable but generally extended over 2 years. By the time of diagnosis most patients have objective neurologic deficits. The symptoms may be difficult to differentiate from those of intramedullary and extradural tumors or nonneoplastic conditions such as a syringomyelia, spondylotic myeloradiculopathy, multiple sclerosis, or spinal arteriovenous malformation.

Pain, either local or radicular, is the most common symptom. Unilateral radicular pain is common with nerve sheath tumors because of their dorsal root origin. Occipital headaches may accompany high cervical or foramen magnum tumors. Local pain is more typical of dural irritation from meningiomas. Symptoms of visceral pain can be seen with tumors in the thoracic spine. Filum terminale ependymomas commonly present with low back pain radiating to one or both legs. Nocturnal pain (pain when laying flat in bed) should alert the examiner to a potential spinal cord tumor.

Segmental sensory or motor root deficits generally appear after pain and prior to myelopathy. The earliest and most common sign of cord compression is corticospinal tract dysfunction. The symptoms may be unilateral or bilateral and include stiffness, gait disturbance, and incoordination of fine hand movement. Sphincter dysfunction is a very unusual sign and tends to occur late. In general the clinical progression is most closely related to tumor location and speed of growth.

Radiographic Diagnosis

Except for occasionally demonstrating foraminal enlargement, bony erosion, or occult instability, plain roentgenograms and plain computed tomography (CT) scans contribute little to the diagnostic evaluation of a patient with an intradural extramedullary lesion. Magnetic resonance imaging (MRI) remains the procedure of choice for localizing and identifying intradural tumors. MRI will generally identify the pathology and define the relationship to the spinal cord and related structures, such as the vertebral artery, and may provide clues as to the histology of the lesion. It may be particularly helpful in dumbbell lesions, by better delineating the extradural component. Meningiomas appear isointense on both T1 weighted and T2 weighted sequences and intensely enhance with the administration of gadolinium contrast. Nerve sheath tumors usually have a higher signal intensity than meningiomas on T2 weighted images. These tumors likewise enhance intensely with the administration of gadolinium.

Myelography, postmyelographic CT scanning, and MRI with gadolinium enhancement are among the most informative diagnostic studies. Myelography is as sensitive as MRI in identifying intradural pathology and may be more sensitive in the lower lumbar region. CT with intrathecal contrast provides excellent delineation of the interface between tumor and spinal cord, as well as superior imaging of bone detail. For suspected meningeal carcinomatosis not apparent on radiographic studies, cytologic examination of cerebrospinal fluid (CSF) obtained by lumbar puncture is essential.

Surgical Therapy

Because most ID-EM tumors are benign, the goal of surgery is complete and total resection. The treatment of intraspinal meningiomas, neurofibromas, and schwannomas is surgical excision. This may include excision of the involved portion of the dura mater (meningioma) or the involved nerve rootlets or entire root (schwannoma, neurofibroma). In nerve sheath tumors arising from the dorsal roots, the nerve root is intimately involved in the tumor and can rarely be separated. Dorsal roots may be sacrificed over a few segments in the thoracic region;

however, very few dorsal rootlets can be safely sacrificed in the cervical or lumbar region. These tumors are rarely adherent to the spinal cord and can easily be separated away from it.

At the level of involvement, neurofibromas and schwannomas typically grow on the dorsal (sensory) root in preference to the ventral (motor) root, and it is generally possible to spare motor function during tumor removal. In neurofibromas, such tumors are part of a more widespread process (neurofibromatosis), in which there are similar tumors on multiple other nerve roots and nerves. Although follow-up surveillance may be needed, a majority of patients with solitary intraspinal lesions (meningioma, neurofibroma, or schwannoma) can be cured with gross total removal of the lesion.

The critical element to successful excision is adequate initial exposure. The posterior midline approach with laminectomy allows adequate access for the majority of these tumors. Even ventrally located lesions can be safely excised via this approach, because the enlarging tumor slowly displaces the spinal cord. The laminectomy must be performed in a nontraumatic fashion to avoid canal compromise. To minimize injury the dura should be opened widely. The arachnoid is initially preserved to prevent spinal cord herniation and to minimize bleeding into the subarachnoid space. Dentate ligament sectioning allows gentle mobilization of the spinal cord. If a posterior root has been sacrificed, this can also be used to rotate the cord. Both anterior and posterior roots from C2 to C4, as well as in the thoracic spine, can be sectioned safely. From C5 to T1 there is minimal deficit if one posterior root is sectioned. Even anterior root section, often required for dumbbell tumor removal, often results in surprisingly minimal deficit. Occasionally large ependymomas or schwannomas may be densely adherent to multiple roots of the cauda equina. These dense attachments may only allow a piecemeal removal of the tumor to minimize the risk of producing a significant deficit.

Small tumors may be removed en bloc, but larger tumors necessitate intracapsular decompression. This can be performed safely with the ultrasonic aspirator. Once the tumor size is reduced, development of the dissection plane can proceed using the reflected arachnoid or the tumor capsule. After the tumor has been removed, it is important to disrupt the arachnoid trabeculae and irrigate out any residual blood products. This will minimize postoperative arachnoid adhesions and intramedullary cyst development from impaired CSF flow. The dura must be closed in a watertight fashion. Sometimes with meningiomas this may require a patch graft and fibrin glue or other sealant. In meningiomas with anterolateral attachments we do not recommend complete excision of the base, but simply extensive cauterization of the dura.

Although anterior approaches have been described, they are only rarely necessary. We prefer to use either a costotransversectomy or a lateral extracavitary approach. This will usually allow access anteriorly, as well as exposure for extradural or pleural extension. One exception to this is for anterior tumors from T1 to T4, where we sometimes use a transthoracic approach, splitting the manubrium and sternum. Adequate dural closure is critical to avoid a CSF-pleural fistula. Fortunately, these cases are rare.

With dumbbell neurofibromas there is usually significant extradural extension out the neural foramina. Single, staged, or simultaneous approaches should be based on the size and location of the tumor. The intra-dural portion should be resected first to minimize spinal cord manipulation during removal of the extradural component. If the patient is elderly, medically unstable, and not symptomatic from the extradural portion, it may not be crucial to remove the extradural tumor. When the nerve root is sectioned laterally, it is important to section it proximal to the ganglion to minimize painful neuralgias postoperatively.

Surgery for metastases within the subarachnoid space is generally not required unless the diagnosis is in question or functional improvement with good life expectancy is felt likely. These are ordinarily managed with radio-therapy and hormonal therapy or chemotherapy.

Results

Surgical results for most intradural, extramedullary benign lesions are quite good, often with rapid improve-ment of neurologic deficits. Final clinical outcome is dependent on the severity of initial deficits, age, and duration of symptoms. Excision of solitary nerve sheath tumors is generally considered curative. For menin-giomas and ependymomas, recurrence rates differ depending on the histology of the tumor. Similarly, angiomas and dermoids are not expected to recur if completely resected.

INTRAMEDULLARY NEOPLASMS

Intramedullary (IM) spinal cord tumors account for 3% of all CNS tumors and about 25% of spinal neoplasms. Astrocytomas and ependymomas are the most common tumors, constituting 45% and 35%, respectively, of intra-medullary lesions (Figures 17-4 and 17-5). The remaining 20% are divided among several different tumor types, including: hemangioblastomas (10%), lipomas (2%), dermoids (1%), epidermoids (1%), teratomas (1%), neuro-blastomas, and mixed tumors.[30] Primary lymphoma, oligo-dendroglioma, cholesteatoma, subependymoma, primary neuroectodermal tumors (PNETs), and intramedullary metastases are extremely rare.[8,27]

Intramedullary spinal cord tumors occur at all ages, predominantly in young or middle-age adults and less commonly in children and the elderly (>60 years old). In children astrocytomas predominate, but in adults ependymomas and astrocytomas occur more equally. An equal distribution between males and females has been reported. Although spinal tumors are more common in the thoracic region, when the incidence is calculated as a function of actual spinal cord length, the distribution is relatively equal.

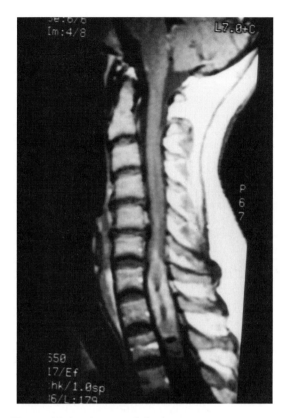

Figure 17-4. Intramedullary tumor—astrocytoma.

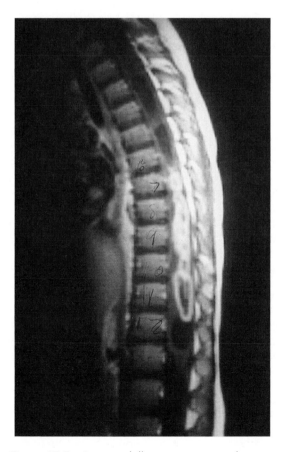

Figure 17-5. Intramedullary tumor—ependymoma.

INTRAMEDULLARY NEOPLASMS

- Astrocytomas 45%
- Ependymomas 35%
- Hemangioblastomas 10%
- Lipomas 2%
- Dermoids 1%
- Epidermoids 1%
- Teratomas 1%
- Neuroblastomas
- Mixed tumors
- Primary lymphomas
- Oligodendrogliomas
- Cholesteatomas
- Subependymomas
- PNETs
- Intramedullary metastases

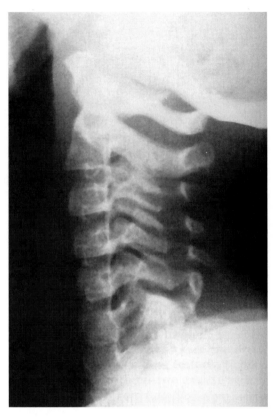

Figure 17-6. Intramedullary tumor—plain films.

Clinical Features of Intramedullary Spinal Cord Tumors

The clinical manifestations of intramedullary spinal cord tumors are not pathognomonic and are identical with many other conditions affecting the spinal cord. The clinical course is variable and dependent upon tumor histology. Patients with malignant tumors typically progress from symptom onset to surgery within 10 months. Intramedullary tumors occur most commonly in adults; however, children also present with these neoplasms. The symptoms in these two groups are similar. However, the majority of intramedullary spinal cord tumors are subtle in symptomatology and only present themselves over a period of years. Patients note slowly developing clumsiness, weakness, or sensory symptoms. Presentation with scoliosis is often noted.

The most common manifestation of intramedullary spinal cord tumors is neck or back pain. Persistent diffuse pain in a dermatomal origin is often indicative of an intramedullary neoplasm. Sensory symptoms typically precede motor dysfunction. Posterior column dysfunction may occur in a slow but progressive fashion. The classic central cord syndrome is a rare presentation for these neoplasms. These symptoms are generally progressive with few remissions or exacerbations. A suspended sensory loss involving the upper extremities or trunk, indistinguishable from that seen with syringomyelia, can be seen. Motor symptoms are less subtle. Patients may have progressive unilateral or bilateral weakness. Children may not complain of weakness, but parents may notice a new gait ataxia or disuse of the involved extremity. Cervical lesions produce paresthesias, dysesthesias, and areas of sensory loss involving one or both upper extremities.

Many patients experience progressive myelopathy. Children may present with abdominal pain as a nonspecific symptom that makes accurate diagnosis particularly difficult. It is not uncommon for these children to undergo an extensive gastrointestinal evaluation prior to diagnosis of an intraspinal neoplasm. Thoracic lesions present with midback pain and radicular symptoms of the trunk and a sensory level consistent with the tumor location. Thoracic spinal cord lesions can also produce spastic paraparesis and bladder dysfunction. Tumors of the conus medullaris characteristically result in sphincter dysfunction with bladder involvement preceding bowel.

Imaging
Plain X-Rays

Fewer than 20% of patients with intramedullary spinal cord tumors have abnormal plain x-rays of the spine. Plain radiographs may reveal some degree of bony erosion but otherwise are of limited value once the diagnosis of an intramedullary spinal cord tumor has been established (Figure 17-6). Widening of the pedicles on the frontal projection may suggest an intraspinal mass, but intramedullary location and a focused differential diagnosis cannot be determined. The use of plain radiographs is otherwise of limited use in the diagnosis of intramedullary tumors.[2] CT-myelography can reveal swelling of the spinal cord but does not delineate the pathology within the cord (Figure 17-7).

Magnetic Resonance Imaging

MRI is the preferred diagnostic modality for the evaluation of intramedullary spinal cord tumors and is generally the only examination necessary for diagnosis (Figure 17-8).[22] Unlike CT-myelography, which visualizes

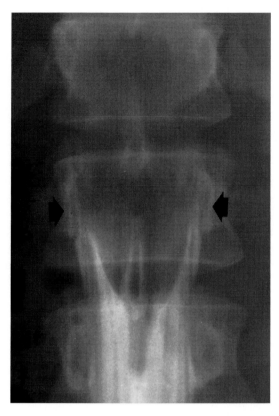

Figure 17-7.   Intramedullary tumor—CT-myelogram.

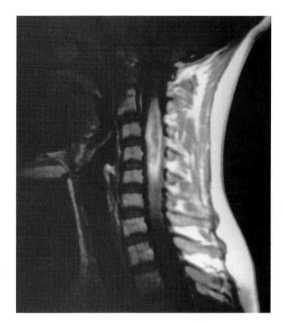

Figure 17-8.   Intramedullary tumor—MRI.

the external configuration of the spinal cord, MRI can image the spinal cord itself with minimal artifact from surrounding osseous structures. It also can define the relationship of the spinal cord to surrounding bone and soft tissue structures. Intramedullary tumors produce fusiform spinal cord expansion with variable signal change on T1 weighted imaging, depending on the histology. Most intramedullary tumors are isointense or slightly hypointense with respect to the surrounding spinal cord on T1 weighted images. There is variability in signal intensity due to tumor cellularity, cysts, edema, calcification, and hemorrhage. However, gadolinium eliminates the confusion of the variable signal intensities. The borders of the tumor may be more clearly identified on T1 weighted images with the administration of gadolinium.

MRI has become increasingly accurate in predicting the histologic tumor type. Sagittal T1 weighted images with gadolinium enhancement are also useful for demonstrating the presence of associated peritumoral cysts, syringomyelia, or edema. MRI provides a three-dimensional view of the neoplasm, which allows accurate differentiation between intramedullary and extramedullary tumors. Although this imaging study is very accurate, occasionally it is difficult to differentiate an inflammatory process such as sarcoidosis, multiple sclerosis, or amyloid angiopathy from neoplasm.

MRI evaluation of the spinal cord should start with imaging of the spinal cord in the sagittal plane with T1 and T2 weighted images. Axial views then should be obtained at the levels of suspected pathology.

Gadolinium-enhanced images define the configuration and extent of the lesion. Intramedullary tumors are often associated with syringomyelia, and any cystic process in the spinal cord must be proven unrelated to a tumor process. Tumor-associated cysts often have a high protein content and may be indistinguishable from the adjacent tumor on nonenhanced studies. These cysts do not enhance with gadolinium and can thus be distinguished from spinal cord widening by tumor.

Imaging patterns, specifically T2 signal characteristics and gadolinium uptake, can help narrow the differential diagnosis by suggesting tumor histology.[27] The majority of astrocytomas have an eccentric location within the cord. The MRI appearance of astrocytomas is variable. T1 weighted images show diffuse spinal cord enlargement with irregular margins and heterogeneous enhancement due to hemorrhage or cystic changes. T2 weighted images demonstrate areas of high signal intensity. T1 weighted sequences following contrast administration help delineate tumor from surrounding edema. Often a cyst can be differentiated from the solid part of the neoplasm. MRI cannot differentiate high-grade neoplasms from low-grade. Although the MRI appearance of astrocytomas and ependymomas can be nearly identical, ependymomas are generally bright on gadolinium-enhanced T1 with sharp borders and moderate uptake of gadolinium.[10]

Despite these patterns, there is enough overlap in appearance that pathologic analysis is required for diagnosis. Postoperatively MRI allows sensitive follow-up for tumor recurrence. This is important because most patients develop radiologic recurrence before they manifest symptoms. In addition to preoperative assessment, a postoperative MRI study can define the extent of resection, hematomas, cyst drainage, and/or CSF collections. Intense gadolinium enhancement with flow voids suggests hemangioblastoma. MRI is invaluable in localizing small hemangioblastomas particularly when associated with a large cyst. Lipomas have a characteristic high signal intensity on T1 weighted images and do not enhance with gadolinium.[36] MRI can be quite helpful in identifying vascular malformations.

Spinal Cord Angiography

Spinal cord angiography is indicated in the evaluation of intramedullary spinal cord tumors only when the clinical history or MRI suggests an arteriovenous malformation or a hemangioblastoma. In both of these entities spinal angiography clarifies the diagnosis and lesion anatomy.

Differential Diagnosis of Intramedullary Spinal Cord Tumors

There are several nonneoplastic lesions that may mimic intramedullary spinal cord neoplasm in their radiographic and clinical presentation. These can be classified as either infectious (tuberculosis [TB], fungal, bacterial, parasitic, syphilis, cytomegalovirus [CMV], herpes simplex virus [HSV]) or noninfectious (sarcoid, multiple sclerosis [MS], myelitis, acute demyelinating encephalomyelitis [ADEM], systemic lupus erythematosus [SLE]) inflammatory lesions, idiopathic necrotizing myelopathy, unusual vascular lesions (amyloid, infarct, isolated intramedullary vascular lesions), or radiation myelopathy. Although biopsy may be indicated in many cases, the mistaken diagnosis of intramedullary neoplasm can often be eliminated preoperatively.[40] MRI facilitates differentiation of intramedullary spinal cord tumors from other entities. Nevertheless, the clinical presentation of two nonneoplastic entities, MS and syringomyelia, can be strikingly similar to that seen with these tumors. Because the MRI may also be misleading in these conditions, MS and syringomyelia warrant particular attention.

Multiple Sclerosis

MS involving the spinal cord can precisely replicate the signs and symptoms of an intramedullary spinal cord tumor.[4,32] Onset of the neurologic deficit is typically more rapid in patients with MS, and remissions and exacerba-

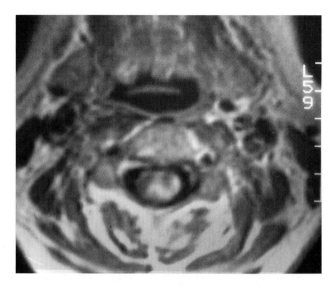

Figure 17-9. Differential diagnosis—multiple sclerosis.

tions are an essential aspect of diagnosis. In contrast, the clinical course of a patient with an intramedullary spinal cord neoplasm is one of relentless progression, although the rapidity of progression can vary from patient to patient (Figure 17-9).

Evaluation of the CSF is often positive for oligoclonal bands, and triple evoked responses may be abnormal. MRI of the brain often identifies lesions consistent with plaques. The MRI appearance of spinal cord lesions caused by MS may bear a superficial resemblance to that of intramedullary spinal cord tumors. The spinal cord lesions of MS are almost always limited in their rostral-caudal extent to one or two spinal segments. Although the signal intensity of the acute MS lesion may be similar to that seen with intramedullary spinal cord tumors and may enhance after administration of gadolinium, spinal cord widening is generally minimal, a sharp contrast to the pattern seen with intramedullary spinal cord tumors. Demyelinating disease can mimic a spinal cord tumor, even on MRI, and must be considered in the differential diagnosis of a symptomatic spinal cord mass.[4]

Syringomyelia

The clinical course of syringomyelia tends to be more indolent than intramedullary spinal cord tumors, but in many other respects the two entities are indistinguishable. Administration of gadolinium is essential to exclude enhancement from a small tumor. Visualization of the cervicomedullary junction in the sagittal plane can be evaluated for a syrinx associated with Arnold-Chiari syndrome in the absence of enhancement (Figure 17-10).

Management Decisions Regarding Intramedullary Spinal Cord Tumors

The presence of an intramedullary spinal cord tumor does not necessarily mandate operative removal. The decision to operate on patients with advanced neuro-

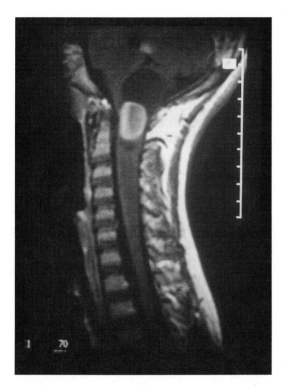

Figure 17-10. Differential diagnosis—syringomyelia.

logic deficits must be made in concert with the patient and the family with realistic expectations. These include a desire to preserve residual sphincter function or to preserve sensation in bedridden patients who are at risk for skin breakdown. Although patients who cannot stand are unlikely to regain enough motor function to ambulate as a result of tumor resection, surgery may maintain the quality of a patient's life by preserving the ability to transfer or to turn in bed. Patients with complete motor and sensory deficits will not improve with surgery and are not operative candidates except when the diagnosis is in doubt.[35]

Ambulatory patients with progressive neurologic deficits are ideal operative candidates. Surgical intervention can halt or slow neurologic deterioration and improve motor and sensory function. Although surgery risks increasing neurologic deficits, once a motor deficit appears, neurologic dysfunction tends to progress relentlessly. Patients with intramedullary spinal cord tumors who forego surgery will inevitably progress to a complete neurologic deficit. Thus the risks of operation are more than outweighed by the natural history of the disease.

Surgery for anaplastic spinal cord astrocytomas does not appear to have lasting benefits except in obtaining an accurate diagnosis. Although a rapid clinical course may strongly suggest the presence of a malignant astrocytoma, only histologic examination of tissue obtained at operation can establish a diagnosis definitively.

Making a decision regarding the patient presenting only with neck or back pain, mild sensory symptoms, and a paucity of objective deficits is more difficult. Many patients with minor symptoms and no significant functional impairment are unwilling to risk neurologic deterioration as a result of an operation. In this situation the patient should be closely followed for the appearance of additional symptoms or an objective deficit. After symptoms progress, patients frequently are more prepared psychologically to face the risks of surgery.

Surgical Technique

The patient should be positioned prone. When the tumor is at or above T2, the patient should be placed in a three-pin head-holder with the neck in a neutral, unrotated position. The horseshoe-shaped headrest should be avoided because skin breakdown of the face or forehead can occur following extended procedures. Antibiotics and steroids, using the spinal cord injury dosing with a gradual taper, are given during the perioperative period. We routinely use SSEP monitoring during spinal cord surgery. Many centers also use motor evoked potentials (MEPs). Whereas SSEPs are mediated principally by the dorsal columns, MEPs monitor the integrity of the descending motor pathways. Though continuous evoked potential response monitoring during spinal surgery is of unproven efficacy, we use it on every case to avoid excessive retraction.

A standard midline approach with a careful, wide laminectomy is performed to completely expose the rostro-caudal extent of the lesion. Tumor-associated cysts are frequently more extensive than the tumor itself. It is unnecessary to extend the laminectomy to include areas of cystic enlargement. The cyst fluid disappears with total tumor removal, and the cyst walls are composed of nonneoplastic tissue, which does not need to be resected. One must remain cognizant of the fact that the underlying spinal cord may be compromised. Placement of instruments under the lamina is contraindicated. A high-speed drill or a double-action rongeur is preferable.

Because of the high incidence of postlaminectomy kyphosis in children, en block removal of the laminae is performed to allow for laminoplastic reconstruction. We do not recommend this in the adult population, because the incidence of postlaminectomy kyphosis is quite low.

Meticulous hemostasis is essential. Bone wax should be applied to the bone edges. Strips of thrombin-soaked Gelfoam are placed along the lateral gutters of the laminectomy site, and moist cotton strips are draped over the adjoining muscle edges. After the laminectomy is performed, ultrasound should be used to confirm the location of solid tumor and any adjacent cysts. We recommend introducing the operating microscope at this point. The dura is opened, and tacking sutures are placed. Sharp dissection of arachnoid from adherent vessels by microsurgical technique is undertaken to avoid vessel avulsion.

Although hemangioblastomas will typically have a pial presentation, most intramedullary tumors do not present on the surface. Hemangioblastoma nearly always reaches the pia at some aspect. It is helpful to search for this site because it will facilitate dissection and isolation of these vascular tumors from the circulation.

Intraoperative ultrasound is very useful for localizing tumor and identifying associated cysts, as well as delineating the extent of resection. The myelotomy should be performed at or near the posterior median septum, preferably at a point where the normal neurologic tissue appears most thinned. When an extensive myelotomy is planned, it is preferable to make a midline myelotomy even when this is not the most attenuated portion of the cord. Being certain of the exact midline is sometimes difficult because the spinal cord anatomy may be distorted by the tumor. Therefore, because normally the midline is midway between the left and right dorsal roots, both the left and right dorsal roots should be identified before initiating the myelotomy. Extension of a myelotomy situated in the area of the dorsal root entry zone can be disastrous. The most common technical error associated with this surgery is inadequate exposure of the tumor poles.

During pial incision all attempts should be made to preserve any large longitudinally oriented veins. If necessary, midline veins or arteries should be cauterized along with the pia-arachnoid by using the bipolar cautery at a low setting. The pia-arachnoid and dorsal surface of the spinal cord then should be incised sharply to a depth of 2 mm to 3 mm over the length of the spinal cord occupied by the solid tumor. Pial and/or arachnoid sutures can be placed and tacked to the dura. The pia-arachnoid and dorsal surface of the spinal cord should be held apart by placing gentle traction on 6-0 sutures placed through the pia-arachnoid on either side of the midline. If the tumor is not immediately visible, dissection within the spinal cord should be continued in a ventral direction until the tumor is encountered. As the myelotomy is performed, the normal spinal tissue will retract laterally with the pia, and the tumor–spinal cord interface will appear with minimal manipulation.

In the case of large nonvascular tumors, internal debulking using the ultrasonic surgical aspirator allows for simpler dissection of tumor margins. Gentle traction on the surface of the tumor serves to expose bridging vessels at the tumor margin that can be cauterized safely. The tumor bed should be carefully inspected under high magnification, because many of these tumors are friable and unencapsulated and small fragments can be left behind inadvertently. When gross total excision is the goal, we believe the first surgical intervention offers the best chance for cure. Delayed reoperation can be difficult, especially in the setting of previous irradiation. The dura is invariably adherent to the underlying cord, and the tumor–spinal cord interface tends to be obscured by scar.

After the tumor resection is completed, the pial sutures should be removed, but closure of the myelotomy is not performed. The dura must be closed in a watertight fashion with interrupted or running sutures. If the dura cannot be closed without undue tension, a dural patch should be used. In addition, if residual tumor is present or the spinal cord remains swollen, a dural graft should be placed to avoid spinal cord constriction. Late neurologic deterioration from arachnoidal adhesions has been observed, and this can be lessened by placement of an adequate dural patch, thereby establishing normal CSF pathways circumferentially. The remainder of the closure should be standard.

Specific Tumor Types
Astrocytoma

Intramedullary spinal cord astrocytomas are usually located several millimeters beneath the dorsal surface of the spinal cord, and although they may be distinguished from the surrounding spinal cord, they blend imperceptibly with the spinal cord at their margins, rendering complete lesion extirpation impossible. Morphologically astrocytomas typically have a gray/whitish yellow, stringy, tough edematous stroma. The lower-grade lesions are relatively avascular and lend themselves to resection with the ultrasonic aspirator. Resection of these infiltrating lesions should be continued until the interface with the spinal cord becomes indistinguishable or until resection produces changes in the evoked potentials. These tumors may infiltrate viable functioning spinal cord pathways at the periphery of the tumor and result in postoperative exacerbation of neurologic deficits, even when the surgeon is confident that resection is confined strictly to grossly apparent tumor. An intramedullary astrocytoma ordinarily cannot be completely removed surgically.[16] However, in some cases, especially at the cervicomedullary junction, cleavage planes can be defined and gross total resection achieved. Gross total resection can result in extended clinical (neurologic) stabilization and effective cure.[6,12]

Tumor cysts may be located rostral or caudal to the tumor. Lack of cyst enhancement in cavities adjacent to tumor suggests the presence of a benign reactive syrinx rather than a frankly neoplastic cyst.

Histologically, compared with the more benign astrocytomas, malignant astrocytomas tend to be more vascular and exhibit a less distinct interface with the spinal cord, making it more difficult to identify a surgical plane between the tumor and normal spinal cord. If biopsy confirms a malignant astrocytoma, further tumor removal is generally unwarranted. There is no evidence that surgical debulking of a malignant astrocytoma is beneficial.

Factors positively influencing the prognosis are low histologic grade of the tumor and good preoperative and postoperative general conditions. Among the grade II astrocytomas the fibrillary and protoplasmatic types present longer survival times regardless of the type of removal performed. In anaplastic astrocytomas the simultaneous presence of certain morphologic features indicative of higher malignancy negatively influence survival. The degree of resection does not influence average survival within each histologic grade.[18]

Because ependymomas cannot be reliably distinguished from astrocytomas by clinical presentation or currently available imaging techniques, all intramedullary spinal cord tumors should be aggressively explored so that curable lesions are not overlooked.[27]

Ependymoma

Ependymomas are the most common intramedullary neoplasm in adults, whereas in children they account for only 12% of all intramedullary tumors. They occur throughout the spinal axis, originating from ependymal rests along the central canal. As they grow from their point of origin, they push the adjacent spinal cord aside and are distinct from the surrounding spinal cord. They are histologically benign and typically have a central location in the spinal cord.[20] Intraoperatively they are firm and have a shaggy reddish purple, gray, or yellow appearance with variable blood supply, which always comes from the anterior spinal artery. At surgery ependymomas appear reddish gray. Ependymomas are well delineated from the surrounding parenchyma and usually can be totally excised. Cysts are frequently found at either or both ends of the tumor and aid in dissection. Ependymomas typically have a clear plane of dissection, and surgical cure is usually possible with preservation of the surrounding spinal cord.

Although smaller lesions often may be removed en bloc, generally the bulk of the tumor should be reduced first in piecemeal fashion to avoid excessive manipulation of adjacent neural structures. If the tumor is highly vascular, tumor reduction can be accomplished by shrinking the surface with the bipolar cautery on a low setting. If the lesion is relatively avascular, the center of the tumor may be debulked with the ultrasonic aspirator. A cleavage plane between tumor and adjacent tissue can be developed by retracting tumor into the residual cavity. As the tumor is lifted out of the spinal cord, its vascular supply can be cauterized and cut and the tumor removed from its bed.

In most patients a total resection is possible. Unfortunately, ependymomas may blend imperceptibly with the spinal cord at their point of origin, and total resection is impossible without injuring the cord. Resection should be stopped when the interface between the tumor and normal spinal cord is indiscernible. Intraoperative findings of arachnoid scarring and cord atrophy are ominous for surgical morbidity.[15] There is typically a portion of the tumor adherent to the anterior median raphe that should be removed sharply to avoid traction injury to the anterior spinal artery. If only a partial resection can be achieved, postoperative irradiation may be required.[41]

Complete removal can be achieved in almost all cases of intramedullary spinal cord ependymomas in children, and the long survival rates justify avoiding postoperative radiation therapy.[26]

Hemangioblastoma

Hemangioblastomas account for 3% to 7% of intramedullary spinal cord tumors and are particularly rare in children.[31] They occur throughout the spinal canal and are most commonly located on the dorsal or dorsolateral surface of the spinal cord (Figure 17-11). On MRI, hemangioblastomas are typically cystic lesions with a strongly enhancing mural nodule. T1 weighted images reveal a well-circumscribed tumor with decreased signal intensity,

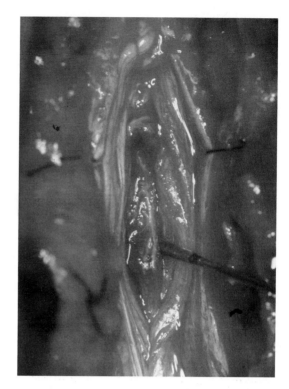

Figure 17-11. Intramedullary tumor—hemangioblastoma.

whereas T2 weighted images reveal hyperintense lesion. Flow voids from a feeding vessel are often discernible.

Hemangioblastomas are typically red and nodular with a clear plane of dissection, and surgical cure is usually possible with maintenance of the surrounding spinal cord. They are immediately apparent on the dorsal surface of the spinal cord, along with a collection of vessels that supply and drain the lesion. They range in size from a few millimeters in diameter to the size of a large grape and are well defined from the surrounding spinal cord.

These lesions are highly vascular, and no attempt should be made to enter these tumors until the vascular supply is interrupted totally because consequent bleeding may be difficult to control. The arterial supply, part of which is visible on the dorsal surface of the spinal cord, should be coagulated and cut and the tumor very slowly reduced in size with bipolar cautery of the feeding vessels and tumor capsule. After this is done, the tumor may be dissected more easily from the adjacent spinal cord. This dissection exposes additional vascular supply, which should be interrupted sequentially, allowing total removal. It is generally advisable to preserve at least one venous pedicle until all feeding arteries are divided.

Hemangioblastomas are curable tumors but may recur as a result of the growth of residual tumor or, as is more commonly the case, growth of additional lesions that were clinically or radiographically unapparent at the time of the first surgery.[7] Hemangioblastomas are relatively benign in their clinical and histologic behavior and can be meaningfully resected by careful microsurgical technique.[33]

Gangliogliomas

Gangliogliomas are benign neoplasms, common in children and young adults. They consist of a mixture of well-differentiated neoplastic neurons and glial elements. The glial elements are usually astrocytes, and the neoplastic neurons are characteristically large and relatively mature. The neurons are readily recognized by their characteristic nuclear and nucleolar features, abundance of cytoplasm, content of Nissl substance, and the presence of argyrophilic neuritic processes. Their expression of neuronal markers such as synaptophysin and neurofilament proteins also serve to identify these abnormal neurons. Most gangliogliomas grow slowly and have an indolent course. Like astrocytomas, these tumors do not have a well-demarcated cleavage plane.

Lipomas

Lipomas of the spinal cord are rare congenital tumors seen most frequently at the level of the conus medullaris.[25] Intramedullary (subpial) lipomas not associated with spinal dysraphism are very unusual. These tumors are not neoplasms; they are histologically identical to normal adipose tissue and are located on the dorsal surface of the spinal cord covered by little or no neural tissue. They increase in size and in relation to fatty tissue elsewhere in the body.

Myelopathic signs and symptoms evolve slowly and generally are first manifest during rapid growth spurts or after excessive weight gain. Preoperative diagnosis is usually possible with MRI.[13] Although distinct from adjacent spinal cord and noninvasive, these lesions adhere densely to normal spinal cord, so total removal is impossible without creating unacceptable neurologic deficits.

The most effective operative strategy consists of subtotal removal, with a rim of tumor left at the interface with the spinal cord. The laser is ideal for removal of lipomas because the fibrous interstices of the lesion make removal with the ultrasonic aspirator difficult. The laser does an excellent job with many of these tumors. Lipomas simply melt away with minimal manipulation of the nerves. These lesions grow slowly, but recurrence may occur as a result of continued growth of residual tumor.

Patients with intramedullary spinal cord lipoma who present with significant neurologic compromise have a very poor prognosis with regard to neurologic function and generally show no improvement with surgical resection.[25]

Intramedullary Metastatic Tumors

Metastases to the spinal cord are rare and represent fewer than 8% of all intramedullary spinal cord tumors (Figure 17-12).[5] Tumors that metastasize to the spinal cord include lung and breast carcinoma. Less commonly lymphoma, colon adenocarcinoma, head and neck carcinoma, and renal cell carcinoma may produce spinal cord metastases. With the availability of more sensitive imaging techniques, these tumors are being diagnosed with increasing frequency.[38] MRI is sensitive

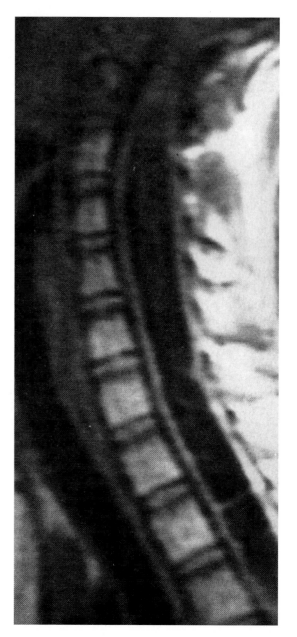

Figure 17-12. Intramedullary tumor—metastatic lesion.

but nonspecific in distinguishing intramedullary spinal cord metastases from primary cord tumors. Urgent biopsy is often necessary prior to definitive treatment. Radiation with chemotherapy significantly prolongs survival.

These lesions tend to be vascular and well defined from the adjacent spinal cord. The most effective operative strategy consists of slow bipolar coagulation of the tumor to reduce the bulk of the lesion, followed by visualization and section of the vascular supply and total removal. Radical subtotal resection may offer additional quality survival, especially in cases of metastatic melanoma with an occult primary.

Intramedullary spinal cord metastasis is a devastating condition, but with appropriate diagnosis and aggressive treatment, selected patients may have sub-

TECHNICAL ADJUNCTS

- Laser
- Ultrasonic aspirator
- Ultrasound
- Evoked potential monitoring

stantially increased survival. Regardless of treatment, many patients survive less than 1 year.[5]

Technical Adjuncts to Intramedullary Spinal Cord Tumor Removal
Intraoperative Spinal Sonography (IOSS) (Ultrasound)

High-frequency sector scanning allows excellent visualization of the spinal canal during surgery on spinal cord tumors. IOSS is performed by filling the operative field with saline solution to maintain an acceptable distance from the probe to the spinal cord. Tumors within the cervical spinal canal are ideal for localization and characterization with IOSS. The only significant exception to this has been with spinal hemangioblastomas, which are often isoechogenic with normal spinal cord. These can be identified with use of intraoperative color flow Doppler ultrasound (CFDU). With vascular tumors, color flow Doppler studies demonstrate the position of high-flow vessels in the region of tumor dissection. IOSS images the tumors, the relationships of the lesions to the spinal cord, and the normal internal structures of the cord itself at the margins. In cases of intramedullary tumors, IOSS defines the extent of the required myelotomy, the presence of syringomyelic cavities caudal and/or cranial to the tumor, and the relationship of tumor depth to the anterior cord surface. Before the dura is opened the overall extent of the tumor is visualized and specific areas of interest such as cysts or calcified regions are defined and localized. This imaging guides the dural opening and often directs the surgeon to a particular location to initiate the myelotomy and exploration. If rostral or caudal cysts are present, the myelotomy is initiated at the cyst-tumor junction. If no cysts are present, the myelotomy is performed over the most voluminous portion of the tumor, where the possibility of damaging functional neural tissue is much less.

In cystic tumors such as astrocytomas or hemangioblastomas, ultrasound will identify the specific mural nodule of tumor. With intramedullary tumors the "central canal" will virtually always be absent to ultrasound imaging. This is helpful in determining the longitudinal extent of tumors. Edema proximal or distal to the tumor will also cause spinal cord widening and loss of the central canal, thus creating some confusion in determining the absolute limits of the tumor. In most cases the tumor border is quite well defined and the edema is less echogenic. The routine use of IOSS during surgery for spinal tumors facilitates determination of the precise locations for biopsy of intramedullary lesions and directs the optimum surgical progression.

Occasionally intraoperative ultrasound is less helpful, only demonstrating widening of the spinal cord with an imaging pattern similar to that of adjacent cord. In this situation the major neoplastic differential diagnostic considerations include astrocytoma and ependymoma.

The diagnosis and intraoperative management of intramedullary spinal cord tumors has been significantly influenced by new diagnostic and surgical tools such as IOSS. With the help of these tools, most intramedullary spinal cord tumors may be diagnosed and treated surgically with significantly decreased risk.[28]

Finally, ultrasound can be extremely useful in monitoring ongoing tumor resection. A persistent abnormal signal or persistent uncollapsed intratumoral cyst encourages continued tumor removal. Thus ultrasound facilitates a radical resection of intramedullary tumors.

Intraoperative ultrasonography should be used routinely during surgery for spinal tumors in order to reduce the extent of the laminectomy, dural opening, and myelotomy. A good correlation exists among signal intensity on T1 weighted images of MRI, the echographic aspect of the tumor, and the pathologic findings at operation.[28]

Ultrasonic Aspirator

This device combines tissue fragmentation, irrigation, and aspiration capability in procedures requiring precise, selective tissue removal with minimal trauma to surrounding tissue. The ultrasonic aspirator emits a variable ultrasonic energy field that emulsifies tissue immediately in front of the unit's tip. A small amount of water is injected into the field to further liquefy the emulsification, and the slurry is then aspirated by the unit. This allows for removal of tissue with little energy being imparted to surrounding tissue (as would happen with simple aspiration, where a pulling force can be exerted).

Placing the aspirator tip in contact with the tumor permits relatively atraumatic tumor resection while avoiding manipulation of adjacent spinal cord. The ultrasonic aspirator allows preservation of blood flow in adjacent white matter within 0.5 to 1 mm of the resection bed. The end result is less injury to surrounding structures. This is particularly helpful with tumors resistant to regular suction. Without the ultrasonic aspirator, tumor removal requires sharp dissection and increased spinal cord manipulation, often resulting in permanent loss of function. The force of the unit can be adjusted so it is unlikely to injure blood vessels adjacent to the tissue being removed.

Laser

The laser is sometimes useful for resecting intramedullary spinal cord tumors. The surgeon can target using the microscope and activate the laser through the microscope. The laser beam is directed through the lens of the operating microscope using a series of mirrors to vaporize tumor. The CO_2 laser is favored for its ability to deliver variable amounts of energy that are highly focused. It is one of the most precise tools for removal of small amounts of tissue and can be used with high precision. The CO_2 laser cauterizes vessels the size of capillaries but will cut through larger vessels with resultant hemorrhage. Its two major drawbacks are the speed at which it works (very slow) and its poor cauterization ability (blood vessels are cut but not sealed, so they bleed). It is helpful in resecting tumors that cannot be removed with the ultrasonic aspirator.

The neodymium-YAG (nd-YAG) laser delivers more diffuse energy to a larger area of tissue around the target point. Tissue surrounding the target is not injured, and there is less associated bleeding because it is more effective at cauterizing blood vessels. The beam is transmitted down a fiberoptic strand to a handheld wand.

Evoked Potential Recordings

Continuous evoked response monitoring is a potentially useful adjunct to surgical therapy.[37] However, the true efficacy of evoked potential (EP) monitoring in improving outcome after operation for intramedullary spinal cord lesions remains unclear. Intraoperative EP monitoring has been demonstrated to provide critical information during spinal surgery. However, EPs may not be as useful for patients with spinal cord tumors because the functional integrity of the sensory and motor pathways may already be disrupted. Nevertheless, intraoperative monitoring of SSEPs during intramedullary spinal cord surgery is commonly employed. Intraoperative monitoring of the functional integrity of the spinal cord during removal of intramedullary spinal cord lesions is an aid in intraoperative decision making and a primary tool for the prediction of neurologic outcome.[22]

Dorsal column and spinothalamic tract injury is reflected in amplitude or latency changes of the recorded waveforms. Patients with profound sensory deficits have evoked responses that are either absent or of such low amplitude that meaningful recordings cannot be obtained. Currently available SSEP monitoring techniques do not provide real-time intraoperative guidance. A delay of up to 60 seconds occurs from the time of injury until changes in the EP waveform are observed. Irreversible damage may occur from operative maneuvers performed before the injury is reflected by changes in the potentials.

Monitoring sensory pathways provides no direct information regarding the integrity of the corticospinal tract. Injury may occur to the motor pathways without any change in the SSEPs. In practice the corticospinal and the spinothalamic tracts are in such close proximity that injury to motor pathways is usually reflected in changes of the sensory EPs. However, false-negative studies do occur.

Several new approaches have been used recently in an attempt to obviate some of the disadvantages of standard EP monitoring techniques. MEPs allow assessment of descending fiber tracts. Morota et al reported that the presence of monitorable MEPs in adults before myelotomy was a better predictor of surgical outcome than is the patient's preoperative motor status.[34]

MEP monitoring has become the neurophysiologic monitoring technique of choice for that purpose. MEPs, elicited with a short train of transcranial electrical stimuli and recorded from limb muscles, reflect the functional integrity of the corticospinal tract. Both epidural and muscle MEPs correlate closely with postoperative neurologic function. Over time both the reliable power of predicting clinical outcome and the practical versatility of the technique have altered the surgical approach in that gross total resections are more readily attempted as long as MEP data indicate the intact functional integrity of the corticospinal tract.[22]

Stimulation and recording of both sensory and motor pathways permit a more complete assessment of spinal cord function. However, it must be recognized that no study has conclusively demonstrated that use of intraoperative EPs, sensory and/or motor, results in an improved clinical outcome.[1,23]

Management

Prior to recent advances the mainstay of therapy for spinal cord tumors was biopsy followed by radiation therapy. Currently standard treatment for intradural spinal cord tumors remains microsurgical resection. Attempts at surgical resection should be performed prior to significant neurologic deterioration. Preoperative neurologic status is the best predictor of functional status postoperatively.

Neurologic outcome in the immediate postoperative period is related most closely to the patient's immediate preoperative neurologic state. Rarely patients who have no motor function may regain a small amount of function after operation, but most likely they will not be able to walk or stand as a result of tumor resection. Similarly, patients who cannot stand are unlikely to be able to walk in the postoperative period.

Complications of Intramedullary Spinal Cord Tumors

Exacerbation of neurologic deficit. Neurologic deterioration is less a function of tumor histology or the extent of surgical resection than preoperative status. Patients with severe preoperative motor deficits have the highest likelihood of sustaining a permanent neurologic deficit postoperatively. Nearly 20% of patients experience a permanent increase in their deficits.

Dorsal column injury will cause loss of proprioception and may occur as a result of the myelotomy. Lateral dissection can injure the spinothalamic tracts and produce sensory dysfunction. Diminution of SSEPs may indicate disturbance or injury to these pathways.

Dysesthesias, hyperesthesias, and hyperpathia are terrible postoperative complications. These entities may render an otherwise functional extremity useless and prevent a patient with minimal or no motor deficit from returning to a former occupation or resuming a normal social life. Frequently these symptoms are present preoperatively from tumor invasion of sensory pathways

---

> ## COMPLICATIONS OF SPINAL CORD TUMOR SURGERY
>
> - Neurologic deficit
> - Wound infection
> - Deformity

---

and persist or are exacerbated as a result of tumor removal.

Neurologic deterioration can occur several days after surgery and has been attributed to too-rapid steroid taper. Subsequent increase in corticosteroid dosage does not always restore neurologic function. Potentially reversible etiologies such as postoperative hematoma and vascular insults must be considered and treated as appropriate.

Operative wound breakdown. Wound breakdown is unusual in patients who have not been previously operated upon. However, in the setting of a previous operation and irradiation, wound dehiscence, CSF fistulae, and meningitis occur commonly, regardless of how meticulously the closure is performed. For this reason the operative incision in the patient who previously underwent operation and irradiation should be closed with rotational flaps of the trapezius or latissimus dorsi muscles from beyond the irradiated field.

Spinal deformities. Postlaminectomy kyphosis and the swan neck deformity are well-recognized complications of surgery for intramedullary spinal cord tumors. Children with intramedullary spinal cord tumors are at risk for the development of these deformities following surgery. Children under 3 years of age, those with preoperative spinal deformity, and those with preoperative neurologic deficits are at greatest risk.[16] In the absence of preoperative kyphosis, development of postlaminectomy kyphosis in adults is extremely rare. Osteoplastic laminotomy is performed to forestall the development of progressive spinal deformity.

In children, deformities of the thoracic and lumbar spine are frequently identified in association with intramedullary spinal cord tumors and often represent the initial manifestation of this condition months or years before the appearance of neurologic signs and symptoms. It is unclear whether the appearance or exacerbation of these deformities in the postoperative period results from the effect of the tumor or from laminectomy. However, in the cervical spine, laminectomy and denervation of the paraspinous muscles likely leads to flexion deformity. Severe, untreated flexion deformity may result in spinal cord compression and progressive neurologic deficit, which may be mistaken for tumor recurrence. Because postoperative spinal deformities commonly occur in children, frequent follow-up is essential. In the cervical spine, early fusion at the first sign of flexion deformity is indicated. In the thoracic and lumbar spine, spinal instrumentation and fusion also are indicated when progressive deformity is recognized.

Adjunctive Treatment of Intramedullary Spinal Cord Tumors

Radiation therapy. No study has demonstrated a beneficial effect of radiation therapy on neurologic function or survival in patients with glial spinal cord tumors.[19] Guidetti et al.[14] did not find any consistent benefit from radiation therapy. Other investigators reported improvement or disappearance of deficits after irradiation, but none of these studies was controlled and no proof exists that the radiation treatment itself resulted in improvement.[19] Although surgery is the treatment of choice for both intramedullary and extramedullary tumors, some authors recommend biopsy and radiation for astrocytomas and ependymomas. The beneficial results of these studies may be related to the effects of the decompressive laminectomy rather than the adjuvant treatment.[12]

The efficacy of radiation therapy is difficult to determine because the natural history of low-grade astrocytomas is unpredictable and long-term survival without radiation may occur. It appears to be reasonable to irradiate all adult patients with spinal cord astrocytomas, regardless of the surgeon's impression of the completeness of removal or the histologic grade of the tumor. Treatment consists of 4500 Gy given in divided doses to the region of the tumor. Garcia[11] noted improved outcomes in patients treated with 4000 Gy compared with those treated with smaller doses. Marsa et al.[29] used doses of more than 5000 Gy, but such treatment is not recommended because of the risk of radiation myelopathy.

Because of the detrimental effect of radiation therapy on development in children, most pediatric patients who are believed to have had a gross total resection of their tumors are not irradiated. However, radiation therapy has been proposed for recurrent low-grade tumors in children or as an initial treatment postoperatively, particularly in patients who have had rapid neurologic deterioration. These patients must be followed with serial MRI scans to detect tumor recurrence.

Patients with ependymomas who are believed to have had complete removal should not be irradiated. Instead they should be followed closely with frequent MRI and treated with reoperation or radiation if recurrence becomes apparent. When removal of an ependymoma is incomplete, local radiation may be given to the area of residual tumor.[39]

Chemotherapy. Adjuvant treatment for intramedullary tumors is based on radiotherapy. The place of chemotherapy in this setting has yet to be determined.[3] For the past decade chemotherapeutic agents such as carmustine (BCNU) have been a standard part of the management protocol for treating patients with brain astrocytomas. However, the efficacy of this and similar agents in managing spinal cord astrocytomas is unknown. Because a large proportion of intramedullary malignancies occur in children, who are more sensitive to the deleterious effects of irradiation, chemotherapy assumes an important role. The efficacy of chemotherapy in patients with intramedullary glial tumors calls for further trials in this setting, especially in young children and patients with metastases.[9] Systemic chemotherapy is reserved for treatment of malignant spinal cord tumors such as glioblastoma multiforme as an adjunct to surgical resection.

Long-Term Outcome of Patients With Intramedullary Spinal Cord Tumors

Long-term survival and postoperative neurologic function are related to tumor histology, the patient's preoperative neurologic status, and the extent of tumor resection.

Most intramedullary spinal cord tumors grow slowly, and long-term survival is the rule. Goh, Velasquez, and Epstein have noted in their series that gross total removal of low-grade spinal cord astrocytomas is associated with no evidence of tumor progression clinically or radiologically for many months.[12] However, higher-grade astrocytomas (anaplastic) often cannot be radically resected due to the infiltrative nature of the tumor. Although the outlook for patients with low-grade astrocytomas is better, slow progression of tumors in the cervical region can result in death from respiratory paralysis. Degeneration of low-grade tumors into malignant ones may occur and further affects the outcome adversely. Patients with malignant astrocytomas have a particularly dismal outcome, and in one report no patient had improvement of neurologic function after operation.[21]

Fortunately, the long-term survival of patients with ependymomas is less bleak than is the case for patients with astrocytomas. Gross total removal of spinal cord ependymomas is associated with extended disease-free survival. Unlike the outcome associated with astrocytomas, the outcome in patients with ependymomas does not appear to be related to histologic grade. Although ependymomas may seed the subarachnoid space, this method of dissemination appears to be the exception rather than the rule.

Hemangioblastomas are benign tumors that are curable if they are removed totally. In practice, hemangioblastomas are found frequently in multiple locations, and the patient's outcome is determined by the behavior of tumors located elsewhere in the nervous system or systemically.

Extent of Tumor Resection

Spinal cord tumors usually grow slowly, so the relationship between outcome and the extent of tumor resection must be examined at an extended interval from surgery. Estimates of the completeness of tumor resection by the operating surgeon are prone to overestimation. Because astrocytomas are infiltrating, complete resection is achieved less frequently than previously believed. Patients with astrocytomas who underwent gross total resection have a high incidence of recurrence and neurologic progression. This finding suggests that complete or nearly complete removal is rarely achieved. The incidence of tumor recurrence is less a function of whether total removal has been achieved than of the length of follow-up. The extent of resection of astrocytomas corre-

lates poorly with the risk of recurrence, patient survival, and neurologic outcome. Unfortunately, systematic follow-up has been lacking from the overwhelming majority of clinical studies.

CONCLUSIONS

Development of new technologies for the diagnosis and treatment of intramedullary tumors, including MRI, the operating microscope, ultrasound, laser, and ultrasonic tissue aspirator, have radically changed the results of surgery, perioperative management, and long-term outcome results. Unsatisfactory outcomes with standard operative therapies prior to the introduction of these new technologies led many surgeons to conclude that the least harmful strategy was limited biopsy with adjuvant postoperative irradiation. These developments have allowed more accurate preoperative diagnosis and safer, more effective operative interventions.

SELECTED REFERENCES

Baleriaux DL: Spinal cord tumors, *Eur Radiol* 9(7):1252-1258, 1999.

Balmaceda C: Chemotherapy for intramedullary spinal cord tumors, *J Neurooncol* 47(3):293-307, 2000.

Constantini S et al.: Radical excision of intramedullary spinal cord tumors: surgical morbidity and long-term follow-up evaluation in 164 children and young adults, *J Neurosurg* 93(Suppl 2): 183-193, 2000.

Deme S et al.: Primary intramedullary primitive neuroectodermal tumor of the spinal cord: case report and review of the literature, *Neurosurgery* 41(6):1417-1420, 1997.

Goh KY, Velasquez L, Epstein FJ: Pediatric intramedullary spinal cord tumors: is surgery alone enough? *Pediatr Neurosurg* 27(1):34-39, 1997.

Hoshimaru M et al.: Results of microsurgical treatment for intramedullary spinal cord ependymomas: analysis of 36 cases, *Neurosurgery* 44(2):264-269, 1999.

Houten JK, Cooper PR: Spinal cord astrocytomas: presentation, management and outcome, *J Neurooncol* 47(3):219-224, 2000.

Innocenzi G et al.: Prognostic factors in intramedullary astrocytomas, *Clin Neurol Neurosurg* 99(1):1-5, 1997.

Isaacson SR: Radiation therapy and the management of intramedullary spinal cord tumors, *J Neurooncol* 47(3):231-238, 2000.

Iwasaki Y et al: Spinal intramedullary ependymomas: surgical results and immunohistochemical analysis of tumour proliferation activity, *Br J Neurosurg* 14(4):331-336, 2000.

Lee RR: MR imaging of intradural tumors of the cervical spine, *Magn Reson Imaging Clin N Am* 8(3):529-540, 2000.

Lonjon M, Goh KY, Epstein FJ: Intramedullary spinal cord ependymomas in children: treatment, results and follow-up, *Pediatr Neurosurg* 29(4):178-183, 1998.

Lowe GM: Magnetic resonance imaging of intramedullary spinal cord tumors, *J Neurooncol* 47(3):195-210, 2000.

Newton HB et al.: Spinal cord tumors: review of etiology, diagnosis, and multidisciplinary approach to treatment, *Cancer Pract* 3(4):207-218, 1995.

Patwardhan V et al.: MR imaging findings of intramedullary lipomas, *Am J Roentgenol* 174(6):1792-1793, 2000.

Schwartz TH, McCormick PC: Intramedullary ependymomas: clinical presentation, surgical treatment strategies and prognosis, *J Neurooncol* 47(3):211-218, 2000.

Schwartz TH, McCormick PC: Non-neoplastic intramedullary pathology: diagnostic dilemma—to Bx or not to Bx, *J Neurooncol* 47(3):283-292, 2000.

REFERENCES

1. Albright AL: Intraoperative spinal cord monitoring for intramedullary surgery: an essential adjunct? *Pediatr Neurosurg* 29(2):112, 1998.

2. Bleriaux DL: Spinal cord tumors, *Eur Radiol* 9(7):1252-1258, 1999.

3. Balmaceda C: Chemotherapy for intramedullary spinal cord tumors, *J Neurooncol* 47(3):293-307, 2000.

4. Braverman DL et al.: Multiple sclerosis presenting as a spinal cord tumor, *Arch Phys Med Rehabil* 78(11):1274-1276, 1997.

5. Connolly ES et al.: Intramedullary spinal cord metastasis: report of three cases and review of the literature, *Surg Neurol* 46(4):329-337, discussion 337-338, 1996.

6. Constantini S et al.: Radical excision of intramedullary spinal cord tumors: surgical morbidity and long-term follow-up evaluation in 164 children and young adults, *J Neurosurg* 93(Suppl 2):183-193, 2000.

7. Cristante L, Herrmann HD: Surgical management of intramedullary hemangioblastoma of the spinal cord, *Acta Neurochir (Wien)* 141(4):333-339; discussion 339-340, 1999.

8. Deme S et al.: Primary intramedullary primitive neuroectodermal tumor of the spinal cord: case report and review of the literature, *Neurosurgery* 41(6):1417-1420, 1997.

9. Doireau V et al.: Chemotherapy for unresectable and recurrent intramedullary glial tumours in children. Brain Tumours Subcommittee of the French Society of Paediatric Oncology (SFOP), *Br J Cancer*, 81(5):835-840, 1999.

10. Fine MJ et al.: Spinal cord ependymomas: MR imaging features, *Radiology* 197(3):655-658, 1995.

11. Garcia MD: Primary spinal cord tumors treated with surgery and postoperative irradiation, *Int J Radiat Oncol Biol Phys* 11(11):1933-1939, 1985.

12. Goh KY, Velasquez L, Epstein FJ: Pediatric intramedullary spinal cord tumors: is surgery alone enough? *Pediatr Neurosurg* 27(1):34-39, 1997.

13. Goyal M et al: Cervical intramedullary lipoma with unusual MRI features: case report, *Neuroradiology* 38(Suppl 1):S117-S119, 1996.

14. Guidetti B, Mercuri S, Vagnozzi R: Long-term results of the surgical treatment of 129 intramedullary spinal gliomas, *J Neurosurg* 54(3):323-330, 1981.

15. Hoshimaru M et al.: Results of microsurgical treatment for intramedullary spinal cord ependymomas: analysis of 36 cases, *Neurosurgery* 44(2):264-269, 1999.

16. Houten JK, Cooper PR: Spinal cord astrocytomas: presentation, management and outcome, *J Neurooncol* 47(3):219-224, 2000.

17. Houten JK, Weiner HL: Pediatric intramedullary spinal cord tumors: special considerations, *J Neurooncol* 47(3):225-230, 2000.

18. Innocenzi G et al.: Prognostic factors in intramedullary astrocytomas, *Clin Neurol Neurosurg* 99(1):1-5, 1997.

19. Isaacson SR: Radiation therapy and the management of intramedullary spinal cord tumors, *J Neurooncol* 47(3):231-238, 2000.

20. Iwasaki Y et al.: Spinal intramedullary ependymomas: surgical results and immunohistochemical analysis of tumour proliferation activity, *Br J Neurosurg* 14(4):331-336, 2000.

21. Jyothirmayi R et al.: Conservative surgery and radiotherapy in the treatment of spinal cord astrocytoma, *J Neurooncol* 33(3):205-211, 1997.

22. Kothbauer K, Deletis V, Epstein FJ: Intraoperative spinal cord monitoring for intramedullary surgery: an essential adjunct, *Pediatr Neurosurg* 26(5):247-254, 1997.

23. Lang EW et al.: The utility of motor-evoked potential monitoring during intramedullary surgery, *Anesth Analg* 83(6):1337-1341, 1996.

24. Lee RR: MR imaging of intradural tumors of the cervical spine, *Magn Reson Imaging Clin North Am* 8(3):529-540, 2000.

25. Lee M et al.: Intramedullary spinal cord lipomas, *J Neurosurg* 82(3):394-400, 1995.

26. Lonjon M, Goh KK, Epstein FJ: Intramedullary spinal cord ependymomas in children: treatment, results and follow-up, *Pediatr Neurosurg* 29(4):178-183, 1998.

27. Lowe GM: Magnetic resonance imaging of intramedullary spinal cord tumors, *J Neurooncol* 47(3):195-210, 2000.

28. Maiuri F et al.: Intraoperative sonography for spinal tumors: correlations with MR findings and surgery, *J Neurosurg Sci* 44(3):115-122, 2000.

29. Marsa GW et al.: Megavoltage irradiation in the treatment of gliomas of the brain and spinal cord, *Cancer* 36(5):1681-1689, 1975.

30. Matsumura A, Nose T, Hori A: Intramedullary subependymoma of the spinal cord, *Neurosurgery* 39(4):879, 1996.

31. McEvoy AW, Benjamin E, Powell MP: Haemangioblastoma of a cervical sensory nerve root in Von Hippel–Lindau syndrome, *Eur Spine J* 9(5):434-436, 2000.

32. Meurice A et al.: A single focus of probable multiple sclerosis in the cervical spinal cord mimicking a tumour, *Neuroradiology* 36(3):234-235, 1994.

33. Miller DJ, McCutcheon IE: Hemangioblastomas and other uncommon intramedullary tumors, *J Neurooncol* 47(3):253-270, 2000.

34. Morota N et al.: The role of motor evoked potentials during surgery for intramedullary spinal cord tumors, *Neurosurgery* 41(6):1327-1336, 1997.

35. Newton HB et al.: Spinal cord tumors: review of etiology, diagnosis, and multidisciplinary approach to treatment, *Cancer Pract* 3(4):207-218, 1995.

36. Patwardhan V et al.: MR imaging findings of intramedullary lipomas, *Am J Roentgenol* 174(6):1792-1793, 2000.

37. Prestor B, Golob P: Intra-operative spinal cord neuromonitoring in patients operated on for intramedullary tumors and syringomyelia, *Neurol Res* 21(1):125-129, 1999.

38. Schiff D, O'Neill BP: Intramedullary spinal cord metastases: clinical features and treatment outcome, *Neurology* 47(4):906-912, 1996.

39. Schwartz TH, McCormick PC: Intramedullary ependymomas: clinical presentation, surgical treatment strategies and prognosis, *J Neurooncol* 47(3):211-218, 2000.

40. Schwartz TH, McCormick PC: Non-neoplastic intramedullary pathology: diagnostic dilemma—to Bx or not to Bx, *J Neurooncol* 47(3):283-292, 2000.

41. Sgouros S, Malluci CL, Jackowski A: Spinal ependymomas: the value of postoperative radiotherapy for residual disease control, *Br J Neurosurg* 10(6):559-566, 1996.

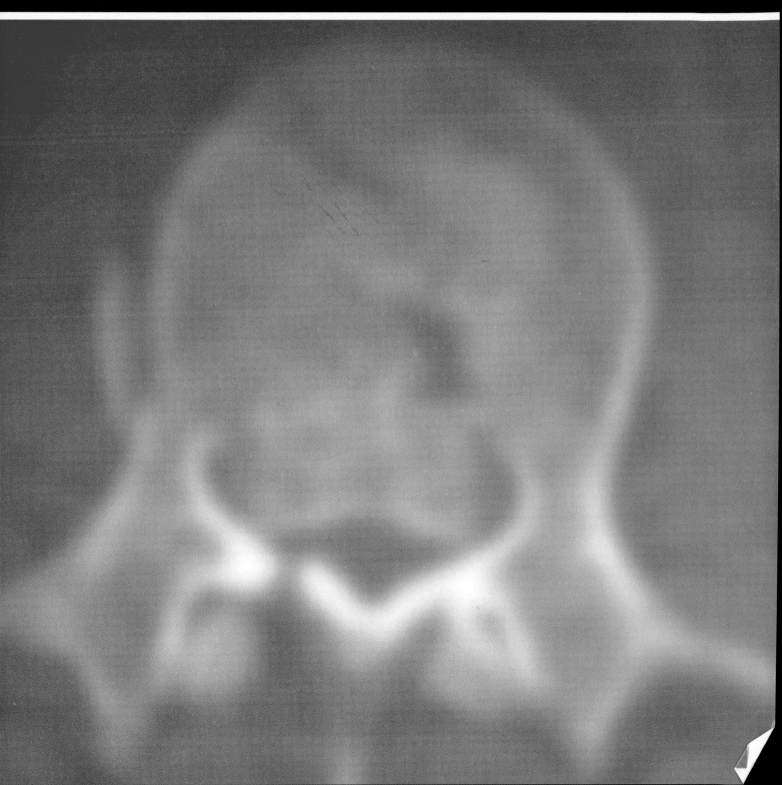

Surgical Techniques IV

Minimally Invasive Techniques of the Cervical Spine

Kenneth S. Yonemura

Minimally invasive surgery has in many ways become synonymous with endoscopic techniques that allow the visualization of deep structures through small portals in the external body wall. This chapter concentrates on the use of endoscopic technology as applied to posterior cervical surgery and illustrates an open anterior approach that may also be considered minimally invasive. There is no doubt that the reduction in approach-related incisional morbidity has been clearly documented in the laparoscopic experience over the past several decades, and in this context, it is a natural progression for this technology to be extended to spinal surgical techniques.

Although cervical disc disease remains one of the most common problems encountered by spine surgeons, there continues to be significant regional variations in surgical treatment strategies. Emphasis is placed on pathology that results in unilateral radiculopathy, which is much more amenable to minimally invasive techniques, rather than on pathology that results in myelopathy. Classic open treatment of cervical spondylosis is divided into anterior and posterior procedures.

Anterior procedures include discectomy with or without fusion, corpectomy with reconstruction, and, more recently, foraminotomy.[3,4] Smith and Robinson[7] initially described the anterior discectomy procedure in 1958. This approach allows direct decompression of osteophytes and disc herniations regardless of the location relative to the dorsally located spinal cord and nerve root. The anterior approach relies on natural cleavage planes in the anterior strap muscles, thus minimizing potential approach morbidity and negating many of the advantages of endoscopic treatment. Anterior percutaneous techniques carry potential risk to the carotid artery, jugular vein, and esophagus, and therefore emphasis is directed to the anterior foraminotomy procedure. This procedure allows for the preservation of a majority of the disc, thus obviating the need for fusion but using a conventional open approach.

Posterior procedures include laminectomy, laminoplasty, and foraminotomy. These posterior procedures generally allow for indirect decompression, with the exception of foraminal disc herniations amenable to direct removal. Approach morbidity from posterior procedures can be significant, and weakening of the posterior elements can lead to instability. Spurling and Scoville[8] initially proposed the posterior approach to cervical disc disease in 1944. Several studies indicated the incidence of postoperative axial neck pain as 18% to 40%,[5,9] whereas one study failed to include this factor in the outcome.[10] The frequently quoted prospective study of anterior and posterior approaches by Herkowitz et al.[2]

PATHOPHYSIOLOGY

- Spondylosis or degenerative processes most common between C5 and C7 vertebral bodies
- Cervical radiculopathy occurs with nerve root irritation from:
  - Herniated nucleus pulposis
  - Osteophytic foraminal stenosis
  - Fractures or dislocations
  - Synovial cysts
  - Tumors
- *Cervical radiculitis*: Correct term for nerve root pain without neurologic findings on the physical examination

---

APPROACHES

- Anterior and posterior open foraminotomy procedures equally effective for relief of unilateral radicular symptoms
- Anterior approaches
  - Allow for direct visualization and removal of ventral canal pathology
  - Routinely combined with interbody fusion
  - Kyphosis and prolonged interscapular pain common with discectomy alone
  - Accelerated junctional spondylosis not uncommon
  - Risk of pseudoarthrosis
- Posterior approaches
  - Eliminate need for concomitant fusion
  - Incisional pain increased from soft tissue dissection
  - Potential for recurrent disc herniation

reported excellent/good results for 90% and 75% of patients, respectively. This study, however, reported an 87.5% rate of excellent or good results for the posterior treatment of radiculopathy, indicating that the major difference was approach-related morbidity from the open surgical technique.

A major technologic innovation that allows minimally invasive procedures is the development of thin glass rod endoscopes with high resolution. These devices allow improved visualization of the deep structures through small portals, thereby minimizing soft tissue trauma. The associated development of various endoscopic delivery systems and instrumentation has provided the means to accomplish minimally invasive surgery in the cervical spine. These innovative procedures will not entirely replace open procedures but provide surgeons with additional options for the treatment of certain specific problems in the cervical spine. The decision to offer an anterior versus a posterior procedure, a single-level versus a multiple-level procedure, and fusion versus decompression alone is not often clear and is reviewed in a subsequent chapter.

EPIDEMIOLOGY

With normal aging of the spine, degenerative changes in the intervertebral disc, apophyseal joints, and ligamentous structures naturally occur. Without these changes, disc herniations or spondylosis will not occur. Although it is speculated that traumatic events may trigger or accelerate the degenerative cascade, there also is a genetic component that determines the strength and dynamic qualities of the spine. The normal aging process is represented by a wide spectrum of progressive pathology, and traumatic events are often superimposed on these preexisting changes.

The most common degenerative changes in the cervical spine occur between the fifth through seventh vertebrae, and this coincides with the sagittal axis of greatest rotation of the head relative to the torso. Cervical radiculopathy, the focus of this chapter, arises from nerve root irritation that may be secondary to compression by a soft disc herniation or by the presence of osteophytes that originate from the joint of Luschka. Both processes result in ventral compression of the nerve root. Ultimately, the original size of the neural foramen is the most important factor in the determination of whether

pathology seen on diagnostic studies is significant in the context of clinical symptoms. Unfortunately, this relative difference in foraminal volume and impact of foraminal pathology is often difficult to quantify on standard two-dimensional radiographic studies. There also can be variations in the length of the afflicted nerve root and postural alignment changes that can be contributing factors.

INDICATIONS

Due to the limited exposure of endoscopic techniques, the pathology should ideally be unilateral and restricted to a single level or to two contiguous nerve root levels. Symptoms include radicular symptoms of pain, numbness, weakness, and reflex changes. Although these techniques are effective for the removal of soft disc herniations, osteophytic foraminal stenosis can also be treated. Compared with standard open surgery, endoscopic foraminotomy has been shown to produce an equivalent or slightly larger decompression.

The anterior foraminotomy procedure was not intended for central lesions, but it can be effectively utilized for central lesions without the need for complete discectomy or fusion. The extensile nature of the anterior approach is less destructive to the surrounding tissues, and the disc-sparing aspect of the foraminotomy warrants its inclusion in this chapter. The ability to preserve a majority of the disc may avoid potential complications from disc space collapse or kyphosis.

Radiculopathy may be associated with significant axial neck pain, which should not be confused with axial neck pain without nerve root or spinal cord symptoms. Referred pain or symptoms of peripheral nerve entrapment are often confused with true radiculopathy. In the author's experience, it is extremely difficult to localize the source of axial neck pain, and the most significant factor is the presence of consistent localized symptoms that occur with specific and limited neck movements or posture. With the use of such restricted criteria, it may be reasonable to consider localization with single-photon emission computed tomography or possibly cer-

---

MINIMALLY INVASIVE PROCEDURES AND ENDOSCOPIC ADVANCES

- For minimally invasive procedures, reduced morbidity associated with operative approach
- Technologic advances in endoscopic equipment
  - Reduced scope profile
  - Improved visual clarity and color balance
  - Hybrid delivery systems no longer require constant irrigation
  - Wide assortment of compatible microinstruments

INDICATIONS AND CONTRAINDICATIONS FOR MINIMALLY INVASIVE ANTERIOR OR POSTERIOR FORAMINOTOMY

- Indications
  - Unilateral radiculopathy
    - Pain
    - Numbness
    - Weakness
    - Reflex
  - Pathology not extended across the midline
- Contraindications
  - Myelopathy
  - Significant signs of peripheral nerve entrapment
  - Primary axial neck pain
  - Segmental instability

vical discography. Too often, the presence of a brachial plexopathy is ignored in favor of cervical disc disease or distal peripheral nerve entrapment, such as the ulnar or median nerve. Shoulder pain with radiation into multiple dermatomal levels, weakness of the hand intrinsics, aggravation with arm elevation, and the absence of significant cervical disc disease should trigger the inclusion of thoracic outlet syndrome into the differential diagnosis.

ANTERIOR CERVICAL FORAMINOTOMY
Technique

Although the effectiveness of open posterior foraminotomy has been well shown, there are definite limitations in dealing with hard osteophytic pathology. The current trend for anterior cervical discectomy resolves this problem but results in complete removal of the disc, necessitating the performance of interbody fusion if the maintenance of cervical lordosis is desired. The anterior cervical foraminotomy procedure allows direct visualization of pathology ventral to the nerve root while motion is preserved. Jho and Kim[3] and Johnson et al.[4] demonstrated the efficacy of this technique.

The approach to the anterior spine is identical to that of an anterior discectomy and fusion. Although a discectomy can be performed with equal efficiency from the right or the left side and is based on the surgeon's preference, the anterior foraminotomy should be approached ipsilateral to the foraminal disease, thus reducing the volume of the discectomy while addressing the foraminal pathology.

A standard retractor is placed into the ipsilateral longus colli muscle with dissection at the lateral border of the vertebral body, at the junction of the transverse process and uncus. A ¼- or ⅜-inch malleable Greenberg-type retractor is then placed between the vertebral body and the vertebral artery that maintains retraction of the longus colli muscle (Figure 18-1).

The exposure allows for direct resection of the uncovertebral joint with a high-speed drill. Removal of the offending pathology, whether disc or osteophyte, is then accomplished with standard curettes or Kerrison rongeurs while a majority of the disc space is preserved.

Results

In the largest reported series of 161 patients, by Jho and Kim,[3] the results are comparable to those obtained with the posterior endoscopic procedure; excellent or good results were obtained in 97% of patients, including 53 patients (33%) with primarily osteophytic spurs. Transient worsening of weakness occurred in two patients, and a transient Horner's syndrome occurred in three patients. One patient had discitis, but postoperative instability or recurrent disc herniation has not been encountered to date.

ANTERIOR CERVICAL FORAMINOTOMY

- Possible to preserve up to 75% of the disc
  - Avoids need for fusion
  - Possible recurrent disc herniation
- Dissection poses risk to vertebral artery
- Standard anterior approach carries low morbidity
  - Limited exposure requires adjustment of surgical technique

---

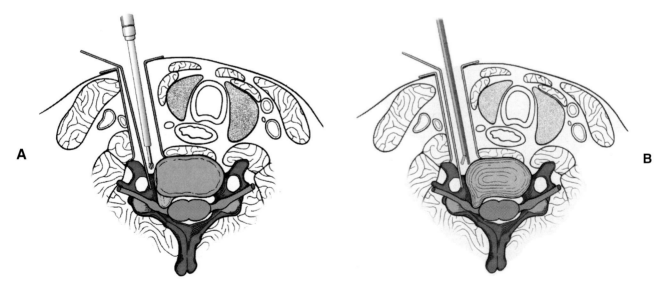

A　　　　　　　　　　　　　　　　　　　　　　　　**B**

Figure 18-1.　**A,** The longus colli muscle is retracted on the ipsilateral side, exposing the lateral vertebral margin. A ribbon retractor is then used to protect the vertebral artery and to allow the use of a high-speed drill to resect the uncinate process. **B,** The disc herniation is removed in a standard fashion without disturbing the central portion of the disc space.

In a series of 21 patients, Johnson et al.[4] noted improvement in radicular symptoms in 19 patients (91%). The remaining two patients required reoperation, one anteriorly with fusion and the other posteriorly with an open foraminotomy. There were no late failures at the 3-year follow-up. No vertebral artery injuries were noted in this series.

POSTERIOR MICROENDOSCOPIC DISCECTOMY/FORAMINOTOMY
Technique

Surgery may be performed with the patient in the prone or supine position. In either instance, a Mayfield device is needed to stabilize the patient's head. The author's series have all been performed with the patient prone, and transverse rolls are utilized rather than a frame to minimize kyphosis over the cervicothoracic junction (Figure 18-2). A fluoroscope is used to localize and ensure that the tubular retractor is centered over the correct spinal level.

A 1.5-cm incision is made approximately 2 cm lateral to the midline. A K-wire is then passed to the appropriate facet joint, and a series of dilators are utilized to create an operative corridor to the spine. The initial dilator is used as a dissector to minimize muscular trauma. A 14-mm tubular retractor is then placed over the last dilator and secured to the operating table with a modified Greenberg articulated table mount (Figure 18-3). Due to the reduced size of the cervical spine, the larger 16-mm tubular retractor has been avoided to prevent excessive resection of the facet joint as demonstrated by Roh et al.[6]

The endoscope is inserted with visualization of the appropriate interlaminar space and facet joint. The inferior margin of the lamina and medial articular process of the superior vertebral segment are then resected with a high-speed drill. Additional resection of the superior laminar margin and medial facet of the inferior vertebral segment is accomplished with the drill or Kerrison ronguer (Figure 18-4).

The epidural space is then entered laterally with resection of the intervening ligamentum flavum and coagulation of the epidural plexus overlying the exiting nerve root. Dissection in the axilla of the nerve root usually uncovers the compressive pathology, but occasionally a disc herniation is found at the shoulder of the

---

POSTERIOR PROCEDURES

- Posterior microendoscopic foraminotomy/discectomy
  ○ Tubular retractor minimizes trauma to paraspinal muscles and ligaments
  ○ Endoscope
    ○ Provides improved visualization of deep structures
    ○ Requires adjustment to two-dimensional video image and 25-degree viewing angle
    ○ Requires significant learning curve
  ○ Preservation of disc space and minimal facetectomy
    ○ Eliminates need for fusion
    ○ Possible recurrent disc herniation

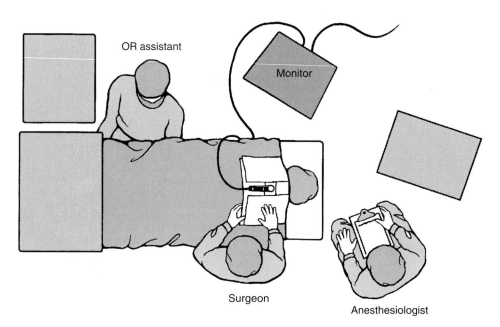

Figure 18-2.   Placement of the patient in the prone position allows the video monitor to be situated directly across from the operating surgeon. A C-arm fluoroscope is used for localization, but it is removed once the tubular retractor is secured over the appropriate disc space.

nerve due to the shape and angulation of the joint of Luschka. The orientation of the endoscopic system and extent of the foraminotomy are demonstrated in Figure 18-5. Once the nerve root has been decompressed, the tubular retractor is removed and the fascia is closed with a single absorbable suture. The 25-degree viewing angle of the endoscope provides a panoramic view of the epidural space and prevents obscuration of the operative field, as can occur if the operating microscopic is used with bayoneted instruments.

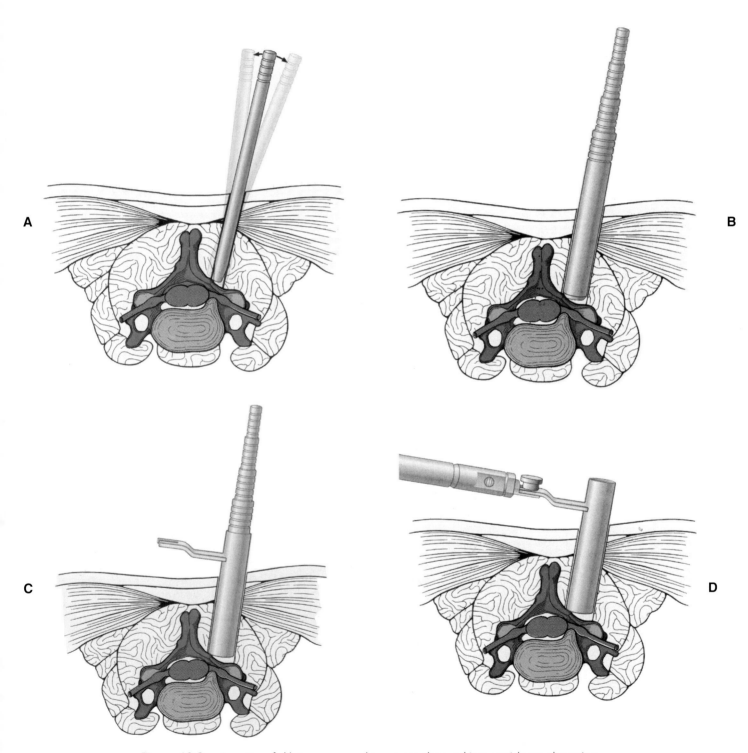

Figure 18-3.   A series of dilators are used to create the working corridor to the spine. **A** to **C,** The first dilator is used as a dissector to minimize soft tissue over the laminar lateral mass junction. **D,** The tubular retractor is secured to the operating room table with an articulated device.

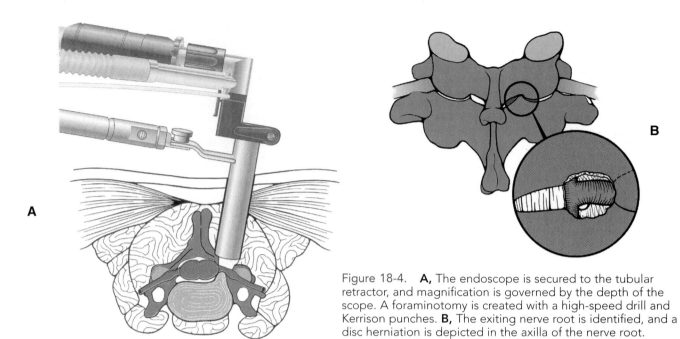

Figure 18-4. **A,** The endoscope is secured to the tubular retractor, and magnification is governed by the depth of the scope. A foraminotomy is created with a high-speed drill and Kerrison punches. **B,** The exiting nerve root is identified, and a disc herniation is depicted in the axilla of the nerve root.

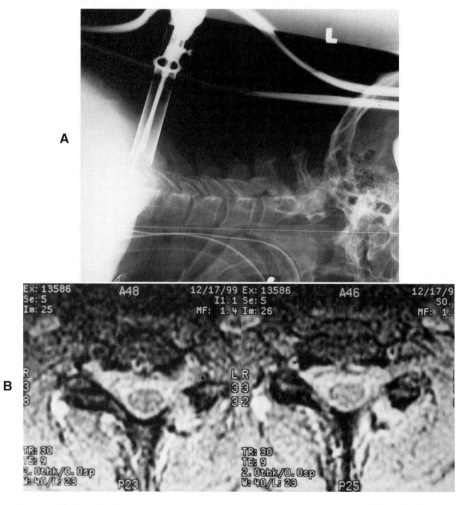

Figure 18-5. **A,** The tubular retractor has been secured over the C6 to C7 facet complex. A probe can be seen within the C7 foramen. **B,** The foraminotomy is well visualized on a postoperative magnetic resonance image.

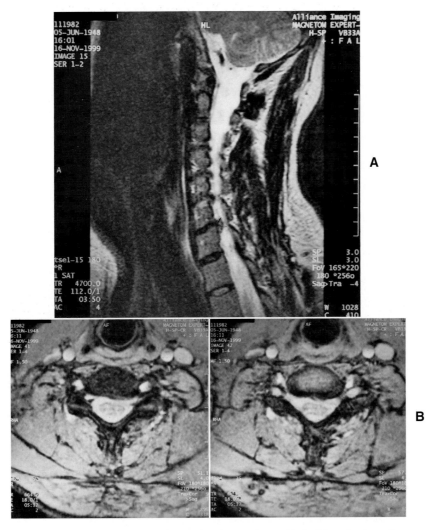

Figure 18-6.   A 52-year-old man presented with a unilateral left C7 radiculopathy. Sagittal **(A)** and axial **(B)** magnetic resonance images demonstrate a C6 to C7 foraminal disc herniation. At surgery, multiple fragments of the nucleus pulposis were recovered from below the nerve root. The patient has had complete relief of radicular pain and only minimal residual sensory loss.

Results

In a series of 24 patients, Adamson and Broome[1] reported complete resolution of radicular arm pain in all patients, as well as discontinuation of the use of pain medications in 22 of 24 patients at 3 weeks. There were no recurrent symptoms during the mean follow-up period of 4 months. All surgeries were performed on an outpatient basis, with discharge 2 to 4 hours after surgery.

In the author's initial series, there were 14 men and women (9 males and 5 females) with a minimum follow-up of 1.5 years. Two patients presented with symptomatic synovial cysts at C7 to T1, and the remainder presented with spondylosis with or without an associated soft disc herniation. Twelve had single-level surgery, and two required double-level procedures. All surgeries were performed on an outpatient basis. Thirteen patients noted complete resolution of radicular symptoms by the first week, and twelve noted the absence of significant post-

operative neck pain (Figures 18-6 and 18-7). By the sixth postoperative week, axial neck pain had resolved in the remaining two patients.

Complications included one patient with recurrent disc herniation, one patient with blood loss of more than 500 ml on one occasion, and one patient with a contralateral neurogenic thoracic outlet syndrome from operative positioning. There also was one patient with open conversion early in the series due to osteophytic foraminal stenosis, which in retrospect had been adequately decompressed from the microendoscopic (MED) procedure.

The Neck Disability Index was utilized to assess outcomes. The patients had a mean entry score of 42.5/65 and a mean score of 12.5/65 at the last follow-up, indicating the absence of any significant disability (Figure 18-8).

This technique results in a definite improvement over historical controls. There was virtual elimination of

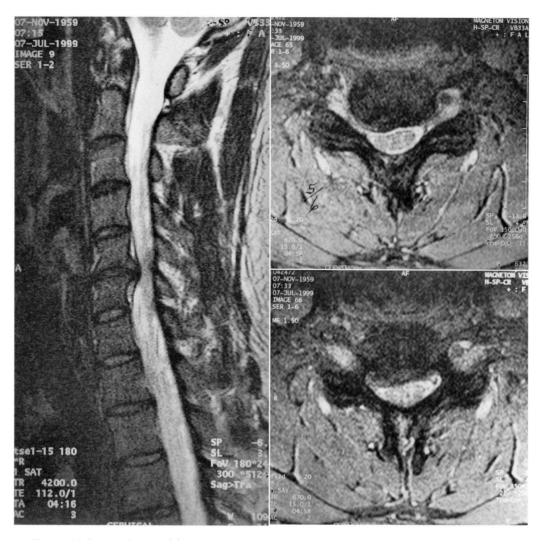

Figure 18-7.   A 40-year-old man presented with a unilateral right C6 radiculopathy. Magnetic resonance images demonstrated the presence of a foraminal osteophytic spur. At surgery, a generous foraminotomy was performed, because a soft disc component was not found. The patient noted complete pain relief and returned to competitive cycling 1 month after surgery.

postoperative axial neck pain and uniform resolution of cervical radiculopathy. There was one open conversion and one recurrent disc herniation that required an anterior fusion. There have been no long-term neurologic deficits, and significant improvement was confirmed with the Neck Disability Index.

CONCLUSIONS

A major question that will be answered in the near future is whether minimally invasive techniques offer any advantages over conventional open procedures. For anterior cervical procedures, there is an extensive track record with proven efficacy for the treatment of unilateral radiculopathy. The ability to preserve a majority of the disc and to avoid the performance of a fusion may be advantageous but may result in an unacceptable rate of recurrent disc herniations. The close proximity of the vertebral artery is also of concern, and any degree of ver-

tebral artery injury would be unacceptable in the treatment of this disease process. Surgeons in Japan have been utilizing both an anterior transvertebral approach to unilateral disc herniations and endoscopic techniques, and both are awaiting validation.

The posterior open approach for unilateral cervical radiculopathy has also been shown to be an effective surgical technique. The approach morbidity for this operation can, however, be significant. The advantages of the microendoscopic approach have been described, but the potential for recurrent disc herniations, the added time for surgery, and the requisite learning curve for endoscopic techniques must be taken into consideration.

Endoscopic equipment has evolved into hybrid systems that create a working corridor that facilitates the recognition of key anatomic structures. For spinal procedures, the ability to identify normal structures is of paramount importance, because an open working space, as in laparoscopic techniques, does not exist in the cervical

Neck disability index

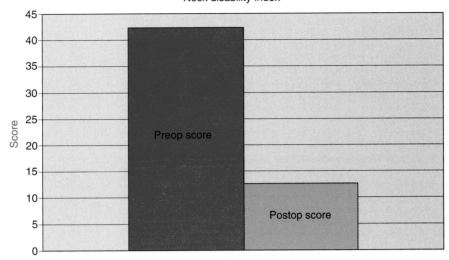

Figure 18-8. Comparison of preoperative and postoperative Neck Disability Index scores. Scores can range from 3 to a high of 65. Lower scores indicate improved function.

spine. Future advances in endoscope design could include the performance of transoral procedures without the need for associated palate or glossal division in difficult cases and may facilitate anterior cervical release procedures for severe kyphosis, such as chin-on-chest deformity in ankylosing spondylitis.

Clearly, the ability to effect a surgical cure with less destruction of normal structures is a desirable goal. New technology has miniaturized the operative field and created a need for greater understanding of both normal and, in particular, normal variant anatomy. Although the acceptance of various minimally invasive techniques may not be universal, the trend remains positive in limiting some of the destructive effects of surgical exposure and has favorably affected many open surgical techniques.

SELECTED READINGS

Adamson TE, Broome AE: Initial experience with endoscopic posterior cervical laminoforaminotomy for the treatment of cervical rediculopathy. American Association of Neurological Surgeons, open paper, Toronoto, 2001.

Herkowitz HN, Kurz LT, Overholt DP: Surgical management of cervical soft disc herniation: a comparison between the anterior and posterior approach, *Spine* 15:1026-1030, 1990.

Johnson JP et al.: Anterior cervical foraminotomy for unilateral radicular disease, *Spine* 25:905-909, 2000.

REFERENCES

1. Adamson TE, Broome AE: Initial experience with endoscopic posterior cervical laminoforaminotomy for the treatment of cervical rediculopathy. American Association of Neurological Surgeons, open paper, Toronto, 2001.
2. Herkowitz HN, Kurz LT, Overholt DP: Surgical management of cervical soft disc herniation: a comparison between the anterior and posterior approach, *Spine* 15:1026-1030, 1990.
3. Jho HD, Kim WK: Anterior cervical microforaminotomy for cervical radiculopathy in 161 patients. Congress of Neurological Surgeons open paper, San Antonio, Tex, 2000.
4. Johnson JP et al.: Anterior cervical foraminotomy for unilateral radicular disease, *Spine* 25:905-909, 2000.
5. Krupp W, Schattke H, Muke R: Clinical results of the foraminotomy as described by Frykholm for the treatment of lateral cervical disc herniation, *Acta Neurochir (Wien)* 107:22-29, 1990.
6. Roh SW et al.: Endoscopic foraminotomy using MED system in cadaveric specimens, *Spine* 25:260-264, 2000.
7. Smith GW, Robinson RA: The treatment of certain cervical-spine disorders by anterior removal of the intervertebral disc and interbody fusion, *J Bone Joint Surg Am* 40:607, 1958.
8. Spurling RG, Scoville WB: Lateral rupture of the cervical intervertebral discs: a common cause of shoulder and arm pain, *Surg Gynecol Obstet* 78:350-358, 1944.
9. Woertgen C, Holzschuh M, Rothoerl RD: Prognostic factors of posterior cervical disc surgery: a prospective, consecutive study of 54 patients, *Neurosurgery* 40:724-728, discussion 728-729, 1997.
10. Zeidman SM, Ducker TB: Posterior cervical laminoforaminotomy for radiculopathy: review of 172 cases, *Neurosurgery* 33:356-362, 1993.

Minimally Invasive Techniques of the Thoracic Spine

Barton L. Sachs

Minimally invasive surgery has experienced explosive development during the past two decades. Factors contributing to this revolution include a societal focus on improving health care, technology advancements employed in every aspect of society, the desire to control the costs of providing health care, and nearly universal access to information on alternative and newer treatment options for illness and disease. This confluence of factors has resulted in new technology and techniques employed for surgical resolution of spinal disease.

The use of technologic advancements in areas of magnification, illumination, visualization, image projection, better anatomic localization, and small tool microsurgery has resulted in a wide range of developments for endoscopic, video-assisted surgical procedures. Each of the specialty disciplines of surgery is moving into more minimally invasive surgery. Urologists have employed endoscopy with illumination and minimally invasive approaches for many decades. For the last 20 years, orthopedic surgeons have popularized the use of arthroscopic surgery for diagnosis and repair of structures of the joints. Over the past 15 years, general surgeons employed endoscopy to treat intraabdominal disease. Thoracic surgeons began to employ video-assisted techniques for surgery in the intrathoracic cavity from the early 1990s.[10]

Noted surgeon champions, which include John Regan, Curtis Dickman, Paul McAfee, Alvin Crawford, Hansen Yuan,[3] Isador Lieberman, and Daniel Rosenthal—leaders in the field of spine surgery—have continued to advance the use of thoracoscopic, video-assisted surgery for the spine. It was synergy and communication among these specialists and thoracic surgeon leaders such as Michael Mack and Peter Geiss that promoted the application of thoracoscopy for the spine.

New video-assisted training techniques, systems for rapid information transfer, and advanced education programs have continued to fuel the interest in thoracoscopic spinal surgery. As young doctors enter medicine with comfortable exposure to video-programming and remote image screen–monitored events, young surgeons create greater demand for the employment of new technology in areas of minimally invasive surgery for the spine.

Consumers have greater demand for new methods of maintaining health and treating disease. Third-party payers and insurance companies look to reducing costs and reducing hospitalization times. Surgeons see the use of technology as a means of meeting both payer and consumer demands.

Additionally, there is greater demand for ethical treatment of patients. This is often inconsistent with providing medical education for students, residents, and practicing physicians. The application of thoracoscopic minimally invasive surgery allows for education and training without subjecting patients to trial-and-error learning during surgery. Actual surgical procedures can be practiced outside of the operating room, where skill levels can be refined and efficiency gained before undertaking surgical procedures on patients. A proctor can more effectively monitor, supervise, and assist a trainee through each step of the thoracoscopic surgical procedure in a manner that best serves the patient.

In general, minimally invasive thoracoscopic surgery is consistent with newer developments of information transfer and technologic surgical advancements of other disciplines of surgery. Thoracoscopic minimally invasive surgery of the spine is dependent on the association of

---

INTRODUCTION

- Advances in technology (magnification, illumination, visualization, image projection, small tool microsurgery) and advanced techniques (video-assisted training)
- Consumer demand for minimally invasive surgery
  - Demand for ethical treatment of patients without trial-and-error learning of surgery
  - Skill assessment for professional certification, licensing, and hospital credentialing
- Combination of advances in several areas
  - Technology
  - Surgical techniques
  - Science and medicine
  - Leaders in spinal thoracoscopy

advances in the following areas: technology, new surgical techniques, science associated with the evaluation of medicine, new methods of education and communication, and the establishment of visionary champions who develop and promote these forms of surgical procedures.

GENERAL PRINCIPLES

The principles for minimally invasive thoracoscopic spinal surgery are based on standard surgical indications and established operative procedures used to treat spinal conditions. Thoracoscopy should be viewed as traditional surgery performed through a different access into the body. That access means a smaller incision and less tissue damage.

The advantages of video-assisted, minimally invasive spinal surgery are reduced surgical time, less tissue damage, decreased blood loss, reduced postoperative pain, improved postoperative respiratory function, shorter hospital stay (ICU and hospital), reduced shoulder dysfunction, improved cosmesis through minimal scars on the torso, and earlier removal of painful postoperative chest tube drains. Additionally, because patients feel better sooner, they are able to return to an earlier stage of rehabilitation as compared with standard open incisional thoracotomy surgery.

Disadvantages of video-assisted thoracoscopic surgery include the requirement for a surgeon to develop the eye-hand coordination of viewing a surgical field on a TV monitor while operating with tools held outside the surgeon's sight line. This requires a learning curve[13] for proficiency and effective adaptation. Additionally, another disadvantage related to thoracoscopic surgery includes inability to easily control major bleeding with direct pressure.

INSTRUMENTATION AND EQUIPMENT

There are five significant categories of instrumentation and equipment needed to perform thoracoscopic surgery.

GENERAL PRINCIPLES

- Standard surgical indications
- Procedures and treatment performed through smaller access into body
- Advantages and disadvantages of video-assisted thoracoscopic surgery
  - Reduced surgical time
  - Less tissue damage
  - Decreased blood loss
  - Reduced postoperative pain
  - Improved postoperative respiratory function
  - Shorter hospital stay (ICU and hospital)
  - Reduced shoulder dysfunction
  - Improved cosmesis from minimal incision scars on torso
  - Earlier removal of painful postoperative chest tube drains
  - Earlier rehabilitation for patient

A specialized operating room table should be radiolucent and allow x-ray image transmission capability. Additionally, a capability for positioning the patient in a lateral decubitus position with the ability to tilt the table during surgery is advantageous. Special pads and stabilization straps should be available to keep the patient in position during the operative procedure.

A second requirement for thoracoscopy includes standard equipment to perform generic types of minimally invasive endoscopic surgical procedures. TV monitors, illumination and light source equipment, and endoscopic visualization and projection equipment are included in this category. The monitors for a thoracoscopic case include a center-mounted main video monitor with "slave" accessory video monitors placed around the room.

A third category includes standard endoscopic access and dissection tools. This includes portals to allow delivery of the instruments from outside the body into the chest cavity. These portals should be soft and flexible so that there is limited pressure applied to the intercostal vessels running adjacent to the rib spaces. Integrated endoscopic suction and irrigation systems are used for thoracoscopic surgery. Retractors must be specialized so that they can completely collapse and enter a small circular portal and then deploy open and angulated to maintain the soft tissue thoracic cavity contents out of the field of visualization during procedure.

A fourth category for thoracoscopy includes spinal endoscopic surgical working tools. These tools include spinal dissection tools, rib dissectors, bone rib-cutter,

---

INSTRUMENTATION AND EQUIPMENT

- Special operating room table
  - Radiolucent
  - Capable of decubitus positioning
- Spinal endoscopic surgical tools
  - Spinal dissection tools
  - Rib dissectors and bone cutters
  - Endoscopic Cobb elevators
  - Microsurgical spinal dissector tools
  - Endoscopic osteotomes and bone gouges
  - Endoscopic micro instruments
- Imaging projection and video equipment
  - Endoscopic visualization
    - 2-D vs 3-D endoscopes
    - 0-, 30-, 45-, 70-degree angled endoscopes
  - Illumination and light source equipment
  - Video recorder system
  - Digital electronic recorder system
- Standard endoscopic access and dissection tools
  - Portals
  - Integrated endoscopic suction system
  - Collapsible retractor
- Hemostatic tools and equipment:
  - Bipolar cautery
  - Monopolar cautery
  - Chemical agents
  - Ultrasonic scalpel
  - Power equipment for bone resection

endoscopic Cobb (periosteal) elevators, microsurgical spinal dissectors, endoscopic osteotomes and bone gouges, and endoscopic microinstruments such as Penfield dissectors, nerve hooks, and microcurettes. These instruments are all manufactured with a long, consistent diameter shaft throughout their length. Each tool should have a comfort-grip handle and a small working end, which will fit within the surgical access portal.

The last category of equipment includes power instrumentation for bone resection. Power instruments relate to burrs, which are manufactured specifically with long, consistent diameter lengths of the shaft.

Additionally, other tools that are helpful during surgery include hemostatic tools and equipment, such as long specialized bipolar cautery instruments, monopolar specialized cautery instruments, ultrasonic scalpels, and chemical agents to control bleeding, such as gel foam and Avitene. Defogging and lens-cleaning material to keep the endoscope clean are very beneficial. These materials include sterile surfactant, lens spray irrigation systems, and endoscopic warmers.

As an option, if the surgeon is working with limited assistance, endoscopic holders, which are stationary (mounted on the table) or mobile (such as robotic style equipment), are necessary to complete surgical thoracoscopic procedures. In the age of information transfer and medical documentation, permanent image recording and capture systems have been much promoted. Those systems include megagraft image printers, video recorder systems, and digital electronic recorder systems.

SURGICAL ANATOMY

The anatomy of the thoracic spine must be thoroughly understood before considering an anterior minimally invasive technique for thoracoscopic surgery. A surgeon must study the unique complexities of the spinal region. A surgeon's ability to successfully perform complex surgery is directly related to an understanding and knowledge of anatomic structures. Any successful surgery involves being able to approach an area of disease—with minimal intrusion and minimal damage to surrounding anatomy—to repair the problematic area, and to exit from the body while repairing the entry approach.

SURGICAL ANATOMY

- Bony architecture
  - Articulations between vertebrae and ribs
  - Ligament attachments
- Neurovascular elements
  - Segmental vascular bundles
  - Intercostal bundles
- Location of great vessels
- Shape of spinal canal

Thoracoscopic surgery involves utilizing a potential body cavity and creating working room around the spinal column while protecting other major thoracic anatomic structures. Those structures are the mediastinum, the lungs, the sympathetic nerve trunk, and the great vessels of the chest cavity. Surgical access portals must be appropriately placed so as not to damage underlying anatomy. Only the first surgical portal is placed through a small incision with blunt finger dissection and penetration into the chest cavity. After that portal is positioned, the endoscope is placed and all subsequent portals are placed under direct visualization while protecting anatomic structures within the thorax. Most portals are placed with a working area between the anterior and middle axillary lines. The visualization field occurs between the middle and posterior axillary lines.

While the surgeon is viewing the chest cavity, the lungs, mediastinum, and great vessels are retracted ventrally away from the spinal column. Parietal pleura is split longitudinally and peeled away from the spinal vertebral body elements. It is important to know where the segmental vertebral vessels reside in the center of each vertebra. These vessels must be dissected and ligated with cautery, suture ligation, or hemoclip control.

Also, it is important to know that the sympathetic chain runs parallel to the spinal column along the rib heads at the location of rib attachment to the costotransverse joints. The other unique aspect of thoracic spinal surgical anatomy as it relates to thoracoscopy is the unique attachment of the rib heads with the transverse process of the vertebral body as related to the intervertebral disc space. The articulations of the ribs are important because rib heads and articulations have to be excised during thoracoscopic surgery to be able to visualize disc space. The vertebral pedicle allows for location and entry access into the spinal canal. In the upper part of the thoracic spine, the ribs attach at the corresponding level of the disc space (e.g., the fourth rib attaches at the T3 to T4, and the eighth rib attaches at the T7 to T8 level). In the inferior part of the thoracic spine, the corresponding rib attaches below the level of the corresponding disc level (e.g., the rib head of T12 attaches below the T11 to T12 disc space). These aspects of unique anatomy for the thoracic spine must be thoroughly understood to allow for successful thoracoscopic spine surgery.

ANESTHETIC CONSIDERATIONS

In order to perform video-assisted thoracoscopic surgery, the surgeon and anesthesiology team must work collaboratively. The surgical team needs adequate exposure in the chest cavity to be able to maintain direct visualization of the spinal column at all times. Space must be created to allow working tools to be placed and manipulated while illumination and visualization is maintained in concert with protecting intrathoracic structures.

Thoracoscopic surgery is best performed with bilumen endotracheal tube placement and single lung ventilation. The lung that is deflated is maintained with

---

ANESTHETIC CONSIDERATIONS

- Bilumen endotracheal tube
- Single lung ventilation
- Hemodynamic monitoring and control

OPERATING ROOM SETUP

- Patient positioning
- Surgeon positioning
- Video monitor placement
- Scrub assistant location
- Table for surgical tools
- Image intensifier fluoroscopy

---

retraction or collapse. The anesthetic team must be fully aware of this before starting surgery. Many times it is advisable to perform flexible bronchoscopy for placement of the bilumen endotracheal tube.

When one lung is deflated, the anesthesiologist must maintain appropriate mean intracircular oxygenation levels and maintain end tidal CO_2, between 35 and 38 mm Hg by using adjusted respiratory rate, bronchial blockers, peak inspiratory airway pressure between 20 cm and 40 cm H_2O, and appropriate ventilator settings with inspiratory FiO_2 and actual arterial blood gas levels.

Hemodynamic stability and renal functional perfusion must be monitored, and close consideration must be given to intraoperative blood loss and transfusion. To this end, the preoperative evaluation for the anesthesia team should include not only a standard hemoglobin/hematocrit level but also evaluation of coagulopathy problems by a check of platelet levels, serum chemistry levels of sodium, potassium, and calcium, and partial thromboplastin time and prothrombin time levels. The anesthesia team must have available appropriate levels of packed red blood cells that are typed and crossed specifically for the surgical patient. Intraoperative access lines should be placed prior to commencing surgery, which allows for monitoring electrocardiogram, heart rate, pulse oximetry, noninvasive blood pressure, and rectal temperature. In summary, the anesthesiology team becomes an integral part of the surgical success for thoracoscopy.

OPERATING ROOM SETUP AND PATIENT POSITIONING

Minimally invasive thoracoscopic surgery is performed with the patient in the lateral decubitus position. The patient should have an axillary roll placed under the recumbent arm to relieve pressure on the brachial plexus. A beanbag or bolsters are placed on both sides of the patient to maintain the lateral recumbency. The upper arm is elevated at the axilla, abducted above the head, and placed on an armrest or bolsters to be maintained out of the direct operative field on the side of the chest. It is easier to approach from the right side of the chest, where the hemi-azygous vein exists and there is no interference from the beating aorta. In cases where the specific pathologic entity is located within the left chest cavity or in situations where the right chest has already been entered for previous surgery, a left-sided approach may be necessary.

Surgeons stand ventral to the patient with a scrub assistant at the foot of the table on the same side as the surgeon team. Visual TV monitors are placed in direct visual line across from the surgical team. A second "slave" monitor may be placed in a direct visual line either for the anesthesiology team, for the second surgical scrub assistant, who may be on the opposite side of the table from the primary surgeon, or to allow the primary scrub assistant to maintain better visual access to the operative procedure. If a fluoroscopic image C-arm is to be used during the procedure, it is to be draped sterilely and kept toward the head or the foot of the table. The C-arm may be moved into position when it is specifically indicated for bony localization. Before beginning the operative procedure and after the patient is positioned on the table, it is often advantageous to use a skin marker and outline the position of the patient's scapula border, line of spinous processes, and anterior and midaxillary lines along the body.

THORACOSCOPIC ACCESS STRATEGIES
Portal Placement

Some general principles guide positioning of portals for surgical access. First, the portals should be spread far enough apart over the surface area of the chest so that the surgeon's hands are neither placed too close together nor too close to the endoscope. The surgeon should not have to "sword fight" or "fence" with the tools in an attempt to perform surgery. The surgeon should stand anteriorly facing the patient's chest during spinal thoracoscopy. The working portals for the insertion of tools, retractors, and suction devices are best positioned anterolaterally in the zone between the anterior and middle axillary lines. The portal for the endoscope is best positioned posterolaterally between the middle and posterior axillary lines within the "viewing zone" for the spine.

The positions of the working portals are triangulated. They should be spaced evenly, rostrally, and caudally to the surgical target. The portal configuration has been referred to as a "baseball diamond" with the surgeon positioned at home plate, the target pathology at second base, and the working portals at first and third base. If a 0-degree angled endoscope is used, the portal must be positioned directly over the spinal segment where the pathology is located. If a 30-degree angled endoscope is used, the portal may be positioned offset, above or below the level of the pathology, and the endoscope is angled obliquely to provide a direct view of the spine. Using a 30-degree angled endoscope brings the end of the endoscope camera away from the working portals, which allows the surgeon's hands more working room on the surface of the chest.

THORACOSCOPIC ACCESS STRATEGIES

- Portal placement
  - Triangulation of instruments
  - Endoscope for direct visualization
  - Parallel portal placement
  - Triangular placement of portals
  - "C-curve" placement of portals
  - Portal placement for percutaneous implants
- Spinal exposure and pleural dissection techniques
  - Spinal exposure and lung mobilization
- Pleural mobilization
- Vascular mobilization and ligation
- Surgery at cephalad portion of thoracic cavity
- Multiple discectomies over longer spine segments

SPINAL LOCALIZATION

- Rib articulation with vertebral body
- Spinal radiograph
- Lung and diaphragm retraction
- Segmental vessel dissection and surgical control

CLOSURE AND POSTOPERATIVE MANAGEMENT

- Chest tubes
- Layered tissue closure
- Aggressive pulmonary physiology routine

Flexible portals are used for thoracoscopy rather than rigid portals that contuse or compress the intercostal nerves and cause intercostal neuralgia postoperatively. The diameter of the flexible thoracoscopic portal must be able to accommodate the size of the tools or objects that will pass through the portal. An 11-mm or a 15-mm portal will be adequate for most purposes during thoracoscopy, because they will fit the endoscope and most tools. A 20-mm-diameter portal is needed if bone grafts or screws and plates are to be placed.

The configuration of the portals can vary depending on the surgeon's preferences, the patient's body habitus, the type of pathology, the type of spinal procedure performed, and the location of the spinal pathology. Most simple spinal procedures can be performed with three portals. Four portals may be needed for more complex procedures such as tumor resections, multilevel anterior release, or screw plate fixation or when a diaphragm retractor is required.

Spinal Exposure

The decision to approach the spine from the left or right side depends on several factors, including the location, lateralization, and extent of pathology. A right-sided approach is most commonly used for benign lesions, because more spinal surface area tends to be available behind the azygous vein than behind the aorta. If a lesion is lateralized to the left, a left-sided approach is more appropriate. If a lesion is located below T9, a left-sided approach is also preferred because at this level, the diaphragm rides higher on the right side. Exposure from T1 to T2 to T12 to L1 interspace[2] is possible via the thoracoscopic approach.

SPINAL LOCALIZATION

Identification of the appropriate spinal level can often be difficult. Counting the ribs endoscopically from within the thoracic cavity is the best way to initially localize the proper level. The first visible rib at the apex of the thoracic cavity is usually the second rib. Each subsequent rib is directly visualized, palpated, and counted.

A long blunt-tipped needle may be inserted into the disc space of question for surgery and a radiograph obtained. Anteroposterior images are best for enabling a reliable rib count on the x-ray.

To expose the spine, the nonventilated lung may be retracted manually or with gravity by rotating the patient anteriorly. Mechanical retraction of the lungs should be performed in an attempt to avoid any further injury to lung tissue. The diaphragm may need to be retracted to access the lower thoracic disc spaces. Once retraction and spinal localization have been performed, pleural mobilization and great vessel mobilization can be performed. If the segmental vessels are to be dissected and divided, the vessels must be ligated individually with endoscopic hemoclips or suture ligatures. Exposing the spinal canal with the contents of the spinal cord must be performed very delicately. This should be undertaken only after advanced training by the surgeon.

WOUND CLOSURE AND POSTOPERATIVE MANAGEMENT

After completion of the thoracoscopic operation, the thoracic cavity is thoroughly irrigated to remove pooled blood and tissue debris. The thoracoscope is used to inspect the lung and thoracic cavity. Before lung reinflation, chest tubes are placed through preexisting portal incisions. The insertion of the chest tubes is visualized with the thoracoscope to ensure the best position. An apical chest tube is used to help reinflate the lung, and a posterior-inferior tube is used to facilitate fluid drainage.

Wounds are closed in a layered fashion with absorbable suture material. Skin is closed using subcuticular sutures. Chest tubes are placed to water suction, and entry sites are covered with sterile occlusive dressings. Patients are usually extubated at the end of the operative procedure and chest and spine radiographs obtained to assess the spine and exclude pneumothorax. Postoperatively, patients are placed on an aggressive pulmonary physiotherapy routine.

SPECIFIC THORACOSCOPIC OPERATIVE PROCEDURES (INDICATIONS AND APPLICATIONS)

Diagnostic Indications for Thoracoscopic Spine Surgery

Thoracoscopic spine surgery can be employed for seven different categories of diagnostic conditions. Those conditions include sympathetic dystrophy related disorders, spinal deformities, vertebral spinal infections, vertebral neoplasms, prolapsed thoracic discs, degenerative thoracic disc disease, and traumatic spinal fractures.

Sympathectomy

Thoracoscopy is the most efficient and least traumatic surgical method for direct visualization of the upper sympathetic chain. In this fashion of surgical access, removal of the upper sympathetic ganglia may readily be performed. Thoracic sympathectomy is indicated to surgically treat palmar hyperhidrosis, axillary hyperhidrosis, reflex sympathetic dystrophy affecting the upper extremities, or ischemic syndromes of the hands such as Raynaud's disease.

The sympathetic chain usually courses superficially to the segmental and intercostal arteries and veins in the upper chest cavity. To remove the sympathetic chain, the surgeon will find that dissection is most easily begun at the level of T4 to T5 and continued in a cephalad direction. Multiple rami to each ganglion are transected to mobilize the sympathetic trunk; the trunk is transected just caudal to the stellate ganglion, which lies over the first rib. The specimen is removed as a single piece.

Thoracoscopy for a sympathectomy provides excellent excision of the thoracic sympathetic chain or its tributaries.[15] This technique reduces approach-related morbidity and facilitates recovery. The technique provides a reliable way of achieving physiologic sympathectomy.

Anterior Release for Spinal Deformity

Anterior release refers to the transection of anterior spinal soft thoracic tissue attachments such as the disc annulus and the anterior longitudinal ligament. This allows for correction of hyperkyphotic disease or scoliotic curves. The thoracoscopic release technique consists of multilevel discectomies[9,12] performed only through four portals in the anterior axillary line.

The pleura is incised over the disc spaces of interest. The spinal canal and dura are not required to be exposed and the rib heads are not removed unless a thoracoplasty is to be performed in conjunction with correction. At each disc space, the annulus is incised, disc material is removed with curette and rongeurs, and the endplates are decorticated with curettes or drills. After the anterior release is performed, bone graft that is taken from associated ribs or iliac crest is packed into the intervertebral disc spaces to provide a long-term arthrodesis after deformity correction. After the release, the curvature is reduced and stabilized with associated specialized anterior implant corrective instrumentation[15] or with a second-stage posterior operative procedure with instrumentation and implant fixation plus arthrodesis.[4]

Thoracoscopy has significant advantages compared with thoracotomy for anterior deformity release. It provides better visualization, wider exposures, and greater access to multiple levels that cannot be reached through a single thoracotomy incision. Also, it is associated with better cosmetic outcomes,[9,12,13] less pulmonary and shoulder dysfunction, shorter hospital stays, and faster recovery times. Therefore thoracoscopy is a major advance in the surgical armamentarium for treating patients with spinal deformities.

Endoscopic Anterior Correction of Thoracic Scoliosis

There have been early reports of endoscopic scoliosis correction and implant stabilization for small numbers of patient series.[7] Because this is a very advanced skill technique, it requires a surgeon who has extensive experience with standard operative treatment of spinal deformities and acquired experience with anterior endoscopic thoracic surgery. If the deformed spine can be made more flexible with anterior release, then corrective stabilization may be carried out through four to six small endoscopic portal incisions. The disadvantages associated with posterior fusion are eliminated.

ENDOSCOPIC ANTERIOR CORRECTION OF DEFORMITY WITH IMPLANTS

- Special implant instruments
- Corrective techniques
- Advantages
  - Smaller scars
  - Less postoperative pain
  - Decreased hospitalization

THORACOSCOPIC MICRODISCECTOMY

- Safe decompression of spinal cord
- Excellent visualization
- Less morbidity compared with thoracotomy
- Treatment
  - Herniated thoracic discs
    - Discectomy with or without PLL resection
  - Painful degenerative disc disease
    - Discectomy with arthrodesis
    - Discectomy with implant instrumentation fusion device

The spine is usually approached along the convex, right side surface of the deformity. Screws are placed into the vertebral bodies and inserted just anterior to the head of the rib at each vertebral level. The screws are then connected to a rod, and all components are linked. Intraoperative fluoroscopic imaging is used to observe trajectory and depth of screws during instrument implantation technique.

Regan et al.[15] have independently reported excellent results with scoliosis and spinal hyperkyphosis treated by anterior longitudinal ligament release, multiple level discectomy combined with a second-stage posterior spine implant corrective instrumentation.

Blackman and Luque have reported early experience with 20 patients treated using endoscopic anterior instrumentation for curves reaching from 41 to 98 degrees with the majority falling between 60 and 65 degrees. The mean correction of the curve was 61%, which was 30% greater than the correction achieved with bending radiographs. Most patients' rib deformities improved significantly with correction. Instrumentation was not extended below T12 to spare the mobility of the lumbar spine. Patients were able to resume light activities within 10 days, such as walking and visiting classmates. School children returned to school by the fourth week after surgery; adult patients began remunerative work between 6 and 8 weeks after surgery. Patients no longer needed intravenous narcotics within 48 hours after surgery due to reduced discomfort compared with that of open standard spine deformity operations. The endoscopic technique of instrumentation adds the advantages of smaller scars, less postoperative pain, and decreased duration of hospitalization.

Thoracoscopic Microdiscectomy

Thoracoscopic microdiscectomy[8] is a reliable surgical technique that can be performed safely with control and an acceptable rate of morbidity and scientific efficacy. The technique is indicated for herniated thoracic discs that compress the spinal cord and spinal nerves with classic myelopathy and/or thoracic radicular pain. Authors such as Mack et al.[10] Dickman and Mican,[6] and Rosenthal et al.[17] have shown excellent clinical and neurologic outcomes associated with thoracoscopic microdiscectomy. Compared with the posterolateral approaches to the thoracic spine, thoracoscopy provides more complete visualization

and access to the ventral surfaces of the spine and spinal cord. Furthermore, midline and calcified discs can be resected more completely. Compared with thoracotomy, thoracoscopy offers identical visualization and exposure of the spine and is associated with significantly less operative morbidity. Patients experience less pain and decreased duration of hospitalization and recovery.[1]

Degenerative thoracic disc disease, similar in diagnosis to lumbar degenerative derangement, can be treated in similar fashion through thoracoscopic minimally invasive surgical approaches.[6] In patients with unremitting thoracic back pain with or without radicular pain, an endoscopic discectomy and distraction of disc space with arthrodesis using bone graft has been very successful.

Thoracoscopic Corpectomy

Thoracoscopic corpectomy can be used to treat unstable thoracic fractures, to resect thoracic tumors, to debride vertebrae infected with osteomyelitis, to drain epidural abscesses, to resect hemivertebrae, and to remove large herniated thoracic discs. Pathology affecting the spine may cause symptomatic myelopathy, myeloradiculopathy, radiculopathy, or mechanical pain. Overt structural instability of the thoracic spine tends to be associated with spinal cord dysfunction. Therefore thoracoscopy is an excellent method for performing a single or multiple level corpectomy. The technique is very similar to techniques used for microdiscectomy. More bone must be resected, and a more extensive reconstruction is required. Technically, the corpectomy can be easier to perform than a thoracoscopic microdiscectomy because the larger operative field provides more mobility and visibility for the surgeon.

Neoplastic Disease Resection

Thoracoscopy can be used to biopsy vertebral lesions in the thoracic spine efficiently with minimal complications, and it produces a high diagnostic yield. Thoracoscopic biopsy is relatively easy to perform. It is an ideal procedure for surgeons to gain initial experience with thoracoscopic surgery. Lesions between T2 and T12 can be accessed readily using standard thoracoscopic techniques. Most radiologists are reluctant to

THORACOSCOPIC CORPECTOMY

- Vertebral neoplasms
  - Simple biopsy of extradural neoplasm
  - Resection of neoplastic lesion
    - En bloc complete removal
    - Debulking of neoplastic lesion
- Vertebral spine infections (with or without localized abscess)
  - Drainage of infection
  - Resection of necrotic tissue

TRAUMATIC SPINAL FRACTURES/THORACOSCOPIC SPINAL RECONSTRUCTION

- Neurologic compressive disease requiring decompression
  - Discectomy and vertebral corpectomy
- Unstable spinal conditions requiring stabilization
  - Bone graft arthrodesis alone
  - Implant instrumentation

pass a needle into the thoracic spine percutaneously for fear of causing a pneumothorax. Additionally, the diagnostic yield from a needle aspiration procedure performed at the thoracic spine is low. Endoscopic biopsy is used to establish a tissue diagnosis and plan further surgical procedures.

Transthoracic endoscopic surgery provides an excellent alternative for the resection of benign thoracic or well-localized neoplastic lesions. Primary spinal tumors such as Schwannomas,[5] neurofibromas, or other neurogenic tumors are well treated in this manner. The operative technique used for endoscopic resection of intrathoracic nerve sheath tumors is similar to the dissection technique used to resect these tumors with open surgery. Thoracoscopy provides an excellent alternative to thoracotomy for removing tumors from the thorax and thoracic neural foramina area. Currently, thoracoscopy is not well suited for treating intradural tumors that compress the spinal cord because achieving an endoscopic watertight dural closure is technically difficult.

Metastatic[11] and malignant tumors are approached differently from benign nerve sheath tumors. If bone destruction is minimal and only diagnosis is needed, a limited biopsy can be performed without performing a resection and reconstruction. This is best performed when the tumor is highly radiosensitive. A vertebrectomy should be performed for metastatic tumors that have destroyed the vertebral body. The vertebral body can be reconstructed with bone grafts or methylmethacrylate. If internal fixation is needed, an anterior plate can endoscopically be inserted and the patient may or may not undergo a subsequent open posterior segmental fixation.

Traumatic Spinal Fractures

Rosenthal has promoted the concept of treating traumatic unstable spinal fractures through thoracoscopic minimally invasive techniques.[17] Neurologic compressive disease can be managed with a decompression discectomy or vertebral corpectomy. Additionally, in the unstable spinal conditions that require stabilization, a bone graft arthrodesis alone or a bone graft with instrumentation can be performed. These procedures require great skill levels and advanced training by the operating surgeon.

Thoracoscopic Spinal Reconstruction

Thoracoscopy provides an alternative approach to large thoracotomy incision for interbody fusion and vertebral body resection.[4] The goals of anterior spine reconstruction are to fill structural defects, to achieve mechanical stability, to restore axial load bearing, to prevent spinal deformity from developing, and to achieve arthrodesis at the involved spine segment. Fusion across a single disc space or across multiple disc levels may be desired. In case of a "moderate-size" cavity, a vertebral stabilization and fusion procedure is most desirable. If a tumor is to be resected or if the spine is rendered unstable due to traumatic fracture, reconstruction can be performed.[3] Internal fixation of the unstable thoracic spine may be performed with spinal instrumentation using methylmethacrylate, large allograft segments of bone, or combinations of screws with plates or screws with rods.

These reconstruction instruments are inserted into the vertebral bodies through the endoscopic portals. The screws can be anchored to bone and linked together with plates or rods to restore spinal stability.[7] The fixation devices restrict spinal motion and maintain positions of bone grafts. Also, implant devices prevent displacement of the spine. Fluoroscopy and direct inspection with the endoscope throughout the procedure are required to provide accurate guidance and trajectory for thoracoscopic hardware placement in the vertebral bodies.

Anterior spinal fixation devices can be applied endoscopically to restore spinal stability and to correct spinal deformities, with techniques as performed by Rosenthal et al.[17] and Picetti et al.[14] The tools to endoscopically insert the hardware must be long enough for percutaneous use. Each of the preceding authors has shown clinical experience with excellent results after endoscopic spine stabilization. They have achieved levels of stabilization similar to those of open techniques of anterior fixation of the thoracic spine.

CONTRAINDICATIONS AND LIMITATIONS

Contraindications to thoracoscopic surgery include conditions such as hypercoagulopathy, inability to tolerate single lung ventilation, irrecoverable terminal illness, severe cardiac or pulmonary disease, or extensive pleural adhesions from prior chest trauma or prior thoracotomy. The other anterior surgical alternatives to

---

CONTRAINDICATIONS AND LIMITATIONS

- Medical conditions
- Previous thoracic surgery
- Posterior anatomic location of the pathology
- Limited number of surgeons and geographic centers

ADVANCING SURGICAL TECHNOLOGY: FUTURE DIRECTIONS

- Visualization, optical magnification, image projection, monitoring
- Endoscopes and cameras
- Robotic tool systems for conducting surgery
- Remote site execution for surgery
- Image guidance surgery
- Virtual reality equipment to localize spinal anatomy
- Tools and implants
  - Soft tissue intracavitary retractors
  - Vertebral realignment and reduction equipment
  - Implant spinal instrumentation made for endoscopic surgery
  - Shape memory metal implants
- Competency standards
  - Objective assessment of surgical technique: Credentialing, licensing, hospital privileging, and recertification
- Improved education using endoscopic visualization and distance video projection surgery

---

anterior thoracoscopic surgery include standard thoracotomy, sternotomy, or costotransversectomy. Because thoracoscopic approaches expose only the anterior and anterolateral areas of the spinal vertebral column, the approach is not employed for lesions of posterior elements. Therefore posterior extradural lesions or extensive intradural lesions are best treated through standard posterior surgical thoracic approaches.

At present, another limitation for thoracoscopic surgery is the limited number of physicians with appropriate experience and the limited number of clinical centers that are equipped to perform such highly technical procedures. There is a significant cost for equipping an endoscopic surgical theater. The application of new surgical techniques requires surgeon patience; a dedicated laboratory to allow the surgeon to practice, acquire, and maintain basic skill levels; and a complete team of hospital staff dedicated to support the advanced operative techniques. Additionally, technically good clinical outcomes require that surgeons perform these procedures on a regular basis to maintain proficiency and skill.

ADVANCING SURGICAL TECHNOLOGY: FUTURE DIRECTIONS

Advancements in the area of minimally invasive surgical procedures are consistent and commensurate with advancements of technology. Advanced visualization produced from optical magnification, image projection, and monitored viewing of surgery continues to improve. Small endoscopic cameras (either rod-lens or fiber-optic) allow wonderful visual clarity in very confined spaces. However, image projection equipment is still maintained through direct cable hook-ups to TV monitors. In the future, we can expect that cables will be replaced by radio frequency projection to image monitoring screens. These screens may be in the immediate location or in a more distant place. These broadcast advancements will allow for improved education and better teaching of anatomy and physiology and may evolve into participatory endoscopic surgical procedures.

Robotics

Other future developments include the field of robotics. Engineers have created robots that can control the operating-room atmosphere, lights, temperature, and even environmental aeration. Other robots act as endoscope holders. These robots respond to manual or voice activation. The most advanced area includes robotic systems, which literally perform operative surgical procedures. At present these robots act as extensions for surgeon capability in performing repetitive tasks in a confined space. Today, the surgeon is still in total control of the robotic arms, which hold the working tools. Future developments are already under way whereby robots will not only act as assistive devices but also perform independently after the surgeon has relinquished control.

Image Guidance

Virtual reality equipment has been incorporated into surgery. This type of equipment allows for localization of spinal anatomy from outside the body. The localization has taken place by radio frequency controls and recently by fluoroscopic x-ray incorporation. Information is fed to a computer, which allows for direct localization to a point inside the body. Precise localization allows for tracking of instruments with greater safety when working around neurologic tissue.

Tools and Implants

Newer developments of specialized working tools and spinal implant devices continue. Specialized soft tissue intracavitary retractors have been developed that allow for creating a safe and protected intracavitary surgical field. Specialized vertebral alignment systems and reduction retractors are now being employed that allow for reshaping the position of the spine from outside the body. Additionally, specialized implant spinal instrumentation[7] will be fashioned specifically for endoscopic anterior minimally invasive spinal surgery. With this instrumentation the construct is actually built inside the body cavity. These types of specialized implants include component pieces with modularity of design. The components are small enough to be placed through the access portals into the body cavity. Then components can be fitted to the spine, locked together, and stabilized in position. Some of these constructs will include shape-memory metal implants combined with specialized vertebral alignment systems.

Competency Standards

Advancements in data capture and information transfer will combine with the use of objective assessment of a surgeon's surgical skill and proficiency. Such analytic review may in the future be used for medical licensing, hospital privileging, special credentialing, and recertification. As better means of objective assessment are developed, the information captured can be used for developing standards of competency of surgeons who perform thoracoscopic minimally invasive surgical procedures.

CONCLUSIONS

Thoracoscopic spinal surgery has been shown to be technically feasible, and it can be performed safely with acceptable rates of morbidity and excellent clinical and neurologic results. The minimal incision access allows for similar results when compared with outcomes of thoracotomies for complete spinal exposure. The endoscopic anterior surgery allows for better visual exposure, standard anatomic dissections, neurologic decompressions, and vertebral reconstructive operations as compared with other more invasive surgical techniques.

Advantageously, minimally invasive thoracoscopic surgery provides more complete access to all aspects of the ventral area of the spine and spinal cord compared with thoracotomy or costotransversectomy. When thoracotomy is used, visualization is good only in areas directly below the incision or up to two levels cephalad and caudad. Additionally, thoracoscopy allows for less postoperative morbidity, reduced pain, and improved recovery times for patients.

Thoracoscopic anterior surgical spine techniques have been performed for a wide range of surgical procedures including biopsy, discectomy, vertebrectomy and corpectomy, vertebral reconstruction, and application of internal implant spinal fixation devices to treat various pathologic spinal conditions. The techniques for these surgical procedures are initially difficult to master. A surgeon must develop specialized psychomotor skills and adapt to new forms of hand-eye coordination, as well as consider new perceptions of operative anatomy. Therefore steep learning curves must be mastered prior to clinical applications. Before a surgeon commences techniques of thoracoscopic surgery, she or he should devote time to instructional seminars, surgical hands-on skill laboratories, and clinical preceptor programs.

In summary, minimally invasive thoracoscopic surgery has advanced through the combination of scientific assessment of outcomes of medical care, modern technologic developments, alternative surgical techniques, and dissemination of surgeon experience through an educational format.

SELECTED REFERENCES

Burgos J, Rapariz JM, Gonzalez-Herranz P: Anterior endoscopic approach to the thoracolumbar spine, *Spine* 23(22):2427-2431, 1998.

Connolly PJ et al.: Video-assisted thoracic corpectomy and spinal reconstruction: a biomechanical analysis of open versus endoscopic technique, *J Spinal Disord* 9(06):453-459, 1996.

Cunningham BW et al.: Video-assisted thoracoscopic surgery versus open thoracotomy for anterior thoracic spinal fusion, a comparative radiographic, biomechanical, and histologic analysis in a sheep model, *Spine* 23(12):1333-40, 1998.

Dickman CA, Mican CA: Multilevel anterior thoracic discectomies and anterior interbody fusion using a microsurgical thoracoscopic approach, *J Neurosurg* 84:104-109, 1996.

Newton PO, Shea KG, Granlund KF: Defining the pediatric spinal thoracoscopy learning curve, *Spine* 25(8):1028-1035, 2000.

Newton PO et al.: Anterior release and fusion in pediatric spinal deformity, *Spine* 22(12):1398-1406, 1997.

REFERENCES

1. Broc GG et al.: Biomechanical effects of transthoracic microdiscectomy, *Spine* 22(06):605-612, 1997.
2. Burgos J, Rapariz JM, Gonzalez-Herranz P: Anterior endoscopic approach to the thoracolumbar spine, *Spine* 23(22):2427-2431, 1998.
3. Connolly PJ et al.: Video-assisted thoracic corpectomy and spinal reconstruction: a biomechanical analysis of open versus endoscopic technique, *J Spinal Disord* 9(06):453-459, 1996.
4. Cunningham BW et al.: Video-assisted thoracoscopic surgery versus open thoracotomy for anterior thoracic spinal fusion, a comparative radiographic, biomechanical, and histologic analysis in a sheep model, *Spine* 23(12):1333-1340, 1998.
5. Dickman CA, Apfelbaum RI: Thoracoscopic microsurgical excision of a thoracic schwannoma, *J Neurosurg* 2112:88(5):898-902, 1998.
6. Dickman CA, Mican CA: Multilevel anterior thoracic discectomies and anterior interbody fusion using a microsurgical thoracoscopic approach, *J Neurosurg* 84:104-109, 1996.
7. Ebara S et al.: A new system for the anterior restoration and fixation of thoracic spinal deformities using an endoscopic approach, *Spine* 25(7):876-883, 2000.
8. Horowitz MB et al.: Thoracic discectomy using video-assisted thoracoscopy, *Spine* 19(9):1082-1086, 1994.
9. King AG et al.: Video-assisted thoracoscopic surgery in the prone position, *Spine* 25(18):2403-2406, 2000.
10. Mack MJ et al.: Video-assisted thoracic surgery for the anterior approach to the thoracic spine, *Ann Thorac Surg* 59(5):1100-1106, 1995.

SUMMARY

- Thoracoscopic spinal surgery: Technically safe and feasible
- Advantages
  - Excellent visualization of anatomy
  - Wide exposure for length of thoracic spine
  - Reduced patient morbidity
  - Improved patient recovery period
  - Application for many surgical procedures
- Disadvantages
  - Steep surgeon learning curve
  - Requires expensive commitment to technology
- Combination of advances in various fields
  - Education
  - Scientific assessment
  - Technologic developments
  - New surgical techniques

11. McLain RF, Lieberman IH: Endoscopic approaches to metastatic thoracic disease, *Spine* 25(14):1855-1858, 2000.
12. Newton PO, Shea KG, Granlund KF: Defining the pediatric spinal thoracoscopy learning curve, *Spine* 25(8):1028-1035, 2000.
13. Newton PO et al.: Anterior release and fusion in pediatric spinal deformity, *Spine* 22(12):1398-1406, 1997.
14. Picetti G III et al.: Anterior endoscopic correction and fusion of scoliosis, *Orthopedics* 21(12):1285-1287, 1998.
15. Regan JJ, Mack MJ, Picetti GD: A technical report on video-assisted thoracoscopy in thoracic spinal surgery, *Spine* 20(7):831-837, 1995.
16. Robertson DP et al.: Video-assisted endoscopic thoracic ganglionectomy, *J Neurosurg* 79(2):238-240, 1993.
17. Rosenthal D, Rosenthal R, Simone A: Removal of protruded thoracic disc using microsurgical endoscopy, *Spine* 19(9):1087-1091, 1994.

Minimally Invasive Techniques in Lumbar Spine Surgery

John J. Regan

There is considerable enthusiasm regarding minimally invasive surgical techniques. Laparoscopic surgical approaches have dramatically altered the field of general surgery. The advantages of transperitoneal laparoscopic surgery for the patient include smaller incisions with reduced postoperative pain, lack of postoperative ileus, and early hospital discharge. For the surgeon, it offers improved visualization of the surgical anatomy and greater participation for the entire operating team, which can watch the monitor during the surgical procedure. Laparoscopic platform technology is merging with robotics and image guidance systems, which will likely lead to improved surgical accuracy and lower patient morbidity.

Spinal fusion has been used to treat various spinal disorders for most of the twentieth century. However, it was not until 1992, with the introduction of threaded spinal fusion cages, that the opportunity arose to combine the benefits of laparoscopy with the latest in fusion technology. A collaborative team consisting of the general surgeon and the spine surgeon has become essential for success. Ultimately, the acceptance of laparoscopic spinal techniques will be based on technical factors and improved patient outcomes.

Transabdominal and retroperitoneal approaches for anterior lumbar interbody fusions are widely accepted, effective tools for the management of painful degenerative disc disease unresponsive to nonoperative measures. Recent advances in interbody fusion cage technology have generated a great deal of interest in their application by laparoscopic techniques. There are several potential advantages of a spinal fusion system that can be inserted using a laparoscopic technique. This approach avoids posterior incisions with associated trauma to the paraspinal musculature. Epidural scarring, traction on nerve roots, and dural lacerations are avoided with the anterior approach.

A team approach is essential to the success of this technology. The general and spinal surgeon must work together from preoperative consultation through the surgical procedure, as well as early postoperative care, to realize the full benefits of these surgical procedures. Appropriate patient selection is vital to success. The ideal candidate is a patient with discogenic pain related to isolated disc space collapse following a previous laminectomy. Assessment of vascular anatomy on preoperative magnetic resonance imaging (MRI) scans and identification of anomalies or vascular disease is essential. Monopolar cautery is avoided during surgery, and blunt dissection is used to avoid injury to the superior hypogastric plexus. The laparoscopic experience should begin at the L5 to S1 disc space. Fusion success is improved by excluding patients with osteoporosis. Achieving appropriate distraction with the cages and packing bone anterior to the cages so that a sentinel fusion sign can be identified on plain x-rays are also essential for a successful outcome.

ADVANTAGES OF LAPAROSCOPIC SPINE SURGERY

- Avoids posterior incisions with associated trauma to paraspinal musculature
- Avoids epidural scarring, nerve root traction, and dural laceration

---

IDEAL SURGICAL CANDIDATE FOR LAPAROSCOPIC SPINE SURGERY

- Discogenic pain related to isolated (single-level) disc collapse
- Young patient (<45 years old) with normal MRI disc intensity signal at adjacent levels
- Single or multilevel posterior pseudarthrosis
- Stable symptomatic grade I spondylolisthesis
- Radiographic evidence of disc space narrowing, end-plate sclerosis, and osteophyte formation

INTERBODY FUSION CAGES

Interbody fusion cages offer the surgeon an alternative approach to fusion for discogenic pain syndromes. Arthrodesis is obtained by achieving immediate stability and long-term support with the ability to heal under compressive loads through and around the implant. Brantigan and Stefee developed a carbon fiber cage used with autogenous bone grafting. Bagby[1] and Kuslich successfully introduced the first threaded titanium interbody cage (BAK; Spinetech, Inc., Minneapolis, Minn.). A 91% clinical success and fusion rate has been reported with this cage. In spite of the subsequent proliferation of interbody fusion devices, the threaded fusion cage remains the only interbody fusion device approved by the U.S. Food and Drug Administration as a stand-alone device. The BAK device was also the first interbody cage to be implanted using a laparoscopic technique in 1994.

Obenchain, who reported the first laparoscopic lumbar discectomy, first described anterior endoscopic spinal surgery.[9] Mack et al.[3] reported the application of thoracoscopy for disease of the spine in 1993. In 1995 Mathews et al.,[6] Zucherman et al.,[17] and Regan et al.[11] reported the technique and preliminary results of laparoscopic lumbar fusion. Instruments have been designed to be placed laparoscopically for the purpose of disc space distraction, centering of the implant, and placement of two threaded titanium cylinders that engage both endplates of the disc space to be fused. These cylinders are packed with iliac crest bone graft.

INDICATIONS

Laparoscopic fusion techniques are indicated for use in patients with single-level symptomatic degenerative disc disease, internal disc disruption, and pseudarthrosis. Surgeons with experience may consider stable grade I spondylolisthesis and two-level degenerative disc disease. The ideal patient for laparoscopic fusion is one who has radiographic degenerative disc changes. These include disc space narrowing, endplate sclerosis, and osteophyte formation. This disease can be diagnosed in a patient with a strong history of mechanical back pain who has isolated changes at one level on radiographs and an MRI scan. This diagnosis is best made in a young patient (younger than 45 years) with a normal disc intensity signal on the MRI scan at adjacent discs. In older patients the diagnosis may be less clear owing to the naturally occurring degenerative changes in the intervertebral discs.

In a patient with single-level disc disease and Modic changes confirmed on MRI, discography is not always necessary.[8] Patients with a strong mechanical back pain history who have conformed to a physical therapy program for 4 months without relief are good candidates for the procedure. Patients who have overlying psychologic conditions, individuals with positive Waddell's signs, and habitual narcotics users are not candidates for fusion surgery.

Internal disc disruption patients who are not ideal candidates for laparoscopic fusion include patients who have relatively normal radiographic examinations,

a semi-decreased signal on MRI, concordant pain response and morphology on discography, and relatively preserved disc space height. These patients can be treated with laparoscopic techniques, but because of a tall disc height, it is more difficult to obtain the disc distraction required for stability. Anatomic fit is more difficult because larger cages are required. The BAK proximity cage (Sulzer-Spinetech, Minneapolis, Minn.) has improved the anatomic fit with cages that can be placed closer together. This decreases the chance of lateral cage extrusion and nerve root irritation.

Patients with extensive peritoneal adhesions from previous surgery or inflammatory or infectious diseases affecting the peritoneum should be excluded from the laparoscopic transperitoneal approach. Radiographs and MRI scans should also be examined for vascular calcifications, aneurysms, and anomalies, which may exclude the anterior approach altogether.

SURGICAL TECHNIQUE
L5 to S1 Approach

A "four-stick" technique is used with one periumbilical Hasson trocar placed for the 0-degree endoscope followed by placement of two 5-mm trocars lateral to the inferior epigastric arteries, which run along the ventrolateral border of the rectus abdominus muscle (Figure 20-1). A 5-mm portal is placed in the suprapubic location after establishing the appropriate trajectory to the L5 to S1 disc space by using lateral C-arm fluoroscopy. The suprapubic trocar is placed above the bladder, which can be visualized endoscopically after it has been drained by Foley catheter insertion. After insertion of the Hasson trocar and establishment of a pneumoperitoneum, other trocar placements are made under

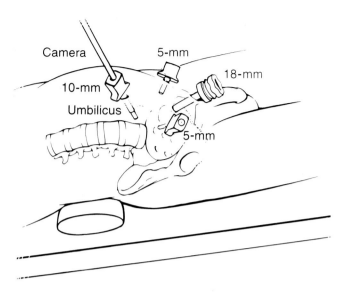

Figure 20-1. Trocars are positioned at the periumbilical site for camera with two 5-mm trocars inserted lateral to the inferior epigastric arteries midway between umbilicus and pubis. An 18-mm trocar is placed above the pubis symphysis. The suprapubic trocar is placed in line with the disc space to be fused.

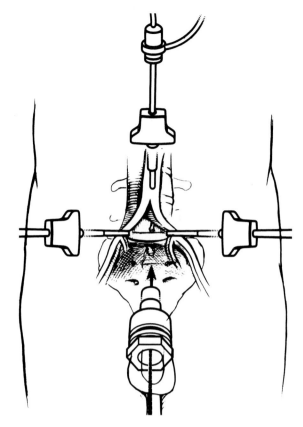

Figure 20-2. Anterior view of abdomen showing four-trocar strategy used to expose L5 to S1 disc space. The middle sacral artery is ligated and 5-mm vein retractors are used to mobilize the iliac vessels.

LAPAROSCOPIC SURGICAL APPROACH L5 TO S1 INSTRUMENTS

- Use "four stick" technique.
- Place single periumbilical Hasson trocar for 0-degree endoscope.
- Place two symmetrical 5-mm trocars lateral to inferior epigastric arteries, which run along the ventrolateral border of the rectus abdominus muscle.
- Place 5-mm portal in suprapubic location after identifying appropriate trajectory by lateral C-arm fluoroscopy.

---

direct vision. The patient is positioned in 20 to 30 degrees of Trendelenburg, and graspers are placed in the 5-mm ports to facilitate packing the intestines into the superior portion of the abdomen. The location of the aortic bifurcation is identified, and the sigmoid colon mesentery is approached from the right side. The right ureter coursing over the right iliac artery must be identified prior to making this incision in the posterior peritoneum. Electrocautery is not used in making the incision to avoid injury to the superior hypogastric plexus. Blunt dissection using Kidner wands is then used to sweep the retroperitoneal tissue from right to left. The sigmoid colon may travel close to the midline, requiring retraction. Preoperative laxatives and a light dinner the day before surgery should result in colon evacuation, which will improve handling of the bowel. In some situations, a Keith needle is inserted from the left lower quadrant percutaneously. The suture is passed through the cut edge of the peritoneum to provide a

sling for the colon. The needle and suture are then passed back out through the skin and tied with the appropriate tension.

After incising the peritoneum and mobilizing the sigmoid colon, the L5 to S1 disc space is visualized with the middle sacral vessels traveling close to the midline across the disc space. The median sacral vein and artery can be ligated with clips, but the author prefers using endoscopic chromic ties (Endoloops; Ethicon Endosurgery Inc., Cincinnati, Ohio) to avoid clip loosening, which can occur during cage insertion. Sharp dissection and cautery are avoided to prevent injury to the hypogastric plexus. Kitner wands and endoscopic vascular retractors are used to retract the iliac vessels on either side. The vessels are mobilized until the sympathetic plexus can be seen on either side (Figure 20-2). This broad visualization of the disc space combined with a true anteroposterior (AP)-lordotic fluoroscopic image of the L5 to S1 disc space is essential in locating the true midline of the disc space. The midline is marked with a Steinmann pin, and an AP and lateral x-ray is obtained. Once the center point is established, a trephine is used to enlarge the center hole. The appropriate size drill alignment guide determined from use of a preoperative template is used to create pilot holes on either side of midline.

The process of disc evacuation has been a source of debate. Although it is clear that simple channel

SURGICAL APPROACH L5-S1

- Establish pneumoperitoneum.
- Place other trocars under direct vision.
- Place patient in 20- to 30-degree Trendelenburg position; use graspers in 5-mm port to facilitate packing intestines into superior portion of abdomen.
- Identify aorta bifurcation; approach sigmoid colon from right side.
- Identify right ureter coursing over right ilial artery before incising posterior peritoneum.
- Use blunt dissection with Kidner wands used to sweep retroperitoneal tissue from right to left.
- Visualize L5 to S1 disc space; ligate median sacral vein and artery.
- Move ilial vessels to each side until the sympathetic plexus can be seen on either side.

TECHINIQUE OF DISC REMOVAL

- Mark midline with Steinmann pin, followed by AP and lateral images.
- Use trephine to enlarge center hole.
- Determine appropriate size drill alignment guide from preoperative template; use to create pilot holes on either side of midline.
- Remove disc with ring curettes and angled and straight pituitary rongeurs.

EXPOSURE OF L4 TO L5 DISC SPACE

- Use preoperative MRI scan to determine location of vascular bifurcation.
- Identify L5 to S1 disc space as previously described; carry dissection in a cephalad direction between the bifurcation.
- Alternatively, approach the L4 to L5 by retracting the left iliac artery and vein from left to right or by going between the left iliac artery and vein.

DISSECTION ABOVE THE BIFURCATION OF THE ILIAC VESSELS

- Identify and divide the ascending iliolumbar vein or veins.
- Note that dissection is complete when the sympathetic plexus is seen on patient's right side.

reaming without thorough disc removal may lead to a higher rate of pseudarthrosis, it may not be necessary or desirable to remove the entire anterior annulus and anterior longitudinal ligament. Disc removal can be accomplished using ring curettes and angled and straight pituitary rongeurs. Coblation technology (Arthrocare, Sunnyvale, Calif.) can also be used to ablate the disc prior to reaming (Figure 20-3).

Technique for L4 to L5 Exposure

The L4 to L5 disc space is visualized by making an incision in the posterior peritoneum to the right of the sigmoid mesocolon after visualizing the bifurcation of the aorta and vena cava. Preoperative MRI scans are evaluated to determine the location of the vascular bifurcation. The sigmoid colon is gently moved to the left of the midline and if necessary, it can be further retracted by placing a suture through the sigmoid mesocolon and bringing it through the anterior abdominal wall in the left lower quadrant. The L5 to S1 disc space is identified, and the dissection is carried in a cephalad direction between the bifurcation. It may be possible to approach the L4 to L5 disc from below the bifurcation, which can be determined at this time. Depending on the vascular anatomy, the L4 to L5 disc may be approached by retracting the left iliac artery and vein from left to right or by going between the left iliac artery and vein.

Above the Bifurcation of the Vessels

This approach should be feasible in most patients, unless the bifurcation of the vessels is extremely high. The issue of autonomic nerve dysfunction is a concern with this approach. One critical step in successfully achieving visualization of the interspace is to identify and divide the ascending iliolumbar vein, which may be a single large vessel taking off obliquely from the left iliac vein or vena cava above or below the L4 to L5 disc space or up to three or four small venous branches arising from the left iliac vein. The preferred method in dealing with the ascending iliolumbar vein is to apply a 5-mm clip to the vein and then protect the iliac vein side with an Endoloop. Loss of control of segmental vessels can often be recovered, but loss of control of the ascending lumbar vein often requires suture-ligature closure and may lead to conversion of the procedure to open surgery. The dissection is complete when the sympathetic plexus is seen on the patient's right side. In 1999 Regan et al. reported results of the laparoscopic approach to L4 to L5 in 58 consecutive patients.[14] This approach was used in 50% of patients in this series (Figure 20-4).

Below the Bifurcation of the Vessels

This approach provides the easiest access to the L4 to L5 disc; however, it involves the most dissection and possibly retraction in the area of the superior hypogastric plexus. All dissection is done with scissors, and no monopolar cautery is used at any time. The bifurcation is elevated, and retraction of the left and right iliac vessels is performed using a 5-mm vessel retractor. It is helpful to elevate the vessels off the surface of the vertebral body to facilitate drill tube insertion. In the aforementioned Regan series from 1999,[14] the surgeons were able to approach the L4 to L5 disc by going under the bifurcation 33% of the time.

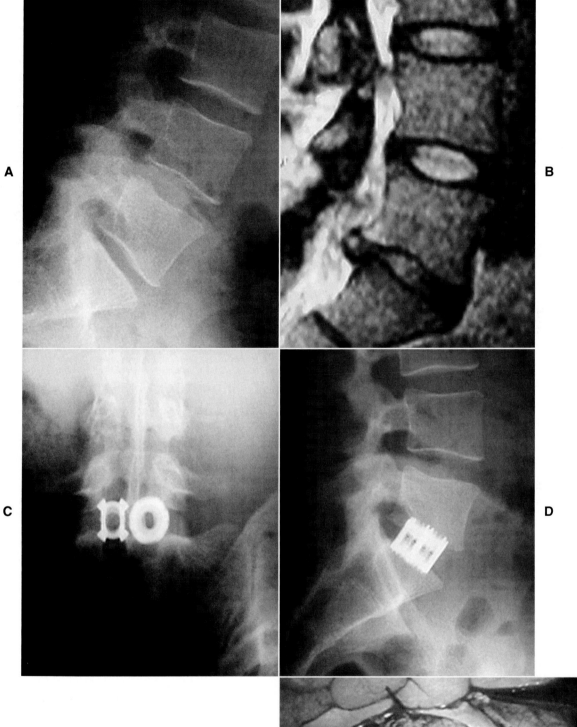

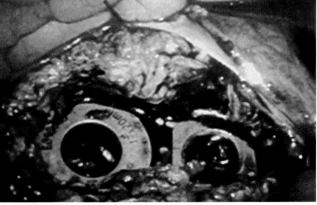

Figure 20-3. This 42-year-old man presented with gradual onset mechanical back pain lasting 6 years following a successful discectomy for sciatic pain. **A,** Plain radiographs demonstrate disc space collapse with degenerative osteophytes. **B,** MRI demonstrates Modic changes on T1 weighted images. **C** and **D,** The patient underwent laparoscopic fusion at L5 to S1 with restoration of disc space height using BAK cylindrical and BAK Proximity cages. **E,** Intraoperative view shows cages in position after discectomy.

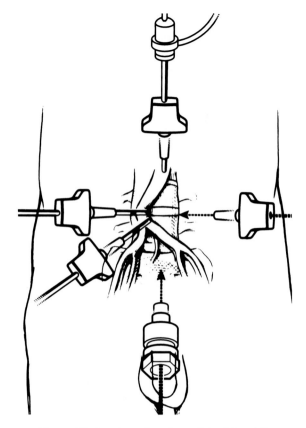

Figure 20-4. Anterior view of the L4 to L5 exposure, which is obtained in this example by retracting the left iliac artery and vein from left to right. In most situations the iliolumbar vein arises from the origin of the left common iliac vein and must be ligated to facilitate the exposure.

> ### LATERAL ENDOSCOPIC FUSION L1 TO L5
>
> - Advantages of retroperitoneal approach
>   - Avoids risk of small bowel obstruction
>   - Potentially reduces risk of retrograde ejaculation
> - Advantages of lateral approach
>   - Easy to place on orthogonally directed cage
>   - Minimal risk of neural injury
>   - Minimal mobilization of great vessels, especially at L4 and L5

> ### LATERAL ENDOSCOPIC FUSION TECHNIQUES L1 TO L5
>
> - Position patient in straight lateral decubitus position on a radiolucent graphite table.
> - Make a 1-cm incision at the anterior portion of the twelfth rib to approach the L1 to L2 disc.
> - Use fluoroscopy below L2 to identify the level of approach.
> - Use a dissecting trocar (Optiview) with 10-mm laparoscope to dissect three muscle layers to retroperitoneal space.
> - Insufflate retroperitoneal space via dissecting balloon or CO_2 insufflation.
> - Place additional trocars after dissecting the peritoneum toward the midline.
> - Reflect sympathetic ganglion in an anterior direction with ureter and great vessels.
> - Split the anterior portion of the psoas to facilitate lateral exposure of disc space.

Between the Artery and Vein

This dissection is much easier than one would think, and it gives excellent exposure with minimal retraction on the iliac artery. The only area of concern arises during the fusion portion of the procedure, where two vessels can be injured instead of just one. Therefore, this approach requires more diligence than the others. In cases of diseased arteries or difficult exposure, this approach is an option that minimizes traction on the left iliac artery. This approach was used 16% of the time in the series reported by Regan et al.[13]

Lateral Endoscopic Fusion L1 to L5

Retroperitoneal lumbar fusion and stabilization offers several advantages over conventional anterior transperitoneal laparoscopic approaches to the lumbar spine. Retroperitoneal approaches obviate the risk of small bowel obstruction. Additionally, there may be reduced risk of retrograde ejaculation compared with that risk with transperitoneal techniques. With the straight lateral position, it is easier to place an orthogonally directed fusion cage rather than one that courses anterior to posterior. There is minimal risk to nerve injury

because the drilling and reaming is directed to the psoas on the opposite side as compared with conventional anterior surgery, where the drilling is directed toward the spinal canal. There is minimal mobilization of the great vessels, especially at the L4 to L5 disc space. The major difficulty in placing a lateral fusion cage is the psoas muscle. The psoas muscle, which contains the lumbosacral nerve plexus, must be split at the lower lumbar levels to provide access for a laterally directed fusion cage. The genitofemoral and ilioinguinal nerves, which lie on the belly of the psoas muscle, must not be stretched during this procedure.

The surgical approach is facilitated with the patient in the straight lateral decubitus position on a radiolucent graphite table. A 1-cm incision is made at the anterior portion of the twelfth rib to approach the L1 to L2 disc space. Below L2, a lateral fluoroscopic image is obtained with a metal marker placed on the patient's back overlying the appropriate disc. A dissecting trocar called an Optiview (Ethicon Endosurgery, Cincinnati, Ohio) is used with a 10-mm laparoscope to dissect through the three muscle layers to the retroperitoneal space. Insufflation of the retroperitoneal space is accomplished using a dissecting balloon or CO_2 insufflation. Additional trocars are

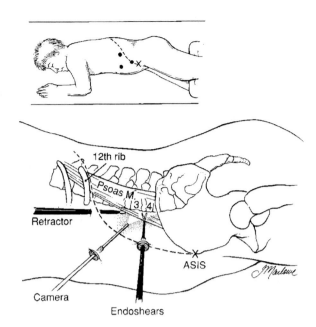

Figure 20-5. This illustration depicts the endoscopic retroperitoneal access for placement of lateral cages at L2 to L3. The patient is placed in the lateral decubitus position. The initial trocar is placed in the midaxillary line just below the twelfth rib. Three additional trocars are placed. One is placed inferior and anterior to the disc space for the camera. A third trocar is placed anterior to the disc space for retraction and suction, and a fourth trocar is placed in the posterior axillary line to retract the psoas muscle.

placed after dissecting the peritoneum toward the midline. Once this space is created, our preference is to continue CO_2 insufflation during the entire case. Manual traction can also be utilized by increasing the size of the incision from 10 mm to 45 cm. The sympathetic ganglion is reflected in an anterior direction with the ureter and great vessels. The anterior portion of the psoas will need to be split to facilitate lateral exposure of the disc space. If a single-level cage fusion is to be done, the segmental vessels can be protected (Figures 20-5 and 20-6).

RESULTS AND COMPLICATIONS

Patient stays following laparoscopic fusion have been dramatically shortened. In the Mahvi and Zdeblick series,[5] the mean hospital stay was 1.7 days, ranging from 0 to 2 days in 20 consecutive patients. Nine of the last 18 patients' surgeries have been performed on an outpatient basis. Operative time averaged 125 minutes (ranging from 70 to 160 minutes). Zdeblick prospectively compared the results of laparoscopic fusion (Group I) with posterolateral fusion with pedicle screws (Group II) and posterior interbody fusion with pedicle fixation (Group III).[15,16] Thirty-nine patients were randomly assigned to these three groups in a prospective randomized protocol for the treatment of L5 to S1 degenerative disc disease. The hospital stay was 1.8 days for Group I, 5 days for Group II, and 5.1 days for Group III. The average

return to work in Groups II and III was 21 weeks and 23 weeks, respectively, compared with 11 weeks for the laparoscopic group. Good to excellent clinical results were reported in 100% of the laparoscopic group compared with 73% for Group II and 91% for Group III.

Hisey et al.[2] reported long-term survivability of threaded fusion devices implanted as stand-alone devices at one or two levels at one medical center by five surgeons. In a retrospective analysis of 190 patients with average follow-up of 33 months (range: 24-61 months) operated on between 1994 and 1997, there were only three cases (1.6%) requiring posterior revision for pseudarthrosis and three cases (1.6%) with cage removal for nerve impingement by cage or displaced disc material. A total of 3.2% required revision surgery at the same level, and six patients (3.2%) had procedures at adjacent levels. There was no statistically significant difference in the revision rate of the laparoscopic group, which consisted of 80 patients (42%), and that of patients who underwent open surgery.

A prospective multimember study evaluating open and laparoscopic lumbar fusion in more than 500 patients was reported by Regan et al.[13] in 1999. There were no major complications (i.e., great vessel damage, pulmonary embolism, implant migration, or death) in the laparoscopic group, which consisted of 215 patients treated by 19 surgeons at 10 medical centers. Preliminary experience indicated a small conversion rate to open surgery resulting from preoperative scarring, bleeding, and poor visualization. Instruments and technique changed from the earliest experience, and no further conversions occurred. Intraoperative disc herniation from reaming and lateral cage placement with nerve irritation requiring posterior surgery was reported in 3.2% of the laparoscopic cases. Postoperative ileus was 4.7%, and incisional hernia did not occur in this group. Retrograde ejaculation occurred in 5.1% of laparoscopic cases, twice the rate of open cases. Most all of these cases occurred early in the series as a result of monopolar cauterization. The elimination of monopolar cautery and use of blunt dissection after incising the peritoneum to the right of the midline has almost eliminated this problem (Table 20-1).

CONCLUSIONS

Minimally invasive spine surgery has experienced significant gains in the past decade, primarily in anterior procedures as a result of laparoscopic surgery. Improvements in camera equipment, navigation systems, and robotics have enhanced this surgical approach. Ultimately, for success with minimally invasive surgery one must show improvements in the quality of the patients' life with less pain, lessened complications, and a faster return to normal activity. Surgical training must keep up with the fast pace of technology advancements if these procedures are to have a broad appeal. At this time the surgical team approach has resulted in success, with reduction of hospital time and a quicker return to work. Progress in spine surgery will come in small steps with the refinement of less-invasive surgical technique making the procedures both safer and more beneficial to patients.

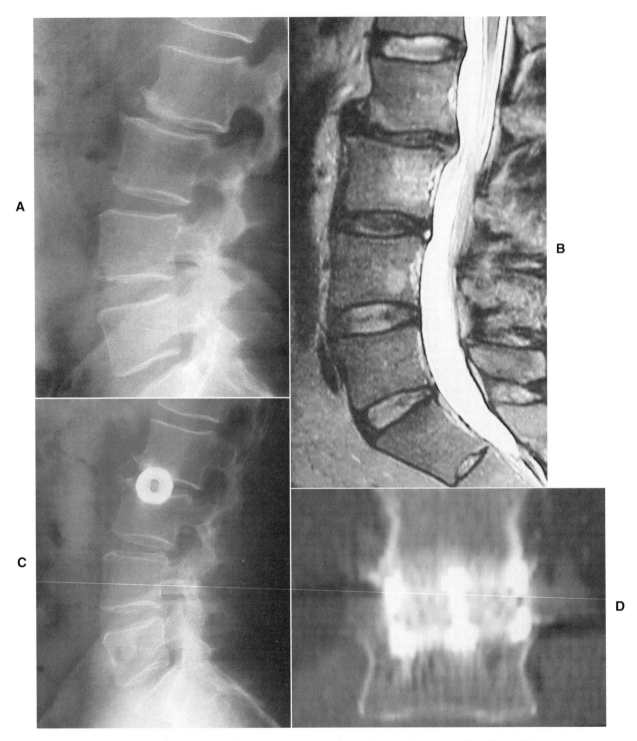

Figure 20-6.   This 45-year-old woman presented with thoracolumbar pain with radiation into the anterior thigh. **A,** Radiographs indicated severe degenerative collapse at L2 to L3 with slight retrolisthesis without significant nerve root compression. **B,** MRI scan confirms disc desiccation and minimal bulge into canal with minimal foraminal stenosis. **C** and **D,** A lateral BAK fusion cage 17 × 36 was placed through a lateral retroperitoneal approach after the appropriate disc preparation was done. CT images obtained 2 years after surgery indicate fusion in and around the fusion cage. The patient had an excellent clinical result with resolution of pain.

Table 20-1	Postoperative Complications for One-Level Cases				
	BAK Open (N = 305)	(%)	BAK Laparoscopic (N = 215)	(%)	P*
Infection	6	2.0	3	1.4	NS
Ileus	10	3.3	10	4.7	NS
Implant migration	4	1.3	1	0.5	NS
Leg pain	2	0.7	1	0.5	NS
Hematoma/seroma	3	1.0	0	0.0	NS
Retrograde ejaculation	7	2.3	11	5.1	NS
Atelectasis/pneumonia	2	0.7	2	0.9	NS
Urologic	3	1.0	0	0.0	NS
Wound dehiscence/incisional hernia	3	1.0	0	0.0	NS
Thrombosis/thrombophlebitis	0	0.0	1	0.5	NS
Disc herniation	0	0.0	6	2.8	0.005
Spondylosis (fractures)	0	0.0	3	1.4	NS
Other	3	1.0	3	1.4	NS
TOTAL	43	14.1	41	19.1	NS

NS, Not significant.
*Fisher exact.

SELECTED REFERENCES

Bagby G: Arthrodesis by the distraction-compression methods using a stainless steel implant, *Orthopedics* 11:931-934, 1988.

Mack MJ et al.: Video assisted thoracic surgery (VATS) for the anterior approach to the thoracic spine, *Ann Thorac Surg* 59:1100-1106, 1995.

McAfee PC et al.: The incidence of complications in endoscopic anterior thoracolumbar spinal reconstructive surgery, *Spine* 20(14):1624-1632, 1995.

McAfee PC et al.: The incidence of complications in endoscopic anterior thoracolumbar spinal reconstructive surgery: a prospective multicenter study comprising the first 100 consecutive cases, *Spine* 20:1624-1632, 1995.

Zucherman JF et al.: Instrumented laparoscopic spinal fusion: preliminary results, *Spine* 20(18):2029-2035, 1995.

REFERENCES

1. Bagby G: Arthrodesis by the distraction-compression methods using a stainless steel implant, *Orthopedics* 11:931-934, 1988.
2. Hisey M et al.: Long term survivability of cages as stand alone devices. Proceedings of the North American Spine Society, Chicago, Oct 1999.
3. Mack MJ et al: Applications of thoracoscopy for diseases of the spine, *Ann Thorac Surg* 56:1100-1106, 1993.
4. Mack MJ et al.: Video assisted thoracic surgery (VATS) for the anterior approach to the thoracic spine, *Ann Thorac Surg* 59:1100-1106, 1995.
5. Mahvi DM, Zdeblick TA: A prospective study of laparoscopic spinal fusion: technique and operative complications, *Ann Surg* 224:85-90, 1996.
6. Mathews HH et al.: Laparoscopic discectomy with anterior lumbar interbody fusion, *Spine* 20(16):1791-1802, 1995.
7. McAfee PC et al.: The incidence of complications in endoscopic anterior thoracolumbar spinal reconstructive surgery, *Spine* 20(14):1624-1632, 1995.
8. Modic MT et al.: Degenerative disc disease: assessment of changes in vertebral marrow, *Radiology* 166:193-199, 1988.
9. Obenchain TG: Laparoscopic lumbar discectomy: a case report, *J Laparoendosc Surg* 1:145-149, 1991.
10. Regan JJ, Mack M, Picetti G: A technical report on video assisted thoracoscopy in thoracic spine surgery, *Spine* 20(7):831-837, 1995.
11. Regan JJ, Mack M, Picetti G: A technical report on video assisted thoracoscopy in thoracic spinal surgery: preliminary description, *Spine* 20:831-837, 1995.
12. Regan JJ, McAfee PC, Mack MJ: *Atlas of endoscopic spine surgery*, St. Louis, 1995, Quality Medical Publishing.
13. Regan JJ, Yuan H, McCullen G: Minimally invasive approaches to the spine, *Instr Course Lect* 46:127-141, 1997.
14. Regan JJ, Yuan H, McAfee PC: Laparoscopic fusion of the lumbar spine: minimally invasive spine surgery, *Spine* 24(4):402-411, 1999.
15. Zdeblick TA: A prospective randomized study of lumbar fusion: preliminary results, *Spine* 18(8):983-991, 1993.
16. Zdeblick TA: A prospective randomized study of the surgical treatment of L5-S1 degenerative disc disease. Presented at the Tenth Annual Meeting of the North American Spine Society, Washington, DC, Oct. 20, 1995.
17. Zucherman JF et al.: Instrumented laparoscopic spinal fusion: preliminary results, *Spine* 20(18):2029-2035, 1995.

Minimally Invasive Approaches to the Lumbar Spine

Alexander R. Vaccaro, Kern Singh,
John S. Thalgott, Jim Giuffre, John J. Regan

Endoscopic techniques have been successfully used in many surgical specialties to access anatomic structures, to excise pathology, and to repair dysfunction. Minimally invasive techniques potentially reduce the cost and length of hospitalization, as well as the amount of iatrogenic trauma to the patient. They also allow for earlier return to normal activities for those being treated. Only recently have great strides been made in the application of minimally invasive techniques to spinal surgery. The use of endoscopes in transperitoneal and retroperitoneal approaches to the lumbar spine is an expanding discipline well performed by only a few specialists.

TRANSPERITONEAL APPROACH

The minimally invasive transperitoneal approach to the lumbar spine has been successfully employed most frequently to access the L5 to S1 disc space from a direct anterior route. Preparation before surgery is important, and routine mechanical large bowel preps are a necessity. Having the sigmoid colon evacuated is extremely important to ensure adequate exposure of the retroperitoneal space. A small incision is made at the umbilicus, and an insufflator needle is inserted, distending the abdominal cavity with a pressure of approximately 15 mm Hg. The initial port for the endoscope is placed 5 to 10 cm cephalad of the umbilicus in the midline 10 mm. Alternatively, a periumbilical port may be used. The patient is then placed into a steep Trendelenburg position. The abdominal wall is visualized endoscopically and two working portals are placed just lateral to the epigastric vessels, opposite the level or levels to be fused. It is advantageous to stagger the portals slightly from direct opposition to each other. Retractors are inserted through these ports, sweeping the small bowel superiorly out of the pelvis. The sigmoid colon is pulled out of the pelvis and held laterally with the left fan retractor (Figure 21-1).

The posterior peritoneum overlying the L5 to S1 disc space is incised longitudinally with endoshears for the desired exposure. Using opposing fan retractors as blunt dissectors, the surgeon sweeps the soft tissue underlying the parietal peritoneum, laterally exposing the anterior annulus of the intervertebral disc. This usually exposes the sacral artery and vein, which can then be individually ligated with hemoclips. If additional working portals are necessary for exposure, a 5-mm midline port can be placed for the suction irrigation catheter. The lumbar sympathetics should be protected by gentle blunt dissection. If necessary, only bipolar cautery should be used at a minimum. Monopolar cautery should never be used due to the risk of retrograde ejaculation. One should also avoid dissection of the adventitial tissue anterior to the left common iliac vein and artery.

For the L4 to L5 level, the posterior peritoneum is incised 3 cm more proximal than the L5 to S1 level. The left fan retractor is used to retract the colon laterally. Careful blunt dissection with a Kitner is used to expose the aorta anteriorly at the bifurcation. The L4 to L5 disc is usually right below this point. Left lateral dissection is done next to the left common iliac vein and artery, gently retracting these vessels to the right. At this point, if the patient is hyperextended, the legs may need to be straightened and the lumbar roll removed. Otherwise, the vessels may be stretched over the spine, making ligation difficult. Once the disc is exposed, it is necessary to align the abdominal entry operating trocar portal site such that the operating trocar is parallel to the

THREE-PORTAL TECHNIQUE

- Endoscopic portal: 5 to 10 mm cephalad to umbilicus in the midline
- Two working portals: Place endoscopically just lateral to the epigastric vessels
- Advantageous to stagger portals slightly from direct opposition

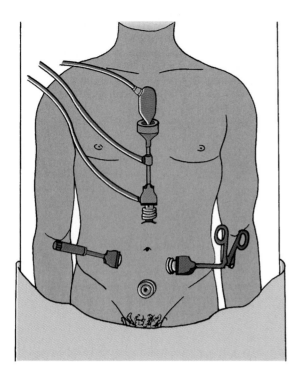

Figure 21-1. Anterior view of abdomen. The endoscope is positioned through a supraumbilical port. Endoshears and endodissector or retractor are inserted through the right and left lower quadrants.

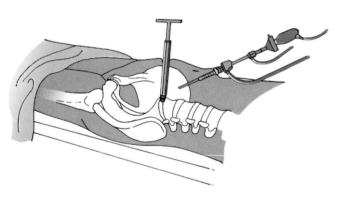

Figure 21-2. Lateral view of abdomen. The camera is directed toward the L5 to S1 disc while a protective operating trocar is placed in the disc space.

end- plates of the disc in the sagittal plane. The entry point is estimated, and a small Steinmann pin is placed in the interspace and is verified with fluoroscopy. A 1.5- to 2.5-cm incision is made for placement of the operating trocar. The blunt introducer is placed over it under endoscopic visualization (Figure 21-2).

RETROPERITONEAL APPROACH IN THE LATERAL POSITION

The lateral position offers several distinct advantages over the supine position used in the direct anterior transperitoneal approach to the spine. In the lateral decubitus position, the intra-abdominal contents fall

---

ADVANTAGES AND DISADVANTAGES OF LATERAL APPROACH

ADVANTAGES
• Intraabdominal organs fall away from operative field
• Reduced risk of retrograde ejaculation
• Easier to place instrumentation orthogonally to disc space
• Able to correct lordosis and small degrees of scoliosis
• Disc space preparation and instrumentation directed away from canal

DISADVANTAGES
• Exposure of L4 to L5 disc space may require removal of part of the iliac crest
• Prolonged retraction may cause genitofemoral neuropraxia

---

anteriorly away from the spine, facilitating exposure. The lateral approach to the disc space minimizes retraction of the great vessels and in cases of single level fusion, the segmental vessels and sympathetic plexus can be spared, thereby reducing the risk of retrograde ejaculation. It is also easier to get orthogonal to the disc space and spine with laterally directed placement of interbody threaded fusion cages. The surgeon can also "dial in" the lordosis by using a drill tube with lordosis-producing paddles. Small degrees of scoliosis can also be corrected with distraction plugs. With the lateral approach, the disc space preparation and cage insertion are directed toward the contralateral psoas muscle rather than the spinal canal as in the transperitoneal approach.

There are also several potential disadvantages of the lateral approach. Particularly at the L4 to L5 level, it may be necessary to remove part of the iliac crest or place the docking portal through the iliac wing in order to be orthogonal to the L4 to L5 disc space. In addition, a large psoas muscle containing the lumbosacral roots may need to be mobilized laterally. Prolonged retraction may cause neuropraxia of the genitofemoral nerve. Ultimately, the surgeon must decide if this approach is preferable to the transperitoneal approach to L4 to L5, which requires mobilization of the left iliac artery and vein.

Technique

The patient is placed in a lateral decubitus position on a radiolucent Jackson table (Figure 21-3). A 1-cm incision is made at the anterior portion of the twelfth rib for approaching from L1 or L2. Below L2, a lateral C-arm fluoroscopic image is obtained with a metal marker overlying the skin of the patient in the midaxillary line. This method optimizes the placement of the working portal directly over the unstable disc or vertebral segment.

Three techniques are used to dissect the retroperitoneal space: finger dissection, balloon insufflation, or the use of an optical, transparent dissecting trocar. If a trocar is selected, following the skin incision, the trocar

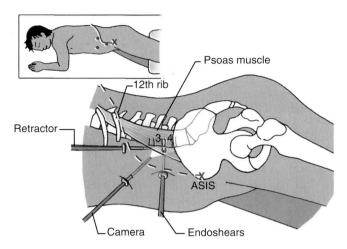

Figure 21-3. Schematic diagram for the lateral position. *X* marks the anterior superior iliac spine, and the three portals are shown in the insert *(black dots)*.

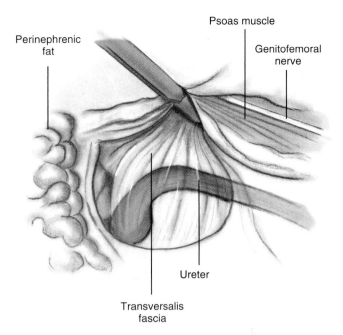

Figure 21-4. Schematic diagram depicting the laparoscopic view through the transversalis fascia at the L3 to L4 intervertebral disc.

is used to penetrate down to the level of the abdominal muscular layer. A 10-mm laparoscope is then inserted into the dissecting trocar and refocused once the trocar enters the subcutaneous tissue. The three abdominal muscular layers overlying the peritoneum are penetrated in sequence under direct visualization until the preperitoneal fat is encountered. The trocar is used to create a potential space that is superficial to the peritoneum until the laterally oriented fibers of the psoas major muscle are visualized. If desired by the surgeon, carbon dioxide (CO_2) insufflation can be forced into the retroperitoneal cavity up to a pressure of 20 mm Hg to create a working space for triangulation.

Three secondary trocars are placed after the peritoneum is dissected away from the anterior abdominal wall. The endoscope is inserted into the anterior inferior site. An anterior superior site is used for exposing the lumbar spine and it serves as a portal for delivery of pituitary rongeurs, curets, a high-powered bur, as well as a Kerrison punch. A posterior portal is used for retraction of the psoas muscle. The ureter, aorta, and vena cava are identified and are dissected anterior to the spine. Retraction of these structures is not necessary. The sympathetic plexus can be mobilized anteriorly and the anterior portion of the psoas muscle is split if necessary to access the lateral aspect of the disc space. The genitofemoral nerve is identified on the surface of the psoas, and retraction is avoided to prevent neuropraxia, which will result in dysesthesia of the anterior thigh and groin. Segmental vessels can be protected when a drill tube is used for lateral cage placement at the disc space (Figure 21-4). Long distraction plugs produce symmetric distraction and will correct a minor degenerative scoliosis. They can also be used as an anterior step in the correction of a kyphotic deformity. Occasionally, a fourth 10-mm portal is used for suctioning in highly vascular cases requiring corpectomies for tumors or infections. Additionally, for longer strut grafts or instrumentation, the 10-mm working portal may be extended in size to as much as 5 cm.

TROCAR PLACEMENT AND APPROPRIATE USAGE

- Anterior inferior: Endoscope
- Anterior superior: Pituitary rongeur, curet, high-powered bur, Kerrison punch
- Posterior: Retractor for the psoas muscle
- Optional fourth portal: Suction

THE BALLOON-ASSISTED RETROGRADE (BERG) APPROACH

Given the limitations of reliable direct anterior access to L4 to L5 and above, the gas-mediated transperitoneal endoscopic approach is somewhat inadequate for the treatment of a wide variety of patients in need of anterior lumbar reconstruction. In addition, CO_2 insufflation of the abdomen can present a number of complications. These include but are not limited to hypercarbia, the inability to use adequate suction, loss of operative exposure due to loss of the pneumoperitoneum, the inability to perform large tissue removal, limited access for large instruments, and spatial constraints with regard to bone grafts or devices. A gasless approach eliminates these roadblocks to anterior lumbar surgery and allows for the use of standard anterior instruments normally reserved for an open approach.

The retroperitoneal approach allows consistent and safe access of the anterior lumbar spine from L5-S1 up to L1 to L2.

LIMITATIONS

TRANSPERITONEAL APPROACH
- Gas-mediated approach
- Problems with suction removing CO_2
- Difficult bowel retraction
- Instrumentation limited to specificity of valved ports

GAS-MEDIATED APPROACH
- Unable to address large discs successfully
- Unable to totally remove disc and end plate
- Unable to use standard instrumentation
- Unable to do multiple levels consistently
- Unable to access retroperitoneum
- Dictates transperitoneal approach
- Unable to instrument with plates, screws, rods
- Limits implant choice to cylindrical cages

BERG APPROACH

BENEFITS
- Gasless: No pneumoperitoneum to maintain vertebral exposure
- Reliable access from L2 to S1 and L1 in most cases
- Ability to use instruments and implants normally reserved for open anterior procedures
- Ability to perform vertebrectomies and reconstruction

INDICATIONS
- Degenerative disease of the spine
- One to three affected levels between L1 and S2 as a method of performing anterior lumbar reconstructive surgery

RELATIVE CONTRAINDICATIONS
- Obesity
- Prior left-sided abdominal surgery
- Prior grafting of major abdominal vessels
- Prior retroperitoneal approach to the spine

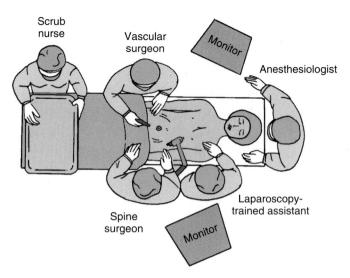

Figure 21-5. The operating room setup for the BERG approach.

TECHNIQUE

- Presence of access surgeon, spine surgeon, technicians.
- Use supine position.
- Make 2-mm left flank incision above the iliac crest and perform balloon dissection.
- Use anterior working/retraction port fashioned lateral to rectus sheath.
- Using fan retractor and mechanical lifting arm, distend abdomen.
- With "helping hand" retractor, push peritoneal sac to right side.
- Difficult learning curve, especially for those not already trained in endoscopic procedures.

SURGICAL TECHNIQUE

The surgical team setup consists of one spine surgeon, one general/vascular surgeon, one endoscopically trained technician, and one surgical technician (Figure 21-5). A well-trained general/vascular surgeon is recommended when selecting this approach. Such advanced training is extremely invaluable if an inadvertent vessel laceration occurs during the case.

The patient is placed in the supine position and draped and prepped in the standard fashion. The appropriate surgical levels are identified with fluoroscopy. The skin is marked, identifying the angle of the disc spaces to be addressed. An initial 2-cm transverse incision is made in the left flank just above the iliac crest in the midaxillary line. Dissection is performed via a Visiport (U.S. Surgical, Norwalk, Conn.) trocar under direct endoscopic vision through the abdominal muscles and the peritoneal fat layer. Great care should be taken not to tear the peritoneum. A deflated balloon-dissector is then introduced through the initial incision. A 0-degree endoscope is placed through a cannula attached to the balloon and the balloon is inflated under direct vision to a volume of approximately 1 liter. As the balloon inflates, it moves the peritoneum off the abdominal wall.

Once the balloon is completely inflated, the peritoneal reflection at the rectus sheath is identified. The anterior working/retraction portal is created with a 2- to 3-cm paramedian incision lateral to the peritoneal reflection and in line with the preoperative skin markings. The balloon is removed and replaced by a flexible, nonvalved port. A fan retractor is introduced into the same left flank incision but *above* the nonvalved port. The fan retractor is attached to a mechanical lifting arm. The arm/retractor combination is lifted, distending the abdominal wall, thereby creating the operative space, without the use of gas insufflation (Figure 21-6). A malleable, long-handled, "helping hand" retractor with an inflatable end is introduced through the port. Following inflation, the retractor is used to push the peritoneal contents to the right side, clearing access to the anterior lumbar spine.

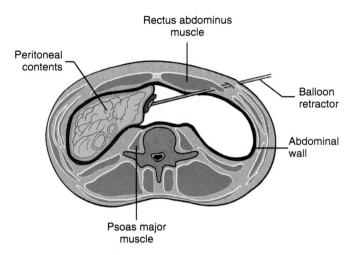

Figure 21-6. Retraction of the peritoneal sac with the aid of the "helping hand" retractor.

The anterior working/retraction port is used for vessel and soft tissue retraction, as well as access for anterior working instruments such as end-plate cutters, curets, rongeurs, and osteotomes. Instruments for vessel retraction may be placed through the left flank port, which is also the entry port for the endoscope. The psoas muscle is bluntly dissected off the anterior lateral lumbar spine, allowing direct access for the intended spinal procedure.

As with any type of anterior lumbar surgery, a key component to success is vessel management. L5 to S1 vessel retraction is performed by mobilizing the iliac veins and by retracting the fascia and presacral veins (Figure 21-7). Retraction of the vessels at L4 to L5 is more complex. The vena cava and/or left iliac vein is retracted and placed on tension. The iliolumbar vein is identified and ligated using vascular clips (Figure 21-8). L3 to L4 vessel retraction is performed similarly to that for L4 to L5 but without the need to ligate the iliolumbar vein.

The intended levels to be operated on are verified with fluoroscopy following vessel retraction. Once the correct levels have been identified and abdominal, peritoneal, and vascular retractors are in place, a discectomy is performed in the standard fashion. Following a complete discectomy and end-plate preparation, subsequent interbody space reconstruction can then proceed. Unlike the gas-mediated transperitoneal approach, the BERG approach does not limit the size of the implant the surgeon may use.

Following placement of the graft or cage, the implant position is verified by fluoroscopy and the incisions are closed in the standard fashion. Should posterior instrumentation and fusion be indicated, the patient may now be placed in the prone position for the subsequent procedure.

CONCLUSIONS

The BERG approach is safe and effective for accessing the lumbar spine; however, the learning curve can be arduous. It allows for reliable access up to L2 and in many cases L1. Standard anterior instruments can be

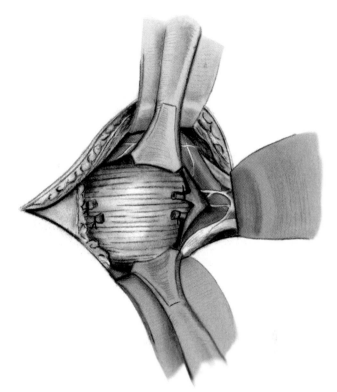

Figure 21-7. Retraction of the vessels at L5 to S1.

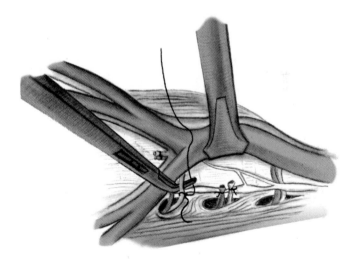

Figure 21-8. Retraction of the vessels at L4 to L5 with ligation of the iliolumbar vein.

used for the discectomy and there is no limitation on implant size. Hospital stays are short and blood loss is minimal.

DISCUSSION

Retroperitoneal approaches to the lumbar spine offer several distinct advantages over the traditional transperitoneal approach. These advantages include the prevention or decrease in the incidence of intraperitoneal adhesions and the potential for small bowel obstructions.

POTENTIAL COMPLICATIONS

VASCULAR
- Vessel laceration with blood loss
- Venous thrombosis
- Pulmonary embolus
- Arterial thrombosis
- Arterial thromboembolism

BOWEL/BLADDER
- Bowel injury
- Ileus/atelectasis
- Bowel ischemia
- Bladder incontinence
- Bladder obstruction

WOUND/NEUROLOGIC
- Hematoma
- Infection (superficial and deep)
- Hernia
- Dyskinesis
- Reflex sympathetic dystrophy
- Retrograde ejaculation
- Impotence

DOCUMENTATION IN LITERATURE

50-PATIENT SERIES WITH 2-YEAR FOLLOW-UP*
- Mean operative time, 1-level: 125 min
- Mean operative time, 2-level: 151 min
- Mean hospital stay: 2.02 days
- Mean anterior blood loss: 155 ml
- Fusion rate (anterior/posterior): 93.3%
- Good/excellent clinical outcome: 75.5%
- Return to work: 47%
- Mean return to work time: 3.3 mo private, 10 mo industrial

Perioperative Complications
- Vessel laceration: 1
- Conversions to open procedure: 0

Postoperative Complications: None

202-PATIENT SERIES WITH LIMITED FOLLOW-UP†
- Mean operative time, 1-level: 101 min
- Mean operative time, 2-level: 129 min
- Mean hospital stay: 1.95 days
- Mean anterior blood loss: 201 ml

Perioperative Complications
- Requiring conversion: 34
  - Vessel laceration: 15
  - Retroperitoneal scarring: 8
  - Obesity: 5
  - Nerve lying on disc space: 2
  - Inadequate bowel retraction: 2
  - Thin peritoneum: 2
- Not requiring conversion
  - Vessel laceration (fixed endoscopically): 6
  - Ruptured diverticulum: 1

Conversion Rate
- First 101 cases: 24%
- Second 101 cases: 10%

Postoperative Complications
- Retrograde ejaculation: 1
- Deep venous thrombosis: 1

*Thalgott JS et al.: *Eur Spine J* 9(S1):551-556, 2000.
†Thalgott JS et al.: *Surg Endosc* 14:546-552, 2000.

Additionally, there is a reduced risk of retrograde ejaculation because the autonomic plexus in not dissected. With the patient in the lateral position, gravity helps to retract the abdominal contents away from the operative site. Furthermore, it is easier to get orthogonal to the disc space and vertebral body in the lateral position. Dissection also does not involve violating the anterior longitudinal and posterior longitudinal ligaments. With the lateral retroperitoneal approach, drilling, reaming, tapping, and cage insertion are directed toward the contralateral psoas muscle instead of the spinal canal.

There are several potential disadvantages of the minimally invasive, retroperitoneal approach. The most obvious disadvantage is the learning curve associated with performing these procedures both for the spine surgeon and the general surgeon. Particularly at L4 to L5, it may be necessary to remove part of the iliac crest or place the docking portal through the iliac wing to be orthogonal to the L4 to L5 disc space. In addition, a large portion of the psoas muscle containing the lumbosacral nerve roots may need to be mobilized laterally.

Both the BERG approach and the straight lateral approach through the psoas muscle have the advantage of not relying on any gas insufflation. CO_2 insufflation can cause significant physiologic and hemodynamic changes. In addition, the gaseous environment does not allow for large tissue removal or large instrument access to the spinal column. Suctioning to remove blood is limited because it also removes CO_2 from the abdomen, leading to the loss of exposure. When the surgeon is using gas insufflation, valved ports are required, placing the instrument fulcrum far away from the operative field and making the operation more difficult. The gasless environment does not limit the size or number of standard anterior instruments or implants that may be used.

SELECTED REFERENCES

Henry LG et al.: Laparoscopically assisted spinal surgery, *J Soc Laroensoc Surg* 1:341-344, 1997.

Mathews HH et al.: Laparoscopic discectomy with anterior lumbar interbody fusion: a preliminary review, *Spine* 20:1797-1802, 1995.

McAfee PC et al.: Minimally invasive anterior retroperitoneal approach to the lumbar spine: emphasis on the lateral BAK, *Spine* 23:1476-1484, 1998.

McAfee PC et al.: The incidence of complications in endoscopic anterior thoracolumbar spinal reconstructive surgery: a prospective multicenter study comprising the first 100 cases, *Spine* 20:1624-1632, 1995.

Obenchain TG: Laparoscopic lumbar discectomy: a case report, *J Laparoendosc Surg* 1:145-149, 1991.

Olsen D, McCord D, Law M: Laparoscopic discectomy and anterior interbody fusion of L5-S1, *Surg Endosc* 10:1158-1163, 1996.

Regan JJ, Yuan H, McAfee PC: Laparascopic fusion of the lumbar spine: minimally invasive spine surgery: a prospective multicenter study evaluation of open and laparoscopic lumbar fusion, *Spine* 24:402-411, 1999.

Slotman GJ, Stein SC: Laparascopic lumbar discectomy: preliminary report of a minimally invasive anterior approach to the herniated L5-S1 disc, *Surg Laparosc Endosc* 5:363-369, 1995.

Thalgott JS et al.: Gasless endoscopic anterior lumbar interbody fusion utilizing the B.E.R.G. approach, *Surg Endosc* 14:546-552, 2000.

Thalgott JS et al.: Minimally invasive 360 degrees instrumented lumbar fusion, *Eur Spine J* 9(S1):S51-S56, 2000.

Zelko JR et al.: Laparoscopic lumbar discectomy, *Am J Surg* 169:496-498, 1995.

Zucherman J et al.: Instrumented laparoscopic spinal fusion: preliminary results, *Spine* 20:2029-2035, 1995.

Posterior Minimally Invasive Techniques

Hallett H. Mathews, Brenda H. Long

Throughout the historical evolution of spine surgery, the goal has been to develop tools and techniques to address the broadest range of spinal pathology while minimizing surgical morbidity. In recent decades, great strides have been made in ongoing efforts to achieve this goal. Improved imaging and fiberoptic technology have led to a better understanding of both spinal anatomy and pathology. A succession of techniques has targeted pathology, particularly for the herniated lumbar nucleus pulposus. The application of these techniques has fostered increasingly refined patient selection criteria and surgical contraindications. Innovative techniques, associated tools, and technology have built one upon the other to create a surgical armamentarium designed for selective techniques for a variety of pathologic presentations. Advancements in minimally invasive spine surgery are a sustained "work in progress."

The evolution of surgery for the herniated nucleus pulposus in the lumbar spine has spanned years of various focus and controversy. The focus has ranged from refining patient selection for decompressive procedures to visually targeting the pathology and anatomic structures at risk. Contemporary methods, spurred by continued refinement of techniques and instrumentation, make minimally invasive spine surgery the mantra for this millennium. This process has always had a sustained goal: to surgically address the herniated disc with the least amount of morbidity, limiting the paradoxic surgical effects of segmental destabilization and postoperative scarring.

Removal of a herniated lumbar disc was first described in the United States by Dandy in 1929.[8] Minimally invasive techniques, however, began with percutaneous methods. Chemonucleolysis, the only minimally invasive method validated by numerous cohort[3,37,38] and three double-blind studies,[7,12,13,18] is the benchmark for comparison purposes. Percutaneous nucleotomy, automated percutaneous nucleotomy, and laser disc decompression, although still being utilized on a limited basis, have fallen from favor because they could not match the success and visualization afforded by the traditional procedure. Their success depended on very rigid patient selection that was difficult to adhere to because of the inadequacies of traditional imaging

> ### MINIMALLY INVASIVE SPINE SURGERY
>
> - Goal: To surgically address the herniated nucleus pulposus with least morbidity.
> - Early reports and techniques include chemonucleolysis, percutaneous manual/automated nucleotomy, laser disc decompression.
> - Now less favored due to lack of operative visualization, rigid selection criteria, and inadequacies of imaging studies.
> - Evolution of endoscopic percutaneous procedures has provided for refined visualization as a basis for contemporary minimally invasive techniques.

studies, the inability to clearly visualize the pathology, and the tendency for clinicians to stretch surgical indications. Endoscopic percutaneous nucleotomy and discoscopy address the visualization obstacle and now provide the basis for endoscopic techniques that remain viable in contemporary minimally invasive methods.

The philosophy for perpetual investigation into improved percutaneous surgical options and tools has been well stated by Mayer and Brock. They propose that:

> . . . reducing lumbar disc surgery to a mere "nerve root decompression procedure" falls short of the standards set by modern surgical philosophy, since failure not only arises from persisting or recurring neurological symptoms but also from anatomical and biomechanical disturbances caused by the surgical approach itself.[35]

The principal objective of this chapter will be to examine the current minimally invasive surgical techniques for herniated lumbar discs. New percutaneous procedures to address compression fractures in the thoracic and lumbar spine warrant mention because they utilize many of the same surgical skills as endoscopic discectomy.

EPIDEMIOLOGY

Back pain and sciatica represent a tremendous challenge to health care delivery systems. They also affect

---

LOW BACK PAIN EFFECTS

- Effects of low back pain and sciatica on workforce include lost time and expense
- Lost work time: 149.1 million days (1988)
- Cost of low back pain disorders: $25 billion to $85 billion (1990)
- Account for one fourth of workers' compensation claims (1995)

PATHOPHYSIOLOGY OF LOW BACK PAIN AND RADICULOPATHY

- Histochemical factors
- Compression of nerve root nociceptors
- Herniated nucleus pulposus (HNP) with annular tear: Leakage of products of nuclear degradation with nerve root inflammatory response
- Phospholipase A_2 and nitric oxide from free fragments—noxious effects on nerve rootlets
- HNP promotes increase of matrix metalloproteinase, nitric acid, prostaglandin E_2, and interleukin-6
- Free glutamate in HNP may affect dorsal root ganglion

---

the workforce in lost time and direct expenses. In 1997 Schwartz and Schafer reported that "up to 80% of the population of industrialized nations at some point complain of low back pain."[41] In 1988 22.4 million cases of low back pain resulted in lost work time of 149.1 million days. The report citing these statistics further notes that in the United States about one fourth of workers' compensation claims can be attributed to back pain.[15] Relative to the cost of low back pain in the United States, Frymoyer reported that in 1990 the cost of low back disorders ranged from $25 billion to $85 billion.[10] A 1998 report by Argoff and Sheeler quantified spine and radicular pain. Both generated economic costs and disability of epidemic proportions.[1] Although these reports do not subdivide causes to diagnostic subcategories such as herniated disc, degenerative disc disease, instability, or stenosis, they still provide statistical information relative to the ever-increasing scope of spinal disorders affecting patients in search of definitive and efficacious intervention.

Management strategies must be based on a comprehensive holistic approach in the evaluation of every patient. Variables include a well-defined pathology, a previous spine history (conservative and/or operative), and general health status. Psychosocial factors, compensation, litigation, and pain control issues must also be factored into the equation. In the well-selected patient, minimally invasive spine surgery for herniated disc pathology offers a less traumatic intervention that is likely to be of lesser cost, taking into consideration outpatient hospitalization and reduction in recovery costs associated with pain medication, in-home assistance, and rehabilitation. A timely return to work and recreational activities results in increased satisfaction in patients with a more realistic outlook on their spinal condition.

PATHOPHYSIOLOGY

The pathophysiology of low back pain with associated radiculopathy is a discovery in progress. Simple compression of nerve root nociceptors may generate radicular pain.[17] In the presence of an annular tear associated with a herniated nucleus pulposus, leakage of products of nuclear degradation may initiate an inflammatory response at the nerve root as an initiator of radiculopathy.[39] The release of phospholipase A_2 and nitric oxide has been demonstrated to be induced by free fragments yielding noxious effects on the posterior root and its extension.[26]

Herniated discs have been noted to promote an increase in matrix metalloproteinase, nitric acid, prostaglandin E_2, and interleukin 6, which have been postulated as being involved in disc degeneration and radiculopathy.[25] Quite recently, it has been observed that free glutamate exists in the herniated disc and may have an impact on the dorsal root ganglion relative to radicular pain.[16]

Ongoing investigation seeks to succinctly explain the etiology of radiculopathy associated with herniated nuclear pathology. This summary does not begin to address all of the possible pathophysiologic and histochemical factors but aims to present some of the most recent findings that may contribute to the ultimate understanding of radiculopathy associated with disc herniations and allow for expanded options for treatment beyond just the removal of compressive nuclear pathology.

DIAGNOSTIC IMAGING

Magnetic resonance imaging (MRI) is probably the best single study for the radiologic diagnosis of the herniated disc, although computed tomography (CT) is still the most used worldwide. MRI provides information on disc location and deformation and can identify free or sequestered fragments, as well as annular tears, represented by a high-intensity zone.[52]

Discography, although controversial, may provide a relevant adjunctive study in the hands of physicians who know how to use it. When there are multiple bulges and/or herniations, pain provocation at the time of the study can identify the pain generator(s) to which surgical intervention should be directed. If followed by CT, details relative to annular fissures or tears can further contribute to the surgical planning. Discography will give additional information on annular tears not detected by MRI. Discography therefore is believed by some proponents of minimally invasive spine surgery to be an integral part of endoscopic spine procedures.[27,30,34,43,50]

Myelography with CT is usually reserved for morbidly obese patients that the average MRI scanner cannot support or for older patients with suspected stenosis or osteophytes in addition to disc herniation.

An important factor in diagnostic imaging is the surgeon's ability to interpret imaging studies. Whereas

---

IMAGING STUDIES

- MRI best study for herniated nucleus pulposus diagnosis
- CT still most used worldwide
- Discography: Relevant adjunctive study
- Discography/CT scan for annular pathology
- Myelography/CT: Age, co-pathology
- Important factors
  - Surgeon ability to interpret own studies
  - Images in operative suite
  - Imaging: A tool that can correlate pain with pathology

CONSERVATIVE CARE

- Contraindications to conservative care
  - Acute herniated nucleus pulposus with significant and progressive neurologic deficit
  - Cauda equina syndrome
- Trial of conservative care imperative because significant percentage of symptomatic disc herniations resolve conservatively

---

GENERALLY ACCEPTED PATIENT SELECTION CRITERIA FOR MOST PERCUTANEOUS LUMBAR PROCEDURES

- Symptoms
  - Leg pain greater than back pain
  - Positive straight leg raise test
- Imaging studies correlating symptoms
- Failure of conservative care
- Preferred: Previously nonoperated disc pathology

---

be conservatively resolved with selected modalities and a "tincture of time." The experience of a surgeon with specific herniation types and clinical presentations at times warrants shortening the conservative treatment period, especially with the newer minimally invasive techniques that limit the paradoxic effects of surgical intervention.

PATIENT SELECTION: A GENERAL OVERVIEW

Although there may be unique selection criteria for some of the newer endoscopic procedures, the procedure chosen depends heavily on the endoscopic surgeon's experience and success with each herniation type.

Patients typically have greater leg pain than back pain. Symptoms are usually reported to have been present for 3 to 6 weeks. Positive straight leg raising is a common physical finding, and a significant percentage of patients can pinpoint the initiating event such as a workers' compensation injury, an accident such as a fall or a motor vehicle accident, or any activity of daily living recreation during which the patient describes hearing and/or sensing a "pop" with acute onset of symptoms. Description of radicular symptoms may range from frank pain to other neuropathic symptoms such as numbness, tingling, burning, aching, or weakness. There may be diminished sensation to light touch or pinpricks and pseudoclaudication that imaging studies may or may not detect. Lateral recess stenosis, inflammatory nerve irritation from annular tears, and relative canal compromise are extremely difficult to detect by traditional imaging studies.

In most procedures, previously nonoperated disc pathology is preferred with regard to optimum surgical outcome and patient satisfaction. Previous surgery, by virtue of its effect on neural tethering and segmental stability, may decrease the degree of satisfaction described by the patient when evaluating the efficacy of these percutaneous procedures. Confronted with extrusion of disc material and potential free fragments that may have migrated and become sequestered, these can be addressed only by the most experienced endoscopic surgeons. The same is true for the size of the herniation and the degree of canal compromise.

The location of the herniation and associated pathologies may dictate the ideal percutaneous approach. It is therefore appropriate at this point to

most radiologists review a broad range of radiologic tests on any given day, the seasoned spine surgeon develops an eye for subtle pathology. Therefore it is essential that the spine surgeon interpret his or her own studies in the patient evaluation process. Never should a surgical plan be pursued based on a radiology paper report. Of the utmost importance is that the diagnostic images themselves be present in the operative suite at the time of surgery for the surgeon's review. Imaging studies are relevant to surgical planning because they present a tool that can correlate pain with the pathology that is being addressed.

CONSERVATIVE CARE

In a managed care environment, conservative care has become defined by time and by an ever-lengthening list of required conservative treatment regimens. Because the indications for minimally invasive disc surgery often serve as a bridge between conservative and traditional surgical treatment, controversy can result when authorization is needed from the insurer.

It is almost universally expected that the patient's symptoms and conservative treatment must be present for a minimum of 6 weeks before consideration for surgical intervention. Certainly there are instances in which conservative care is not indicated and may in fact endanger the patient. An example of such a circumstance could be an acute herniation with significant canal compromise in the presence of a cauda equina syndrome.

Nevertheless, a trial of conservative care is always preferred in the majority of patients because a significant percentage of symptomatic disc herniations can

proceed to a description of contemporary posterior percutaneous techniques. Attention will be given to unique patient selection criteria and associated indications and contraindications to surgical intervention.

SURGICAL PREPARATION

As with any new procedure, informed consent should be thorough and clearly spelled out. Because patients are often attracted to the concept of minimally invasive procedures, it is imperative that the indications, outcomes, and treatment options available, as well as the risks, are specifically addressed with each patient. When surgeons educate their patients about the entire process from diagnosis to recovery, the informed patients gain confidence in their surgeon and are willing and active participants in their recovery.

SURGICAL TECHNIQUES
Arthroscopic Microdiscectomy

Arthroscopic microdiscectomy was introduced in the United States by Dr. Parviz Kambin, with reports of the technique dating back to the early 1980s.[23] This technique is the backbone of newer systems that build on the concept of visualization.

Patient selection features the generally accepted indications, including conservative care failure, leg pain greater than back pain, evidence of neurologic deficits, and correlation with imaging studies. Contraindications

as determined by Kambin are fairly universally acknowledged: low back pain only, cauda equina syndrome, disc recurrence, and the likelihood of scar interfering with the approach and setting up the potential for dural insults. Other contraindications include severe ligamentous or bony stenosis, multilevel degenerative disc disease, and anatomic barriers to the L5 to S1 disc, albeit the latter is a relative contraindication. Newer advanced techniques are designed to overcome some of these contraindications and make them "relative," limited only by the endoscopic surgeon's ability and experience.

Arthroscopic microdiscectomy is performed either uniportally or biportally (Figure 22-1), depending on the offending pathology. The uniportal approach is indicated for paramedian and small central discs. Additional acceptable targets are foraminal and extraforaminal herniations. Large central herniations and subligamentous or extraligamentous sequestered herniations are best addressed with a biportal approach allowing continuous visualization.

The surgical technique for intradiscal work begins with a posterolateral approach approximately 9 to 12 cm off the midline. Slight lateralization of the approach may be necessary to access foraminal pathology or for canal inspection. A careless needle approach can be a setup for surgical misadventure and serious complications. Too vertical an entry threatens the bowel and vascular structures, whereas an excessively far lateral approach can invade the abdominal cavity with potential visceral injury.

The needle is introduced via a posterolateral approach. Needle position is extremely important because the obturator and cannula that follow should be close to the

---

SURGICAL PREPARATION

- Clear and thorough informed consent
- Delineation of indications, risks, expected outcomes, and options to procedure

---

SURGICAL TECHNIQUE

- Generally accepted contraindications for minimally invasive procedures
  ○ Primary low back pain
  ○ Cauda equina syndrome
  ○ Disc recurrence, the presence of significant scarring
  ○ Severe ligamentous/bony stenosis
  ○ Multilevel degenerative disc disease
  ○ Physical barriers to access the L5 to S1 interspace
- Surgical approaches: Uniportal; biportal
- Specific techniques
  ○ Posterolateral approach
  ○ Fluoroscopic guidance
  ○ Needle K-wire placement followed by cannulated obturator, access cannula, and finally annular docking and fenestration
  ○ The endoscope is delivered and operative excursion is assessed to see if adequate to address pathology

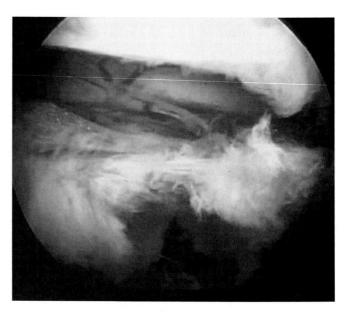

Figure 22-1. Foraminal view of L3 to L4 after extraction of a large subligamentous paracentral disc herniation. The posterior longitudinal ligament (PLL) is still intact. The anatomic structures seen from top to bottom are the foraminal ligament, the traversing nerve, the PLL, and the disc cavity.

herniation at the foramen. Anteroposterior and lateral fluoroscopy should confirm needle positioning at the midpedicular line and posterior to annular fibers, respectively. For extraforaminal work, fluoroscopic landmarks should be lateral to the pedicle at the dorsolateral corner of the annulus.

Proceeding with uniportal intradiscal intervention for paramedian and small central disc pathology, a K-wire replaces the stylet of the needle. A cannulated obturator is then passed over the K-wire, which is then removed. An access cannula is then passed through the obturator with firm, sustained docking on the annulus to aid in the reduction of bleeding. With the removal of the obturator, annular fenestration is afforded using an appropriate sized trephine. Annular topical anesthesia is required for this painful portion of the procedure. A pathway has now been created for delivery of an arthroscopy or working channel endoscope fashioned with irrigation and suction portals. In this instance a 0- to 30-degree endoscope can provide for visualized inspection and protection of at-risk structures while manual and automated surgical tools are introduced through the working channel for resection of the disc and disc fragments, resulting in decompression of the nerve root. Operative excursion is confined in a triangular working zone defined by the exiting nerve root anteriorly, the traversing root and thecal sac medially, and the inferior (caudal) vertebral end plate. Kambin prefers to be on the asymptomatic side for his approach, reaching across the patient to operate on the symptomatic side.

For the biportal approach to the disc, usually considered for large central, subligamentous, and extraligamentous (sequestered) herniations, the arthroscope is introduced from one side while the working channel scope is introduced contralaterally. Larger scopes (6.4-mm outer diameter) and oval cannulas are usually used in this technique for maximum excursion of articulating instruments to address the pathology.

A key element to this and all visualized endoscopic techniques is the need for high–optical resolution rod-lens scopes with variable-angle lenses. Multiple sizes help with special situations in which the standard size is not appropriate. A local anesthetic and IV sedation should be employed. Although Kambin has used general or spinal anesthesia, local anesthesia is preferred. General anesthesia takes away the surgeon's ability to communicate with the patient regarding sensations suggestive of nerve root encroachment or sensory response to successful nerve root decompression. Critical to this technique and all other visualized endoscopic techniques is hand-eye coordination and spatial orientation, as well as an understanding of neurovascular anatomy and structures at risk. These techniques mandate mastery of a steep learning curve and proficiency maintained by regular surgical practice.

As we proceed to describe other techniques, the advantages of these endoscopic techniques are similar. Surgical morbidity is low, recovery time is speedy, and extensive rehabilitation is not usually necessary. Postoperative pain is minimal, and return to preoperative lifestyle is timely and satisfying.[21-24]

Foraminal Epidural Endoscopic Discectomy

The foraminal epidural endoscopic approach to herniated nuclear pathology was the next step forward in advancing and expanding surgical options for herniated nuclear pathology. With this technique, established indications for endoscopic spine surgery were expanded. A technique to address preferred previously nonoperated, single-level paramedian, foraminal, or extraforaminal herniated discs now allowed for access to contained or noncontained fragments of equal to or less than 50% of the spinal canal diameter if the fragments fall within the confines of the axilla and the pedicle.

Contraindications and the importance of correlating the patient's clinical symptoms with imaging studies essentially mirror the list already annotated. Advantages of the technique virtually parallel those of arthroscopic microdiscectomy.

For foraminal epidural endoscopic discectomy, the patient is placed on a padded radiolucent frame with standard prepping and draping. The surgeon is positioned on the side of the offending pathology with the endoscopic monitor and light source at the foot of the surgical table. Fluoroscopy equipment is placed to allow unrestricted anteroposterior and lateral imaging throughout the procedure. Prophylactic broad-spectrum antibiotics are administered preoperatively.

Anesthesia is twofold. A local anesthetic is administered at the skin level and in the musculature of the approach trajectory, taking care not to advance to the point of anesthetizing the neural structures at the foramen. Monitored anesthesia care provides for the delivery of light IV sedation only to the extent that patient-physician dialogue can be maintained relative to procedural sensations. The presence of anesthesia professionals also allows for timely conversion to an open procedure if necessary.

At the commencement of the surgical intervention, a K-wire placed at the surgical level allows for fluoroscopic verification of accuracy. If there is equivocation relative

---

FORAMINAL EPIDURAL ENDOSCOPIC DISCECTOMY

- Unique indications
  - Paramedian, foraminal, or extraforaminal herniation.
  - Access to contained/noncontained fragments greater than 50% canal diameter.
  - Confined to the axilla of the nerve root or within the confines of the pedicle.
- Technique: Discography
  - Needle approach 9 to 13 cm off midline.
  - Under fluoroscopic guidance.
  - Direct needle to interarticularis and then pass medially to contact pars foraminal ligament in foramen.
  - Pass a cannula over the needle.
  - Remove the needle.
  - Deliver an endoscope to the foramen for intradiscal/epidural access.
- Adjunct: Cool free-flow irrigant.

to the pain generator in a suspected multilevel pathology or if there is question as to the state of containment or fragmentation of the nuclear material, discography may precede the actual procedure.

The surgical approach at approximately 9 to 13 cm from the midline and a discogram-type needle is advanced to the pars interarticularis and then directed medially to the foraminal ligament, an extension of the ligamentum flavum. At this point, the needle is positioned at the foramen. In the foraminal approach, a cannula is passed over the needle, the needle is removed, and the rod-lens working channel endoscope is then passed through the cannula with delivery to the foramen, from which intradiscal or epidural access can proceed. The optics and lighting provide for clarity of visualization to identify, inspect, and avoid critical structural anatomy and pursue the pathology. Approach structures may dictate the size and sturdiness of the endoscope with a working channel diameter that can accommodate surgical tools appropriate to the targeted pathology.

Within the safe neural working zone of the epidural space, manipulation of the endoscope allows delivery of instruments designed to address the pathology at distances from and angles to the scope. This safe working zone is defined by the offending levels exiting the nerve root, the traversing nerve root that courses along the pathologic disc and exits at the caudal foramen, and the intervertebral disc itself (Figure 22-2).

As visualized dissection ensues, a cool (62° F) free-flow irrigant via the endoscope disperses debris from the operative field, promotes hemostasis and analgesia, and also provides a safety factor. Bubbles generated by irrigation aid in spatial orientation because they exclusively migrate posteriorly. The irrigant also maintains an expanded work space for facilitation of surgical dissection and video documentation of operative success by way of visual inspection.

Upon conclusion of the procedure, sterile adhesive strips and elastic bandages are applied. The patient is placed in a Neoprene corset with an ice pocket. Ice addresses postoperative pain and swelling.

Postanesthesia care concludes when the patient is safely ambulating and demonstrates no negative anesthesia effects such as nausea and vomiting or vital sign instability.

Return to activities begins with walking and the avoidance of bending, twisting, lifting, as well as long periods of sitting and high-impact recreational activities. Follow-up at 1 week allows planning for return to work and other activities that may take place at the 1-week point or may extend up to 6 weeks for patients with more demanding work or lifestyles.

Complications in addition to those related to malpositioned approach trajectory can include nerve root impingement, although this is unlikely in the awake patient, epidural hematoma, discitis, or recurrent herniation usually related to failure to adhere to postoperative activity guidelines. Postprocedure headache has been observed in the absence of dural insult.[28,29,31,33,34]

Laser-Assisted Foraminal Discectomy

Casper and Stoll have integrated a rod-lens working channel endoscope, with the right-angle (side-firing) HoYag laser wavelength of 2.1 m delivered via the foraminal approach, as previously described. Indications for this technique are intradiscal and/or epidural disc herniations and fragments that can be visualized via angled endoscope lenses and addressed with a steerable laser fiber, the wavelength of which is cool and well tolerated by hydrated tissues (Figure 22-3).[6] Laser energy serves to

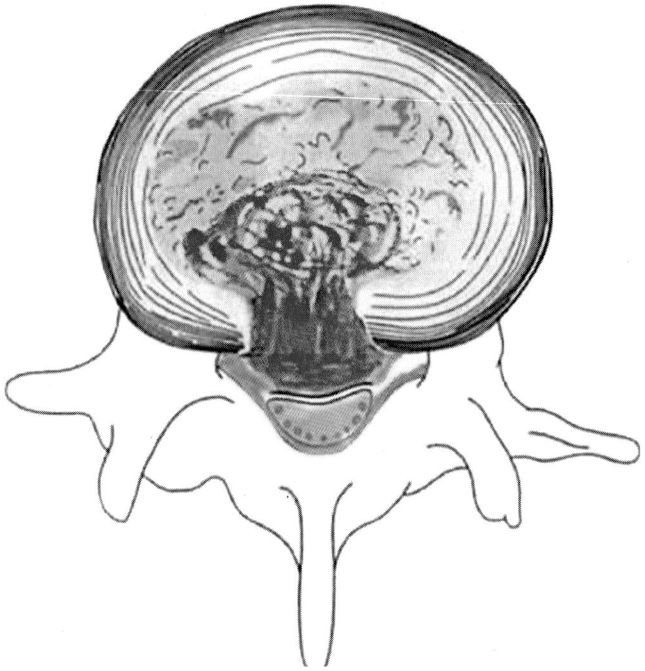

Figure 22-2. Schematic drawing of a large central disc herniation that has disrupted all the layers of the annulus. *(Courtesy Paul Tsou, MD.)*

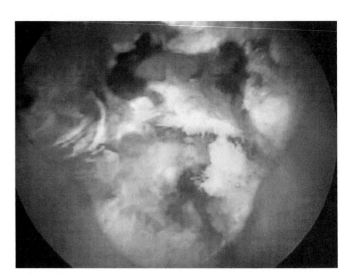

Figure 22-3. Foraminal view (20-degree YESS scope) of grade V annular tear after removal of a paracentral disc herniation. Note the residual indigo carmine-stained annular fibers and disc material. *(Courtesy Anthony T. Young, MD.)*

ablate the offending pathology. Flexible grabbing instruments adaptable to the working channel also aid in selective discectomy.

Contraindications to this technique include previous-procedure scarring, severe lateral recess or central stenosis, or a posterior herniated disc medial to the facet joint. Satisfactory outcome is seen in both single-level and multilevel interventions.

Relative to intradiscal work, this combination technique features a 5-mm outer diameter fiberoptic endoscope with a working channel of 1.5 to 1.8 mm. Lateral and posterolateral herniations are best addressed by this technique with 5 second on/5 second off intervals for laser delivery up to 20,000 joules. Holmium laser energy may also be used for foraminal bony decompression to assist in lateral recess stenosis procedures.

Complications for this procedure are low due to visualization and controlled, cool laser energy. Potential complications include discitis and transient dermatomal discomfort or nerve block.

This procedure is done under local anesthetic with light IV sedation, with a high level of patient satisfaction and clinical success.[2-6,42]

Microendoscopic Discectomy

Microendoscopic discectomy was introduced by Foley and Smith in the late 1990s. Of all the posterior percutaneous procedures described, this technique most closely resembles an open microdiscectomy in its capabilities. It features an interlaminar approach to herniated disc pathology via successively delivered dilators through the paraspinous musculature with the final dilator providing for insertion of a tubular retractor that provides a corridor for insertion of a working channel endoscope (Figure 22-4). The approach allows for selective operative exposure based on the choice of dilators. Broader exposure allows for attention to both disc and bony pathology that may be the cause of neural compressive symptomatology. Lateral recess stenosis and/or foraminal stenosis can also be addressed by microendoscopic capabilities.

Instruments unique to this system in conjunction with the retractor and endoscope allow for both intradiscal and extradiscal intervention spanning from pedicle to pedicle. Irrigation maintains a clear lens and diverts operative debris from the surgical field. Upon conclusion of the procedure, removal of the retractor allows for spontaneous closure of the surgical corridor and the 12-mm incision that facilitates this technique is closed with a single suture.

In a preliminary report, these surgeons report 100% good to excellent results for far lateral herniations and herniations within the spinal canal, as well as free-fragment pathology. This outpatient procedure with timely recovery and return to premorbid activity levels has demonstrated only one complication in the 41 patients, that being a self-limited cerebrospinal leak.

Microendoscopic discectomy offers a system with broadened endoscopic indications and low morbidity with satisfying clinical outcomes. Because of its ability to mimic open microdiscectomy through a tubular retractor, this endoscopic minimally invasive procedure offers most surgeons the comfort of familiar anatomy and a gradual transition to a fully endoscopic approach from a posterolateral portal. It may also offer the most flexibility because it can easily be converted to an open traditional procedure if more exposure is needed.[11]

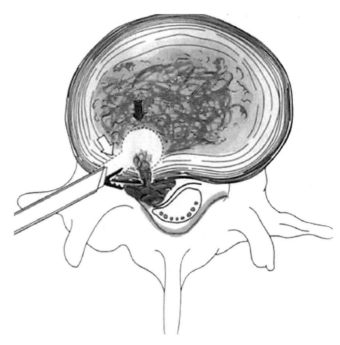

Figure 22-4. Schematic drawing of an extruded disc fragment trapped by a collar of annular tissue. Illustrates the YESS "inside-out" technique. The nucleus is first extracted, creating a working cavity within the disc. The epidural space is explored for extruded fragments. If an extruded fragment is seen trapped by the annulus, the collar is released or resected, and the fragment is pulled back into the disc cavity and extracted through the foramen. (*Courtesy Paul Tsou, MD.*)

LASER-ASSISTED FORAMINAL DISCECTOMY

- Surgical tools: Working channel endoscope; right-angle side-firing HoYag laser
- Action: Laser ablation of offending pathology
- Unique contraindications
  - Previous procedure scarring
  - Severe lateral recess/central stenosis, posterior Herniated nucleus pulposus medial to facet joint
- Technique
  - Foraminal approach
  - 1.5- to 1.8-mm inner diameter working channel endoscope
  - Laser delivery 5 seconds on/5 seconds off at intervals up to 20,000 joules
- Potential complications
  - Discitis
  - Transient dermatomal discomfort or nerve block

MICROENDOSCOPIC DISCECTOMY

- Most closely resembles open microdiscectomy.
- Indications: Disc and bony pathology, including lateral recess/foraminal stenosis.
- Technique: Interlaminar approach through paraspinous musculature.
  - Progressively deliver dilators with final placement of a tubular retractor.
  - Insert working channel endoscope with room to allow placement of adjunctive working instruments.
- Benefits
  - Broadened endoscopic indications.
  - Low morbidity.
  - User friendly to surgeons.
  - Ease in conversion to open traditional procedure as needed.

YEUNG ENDOSCOPIC SPINE SURGERY SYSTEM

- Broadened indications
  - Discogenic back pain
  - All disc pathology contiguous with disc space
  - Endoscopic bone removal—access to free/migrated fragments
  - Allows for neurolysis
  - Allows for foraminotomy
- Technique
  - Similar to discography
  - Posterolateral approach with a needle
  - Placement with fluoroscopy
  - Pass wire through the needle
  - Place dilators over the needle, locking on the annulus
- Place trephine-cannula into disc
- Place 2.8-mm working channel endoscope through trephine-cannula
- Adjuncts: HoYag laser, electrothermal probe, cool irrigant
- Potential complications: Neurovascular trauma, hematoma, dysesthesias

Selective Endoscopic Discectomy

Bringing together the best elements of contemporary techniques, Dr. Anthony Yeung introduced selective endoscopic discectomy. The broad applicability of this technique is based on a specially designed system of endoscopes and instruments known as YESS (Yeung Endoscopic Spine Surgery System, Richard Wolf Medical Instrument Corp).

The system is capable of addressing discogenic back pain, as well as all types of disc pathologies, as long as they are contiguous with the disc space. More recent advancements that give the surgeon the ability to remove bone endoscopically have allowed for improved surgical access *and* success with free and migrated fragments. Further technical advancements combined with surgeon experience allow surgical interventions such as neurolysis and/or foraminotomy even in previously operated patients.

As with all percutaneous procedures, success is based on patient selection and the surgeon's clear understanding of neurovascular anatomy and pathology, as well as mastery of the technique through education, proctoring, and frequent application. In the patient selection process, the surgical approach has to be uniquely tailored to the individual patient. An adjunct for surgical planning is careful study of the MRI to ensure that the disc space and/or spinal canal is accessible. Lack of accessibility and/or failure to achieve the learning curve pinnacle are the main relative contraindications to this technique. Yeung feels these skills are transferable and within the grasp of most dedicated spine surgeons willing to overcome the steep learning curve.

The YESS system features a variety of scopes and instruments so that the surgical technique can be tailored to the anatomy to be inspected or the targeted pathology.

The most broadly applicable scope has been a rod-lens endoscope with a 2.8-mm working channel. Additional channels for irrigation inflow, outflow, and suction control visualization and capillary bleeding by hydrostatic pressure.

Discography with a dye contrast precedes the procedure to verify the disc pathology through symptom provocation and to identify potential extrusions or the presence of annular fissures or tears. The dye contains a nonionic contrast agent (Isovue 300M) and a vital dye (indigo carmine) to stain degenerated tissue in contact with the dye.

The posterolateral approach is preferred, and the technique for discectomy is performed under continuous intermittent fluoroscopy. A needle is directed to the disc, and the position must be confirmed as consistent with the pathology and surgical plan because subsequent instrumentation will follow the trajectory of the needle. The needle further provides for palpation and penetration of the annulus.

Subsequent steps in the procedure begin with placement of a sturdy wire directed through the needle to the annulus. With removal of the needle, a dilator is delivered to the annulus. The dilator has an accessory channel that can be used for probing or anesthetizing structures adjacent to the central hole of the dilator. A cannula is then placed into the disc, through which an endoscope is passed, followed by removal of the dilator and cannula.

Inspection via the endoscope ensures that no neurovascular at-risk structures are in harm's way. The working channel endoscope can then be advanced to inspect and address the visualized pathology. With irrigation, suction, and the adjunct channel now attached, a trephine facilitates an opening in the disc that allows for the use of mechanical and motorized instruments appropriate to the disc location to achieve the discectomy goal. Discoscopes with varied optical angles may be required to best view the pathology to facilitate the surgical steps (Figure 22-5).

If annular tears or adherence of nuclear fragments to end plates or nerves is identified, adjuncts such as the HoYag laser or a high-frequency (4 MHz) flexible steer-

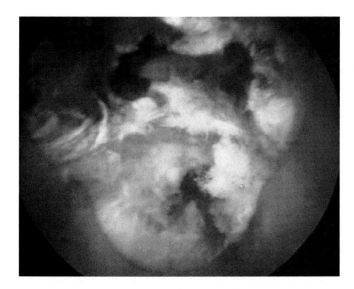

Figure 22-5. Surgical pathology, approach, and technique for selective endoscopic discectomy. *(Courtesy Anthony T. Yeung, MD.)*

able electrothermal probe (Ellman) can be employed for thermal tissue modulation, as well as hemostasis. These modalities may assist in completion of the discectomy. Furthermore, these modalities, along with cool irrigant to which has been added epinephrine and gentamicin, aid in hemostasis.

Potential complications parallel those of other percutaneous techniques, including neurovascular trauma, hematoma, and dysesthesias.

Having treated more than 1000 patients in a 9-year time span dating from 1991, an initial patient satisfaction of 86.4% in the first 500 patients has continued to rise concurrent with diligence in the refinement of indications, techniques, and adjuncts.[45-49,51]

Kyphoplasty and Vertebroplasty

Advances in minimally invasive techniques have redefined the treatment of many spinal disorders. The application of these technologies to compression fractures is demonstrating efficacy and bears inclusion in the discussion of posterior percutaneous procedures. Kyphoplasty will be described, followed by a comparison with vertebroplasty.

This technique is designed for the surgical stabilization of thoracic and/or lumbar osteoporotic vertebral body compression fractures that are 3 months old or less. This is the key indication for patient selection. Up to three fractures may be treated at one time in an individual patient. A summary of contraindications include high-velocity burst fractures, bony tumor, and concomitant medical illnesses or neurologic deficits. Severe kyphosis, three-column injury with instability, and vertebral body arteriovenous malformations are also stringent contraindications.

Patients present with acute onset of back pain that can often be pinpointed to a specific time or event. Kyphosis may be evident.

KYPHOPLASTY/VERTEBROPLASTY

- Indication: Thoracic and/or lumbar osteoporotic vertebral compression fractures less than three months old.
- Contraindications: High-velocity burst fractures, bony tumor, medical illnesses, neurologic deficits, severe kyphosis, three-column injury with instability, arteriovenous malformations.
- Radiologic diagnostic confirmation: Plain films with or without a bone scan and CT scan with sagittal reconstructions.
- Technique
  - Under fluoroscopic control place the needle through the pedicle into the anterior vertebral body.
  - Place a dilator over the needle, then place the cannula.
  - Place a balloon inflation device through the cannula.
  - Inject methylmethacrylate under continuous fluoroscopy until the bone void is filled.
- **Caution:** During the injection procedure, continuous fluoroscopic visualization is required to prevent extravasation of methylmethacrylate, which can cause potential serious results from thermal effects or embolization.
- Postulated mechanism of action: Immediate stabilization of vertebral body fractures along with the exothermic effect of methylmethacrylate leading to denaturization of periosteal nerve receptors.

Following evaluation of plain radiographs, the ideal study to confirm the diagnosis is either a bone scan and/or a CT scan with sagittal reconstruction. An MRI often is not helpful in assessing posterior vertebral body involvement.

The surgical intervention follows prone placement of the patient on a radiolucent table with postural reduction. Anteroposterior and lateral fluoroscopy should be accessible throughout the procedure. Depending on the pain level of the patient, general anesthesia versus local with IV sedation is selected.

Under fluoroscopic guidance, a guidewire is directed through the pedicle or along the lateral border of the pedicle and into the anterior portion of the vertebral body. Variation in approach may be necessary in upper thoracic vertebrae due to small pedicles. A dilator followed by a cannula is placed. A balloon device is then delivered to the surgical site within the vertebral body. The balloon is inflated to compress cancellous bone, thus creating a void within the selected vertebral body. A bone void nozzle is placed into the void, and barium-impregnated methylmethacrylate with or without an antibiotic is gently and slowly injected under fluoroscopic visualization until the void is filled (Figure 22-6). The technique may be reproduced contralaterally for maximum vertebral stabilization. During the injection phase of the procedure, there must be continuous fluoroscopic visualization to ensure that cement does not migrate through the foramen, through a posterior vertebral body wall fracture, or anterior to the vertebral

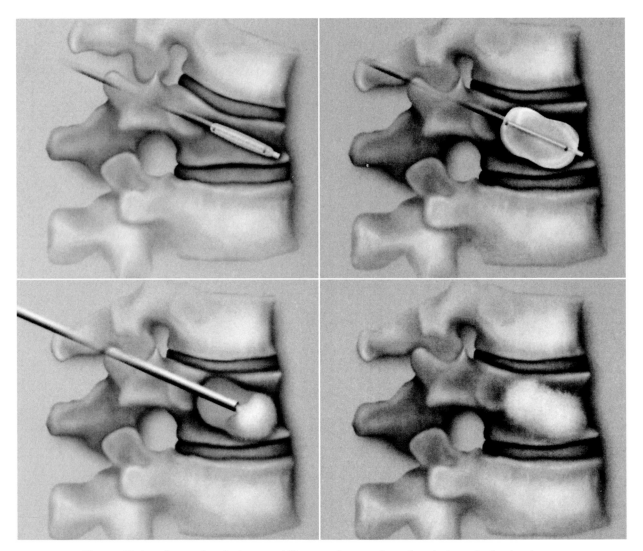

Figure 22-6.   Surgical technique and illustrated correction of pathology for kyphoplasty.
(Courtesy Kyphon Inc. © 2000 Kyphon Inc.)

body. Cement extravasation may lead to significant complications such as neurologic or vascular or distant cement embolization. With even a hint of cement migration, the procedure should be aborted.

Patients usually get immediate relief of symptoms. The mechanism of action for kyphoplasty is postulated to be immediate stabilization of the vertebral body fracture along with the exothermic effect of methylmethacrylate leading to denaturation of the periosteal nerve receptors.

By comparison, vertebroplasty seeks to stabilize the vertebral body compression fracture in its static state rather than attempting to restore vertebral body height and integrity. The technique simply involves use of a bone access needle placed via a posterior transpedicular approach into the anterior half of the vertebral body. The methylmethacrylate is then injected incrementally using a 1- to 3-ml syringe. This procedure also can be done biportally and carries the same risks and benefits. However, due to pressurization and the potential for overfilling of

the vertebral body, the embolization risk may increase specifically to the lungs.

Critical to the satisfactory outcome of both procedures is, as always, patient selection.[14,19,20,32,44]

CONCLUSIONS

John A McCulloch, MD, has quoted a 1913 statement of William Halstead that seems to validate the ongoing refinement of minimally invasive spine surgery tools and techniques. Says Halstead, "I believe that the tendency will always be in the direction of exercising greater care and refinement in operating, and that the surgeon will develop increasingly a respect for tissues; a sense which recoils from inflicting, unnecessarily, insult to structures concerned in the process of repair."[36]

This challenging observation certainly demonstrates great foresight, and the authors believe that the techniques described in this chapter have certainly risen to the challenge.

Minimally invasive spine surgeons must now remain focused on continuing efforts toward the least surgically traumatic procedures, prospectively evaluated for clinical efficacy, a high level of patient satisfaction, and proven cost-effectiveness. Through physician collaboration, crossing this threshold is close at hand.

ACKNOWLEDGMENTS

The authors acknowledge with appreciation the assistance of the following individuals and organizations in the preparation of this publication: G. David Casper, MD, James E. Stoll, MD, Anthony T. Yeung, MD, Robert Edwards, illustrator, Kyphon, and Medtronic Sofamor Danek.

SELECTED REFERENCES

Casper GD: Results of a prospective clinical trial of the Ho:YAG laser in disc decompression utilizing a side-firing fiber: four year results. International Intradiscal Therapy Society, San Antonio, Texas, May 1998.

Foley KT, Smith MM: Microendoscopic discectomy, *Tech in Neurosurg* 3:301-307, 1997.

Jensen ME, Dion JE: Percutaneous vertebroplasty in the treatment of osteoporotic compression fractures: percutaneous vertebroplasty in the treatment of osteoporotic compression fractures, *Neuroimaging Clin North Am* 10:547-568, 2000.

Jensen ME et al.: Percutaneous polymethylmethacrylate vertebroplasty in the treatment of osteoporotic compression fractures: technical aspects, *Am J Neuroradiol* 18:1897-1904, 1997.

Kambin P: Diagnostic and therapeutic spinal arthroscopy, *Neurol Clin* 7:65-76, 1996.

Savitz MH, Chiu JC, Yeung AT, eds: *The practice of minimally invasive spinal technique*, Richmond, Va, 2000, AAMISMS Education LLC.

Tehranzadeh J: Discography 2000, *Radiol Clin North Am* 36:463-495, 1998.

Wilson DR et al.: Effect of augmentation on the mechanics of vertebral wedge fractures, *Spine* 15:158-165, 2000.

Yeung AT: The evolution of percutaneous spinal endoscopy and discectomy: state of the art, *Mt Sinai J Med* 67:327-332, 2000.

REFERENCES

1. Argoff CA, Sheeler AH: Spinal and radicular pain disorders, *Neurol Clin* 16:833-850, 1998.
2. Casper GD: Personal communication. 2000.
3. Casper GD: Results of a prospective clinical trial of the Ho:YAG laser in disc decompression utilizing a side-firing fiber: four year results, International Intradiscal Therapy Society, San Antonio, Texas, May 1998.
4. Casper GD, Hartman VL, Mullins LL: Results of a clinical trial of the Holmium:YAG laser in disc decompression utilizing a side-firing laser: a two-year follow-up, *Lasers Surg Med* 19:90-96, 1998.
5. Casper GD, Mulling LL, Hartman VA: Laser-assisted disc decompression: a clinical trial of the holmium YAG laser with side-firing fiber, *J Clin Laser Med Surg* 13:27-31, 1995.
6. Casper GD, Stoll JE: *Endoscopic laser foraminotomy*, International Intradiscal Therapy Society, San Antonio, Texas, May 1998.
7. Dabezies EJ, Langford K: Safety and efficacy of chymopapain (Discase) in the treatment of sciatica due to a herniated nucleus pulposus: results of a randomized, double-blind study, *Spine* 13:561-565, 1988.
8. Dandy WE: Loose cartilage from intervertebral disk simulating tumor of the spinal cord, *Arch Surg* 19:660-672, 1929.
9. Deutman R: 2000 chemonucleolysis procedures in 20 years, International Intradiscal Therapy Society, Williamsburg, Va, June 2000.
10. Dvořák J, Bell G: *The International Society for the Study of the Lumbar Spine*, Philadelphia, 1996, WB Saunders, pp. 8-16.
11. Foley KT, Smith MM: Microendoscopic discectomy, *Tech Neurosurg* 3:301-307, 1997.

12. Fraser RD: Chymopapain for the treatment of intervertebral disc herniation: a preliminary report of a double blind study, *Spine* 7:608-612, 1982.
13. Fraser RD: Chymopapain for the treatment of intervertebral disc herniation: a preliminary report of a double blind study, *Spine* 9:815-818, 1984.
14. Garfin SR et al.: Vertebroplasty and kyphoplasty. In Savitz MH, Chiu J, Yeung AT, eds: *The practice of minimally invasive spinal technique*, Richmond, Va, 2000, AAMISMS Education, pp. 249-260.
15. Guo H et al.: Back pain among workers in the United States: national estimates and workers at high risk, *Am J Ind Med* 28:591-602, 1995.
16. Harrington JF et al.: Herniated lumbar disc material as a source of free glutamate available to affect pain signals through the dorsal root ganglion, *Spine* 25:929-936, 2000.
17. Hayashi N, Lee HM, Weinstein JN: The source of pain in the lumbar spine. In Bridwell KH, DeWald RL, eds: *The textbook of spinal surgery*, ed 2, Philadelphia, 1997, Lippincott-Raven, pp. 1503-1514.
18. Javid MF, Nordby EJ: Safety and efficacy of chymopapain (Chymodiactin) in herniated nucleus pulposus with sciatica: results of a randomized, double-blind study, *JAMA* 249:2489-2494, 1983.
19. Jensen ME, Dion JE: Percutaneous vertebroplasty in the treatment of osteoporetic compression fractures, *Neuroimaging Clin North Am* 10:547-568, 2000.
20. Jensen ME et al.: Percutaneous polymethylmethacrylate vertebroplasty in the treatment of osteoporotic compression fractures: technical aspects, *Am J Neuroradiol* 18:1897-1904, 1997.
21. Kambin P: Arthroscopic microdiscectomy. In Mayer HM, ed: *Minimally invasive spine surgery*, Berlin, 2000, Springer-Verlag, pp. 187-199.
22. Kambin P: Diagnostic and therapeutic spinal arthroscopy, *Neurol Clin* 7:65-76, 1996.
23. Kambin P, Gellman H: Percutaneous lateral discectomy of the lumbar spine: a preliminary report, *Clin Orthop* 174:127-132, 1983.
24. Kambin P, Savitz MH: The advent of arthroscopic microdiscectomy. In Savitz MH, Chiu J, Yeung AT, eds: *The practice of minimally invasive spinal technique*, Richmond, Va, 2000, AAMISMS Education LLC, pp. 105-114.
25. Kang JD et al.: Herniated lumbar intervertebral discs spontaneously produce matrix metalloproteinases, nitric acid, prostaglandin E2 and interleuken-6, *Spine* 21:271-277, 1996.
26. Kawakami M et al.: Possible mechanism of painful radiculopathy in lumbar disc herniation, *Clin Orthop* 351:241-251, 1998.
27. Kinard RE: Diagnostic spinal injection procedures, *Neurol Clin* 7:151-165, 1996.
28. Mathews HH: Endoscopic discectomy. In Vaccaro AR, Albert TJ, eds: *Tricks of the trade in spine surgery*, New York, 2000, Thieme (in press).
29. Mathews HH: Foraminal epidural endoscopic discectomy. In Fessler R, Sekhar T: *Atlas of neurosurgical techniques*, New York, 2000, Thieme (in press).
30. Mathews HH: Spinal endoscopy: evolution, foundations, and applications. In Bridwell KH, DeWald RL: *The textbook of spinal surgery*, ed 2, Philadelphia, 1997, Lippincott-Raven, pp. 2297-2311.
31. Mathews HH: Transforaminal endoscopic microdiscectomy, *Neurol Clin* 7:59-63, 1996.
32. Mathews HH: Vertebroplasty. In Vaccaro AR, Albert TJ, eds: *Tricks of the trade in spine surgery*, New York, 2000, Thieme (in press).
33. Mathews HH, Long BH: Minimally invasive techniques for treatment of intervertebral disc herniations. In *Update of new technology on lumbar intervertebral disc surgery*, JAAOS, 2000, (in press).
34. Mathews HH, Mathern BE: Percutaneous procedures in the lumbar spine. In An HS, ed: *Principles and techniques of spine surgery*, Baltimore, 1998, Williams and Wilkins pp. 731-745.
35. Mayer HM, Brock M: Percutaneous endoscopic discectomy: surgical technique and preliminary results compared to microsurgical discectomy, *J Neurosurg* 78:216-225, 1993.
36. McCulloch JA: Microsurgery for lumbar disc disease. In An HS, ed: *Principles and techniques of spine surgery*, Baltimore, 1998, Williams & Wilkins, pp. 747-764.
37. Nordby E, Fraser R, Javid M: Spine update chemonucleolysis, *Spine* 21:1102-1105, 1996.
38. Nordby EJ, Javid MJ: Continuing experience with chemonucleolysis. *Mt Sinai J Med* 67:311-313, 2000.
39. Saifuddin A, Mitchell R, Taylor BA: Extradural inflammation associated with annular tears demonstrated with gadolinium-enhanced lumbar spine MRI, *Eur Spine J* 8:34-39, 1999.

40. Savitz MH, Chiu JC, Yeung AT, eds: *The practice of minimally invasive spinal technique*, ed 1, Richmond, Va, 2000, AAMISMS Education LLC.
41. Schwartz DG, Schafer MF. Low back pain in athletes. In Bridwell KH, DeWald RJ, eds: *The textbook of spinal surgery*, ed 2, Philadelphia, 1997, Lippincott-Raven, pp. 1515-1531.
42. Stoll JE: Personal communication, 2000.
43. Tehranzadeh J: Discography 2000, *Radiol Clin North Am* 36:463-495, 1998.
44. Wilson DR et al.: Effect of augmentation on the mechanics of vertebral wedge fractures, *Spine* 15:158-165, 2000.
45. Yeung AT: Personal communication, 2000-2001.
46. Yeung AT: Minimally invasive disc surgery with the Yeung endoscopic spine system [YESS] In *Surgical technology international VIII*, San Francisco, 1999, Universal Medical Press (reprint 1-11).
47. Yeung AT: Selective discectomy with the Yeung endoscope spine system. In Savitz MH, Chiu JC, Yeung AT, eds: *The practice of minimally invasive spinal technique*, ed 1, Richmond, Va, 2000, AAMISMS Education LLC, pp. 115-122.
48. Yeung AT: Selective endoscopic discectomy with a multi-channel, flow-integrated spine scope (YESS system) for the treatment of herniated discs, back pain and sciatica, Williamsburg, Va, 2000, International Intradiscal Therapy Society.
49. Yeung AT: The evolution of percutaneous spinal endoscopy and discectomy: state of the art, *Mt Sinai J Med* 67:327-332, 2000.
50. Yeung AT: The role of provocative discography in endoscopic disc surgery. In Savitz MH, Chiu JC, Yeung AT, eds: *The practice of minimally invasive spinal technique*, ed 1, Richmond, Va, 2000, AAMISMS Education LLC, pp. 231-236.
51. Yeung AT: *Tips on selective endoscopic discectomy: the YESS technique*, www.dryeung@amdaz.com, 1996-2000.
52. Yussen PS, Swartz JD: The acute lumbar disc herniation: imaging diagnosis, *Semin Ultrasound CT NR* 14:389-398, 1993.

Surgical Approaches and Reconstruction of the Sacrum

Stephen I. Esses, Richard R. Frances

The sacrum is often given much less attention in the literature than other parts of the axial skeleton. Surgical approaches to the sacrum and reconstruction can be challenging, emphasizing the importance of a sound knowledge of these principles. An appreciation of sacral anatomy with its variations and a knowledge of how it functions as part of the skeleton are key to grasping these concepts. Traumatic injuries, neoplastic conditions, and to a lesser extent sacral infections often provide the reason for surgical intervention. Thorough familiarity with the details of these conditions forms the foundation for proper decision making.

SURGICAL ANATOMY

The sacrum is formed from the fusion of five sacral vertebrae and their costal elements.[26,34] The costal elements form the lateral mass of the sacrum, which is found lateral to the transverse tubercles on the back of the sacrum. The auricular surface for the sacroiliac joint lies wholly on the lateral mass, so in morphologic terms the pelvis articulates with ribs, not with the centra of vertebrae.

The sacrum bears the whole weight of the body. It articulates above with the lumbosacral facet joints and laterally with the pelvis to form the sacroiliac joint. Below this, it tapers down to its apex. It is therefore a triangular dish-shaped bone, with its concavity found anteriorly. The sacroiliac joint is non–weight bearing; the ligaments above and behind the joint carry the body weight.

There are two surfaces, a pelvic surface and a dorsal surface (Figure 23-1). The pelvic surface is smooth and concave. Fusion of the five sacral bodies leaves behind four persisting transverse ridges, which mark the position of the intervertebral discs. On each side, four large anterior sacral foramina are found, diminishing in size from above downward. The mass of bone lateral to the foramina is the lateral mass. The piriformis muscle arises from the three ridges that separate the four anterior foramina and also from the adjacent lateral masses.

Medial to each anterior foramen is the sacral sympathetic trunk; in the midline of the sacral hollow is the median sacral artery and vein. Lateral to the foramina, the sacral plexus lies on the piriformis muscle.

The prominent anterior lip of the first sacral body is the sacral promontory. Below this, peritoneum is draped over the first two sacral bodies. Inferior to S2, however, the retroperitoneal rectum lies directly against the lower three bodies. Between the rectum and peritoneum in front and the sacrum behind lie Waldeyer's fascia and the superior rectal vessels.

The dorsal surface is convex, irregular, and rough (Figure 23-2). Superiorly, ligamentum flavum fills in the gap between the first sacral and fifth lumbar laminae. Below this, the sacral laminae fuse in the midline to give a prominence known as the median sacral crest. This represents fused adjacent spinous processes. Inferiorly, failure of fusion of the laminae of S5 and sometimes S4 leaves a gap known as the sacral hiatus (Figure 23-3). The fibrous tissue that closes this gap is known as the superficial sacrococcygeal ligament. It is also the site of an intervertebral disc between the end of the sacrum and the base of the coccyx.

The sacrococcygeal joint is a symphysis between the end of the sacrum and the base of the coccyx and is prone to injury. Both bones are united by a disc of fibrocartilage and by ventral, dorsal, and lateral sacrococcygeal ligaments. The fibrocartilage is a thin disc that intervenes between both bones. Occasionally the coccyx is freely movable and articulates with the sacrum by a synovial joint. A good deal of motion is possible in this articulation, but only flexion and extension. There is no side-to-side movement. At an advanced age the joint between the sacrum and coccyx becomes obliterated.

Ligaments reinforce the sacrococcygeal symphysis, a single ventral ligament and two dorsal ligaments, one deep and one superficial. The latter closes over the sacral hiatus at the lower end of the sacral canal. On each side a lateral sacrococcygeal ligament runs from the tip of the coccyx to the inferolateral angle of the sacrum, so forming an inferior boundary for the anterior ramus of the fifth sacral nerve. This ligament may become ossified so that the sacrum appears to have five foramina on one or both sides.

The transverse processes of the sacral vertebrae fuse to form the longitudinal lateral sacral crest. Between the median sacral crest in the midline and the lateral sacral crest is the intermediate crest. This is a line of irregular

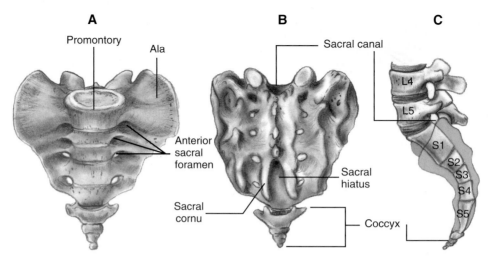

A

Promontory

Ala

B

Sacral canal

C

L4

L5

S1

S2

S3

S4

S5

Anterior
sacral
foramen

Sacral
cornu

Sacral
hiatus

Coccyx

Figure 23-1.   The sacrum and coccyx. **A,** Anterior view. **B,** Posterior view. **C,** Midsagittal view.

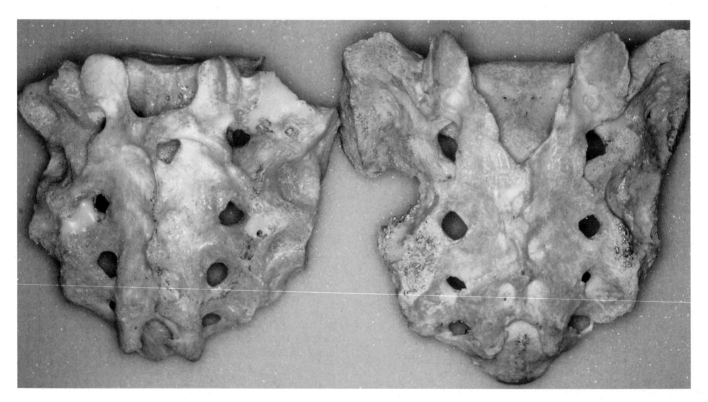

Figure 23-2.   The dorsal surface of the sacrum showing four large foramina.

tubercles that represent fusion of adjacent articular processes of the sacral vertebrae. The posterior sacral foramina lie between the intermediate and lateral crests. However, the groove between the median and intermediate crests is filled by erector spinae, and the posterior layer of lumbar fascia that covers it is attached to both crests.

The lateral border of the sacrum that forms the sacroiliac joint is the irregular auricular surface. It is broad above and narrow below. Between the lateral crest and the auricular surface are three or four deep fossae that give an undulating appearance to the lateral mass.

The whole of this area gives attachment to the weight-bearing sacroiliac ligaments.

The ala of the sacrum is the transverse process of the first sacral vertebra. It projects laterally from the upper surface of the S1 vertebra so that its margin forms the brim of the pelvis. The sympathetic trunk crosses the base of the ala. Lateral to this, on the ala, lie the lumbosacral trunk medially, the obturator nerve laterally, and the iliolumbar artery between them (Figure 23-4).

The sacral canal is triangular in cross-section. It accommodates the meninges that extend down to the S2 vertebra. Below this the filum terminale runs down to

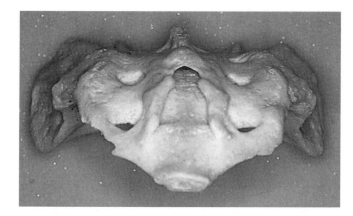

Figure 23-3. The dorsal surface of the sacrum is convex and rough. The sacral hiatus is the result of failure of fusion of the laminae of S5 and sometimes S4.

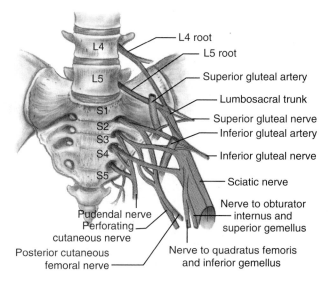

Figure 23-5. The sacral plexus.

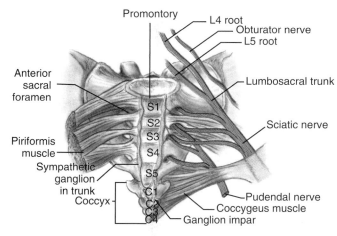

Figure 23-4. The two major branches of the solar plexus are shown in red.

join the periosteum on the back of the coccyx. The space between the dura mater and its nerve root prolongations is filled with loose fat and the internal vertebral venous plexus.

The sacral pedicles lie laterally, projecting from the upper half of each sacral body, forming four intervertebral exit foramina as in the rest of the vertebral canal.

The lumbosacral articulation is the most variable portion of the spine. Bertolotti et al.[4] have described and classified assimilation of the fifth lumbar vertebra into the sacrum. This is known as sacralization and may take various forms.[6] Six sacral vertebrae may also be present due to incorporation of the first coccygeal vertebra. Less commonly there is a reduction in the constituents of the sacrum. This lumbarization of the first sacral segment may be partial or complete. The sacral hiatus is normally located at the level of the S4 vertebral body but is often found much higher. In 5% of the population the hiatus is rudimentary, with an opening smaller than 2 mm.[9,31] A considerable part of the dorsal wall of the sacral canal may be deficient due to imperfect development of the laminae and spines. There are differences

in the shape of the sacrum based on sex, weight, and race. The body of the first sacral vertebra in the male is cross-sectionally wider and larger in the sagittal plane than in females, while the width of the sacral alae, but not the thickness, is greater in the female.[14]

Neural Anatomy

The sacral spinal nerves each split into anterior and posterior rami. The anterior rami exit the anterior foramina while the posterior rami emerge through the dorsal foramina. The anterior rami of S1, S2, and S3 rest on the surface of periformis muscle as they curve laterally to meet the lumbosacral trunk and so form the sacral plexus (Figure 23-5). The union of the L4 and L5 anterior rami forms the lumbosacral trunk. The anterior ramus of L4 descends to the middle of the ala just superior to the first sacral foramen, where it joins L5 as it travels laterally across the ala. Lateral to the lumbosacral trunk is the obturator nerve formed from contributions from second, third, and fourth lumbar roots. It emerges on the medial border of the psoas muscle and runs in a caudal direction to the superior surface of the sacroiliac joint. From there it runs laterally to the pelvic brim. The sacral sympathetic trunk runs longitudinally, medial to the anterior sacral foramen to form the ganglion impar on the surface of the coccyx.

Vascular Anatomy

The bifurcation of the aorta is variable in position[42] but most times is found on the left anterior surface of the fourth lumbar vertebral body. Just proximal to the bifurcation, the aorta gives off the middle sacral artery. This runs distally in the midline over the lower lumbar vertebra, sacrum, and coccyx. It runs posterior to the venous system and anastomoses with the lateral sacral artery. In general, however, the important vascular structures related to the anterior sacrum are arranged so that the venous system is placed closer to bone than the arterial

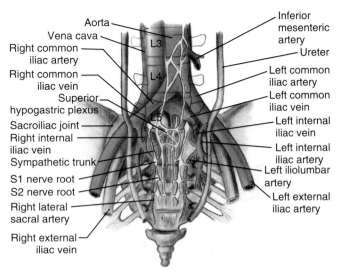

Figure 23-6.   Vascular anatomy.

system. The common and internal iliac veins are located posterior and lateral to the corresponding arteries. In fact, the internal iliac veins course in a superior and medial direction in the connective tissue along the anterior sacral surface. Their course runs either directly over the sacroiliac joint or medial to that position on the anterolateral surface of the sacral ala.

The common iliac arteries arise from the bifurcation of the aorta and run caudally and laterally to the inferior edge of the lumbosacral disc, lateral to the sacroiliac joint, where they divide into the internal and external iliac arteries. The first branch of the internal iliac artery is the iliolumbar artery, but it may also originate from the common iliac artery. For part of its course it overlies the superior aspect of the sacroiliac joint. The second branch of the internal iliac artery is the lateral sacral artery, which alternately may be a branch of the superior gluteal artery. There may be two lateral sacral arteries for each internal iliac artery, a superior and an inferior branch. Each crosses the sacroiliac joint to anastomose with the middle sacral artery, after which branches are sent to the upper and lower sacral foramina (Figure 23-6).

The superior gluteal artery is the largest branch of the internal iliac. The inferior gluteal artery comes off below it. The S1 nerve root often separates the gluteal arteries, although at times the inferior gluteal artery may course between S2 and S3 rather than S1 and S2.

In general terms the venous anatomy is analogous to the arterial anatomy. The internal and external iliac veins join at the sacroiliac joint, so forming the common iliac vein. Both common iliac veins slope upward behind their corresponding arteries, uniting to form the inferior vena cava behind the right common iliac artery. The inferior vena cava is to the right of the midline, so the left common iliac vein is longer than the right, joining its fellow almost at a right angle. The middle sacral vein, which is often double, drains into the left common iliac vein and not the inferior vena cava, because the inferior vena cava is to the right of the spine. The iliolumbar vein may be quite large. It usually drains into the posterior

part of the common iliac vein but occasionally may be the first tributary of the internal iliac vein. It is important to note its posterior position at the level of the common iliac vein.

SURGICAL APPROACHES

Surgical approaches to the sacrum must be selected principally on the basis of access to the lesion being treated. The purpose of the planned procedure, the relevant anatomy, and the size, location, and extent of the pathology are important. In general, anterior approaches expose the anterior concavity of the sacrum, laying bare the vertebral bodies, discs, anterior foramina, and lumbosacral plexus, as well as the retroperitoneal space immediately anterior to the sacrum. Posterior approaches expose the posterior elements and sacral spinal canal.

Posterior Approaches

A posterior approach is most commonly used for the sacrum. After induction of general anesthesia, the patient is rolled in a controlled manner to the prone position. Appropriate prone positioning will contribute to adequate visualization of the surgical site by the surgeon and assistant, the avoidance of pressure complications, and minimizing blood loss. Batson[3] documented an intricate system of sinusoidal channels surrounding the spine throughout its entire length. The system drains into the superior vena cava via a valveless channel.[43] Under physiologic conditions, flow is directed toward the caval system. With obstruction or pressure on the caval system, the direction of flow can be reversed, leading to engorgement of the venous plexus surrounding the spine. This may produce unnecessary blood loss. Increased thoracic pressure or abdominal pressure created from improper positioning will partially or completely obstruct the vena cava, causing the same effect. Every effort must be made to minimize chest and abdominal pressure by allowing the abdomen to hang as freely as possible when the patient is prone. There are three styles of devices for prone positioning. Lateral bolsters placed longitudinally from the chest to the iliac crest or use of a fixed device such as the Wilson frame is one type. This type has high abdominal and vena cava pressures compared with the other two devices. The second requires strategically placed bolsters under the chest and pelvis with the abdomen hanging free. The Relton-Hall or four-poster frame is a commonly used example. It places pressure on the chest and both iliac crests, allowing the entire abdomen to hang free. The third type employs the knee-chest position or one of its modifications. The Andrews frame is popular as a knee-chest positioning device. It places the patient's torso and thighs at 90 degrees to each other. The abdomen hangs freely, with weight bearing shared between the chest, knees, and buttocks. The last two devices allow minimal abdominal pressure, which results in reduced intraoperative blood loss and better visualization.[8]

Special care should be taken to protect the eyes. Direct pressure on the eye, especially as a result of patient malposition in a horseshoe type of headrest, has been cited in several published reports as a factor contributing to visual loss.* The incidence of significant visual complications after spine surgery is of the order of 1 case per 100 spine surgeons per year.[36] Most cases occur in patients with no identified risk factors, although hypertension, smoking, diabetes, and vascular disease lead to increased risk. Long operative times and substantial intraoperative blood loss are contributory factors. A padded Mayfield headrest may not be appropriate for all patients undergoing spinal surgery, because exophthalmos or a flattened nasal bridge may allow transmission of pressure to the globe. Alternatively, a Gardner three-pronged head holder, which keeps the face completely free of all pressure, may be used. Most postoperative visual defects will show no significant improvement with time.

Lower limb compartment syndrome as a complication of prolonged surgery in the prone position has been reported,[2,20] as has upper limb compartment syndrome associated with the lateral decubitus position.[37] The need to avoid pressure to the extremities in all positions selected cannot be overemphasized.

A longitudinal midline incision over the area to be operated on is scratched unto the skin. The subcutaneous tissues are infiltrated with a mixture of 1:500,000 epinephrine to cause vasoconstriction and reduce bleeding. The subcutaneous tissues are then incised directly down to the lumbodorsal fascia, which is incised and exposed through the midline. On each side a Cobb elevator and electrocautery are used to subperiosteally dissect the soft tissues from the distal lumbar spinous processes and from the posterior midline crest of the sacrum. In the case of the facet joint between L5 and S1, the Cobb elevator can be hooked around the joint to lift the muscles over, while preserving the capsular integrity of the joint. The posterior foramen must be carefully approached to prevent bleeding from its vessels. If this occurs, then bipolar electrocautery will achieve hemostasis.

The bony landmarks may be identified in three ways. First and foremost, a lateral intraoperative x-ray exami-

nation with a suitable marker in place identifies the sacrum. This is a mandatory part of the procedure. Second, the sacrum has a hollow sound when tapped with a blunt instrument. Third, a towel clip applied to the spinous process of L5 will demonstrate motion. That is to say, it identifies the last mobile segment, indicating that the sacrum is immediately adjacent. No motion is seen at the sacrum.

Posterior Sacrospinalis-Splitting Approach

Wiltse et al.[50] described the paraspinal sacrospinalis-splitting approach to the lumbar spine. It provides access to the transverse process of L5 and to the ala of the sacrum. This incision may be carried further distally to expose the whole sacrum either on one or both sides. The patient is placed in the prone position as described previously. Two longitudinal incisions are made starting medial to the posterior superior iliac spine, with a slight medial curve to the incision at its distal extent. The subcutaneous tissues are incised down to the deep fascia overlying the sacrospinalis muscle. Alternatively a single midline incision may be used. In this case a full-thickness flap is lifted on each side at the level of the deep fascia to expose the paramedian tissues. On each side the muscle is split bluntly to avoid bleeding and the bony tissues identified in the floor of the wound. The approach is ideal for lumbosacral fusions as exposure of the lateral gutter is excellent. A separate incision in the deep fascia is used for harvesting bone graft from the iliac crest.

Retroperitoneal Approaches

Retroperitoneal approaches to the sacrum may be performed through either an anterior paramedian incision with the patient supine or an oblique incision with the patient in the lateral decubitus position. Retroperitoneal approaches have the advantage of avoiding contact with the intraperitoneal contents. Usually a postoperative ileus can be avoided.

The anterior paramedian approach affords good access to both sides of the sacrum and avoids having to completely mobilize the iliac arteries. The patient is positioned supine with a sandbag beneath the lower lumbar spine. A left paramedian incision is made based over the lateral border of the left rectus abdominis muscle. Subcutaneous tissue is incised down to the anterior rectus sheath, which is also incised in the line of the skin incision. This reveals the left rectus abdominis muscle, which is then either retracted toward the midline or from the midline to reveal the posterior rectus sheath. The inferior epigastric vessels are usually identified and cauterized as this is done. Careful sharp dissection is used to open the posterior rectus sheath to reveal the thin peritoneum beneath. A sponge is then used to peel the peritoneum circumferentially from the abdominal wall and so open up the retroperitoneal space. The peritoneum, with its contained abdominal contents, along with the ureter, is now retracted to the right. Blunt dissection over the anterior promontory of

---

*References 23, 27, 29, 30, 36, 46, 49, 51.

the sacrum will reveal the middle sacral vessels, which are ligated if needed.

An oblique incision for this approach allows the more cranial part of the lumbar spine to be exposed. If used, the muscle fibers of the external oblique, internal oblique, and transverse abdominis muscles are incised to expose the peritoneum.[16,28] The peritoneum is dissected from the abdominal wall as described. Fraser[17] has modified this approach by splitting each muscle layer in the line of its fibers. At no point are the muscle fibers cut, so theoretically bleeding should be decreased. The anterior retroperitoneal approach can also be performed with the patient lying on the side. In this case a flank incision is made halfway between the iliac crest and the twelfth rib. The muscle layers of the abdominal wall are incised and the peritoneum identified in the midaxillary line. The retroperitoneal space is then exposed in the manner described.

Anterior Transperitoneal Approach

The anterior transperitoneal approach to the lumbar spine is performed with the patient supine on the operating table. It is suitable for sacral resections, which in most cases will be done for tumors. The bowel should be cleansed prior to surgery. A nasogastric tube is passed first at the time of surgery because postoperative ileus is common. The bladder should be emptied with a urinary catheter. A small bolster or rest placed underneath the small of the back hyperextends the lumbosacral junction, so allowing easier access. Alternatively the table may be broken to achieve the same effect.

The incisions used can be either a vertical midline,[17] left paramedian,[41] or a Pfannensteil horizontal "smile" incision. Where sacral resection is to be done, a wide exposure is necessary, and for this the horizontal smile incision is extended upward. After incising skin and subcutaneous tissue, the rectus abdominis muscles are divided close to their insertion and lifted up superiorly to reveal the peritoneum. When a vertical midline approach is used, the incision is taken sequentially through skin, subcutaneous tissue, the linea alba, and the peritoneum. Bowel is packed off superiorly and laterally. Tilting the patient into the Trendenlenburg position facilitates this. The posterior peritoneum can now be opened over the sacral promontory with due care being taken to control the middle sacral vessels. It is important not to use diathermy because this procedure can damage the presacral nerves. Blunt dissection, starting from the midline and going laterally, seems to be the least traumatic to these nerves. More proximal access requires taking the large vessels to the right side. This can only be achieved by ligating their tethers, that is, the segmental vessels and the large iliolumbar vein.

Any exposure done immediately above the sacral promontory must be done carefully to avoid damage to the hypogastric plexus. Blunt dissection is preferred in favor of electrocauterization and gives the best chance of preserving nerve function. It is facilitated by first infiltrating the retroperitoneal tissues with adrenaline mixed with saline.[18,19] The superior hypogastric plexus is

> ### SURGICAL APPROACHES
>
> - Surgical exposures to the sacrum are selected sensibly based on the access desired.
> - The posterior midline or paramedian approaches grant access to the dorsum of the sacrum.
> - Access to the anterior sacrum may be gained through a retroperitoneal or transperitoneal approach.
> - Be on guard for hypogastric plexus injury or vascular injury. The iliolumbar vein, segmental vessels, and median sacral vessels should be identified and ligated.

formed from the sympathetic nervous system and lies in the bifurcation of the aorta. It is responsible for bladder neck closure during ejaculation and spermatozoa transport through the vas deferens.[32] Damage to the plexus may cause retrograde ejaculation in the male. The reported incidence of retrograde ejaculation and sexual dysfunction is inconsistent. Flynn and Hoque[16] reported an incidence of 0.42% and 0.44%, respectively. Recently Parazon[39] reported a series in which the incidence was low and any dysfunction not permanent.

When exposing the upper part of the sacrum anteriorly, vessel retraction is important for access. Steinmann pins placed into bone will effectively retract the large vessels and soft tissues. Care must be taken that there is a pulse distal to any vessel retracted to prevent ischemic injury. When removing these pins, vascular injury is possible from the sharp pin tips. The author's preference is to seat a flexible rubber tubing over the lower half of the Steinmann pin. When removing the pin, gentle downward pressure on the encircling tube ensheaths the tip so that it cannot damage the vasculature.

Sacral Tumors

Sacral tumors are uncommon. Primary sacral tumors may be benign or malignant. Benign ones include giant cell tumors (GCTs), aneurysmal bone cysts, neurofibromas, and schwannomas. Chordomas and chondrosarcomas are the most common primary malignant sacral tumors but, when placed in perspective, are still relatively rare. Their prominence in the literature is because of the unique difficulty in their management. Despite surgical resection, adjuvant radiation therapy, and chemotherapy, recurrence is common. The literature also reports other forms of primary malignant sacral tumors that are even less frequently seen; these are the osteosarcomas, Ewing's sarcomas, and hemangiopericytomas of the sacrum. Secondary sacral tumors arise from the breast, thyroid, lungs, kidneys, testes, and prostate. By far, breast carcinoma is the most common. In general the patients who come to surgery are those with malignant, large benign, or aggressive benign tumors. The key issue in the management of sacral tumors is to make the appropriate decision, surgical or otherwise, based on the biologic behavior of the tumor.

Application of the correct principles leads to a high standard of care. Adequate excision and reconstruction of the sacrum for neoplastic processes requires an understanding of the evaluation and staging of sacral neoplasm. The staging system of the Musculoskeletal Tumor Society[11,12] (Enneking et al.) is widely used, although the system has never been subjected to statistical validation tests. It was described before advanced imaging appeared and before the widespread use of adjuvant therapy. Additionally, this system was developed specifically for the long bones, with later application to the spine. Despite these criticisms it is useful as an oncologic staging system because it has prognostic value and defines the biologic behavior of primary tumors to facilitate planning and evaluation for surgery.

The Enneking staging system divides benign tumors into three stages and localized malignant tumors into four stages. It is based on a complete preoperative workup of the patient and includes clinical features, the radiographic, computed tomography (CT), and magnetic resonance imaging (MRI) data describing tumor extent, its peculiar imaging and the relationship with the neighboring tissues, an isotope bone scan, and histologic findings obtained by biopsy.

Oncologic Staging of Benign Bone Tumors

The staging is based on the biologic behavior of these tumors as suggested by radiographic findings. A stage 1 latent tumor is asymptomatic and commonly discovered incidentally on radiographs. Thick, dense reactive bone is present on both plain radiographs and CT scans. These lesions remain dormant or heal spontaneously. They include fibrous cortical defects, nonossifying fibromas, and osteoid osteomas.

Stage 2 benign tumors are actively growing and enlarging and therefore may be associated with physical signs and symptoms. A thin rim of bone outlines the perimeter, but the tumor remains intracompartmental. Pathologic fracture of the cortex may occur, however. Examples include slowly expanding aneurysmal bone cysts and chondroblastomas. Operative curettage and bone grafting are sufficient for these.

Stage 3 benign tumors are locally invasive. Their growth is progressive and not limited by barriers. There is little associated reactive bone, and the tumor often breaks through the bone cortex. Clinically and radiologically they are locally invasive. Pain, tenderness, and the presence of a mass are common. Imaging shows extension into surrounding tissues. These include GCTs and rapidly expanding aneurysmal bone cysts. Treatment is difficult and depends on the location of the tumor. In the long bones curettage with bone grafting or insertion of polymethyl methacrylate cement may be sufficient. In the spine a marginal resection is more appropriate.

Oncologic Staging of Malignant Bone Tumors

The staging of malignant bone tumors is based on three parameters:
1. Histologic grade (G)
2. Anatomic site (T)
3. The presence or absence of metastases

The grade is assigned on the basis of histopathologic criteria. There are two possibilities: low grade or high grade. Low-grade tumors have an estimated risk of metastasis of less than 25%. High-grade tumors have a risk exceeding 25%.

The anatomic site may be intracompartmental (A) or extracompartmental (B), with the designation "A" or "B" affixed to the stage. Intracompartmental tumors are bounded by natural barriers to extension, such as bone, fascia, synovial tissue, periosteum, or cartilage; that is, they remain within the vertebra. Extracompartmental tumors may be primary (occurring in an extracompartmental location) or secondary (i.e., an intracompartmental tumor that has penetrated into an additional compartment such as the paravertebral compartments by means of natural extension, fracture hemorrhage, or contamination at surgery).

Tumors that have not metastasized are assigned the designation M0. Those that have are designated M1.

Stage I tumors have metastatic potential of 25% or less. Therefore these are all G1 tumors. They are low-grade malignant tumors.

Stage II tumors have a metastatic potential of more than 25%. These are the G2 tumors. They are high-grade malignancies. With such rapid growth the host has no time to form a continuous reactive tissue layer. These tumors can have neoplastic nodules at some distance from the main tumor mass (skip metastases). Adjuvant courses of radiation and chemotherapy must be considered for local control and in an attempt to control distant spread.

Stage III tumors are those with metastases.

Staging of any tumor, whether benign or malignant, is critical, since this determines how the tumor will be managed. An intralesional resection is essentially a curettage or debulking of the tumor. It is appropriate for stages 1 and 2 benign bone tumors, as well as stage 3 when combined with adjuvant treatments.

A marginal resection is one that is done through the pseudocapsule or perilesional zone surrounding the tumor. It is appropriate for stage 3 benign bone tumors with adjuvant therapy and for selected low- and high-grade sarcomas after successful preoperative adjuvant chemotherapy and radiation therapy.

A wide excision is appropriate for recurrent stage 3 benign bone tumors and for most low- and high-grade bone sarcomas with or without adjuvant treatment. The resection is done through normal tissue outside the capsule.

A radical resection is one in which the entire compartment of tumor origin is excised. In the long bones this is suitable for recurrent sarcomas, for sarcomas whose extent cannot be determined, and where there is a displaced pathologic fracture through bone sarcomas. A tumor arising in the tibia that is treated by an above-knee amputation has by definition been radically resected. It is important to emphasize, however, that it is absolutely impossible to achieve a truly radical excision anywhere in the spine. Even if the spinal cord is sectioned above and below, the epidural space represents a huge compartment extending from the skull to the coccyx that cannot

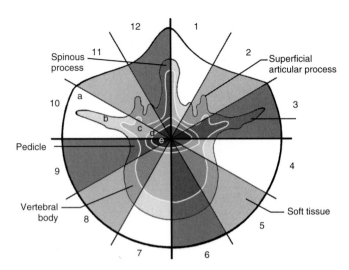

Figure 23-7. The Weinstein-Boriani-Biagini surgical staging system. The transverse extension of the vertebral tumor is described with reference to 12 radiating zones (numbered *1* to *12* in clockwise order) and to five concentric layers (*a* to *e*, from the paravertebral extraosseous compartments to the dural involvement). The longitudinal extent of the tumor is recorded according to the levels involved.

be excised. The best that can be done is a proper wide excision.

Surgical staging follows oncologic staging. Weinstein, Boriani, and Biagini[5] proposed a staging system that has been clinically evaluated (Figure 23-7). In the transverse plane the vertebra is divided into 12 radiating zones and 5 layers. The radiating zones are numbered 1 to 12 in a clockwise order and the 5 layers labeled a to e, from the paravertebral extraosseous region to the dura. The longitudinal extent of the tumor is recorded by spine segments involved. CT scanning, MRI, and sometimes angiography are needed to assign a designation. The system was designed to facilitate decision making about how to properly achieve an en bloc resection (wide excision) in the thoracolumbar spine, whether by vertebrectomy, sagittal resection, or posterior arch resection. Its importance in the sacrum is that it emphasizes the importance of approaching malignant tumors both anteriorly and posteriorly in order to achieve a wide excision.

Surgical Approaches to Sacral Tumors

Appropriate preoperative investigations include CT scans of the pelvis and sacrum, myelography plus CT of the lumbosacral spine, urography, angiography, and a barium enema examination. Neurologic status has to be investigated and documented with respect to sphincter function, perineal sensitivity, and motor power and sensation in the lower limbs. The role of plain radiography as a diagnostic tool is not to be underestimated. An early presumptive diagnosis of the common sacral tumors can be made on the basis of their radiographic characteristics.

Chordomas are characterized by osteolysis in the sacrococcyx, diminishing the outlines of the bone and

sacral foramina. The lesion occupies the midline, because the tumor arises from the remnants of the midline notochord. Extraosseous extension (either anteriorly or posteriorly) may be visible on x-ray examination, although it is better seen on MRI (Figure 23-8). The lesion may contain nonstructural and faded radiopaque spots that correspond to intratumoral calcifications. This is important, because it makes radiographic distinction between a chordoma and chondrosarcoma impossible. A central chondrosarcoma, however, is a rare occurrence in the sacrum, and at any rate its treatment is the same as that of a chordoma.

A GCT is unusual in the sacrum. In 90% of cases it is observed in the long bones, typically in the meta-epiphyseal segment. When in the sacropelvic region it is usually eccentric in position and may cross the sacroiliac joint to affect the ilium. The lesion is both expansive and osteolytic, with neither ossification nor calcification seen. Its boundaries with the surrounding bone are regular and clearly defined. Some GCTs grow rapidly and aggressively. These may show such rapid osteolytic expansion that the boundaries with the cancellous bone become unclear. Depending on the radiographic appearance, it is even possible to distinguish three categories of GCT, consistent with Enneking's stages for benign tumors.

Chondroblastomas are infrequent tumors and are distinctly rare in the sacropelvis. They are tumors of chondroblasts and so arise in an epiphysis or apophysis. In the sacropelvis they are found mostly around the triradiate cartilage but can involve the sacrum. As with GCTs these tumors are eccentrically positioned and characteristically have considerable calcification within the lesion. The borders are well defined and may at times be marked by a thin rim of osteosclerosis.

CT-guided biopsy provides a preoperative histologic diagnosis; however, the biopsy site has to be planned so that the biopsy scar can be removed en bloc with the surgical specimen. This emphasizes the importance of proper preoperative planning with a team approach. Occasionally a biopsy may be performed at an inappropriate site that makes surgical excision of the track difficult or impossible. This is seen when the procedures are done at different institutions or when the diagnosis is not considered at the time of biopsy. Prophylactic irradiation to the site is suggested as a method of gaining control. An intraoperative biopsy should always be avoided, because it is inadvisable to open the tumor in the surgical field.

Historically, various approaches have been proposed for excision of sacral tumors. Single posterior and combined anterior-posterior procedures have been described. In general, few truly large series with proper long-term follow-up exist.

Kaiser[33] reported the results from the Mayo Clinic of 63 patients who underwent an en bloc excision by a single posterior approach for malignant and aggressive benign sacral tumors. Even when the tumor appeared to have been removed en bloc, the recurrence rate was 28%. When the tumor was entered at surgery, the recurrence rate was 64%.

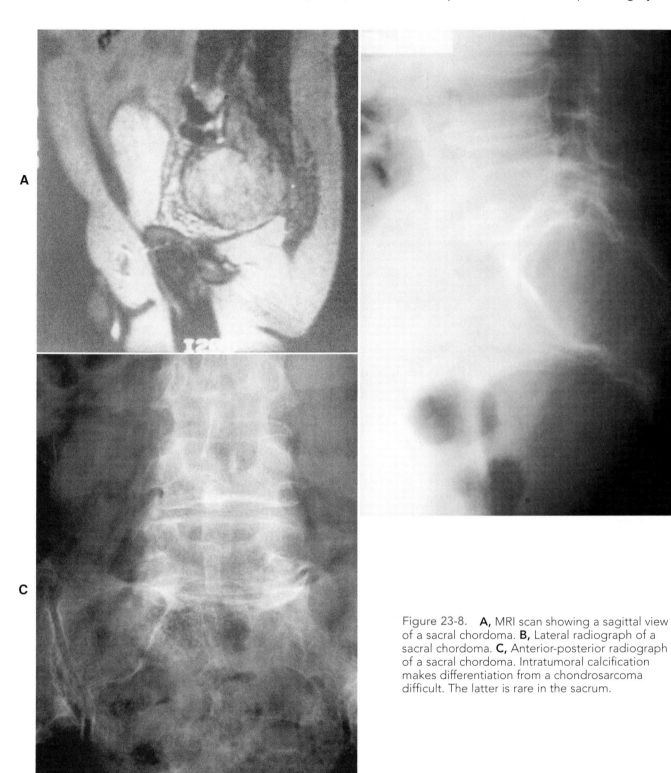

Figure 23-8. **A,** MRI scan showing a sagittal view of a sacral chordoma. **B,** Lateral radiograph of a sacral chordoma. **C,** Anterior-posterior radiograph of a sacral chordoma. Intratumoral calcification makes differentiation from a chondrosarcoma difficult. The latter is rare in the sacrum.

Gennari et al.[21] described a single posterior approach in eight patients for radical excision of sacrococcygeal chordomas, by a high resection through S2. They proposed this as an easier alternative to the combined abdominosacral approach. However, this was really only a marginal excision, based on the classification of Enneking, Spanier, and Goodman.[13] Four patients had recurrences around the rectum and lower buttock.

York et al.[52] reported their 40-year experience at a major cancer center. Over this period 40 patients had surgical resection, and, based on microscopic analysis of the margins, they were categorized as having either a radical resection or total excision. Many of these procedures were done through a single approach. The overall disease-free interval for patients undergoing a wide resection was 2.27 years compared with 8 months for patients having a subtotal excision. The addition of radiation after subtotal resection was found to improve the disease-free interval, but radiation therapy in general can be given only once.

Stener and Gunterberg[47] published a technique of near total resection of the sacrum but sparing either all or part of S1. Combined anterior and posterior approaches are required. If the rectum must be sacrificed, the surgery is done in three stages, starting anteriorly, then posteriorly, and finishing anteriorly with a colostomy. If the rectum can be saved, the operation is started anteriorly and completed posteriorly. This method has the lowest rate of recurrence in the literature. A dual anterior-posterior approach is now regarded as the accepted standard for excision of malignant or aggressive benign tumors.

Reports of a total sacrectomy exist in the literature. Edwards[10] reported two cases of complete resection of the sacrum, but he did no reconstruction. Shikata et al.[43] described their technique of total sacrectomy followed by reconstruction with Harrington instrumentation, sacral bars, and a massive bone allograft. Neither case had a sufficient number of patients to perform an adequate analysis of results.

Surgical Technique: Partial Sacral Resection

On the day before surgery, bowel preparation with repeated enemas should be done. Just prior to surgery, a vaginal pad inserted into the rectum allows identification of the rectum during surgery. Identifying the rectum in males can be difficult intraoperatively since males have a narrow angular path between the rectum and tumor.

A wide resection is done in normal tissue around the perimeter of the capsule of a tumor. At no time is the tumor or capsule exposed. Obtaining adequate surgical margins is of significant importance in avoiding recurrence. Considerations of preservation of bladder and bowel innervation and pelvic stability after surgery are important but secondary to the above considerations.

Conceptually, a true radical resection is a resection of the entire compartment of tumor origin. A marginal resection is one that is done through the pseudocapsule or perilesional zone surrounding a tumor. An intralesional resection is a curettage or debulking of a tumor, with certain risk of recurrence if it is malignant. It is only suitable for stage 1 and stage 2 benign bone tumors (i.e., latent or active benign tumors such as a GCT).

Even more important than the technical details of a given procedure are the principles included in sacral resection. This chapter will emphasize these points. The ardent reader is referred to more detailed tumor texts for precise detail.

The current standard for excision of malignant and aggressive benign sacral tumors is a combined anterior and posterior approach, starting anteriorly and finishing posteriorly. If it is necessary to excise the rectum, then a third anterior stage is added.

The patient is first placed in the lithotomy position and the rectum sutured closed. A curved lower abdominal skin incision is made in the suprapubic region; it is directed upward on each side far enough to get adequate exposure. Dissection deep to the subcutaneous tissues reveals the tendons of the rectus abdominis muscle. These are divided approximately 1 cm above the pubic bone so that a small cuff is left for repair. The lateral border of the aponeurotic sheath of the rectus abdominis is cut through so that the recti can be lifted upward. This approach reveals the parietal peritoneum. Where the rectum is to be preserved, the dissection is kept in the retroperitoneal plane. On either side the parietal peritoneum is dissected bluntly with sponges in a circumferential manner until the common iliac vessels are reached. From this point, the posterior parietal peritoneum is lifted up with further blunt dissection, taking with it the ureter and branches from the superior hypogastric nerve plexus. Both dissections will meet behind the rectum, so exposing the sacral promontory and the superior part of the sacrum. At this point the internal iliac artery and vein are divided separately and the cut ends secured by suture ligatures. The lateral and median sacral vessels are also divided and ligated. For high amputations through the S1 vertebra, it is advisable to also divide and ligate the iliolumbar vessels.

Usually the anteriorly protruding part of the tumor is covered with periosteum and presacral fascia. It is therefore necessary to strip the periosteum from the sacral promontory downward to the level selected for division of the sacrum. The sacrum should be resected to the extent necessary to provide a suitable margin for tumor excision. If the proximal extent lies between S1 and S2, then two thirds of the sacroiliac joint with the attached ligaments and both S1 nerves can be preserved. Sacral amputation at this level weakens the posterior arch of the pelvis by approximately one third.[7] If the proximal extent goes through the S1 vertebra, then the S1 nerves will have to be sacrificed, because the S1 foramen lies at the level of the S1 to S2 disc space. Under these circumstances only about half of the sacroiliac joint with corresponding ligaments will be left behind. This weakens the pelvis by approximately 50%. Because the sacral canals run in an anteroinferior direction, the osteotomy will be oblique, with more of the vertebra being preserved anteriorly compared with posteriorly.

Loss of all the sacral nerves, as in a high amputation through the S1 vertebra, leads to loss of the motor and sensory function of S1 and loss of all functions of S2 to S4 nerves. The parasympathetic, voluntary motor, and sensory innervation of the pelvic viscera are mediated by S2 to S4. If they are lost, one can expect denervation of the urinary bladder and urethral sphincters, impaired genital function, and bowel incontinence from loss of anorectal function. It is, however, still possible to maintain good motor function in the leg because the innervation by L5 can provide plantar flexion of the foot. Sympathetic innervation to the pelvic viscera is through the superior hypogastric plexus and in theory is un-affected whether all sacral nerves are sacrificed or S1 is preserved. If all the sacral nerves are sacrificed on one side only, there will be practically no deficit of the uro-genital or anorectal function.[47]

Placement of the osteotomy at the S1 to S2 junction, would mean cutting through the S1 canals on the ante-rior side. With a suitable osteotome the anterior cortical wall of the sacrum is divided transversely, ensuring that the osteotomy extends laterally past the sacroiliac joints on each side. This makes it easier to feel for the position of the osteotomy track when the posterior exposure is performed. Prior to starting the anterior osteotomy, however, always remember to mobilize and protect the lumbosacral trunk (L4 and L5).

If a decision to sacrifice the rectum has been made, then the anterior approach has to be transperitoneal. For this an inferior midline incision is more appropriate. The superior and middle rectal vessels are divided and ligated on each side, the bowel is cut through at the rectosigmoid junction, and both ends are closed by invagination. The rectovesical/rectouterine pouch is divided so that the rectum can be released as far distally as possible. With the patient in the lithotomy position, an inverted "U" incision is made around the anus, and the anal canal and rectum are dissected free anteriorly as far as possible working from below.

The posterior procedure is performed with the patient prone. The posterior incision should extend proximally to allow good exposure of the posterior elements of L5. Proximally, a flap of skin and subcutaneous tissue must be raised to expose and allow transection of the gluteus maximus muscle well away from the sacrum and sever-ance of the underlying piriformis muscle at its musculo-tendinous junction. Distally, it is important to include in the specimen the skin and the underlying subcutaneous layers over the lower part of the sacrum. This includes the tissues over the hiatus of the sacral canal through which the tumor might have penetrated. Any biopsy tract is widely excised, and while doing so, the knife must be directed obliquely away from the tract as it goes through the subcutaneous tissues. All skin and subcuta-neous tissue around the inferior part of the sacrum must be removed so that the sacral hiatus, through which tumor may have penetrated, is not breached. As the tumor grows, it extends through the sacral canal and may emerge through the posterior sacral holes. Because of this, exposure of the posterior sacrum would expose the tumor and breach the margin of resections. A margin of healthier tissue consisting of sacrospinalis muscle and a good portion of gluteus maximus on each side should accompany the specimen. The gluteus maximus is transected well away from the sacrum, and the piri-formis muscles are divided at their musculotendinous junction close to the piriformis fossa so that they are taken with the specimen. The superior and inferior gluteal vessels are divided and ligated, but it is impor-tant to preserve the superior gluteal nerve since it inner-vates the gluteus medius, gluteus minimus, and the tensor fascia lata. The sacrotuberous ligament is severed close to the ischial tuberosity. The sacrospinalis liga-ment is released by osteotomizing the ischial spine. When the rectum is to be sacrificed, the inferior skin incision is taken distally to meet the previously made inverted "U." The levator ani are transected on each side as part of the posterior dissection. In all cases the midline dissection must extend far enough superiorly to expose the posterior elements of L5 and the sacrospinalis muscles.

The level of the osteotomy determines whether the S1 nerve is preserved. If it is to be preserved, a partial laminectomy of L5 is performed and the dural sac ligated and divided below the S1 nerve root, which comes off at the level of the lumbosacral disc. If the S1 nerve is to be sacrificed, a complete laminectomy of L5 is done and the sac transected above S1. As a rule, the contents of the sacral canal should be divided as far proximally as the amputation permits, since tumor may extend up the canal further proximally than the ra-diographic limit in the bone suggests. The posterior osteotomy is done using the previous anterior cut for reference; this is easily palpated with the finger. When the S1 nerve is preserved, the osteotomy is made between the S1 and S2 vertebrae; the inferior half of each S1 canal is included in the specimen. When S1 is sacrificed, the entire canals of these nerves must be included in the specimen. Because the canals run obliquely in the sagittal plane, the sacral body is always divided obliquely, with more of the sacrum being pre-served anteriorly than posteriorly. The posterior parts of the iliac wings that protrude posterior to the sacrum should be included in the resection, because this area may be involved by the tumor as it spreads laterally under the sacrospinalis musculature.

When the osteotomy is completed, all the sacral con-tributors to the sciatic nerves bilaterally are severed at the level of the greater sciatic foramen. The specimen is now removed. After securing hemostasis, the posterior stage of the operation is completed by suturing the skin flaps in the midline. Distally an opening is left for drainage and a compression bandage applied.

If the rectum is to be included in the specimen, the patient is turned prone and the abdominal wound reopened. The sigmoid colon is released from its mesen-tery and a colostomy fashioned. The released mesentery, with its preserved vascular supply, can be used to create a pelvic closure of the peritoneal cavity. The periphery of the mesentery is sutured to the edge of the peritoneum, where it was cut in the rectovesical pouch (rectouterine pouch in females). The abdominal wound is then closed.

We believe the only way of achieving a true wide resection for a malignant sacral tumor is by approaching it anteriorly and posteriorly. The anterior approach allows visualization of every aspect of the dissection, which should only take place through healthy tissue with no exposure of the tumor. Simpson[45] has reported a series of 12 patients in whom an extended ilioinguinal approach was used in conjunction with a posterior midline approach. This widely extensile procedure permits simultaneous visualization of the anterior and posterior aspects of the sacrum at the time of oste-otomy. A solitary posterior approach cannot guarantee en bloc tumor excision, and as such I do not recommend it for malignant sacral tumors. The results in the literature from this procedure are inconsistent and in some instances unacceptable. A single posterior approach should only be used when a marginal excision is an acceptable method of treatment.

Rectal excision is only indicated in two circumstances: (1) involvement of the rectum by tumor and (2) when a transrectal biopsy has been performed in the presence of a malignant tumor. Such a biopsy through the rectal wall transgresses the anterior fibrous barrier for the tumor, with contamination of the retrorectal space and rectal wall with tumor cells. A transrectal biopsy of a sacral tumor is always a mistake. Under these circumstances the rectum must be included in the specimen in order to obtain clearance.

If the rectum is to be spared, surgery starts anteriorly and finishes posteriorly. The anterior dissection is extraperitoneal, which gives good exposure. When the rectum is to be sacrificed, a colostomy will be necessary. The surgery starts anteriorly, continues posteriorly, and finishes anteriorly.

Surgical Technique: Total Sacrectomy

Total sacrectomy is reserved for extensive tumors, the size of which would not allow preservation of the S1 vertebra with en bloc tumor resection. Whereas partial sacral amputation does not destabilize the pelvis, total sacrectomy does do so and requires extensive reconstruction of the pelvic ring, with establishment of bilateral union between the lumbar spine and ilium. Additionally, because all sacral roots are removed, urinary bladder, rectosigmoid colon, and sexual function are markedly altered, although functional impairments are manageable with rehabilitation.

The surgery is performed in two stages.[24] The first stage is an anterior transperitoneal procedure. The goal here is to mobilize the visceral and vascular structures from the anterior aspect of the lumbosacral spine. The rectosigmoid colon is dissected from the presacral area to the coccyx. The internal iliac arteries and veins and the lateral and median sacral vessels are divided at their origin to expose the first and second anterior sacral nerve roots. The common iliac vessels, distal vena cava, and aorta are also mobilized laterally by dividing their posterior branches. This allows a clear view of the L5 disc space and also allows visualization of the lumbosacral trunk (L4 and L5 nerve roots). Once this trunk is found, the sacroiliac joint will be lateral to it. Bilateral partial ventral sacroiliac osteotomies are performed. The lumbosacral disc is excised and the S1 to S3 ventral sacral roots divided at their foramina. Because the second stage may be delayed, a Silastic sheath should be placed dorsal to the viscera and vascular structures to prevent adhesion formation that would make the second stage difficult.

The second stage involves reopening the initial incision, then mobilizing a unilateral myocutaneous flap fed by the inferior epigastric vessels. It is placed dorsal to the rectosigmoid colon but ventral to the Silastic sheath

close the defect in the pelvic floor. The abdominal incision is closed and the patient placed prone.

The posterior procedure requires exposure of L2 to the coccyx. The midline structures are exposed distally as far as L5, and at this level a total laminectomy is performed. The posterior iliac crests, greater sciatic foramen, and sciatic nerves are exposed bilaterally, but skin, subcutaneous tissue, and muscle over the sacrum are left intact to facilitate en bloc tumor removal. This means that the incision becomes elliptical in its distal aspect. Once the L5 laminectomy is done, the thecal sac and cauda equina become exposed. All the sacral roots are divided and the thecal sac closed. The posterior-superior iliac spines are removed so that osteotomy cuts can be made lateral to the sacral ala and parallel to the sacroiliac joints, so completing the anterior osteotomy cuts made previously. The sacrospinous and sacrotuberous ligaments must be divided and the rectum carefully separated from the distal sacrococcygeal attachments. The entire sacrum is then removed en bloc.

The sacral area is reconstructed using two vertical L-shaped rods. These are fixed to the L3 to L5 pedicles with screws and into the ilia using the Galveston technique. Two or three cross-connecting rods are used to create a rigid quadrilateral frame. A transverse threaded rod (transiliac bar) is used to bridge opposing iliac bones and prevent axial rotation of the lumboiliac union. An autograft from the posterior iliac crest and an allograft are used for the posterolateral intertransverse fusion. A tibial allograft strut is used to close the space between the two ilia. The rectus abdominis myocutaneous flap is now advanced through the pelvis, positioned over the reconstructed area, and secured to muscle and skin after placement of drains.

SUMMARY OF SURGICAL PROCEDURES

- Appropriate staging of all benign and malignant sacral tumors should precede any decision concerning treatment.
- A marginal resection is done through the pseudocapsule or perilesional zone surrounding the tumor. This technique is inappropriate for malignant sacral tumors but suitable for aggressive benign ones (e.g., giant cell tumors).
- A wide resection or en bloc excision is one done through normal tissue surrounding the tumor. This gives the least risk of recurrence. At no time during the dissection should the tumor be breached or visualized.
- It is impossible to achieve a radical resection in the spine.
- A combined anterior and posterior procedure gives the best chance of achieving a wide resection in the sacrum. Solitary posterior approaches have high recurrence rates.
- A transrectal biopsy of a malignant sacral tumor is a mistake. It commits the patient to having a rectal excision in order to obtain adequate clearance.

Extensive rehabilitation is required following this procedure. Patients remain in bed for 8 weeks of progressive ambulation. Ambulation may be difficult due to weak hip extensors and plantar flexors of the feet, but this improves with time.

Voluntary bowel and bladder control is permanently lost due to sectioning of the S2 nerve roots. Bowels are managed by use of a constipating diet along with regularly timed laxatives and evacuations. The bladder will require intermittent catheterization, usually at 6-hour intervals.

TRAUMA

Sacral fractures are distinctly uncommon and require a high degree of suspicion for associated diagnoses. There are two main types:

1. Isolated sacral fractures account for only 5% to 10% of these types of injuries.
2. Sacral fractures associated with pelvic injuries are more commonly seen. They are potentially serious injuries resulting from medium- to high-energy trauma.

The easiest and perhaps most common way in which sacral fractures are classified is according to the direction of the fracture line within the sacrum. Hence these fractures may be vertical, oblique, or transverse (Figure 23-9) and occur at any level in the sacrum.

Denis et al. provided the most comprehensive analysis of sacral fractures, based on both clinical and cadaveric data.[7] Their classification system, made on this basis, correlates with neurologic injuries and the treatment recommendations. Three vertical zones are identified (Figure 23-10):

- Zone I Alar fractures; that is, they occur lateral to the sacral foramina.
- Zone II—Involve all four neural foramina.
- Zone III—Involve the central sacral canal.

A given fracture is classified based upon the highest zone that it transverses. Therefore a transverse sacral fracture would be a zone III injury because it involves the central canal.

Zone I fractures may be either minimally displaced or severely displaced. The former is seen in association with open book or lateral compression fractures of the pelvis. The latter is seen in vertical shear pelvic fractures. It is unusual for a zone I fracture to have a neurologic deficit. It is only seen in 6% of such cases, and when it occurs, it typically is either a sciatic nerve injury or involves the L5 nerve root. Unless seen in association with a serious pelvic injury, these fractures can be treated by bed rest and early mobilization. Deficits caused by root compression at the level of the sacral foramen or traumatic "far-out" lesions of L5 are treated by decompression with open reduction and internal fixation.

Zone II injuries have accompanying neurologic injury in 30% of patients, typically unilateral L5, S1, or S2 nerve deficits. Absence of central canal involvement means bowel and bladder function are spared. Vertical fractures involving zone II are managed operatively with direct screw fixation; however, compression of the fracture site is not desirable.

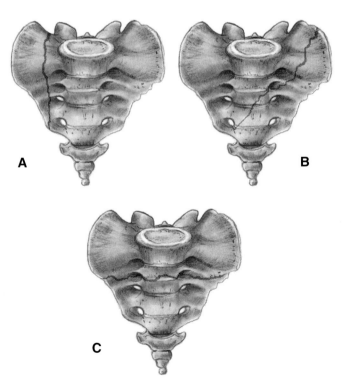

Figure 23-9. Classification of sacral fractures.
A, Vertical. **B,** Oblique. **C,** Transverse.

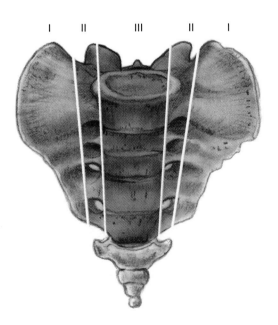

Figure 23-10. Classification of sacral fractures according to Denis et al.[7] Three zones of injury are differentiated: zone I, sacral ala; zone II, foraminal region; zone III, spinal canal. The most medial fracture extension is used to classify an injury.

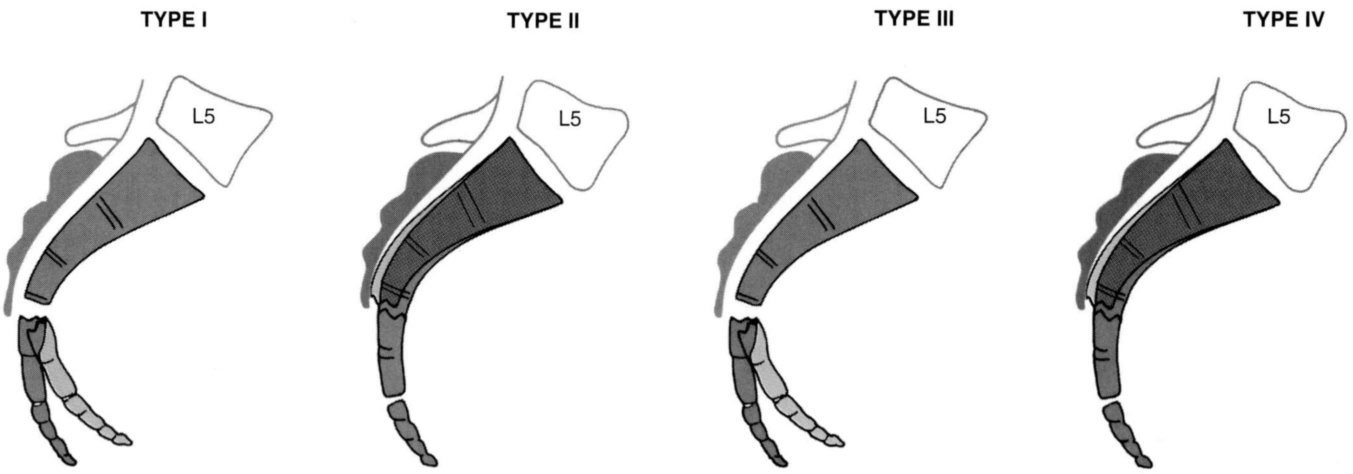

TYPE I	TYPE II	TYPE III	TYPE IV

Figure 23-11. Classification of transverse sacral fractures by Roy-Camille and associates as modified by Strange Vognsen and Lebech: Type I, flexion fracture without translation; type II, flexion fracture with posterior displacement; type III, extension fracture with anterior displacement; type IV, segmental comminution of the upper sacrum.

Zone III fractures have an overall 57% incidence of neurologic injuries. In the series of Denis et al.,[7] 76% of patients presented with bowel or bladder and sexual functional deficits. Upper sacral fractures (S1 to S3) are more frequently associated with bladder dysfunction when compared with lower sacral fractures (S4 and S5).

Transverse sacral fractures are really Denis type III injuries. Roy-Camille and associates classified these into three types; Strange Vognsen and Lebech later added a fourth category[48] (Figure 23-11):

1. Type I—Flexion fractures without translation
2. Type II—Flexion fractures with posterior displacement
3. Type III—Extension fractures with anterior displacement
4. Type IV—Segmental comminution of the upper sacrum

Transverse fractures with neurologic deficits may be treated by direct decompression and stabilization. Overall, neurologic recovery ranges from 50% to 100%.[48] The series reported by Denis et al.[7] showed that all patients with loss of bowel and bladder function had full return of function when treated operatively. Nonoperatively treated patients had either partial or no return of the function; these findings are also supported by the work of Gibbons et al.[22] and Albert et al.

Imaging is important for precisely identifying the fracture pattern and determining the surgical approach if needed.

Radiographs

Plain anteroposterior (AP) radiographs may not always show a fracture because there is a 45-degree posterior inclination of the sacrum due to the lumbosacral lordosis. Additionally, detail is obscured by the overlying soft tissues and gas. A Ferguson AP view helps; this is a 30-degree AP view with cranial projection meant to eliminate the effect of the lordosis. All suspected cases of

---

> **INDICATIONS FOR SURGICAL TREATMENT OF SACRAL FRACTURES**
>
> - Neurologic deficit
> - Pelvic ring instability
> - Lumbosacral junction instability
> - Major angular or translational deformity

sacral fracture should have a coned-down lateral sacral view and inlet and outlet views of the pelvis. It is important to search for associated injuries to the pelvis and fractures of the transverse process of L5.

Computed Tomography

The purpose of CT is to define the anatomy of the injury and the position of the fracture fragments and to plan reduction techniques. Narrow-section CT and sagittal and coronal reconstructions give good anatomic detail of fractures. Axial CTs on their own are inadequate because their cut may pass through the fracture and remain unseen.

Magnetic Resonance Imaging

MRI is inferior to CT scanning for the resolution of detail in comminuted fractures but is of value in demonstrating neural element compression when there is a neurologic deficit. Direct images in the coronal and sagittal planes can be obtained. There is no need for reconstructing images as is necessary when CT scanning is done.

The goal of treatment is to reestablish a pain-free stable pelvic ring with optimal neurologic function. The indications for surgical treatment of sacral fractures are listed in the box.

Gibbons et al.[22] showed that patients with neurologic deficit benefit from decompression. In his study 88% of

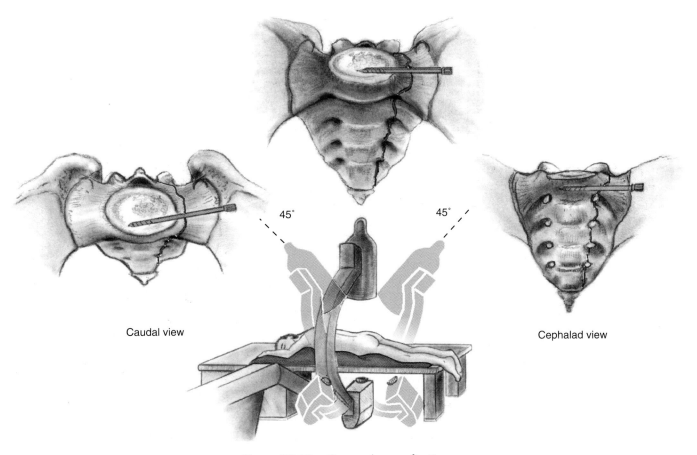

Caudal view

45°   45°

Cephalad view

Figure 23-12.   Iliosacral screw fixation.

patients with neurologic deficit improved after decompression, compared with 20% of nonsurgically treated patients.

There are two methods for achieving decompression. Indirect techniques rely on realignment of a displaced neural canal or neuroforamen. Direct techniques involve sacral laminectomy and a ventral sacral foraminotomy if needed. Pelvic ring instability is dealt with either indirectly by external fixation or directly by open reduction and internal fixation. Decompression should always be followed by surgical stabilization if there is pelvic ring instability. Methods of sacral stabilization include sacroiliac joint plating anteriorly or posteriorly, sacral bars fixation using compression rods placed through the posterior iliac crest, and percutaneous iliac sacral screw fixation.

Surgical Technique: Iliosacral Screw Fixation

This technique is used for displaced vertical fractures in zone I and zone II with pelvic involvement. Iliosacral screw fixation is preferable to the use of sacral bars. When needed, compression is achieved directly across the fracture site. Sacral bar fixation may lever open the anterior part of the sacral fracture because the point of compression is posterior to the sacral line.

The technique allows the operator to vary the amount of compression applied. A partially threaded 6.5-mm

cannulated screw will appropriately compress vertical zone I fractures. Compression is undesirable in foraminal zone II fractures since this would cause impingement of the local nerve roots. Use of a fully threaded screw gives the option of minimal or no compression.

Debate in the literature concerning the use of one or two screws continues. The work of Simonian et al.[44] shows little difference between one or two iliosacral screws.

Iliosacral screw fixation is done under general anesthesia with the patient in either the prone or supine position using imaging intensification to verify fracture reduction and guide pin position prior to definitive screw placement. Whether supine or prone positioning is used depends on the surgeon's preference. The prone position facilitates the initial access when one is dealing with an obese patient. The image intensifier is placed opposite the surgeon transversely so that it may be swung to provide the direct lateral, 45-degree caudal, and 45-degree cephalad view needed to visualize the lateral sacrum, and the pelvic inlet/outlet views, respectively (Figure 23-12). It is imperative that the fracture is reduced prior to starting, and this is done by means of skeletal traction applied at surgery via a femoral transcondylar Steinmann pin. An assistant pulls on the traction device to achieve the desired amount of fracture reduction. The first view taken is a direct lateral view of the lumbosacral area. Its purpose is to identify the starting point for passage of the guide wire. The superior aspect of the

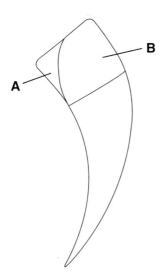

Figure 23-13.   Lateral view of the sacrum showing the safe zone for iliosacral screw fixation. **A,** Unsafe zone. **B,** Safe zone for screw insertion. This area represents the body of S1.

sacrum shows a curved condensation, which represents the corticated upper surface of the sacral ala. It is important not to transgress the triangular area in front of this because the L5 nerve root courses here and would be penetrated[40] (Figure 23-13). At all times the guide wire and screw should be within the sacral ala.

Screw Placement

The starting point also coincides approximately with the intersection of a line from the midpoint of the sciatic notch and one from the posterior superior iliac crest. A small skin incision is made and the guide wire advanced to the lateral wall of the ilium. Another direct lateral view confirms that the starting point is within the confines of the safe zone of the ala as described. Repeated identification of this alar safe zone following fracture reduction is the most important part of the procedure. The author's preferred method is to gently tap the guide wire across the ilium, the sacroiliac joint, and into the body of S1 while swinging the imaging intensifier alternately between the pelvic inlet and outlet views to ensure safe guide wire passage. The pelvic outlet view shows the position of the S1 foramen at all times because the guide wire must be above this to prevent S1 nerve root injury. It is often easier to identify this foramen on the opposite uninjured side in order to appreciate its position on the ipsilateral injured side.

The pelvic inlet view shows the position of the cauda equina. This is really a bird's-eye view of the sacral spinal canal. To be safe, the operator must be below this circle to avoid injury to the sacral nerve roots (see Figure 23-12).

Definitive screw fixation with a 6.5-mm cancellous screw over a washer is then done. For zone I injuries it is sufficient to achieve a depth of penetration to the midline. Zone II injuries require fixation across the midline, and zone III injuries require fixation as far as the contralateral ala (Figure 23-14).

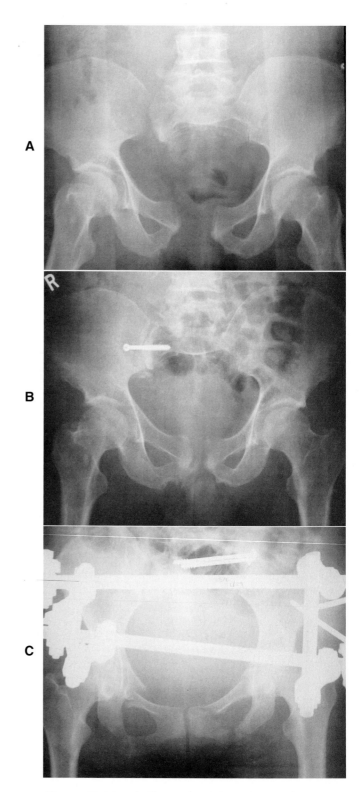

Figure 23-14.   **A,** External rotation injury to the pelvis. The symphysis pubis and the right sacroiliac joint are both disrupted. **B,** Sacroiliac screw in place. **C,** Two sacroiliac screws in place.

INDICATIONS FOR SACRAL PLATING

- Unstable fractures, oblique or transverse injuries
- Significant deformity
- Neurologic deficit

PEDICLE SCREW FIXATION

- Ideal pedicle screw placement in S1 pedicle parallel to superior sacral end plate and directed slightly medially.
- Large overhanging ilium may dictate laterally directed screw. Again placement should be parallel to end plate but directed 30 degrees laterally. Lateral placement has a smaller margin for error than does medial placement.
- Be especially careful on the left side, where the left iliac vein is easily injured. Remember, it is closely applied to the anterior sacral surface.

The use of CT with multiplanar reconstruction improves accuracy in determining the sacroiliac screw position relative to the neural foramen . The assessment of screw position may be facilitated using titanium screws.[25]

Sacral plating is done with the patient prone on a slightly flexed radiolucent table. Image intensification may be used to establish correct screw positioning.

A midline posterior incision done from L4 to S5 will give wide exposure. It is important to dissect laterally in a subperiosteal manner beyond the sacral foramina to get adequate space for plate positioning. Meticulous attention must be paid to hemostasis. It is important to avoid worsening the neurologic deficit by undue motion of the sacral fragments. Proximally the L5 to S1 facet joints must be preserved by dissecting around them onto the sacral alae. At this stage a wide sacral laminectomy should be done, starting proximally and extending distally. The lateral extent is the medial wall of the vestigial sacral pedicles. Starting proximally has the advantage of exposing the wider part of the sacral canal first, which is technically easier, as well as being above the neurologic deficit. This approach allows the surgeon to work from an area of normal nerve root tissue to an area of abnormal compressed tissues. It exposes the area of maximum deformity, giving better visual identification and orientation.

Fracture reduction usually can be done with a Cobb elevator (Figure 23-15). This instrument is carefully inserted into the fracture site and the fragments gently levered back into place. For transverse fractures this is usually sufficient. Oblique fractures, however, tend to foreshorten with impaction of the cancellous bone at the fracture site. A useful technique for reduction is to insert a bicortical screw in the sacral ala proximally and another distal to the fracture. Pelvic reduction clamps placed over both screws allow distraction with disimpaction of the fracture fragments so that realignment is possible. Occasionally even after fracture reduction, a large fragment of bone protrudes dorsally into the sacral canal with nerve root compromise. This is best dealt with by decancelization of one or both sacral alae to give access via an oblique lateral exposure. A pituitary rongeur can be used to remove the fragments. This is a safe technique. No attempt should be made to tamp the fragments back into place.

Two pelvic reconstruction plates are contoured and placed dorsally in a line directly over the dorsal foramina. Either a 3.5- or 4.5-mm plate may be used, depending on hole spacing and the size of the sacrum. The proximal part of the sacrum is preferably fixed with two screws. The more proximal screw is introduced at the lateral part of the S1 superior facet and directed medi-

ally. The lower screw, at the inferior edge of the S1 facet, is directed 30 degrees laterally into the sacral ala and parallel to the sacral end plate. More distally, the screws are inserted at S2, S3, and S4. These are progressively shorter screws that are directed laterally at a trajectory of 20 to 35 degrees in order to be parallel to the sacroiliac joint. This allows for maximum screw length. Screws are placed at every hole that does not fall directly over a dorsal foramen. For maximum pullout strength, pairs of adjacent screws should converge in the caudocephalad direction.

Surgical Technique: Pedicle Screw Fixation

Pedicle screw devices have become an important reconstructive tool in surgery of the lumbosacral spine. It facilitates sacral fixation and fusion to the lumbar spine. The complex interdigitation of neurovascular, visceral, and urogenital structures anterior to the sacrum constitutes a significant risk factor should the anterior surface of the sacrum be penetrated.

When placing pedicle screws in the sacrum, it is unnecessary in most circumstances to achieve fixation to the anterior cortex. On a theoretical basis, then, the risks provided by these anatomic structures may not seem to matter. However, the desire to use the best available bone stock, the risk of inadvertent penetration of the anterior cortex of the sacrum, and the need to gain bicortical purchase where bone stock is poor or after a failed attempt at screw insertion mean that anatomic guidelines are important.

Variations in the bony architecture of the sacral canal have been well documented.[9] The shape of the sacral foramina is variable and their position in three dimensions inconsistent.[31] In particular, the morphology of the posterior crest of the ilium is highly variable with respect to its thickness and proximity to the midline. This affects any proposed trajectory for sacral screw fixation. The lumbosacral plexus is firmly attached to the anterior bony sacral surface where the roots exit the sacrum and travel lateral to the foramina. Any implant that penetrates the anterior bony sacrum lateral to the foramen would endanger the integrity of the sacral roots inferior to the first sacral foramen and endanger the L5 root at the level of the first sacral foramen.

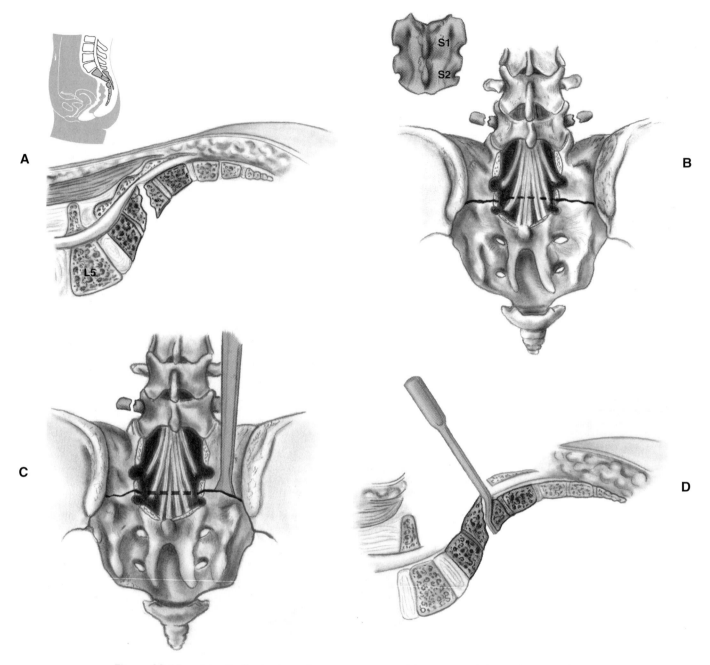

Figure 23-15. **A** to **G,** Illustration of a transverse sacral fracture and the technique of reduction and fixation.

Continued

The common iliac veins lie close to the anterior sacral surface. A screw placed internally at or above the level of the first sacral foramen could easily penetrate the iliac vein, particularly on the left side.[15]

Biomechanical studies[1] indicate that the maximum shearing stress is obtained for screws directed obliquely medially, less for screws placed straightforward, and least for screws directed laterally.

Esses et al.[15] have shown that radiographic examination with CT scanning before surgery is a simple means

of unveiling potentially disastrous anatomic variations in the lumbosacral region. CT should be performed with the scanner gantry tilted parallel to the superior sacral end plate. CT scans in individually tilted planes also allows one to assess the quality of cancellous bone in the lateral masses of the sacrum, as well as the thickness of cortical bone.

When all the anatomic and biomechanical data are considered, it seems that a safe course for screw implantation in the sacrum would involve starting above the

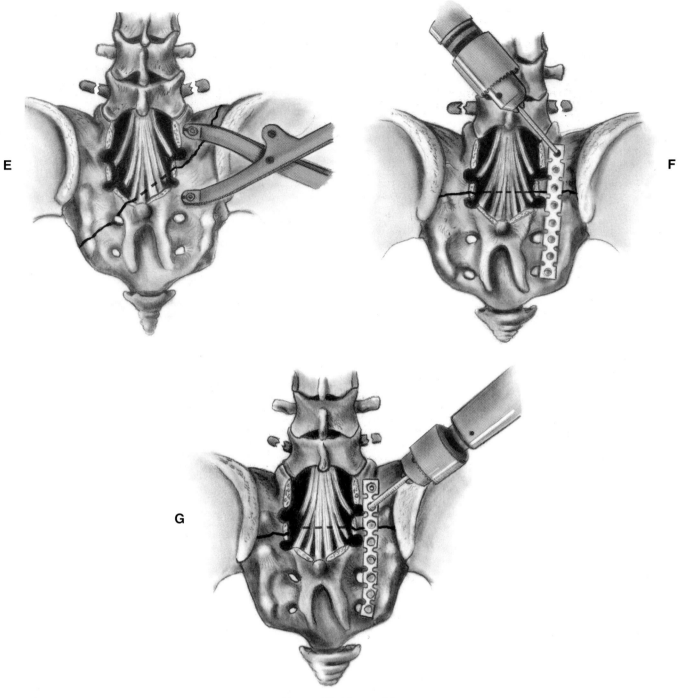

Figure 23-15, cont'd.

level of the first sacral foramen, directing the screw parallel to the superior sacral end plate to ensure that the screw tip does not violate the first sacral foramen. The screws are best directed medially toward the promontory to optimize pull-on strength and to avoid the common iliac vein on the left. The iliac vein can be injured if the screw on this side is directed straight ahead. Optimally, then, the screw should be directed medially in the axial planes and parallel to the lumbosacral disc in the sagittal plane, with no penetration of the anterior cortex.

It is possible to direct the screws laterally in a safe manner. This becomes necessary when a prominent and medially overhanging ilium precludes a medial trajectory. Cadaveric studies[35] have determined that a "safe zone" exists lateral to the lumbosacral trunk and medial to the sacroiliac joint. This safe zone is smaller with less margin for error when compared with a similar zone for medial screw placement. It dictates that any laterally directed screw is best angled downward 25 degrees to the sagittal plane (to be parallel to the superior sacral end plate) and directed 30 degrees laterally. Bicortical purchase is unnecessary. A screw with a blunt tip and tapered distal threads is preferred to push away any neurovascular structures that may be encountered.

The pedicle of S1 can often accommodate a screw of larger thread diameter such as a 7.5-mm screw. The larger diameter screw will find use in osteopenic bone or where the initial hole drilled in the bone has been inadvertently enlarged.

Sacral Infection

Pyogenic infection of the sacrum is not frequently seen. It is more common in adults, with an average age of presentation in the fourth to fifth decade. A higher incidence occurs among patients with an impaired immune system secondary to diabetes mellitus, alcoholism, the use of corticosteroids, chemotherapy for cancer, rheumatic or immunologic disease, renal or hepatic failure, malnutrition, or myelodysplasia. Sepsis from a distant site provides an increased risk of infection; local infections and operative interventions may facilitate contiguous spread. Prolonged surgery, a high volume of personnel moving through the operating room, prolonged bed rest, obesity, previous spinal surgery, and smoking are additional risk factors.

The most common bacterial organism is still *Staphylococcus aureus*. Gram-negative and low-virulence atypical organisms are increasingly isolated. Gram-negative aerobic bacilli may have their origin in genitourinary infections, and, in particular, *Pseudomonas* sp. is commonly seen in association with intravenous drug use.

Streptococcus sp. may also account for pyogenic osteomyelitis of the sacrum. Group B streptococcus will be seen in immunocompromised or debilitated adults. *Streptococcus pneumoniae* may be the etiologic agent in some patients with hemoglobinopathies, bone trauma, and advancing years. *Streptococcus bovis* and group G streptococci may also produce vertebral infection. Salmonella often causes sacral osteomyelitis in patients with sickle cell anemia.

Mycobacterium sp. has seen a resurgence among the immunocompromised. As in other areas of the spine, it causes a spondylitis of the sacrum, which can later progress to abscess formation either anteriorly or posteriorly. The epidural space may be the site of an epidural abscess.

Fungal infections are rare but include aspergillosis, blastomycosis, coccidioidomycosis, and cryptococcosis.

These are seen in immunocompromised hosts and in areas where these fungi are geographically endemic. *Candida albicans* osteomyelitis and other opportunistic fungi such as *Pseudallescheria boydii* or *Phialemonium obovatum* occur opportunistically. *Actinomyces israelii* has been reported as a cause of infection. *Coccidioides immitis* may produce lesions in more than one area simultaneously.

Sacral osteomyelitis may be treated conservatively or operatively. The mainstay of conservative treatment is parenteral antibiotic therapy. Ideally this follows the culture of a sample obtained by CT-guided biopsy, with culture and in vitro antibiotic sensitivity testing. The duration of treatment is controversial, but 6 weeks seems acceptable to most authorities. The addition of surgery is only mandatory for the treatment of complications of sacral osteomyelitis (e.g., paraspinal abscess or progressive paraplegia) and for neurologic impairment. Failure to obtain an appropriate sample for testing via CT-guided biopsy is an indication to proceed to open biopsy, at which time debridement and stabilization can be carried out. Chronic osteomyelitis of the sacrum means that dead bone is present and mandates debridement. Surgical debridement is also indicated when parenteral antibiotics have failed.

Postoperative deep infections are treated by irrigation and debridement. A bone graft, with or without instrumentation, should be allowed to remain in situ unless the graft is grossly suppurative or necrotic. Instrumentation should be left in situ to avoid the risk of pseudarthrosis. The instability created by removing the instrumentation will compromise resolution of the infection. The wound may be closed over one or more suction drains, but in some circumstances it may be more appropriate to pack the wound open and opt for delayed primary closure.

SELECTED REFERENCES

Denis F, Davis S, Comfort T: Sacral fractures: an important problem, *Clin Orthop* 227:67, 1988.

Fraser RD: A wide muscle-splitting approach to the lumbosacral spine, *J Bone Joint Surg Br* 64:44-46, 1982.

Gibbons KJ, Soloniuk DS, Razach N: Neurological injury and patterns of sacral fractures, *J Neurosurg* 72:889, 1990.

Wiltse LL et al.: The paraspinal sacrospinalis- splitting approach to the lumbar spine, *J Bone Joint Surg Am* 50:919-926, 1968.

REFERENCES

1. Argenson C: Tearing stress of pedicle screws. Poster session at Scoliosis Research Society, Amsterdam, Sept 1989.
2. Aschoff A et al.: Lower lumbar compartment syndrome following lumbar discectomy in the knee-chest position, *Neurosurg Rev* 13(2):155-159, 1990.
3. Batson OV: The function of the vertebral veins and their role in the spread of metastases, *Ann Surg* 112:138-149, 1940.
4. Bertolotti M: Contributo alla conoscenza dei vizi didderenzazione regionle del rachid con speciale riguardo all'assimilazione sacrale adlla v lombare, *Radiol Med* 4:113-144, 1917.
5. Boriani S, Weinstein JN, Biagini R: Primary bone tumors of the spine: terminology and surgical staging, *Spine* 22(9):1036-1044, 1997.
6. Castellvi AE, Goldstein LA, Chan DP: Lumbosacral transitional vertebrae and their relationship with lumbar extradural defects, *Spine* 9(5):493-495, 1984.

SACRAL INFECTION

- Pyogenic infections of the sacrum are uncommon.
- The most common organism is *Staphylococcus aureus*.
- Immunocompromised patients develop unusual infections with *Streptococcus* sp., mycobacteria, and fungi.
- Surgical treatment is reserved for the complications of sacral osteomyelitis.

7. Denis F, Davis S, Comfort T: Sacral fractures: an important problem, *Clin Orthop* 227:67, 1988.

8. Distefano DJ et al.: Intraoperative analysis of the effects of position and body habitus on surgery of the low back, *Clin Orthop* 99:51, 1974.

9. Ebraheim NA et al.: Evaluation of the upper sacrum by three-dimensional computed tomography, *Am J Orthop* 28(10):578-582, 1999.

10. Edwards CC: Spinal reconstruction in tumor management. In Uhthoff HK: *Current concepts of diagnosis and treatment of bone and soft tissue tumors*, New York, 1984, Springer pp. 329-349.

11. Enneking WF: *Musculoskeletal tumor surgery*, New York, 1983, Churchill Livingstone, pp. 9-122.

12. Enneking WF: Staging of musculoskeletal neoplasms. In Sundaresan N et al., eds: *Tumors of the spine: diagnosis and clinical management*, Philadelphia, 1990, WB Saunders, pp. 22-23.

13. Enneking WF, Spanier SS, Goodman MA: A system for the surgical staging of musculoskeletal sarcoma, *Clin Orthop* 153:106-120, 1980.

14. Esses SI, Botsford DJ: Surgical anatomy and operative approaches to the sacrum. In Frymoyer JW, ed: *The adult spine: principles and practice*, New York, 1991, Raven Press, pp. 2095-2106.

15. Esses SI et al.: Surgical anatomy of the sacrum: a guide from rational screw fixation, *Spine* 16(6) Suppl:S282-288, 1991.

16. Flynn JC, Hoque MA: Anterior fusion of the lumbar spine: end-result study with long term follow up, *J Bone Joint Surg Am* 61:1143-1150, 1979.

17. Fraser RD: A wide muscle-splitting approach to the lumbosacral spine, *J Bone Joint Surg Br* 64:44-46, 1982.

18. Freebody D: Treatment of spondylolisthesis by anterior fusion via the transperitoneal route, *J Bone Joint Surg Br* 46:788, 1964.

19. Freebody D, Bendall R, Taylor RD: Anterior transperitoneal lumbar fusion, *J Bone Joint Surg Br* 53:617-627, 1971.

20. Geisler FH et al.: Anterior tibial compartment syndrome as a positioning complication of the prone-sitting position for lumbar surgery, *Neurosurgery* 33(6):1117, 1993.

21. Gennari L, Azzarelli A, Quagliuolo V: A posterior approach for the excision of sacral chordoma, *J Bone Joint Surg Am* 69:565-568, 1971.

22. Gibbons KJ, Soloniuk DS, Razach N: Neurological injury and patterns of sacral fractures, *J Neurosurg* 72:889, 1990.

23. Givner I, Jaffe N: Occlusion of the central retinal artery following anaesthesia, *Arch Ophthalmol* 43:197-201, 1950.

24. Gokaslan ZL et al.: Total sacrectomy and Galveston L-rod reconstruction for malignant neoplasm, *J Neurosurg* 87(5):781-787, 1997.

25. Goldberg BA et al.: Imaging assessment of sacroiliac screw placement relative to the neuroforamen, *Spine* 23(5):585-589, 1998.

26. *Grays anatomy*, ed 36, New York, 1980, Churchill Livingstone.

27. Grossman W, Ward WT: Central retinal artery occlusion after scoliosis surgery with a horseshoe headrest, *Spine* 18:1226-1228, 1993.

28. Hodgson AR, Wong SK: A description of a technique and evaluation of results in anterior spinal fusion for deranged intervertebral disc and spondylolisthesis, *Clin Orthop* 56:133-162, 1968.

29. Hollenhorst RW, Svien HJ, Benoit CF: Unilateral blindness occurring during anaesthesia for neurosurgical operations, *Arch Ophthalmol* 52:819-830, 1954.

30. Hoski JJ, Eismont FJ, Green BA: Blindness as a complication of intraoperative positioning, *J Bone Joint Surg Am* 75:1231-1232, 1993.

31. Jackson H, Burke JT: The sacral foramina, *Skeletal Radiol* 11:282-288, 1984.

32. Johnson RM, McGuine ES: Urogenital complications of anterior approaches to the lumbar spine, *Clin Orthop* 154:114-118, 1981.

33. Kaiser TE, Pritchard DJ, Unni KK: Clinicopathologic study of sacrococcygeal chordoma, *Cancer* 53(11):2574-2578, 1984.

34. *Lasts anatomy: regional and applied*, ed 8, New York, 1990, Churchill Livingstone.

35. Mirkovic S et al.: Anatomic consideration for sacral placement, *Spine* 16(6 Suppl):S289-S294, 1991.

36. Myers MA et al.: Visual loss as a complication of spine surgery: a review of 37 cases, *Spine* 22(12):1325-1329, 1997.

37. Nambisan RN et al.: Axillary compression syndrome with neurapraxia due to operative positioning, *Surgery* 105(3):449-454, 1989.

38. Norgore M: Clinical anatomy of the vertebral veins, *Surgery* 17:606-615, 1945.

39. Parazon SJ: Incidence of sexual dysfunction with anterior lumbar surgery. *Proceedings of the 14th Annual Meeting of the North American Spine Society*, 1999.

40. Rout ML Jr et al.: Radiographic recognition of the sacral alar slope for optimal placement of iliosacral screws: a cadaveric and clinical study, *J Orthop Trauma* 10(3):171-177, 1996.

41. Sacks S: Anterior interbody fusion of the lumbar spine, *J Bone Joint Surg Br* 47:211-223, 1965.

42. Shah PM, Scarton HA, Tsapogas MJ: Geometric anatomy of the aortic-common iliac bifurcation, *J Anat* 126:451-458, 1978.

43. Shikata J et al.: Total sacrectomy and reconstruction for primary tumors, *J Bone Joint Surg Am* 70:122-125, 1988.

44. Simonian PT et al.: Internal fixation for the transforaminal sacral fracture, *Clin Orthop* 323:202-209, 1996.

45. Simpson AH, Porter A, Davis A: Cephalad sacral resection with a combined extended ilioinguinal and posterior approach, *J Bone Joint Surg Am* 77(3):405-411, 1995.

46. Slocum HC, Oneal KC, Allen CR: Neurovascular complications from malposition on the operating table, *Surg Gynecol Obstet* 86:729-734, 1948.

47. Stener B, Gunterberg B: High amputation of the sacrum for extirpation of tumors: principles and technique, *Spine* 3(4):351-366, 1978.

48. Strange Vognsen HH, Lebech A: An unusual type of fracture in the upper sacrum, *J Orthop Trauma* 5:200-203, 1991.

49. West J et al.: Loss of vision in one eye following scoliosis surgery, *Br J Ophthalmol* 74:243-244, 1990.

50. Wiltse LL et al.: The paraspinal sacrospinalis-splitting approach to the lumbar spine, *J Bone Joint Surg Am* 50:919-926, 1968.

51. Wolfe SW, Lospinuso MF, Burke SW: Unilateral blindness as a complication of patient positioning for spinal surgery, *Spine* 17:600-605, 1992.

52. York JE et al.: Sacral chordoma: 40-year experience at a major cancer center, *Neurosurgery* 44(1):74-79, 1999.

Cervical Degenerative Disc Disease

S. Tim Yoon, Howard S. An

Cervical degenerative disc disease refers to a variety of distinct degenerative conditions, including herniated disc and spondylotic disease, that can lead to radiculopathy and myelopathy. Clinical manifestations of neck pain, radiculopathy, and myelopathy may be present in isolation or in combination. The etiology of the pathology is varied and determines the natural history.[26,28,29] For example, radiculopathy from herniated disc often resolves with nonoperative treatment, while spondylotic myelopathy is either static or progressive. When nonoperative treatment fails, surgical intervention should be planned with careful consideration of the history, physical findings, and imaging studies. Surgical intervention consists of decompression, stabilization, or both. The anterior surgical approach is most often used in degenerative cervical disc disease, but posterior approaches are also frequently used. The combined anterior and posterior approaches are much less often used but can be useful in certain situations.

The rubric of degenerative cervical disc disease covers an array of clinical entities. These entities should be differentiated from degenerative anatomic changes that are often seen with the aging process. Many individuals with degenerative changes are asymptomatic, and only a subset of them go on to develop significant clinical pathology. This includes axial pain, deformity, radiculopathy, myelopathy, or a combination. Proper management of cervical disc disease is based on a thorough understanding of the anatomy, the natural history, and the available therapeutic options. In this chapter, we review the pathophysiology of degenerative cervical changes (spondylosis) and relate it to the development of clinical manifestations. Then we discuss the clinical evaluation and imaging methods. Indications and techniques of anterior, posterior, and combined approaches are presented.

PATHOANATOMY

By understanding the anatomy of the normal and pathologic cervical spine, better management of the symptomatic individual with cervical disc disease is possible.

There are seven cervical vertebrae (Figure 24-1). The first two levels (C1 and C2) have unique anatomy and are rarely involved in the usual degenerative process; instead they are more commonly affected by inflammatory processes such as rheumatoid arthritis. The subaxial spine is composed of the third through seventh vertebrae. They have a more typical anatomy with significant similarities among themselves.

The typical normal cervical spine has a lordotic sagittal contour. This is achieved through the shape and configuration of the intervertebral disc. The discs make up nearly 22% of the overall length of the cervical spine. They are thicker in height in the anterior aspect of the intervertebral space, supporting the lordotic curvature. The intervertebral discs increase range of motion between the vertebral bodies and distribute forces over the length of the spine.

The neuroforamina are confined zones for the exiting nerve roots, bordered anteriorly by the lateral aspect of the intervertebral disc and uncovertebral joint, superiorly and inferiorly by the pedicles, and posteriorly by the articular masses, notably the superior articular facet.[15] Pathologic conditions involving these structures can lead to critical stenosis of the foramen and nerve root compression.

Disc dehydration leads to loss of height. There is relatively more height loss in the anterior disc space because the uncovertebral joints resist height loss posteriorly. The combined effect leads to the characteristic loss of cervical lordosis on lateral plain radiographs.

Approximation of the vertebral bodies alters the biomechanical forces placed on the uncovertebral joints and articular facet joints. Osteophytic spurring, often referred to as "hard disc," may develop, leading to encroachment on the neuroforamina. Similarly, reactive bone forms along the posterior vertebral bodies as the margins come into greater contact when higher forces are applied. A spondylotic transverse bar may subsequently form, combined with bulging of the posterior disc and stretching of the posterior longitudinal ligament. Further collapse of the anterior column height leads to buckling of the ligamentum flavum into the spinal canal, most notably during neck extension. This combination of events may lead to spondylosis-induced compromise of the anterior-posterior diameter of the canal.

As the cervical discs degenerate, there are several potential sources of pain. Distortion of the intervertebral disc may lead to stretching or compression of the sinu-vertebral nerve and finer nerve endings with subsequent symptoms. Additionally, distortion or injury of inner-vated areas such as the apophyseal facet joints, liga-mentous structures, and posterior musculature may produce pain.

There are several sites within the spinal canal where neurocompression may occur. Radiculopathy may occur

from posterolateral soft disc herniation (Figure 24-2) either contained by the posterior longitudinal ligament (PLL) or free material extruded into and sequestered within the canal. In addition, foraminal stenosis from the changes previously described may also lead to impingement on the exiting nerve root. The pathophysi-ology of myelopathy involves many factors. The stenotic

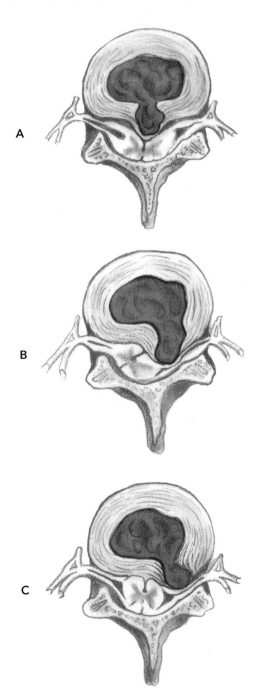

Figure 24-2. Depiction of types of "soft disc" herniation causing impingement on the exiting nerve root or spinal cord. **A,** Central herniation causes spinal cord compression. **B,** Posterolateral herniation can cause a combination of spinal cord and nerve root compression. **C,** Intraforaminal herniation causes nerve root compression.

PATHOANATOMY

CERVICAL VERTEBRAE
- Most often involved: Subaxial cervical spine, C3 to C7

CERVICAL LORDOSIS
- Largely due to lordotic shape of disc

CERVICAL DISC DISEASE
- Associated with disc dehydration, decreased disc height, and loss of lordosis
- Disc derangement and biomechanical changes may lead to neck pain
- With loss of disc height: Narrowing of neuroforamen
- With altered biomechanics: Promotes osteophyte formation, which can cause canal and neuroforaminal stenosis
- Herniated disc: Can cause myelopathy or radiculopathy

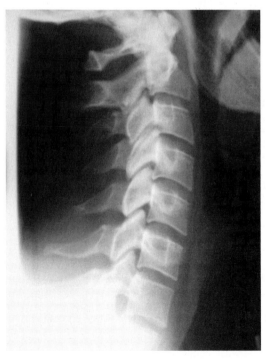

Figure 24-1. Lateral view of a normal cervical spine. Note the typical lordosis.

spinal canal may lead to neurologic dysfunction via compression of the anterior spinal artery with cord ischemia or mechanical deformation of the spinal cord from direct pressure and/or dynamic compression.[32] Hyperextension may cause the lax and hypertrophied ligamentum flavum to buckle, compressing the spinal cord against the anterior spondylotic bar.[32] Another mechanism of dynamic compression occurs in flexion, where the spinal cord is stretched over the anterior bony prominences. Occasionally a midline soft disc herniation may cause cord compression and myelopathy combined with a degree of nerve root compression, leading to a myeloradiculopathy (see Figure 24-2).

NATURAL HISTORY OF CERVICAL DISC DISEASE

The prognosis for a patient with neck pain varies in part due to the fact that there are numerous etiologies that can produce neck pain. The natural history of neck pain has been evaluated by Gore et al.[13] They performed a retrospective review of patients with neck pain followed clinically and radiographically over a 10-year period. Seventy-nine percent of patients had diminished pain, while 43% had nearly complete relief of symptoms. However, nearly one third of the study group reported persistent moderate to severe pain. Outcome could not be correlated with radiographic or clinical findings, making outcome projections difficult for patients with neck pain.

The natural history of cervical radiculopathy has been well described previously.[12,19,25] Lees and Turner reported on the long-term follow-up of patients with spondylosis and confirmed that 30% experienced intermittent radicular symptoms while 25% had persistent pain.[25] Progression from radiculopathy to myelopathy is unusual, and it appears that these are distinct entities. In general there is agreement that nonoperative treatment may alleviate symptoms of cervical spondylotic radiculopathy (CSR) in the short term, but over a long period of time symptoms frequently recur. Gore et al. retrospectively reviewed patients with cervical radiculopathy treated conservatively and noted 50% with persistent symptoms at 15-year follow-up.

Cervical spondylotic myelopathy (CSM) is associated with an insidious onset of symptoms, and in general, neurologic function undergoes episodes of worsening with intervening stable periods.[2,3,10,22] However, there are no pathognomonic findings to predict the progression of symptoms. Clarke and Robinson[8] evaluated the natural history of CSM prior to treatment and concluded that 75% in their cohort experienced episodic worsening of symptoms, 20% showed slow, steady progression without intervening stabilizing periods, and 5% experienced rapid onset of the disease process and progression. Progression to total disability is unusual, although slight incremental neurologic deterioration may occur with time, resulting in upper and lower extremity functional deficits. As the neurologic deficit worsens, improvement in disability becomes more unlikely and complete recovery even less so.

CLINICAL EVALUATION

The clinical evaluation of patients with cervical degenerative disorders requires interpretation of a patient's complaints, a meticulous examination, and appropriate selection of diagnostic tests. To perform a complete evaluation of a patient's complaints, the clinician must first determine if the problem involves neck pain, arm pain, myelopathy, or a combination of these components. A detailed history is the initial step in evaluating a patient with cervical degenerative disc disease. A complete description of the symptomatology is sought, including the onset, quality, and location of pain; inciting and alleviating factors; temporal nature; degree of impairment; and any associated symptoms. Axial neck pain may be discogenic or musculogenic in origin, or it may be related to shoulder, occipitocervical, myofascial, or visceral pathology. On occasion, it may be due to C4 radiculopathy.[20] To differentiate the potential multiple sources of neck pain, it is necessary to establish whether the symptoms are mechanical (increased with activity and diminished with rest or positioning) or nonmechanical (no relief with positional changes or rest). Nonmechanical neck pain may be related to tumor or infection, and such processes should be carefully sought.

Mechanical neck pain is commonly discogenic in origin and exacerbated with neck extension and rotation toward the side that is more symptomatic.[27] Patients may describe pain referred to the shoulder, upper arm region, or interscapular area. Patients with upper cervical degeneration may also experience occipital or temporal pain, or retro-ocular headaches. Musculogenic pain, as from an acute or chronic muscle strain, is more often exacerbated with neck flexion and rotation, leading to increased symptoms on the opposite side of head rotation.

Radicular symptoms may be caused by a soft lateral disc herniation, chronic disc degeneration with osteophytic spurring, or segmental instability. The majority of patients present with a monoradiculopathy, although several roots can be involved. Symptoms consist of

---

NATURAL HISTORY OF CERVICAL DISC DISEASE

DIFFERS BY PATHOANATOMY

NECK PAIN
- Has variable outcome
- Usually gets better with time
- Outcome strongly influenced by psychosocial factors

SPONDYLOTIC RADICULOPATHY LONG TERM
- 30% have intermittent pain
- 25% have persistent pain

SPONDYLOTIC MYELOPATHY LONG TERM
- 75% have episodic progression
- 20% have slow, steady progression
- 5% have rapid progression

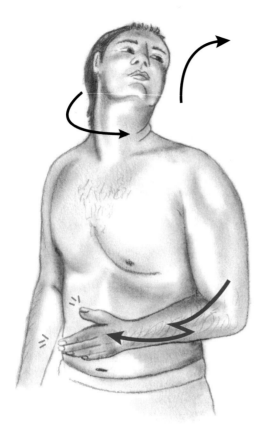

Figure 24-3.   Spurling's sign: Extension of the neck coupled with lateral rotation towards the affected arm will exacerbate cervical radiculopathy by further narrowing the neural foramina.

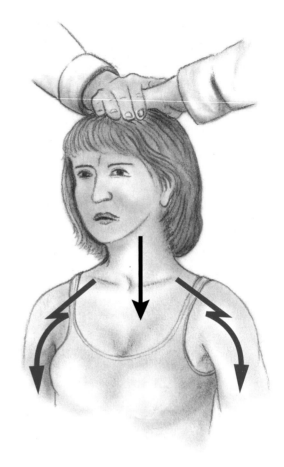

Figure 24-4.   Axial cervical compression testing may also reproduce cervical radicular symptoms by narrowing the neuroforamina. Distractive forces may relieve root compression.

sharp, lancinating, radiating arm pain associated with various degrees of dysesthesias, paresthesias, and numbness along a dermatomic pattern consistent with distribution of the involved nerve root. The symptoms may be exacerbated or relieved by several provocative tests. Typically patients describe an increase in pain with valsalva activities and with neck extension or turning the head toward the symptomatic side. Spurling's sign is indicative of radiculopathy. This is elicited by neck hyperextension and rotation toward the symptomatic side, resulting in reproduction of the patient's pain (Figure 24-3). This maneuver serves to diminish the available area in an already compromised neuroforamen, leading to further nerve root compression. A less reliable provocative sign is the axial compression test, where compression on the vertex of the skull may diminish the height of the foramen and reproduce symptoms (Figure 24-4). The shoulder abduction sign is a test that relieves symptoms of compression by lessening nerve root stretch with placement of the ipsilateral hand on top of the head. Patients may present with this as the only upper extremity position that provides relief or comfort.

The history and examination identify the level of radiculopathy. The patterns of pain distribution that are classically described are often imprecise because of anatomic variations, involvement of multiple levels, or the presence of chronic conditions. Upper cervical nerve

root compression is less common than lower levels; however, it must be considered in the differential diagnosis of recalcitrant neck pain.[20]

The symptoms of cervical myelopathy are variable and complaints may be vague, so that myelopathy is not easily picked up on the initial examination. Symptoms and findings can include gait difficulties, spasticity, decreased manual dexterity, paresthesias in the extremities, urinary urgency or frequency, and specific extremity or generalized weakness.[7,23] In contrast to cervical radiculopathy, pain is not a common presenting finding. Depending on the site of anatomic spinal cord compression, the symptoms may be quite variable.

The gait disturbance may be an early presenting complaint. Stumbling or generalized gait disturbances are usually insidious and slowly progressive. Patients may initially become aware of these changes from family members who note a shuffling gait or frequent falls. The characteristic stooped, wide-based gait of the elderly is the common end result. Involvement of the upper extremities may occur concomitantly or follow the gait changes with complaints of clumsy or numb hands. Weakness of the hand manifests as decreased grip strength. Manual dexterity will often suffer and progress until the patient lacks the ability to complete routine activities such as buttoning a shirt, counting change, or

CLINICAL EVALUATION

NECK PAIN
- Mechanical vs nonmechanical
- Discogenic
- Musculogenic
- Neurogenic—C3 or C4 radicular pain

RADICULAR PAIN
- Level identified with history and examination
- Spurling's test
- Axial compression test
- Shoulder abduction test

MYELOPATHY
- Lower-extremity clonus
- Babinski test
- Hyperreflexia
- Hoffmann's sign
- Inverted brachioradialis reflex
- Scapulohumeral reflex
- Lhermitte's sign

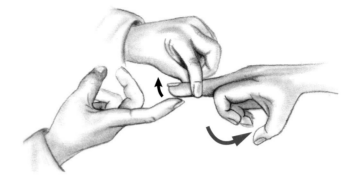

Figure 24-5. Hoffmann's sign is indicative of cervical cord impingement. The reflex is positive if the fingers and thumb react in flexion when the long-finger distal interphalangeal joint is tapped in extension.

writing. Several authors have noted characteristic hand dysfunction in cervical myelopathy. Ono et al.[30] reported on the myelopathic hand syndrome, in which the finger escape sign and grip and release test were described. The finger escape sign is positive when the patient is asked to hold all the digits of the hand in an adducted and extended position and the two ulnar digits fall into abduction and flexion with time. In the grip and release test, the patient is asked to rapidly form a fist and then release all digits into extension repeatedly. A patient without myelopathy should be able to perform this test 20 times in a 10-second period.

Physical examination of a myelopathic patient consists of thorough neurologic examination, as well as other special testing. The presence of lower extremity clonus and Babinski extensor plantar responses should be noted. Hoffmann's reflex (finger and thumb interphalangeal flexion with sudden long-finger distal interphalangeal joint extension) when present and especially when asymmetric is strongly suggestive of cervical myelopathy (Figure 24-5). Other tests that may be noted include an inverted radial reflex, scapulohumeral reflex, and Lhermitte's sign (Figure 24-6).

DIAGNOSTIC TESTING

Improved neuroradiologic imaging has led to a better understanding of the pathologic process of cervical radiculopathy and myelopathy. Several techniques are available for the evaluation of the symptomatic patient. Each modality has its own inherent strengths and weaknesses, and often combinations of examinations are required.

For initial radiographic evaluation, anteroposterior (AP) and lateral views are necessary. Oblique views are useful to evaluate bony narrowing of the foramina. Flexion-extension views are useful when instability is suspected or when evaluating the rigidity of sagittal

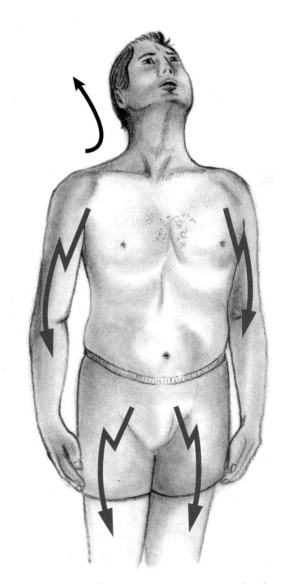

Figure 24-6. Lhermitte's sign is associated with spinal cord compression. With certain provocative positions of the head and neck, the patient experiences an electric "shock" sensation throughout the body.

DIAGNOSTIC IMAGING

PLAIN RADIOGRAPHS
- Cost-effective initial imaging
- Evaluates deformity—global balance, contour, subluxation, instability
- Degenerative changes—disc height loss, osteophyte formation, bony sclerosis
- Developmental canal stenosis or congenital malformations seen

MYELOGRAPHY AND CT SCAN
- Excellent bony detail (e.g., neuroforaminal osteophytes)
- Can evaluate compression on neural structures, but not directly identify the etiology of the compression

MRI
- Directly visualize compressive structures
- Excellent view of spinal cord and nerve roots
- Less sensitive than CT scan in detecting foraminal stenosis and cortical margins

EMG/NCS
- Used for confirming or refining radicular findings
- Differentiates root compression from peripheral neuropathy

plane deformity. Findings such as disc space narrowing, developmental canal stenosis, subluxations and malalignments, and vertebral osteophtye formation must be evaluated in light of symptoms. Abnormal findings on plain radiographs may not be the cause of the clinical picture; therefore further correlative studies may be necessary prior to recommending specific treatment. Changes on plain radiographs may also confirm the clinical suspicion of typical degenerative disease and reassure the clinician and the patient that appropriate therapy is being followed.

Water-soluble myelography has been used to evaluate cervical radiculopathy and myelopathy. The AP view demonstrates the exiting nerve roots to the level of the pedicle. A filling defect is a typical finding of nerve root compression. The lateral view may detect spinal cord compression by the disc or posterior vertebral osteophytes and/or hypertrophied ligamentum flavum. Current practice includes myelography followed by computed tomography (CT), which permits visualization of osseous compressive structures. Forty-five–degree oblique reconstruction views are especially helpful in visualizing the neuroforamina. CT-myelography, however, infers neural compression by deformity of the dural sac or nerve roots and cannot directly determine the etiology of contrast blockade.

Magnetic resonance imaging (MRI) does provide direct information about nerve root or spinal cord compression. The advantage of MRI in detecting direct compression is the intrinsic "contrast" available from the cerebrospinal fluid (CSF) as seen on T2 weighted images. This is the most sensitive modality for assessing the morphology of the spinal cord and its relation to the spinal canal. MRI also shows intramedullary cord changes that may relate to disease prognosis. However, MRI is less sensitive in detecting foraminal stenosis and does not demonstrate cortical margins as well as CT-myelography. Forty-five–degree oblique reconstruction views provide improved view of the neuroforamina.

Electromyography/nerve conduction studies (EMG/NCS) may be utilized to confirm suspected radiculopathy or may be used as an additional modality to further elucidate the cause of symptoms in a patient with atypical findings. These tests may be most useful when attempting to differentiate root compression and a peripheral neuropathy. Nuclear medicine bone scanning, local diagnostic injections, discography, and CSF analysis have a limited role in the diagnostic process.

NONOPERATIVE TREATMENT

Most patients with symptoms of neck pain with or without radiculopathy can be managed nonoperatively. The initial treatment of moderate to severe symptoms should consist of a soft collar, nonsteroidal anti-inflammatory drugs (NSAIDs), and physical therapy modalities including traction, particularly when radicular signs are present. The limited use of a soft collar may help to decrease the dynamic compression of an irritated nerve root and permit the pain from fatigue or spasm in the paraspinal muscles to resolve. Prolonged use of a collar is not recommended due to paraspinal muscle atrophy. Restrict activities to avoid neck extension and heavy lifting during the acute period. Aspirin, ibuprofen, or NSAIDs may provide pain relief. Narcotic pain medications should be used sparingly, especially in elderly patients. Occasionally a brief, tapered course of oral cortisone may alleviate symptoms of radiculopathy. Physical therapy modalities such as heat and ultrasound may improve acute symptoms, but it is unclear whether they have any effect on natural history. Manual or home traction may provide relief of nerve root compression through distraction of the intervertebral foramen.

As in the lumbar spine, epidural steroid injections (ESIs) may be recommended for treatment of the inflammatory component of cervical radiculopathy. The role of ESIs is controversial, and the literature lacks well-designed studies documenting their efficacy. Before recommending their use, the short-term relief of symptoms must be weighed against possible risks and complications of needle placement.

Patients with symptoms of myelopathy may be immobilized in a soft collar to prevent dynamic spinal cord compression. However, this is a temporizing measure only and is not definitive treatment.

OPERATIVE MANAGEMENT
Indications

The indications for surgery in patients with neck pain secondary to spondylosis, canal stenosis, or discogenic neck pain are limited. Whitecloud and Seago[41] reported 70% good to excellent results from anterior interbody fusion for patients with concordant neck pain on discography.[9] Palit et al.[31] reported 79% of patients satisfied with results and improved Oswestry scores at long-term follow-up. However, others have found that fusion for discogenic neck pain based on provocative testing yields results not much improved from the natural history of the disorder. The conservative management for these individuals remains the treatment of choice. Recalcitrant neck pain from degenerative spondylolisthesis or retrolisthesis is rare in the cervical spine. Instability suggested on dynamic flexion-extension radiographs may be managed by either anterior or posterior segmental fusion.

The indications for operative intervention in cervical radiculopathy include (1) failure of a 3-month trial of nonoperative methods of treatment to relieve persistent or recurrent radicular arm pain with or without neurologic deficit and (2) a progressive neurologic deficit. Neuroradiographic findings must be consistent with the clinical signs and symptoms, and the duration and magnitude of symptoms must be sufficient to justify surgery.[6]

The surgical indications for the treatment of cervical myelopathy are not as well defined as they are for the treatment of radiculopathy.[2] A patient with mild, nonprogressive myelopathy that is long-standing and does not cause significant disability can be observed closely. Operative intervention is recommended in the following situations: (1) progressive myelopathy, (2) moderate or severe myelopathy that is stable and of short duration (less than 1 year), and (3) mild myelopathy that affects routine activities of daily living. The age of the patient or severity of the disease should not serve as a contraindication for surgery, but the goal of surgery to prevent neurologic worsening must be conveyed to the patient. However, the majority of patients with myelopathy have improved neurologic function after surgical decompression.

ANTERIOR APPROACH
Positioning and Exposure

Surgical exposure of the anterior aspect of the cervical spine is a relatively safe procedure and takes advantage of normal anatomic fascial planes during the approach. The patient is positioned in the supine position with either halter or skeletal traction. Reverse Trendelenburg's position can be used to reduce venous bleeding if needed. The superficial anatomic landmarks for incision include the hyoid bone overlying C3, thyroid cartilage overlying the C4 to C5 interspace, and cricoid cartilage overlying the C6 level. The incision can be either transverse or longitudinal. Use the transverse incision when one to three discs are to be exposed. Use the longitudinal incision when four or more levels are approached. A longitudinal incision along the anterior border of the sternocleidomastoid muscle is recommended. The transverse incision has better cosmetic appeal and access to the anterior spine, while the longitudinal incision has better visualization of the region over multiple levels and avoids excessive retraction that may otherwise be necessary.

The anterior approach places several structures at risk. The superior and inferior thyroid arteries extend

> ## ANTERIOR CERVICAL EXPOSURE
> - Skin incision—undermine skin, subcutaneous tissue
> - Divide platysma, separate deep cervical fascia between sternocleidomastoid laterally and strap muscle medially
> - Dissect through pretracheal fascia (carotid sheath laterally, trachea and esophagus medially)
> - Mobilize longus colli muscles laterally

through the pretracheal fascia from the carotid artery to the midline. The superior and inferior thyroid arteries travel at the C3 to C4 and C6 to C7 levels, respectively. The intervening area provides a relatively avascular plane for dissection. The recurrent laryngeal nerves are also at risk during the anterior approach. The right recurrent laryngeal nerve ascends in the neck after passing around the subclavian vessels and courses medially and cranially at the C6 to C7 level, often along with the inferior thyroid artery. The left recurrent laryngeal nerve ascends after curving around the aortic arch along the tracheoesophageal groove in a more midline and protected position. A left-sided procedure may be safer, especially when lower cervical segments are approached. However, the thoracic duct is often visible on the left at the C7 to T1 level and must be protected.

After the skin incision the anterior approach is performed by undermining the skin and subcutaneous tissue and dividing the platysma. The deep cervical fascia is divided between the strap muscles (medially) and the sternocleidomastoid muscle (laterally), and blunt dissection is used to go through the pretracheal fascia. The carotid sheath is palpable laterally, and the trachea and esophagus are swept medially. After the exposure a localizing lateral radiograph should be taken. The longus colli muscles are mobilized laterally with a Cobb elevator or curette. The disc is more prominent than the vertebral body.

Anterior Cervical Discectomy and Fusion

The success of anterior cervical discectomy and fusion (ACDF) as a procedure is demonstrated by the frequency of its use in the cervical spine.* Discectomy is performed by sharply incising the anterior annulus and removing the disc with a rongeur and curette. The discectomy should go to the uncovertebral joints laterally and to the PLL posteriorly. The PLL is removed in cases of myelopathy or extruded disc herniation. Direct decompression of the nerve root can be accomplished with a small Kerrison rongeur or curette.

Several techniques of anterior interbody fusion in the cervical spine have been described, each differing by the graft configuration. The Robinson interbody fusion technique involves the placement of a tricortical iliac crest wedge graft into the disc space for bony healing[34] (Figure 24-7). This is the most common method of fusion at the

---

*References 33, 35, 37, 40, 42, 45, 49.

Iliac crest graft

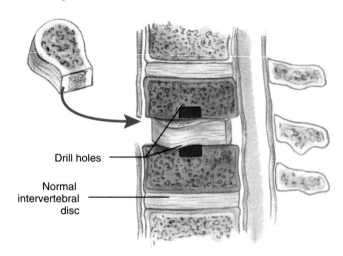

Drill holes

Normal intervertebral disc

Figure 24-7. Anterior cervical discectomy and fusion using the Robinson technique. The interspace is distracted and discectomy is performed to the PLL. Fusion is performed with tricortical iliac crest bone.

ANTERIOR CERVICAL DISCECTOMY AND FUSION

- Incise anterior annulus fibrosus.
- Remove disc with a rongeur and curette.
- Carry discectomy out laterally to uncovertebral joints and PLL posteriorly.
- Perform nerve root decompression with a small Kerrison rongeur or curette.

---

present time and is described in more detail.[4] The graft height should be 2 mm greater than the preexisting disc height or at least 5 mm to obtain adequate compressive strength and to enlarge the neural foramina.[1] Overdistraction of the disc space by greater than 4 mm of the preexisting height may result in graft collapse and pseudarthrosis by overly increasing the graft load.[1,5] Disc space distraction is achieved with skull traction, laminar spreader, vertebral screws, or a combination of these. The end plates are burred to create a flat surface on both sides of the intervertebral space. Additionally, a 3- to 4-mm hole may be created in the middle of the end plates to promote vascularization of the graft. After measuring the depth and width of the disc space, the tricortical graft is harvested from the anterior iliac region. The graft is obtained with an oscillating bone saw as graft weakening has been associated when osteotomes are utilized.[21] The graft is contoured to fit into the disc space and inserted with the leading cortical edge anteriorly and inset 2 mm beyond the vertebral bodies. The graft should be stable with compression following removal of all traction devices.

The alternative fusion techniques are described for historical interest. The Cloward technique utilizes a bicortical dowel-shaped graft. The technique requires the use of specialized instruments including drills, guards, and a dowel cutter. The Simmons technique for interbody fusion utilizes a keystone-shaped graft. The Bailey and Badgley technique involves developing an anterior trough in the vertebral bodies to accomplish fusion. The Cloward, Simmons, and Bailey and Badgley techniques have as a disadvantage no direct nerve root decompression and thus are seldom used today.

Since iliac crest bone harvesting has an associated morbidity, the use of allograft bone has become a popular method of interbody fusion.[12, 24] In one study, although nonunion rates and graft collapse were more common in ACDF with freeze-dried tricortical iliac crest allograft, the clinical results were similar to ACDF with autogenous bone graft.[47] Fibular allograft has also been shown to provide results similar to autograft with acceptable single-level fusion rates and the absence of donor site pain.[44] Other studies have found a higher radiographic nonunion rate with allograft and greater clinical improvement when autograft is used. Therefore the results of using allograft bone are difficult to evaluate. One-level fusion with allograft may be acceptable.

The presence of fusion following discectomy has not been uniformly correlated with a favorable clinical outcome, nor has nonunion consistently resulted in a clinical failure. The fact that a pseudarthrosis may be associated with a good clinical result led to the concept of anterior cervical discectomy without fusion (ACD). A major advantage of ACD is the lack of donor site complications. However, the disadvantage is postoperative neck pain, which may become severe and is more common than in ACDF. Postdiscectomy collapse and angular kyphosis may also occur, leading to recurrent nerve root compression if posterior osteophytes are not widely resected at the index procedure. Bilateral foraminotomies must be performed to prevent contralateral radiculopathy due to resultant disc space collapse. If ACD is to be performed, it most likely should be limited to soft disc herniations and avoided in patients with evidence of spondylosis who require disc space distraction.

Anterior Cervical Corpectomy and Fusion

Single-level or multilevel corpectomies and strut graft fusion (ACF) have been recommended by many authors for multilevel spondylotic myelopathy and myeloradiculopathy.* A partial or complete corpectomy and fusion may be necessary in situations where access to the posterior aspect of the vertebral body is needed, for example, a disc herniation with a sequestered fragment that has migrated behind the vertebral body. A significant advantage of corpectomy and strut grafting over multilevel ACDF is the reduction of the number of surfaces that must fuse. With each additional level that needs to fuse in multilevel ACDF, there is increased risk of failure of fusion.

The technique of corpectomy and fusion can be accomplished in the following manner. Anterior cervical discectomy above and below the vertebra in question is performed. Then the vertebral body is excised with

---

*References 2, 14, 19, 36, 43, 45.

ANTERIOR CERVICAL CORPECTOMY AND FUSION

- Perform anterior cervical discectomy above and below the vertebra in question.
- Excise vertebral body with rongeurs or a high-speed burr to the posterior cortex.
- Remove posterior cortex with angled curettes.
- Remove at least one third of vertebral body to within 5 mm of the transverse foramen.

rongeurs or a high-speed burr to the posterior cortex. Next the posterior shell is removed with angled curettes directed away from the dura. Approximately one third of the vertebral body should be removed to provide adequate cord decompression in a safe manner. Preservation of the lateral aspect of the vertebral body has the advantage of maintaining some structural integrity. The corpectomy may be carried to within 5 mm of the transverse foramen. Traction or distraction may then be applied to restore sagittal plane alignment at the decompressed level. A structural graft is crafted and inserted into the prepared end plates. Fibular autograft, tricortical iliac crest autograft, allograft, and cages filled with bone have all been used successfully. The graft is countersunk slightly into the vertebral bodies. The stability of the graft is assessed with traction released. Internal fixation with an anterior plate can be used to increase stability. External stabilization with rigid orthosis or halo should be considered when appropriate.

Anterior Instrumentation

The use of anterior plate fixation in cervical spine surgery for degenerative conditions has increased.[36,46] It is most often used in multilevel ACDFs, and some surgeons are also using it in single-level ACDF. It is used in one- to two-level corpectomies. When more than two corpectomies are performed, it is the authors' preference to instrument posteriorly with lateral mass plates. Whenever possible, segmental instrumentation should be used. This can be accomplished by performing corpectomies at only the most severely involved levels in multilevel disease and performing ACDFs at the less involved areas (Figure 24-8). This allows for another segment of fixation and avoids the biomechanical problems of a long plate secured only at the bottom and top.

The technique of anterior plating starts with the usual anterior approach as described above. The appropriate size plate must be chosen: The plate must extend from the middle or proximal portion of the superior vertebrae to the middle or distal portion of the inferior vertebrae. The plate should make maximal contact with the anterolateral surface of the spine. Smooth the bed for the plate by removing osteophytes with a burr or rongeur. The plate is fixed to the spine with screws. The screw holes are drilled roughly parallel to the end plate and slightly toward the midline. Newer instrumentation systems provide for a mechanism to lock the screws to the plate,

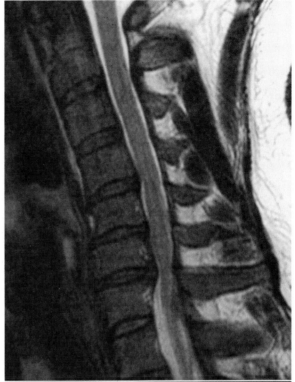

A

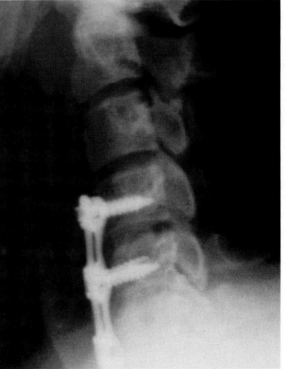

B

Figure 24-8. **A,** An MRI of a myelopathic patient with severe cord compression at C5 to C6 and C6 to C7 and moderate cord compression at C4 to C5 is shown. In this case corpectomy of C6 is performed, and discectomy at C4 to C5 is performed, and plating is achieved with screws at C4, C5, and C7, which is more stable than strut grafting from C4 to C7 with plating with screws only at C4 and C7. **B,** Post op lateral x-ray with corpectomy of C6 and plate from C4, C5, and C7 are shown.

ANTERIOR SURGERY SUMMARY

ACDF
- Most frequent cervical procedure
- Increasing number of levels increases pseudarthrosis rate
- Appropriate graft size improves fusion rate
- Plate stabilization increases fusion rate in multilevel fusion
- Adjacent segment degeneration rate: 3% per year

ACD
- Controversial
- Higher incidence of neck pain and kyphosis postoperatively

ACF
- Used in multilevel fusion
- Does not increase number of fusion surfaces (i.e., chance of pseudarthrosis)
- Rigid anterior instrumentation difficult to maintain with long strut graft

---

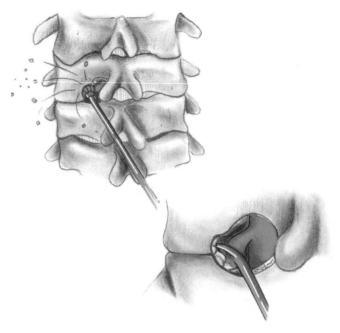

Figure 24-9. Posterior laminotomy and foraminotomy depicting thinning of the lamina and facet joint and nerve root decompression.

which increases the overall rigidity of the instrumentation. The choice of static or dynamic instrumentation systems exists for the surgeon.

Results of Anterior Surgery

Postoperative results of surgical treatment of cervical radiculopathy and myelopathy vary depending on the type of approach utilized and severity of the disease. Limitations in drawing firm conclusions from previous reports stem from the lack of uniform patient population, inclusion of different disease processes in the same analysis (soft vs hard disc), and inconsistency of establishing successful results. Overall, the surgical treatment of radiculopathy yields satisfactory results in greater than 90% of patients. Although controversial, it appears that patients who attain a solid fusion do have better outcomes than those with a pseudarthrosis. The results of treatment of myelopathy also are variable as depicted by the numerous techniques utilized to decompress the spinal cord. Overall, patients with greater neurologic deficits tend to experience less improvement in symptoms following surgery than those with more acute and less severe neurologic findings.

POSTERIOR APPROACH
Positioning and Exposure

Careful patient positioning is required to minimize the risk of neurologic injury and to maximize exposure of the required level. The head is stabilized in the prone position with Mayfield skull tongs, leaving the face free without sources of pressure. The reverse Trendelenburg's position promotes epidural venous drainage. The posterior approach to the cervical spine utilizes an internervous plane in the midline that separates the muscles from the segmental innervation sup-

plied by the right and left posterior rami of the cervical nerves. The ligamentum nuchae is incised in the midline, and the subperiosteal dissection is carried down the spinous processes and corresponding laminae. In the cervical spine the laminae do not override each other as much as in the thoracic spine; therefore the interlaminar space may be inadvertently penetrated if caution is not taken during the exposure. The dissection is carried out to the lateral edge of the lateral masses, and the facet joint capsule is preserved if no fusion is required or anticipated.

Keyhole Foraminotomy

The primary indication for keyhole foraminotomy is unilateral pure radiculopathy at one or more levels. The presence of neck pain or bilateral involvement would favor an anterior approach. The technique begins with a posterior approach only on the symptomatic side. Then portions of the inferior and superior lamina at the level of the specific nerve root compression are removed, and partial facetectomy is performed with a high-speed burr (Figure 24-9). To prevent iatrogenic instability, no more than 50% of the facet should be removed.[48] The lamina and thinned bone should be gently lifted off the nerve and spinal cord with small angled curettes. The foraminotomy is assessed by placing a blunt probe or Woodson dental instrument into the neuroforamen to judge its patency. If disc removal is deemed necessary, the nerve root is exposed, and the surrounding venous plexus is cauterized. The nerve root is gently retracted cephalad, and the disc tissue removed.

Excellent results can be achieved with this procedure. Up to 96% good outcome has been reported without disc

---

KEYHOLE FORAMINOTOMY

- Use posterior cervical approach.
- Remove portions of inferior and superior lamina at level of nerve root compression.
- Perform partial facetectomy with high-speed burr.
- Elevate lamina and thinned bone with small angled curette.
- For disc removal, cauterize venous plexus. Retract nerve gently cephalad to expose disc.

LAMINECTOMY

- Thin cortex at junction of laminae and lateral masses bilaterally with power burr.
- Use small Kerrison rongeur to complete cut and small angled curette to elevate the laminae.
- Cauterize underlying venous plexus.
- Perform foraminotomies if needed.

---

removal. In a small comparative prospective study between ACDF and foraminotomy for soft disc herniation, Herkowitz et al.[17] were unable to show a statistical difference in outcome between the two procedures.

Laminectomy

This is an option for treating multilevel spondylotic myelopathy with or without radiculopathy or patients with congenital spinal canal stenosis. It is indicated in patients with preserved cervical lordosis or can be combined with lateral mass fusion and instrumentation in patients with a flexible loss of lordosis. This procedure increases the space available for the cord by removing the offending ligamentum flavum and bony lamina. Indirect decompression is achieved by the posterior translation of the cord in a lordotic spine. Laminectomy should be combined with lateral mass fusion if there is instability or deformity.

Laminectomy is performed by thinning the cortices at the junction of the laminae and lateral masses bilaterally with a power burr. Then a small Kerrison rongeur is used to complete the cut, and a small angled curette is used to elevate the laminae. The adherent underlying venous plexus is cauterized to minimize epidural hematoma formation. Foraminotomies can be added to the procedure when indicated by radicular pathology.

The literature reports varying degrees of success with laminectomy for spondylotic myelopathy. Approximately 68% to 85% of patients undergoing laminectomy for spondylotic myelopathy or myeloradiculopathy have good to excellent results. In comparing anterior decompression and fusion to laminectomy for the treatment of multilevel spondylotic radiculopathy, Herkowitz[16] found 66% good to excellent results with laminectomy vs 92% with anterior fusion. Significant complications of postlaminectomy kyphosis (25%) and anterior subluxation (40%) compromised the results of laminectomy. These complications seem to be related to foraminotomies required for adequate decompression. Loss of the posterior structural support of the bony elements may increase the risk of these complications. Facetectomy (partial or full) has been linked to development of instability in both clinical and biomechanical studies. The complication rate of postlaminectomy kyphosis and subluxation can be extremely high in younger patients. The surgeon should consider fusion at the time of decompression in these cases.

The lateral mass, a structure unique to the cervical spine, can be used for fusion if indicated in conjunction with laminectomy. The fusion is accomplished by destroying the interarticular facet capsule and decorticating the facet joint. The most stable internal fixation is obtained by lateral mass screws and plates. Techniques for screw placement differ by start site and angulation of screw placement on the lateral mass. An et al.[1] described a technique that provides the largest clearance of the nerve root and facet joint. This technique consists of starting 1 mm medial to the center of the lateral mass and angulating the screw 15 degrees cephalad and 25 to 30 degrees lateral.

Laminoplasty

Laminoplasty is indicated in the treatment of multilevel spondylotic myelopathy, myeloradiculopathy, or multilevel radiculopathy.[16,18] While multilevel bilateral radiculopathy can be addressed with laminoplasty, many authors prefer an anterior approach with bilateral radicular disease. The critical difference between laminectomy and laminoplasty is the preservation of posterior bony elements that significantly reduce postoperative instability and deformity. Therefore laminoplasty is preferred in younger patients and those who have some preoperative instability. Similar to laminectomy, cervical lordosis is necessary to provide spinal cord decompression.

Several methods of laminoplasty exist; they vary by location of the hinge and means of maintaining the open position. The open-door laminoplasty (Figure 24-10) is performed by thinning the cortex at the lamina and lateral mass junction with a high-speed burr bilaterally to the inner cortex. The hinged side is thinned without completing the cut while the osteotomy is completed on the opening side. The more symptomatic side is chosen as the open side. The lamina is gently opened either with towel clips placed through the respective spinous processes or with a vertebral spreader placed into the defect. The thinned inner cortex of the hinged side is plastically deformed, and the posterior elements are held open by a variety of different methods. The authors prefer to use bone graft at the open side to hold the posterior elements in position (Figure 24-11).

The results of laminoplasty have been relatively good. While the risk of instability problems still remains, it is significantly reduced in laminoplasty as compared to laminectomy. In a comparison between laminoplasty

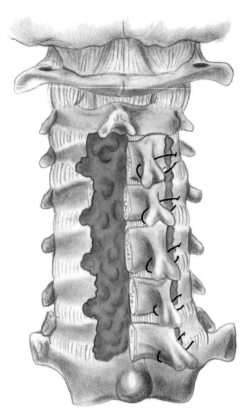

Figure 24-10. Open-door laminoplasty depicting hinged lamina and spinal canal decompression.

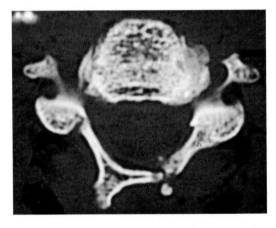

Figure 24-11. The axial CT scan of a patient who has had cervical laminoplasty for cervical myelopathy is shown. The hinge-side thinned cortex is seen on the right lamina, and the bone graft on the "open" side is seen on the left.

OPEN-DOOR LAMINOPLASTY

- Thin cortex at lamina and lateral mass junction bilaterally with high-speed burr to inner cortex.
- Thin hinged side without completing cut, and complete osteotomy on opening side.
- Make more symptomatic side the open side.
- Gently open lamina.
- Hold lamina open (various techniques).

POSTERIOR APPROACH SUMMARY

FORAMINOTOMY
- Useful in decompressing nerve root
- Removal of herniated disc not needed
- Remove less than 50% of the facet joint
- Preserve remaining facet capsule

LAMINECTOMY
- Useful in multilevel canal stenosis
- Can be combined with foraminotomy
- High rate of instability/subluxation in young patients
- Requires lordotic spine to decompress spinal cord

LAMINECTOMY AND INSTRUMENTED LATERAL MASS FUSION
- Indicated in patients who need laminectomy and have the following associated factors
  ○ Young patients who are likely to fall into kyphosis
  ○ Instabilities such as spondylolisthesis
  ○ Supple kyphosis or loss of lordosis
  ○ Neck pain
- Choose over laminoplasty given the following factors
  ○ Neck pain
  ○ Bilateral radiculopathy

LAMINOPLASTY
- Preserves bony anatomy and increases stability postoperatively
- Higher incidence of neck pain
- Hinge on less painful side
- Requires lordotic spine to decompress spinal cord

---

and laminectomy for the treatment of myelopathy or myeloradiculopathy, Herkowitz et al.[16] reported that laminoplasty had 86% good to excellent results as compared to 66% for laminectomy. Interestingly, in patients with bilateral disease, bilateral foraminotomies after laminoplasty may not be necessary as the radicular pain on the hinged side seems to abate without foraminotomies. While the mechanism for this is not proven, improved vascular supply to the nerve root after decompression may be involved.

COMBINED APPROACH

The combined approach in treating degenerative disc disease is less common. However, there are situations where both anterior and posterior surgery are warranted either on the same day or staged by some time interval. Previous surgery on one side may suggest surgery on the opposite side to avoid scar and reduce risk. Combined approach may be needed in situations where inadequate fixation was obtained. This can occur when the bone quality is excessively poor or when there are technical problems during surgery on one side and adequate stabilization could not be obtained. A type of inadequate fixation is anterior plating to stabilize a long strut grafting across multiple levels. The biomechanics of that situation is very unfavorable for the plate, and the surgeon may elect to add posterior surgery to supplement the fixation and fusion surface. This is particularly useful in patients who cannot tolerate external stabilization (brace or halo). When treating severe spinal cord compression, inadequate decompression may be obtained with the posterior approach due to compressive pathology anterior to the cord (large osteophytes, DISH, or OPLL). The addition of anterior decompression is indicated in this situation. Deformity of the cervical spine may force the surgeon to reconstruct the spine anteriorly and combine that with further decompression posteriorly. For these situations, combined procedures are indicated and have been successful.

CONCLUSIONS

Cervical degenerative disc disease presents a complex diagnostic and therapeutic challenge. The clinician must determine the relative contributions of neck pain, radicular pain, and myelopathy in the patient's presentation. Diagnostic studies such as x-ray, CT scan, or MRI must be ordered and interpreted within the context of the clinical presentation. Once the diagnosis is established, an individualized treatment plan should be formulated. Nonoperative treatment may be successful in many situations, but when the problem is refractory or recurrent, operative treatment can be considered. Patients with cervical spondylotic myelopathy should be treated more aggressively to prevent permanent loss of neurologic function. The surgical options include anterior, posterior, or combined approach. The surgical treatment is individualized based on the patient's symptoms, location of pathology, levels of involvement, sagittal alignment, and surgeon's preference.

SELECTED REFERENCES

Clarke E, Robinson P: Cervical myelopathy: a complication of cervical spondylosis, *Brain* 79:483-510, 1956.

Gore D et al.: Neck pain: a long term follow-up of 205 patients, *Spine* 12:1-5, 1987.

Lees F, Turner J: Natural history and prognosis of cervical spondylosis, *Br Med J* 2:1607-1610, 1963.

Ono K et al.: Myelopathy hand: new signs of cervical cord damage, *J Bone Joint Surg* 69B:215-219, 1987.

Simpson J, An H: Degenerative disc disease of the cervical spine. In An H, ed: *Surgery of the cervical spine*, Baltimore, 1994, Williams & Wilkins, pp. 181-226.

REFERENCES

1. An H et al.: Ideal thickness of Smith-Robinson anterior cervical fusion, *Spine* 18:2043-2047, 1993.
2. Bohlman H: Cervical spondylosis and myelopathy, *Instr Course Lect* 44:81-97, 1995.
3. Bohlman H, Emery S: The pathophysiology of cervical spondylosis and myelopathy, *Spine* 13:843-846, 1988.
4. Bohlman H et al.: Robinson anterior cervical discectomy and arthrodesis for cervical radiculopathy, *J Bone Joint Surg Am* 75:1298-1307, 1993.
5. Brower R, Herkowitz H, Kurz L: Effect of distraction on the union rate of Smith-Robinson type anterior cervical discectomy and fusion. Presented at the Cervical Spine Research Society Annual Meeting, Palm Desert, Calif, 1992.
6. Chestnut R, Abitol J, Garfin S: Surgical management of cervical radiculopathy: indications, techniques, and results, *Orthop Clin North Am* 23:461-474, 1992.
7. Clark C: Cervical spondylotic myelopathy: history and physical findings, *Spine* 13:847-849, 1988.
8. Clarke E, Robinson P: Cervical myelopathy: a complication of cervical spondylosis, *Brain* 79:483-510, 1956.
9. Connor P, Darden B: Cervical discography complications and efficacy, *Spine* 18:2035-2038, 1993.
10. Crandall P, Batzdorf U: Cervical spondylotic myelopathy, *J Neurosurg* 25:57-66, 1966.
11. Dillin W et al.: Cervical radiculopathy: a review, *Spine* 11:988-991, 1988.
12. Fischgrund J, Herkowitz H: Anterior surgical procedures for cervical spondylotic radiculopathy and myelopathy. In An H, ed: *Surgery of the cervical spine*, Baltimore, 1994, Williams and Wilkins, p. 195.
13. Gore D et al.: Neck pain: a long term follow-up of 205 patients, *Spine* 12:1-5, 1987.
14. Hanai K, Fujiyoshi F, Kamei K: Subtotal vertebrectomy and spinal fusion for cervical spondylotic myelopathy, *Spine* 11:310-315, 1986.
15. Hayashi K, Yabuki T: Origin of the uncus and of Luschka's joint in the cervical spine, *J Bone Joint Surg Am* 67:788, 1985.
16. Herkowitz H: A comparison of anterior cervical fusion, cervical laminectomy, and cervical laminoplasty for the surgical management of multiple level spondylotic radiculopathy, *Spine* 13:774-780.
17. Herkowitz H, Kurz L, Overholt D: Surgical management of cervical soft disc herniation: a comparison between the anterior and posterior approach, *Spine* 15:1026, 1990.
18. Hirabayashi K et al.: Expansive open-door laminoplasty for cervical spinal stenotic myelopathy, *Spine* 8:693-699, 1983.
19. Isomi T et al.: Stabilizing potential of anterior cervical plates in multilevel corpectomies, *Spine* 24:2219-2223, 1999.
20. Jenis L, An H: Neck pain secondary to radiculopathy of the fourth cervical root: an analysis of 12 surgically treated patients, *J Spinal Disord* 13:345-349, 2000.
21. Jones A et al.: Iliac crest bone graft: osteotome versus saw, *Spine* 18:2048-2053, 1993.
22. LaRocca H: Cervical spondylotic myelopathy: natural history, *Spine* 13:854-855, 1988.
23. Law M, Bernhardt M, White A: Evaluation and management of cervical spondylotic myelopathy, *Instr Course Lect*, 44:99-110, 1995.
24. Lee S et al.: Anterior cervical fusion using allograft versus autograft bone. Presented at the annual meeting of the Cervical Spine Research Society, Baltimore, 1994.
25. Lees F, Turner J: Natural history and prognosis of cervical spondylosis, *Br Med J* 2:1607-1610, 1963.
26. Lestini W, Weisel S: The pathogenesis of cervical spondylosis, *Clin Orthop* 239:69-93, 1989.
27. McNab I: Symptoms in cervical disc degeneration. In Sherk H, ed: *The cervical spine*, ed 2, Cervical Spine Research Society, Philadelphia, 1989, Lippincott, pp. 599-606.
28. Montgomery D, Brower R: Cervical spondylotic myelopathy: clinical syndrome and natural history, *Orthop Clin North Am* 23:487-492, 1992.
29. Nurick S: The pathogenesis of the spinal cord disorder associated with cervical spondylosis, *Brain* 95:87-100, 1972.
30. Ono K et al.: Myelopathy hand: new signs of cervical cord damage, *J Bone Joint Surg Br* 69:215-219, 1987.
31. Palit M: Anterior discectomy and fusion for the management of neck pain, *Spine* 24:2224-2228, 1999.
32. Parke W: Correlative anatomy of cervical spondylotic myelopathy, *Spine* 13:831-837, 1988.
33. Riley L, Robinson R, Johnson K: The results of anterior interbody fusion of the cervical spine, *J Neurosurg* 30:127, 1969.
34. Robinson R, Riley L: Techniques of exposure and fusion of the cervical spine, *Clin Orthop* 109:78-84, 1975.
35. Robinson R et al.: The results of anterior interbody fusion of the cervical spine, *J Bone Joint Surg Am* 44:1569-1587, 1962.

36. Saunders R et al.: Central corpectomy for cervical spondylotic myelopathy: a consecutive series with long term follow-up evaluation, *J Neurosurg* 74:163-170, 1991.

37. Simpson J, An H: Degenerative disc disease of the cervical spine. In An H, ed: *Surgery of the cervical spine*, Baltimore, 1994, Williams and Wilkins, pp. 181-226.

38. Waldman S: Complications of cervical epidural nerve blocks with steroids: a prospective study of 790 consecutive blocks, *Reg Anesth* 14:149-151, 1989.

39. Wang J et al.: Increase fusion rates with cervical plating for two-level anterior cervical discectomy and fusion, *Spine* 25:41-45, 2000.

40. White W, Southwick W, Deponte R: Relief of pain by anterior cervical spine fusion for spondylosis, *J Bone Joint Surg Am* 55A:525-534, 1973.

41. Whitecloud T, Seago R: Cervical discogenic syndrome: results of operative intervention in patients with positive discography, *Spine* 12:313-316, 1987.

42. Yamamoto I et al.: Clinical long term results of anterior cervical discectomy without interbody fusion for cervical disc disease, *Spine* 16:272-279, 1991.

43. Yang K et al.: Cervical spondylotic myelopathy treated by anterior multilevel decompression and fusion, *Clin Orthop* 221:161-164, 1987.

44. Young W, Rosenwasser R: An early comparative analysis of the use of fibular allograft versus autograft iliac crest graft for interbody fusion after anterior cervical discectomy, *Spine* 18:1123-1124, 1993.

45. Zdeblick T, Bohlman H: Cervical kyphosis and myelopathy: treatment by anterior corpectomy and bone grafting, *J Bone Joint Surg Am* 71:170-182, 1989.

46. Zdeblick T et al.: Anterior cervical discectomy, fusion, and plating: a comparative animal study, *Spine* 18:1974-1983, 1993.

47. Zdeblick T, Ducker T: The use of freeze-dried allograft bone for anterior cervical fusions, *Spine* 16:726-729, 1991.

48. Zdeblick T et al.: Cervical stability after foraminotomy: a biomechanical in-vitro analysis, *J Bone Joint Surg Am* 74:22-27, 1992.

49. Zhang Z et al.: Anterior intervertebral disc excision and bone grafting in cervical spondylotic myelopathy, *Spine* 8:16-19, 1983.

Thoracic Degenerative Disc Disease

Hugh L. Bassewitz, Jeffrey S. Fischgrund

Uncommon and difficult to diagnose and treat, a symptomatic thoracic disc herniation presents a challenging problem to the spinal surgeon. The symptoms can be varied and vague, from back pain to florid cord compression and from a chronic time course to an acute presentation. The use of the myelogram with a computed tomography (CT) scan and the use of magnetic resonance imaging (MRI) have both helped in the diagnostic imaging of thoracic disc herniations, as well as sometimes complicating issues by being too sensitive. In contrast to the classic principles of concordance of symptoms, physical findings, and myelographic findings that are applicable with relative ease in the lumbar spine, thoracic disc herniations are far more challenging. When the clinician has concluded that surgery is indicated, a number of surgical options are available.

Thoracic disc herniations have long been considered a difficult clinical entity to both diagnose and treat. In 1838 Key described the first report of a thoracic herniated disc causing spinal cord compression.[13] In 1911 Middleton and Teacher described a patient who developed paraplegia secondary to a traumatic thoracic disc herniation.[21] In 1922 Adson performed a laminectomy to remove a herniated disc, while in 1934 Mixter and Barr described four cases of thoracic disc herniation.[22] Three of these four patients had a laminectomy, and two became paraplegic after the surgery.

Over the years many authors have recommended other approaches to surgically treat thoracic herniated discs, given the poor outcome of laminectomies. In 1960 Hulme reported his experience with the costotransversectomy and demonstrated the relative safety of this approach over the laminectomy.[11] Other authors adopted the approach of Hodgson and Stock[10] to utilize an anterior transthoracic approach for herniated discs and also demonstrated the decreased complication rate yielded by this procedure. Posterolateral, lateral cavitary, and video-assisted thoracoscopic approaches have become popular. Many authors have attempted to delineate the optimal treatment method for this problem.

As will be discussed in this chapter, the difficulty relates to the following challenge. Recent literature has suggested that the incidence of asymptomatic thoracic disc herniation is exceedingly high and that the natural

> ## THE CHALLENGE
> - Variable signs and symptoms
> - Large incidence of asymptomatic disc herniations
> - Benign natural history
> - Thoracic canal is small and unforgiving

history of many thoracic disc herniations may be benign. Given that the clinical presentation of thoracic disc herniations is highly variable, how can the clinical information be used to determine whom to treat and with what treatment (Figure 25-1)?

EPIDEMIOLOGY

The true incidence of all (symptomatic and asymptomatic) thoracic herniated discs is unknown. Most patients present with symptoms in the fourth through sixth decades of life.[1,4] Only 0.15% to 4% of all symptomatic protrusions of a disc are in the thoracic spine.[1] Thoracic disc herniations that require surgery account for only 0.2% to 1.8% of all operations performed on symptomatic herniated discs. Awwad et al.[3] found an 11% rate of asymptomatic thoracic disc herniations, most of which were deforming the spinal cord in some way, as determined by CT-myelograms.[3] With the use of MRI the reported rate of asymptomatic thoracic disc herniations has ranged from as little as 15% to16% to as high as 37% as reported by Wood et al.[35] Wood et al.[35] noted an overall rate of 73% positive findings, which included in addition to the herniation rate, a disc bulge in 53%, annular tear in 58%, and deformation of the spinal cord in 29%.[35] Some authors have suggested that thoracic disc herniation may be common enough to be considered a normal variant on MRI.[33]

ETIOLOGY

Most herniated thoracic discs are degenerative in etiology. The highest incidence of herniation is found in the thoracolumbar spine, where greater motion and

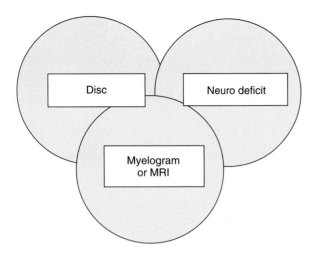

Figure 25-1. Venn diagram for disc surgery. The surgical outcome is considered to be successful if the patient's neurologic status can be explained by an imaging study that confirms the level of the disc herniation.

CLINICAL PRESENTATION

- Back pain
- Neck pain
- Other pain
  - Bandlike "zoster-type"
  - Lower extremity radicular-type
  - Retrosternal
  - Retrogastric
  - Interscapular
  - Flank
- Altered sensation
  - Bandlike
  - Radicular
  - Sensory level
- Altered motor function
  - Weakness in the lower extremities
- Myelopathy
  - Babinski's sign
  - Clonus
  - Spasticity
  - Hyperreflexia
  - Hyporeflexia
- Bowel and bladder dysfunction
- Spinal cord lesions
  - Complete
  - Incomplete
    - Brown-Séquard

---

degenerative changes occur as opposed to the thoracic spine, where less motion occurs.[31] Most commonly, thoracic disc herniations and degenerative changes are found at T8 to T12.[1] Trauma may play a role in a subset of patients, albeit in a smaller population. What is unclear, and the cause for debate, is whether the patients who can relate the onset of symptoms to a traumatic event already had preexistent degeneration or whether the herniation was a new event. This problem will most likely never be satisfactorily resolved, given the high incidence of asymptomatic pathology in the thoracic spine. Scheuermann's disease has also been implicated as a predisposing condition as described by Wood et al.[35] They reported that end-plate changes consistent with Scheuermann's disease were more prevalent in their symptomatic patients than in their asymptomatic patients.

PATHOANATOMY AND PATHOPHYSIOLOGY

As mentioned above, most thoracic disc herniations (75%) occur between T8 and L1. They can be classified as central, centrolateral or paramedian, and lateral. Approximately 70% of herniations are either central or centrolateral. The reported incidence of multiple-level herniations ranges from less than 4% to as high as 16%. The increased rate is likely due to the increased sensitivity of the imaging studies available today. The thoracic spinal canal is relatively small, and the cord occupies most of the available space. The blood supply to the cord is tenuous in this region, especially in the critical zone of T4 to T9. Most thoracic disc protrusions occur centrally rather than laterally, are often calcified, and may adhere to or rarely penetrate the dura. These facts have led to the suggestion that the pathophysiology of a thoracic disc herniation causing neurologic damage is due to direct anterior compression by the disc and with posterior displacement of the spinal cord,

leading to traction and distortion of the neural structures. This compression and displacement may also cause local vascular insufficiency and can explain transitory paresis at adjacent levels.[9]

CLINICAL PRESENTATION AND DIFFERENTIAL DIAGNOSIS

The challenge lies in the difficulty and variety of the clinical presentation of a patient with a herniated thoracic disc. Arce and Dohrmann reviewed the literature in 1985 in an attempt to determine the symptoms of a protruded thoracic disc.[1] Initial symptoms included pain (57%), sensory abnormalities (24%), motor abnormalities (17%), and 2% with bladder difficulties. By the time the patient presented, 61% had both motor and sensory deficits, 9% had a Brown-Séquard syndrome, 15% had sensory symptoms only, 6% had motor symptoms only, 9% had radicular pain only, and 30% had bowel or bladder dysfunction. Symptoms can include pain in the back, leg, and chest; leg weakness; gait disturbance; bowel and bladder dysfunction; spasticity; and numbness. When the herniation is in the midthoracic spine, the patient may present with radiation of pain into the chest or abdomen simulating cardiac or abdominal disease.[32] Pain from a lower thoracic disc herniation may radiate to the groin and simulate ureteral calculi or renal disease. Herniated discs at the lowest thoracic levels can impinge on the distal spinal cord or the cauda equina, with resultant leg pain, mimicking a herniated lumbar disc.[19] The differential diagnosis includes spinal

NONSPINAL CAUSES OF PAIN

MUSCULOSKELETAL
- Infectious
- Neoplastic
- Degenerative
  - Spondylosis
  - Spinal stenosis
  - Degenerative disc disease
  - Facet syndrome
  - Costochondritis
- Metabolic
  - Osteoporosis
  - Osteomalacia
- Traumatic
- Inflammatory
  - Ankylosing spondylitis
- Deformity
  - Scoliosis
  - Kyphosis
- Muscular
  - Strain
  - Fibromyalgia
  - Polymyalgia rheumatica

NEUROGENIC
- Thoracic disc herniation
- Neoplasms
  - Extradural
  - Intradural
  - Extramedullary
  - Intramedullary
- Arteriovenous malformation
- Inflammatory
  - Herpes zoster
- Postthoracotomy syndrome
- Intercostal neuralgia

REFERRED PAIN
- Intrathoracic
  - Cardiovascular
  - Pulmonary
  - Mediastinal
- Intraabdominal
  - Gastrointestinal
  - Hepatobiliary
- Retroperitoneal
  - Renal
  - Tumor
  - Aneurysm

SOCIOPSYCHOGENIC

From Mirkovic S: Thoracic disc herniations. In Garfin SR, Vaccaro AR, eds: *Orthopaedic knowledge update: spine*, ed 1, Rosemont, Ill, 1997, American Academy of Orthopaedic Surgeons, pp. 87-96.

tumors, infections, transverse myelitis, ankylosing spondylitis, fractures, intercostal neuralgia, herpes zoster, and cervical and lumbar herniated discs. Nonspinal causes include disorders of the thoracic and abdominal viscera, amyotrophic lateral sclerosis, multiple sclerosis, and arteriovenous malformations.

IMAGING CAVEATS

- Plain x-rays: 45% to 71% of symptomatic disc herniations have calcification
- Frequency of asymptomatic thoracic disc herniations on myelogram/CT: 11.1% to 13.3%
- Frequency of asymptomatic thoracic disc pathology on MRI: 73%

MRI CHARACTERISTICS OF A HERNIATED THORACIC DISC

- T1: Intermediate signal intensity
  - Low signal intensity if calcified
- T2: Low signal intensity

NATURAL HISTORY

There are few reports in the literature describing the natural history of conservatively treated thoracic disc herniations. In 1992 Brown et al.[6] reported on the 2- to 7-year follow-up of 55 patients with 72 thoracic disc herniations.[6] The most common presenting complaint was anterior bandlike chest pain. Fifty-four were treated initially with conservative measures. Ultimately 15 patients (27%) underwent operation. Of the remaining patients (73% who were treated nonoperatively), all returned to their prior activity. Brown et al.[6] noted, however, that of the 11 patients who initially demonstrated lower-extremity complaints, 9 went on to have surgery. So it appears that in patients with lower-extremity complaints, the natural history of the disorder is one of progression, whereas the patients who present without lower-extremity complaints have a much better chance of resolving with conservative treatment.

DIAGNOSTIC EVALUATION

Radiographic imaging provides useful information when evaluating a patient with a suspected thoracic herniated disc. This fact must be tempered with the knowledge that although MRI may be highly sensitive, the specificity is quite low. On plain lateral radiographs, disc calcification will sometimes suggest the diagnosis of a thoracic disc herniation. Approximately 45% to 71% of symptomatic herniated thoracic discs have intradiscal calcification seen at the corresponding disc level.

Myelograms followed by CT scans are a useful imaging modality. A myelogram alone is difficult to interpret in the thoracic spine because of the superimposing mediastinal structures, as well as the kyphosis of the thoracic spine. With the aid of a CT scan, the canal is easily visualized on transverse sections, and sagittal three-dimension reconstruction can provide useful information (Figure 25-2). Calcified fragments may be identified, as well as soft herniations. The major drawback is the low sensitivity. As noted earlier, Awwad et al.[3]

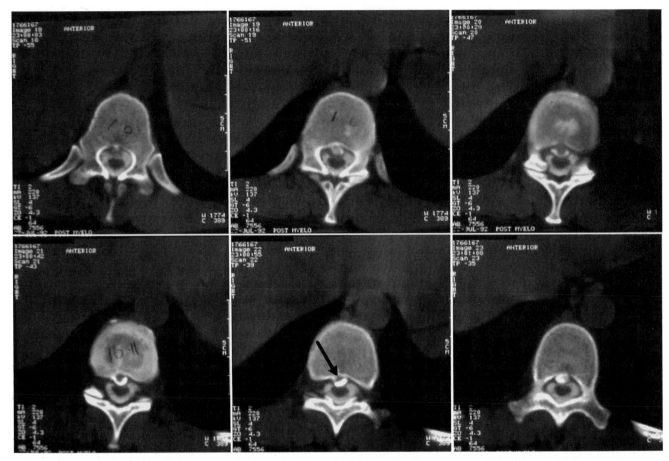

Figure 25-2. Serial axial sections from a postmyelogram CT scan. A calcified herniated T10 to T11 thoracic disc *(black arrow)* is seen centrally compressing the spinal cord.

found the frequency of asymptomatic herniated thoracic disc herniations to be between 11.1% and 13.3%.[3] MRI is fast replacing CT-myelography because of its increasing availability and its noninvasive nature (Figure 25-3).

TREATMENT
Nonoperative Treatment

Most acute thoracic disc herniations should be treated conservatively, because of the wide variety of presenting symptoms in addition to back pain. Relative surgical indications include progressive myelopathy, lower-extremity weakness or paralysis, or chronic radicular pain that is refractory to conservative measures. Given the data from Brown's paper,[6] it is prudent to treat most thoracic disc herniations conservatively, with the exception of the aforementioned indications. Treatment should include a course of nonsteroidal anti-inflammatory medication, rest and modification of activities, physical therapy that focuses on trunk stabilization, and the use of various modalities. An important factor in any treatment plan is education. The gains achieved by explaining to the patient the significance of the findings of a diagnostic test and their true relevance or lack thereof should not be overlooked.

> ### INDICATIONS FOR SURGERY
> • Progressive myelopathy
> • Lower-extremity weakness or paralysis
> • Radicular pain refractory to conservative measures

Surgical Treatment

Indications for Surgery

As the patient is monitored clinically, special attention should be paid to myelopathy and the onset of weakness. If the patient begins to develop lower-extremity weakness, bowel or bladder irregularities, or the long tract signs of myelopathy, surgery is indicated. In the older patient, however, other causes of myelopathy should be ruled out, such as cervical spinal stenosis or a medical myelopathy such as multiple sclerosis. A true sensory level in combination with lower-extremity weakness or paralysis at the corresponding herniation on the imaging test is an absolute indication for surgery.

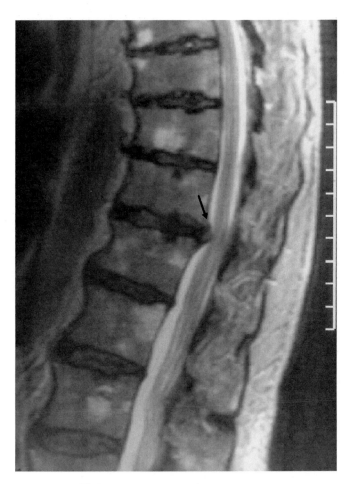

Figure 25-3. Sagittal view of a herniated T9 to 10 herniated thoracic disc (black arrow) seen on a T2 weighted MRI.

The Evolution of Surgical Management

Once the decision has been made to perform a decompression of the spinal cord, a strategy needs to be devised to approach the herniation. Today's surgeons have the benefit of their predecessors, and the evolution of attacking this problem is well detailed in the literature. In this section, a series of surgical options will be presented, along with suggestions for their use.

Laminectomy

Laminectomy was the first surgical approach performed for thoracic disc excision, and the results of this operation have been the benchmark to which other approaches have been compared. For more than 30 years surgeons dealt with poor results and ultimately abandoned the laminectomy because of the risk of neurologic deterioration. In 1934 Mixter and Barr reported that two of the three patients on whom they performed a laminectomy for a herniated thoracic disc developed complete spinal cord lesions postoperatively.[22] Love and Kiefer reported a worsening of neurologic status in 7 of 17 patients,[18] and Logue reported complete paralysis in 5 of 11 patients postoperatively.[17] To further illustrate these poor results,

Arce and Dohrmann reviewed 135 cases of laminectomy for thoracic disc excision and found the following results: 28% of the patients had a worsening of neurologic status, 4% died, 58% improved, and 10% had no change.[2] Disc herniations are generally located anterior to the spinal cord, and when a laminectomy is used, mobilization of the spinal cord is necessary to remove the herniated material and effectively decompress the cord.

Laminectomy may not be the best surgical option for several possible reasons. The blood supply to the cord is tenuous in the compressed situation, and by mobilizing the cord (as opposed to the relatively forgiving cauda equina), there may be additional damage sustained. This mobilization may further decrease the blood flow and oxygenation to the already stressed neural tissues. Another possible reason is that after a laminectomy alone (disc excision is not possible due to the desire to not mobilize the cord) the anterior compression remains, and only the posterior cord is effectively decompressed.

Transthoracic Approach

In 1958 Crafoord et al. first described the use of a thoracotomy approach to decompress a herniated thoracic disc.[7] This approach had been originally used for Pott's disease; investigators were willing to try anything to avoid the devastating complications of a laminectomy. Perot and Munro and Ransohoff et al. described the transthoracic approach for treatment of herniated thoracic discs.[25,26] They and others have demonstrated favorable results with this technique.

The advantages of a thoracotomy include excellent exposure from T4 to T5 to T11 to T12, the ability to easily fuse an unstable level with a rib strut graft, and avoidance of spinal cord manipulation. The obvious disadvantages include the need for a chest tube, the inherent pulmonary morbidity of a thoracotomy, and the possibility of injury to other vital structures such as the great vessels. Recent literature continues to support the efficacy and success of this approach.[14] Otani et al. reported good to excellent results in 18 of 23 cases.[23] Bohlman and Zdeblick reported on the results of 19 patients over a 14-year experience.[5] They found that 16 patients had good to excellent results, 1 fair, and 2 poor. Currier et al. reported in 1994 on 19 patients, of which 3 had a previous laminectomy and 2 had multiple sclerosis.[8] Of the 14 patients who did not have a previous laminectomy or multiple sclerosis, 12 had good to excellent results with a transthoracic approach. In this study all patients were routinely fused with a rib strut autograft. Fusion is recommended when stability is compromised or in cases associated with Scheuermann's disease.

A special consideration when approaching the spine anteriorly is the localization of the segmental blood vessels. Frequently these needed to be ligated to proceed with the approach. At T1 to T3 usually the anterior bodies are free of overlying intercostal arteries. At T3 to T5 the third through the sixth intercostal arteries run vertically over the bodies, and at T6 to T10 they originate on the posterior aspect of the aorta bilaterally. Distally they are below the middle of the vertebral body, then exit through the intervertebral foramen. Another surgical anatomic point is the correlation of rib level with disc level. At T1, T11, and T12 only one rib articulates with the corresponding body. From T2 to T10 each body articulates with two ribs. The rib head overlies the disc space in the lower-numbered body. For example, the tenth rib overlies the T9 to T10 disc space (Figures 25-4 and 25-5).

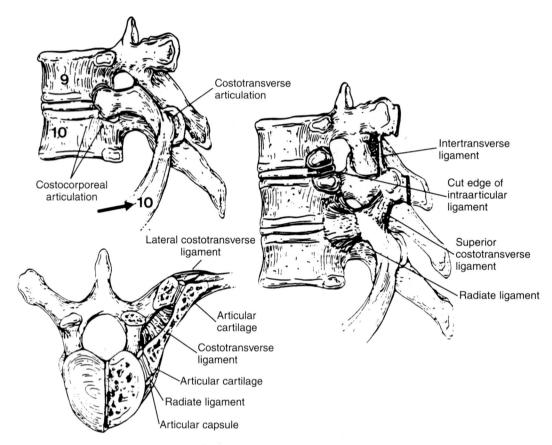

Figure 25-4. Drawing shows that the tenth rib *(black arrow)* overlies the T9 to T10 disc space. When the rib head is removed, the posterior disc space is revealed. *(From Cramer GD, Darby S: Basic and clinical anatomy of the spine, spinal cord, and ANS, p 166, St. Louis, 1995, Mosby.)*

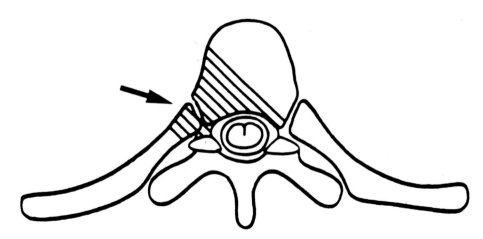

Figure 25-5. The cross-hatched area of bony resection and the angle used in the transthoracic approach for herniated thoracic discs. *(From Cybulski G: Thoracic disc herniation: surgical technique,* Contemp Neurosurg *14[1]:1-6, 1992.)*

Costotransversectomy

Given the problems of the straight posterior approach, surgeons began to look at other ways to attack this problem. In 1960 Hulme adopted the modifications of the original costotransversectomy approach described by Menard for the drainage of spinal tuberculosis. Hulme's results were successful for 4 out of 6 patients.[11] More recently Simpson et al. reported on their experience of 21 patients.[30] Of the 19 patients available for follow-up (mean 4.8 years), 13 were excellent, 6 were good, and 3 were fair. No patients were worse (Figure 25-7).

Lateral Extracavitary Approach

First described by Larson in 1961, this approach provides direct visualization of the posterior margin of the vertebral bodies and disc herniation without the morbidity of a thoracotomy. It can be used at any level of the thoracic spine for both soft and hard disc herniations, either lateral or paramedian. Maiman et al. reported on their series of 23 patients in 1984.[20] They noted improvement in 20 patients, and, most importantly, no patient worsened. The three patients who did not improve had presented with complete motor loss and did not achieve any gains in function (Figure 25-8).

INDICATIONS FOR THE TRANSTHORACIC APPROACH

- Midline disc herniations
- Lateral disc herniations
- T2 to T12 disc herniations

TECHNIQUE: TRANSTHORACIC APPROACH

- Position: Lateral decubitus.
- Approach from side of the disc herniation.
- If disc herniation is central, use the following guidelines:
  - Use left-sided approach for herniations at T4 to T10 (avoids vena cava on right).
  - Use right-sided approach for herniations above T4 (avoids aortic arch at T4).
  - Make incision over rib that is one to two levels above the desired disc space for a wide exposure or over the rib leading to the disc space (tenth rib for a T9 to 10 disc) for a more narrow approach.
  - After the main portion of the rib is resected, incise the pleura and place a rib spreader retractor.
  - Control and ligate the segmental vascular bundle.
  - Remove the rib head at the level of the disc.
  - Identify the disc space, the pedicle above and below, and posterior bodies above and below the disc (Figure 25-6, A).
  - At the level of the superior pedicle, identify the dura and epidural space that orients the surgeon to the posterior margin of the dissection.
  - Perform a discectomy anterior to the herniation, and use a burr to widen the disc space superiorly and inferiorly into the respective bodies.
  - A thin shell of posterior vertebral body cortex is all that remains above and below the disc herniation
  - Create a cavity at the posterior aspect of the superior and inferior bodies and just anterior to the disc herniation.
  - Through this space, pushing fragments from the dura forward into the newly created space completes a posterior-to-anterior resection of the disc material without placing instruments between the compressed spinal cord and the posterior disc protrusion (Figure 25-6, B and C).

INDICATIONS FOR COSTOTRANSVERSECTOMY

- Lateral disc herniation
- Upper thoracic spine (above T5)
- Preexisting pulmonary compromise

TECHNIQUE: COSTOTRANSVERSECTOMY

- Position: Prone or lateral decubitus.
- Incision: Straight midline or lateral muscle splitting.
- Approach: Subperiosteal muscle elevation or paraspinal muscle splitting.
- Identify facet and costotransverse joint.
- Resect rib head and costotransverse joint.
- Identify intercostal nerve and resect the lateral transverse process.
- What should be exposed:
  - Lateral pedicle
  - Vertebral body
  - Disc space
- Portions of the superior and inferior pedicles may need to be removed.
- Perform a discectomy anterior to the herniation, and use a burr to widen the disc space superiorly and inferiorly into the respective bodies.
- Create a cavity at the posterior aspect of the superior and inferior bodies and just anterior to the disc herniation.
- Through this space, pushing fragments from the dura forward into the newly created space completes a posterior-to-anterior resection of the material without placing instruments between the compressed spinal cord and the posterior disc protrusion.

INDICATIONS FOR THE LATERAL EXTRACAVITARY APPROACH

- Soft or hard disc herniations
- Any level
- Lateral or paramedian herniations
- Patients who will have difficulty tolerating a thoracotomy

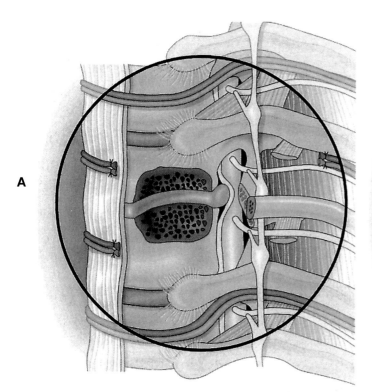

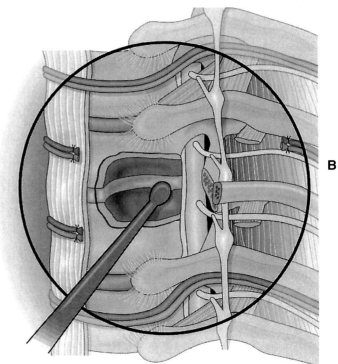

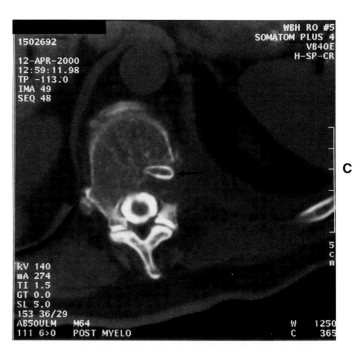

Figure 25-6.   **A,** Drawing of the view obtained after resecting the head of the rib and ipsilateral pedicle. The disc space can now be safely visualized and entered anteriorly. **B,** Drawing showing how a burr may be used to thin the posterior cortex, which may then be pulled anteriorly away from the dural sac with the herniated disc to effect a decompression. After completion of the decompression, the dura can be visualized well across the midline, potentially to the opposite pedicle. **C,** Axial section from a postoperative postmyelogram CT scan after a transthoracic decompression and rib strut autograft fusion was performed for a herniated T10 to 11 disc. The spinal cord is decompressed (*open arrow*) from the anterior compression, and the rib strut is seen anterior to the decompression (*black arrow*). (**A** and **B** *from Zdeblick TA:* Anterior approaches to the spine, *St. Louis, 1999, Quality Medical Publishing,* pp 113-114.)

Pediculofacetectomy

In selected patients, a transpedicular or pediculofacetec-tomy approach may be a useful technique. First described by Patterson and Arbit in 1978, the technique has the advantage of avoiding the medical comorbidities of a thoracotomy.[24] Limitations of the technique include lack of direct visualization, inability to remove central or hard discs, and possible iatrogenic instability. LeRoux et al. reported good results in their series of 20 patients.[16]

They attribute their success in part to early intervention and to the use of specially designed intrapedicular curved curettes. The technique involves using these curettes to work through the pedicle, removing the disc herniation from a posterior to anterior direction. This technique is technically demanding, and most authors recommend the use of the microscope and possibly an endoscope inside the spinal canal to visualize the disc herniation to ensure decompression (Figure 25-9).[12]

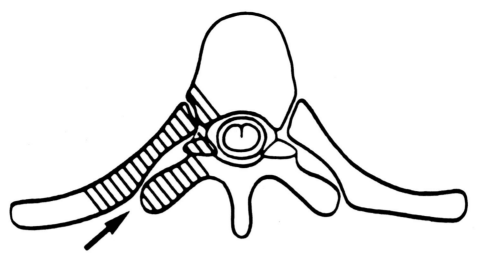

Figure 25-7. The cross-hatched area of bony resection and the angle used in the costotransversectomy approach for herniated thoracic discs. *(From Cybulski G: Thoracic disc herniation: surgical technique,* Contemp Neurosurg *14[1]:1-6, 1992.)*

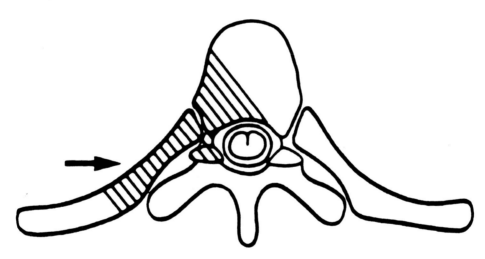

Figure 25-8. The cross-hatched area of bony resection and the angle used in the lateral extracavitary approach for herniated thoracic discs. *(From Cybulski G: Thoracic disc herniation: surgical technique,* Contemp Neurosurg *14[1]:1-6, 1992.)*

TECHNIQUE: LATERAL EXTRACAVITARY APPROACH

- Position: Lateral decubitus.
  - Incision: Short posterior incision over the rib desired (tenth for a T9 to 10 disc herniation).
- Once the rib is removed, separate the pleura from the adjacent ribs and vertebral bodies.
- Remove the remaining rib head, allowing visualization of the bodies and disc space.
- Identify the disc space, the pedicle above and below, and the posterior bodies above and below the disc.
- At the level of the superior pedicle, identify the epidural space, which orients the surgeon to the posterior margin of the dissection.

- Perform a discectomy anterior to the herniation, and use a burr to widen disc space superiorly and inferiorly into the respective bodies.
- A thin shell of posterior vertebral body cortex is all that remains above and below the disc herniation.
- Create a cavity at the posterior aspect of the superior and inferior bodies and just anterior to the disc herniation.
- Through this space, pushing fragments from the dura forward into the newly created space completes a posterior-to-anterior resection of the material without placing instruments between the compressed spinal cord and the posterior disc protrusion.

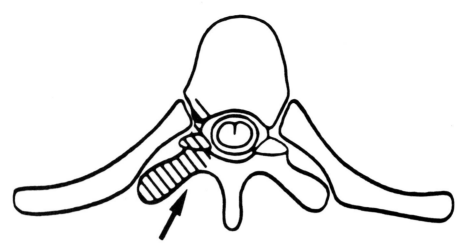

Figure 25-9.   The cross-hatched area of bony resection and the angle used in the pediculofacetectomy approach for herniated thoracic discs. *(From Cybulski G: Thoracic disc herniation: surgical technique,* Contemp Neurosurg *14[1]:1-6, 1992.)*

INDICATIONS FOR PEDICULOFACETECTOMY

- Lateral disc herniations, preferably soft.
- Avoid this approach if the herniation is central and hard, or fusion may be necessary.

INDICATIONS FOR VIDEO-ASSISTED THORACIC SURGERY

- Most important: Technical skills acquired
- High-risk patients
- Most disc herniations

TECHNIQUE: PEDICULOFACETECTOMY

- Position: Prone.
- Incision: Midline approach, unilateral subperiosteal exposure of lamina, transverse process, and facet joint.
- Drill the facet and pedicle inferior to the disc.
- Remove the superior and anterior portion of the pedicle (preserve as much as possible).
- Visualize the exiting nerve root and disc space.
- Create an empty space anterior to the disc herniation with curettes and a high-speed burr.
- Create a cavity anterior to the disc herniation, as well as above and below the herniated disc.
- Through this space, pushing fragments from the dura anteriorly into the newly created anterior space completes the posterior-to-anterior resection of the disc material without placing instruments between the compressed spinal cord and the posterior disc protrusion.

Video-Assisted Thoracic Surgery (VATS)

As technology has advanced in medicine, the natural evolution of thoracic disc surgery is the introduction of video-assisted surgery by Regan and Mack.[28] In 1998 they reported on their preliminary experience with 29 patients who had symptomatic herniated thoracic discs.[27] At 1-year follow-up 75% of the patients were satisfied, 20.1% were unchanged, and 3.4% were dis-satisfied. The complication rate was 13.8%. Advantages of the technique include decreased intensive care unit (ICU) days, chest tube days, and time lost from work when compared with the transthoracic approach.[28,29] The disadvantages include a steep learning curve, the possible need for a thoracic surgeon, and difficulty in performing a strut graft fusion if necessary. The technique is similar to the transthoracic approach after the portals are established and visualization is achieved. However, to become proficient enough to truly benefit the patient, one needs to be thoroughly prepared through animal laboratory work and by performing a high volume of this procedure. The caveat is that realistically it is difficult to achieve technical proficiency when the majority of thoracic disc herniations are asymptomatic, and even in the symptomatic ones, few will need surgery (Figure 25-10).

Other Approaches

For high thoracic disc hernations, an extension of the Smith-Robinson technique can be used for T1 to T2. Occasionally a transsternal, transthoracic,[1] or medial clavicle resection may be used. Described by Kurz et al., the medial clavicle resection avoids splitting the sternum.[15] The incision for this approach is made vertically along the border of the sternocleidomastoid, and then an L-shaped limb is extended distally and laterally at the manubrium and along the clavicle. After developing

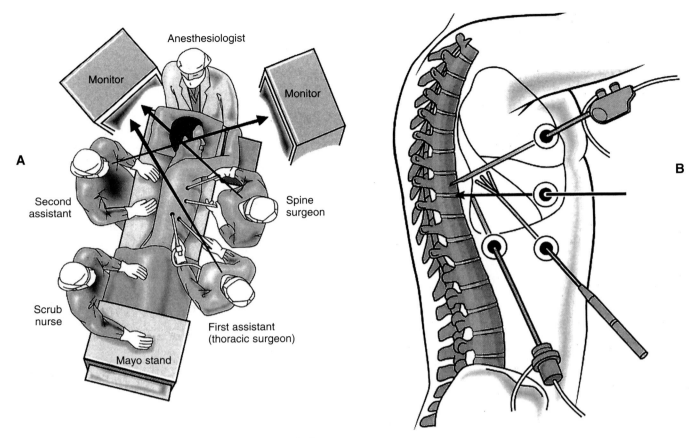

Figure 25-10. **A,** Positioning for thoracoscopy, including position of the surgeon and assistants. The lateral decubitus position is used for thoracoscopy. **B,** Four-portal technique of video-assisted thoracic surgery, which allows for the use of a retractor or suction-irrigation device. *(From Zdeblick TA: Anterior approaches to the spine, St. Louis, 1999, Quality Medical Publishing, pp. 138-140.)*

TECHNIQUE: VIDEO-ASSISTED THORACIC SURGERY

- Position: Lateral decubitus.
- Initial trocar: At the sixth or seventh rib space, at the anterior axillary line.
- Insert a 30 endoscope and deflate the lung with a double-lumen endotracheal tube.
- Add additional two to three portals (anterior axillary line and posterior axillary line) just below the disc space under direct vision. (See Figure 25-10, *A* and *B*.)
- Remove rib head overlying the correct disc (ninth rib for a T8 to T9 disc) with the use of a burr.
- Use a Kerrison rongeur to remove the edge of the superior pedicle.
- The disc space is now exposed.
- Visualize the exiting nerve root and disc space.
- Create an empty space anterior to the disc herniation with curettes and high-speed burr.
- Create a cavity anterior to the disc herniation, as well as above and below the herniated disc.
- Through this space, pushing fragments from the dura back into the newly created space completes a posterior-to-anterior resection of the disc material without placing instruments between the compressed spinal cord and the posterior disc protrusion.

the interval between the sternocleidomastoid and the trachea and esophagus proximally, the sternal and medial clavicle heads of the sternocleidomastoid are elevated subperiosteally. The medial clavicle is then resected and may be used for a strut fusion if needed. The discectomy is then performed similarly to an anterior cervical discectomy and fusion.

CONCLUSIONS

The varied clinical presentation, frequent benign natural history, high incidence of asymptomatic lesions, an unforgiving canal size, and multiple surgical options are what make thoracic disc herniations so challenging to the spinal surgeon. As opposed to the radiculopathy due to lumbar disc herniations or the radiculopathy or myeloradiculopathy of cervical disc herniations, thoracic disc herniations can present with a myriad of symptoms (Table 25-1).

Brown et al. have shown that the natural history of most thoracic disc herniations is benign. Other authors have shown that the incidence of these herniations is quite high. Still other authors have shown that the clinical presentations are rarely clear. Making matters worse for spine surgeons is that the thoracic spinal canal is not large like the lumbar canal, and what resides there, the

Table 25-1	Surgical Approaches for Various Pathologies	
Levels	**Disc Herniation**	**Approaches**
SOFT DISCS		
T1 to T4	Central, centrolateral	Transsternal
	Central, centrolateral	Medial clavisectomy
	Centrolateral, lateral	Costotransversectomy
T4 to T12	Central, centrolateral, lateral	Transthoracic
	Central, centrolateral, lateral	Thoracoscopy
	Centrolateral, lateral	Lateral
	Central, centrolateral, lateral	Costotransversectomy
	Lateral	Transpedicular
CALCIFIED DISCS		
T1 to T4	Central, centrolateral	Transsternal
	Central, centrolateral	Medial clavisectomy
	Lateral	Costotransversectomy
T4 to T12	Central, centrolateral, lateral	Transthoracic
	Lateral	Lateral
	Lateral, centrolateral	Costotransversectomy

From Mirkovic S: Thoracic disk herniations. In Garfin SR, Vaccaro AR, eds: *Orthopaedic knowledge update: spine*, Rosemont Ill, 1997, American Academy of Orthopaedic Surgeons, pp 87-96.

spinal cord, is not nearly as forgiving as the collection of nerve roots that constitute the cauda equina. In the past, posterior approaches have led to many poor clinical results, with iatrogenic paralysis an all too familiar outcome.

Fortunately advances have been made over time in imaging and treatment. We now have a better understanding of the pathoanatomy and physiology. Best of all, newer surgical techniques have improved patient outcomes and greatly decreased the incidence of patients who experience neurologic worsening after surgery. In general, posterolateral techniques are sufficient for lateral lesions and may be the best choice for herniated discs with coexistent stenosis. The transthoracic approach permits the best visualization for central lesions. Upper thoracic central lesions are more difficult to approach through the chest and may be managed best by costotransversectomy. As more experience is gained with VATS, the indications for this procedure will become better delineated.

SELECTED REFERENCES

Awwad EE et al.: Asymptomatic versus symptomatic herniated thoracic discs: their frequency and characteristics as detected by computed tomography after myelography, *Neurosurgery* 28:180-186, 1991.

Bohlman HH, Zdeblick TA: Anterior excision of herniated thoracic discs, *J Bone Joint Surg Am* 70:1038-1047, 1988.

Brown CW et al.: The natural history of thoracic disc herniation, *Spine* 17(Suppl 6):S97-S102, 1992.

Regan JJ, Ben-Yishay A, Mack MJ: Video-assisted thoracoscopic excision of herniated thoracic discs: description of technique and preliminary experience in the first 29 cases, *J Spinal Disord* 11:183-191, 1998.

Wood KB et al.: Magnetic resonance imaging of the thoracic spine: evaluation of asymptomatic individuals, *J Bone Joint Surg Am* 77:1631-1638, 1995.

REFERENCES

1. Arce CA, Dohrmann GJ: Herniated thoracic disks, *Neurol Clin* 3:383-392, 1985.
2. Arce CA, Dohrmann GJ: Thoracic disc herniation: improved diagnosis with computed tomographic scanning and a review of the literature, *Surg Neurol* 23:356-361, 1985.
3. Awwad EE et al.: Asymptomatic versus symptomatic herniated thoracic discs: their frequency and characteristics as detected by computed tomography after myelography, *Neurosurgery* 28:180-186, 1991.
4. Benson MKD, Byrnes DP: The clinical syndromes and surgical treatment of thoracic intervertebral disc prolapse, *J Bone Joint Surg Br* 57B:471-477, 1975.
5. Bohlman HH, Zdeblick TA: Anterior excision of herniated thoracic discs, *J Bone Joint Surg Am* 70:1038-1047, 1988.
6. Brown CW et al.: The natural history of thoracic disc herniation, *Spine* 17(Suppl 6):S97-S102, 1992.
7. Crafoord C et al.: Spinal cord compression caused by a protruded thoracic disc: report of a case treated with anterolateral fenestration of the disc, *Acta Othop Scand* 28:103-107, 1958.
8. Currier BL, Eismont FJ, Green BA: Transthoracic disc excision and fusion for herniated thoracic discs, *Spine* 19:323-328, 1994.
9. Currier BL et al.: Thoracic disc disease. In Herkowitz HN et al., eds: *Rothman-Simeone the Spine*, ed 4, Philadelphia, 1999, WB Saunders, p. 583.
10. Hodgson AR, Stock FE: Anterior spinal fusion: a preliminary communication on the radical treatment of Pott's disease and Pott's paraplegia, *Br J Surg* 44:266-275, 1956.
11. Hulme A: The surgical approach to thoracic intervertebral disc protrusions, *J Neurol Neurosurg Psychiatry* 23:133-137, 1960.
12. Jho HD: Endoscopic microscopic transpedicular thoracic discectomy: technical note, *J Neurosurg* 87:125-129, 1997.
13. Key CA: On paraplegia: depending on disease of the ligaments of the spine, *Guys Hosp Rep* 3:17-34, 1838.
14. Korovessis PG et al.: Transthoracic disc excision with interbody fusion, *Acta Orthop Scand* 68(Suppl 275):12-16, 1975.
15. Kurz LT, Pursel SE, Herkowitz HN: Modified anterior approach to the cervicothoracic junction, *Spine* 16:S543-S547, 1991.
16. LeRoux PD, Haglund MM, Harris AB: Thoracic disc disease: experience with the transpedicular approach in twenty consecutive patients, *Neurosurgery* 33:58-66, 1993.
17. Logue V: Thoracic intervertebral disc prolapse with spinal cord compression, *J Neurol Neurosurg Psychiatry* 15:227-241, 1952.

18. Love JG, Kiefer EJ: Root pain and paraplegia due to protrusions of thoracic intervertebral disks, *J Neurosurg* 7:62-69, 1950.

19. Lyu RK et al.: Thoracic disc herniation mimicking acute lumbar disc disease, *Spine* 24:416-418, 1999.

20. Maiman DJ et al.: Lateral extracavitary approach to the spine for thoracic disc herniations: report of 23 cases, *Neurosurgery* 14:178-182, 1984.

21. Middleton GS, Teacher JH: Injury of the spinal cord due to rupture of an intervertebral disc during muscular effort, *Glasgow Med J* 76:1-6, 1911.

22. Mixter WJ, Barr JS: Rupture of the intervertebral disc with involvement of the spinal canal, *N Engl J Med* 211:210-218, 1934.

23. Otani KI et al.: Thoracic disc herniation: surgical treatment in 23 patients, *Spine* 13:1262-1267, 1988.

24. Patterson RH Jr, Arbit E: A surgical approach through the pedicle to protruded thoracic discs, *J Neurosurg* 48:768-772, 1978.

25. Perot PH Jr, Munro DD: Transthoracic removal of the midline thoracic disc protrusions causing spinal cord compression, *J Neurosurg* 31:452-458, 1969.

26. Ransohoff J et al.: Case reports and technical notes on transthoracic removal of thoracic disc: report of three cases, *J Neurosurg* 31:459-461, 1969.

27. Regan JJ, Ben-Yishay A, Mack MJ: Video-assisted thoracoscopic excision of herniated thoracic discs: description of technique and preliminary experience in the first 29 cases, *J Spinal Disord* 11:183-191, 1998.

28. Regan JJ, Mack MJ, Picetti GD: A technical report on video-assisted thoracoscopy in thoracic spinal surgery, *Spine* 20:831-837, 1995.

29. Rosenthal D, Dickman C: Thoracoscopic microsurgical excision of herniated thoracic discs, *J Neurosurg* 89:224-235, 1998.

30. Simpson JM et al.: Thoracic disc herniation: re-evaluation of the posterior approach using a modified costotransversectomy, *Spine* 18:1872-1877, 1993.

31. Videman T: Magnetic resonance imaging findings and their relationships in the thoracic and lumbar spine, *Spine* 20:928-935, 1995.

32. Whitcomb DC et al.: Chronic abdominal pain caused by thoracic disc herniation, *Am J Gastroenterol* 90(5):835-837, 1995.

33. Williams MP, Cherryman GR, Husband JE: Significance of thoracic disc herniation demonstrated by MR imaging, *J Comput Assist Tomogr* 13:221-224, 1989.

34. Winter RB, Siebert R: Herniated thoracic disc at T1-T2 with paraparesis, *Spine* 18:782-784, 1993.

35. Wood KB et al.: Magnetic resonance imaging of the thoracic spine: evaluation of asymptomatic individuals, *J Bone Joint Surg Am* 77:1631-1638, 1995.

Cauda Equina Syndrome Secondary to Lumbar Disc Prolapse

Mesfin A. Lemma, Andrea S. Herzka,
P. Justin Tortolani, John J. Carbone

The evaluation and treatment of cauda equina syndrome (CES) has been the subject of substantial confusion, controversy, and litigation for several reasons, including lack of definition, rarity of occurrence, slowness of onset, and timing of surgical decompression.

Despite documentation of severe compression of the cauda equina dating back to 1909,[20] CES remains poorly defined. Most investigators agree that the clinical syndrome is characterized by severe low back pain, unilateral or bilateral sciatica, saddle anesthesia, motor weakness (possibly progressing to frank paraplegia), loss or reduction in lower extremity reflexes, and varying degrees of bladder or rectal dysfunction. Importantly, however, none of these criteria, either alone or in combination, have been validated in predicting the diagnosis of CES or response to treatment. Although some clinicians have used the onset of bladder dysfunction or a progressive neurologic deficit to mark the onset of frank CES,[1,10,15] the diagnosis tends to be based more on the physician's clinical suspicion and overall gestalt rather than on objective or measurable factors.

CES is a rare disorder. A spine surgeon in tertiary care practice may see only a few cases per year,[16] and a general orthopedic surgeon may evaluate fewer than five cases throughout his or her career.[15] In the current health care climate, primary care physicians and nurse practitioners are often the first providers to evaluate patients presenting with low back pain.[6] Because CES is so uncommon and its presentation is often insidious, its presence may not be suspected by a general care provider, and therefore performing a complete neurologic history and physical examination (including a determination of sphincter tone, perianal sensation, and volitional sphincter control) may be overlooked at the initial office visit. In a retrospective review, Shapiro[24] reported that in 7 of 20 patients (35%), delay of surgical decompression was a result of initial mismanagement by primary care physicians.

Although CES may present abruptly with the acute onset of symptoms, it more commonly has a slower

---

CAUDA EQUINA SYNDROME

- Poorly defined and rare
- Characteristics
  - Severe low back pain
  - Unilateral or bilateral sciatica
  - Saddle anesthesia
  - Unilateral or bilateral lower extremity weakness
  - Loss or reduction in lower extremity reflexes
  - Varying degrees of bladder or bowel dysfunction
- Presentation may be abrupt, but more commonly has slower onset
- Symptoms mimic typical presentation of a herniated nucleus pulposus
- Timing of surgical intervention controversial—immediate surgical decompression advocated by most clinicians, but outcome may not change with delay

---

onset, with symptomatology that mimics the "typical" presentation of a herniated nucleus pulposus.[10,15] Because a herniated lumbar disc responds well to nonoperative measures, an accurate diagnosis may be substantially delayed or missed completely. The value of repeat examinations and timely follow-up cannot be overemphasized in the evaluation of patients with lumbar disc herniations. It is reasonable and prudent to discuss the signs and symptoms of CES with all patients with herniated nucleus pulposus.

Timing may be critical in the management of CES by surgical decompression. This factor is associated with clinical uncertainty and medical malpractice. Although CES is an indication for surgical intervention in lumbar disc herniation, the timing of that intervention and its relation to outcome remain the subjects of controversy. Most clinicians advocate immediate surgical intervention as a means of improving outcome,[1,23,24] but some studies have demonstrated no change in outcome with delayed surgery.[7,15]

This chapter reviews the epidemiology, pathophysiology, diagnosis, treatment, and outcomes for CES.

HISTORY AND EPIDEMIOLOGY

The first recognized case of compression of the cauda equina was reported in Berlin in 1909.[20] In that study the causative factor was hypothesized to be bone overgrowth in the spinal canal. Not until the seminal work of Mixter and Barr[17] in 1934 were protrusions of the nucleus pulposus considered critical to the development of nerve root or cauda equina impingement. In that study,[17] 6 of 19 cases showed physical signs consistent with CES. Over the ensuing six decades, CES has been the subject of numerous case reports and small case series. To our knowledge there have been no published prospective studies evaluating the prevalence of

this condition in patients with documented herniated nucleus pulposus, although there are at least two retrospective reports in the literature. In one study of 1,011 operations for lumbar herniated discs, Hurme et al.[12] reported 11 cases of CES. The second study reported that of 470 consecutive lumbar laminectomies for disc protrusion, there were 12 cases of CES.[15] Based on these studies, the prevalence of CES in patients with operatively treated lumbar disc herniations has been estimated as 1% to 2%. However, because most cases of herniated lumbar discs are either asymptomatic[2] or respond well to nonoperative measures, the prevalence of CES in all cases of herniated nucleus pulposus is very difficult to measure accurately and is probably substantially lower.

PATHOPHYSIOLOGY AND DIAGNOSIS

Pathophysiology

CES is defined clinically based on history and physical examination. It can be thought of as the result of sacral root injury that causes a neurologic deficit. Although this injury occurs most commonly as a result of direct compression from extruded nucleus pulposus, CES can also occur in association with tumor, vascular insult, or epidural hematoma. It is the disruption of motor and

---

PREVALENCE OF CAUDA EQUINA SYNDROME

- In patients with operatively treated lumbar disc herniations CES approximates 1% to 2%.
- In all cases of herniated nucleus pulposus, CES is probably significantly lower and difficult to measure accurately.

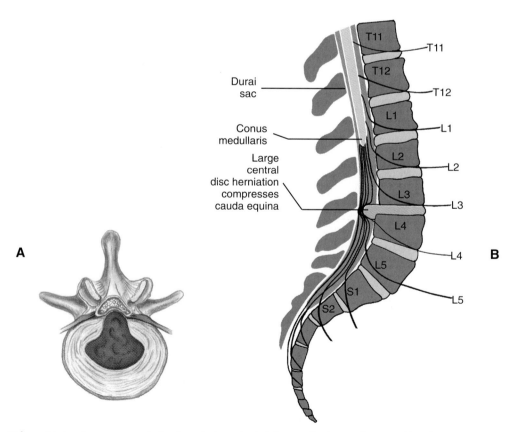

Figure 26-1.   Large central disc herniation. **A,** Axial view. **B,** Sagittal view of lumbar spine. (**A** *modified from Rothman RH, Simeone FA, eds: The spine, ed 2, Philadelphia, 1982, WB Saunders, p 529.*)

sensory function of multiple sacral nerve roots that produces CES.

Figures 26-1 and 26-2 illustrate possible mechanisms of injury that can cause CES.

History and Physical Examination

Although classic CES is associated with a myriad of symptoms, its initial presentation may be subtle. It is paramount that a focused medical history and physical examination be performed to avoid overlooking this diagnosis. CES has been reported in patients who pre-sented with radiculopathy secondary to disc extrusion after migration of a sequestered lumbar disc.[3,10] The clinician must distinguish between an isolated nerve root irritation causing radicular symptoms and compression of the sacral nerves causing CES because the treatments vary dramatically. CES should be ruled out in any patient who presents with signs and symptoms consistent with lumbar radiculopathy.

The clinical presentation of CES can vary, but two distinct modes of presentation have been described: acute and insidious.[15] The acute presentation is characterized by the sudden onset of severe lower back pain, sciatica, urinary retention requiring catheterization, motor weakness of the lower extremities, and saddle anesthesia or hypoesthesia. The insidious presentation is characterized by a history of recurrent episodic backaches with the gradual onset (days to weeks) of sciatica, motor and/or sensory loss, and bowel and bladder dysfunction. In one retrospective study the average times to surgery for acute-onset and insidious-onset patients were 1.1 and 3.3 days, respectively.[15] This delay in treatment was attributed to delay in diagnosis of new-onset urinary retention in patients in the insidious category. These findings emphasize the importance of obtaining a thorough history and maintaining a high index of suspicion for CES in patients at risk.

The history is used to investigate the presence of clinical indicators of CES. In addition to asking questions pertaining to symptoms consistent with lumbar disc prolapse (such as lower back pain and radiculopathy), the clinician should ask the patient about more specific indicators of CES, such as progressive motor weakness, perineal or saddle anesthesia, sexual dysfunction, or bowel or bladder dysfunction. Four types of bladder symptoms secondary to disc derangement have been described: total urinary retention, chronic long-standing partial retention, vesicular irritability, and loss of desire to void associated with unawareness of necessity to void.[14] These symptoms should be sought by specific questioning because patients, particularly those with chronic episodic bladder symptoms associated with progressive spinal stenosis, may not realize the importance of reporting such findings.

In the physical examination the physician should attempt to correlate neurologic physical examination findings with spinal cord or root pathology. A regional spinal examination, including a meticulous neurologic examination, should be performed, and the spinal range of motion should be tested. Findings may include loss of normal lumbar lordosis, paravertebral muscle spasm, or tenderness to palpation over the level of a degenerative

---

ACUTE VERSUS INSIDIOUS PRESENTATION

- Acute syndrome characteristics
  - Sudden-onset severe lower back pain, sciatica
  - Urinary retention requiring catheterization
  - Motor weakness of the lower extremities
  - Saddle anesthesia or hypoesthesia
- Insidious characteristics
  - History of recurrent episodic backaches with the gradual onset of sciatica
  - Motor and/or sensory loss
  - Bowel and bladder dysfunction that developed over days to weeks

---

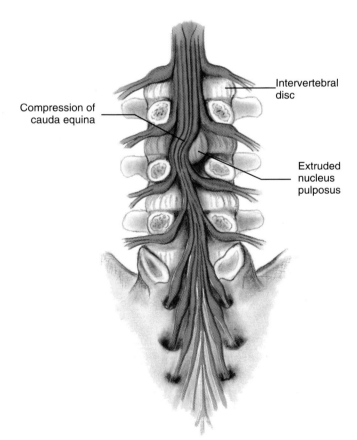

Compression of cauda equina

Intervertebral disc

Extruded nucleus pulposus

Figure 26-2. Coronal view of migrated sequestered lumbar disc.

BLADDER SYMPTOMS

- Total urinary retention
- Chronic long-standing partial retention
- Vesicular irritability
- Loss of desire to void associated with unawareness of necessity to void

Table 26-1	Common Neurologic Findings of Cauda Equina Syndrome
Parameter	Signs/Symptoms
Sensory deficit	Perineal anesthesia, including penile anesthesia in men, or sensory deficits in a dermatomal distribution consistent with lumbar radiculopathy
Motor deficit	Symmetric bilateral lower extremity weakness, flaccid paralysis, weakness in a myotomal distribution
Reflex changes	Loss of deep tendon reflexes below level of lesion: Patellar, Achilles, bulbocavernosus, anal wink
Sexual dysfunction	Loss of reflexogenic erections, ejaculation, orgasm
Pain	Lower back, radicular leg, perineum

Table 26-2	Nerve Root Patterns		
	LOCATION OF FOLLOWING FINDINGS		
Nerve Root	Pain and Numbness	Weakness and Atrophy	Reflex
L4	L4 dermatome, posterolateral aspect of thigh, across patella, anteromedial aspect of leg	Weak extension of knee and quadriceps muscle atrophy	Depression of patellar reflex
L5	L5 dermatome, posterior aspect of thigh, anterolateral aspect of leg	Weak dorsiflexion of foot and toes and atrophy of anterior compartment of leg	None, or absent posterior tibial tendon reflex
S1	S1 dermatome, posterior aspect of thigh, posterior aspect of leg, posterolateral aspect of foot, lateral toes	Weak plantarflexion of foot and toes and atrophy of posterior compartment of leg	Depression of Achilles' reflex

Modified from Rothman RH, Simeone FA, Bernini PM: Lumbar disc disease. In Rothman RH, Simeone FA, editors: *The spine*, ed 2, Philadelphia, 1982, WB Saunders, p 533.

disc, the sciatic notch, or along the course of an irritated nerve root. The common neurologic findings of CES (Table 26-1) should be differentiated from those of isolated radiculopathy (Table 26-2). Pain and numbness in a dermatomal distribution, weakness and atrophy, and/or loss of deep tendon reflex may correspond to a specific spinal root level. Loss of sphincter tone and saddle anesthesia are consistent with CES, although all the neurologic findings of the classic CES need not be present to make the diagnosis.

Tension signs are investigated. A positive straight leg raise test (one that reproduces radicular symptoms) suggests L5 and S1 nerve root pathology. There are many variations of this test. For example, McCulloch and Transfeldt[16] described the bowstring sign as a more reliable sign of root tension than the leg raise. In this maneuver the supine patient's leg is elevated as it is for the standard straight leg raise. Once the radicular pain commences, the knee is bent. This usually alleviates the pain. Finger pressure is then applied to the popliteal fossa over the terminal aspect of the sciatic nerve; if this maneuver reestablishes the radicular pain, it is a positive sign. The contralateral straight leg raise or crossover straight leg raise is performed in the same manner; raising the nonpainful leg reproduces the patient's leg pain in the contralateral leg.

A careful rectal examination is imperative in screening for CES. Saddle anesthesia to light touch and pinprick, loss of anal wink, bulbocavernosus reflex, and volitional sphincter contraction are all consistent with CES.

Radiographic Evaluation

If the history and physical examination findings are consistent with CES, an immediate diagnostic study is indicated. It is necessary to correlate physical examination and radiographic findings when evaluating a patient for CES. Although plain radiographs often are only minimally useful in this setting, they may show evidence of a primary or metastatic tumor or osteomyelitis. Myelography, computed tomography (CT)-myelography, and magnetic resonance imaging (MRI) are modalities commonly used in the evaluation of CES; many clinicians choose MRI rather than CT-myelography as their study of choice.[5,16] One report in particular demonstrates the advantages of MRI in the diagnosis of CES. Coscia et al.[5] described a 30-year-old patient with acute-onset CES whose CT-myelogram showed a congenitally narrow spinal canal at L3 to L4 and L4 to L5 levels and complete myelographic block at the L3 to L4 level with coalescence of the cauda equina cephalad to L3 to L4. Emergent L3 to L4 decompression was performed, but there was no postdecompression intraoperative free flow of dye, a circumstance attributed to intrinsic scarring. A postoperative lumbar MRI showed a large central and posterolateral disc herniation at L4 to L5, for which the patient underwent a second decompression surgery. Intraoperative dural ultrasound after L4 to L5 decompression showed a patent canal. In a similar study, Gindin and Volcan[11] reported variable degrees of filling defects with myelography performed in patients with CES: of six patients, two

> ## EVALUATION OF CAUDA EQUINA SYNDROME
>
> - Imperative to correlate physical examination and radiographic findings
> - Myelography, computed tomography myelography, and magnetic resonance imaging (MRI) commonly employed

> ## TREATMENT
>
> - Cornerstone of treatment is surgical decompression of all involved neural elements.
> - Most advocate wide laminectomy and gentle retraction of the thecal sac followed by discectomy.
> - Microdiscectomy is not advocated because excessive manipulation may lead to permanent neural compromise.

(33.3%) demonstrated only small filling defects and one (16.7%) was reported as normal.

TREATMENT AND OUTCOMES

Sciatica resulting from lumbar disc prolapse is a common and well-recognized clinical entity. Although as many as 95% of disc prolapses resulting in radiculopathy respond to nonoperative management,[9] the onset of discogenic CES should be regarded with surgical urgency. After obtaining a thorough history, clinical examination with careful documentation, CT or MRI results, and (optionally) urodynamic study results,[15] urgent neural decompression should be undertaken.

The cornerstone of treatment for CES is surgical decompression of all involved neural elements. Most authors advocate a wide laminectomy and gentle retraction of the thecal sac followed by a discectomy.* A microdiscectomy is not advocated because, in the presence of a spinal canal narrowed by a combination of a massive disc herniation and stenosis, a small laminotomy followed by excessive manipulation may be dangerous and has the potential for producing a permanent neurologic deficit. Therefore a standard midline approach and a wide laminectomy are preferred. The overhanging, hypertrophied facet is undercut, the lumbar nerve roots are visualized up to their exit foramina, and any additional decompression for concomitant pathology, which is often present, is carried out. Care must be taken to remove any free disc fragments. Schaeffer[21] advocated opening the dura to inspect the nerve roots within to evaluate for intrathecal loose disc fragments. Similarly, Jennett[13] advocated opening the theca in patients with tightly filled spinal canals. In contrast, other studies[23,24] have indicated that such a procedure is not routinely required. Single-level decompressions, performed with care to avoid destabilizing the facet joints, have not resulted in postoperative spinal instability.[4]

The timing of surgical decompression remains controversial. Most authors conclude that the earlier the operative intervention can be accomplished, the better, although some studies have failed to demonstrate any temporal difference in outcomes.[7,15] In a retrospective study of 31 patients, Kostuik et al.[15] reported no significant difference in motor or sensory recovery between patients undergoing surgery at less than 48 hours and those treated after 48 hours. Nevertheless, those authors, like most others,[1,18,19,23,24] continued to advo-

cate early surgery. In a meta-analysis of 42 studies and 322 patients to investigate surgical outcomes of CES secondary to lumbar disc herniation, Ahn et al.[1] reported significantly better sensory, motor, urinary, and rectal function in patients treated within 48 hours compared with those treated after 48 hours. There was no statistically significant difference between those treated within 24 hours and those treated between 24 and 48 hours. Similarly, Shapiro[23,24] reported that compared with patients treated after 48 hours, those treated within 48 hours had a higher likelihood of unassisted ambulation, and those treated within 24 hours had significantly better motor strength and a higher percentage of recovery to normal or near normal strength by 6 to 12 months. Dinning and Schaefer[8] also reported that motor function usually recovers, even in the presence of marked preoperative deficiencies. They postulated that such recovery may be secondary to the fact that the compressive lesion is distal to the anterior horn cells and hence could behave as peripheral nerve neuropraxia, provided that irreversible damage had not occurred.

The time to recovery after surgical decompression can vary greatly. Although most patients improve within the first several months, some may continue to improve for many years after surgery.[18] With respect to the temporal sequence for recovery, Choudhury and Taylor[4] and Shapiro[23] reported essentially complete motor recovery by 1 year. In contrast, Nielsen et al.[18] reported that the temporal sequence for recovery of continence was more variable.

Bladder and bowel recovery tends to be more adversely affected, with slower and more incomplete recovery after surgical decompression. Shapiro[23] reported a more variable temporal sequence for recovery of bowel and bladder function. In a retrospective study of 10 patients, Scott[22] reported no evidence of recovery of complete bladder paralysis at the 6-year follow-up. All patients underwent immediate surgery, but the earliest referral was 3 days after the onset of symptoms. Jennett[13] reported that only 14% (2 of 14) of patients with total paralysis of the bladder regained full control. Several authors have reported that early surgical intervention improves bowel and bladder function. As stated earlier, Ahn et al.[1] used a meta-analysis for 322 patients and showed that urinary recovery and rectal function was significantly better in patients treated within 48 hours than in those treated after 48 hours. Similarly, Nielsen et al.[18] in a study of 26 patients with CES who were evaluated postoperatively with cystometry, reported an

---

*References 1, 4, 15, 21, 23, 24.

improved urologic outcome with early surgery: 8 of 11 patients (72.7%) treated within 48 hours had normal detrusor function. Shapiro[23] reported that of 13 patients presenting with bilateral sciatica, leg weakness, and bladder incontinence, 7 (53.8%) underwent surgery within 48 hours and 6 (46.2%) were treated after 48 hours. Bladder control was regained by all 7 patients (100%) treated within 48 hours but by only 2 of the 6 treated (33.3%) after 48 hours.

Another common sequela of CES is sexual dysfunction (e.g., impotence, loss of coital sensation, and incontinence during intercourse [particularly in women]). The incidence of this sequela also seems to be related to the timing of surgery. Shapiro[24] stated that "unsuccessful intercourse" secondary to vaginal anesthesia and incontinence was reported by 100% (4 of 4) of women who had undergone surgery for CES after 48 hours but by only 14% (1 of 7) of women treated within 48 hours. Interestingly, Scott[22] reported surprisingly good sexual function in men undergoing surgery for CES; only 13% (1 of 8) had no sensible ejaculations. One patient with saddle, penile, and urethral anesthesia and bladder paralysis had normal sexual function.

The severity of the initial symptoms and the acuteness or chronicity of CES has also been shown to influence outcome.[15,19] Kostuik et al.[15] reported that patients with unilateral saddle anesthesia had a better prognosis than those with bilateral sensory loss. In addition, patients with an acute clinical presentation tended to have residual neural dysfunction after surgery. Similarly, O'Laoire et al.[19] reported severity of the preoperative sphincter tone and sensory disturbance as major factors that influenced the outcome of surgery for CES. A complete lack of leg pain carried a particularly poor prognosis, possibly because the diagnosis was delayed in these cases.

Reasons for surgical delay are many and may be multifactorial. In a retrospective study of 44 patients, Shapiro[24] reported that surgical intervention more than 48 hours after the onset of CES was physician-related in 20 of 24 (83.3%; mean time to surgery, 4.3 days) and patient-related in 4 of 24 (16.7%; mean time to surgery, 32.5 days). The delays were attributed to misdiagnosis and initial mismanagement by the primary care physician (35%, 7 of 20), diagnostics (40%, 8 of 20), and surgeon convenience (25%, 5 of 20). He also reported that patients undergoing delayed surgery had a significantly higher chance of persistent bowel and bladder dysfunction, severe motor deficit, and sexual dysfunction.

CONCLUSIONS

In summary, CES is a clinical syndrome with little margin for delay in diagnosis. Operative decompression should be undertaken as soon as possible. Most of the reported literature supports early surgery as a means of improving the outcome for patients with CES. Patients undergoing nonoperative treatment for acute disc prolapse should be closely monitored for the development of saddle area sensory loss, loss of bowel or bladder function, and progressive motor deterioration. Because primary care physicians often see the patient first, special efforts should be made to direct information about early diagnosis and management to those physicians.

SELECTED REFERENCES

Ahn UM et al.: Cauda equina syndrome secondary to lumbar disc herniation: a meta-analysis of surgical outcomes, *Spine* 25(12):1515, 2000.

Bonaroti EA, Welch WC: Posterior epidural migration of an extruded lumbar disc fragment causing cauda equina syndrome: clinical and magnetic resonance imaging evaluation, *Spine* 23(3):378, 1998.

Coscia M, Leipzig T, Cooper D: Acute cauda equina syndrome: diagnostic advantage of MRI, *Spine* 19(4):475, 1994.

Delamarter RB, Sherman JE, Carr JB: 1991 Volvo Award in experimental studies: cauda equina syndrome—neurologic recovery following immediate, early, or late decompression, *Spine* 16(9):1022, 1991.

Dinning TA, Schaeffer HIR: Discogenic compression of the cauda equina: a surgical emergency, *Aust N Z J Surg* 63(12):927, 1993.

Floman Y, Wiesel SW, Rothman RH: Cauda equina syndrome presenting as a herniated lumbar disk, *Clin Orthop* 147:234-237, 1980.

Kostuik JP et al.: Cauda equina syndrome and lumbar disc herniation, *J Bone Joint Surg Am* 68(3):386, 1986.

McCulloch JA, Transfeldt E: *Macnab's backache*, ed 3, Baltimore, Williams & Wilkins, 1997.

Schaeffer HR: Cauda equina compression resulting from massive lumbar disc extrusion, *Aust N Z J Surg* 35(4):300, 1966.

Shapiro S: Medical realities of cauda equina syndrome secondary to lumbar disc herniation, *Spine* 25(3):348, 2000.

REFERENCES

1. Ahn UM et al.: Cauda equina syndrome secondary to lumbar disc herniation: a meta-analysis of surgical outcomes, *Spine* 25(12):1515, 2000.
2. Boden SD et al.: Abnormal magnetic-resonance scans of the lumbar spine in asymptomatic subjects: a prospective investigation, *J Bone Joint Surg Am* 72(3):403, 1990.
3. Bonaroti EA, Welch WC: Posterior epidural migration of an extruded lumbar disc fragment causing cauda equina syndrome: clinical and magnetic resonance imaging evaluation, *Spine* 23(3):378, 1998.
4. Choudhury AR, Taylor JC: Cauda equina syndrome in lumbar disc disease, *Acta Orthop Scand* 51(3):493, 1980.
5. Coscia M, Leipzig T, Cooper D: Acute cauda equina syndrome: diagnostic advantage of MRI, *Spine* 19(4):475, 1994.
6. Deen HG Jr: Diagnosis and management of lumbar disk disease, *Mayo Clin Proc* 71(3):283, 1996.
7. Delamarter RB, Sherman JE, Carr JB: 1991 Volvo Award in experimental studies: cauda equina syndrome—neurologic recovery following immediate, early, or late decompression, *Spine* 16(9):1022, 1991.
8. Dinning TA, Schaeffer HR: Discogenic compression of the cauda equina: a surgical emergency, *Aust N Z J Surg* 63(12):927, 1993.
9. Errico TJ, Lowell TD: The operative treatment of lumbar herniated nucleus pulposus, *Curr Opin Orthop* 4:115, 1993.
10. Floman Y, Wiesel SW, Rothman RH: Cauda equina syndrome presenting as a herniated lumbar disk, *Clin Orthop* 147:234, 1980.
11. Gindin RA, Volcan IJ: Rupture of the intervertebral disc producing cauda equina syndrome, *Am Surg* 44(9):585, 1978.
12. Hurme M et al.: Operated lumbar disc herniation: epidemiological aspects, *Ann Chir Gynaecol* 72(1):33, 1983.
13. Jennett WB: A study of 25 cases of compression of the cauda equina by prolapsed intervertebral discs, *J Neurol Neurosurg Psychiatry* 19:109, 1956.
14. Jones DL, Moore T: The types of neuropathic bladder dysfunction associated with prolapsed lumbar intervertebral discs, *Br J Urol* 45(1):39, 1973.
15. Kostuik JP et al.: Cauda equina syndrome and lumbar disc herniation, *J Bone Joint Surg Am* 68(3):386, 1986.

16. McCulloch JA, Transfeldt E: *Macnab's backache*, ed 3, Baltimore, Williams & Wilkins, 1997.

17. Mixter WJ, Barr JS: Rupture of the intervertebral disc with involvement of the spinal anal, *N Engl J Med* 211(5):210, 1934.

18. Nielsen B et al.: A urodynamic study of cauda equina syndrome due to lumbar disc herniation, *Urol Int* 35(3):167, 1980.

19. O'Laoire SA, Crockard HA, Thomas DG: Prognosis for sphincter recovery after operation for cauda equina compression owing to lumbar disc prolapse, *Br Med J (Clin Res Educ)* 282(6279):1852, 1981.

20. Oppenheim H, Krause F: Ueber Einklemmung bzw: Strangulation der Cauda equina, *Dtsch Med Wochenschr*, 35(16):697, 1909.

21. Schaeffer HR: Cauda equina compression resulting from massive lumbar disc extrusion, *Aust N Z J Surg* 35(4):300, 1966.

22. Scott PJ: Bladder paralysis in cauda equina lesions from disc prolapse, *J Bone Joint Surg Br* 47:224, 1965.

23. Shapiro S: Cauda equina syndrome secondary to lumbar disc herniation. *Neurosurgery* 32(5):743, 1993.

24. Shapiro S: Medical realities of cauda equina syndrome secondary to lumbar disc herniation, *Spine* 25(3):348, 2000.

Lumbar Spinal Stenosis: Nonoperative and Operative Treatment

Christopher L. Hamill, Joseph M. Kowalski

Lumbar spinal stenosis is increasingly being recognized as a cause of disabling low back and lower extremity pain in the adult population. Improvements in living conditions and health care have resulted in a gradual increase in life expectancy. With increased longevity there has been an associated increase in productive years, resulting in more elderly adults continuing with active lives beyond previous generations. Although current imaging techniques may easily identify narrowing of the spinal canal, the diagnosis of spinal stenosis remains a clinical task. The incidence and natural history of spinal stenosis remain unknown, and the ideal treatment remains a matter of debate and has not yet been determined. There have been few prospective or randomized studies comparing the clinical outcomes of patients treated with surgery to those without. Patients with mild symptoms of short duration have traditionally done well with nonsurgical management. People with moderate to severe symptoms experience better results with surgical decompression than those with mild symptoms treated surgically. There remain no predictors for the outcome of surgery regarding the surgical treatment of patients with severe pain or symptoms refractory to conservative measures.

Stenosis of the spinal canal has many causes (Box 27-1). Congenital abnormalities, disc herniations, and other space-occupying lesions cause a decrease in the volume of the spinal canal but are considered separate entities. The clinical syndrome of lumbar spinal stenosis most commonly occurs secondary to the age-related changes in the lumbar spine. These changes occur at the three-joint motion complex in the lumbar spine and are the same age-related changes that occur in other articulations throughout the body. These changes include a decrease in joint cartilage thickness, osteophyte formation, subchondral sclerosis, and joint subluxation at the intervertebral disc and facet joints, resulting in a decrease in the volume of the spinal canal. This results in less space available for the neural elements. Encroachment of the spinal canal in combination with residual motion leads to vascular and conduction

Box 27-1	Classification of Lumbar Spinal Canal Stenosis

DEVELOPMENTAL (CONGENITAL)
- Idiopathic
- Achondroplastic
- Osteopetrosis

ACQUIRED
- Degenerative
  - Central
  - Lateral recess or foraminal
  - Degenerative spondylolisthesis
- Iatrogenic
- Miscellaneous
  - Acromegaly
  - Paget's disease
  - Ankylosing spondylitis
  - Fluorosis
- Traumatic

COMBINATION

changes in the neural elements, thought to be responsible for clinical symptoms. Perturbations of the motion segment can lead to local inflammatory responses, causing local effects. Symptoms related to such events may respond to activity modification, orthosis application, antiinflammatory medications, and the like. The only absolute way to enlarge the spinal canal is to physically decompress the neural elements via surgery.

EPIDEMIOLOGY

The exact prevalence of lumbar spinal stenosis is unknown. The first National Health and Nutrition Examination Survey (NHANES I) of 6913 subjects revealed a 17.7% self-reported prevalence of low back pain. The NHANES II (1976-1980) included 27,801 subjects and reported a 13.8% cumulative lifetime prevalence of low back pain lasting at least 2 weeks. These numbers include multiple diagnoses, of which lumbar spinal stenosis is a small percentage. These surveys found that low back pain was the most frequent cause of activity limitation in patients under 45 years of age, and this decreased to the fourth leading cause in the population 45 to 64 years of age.

Boden and Wiesel[5] have reported that 30% of asymptomatic adults have a major abnormality on a magnetic resonance imaging (MRI) scan of the lumbar spine. These findings increase with age, and essentially all patients over the age of 65 years have significant findings. These findings are consistent with previous studies revealing a 24% rate of abnormal lumbar spine myelograms and a 36% rate of abnormal computed tomography (CT) scans in asymptomatic patients. MRI has been able to detect disc signal change in subjects 15 to 18 years of age. Cadaveric studies have revealed significant disc degeneration in most spines in the fourth decade of life.

Risk factors associated with severe back pain include heavy lifting, use of a jackhammer or machine tool, and the operation of a motor vehicle. Risk factors associated with moderate low back pain include cigarette smoking, jogging, and cross-country skiing. The prevalence of low back pain increases with age and is inversely related to income and level of education. Unfortunately, no data currently exist to report specifically on the prevalence of spinal stenosis.

PATHOPHYSIOLOGY

The anatomy of the spinal canal has a degree of variability. The cross-sectional configuration of the spinal canal is somewhat variable, and a trefoil canal has the smallest cross-sectional area. The arthritic changes that occur in the spine are the same that occur at other articulations throughout the body. These changes occur in the three-joint motion complex, which is the intervertebral disc anteriorly and the facet joints posteriorly. Disc degeneration is commonly the first event in the aging process, although facet arthrosis can precede this. Evidence of degenerative changes is most rapid between the ages of 25 and 35 years, with the lowest two motion segments most frequently affected. Desiccation of the disc results in annular bulging, and the decreased cartilage thickness at the disc space and facet joints results in a decrease in the volume of the spinal canal. Aberrant motion leads to thickening of the ligamentous structures and osteophyte formation, which further compromise the volume of the spinal canal. The decreased volume of the spinal canal reduces the space available for the neural elements. Extension movements of the lumbar spine also decrease the cross-sectional area of the spinal canal, causing dynamic compromise of the spinal canal. This encroachment leads to vascular and conduction changes in the neural elements, thought to be responsible for clinical symptoms. Mechanical irritation of the motion segment can incite a local inflammatory response.

Spinal stenosis can be divided into central and lateral recess stenosis. Central stenosis is commonly found at

---

PATHOPHYSIOLOGY

- Pathophysiology
  - Decreased volume of spinal canal due to osteoarthritis of disc and facet joints.
  - Less space available for neural elements.
  - Mechanical irritation can incite a local inflammatory response.
  - Vascular and conduction changes of neural elements are thought to be responsible for symptoms.
  - Chronic neural compression leads to edema, demyelination, and wallerian degeneration of the afferent and efferent fibers.
  - Substance P has been proposed as a pain modulator related to involvement of the nerve root and dorsal root ganglion.
- Central stenosis
  - Ligamentum flavum buckling or hypertrophy.
  - Superior facet process hypertrophy or osteophyte formation.
  - Intervertebral disc protrusion or osteophyte formation.
- Lateral recess stenosis
  - Entrance zone: Hypertrophy of the superior articular process.
  - Mid zone: Fibrocartilage overgrowth of a pars interarticularis defect.
  - Foraminal stenosis: Pedicular kinking from scoliosis, foraminal disc herniations, or foraminal collapse secondary to collapse of disc space.

---

the intervertebral level and is caused by infolding or hypertrophy of the ligamentum flavum, osteophytes or hypertrophy of the superior facet process, or protrusion of or osteophyte formation from the intervertebral disc level.

Lateral recess stenosis is divided into the nerve root canal and the intervertebral foramen. This kind of stenosis affects the nerve root and therefore commonly presents with signs of radiculopathy. Lee et al.[13] divided the lumbar nerve root canal into three anatomic zones: (1) entrance zone, (2) mid zone, and (3) exit zone (Figure 27-1). The entrance zone is what has been commonly referred to as the lateral recess. This is the subarticular area located anterior to the superior articular process and medial to the pedicle. The mid zone is located underneath the pars interarticularis and below the pedicle. The exit zone is intraforaminal. Lateral recess stenosis most commonly occurs in the entrance zone and is usually secondary to hypertrophy of the superior articular process in the subarticular zone and medial aspect of the pedicle. Stenosis of the mid zone is most commonly caused by fibrocartilage overgrowth of a pars interarticularis defect. Foraminal stenosis is less common and is seen with pedicular kinking from scoliotic deformity or foraminal disc herniations.[5]

Degenerative spondylolisthesis causes a decrease in cross-sectional area as well.[1,2] One or more of the above may predominate, but they commonly occur together.

There have been many attempts to identify the mechanism of symptom production in spinal stenosis, but the precise pathophysiology remains poorly understood. An increase in venous pressure, decreased blood flow, and

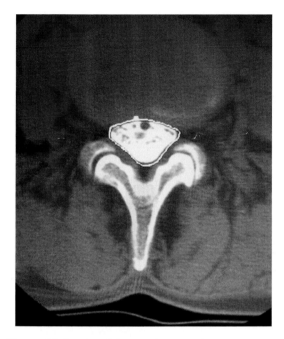

Figure 27-1. Axial CT-myelogram demonstrating normal spinal canal dimension and configuration.

SYMPTOMS AND SIGNS

- Symptoms
  - Low back pain (95%), claudication (91%), leg pain (71%), leg weakness (33%)
  - Exacerbated by walking; relieved by sitting or leaning forward
  - May have radicular pain with herniated disc
- Signs
  - Paucity of neurologic deficits despite profound symptoms
  - May have positive femoral nerve stretch test or straight leg raise with disc herniation
- Cervical and lumbar spinal stenosis can coexist; therefore a detailed examination of both areas and the upper and lower extremities is essential.

decreased axoplasmic flow have all been identified in animal models of spinal stenosis. This results in edema, demyelination, and wallerian degeneration of the afferent and efferent fibers. Compression of a peripheral nerve causes paresthesias, sensory deficits, and motor deficits but does not cause pain. Inflammation is required to cause pain. An irritated or inflamed nerve may be further aggravated by compression, causing pain and symptoms. Substance P has been proposed as a key modulator in symptom production related to involvement of the nerve root and dorsal root ganglion.

SIGNS AND SYMPTOMS

The degenerative process is slow and sometimes relentlessly progressive. Low back pain and stiffness are common complaints, and fortunately few patients with spinal stenosis have significant symptoms warranting medical attention. Most symptoms are mechanical, being aggravated with activity and relieved by rest.

The most common symptoms are low back pain (95%), claudication (91%), leg pain (71%), weakness (33%), and voiding difficulties (12%). Typical symptoms of spinal stenosis, or neurogenic claudication, include pain, numbness, and paresthesias in the posterolateral legs and thighs. It is not uncommon to have a cramping or heaviness sensation in one or both legs. These symptoms may start in the low back and radiate distally or may start in the lower extremities and propagate proximally. The symptoms are classically exacerbated with walking and are commonly asymmetric and inconsistent. Urinary dysfunction is no more common in patients with spinal stenosis than in those without stenosis but needs to be investigated appropriately in this age population.

Extension of the lumbar spine causes a decrease in the cross-sectional area of the spinal canal; therefore symptoms of spinal stenosis are worsened in the upright posture. Symptoms can be relieved with flexion of the lumbar spine such as leaning forward on a shopping cart or walker, and walking uphill may be more comfortable than walking downhill. Riding a bicycle places the spine in flexion and can be helpful in differentiating symptoms of claudication due to vascular disease from those due to spinal disease. Patients with vascular disease will experience leg pain with any form of muscular exertion in the lower extremities, whereas spinal disease will cause symptoms when the spine is held in an upright or extended position. Patients with degenerative spondylolisthesis may actually experience increased symptoms with flexion due to increased slippage with this maneuver. An acute change in symptoms may reflect a disc herniation or fracture.

Despite profound symptoms, the objective physical findings or deficits are few. Nonetheless, a thorough and methodical examination is required to make the diagnosis. Lower motor deficits from lumbar spinal stenosis may mask the typical findings of cervical spondylotic myelopathy, that is hyperreflexia, clonus, and pathologic reflexes in the lower extremities. A detailed examination of the cervical spine is important as well, because 5% to 20% of patients may have concomitant lumbar and cervical spinal stenosis. Local tenderness in the lumbar spine is common, as is loss of lumbar lordosis. Motor weakness is not pronounced. Straight leg raising and other nerve root tension signs are not common unless there is a concurrent disc herniation. Symptoms and even reflex changes may be elicited with extension of the back in the supine position, but this is not consistent.

Other medical conditions can cause low back and lower extremity complaints and need to be considered in the differential diagnosis. Vascular disease is common in this age-group and can present in similar fashion (Box 27-2). Vascular claudication is typically associated with pain in the calf that is aggravated by muscular exertion regardless of the position of the lumbar spine. Therefore walking or bicycling will cause

| Box 27-2 | Differential Diagnosis of Lumbar Spinal Stenosis |

VASCULAR CONDITIONS
- Peripheral vascular disease
- Aortic aneurysm

NEUROLOGIC DISORDERS
- Diabetic neuropathy
- Peripheral compressive neuropathy
- Cervical myelopathy
- Amyotrophic lateral sclerosis (Lou Gehrig disease)
- Demyelinating disease

MUSCULOSKELETAL DISEASE
- Osteoarthritis of hip or knee

OTHER
- Renal disease
- Retroperitoneal disorders
- Psychologic disorders

SPINAL IMAGING

PLAIN RADIOGRAPHY
- Remains essential to survey bone quality, spinal alignment, and arthritic conditions and may reveal destructive lesions
- Disc space collapse, osteophyte formation, and loss of lordosis common

MAGNETIC RESONANCE IMAGING (MRI)
- The technique of choice to evaluate the patency of the spinal canal
- Very sensitive and noninvasive

COMPUTED TOMOGRAPHY (CT)-MYELOGRAPHY
- Next best option if MRI is not available
- Cross-sectional area less than 100 mm^2 suggests spinal stenosis

pain in the affected area, and resting in any position will dramatically relieve the symptoms. Physical examination may reveal decreased peripheral pulses and evidence of vascular insufficiency. An aortic aneurysm can cause severe low back and leg pain, although it is much less common than spinal stenosis.

Osteoarthritis commonly causes pain in the buttock and back. Typical pain from hip osteoarthritis is localized to the groin area and aggravated by hip movement. The patient with hip osteoarthritis will have pain with hip flexion, such as when attempting to tie one's shoes or getting in and out of an automobile with a low seat level. Peripheral neuropathies are common in this age-group and may be secondary to diabetes or dietary deficiencies and typically have a glove-and-stocking distribution of symptoms unrelated to the position of the lumbar spine. Electromyography and nerve conduction studies may be helpful in differentiating peripheral neuropathies and other neurologic disorders as well.

The importance of the clinical examination should not be underplayed in patients with lumbar stenosis. There generally is a paucity of gross motor weakness; however, the examination should include both static and dynamic testing. Observation of ambulation, especially progressive ambulation, may show the patient becoming increasingly pitched forward. This is an attempt to decrease neural compression by increasing canal or foraminal size by flexion of the lumbar spine. These patients will forward flex with ease; however, extension usually is quite limited. The examination should always test lower extremity strength, testing, nerve root tension, deep tendon reflexes, distal pulses, and hip range of motion.

SPINAL IMAGING

Spinal imaging is used to confirm the clinical diagnosis of spinal stenosis. The rate of false-positive imaging studies in an asymptomatic patient population is quite high, with more than 30% of adults having abnormalities on MRI.[6] The judicious use of imaging studies can be cost-effective when these studies affect the treatment plan. Numerous studies have shown that excessive reliance on imaging studies can lead to poor outcomes after spinal surgery when there is failure to correlate the imaging studies with clinical findings.

Spinal imaging begins with anteroposterior and lateral radiographs of the lumbosacral spine. However, the correlation of plain radiographs and clinical symptoms has been poor.[7-9] Plain radiographs give a survey of bone quality, alignment, and underlying arthritis and may reveal evidence of infection or tumor. The presence of scoliosis and other sagittal and coronal plane deformities needs to be recognized. A single-view anteroposterior radiograph of the pelvis to visualize the hip joints may reveal the presence of osteoarthritis and should be part of every screening study for lumbar spine disease.

Stenosis can only be inferred from plain radiographs with attention to sclerotic end plates, osteophyte formation, and facet joint arthropathy. Cadaver studies have shown that a foraminal height less than 15 mm and a posterior disc height less than 4 mm do correlate with nerve root compression.[10] The absolute value for stenosis based on conventional radiographs still does not exist. A postmyelography axial CT scan is useful in determining the degree of stenosis. An anteroposterior diameter of the spinal canal less than 13 mm suggests relative stenosis and less than 10 mm represents absolute stenosis.[3,4] Because the shape of the spinal canal can be variable, a more accurate measure is a cross-sectional area of the canal that is less than 100 mm^2, which suggests spinal stenosis (Figures 27-2 and 27-3).

Flexion and extension lateral radiographs can also help determine the presence or absence of instability. The exact definition of instability in the lumbar spine is still controversial. According to Boden and Wiesel,[5] normal vertebral levels should have less than 3 mm of dynamic anterior-posterior translation. On occasion side-bending films are useful in the case of scoliosis.

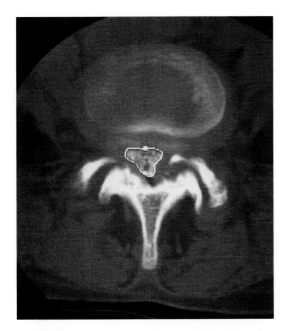

Figure 27-2. Axial CT-myelogram demonstrating spinal stenosis. Note the diffuse disc bulge with facet irregularity and osteophyte formation causing spinal canal encroachment. The cross-sectional area measures 67 mm². Compare with Figure 27-1.

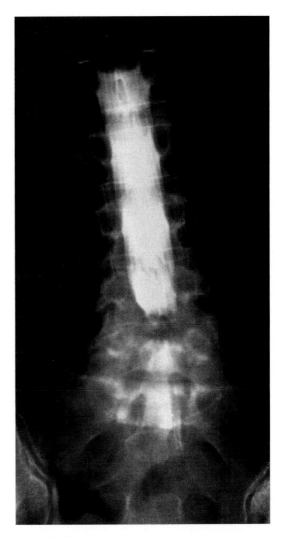

Figure 27-3. Anteroposterior lumbar myelogram demonstrating dye-column cut-off at L4 to L5 indicating spinal canal encroachment.

The use of advanced spinal imaging should be thought of as a preoperative tool to delineate the extent and precise location of pathology. Myelography was the gold standard in the evaluation of lumbar disc disease and spinal stenosis (Figure 27-4). However, this has been supplanted by MRI, which is noninvasive and provides a highly detailed, multiplanar view of the spinal canal (Figure 27-5). MRI has been found to be at least equivalent to CT-myelography for the evaluation of disc disease and spinal stenosis. Because of the tremendous sensitivity of MRI, it should not be used as a screening tool but as a tool to confirm the clinical diagnosis of spinal stenosis. The cerebrospinal fluid on T2 imaging appears similar to a postmyelographic CT image for best diagnosing spinal canal stenosis in the lumbar spine. The central and foraminal areas of the spine are well visualized on both sagittal and axial images. Sagittal images may be better for determining anteroposterior dimension of the spinal canal (Figure 27-6). Axial images may better demonstrate thecal sac compression and narrowing of the lateral recess (Figure 27-7). The lateral recess is more difficult to interpret with MRI than with CT because the osteophyte formation around the facet joints has a low signal intensity on T1 and T2 weighted images. Thus MRI tends to overread the degree of encroachment. Patients with a history of previous surgery, infection, or tumorlike processes require gadolinium to enhance the imaging technique.

CT-myelography is the test of choice when MRI cannot be used to evaluate the spinal canal (see Figure 27-2). One advantage of CT-myelography is the ability to perform dynamic visualization of the spine by obtaining flexion and extension views. CT-myelography is better at visualizing the spinal canal in patients with scoliosis. The disadvantage of this technique is the invasive nature of the procedure and associated risks. The sensitivity and specificity of CT and MRI have been reported to be comparable to that of myelography, with the reported accuracy between 48% and 100%.[12] The most accurate way to determine lumbar stenosis is the cross-sectional area of the thecal sac measured by axial CT-myelography. Although CT without myelography allows for great visualization of bony anatomy, its utility for the evaluation of spinal stenosis is poor, and it is not recommended for routine use.

NONOPERATIVE TREATMENT

The clinical presentation of patients with lumbar spinal stenosis is variable. Classically the patient's discomfort is aggravated by walking and relieved with rest. The severity of symptoms helps dictate the optimum treatment for these patients. The goal of treatment is to

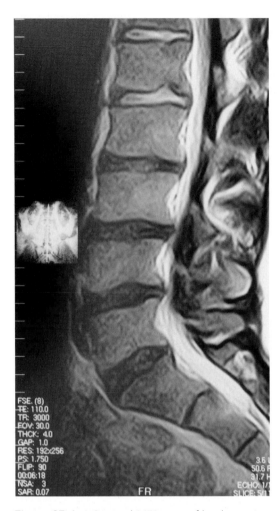

Figure 27-4.   Sagittal MRI scan of lumbar spine demonstrating spinal stenosis.

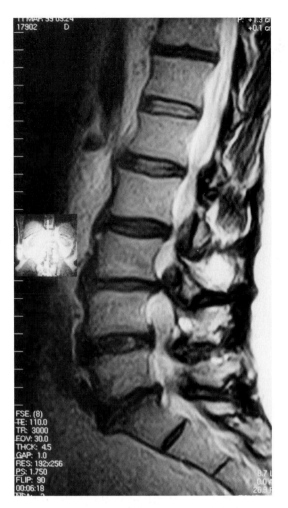

Figure 27-5.   Sagittal MRI scan of lumbar spine demonstrating disc bulging anteriorly, most pronounced at L3 to L4, and to lesser degrees at L4 to L5, L2 to L3, and L5 to S1. Also note enfolding of the ligamentum flavum posteriorly.

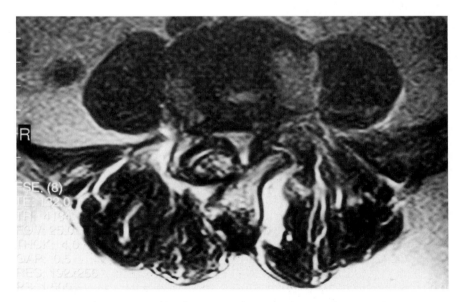

Figure 27-6.   Axial MRI scan of lumbar spine demonstrating a decreased cross-sectional area of the spinal canal. Note the lateral recess stenosis secondary to hypertrophic facet processes, which are greater on the left.

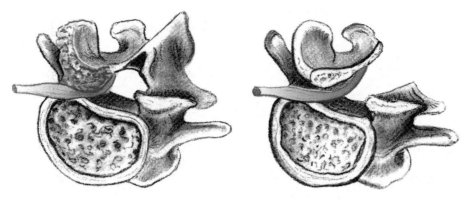

Figure 27-7. Axial view demonstrating thecal, sac compression and narrowing of the lateral recess.

NONOPERATIVE TREATMENT

- Medications: Analgesics, nonsteroidal anti-inflammatory drugs.
- Muscle relaxants, narcotics (short-term).
- Activity modification.
- Exercise to maintain strength and endurance.
- Manipulation by a qualified practitioner may provide significant relief.
- Epidural steroid injection may provide relief.

improve the level of function and decrease lower extremity discomfort. The armamentarium for nonoperative treatment of patients with lumbar stenosis includes a combination of patient education, reassurance, pain control, and physical therapy.

Mild symptoms and symptoms of short duration can be managed with nonsurgical modalities. Pain control can be in the form of analgesics, nonsteroidal anti-inflammatory medications, and even short-term usage of narcotics. Complications secondary to medications are more common in the elderly, and one needs to monitor renal and hepatic function, as well as drug interactions. Narcotic use can cause constipation, which should be anticipated. Greene and Winickoff[9] suggested a drug treatment algorithm for the elderly patient population with spinal stenosis. The use of muscle relaxants in this patient population should be reserved for short-term use because of the significant habit-forming potential of these medications. The benefit of these drugs over narcotic or nonsteroidal medications is unclear.[15]

Exercise is important to maintain strength and endurance, and low-impact or aquatic therapy is well tolerated. Although there is little scientific proof regarding the efficacy of different physical therapy modalities and manipulation, their application by a qualified practitioner may provide significant relief of symptoms in select patients.

The use of epidural steroid injections is on the presumption of an inflammatory etiology as a mechanism for the symptoms. The use of epidural steroid injections in elderly patients with stenosis is common, but the efficacy has not yet been established[16] Abanco et al.[1] found that epidural steroid injections provided more favorable results in older patients than younger patients at 1-year follow-up. The infiltration of epidural steroid injections may provide dramatic pain relief; however, many patients will have recurrent symptoms because the underlying pathology is not removed. The consensus of retrospective studies has found that approximately 60% to 80% of patients with stenosis experience some relief with four or five epidural steroid injections; up to 25% of them report long-term relief.[17,18]

The use of a lumbosacral corset may provide benefit from the increased intraabdominal pressure. This reduces the loads in the lumbar spine through force dissipation into the thoracic spine via the diaphragm.[19] However, the tolerance of the elderly to rigid bracing is poor, and compliance is usually quite low. The addition of significant medical comorbidities also limits the application of bracing in the elderly patient with spinal stenosis.

SURGICAL TREATMENT

Surgery should be considered in those patients with clinical symptoms of spinal stenosis with an unacceptable quality of life after other treatment modalities have been exhausted.

The primary objective of surgery is to decompress the neural elements. The decompressive procedure is directed at relieving symptoms of neurogenic claudication such as leg pain, numbness, tingling, or weakness. The degenerative process is usually not limited to one level or one side. Occasionally a soft disc herniation may occur in a stenotic spine, causing radiculopathy or cauda equina symptoms. Treatment should address all levels that appear to correlate radiographically with the patient's symptoms. The minimum preoperative studies should include an anteroposterior and lateral standing radiograph of the lumbosacral spine. An MRI or CT-myelogram of the lumbosacral spine is also required to show the location and extent of encroachment.

Typically the symptoms of spinal stenosis are worse in extension; therefore patient positioning in the operating room is critical. The surgeon should place the

OPERATIVE TREATMENT

- Laminectomy or limited laminotomy(s)
- Decompression of neural elements
- Decompression and fusion when associated with spondylolisthesis
- Instrumented fusion to maintain correction of deformity or with gross instability

patient prone with the hips extended, recreating the upright standing sagittal alignment. This places more compression on the neural elements and may make them more vulnerable to manipulation during surgical dissection. However, the surgeon can better assess the degree of decompression, ensuring the patency of the spinal canal and course of the nerve roots through the lateral recesses and into the foramina. After the decompression one should be able to pass a dural elevator or seeker along the course of the nerve root without any impedance. The intraoperative complication of an incidental durotomy can be markedly decreased by (1) thinning of the lamina and the hypertrophic bone with a high-speed diamond-tip burr, (2) the use of a blunt probe to release adhesions, and (3) performing the decompression in a caudal to cephalad direction. Headlight illumination and magnification with either loupes or a microscope are also helpful.

The decompression of the stenotic canal associated with a degenerative spondylolisthesis at the L4 to L5 level needs to address both the L4 and L5 nerve roots. Decompression is directed at three areas: centrally, at L4 to L5; laterally, following the course of the L5 nerve root; and into the foramen, following the course of the L4 nerve root. To adequately decompress the L4 nerve root some of the pars interarticularis and/or superior articular facet needs to be removed with undercutting rather than cutting the structures flush. The L5 nerve root is decompressed by undercutting the medial third of the superior articular facet.

Although degenerative changes and deformity are not uncommon in the lumbar spine, the majority of cases requiring decompression are without deformity. The two most common types of deformity associated with the degenerative lumbar spine are spondylolisthesis (sagittal plane deformity) and degenerative scoliosis (a three-dimensional deformity). Degenerative scoliosis is caused by asymmetric facet erosion and disc disease and results in a rotational three-dimensional deformity with stenosis. The concave portion of the curve has a lateral or rotational-listhesis, leading to articular facet compression of the underlying lumbar nerve root. Therefore stenosis secondary to degenerative scoliosis will occur in the lateral recess or foramen. Patients with concomitant deformity or instability may require more than decompression of the neural elements.

Herkowitz and Kurz[12] performed a prospective study comparing the results of decompression and fusion to decompression alone in the treatment of patients with one-level spinal stenosis and spondylolisthesis. The group that had an intertransverse arthrodesis at the time

of decompression had much better results. Therefore it is generally accepted that an arthrodesis be performed when there is associated spondylolisthesis.

It is also important to preserve spinal stability at the time of decompression. The pars interarticularis and facet joint complex must be preserved to maintain spinal stability. Removal of more than 50% of the facet joint complex can lead to postoperative instability. Excessive thinning of the pars interarticularis may lead to postoperative fracture and instability. If spinal instability is suspected prior to surgery or if dissection requires destabilization, then an arthrodesis is recommended at the time of decompression. Limited laminotomies have also been reported to provide good relief of symptoms in a select group of patients. This approach may be best reserved for patients with focal or well-localized disease. One advantage of this technique is the preservation of the interspinous and supraspinous ligaments, which minimizes spinal destabilization.

The use of spinal instrumentation at the time of arthrodesis has been shown to increase the fusion rate. However, there is no agreement on outcomes and the application of internal fixation. The goals of instrumentation in spinal stenosis surgery should be to maintain or balance the spine, perhaps provide a method of indirect neural decompression, as well as providing rigid immobilization of spinal segments to enhance fusion. The effect on this was reported by Fischgrund et al.[7] who studied 67 patients treated with either instrumented fusion or uninstrumented fusion at the time of the decompression. The fusion rate was considerably higher in the instrumented than in the uninstrumented group (82% versus 45%). The clinical success in this patient population was not significantly changed with the achievement of a solid arthrodesis. The use of instrumentation should be reserved for those patients who demonstrate preoperative instability. The instability or imbalance can be over a single segment or multiple levels leading to significant sagittal or coronal imbalance. The indications for instrumentation in those patients undergoing decompression are limited. Indications include progressive deformity, a resection of more than 50% of a facet, or extensive decompression with an underlying deformity.

Another consideration for an instrumented arthrodesis includes significant loss of lordosis or flatback deformity. Sagittal alignment can be restored and stabilized with posterior instrumentation in an attempt to provide a more stable, balanced, and pain-free spine. Use of segmental spinal instrumentation can allow for correction through both distraction and compressive forces being applied to correct the deformity and restore lordosis. The patient with significant radiculopathy associated with neural compromise from within the concavity of the curve can also be considered a good candidate for instrumentation. The need for anterior release and arthrodesis is typically not necessary and should be used judiciously in the older patient population.

CONCLUSIONS

Arthritic changes in the lumbar spine are common. The diagnosis of spinal stenosis remains a clinical task, with

CONCLUSIONS

- Diagnosis is made by history and imaging studies demonstrating neural encroachment.
- Majority of cases respond well to activity modification, therapy, medication, and perhaps epidural steroid injection.
- Surgical treatment is reserved for patients failing above modalities.
- Surgery is directed at nerve root decompression and maintaining a stable and balanced spine.

claudication being a hallmark of the condition. Typically there is a paucity of physical findings. Advanced imaging studies reveal a decreased cross-sectional area of the spinal canal and/or foramina. Treatment is directed at symptom relief. The majority of patients can be successfully managed with activity modifications, structured therapy, and a variety of medications. Epidural steroid injections may provide short-term relief. Surgical treatment is reserved for those patients who have failed the above modalities. Surgery is directed at relief of claudication. Decompression of the nerve roots is necessary, and arthrodesis should be performed if there is associated spondylolisthesis or instability. Instrumentation may be helpful to maintain correction of deformity and may be associated with a higher fusion rate; however, the clinical outcome may be no different.

SELECTED REFERENCES

Boden SD, Wiesel SW: Lumbosacral segmental motion in normal individuals: have we been measuring instability properly? *Spine* 15:571-576, 1990.

Fischgrund JS et al.: Degenerative lumbar spondylolisthesis with spinal stenosis: a prospective randomized study comparing decompressive laminectomy and arthrodesis with and without spinal instrumentation, *Spine* 22:2807-2812, 1997.

Herkowitz HN, Kurz LT: Degenerative lumbar spinal listhesis with spinal stenosis: a prospective study comparing decompression with decompression and intertransverse process arthrodesis, *J Bone Joint Surg Am* 73:802-808, 1991.

REFERENCES

1. Abanco J et al.: Epidural infiltrations in the treatment of lumbar radiculopathy, *Rev Chir Orthop Reparatrice Appar Mot* 80(8):689-693, 1994.

2. Basmajian JV: Acute back pain and spasm: a controlled multi-center trial of combined analgesics and anti-spasm agents, *Spine* 14:438-439, 1989.

3. Bell GR et al.: A study of computer-assisted tomography. II. Comparison of metrizamide myelography and computed tomography in the diagnosis of herniated lumbar disc and spinal stenosis, *Spine* 9:552-556, 1984.

4. Boden SD: The use of radiographic imaging studies in the evaluation of patients who have degenerative disorders of the lumbar spine, *J Bone Joint Surg Am* 78:114-124, 1996.

5. Boden SD, Wiesel SW: Lumbosacral segmental motion in normal individuals: have we been measuring instability properly? *Spine* 15:571-576, 1990.

6. Carrera GF, Williams AL: Current constants in evaluation of the lumbar facet joint, *CRC Crit Rev Diagn Imaging* 21:85-104, 1985.

7. Fischgrund JS et al.: Degenerative lumbar spondylolisthesis with spinal stenosis: a prospective randomized study comparing decompressive laminectomy and arthrodesis with and without spinal instrumentation, *Spine* 22:2807-2812,1997.

8. Frymoyer JW, Newberg A, Pope MH: Spine radiographs in patients with low back pain, *J Bone Joint Surg Am* 66:1048-1055, 1984.

9. Greene JM, Winickoff RN: Cost-conscious prescribing of non-steroidal anti-inflammatory drugs for adults with arthritis: a review and suggestions, *Arch Intern Med* 152:1995-2002, 1992.

10. Hasegawa T et al.: Lumbar foraminal stenosis: critical heights of the intervertebral discs and foramina, *J Bone Joint Surg Am* 77:32-38, 1995.

11. Haughton VM, Syversten A, Williams AL: Soft tissue anatomy within the spinal canal as seen on computed tomography, *Radiology* 134:649-655, 1980.

12. Herkowitz HN, Kurz LT: Degenerative lumbar spinal listhesis with spinal stenosis: a prospective study comparing decompression with decompression and intertransverse process arthrodesis, *J Bone Joint Surg Am* 73:802-808,1991.

13. Lee CK, Rauschning W, Glenn W: Lateral lumbar spinal canal stenosis: classification, pathologic anatomy and surgical decompression, *Spine* 13:313-320, 1980.

14. Liebergall M et al.: The role of epidural steroid injection in the management of lumbar radiculopathy due to disc disease or spinal stenosis, *Pain Clin* 1:35-40,1986.

15. Nachemson A: Towards a better understanding of low back pain: a review of the mechanics of the lumbar disc, *Rheumatol Rehabil* 14:129-143, 1975.

16. Rosen CD, Kahanovitz N, Bernstein R: A retrospective analysis of the efficacy of epidural steroid injections, *Clin Orthop* 228:270-272, 1988.

17. Schönström NSR, Bolender N-F, Spengler DM: The pathomorphology of spinal stenosis as seen on CT scans of the lumbar spine, *Spine* 10:806-811,1985.

18. Surin V, Hedelin E, Smith L: Degenerative lumbar spinal stenosis, *Acta Orthop Scand* 53:79-85,1982.

19. Torgerson WR, Dotter WE: Comparative roentgenographic study of the asymptomatic and symptomatic lumbar spine, *J Bone Joint Surg Am* 58:850-853, 1976.

20. Ullrich CG et al.: Quantitative assessment of the lumbar spinal canal by computed tomography, *Radiology* 134:137-143, 1980.

21. Verbiest H: Significance and principles of computerized axial tomography in idiopathic developmental stenosis of the bony lumbar vertebral canal, *Spine* 4:369-378, 1979.

Surgical Treatment of Lumbar Degenerative Disc Disease: Axial Low Back Pain

Stephen D. Kuslich

The history of interbody fusion is fascinating and instructive. During the past 50 years, surgeons and device developers have created a confusing variety of methods, tools, and implants. The rate of progress (or at least change) is accelerating. We are beginning to emerge from decades of pessimism and nihilism with respect to the treatment of discogenic low back pain. Many aspects of this field are highly controversial. We know that many, if not most, cases of chronic mechanical low back pain are discogenic. We know that a solid interbody fusion can relieve the pain, but only when the indications are appropriate and the surgery is performed expertly. And we know that we have not yet reached the end of our struggle to achieve a simple, safe, effective, and universally accepted method of treatment.

This chapter explores the historical landscape of interbody fusion surgery. The principal accomplishments and milestones of the past and present will be highlighted. At the end are cautious predictions about the likely course of future events.

What is the best treatment for chronic discogenic back pain, and does spinal fusion have a place in the treatment of that condition?

After decades of acrimonious debate, part of that question has been settled. The Swedish Spine Study Group presented their multicenter, prospective, randomized, controlled trial at the 2000 Eurospine meeting in Antwerp.[29] Their results showed clearly that fusion was superior to conservative treatment.[29] The authors concluded that "evidence-based medicine" now confirms the assertion that spinal fusion is an effective form of treatment for discogenic back pain. The Swedish study used posterolateral fusion with or without pedicle fixation.

In 1996 Rolander showed that posterior fusion techniques do not completely unload the disc.[71] Many authorities are convinced that a properly performed interbody fusion is superior to posterolateral fusion in terms of biomechanical stability and/or safety and efficacy.*

THE PAST

The history of lumbar interbody fusion is fascinating and instructive. In its principal characters and events we find the entire spectrum of human behavior: ingenuity, courage, resourcefulness, curiosity, altruism, and stubborn determination. Unfortunately, we also uncover less desirable features of character: stubbornness conservatism, pessimism, provincialism, professional envy, greed, and sloppy follow-up. During the past few decades, a great deal of change has taken place. Optimists might even call it progress.

The process of changing long-entrenched cultural, religious, or medical customary practices has always been fraught with difficulties and dangers. A recently published book by Roy Porter entitled *The Greatest Benefit to Mankind: A Medical History of Humanity* describes in poignant detail the struggles encountered by medical innovators:

> Nothing better describes the modern medical environment than the vision of the struggle conjured up by Darwin's *Origin of Species* (1859): a competitive arena in which adaptation produces niches in which some flourish, develop, innovate or adapt while other thinkers and practices fall by the

---

> **SPINAL FUSION**
> - Effective treatment for chronic discogenic back pain
> - Superior to conservative treatment
> - Interbody fusion is believed to be superior to posterolateral fusion in terms of biomechanical stability and/or safety and efficacy

---

*References 5, 11, 17, 19, 30, 35, 39, 42, 44, 48, 51, 62, 70, 79, 80.

365

wayside; nothing is preordained in fulfillment of some over-riding transcendental scheme. As with Darwin's vision of nature, the panorama of medicine is as an arena of waste, pain, death and imperfect mechanisms—but also remarkable developments.[68]

The "niches" of low back pain and interbody stabilization fit into this competitive scenario. Many unanswered questions invite experimentation, innovation, challenges, controversy, and struggle. If Darwin and Porter are correct, only the fit will survive. Unfortunately, fitness in this rapidly changing field is difficult to define and accomplish. Perhaps the best we can do is to create reasonable hypotheses and test those hypotheses using acceptable methodology. Innovation and peer-reviewed clinical trials, combining the experience of many practitioners, provide our best hope for achieving correct solutions and conclusions.

Discogenic Pain: Evolution of a Concept

Some "authorities" continue to support a doctrine of ignorance regarding the tissue origin of low back pain, repeating the often-published opinion that the causes of back pain are unknown and, worse yet, unknowable. This nihilistic viewpoint is particularly prominent in the writings of three groups of authors. The first group comprises non–medical-practicing public health professionals whose "experience" consists of literature reviews, interviews, and statistical surveys. The second group consists of retired academic physicians (often funded by governmental agencies or insurance conglomerates) who have not practiced for several years but continue to write review articles based on their experiences from previous decades. The third and final group consists of physicians or other health professionals who practice in environments that lack easy access (because of restrictive socialistic health care programs) to modern diagnostic technology such as magnetic resonance imaging (MRI), discography, and selective tissue injection procedures. After practicing exclusively in the field of low back pain and sciatica for the past 20 years, in an environment that allowed easy access to the best and most modern diagnostic technology, and having specifically studied the origin of spinal pain, I heartily disagree with this pessimistic outlook. In fact, it has been my experience that if a concerted search is made for tissue pathology, by means of physical examination, x-ray, MRI, blood tests, and carefully and expertly performed injection techniques, most cases can be diagnosed.

Sore muscles have always been, and continue to be, implicated as an important cause of low back pain. This notion maintains its popularity in spite of the fact that there is *no pathologic evidence* to support the claim. Unless all back pain is psychogenic (an extremely unlikely proposition), some other tissue or tissues must be the true cause or causes.

Many medical historians credit Goldthwait with the suggestion that lumbar intervertebral discs are somehow involved in the production of back pain.[36] Danforth and Wilson are also cited in this regard.[20] Mixter and Barr are most commonly credited with the

discovery that herniated discs cause sciatica and with proving that disc hernia excision relieves sciatica.[57] Hirsch was one of the first to demonstrate conclusively that mechanical stimulation of the outer disc produces the typical symptoms of clinical low back pain.[41] The elegant experiments of Falconer et al.; Murphy; Smyth and Wright; and Wiberg helped define our understanding of the tissue origin of back pain.[24,59,72,78]

The work of the aforementioned authors stimulated the author and colleagues to perform experiments on a large series of patients during spinal operations under local anesthesia. The experiments proved that the outer disc is the primary tissue involved in mechanical low back pain and that the compressed or inflamed nerve root causes sciatica. Remarkably, they determined that most other tissues in the spinal region are insensitive to mechanical or electrical stimulation.[45,47] Nystrom later confirmed these findings.[61] Recent histopathologic studies of the disc also support the conclusion that the degenerated disc is neurologically "wired" to transmit the sensation of back pain.[28] Discography, beginning with Lindblom and continuing with the work of many researchers, including Aprill and Bogduk; Bogduk; Weinstein et al.; and many others, demonstrated that discs can and do cause back pain when they are inflated with fluid pressure.[2,9,52,77] Kuslich and Ulstrom determined that about two thirds of degenerated discs are painful and the other one third are painless, thereby explaining the apparent inconsistency in the correlation between MRI findings and the presence or absence of back pain.[47] Furthermore, they discovered that epidural scar tissue is not itself painful but, rather, that it induces pain by tethering nervous elements within the spinal canal.[47] Recent investigations refined this understanding of mechanical and inflammatory back pain.[31,56,65] The causes of sciatica are also more completely understood, but controversy still exists on the subject of whether the primary causes are compression and its resultant ischemia, chemically induced inflammation, or both (Figure 28-1).

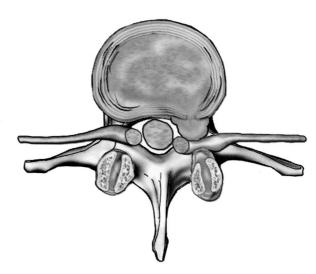

Figure 28-1. The primary tissues causing back and leg pain.

It is now abundantly clear that although psychosocial factors do not cause tissue pathology, these nonorganic conditions predominate as the main cause of disability.*

The epidemiology, natural history, and pathophysiology of low back pain are now reasonably well understood.[1,4] The condition is so common that most adults are familiar with its symptoms. A majority of patients suffer from the acute or subacute varieties of low back pain and require only comfort measures and reassurance.[23,60,75] The symptoms usually resolve, with or without treatment, and sometimes in spite of treatment.

About 5% to 10% of patients, however, develop a chronic form of the condition, wherein disabling pain continues despite the passage of time, activity modification, and the application of extensive conservative treatment. Most commonly, the condition affects only one or two lower lumbar levels, usually L4 to L5, L5 to S1, or both. Multilevel cases are usually not surgically treated, except in unusual circumstances and by unusual surgeons.[21,26] However, in one- and two-level cases—when psychosocial factors have been evaluated and managed, nonorganic pain syndromes have been excluded, and the pathology is discogenic and mechanical—the only remaining treatment may be surgery. Although posterior and posterolateral fusions continue to be popular in some surgical practices, the recent literature demonstrates several advantages for interbody techniques in terms of both safety and efficacy.

A Review of Pre-Cage Interbody Methods

A variety of interbody fusion methods have been described in the literature.[33,34] Capner was the first to publish an account of anterior interbody fusion (ALIF) in 1932.[14] Burns described his technique in 1933.[12] Moore reported his "self-locking bone prop" in 1945.[58]

The pioneering work of Cloward; Crock; Freebody; Goldner et al.; Hodgson and Stack; O'Brien et al.; Wiltberger; and many others demonstrated that interbody fusion using bone graft can, under certain circumstances, provide effective and long-lasting relief from discogenic pain.*

Ralph Cloward must be prominently acknowledged within this group. His early (1945) appreciation of the fact that the disc was the principal site of the pain is noteworthy in itself, but it was his unique methods for dealing with the degenerative disc that deserve mention here. Cloward's posterior lumbar interbody fusion (PLIF) method using bone graft alone proved successful in the hands of many surgeons (Figure 28-2). However, the operation never became the standard of care, perhaps because the technique requires a degree of surgical skill that is beyond the capabilities of most practitioners, or perhaps because the bone graft sometimes displaced or collapsed, thereby reducing segmental distraction and increasing instability.[49] There is no doubt, however, that Cloward's PLIF was fundamentally sound and that many patients benefited from its performance.[17]

Bagby's Unique Contribution

In the early 1970s George Bagby originated a new concept in the field of interbody fusion. Bagby invented

---

PSYCHOSOCIAL FACTORS

- Discogenic pain: Outer disc is primary tissue involved in mechanical low back pain, and a nerve root that is either compressed or inflamed causes sciatica.
- Although psychosocial factors do not cause tissue pathology, these nonorganic conditions predominate as main cause of disability.
- After psychosocial factors have been evaluated and managed and nonorganic pain syndromes excluded, surgical treatment may be appropriate in patients with chronic disabling pain attributable to one- to two-level discogenic/mechanical pathology.

BAK SYSTEM

- The original interbody fusion cage, introduced by George Bagby, was a bone graft–filled device that successfully stabilized and achieved fusion.
- The BAK System was the first interbody fusion implant approved for human use in the United States by means of all surgical approaches (open posterior, open anterior, and laparoscopic).
- Currently many cage systems are on the market, and up to 89% of spine surgeons report using the technology.
- Rectangular carbon fiber devices are being used with and without posterior fixation, apparently with good results.

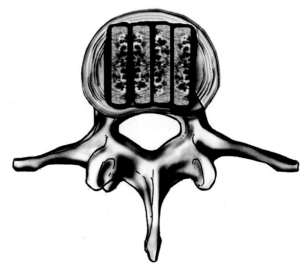

Figure 28-2.   The Cloward PLIF.

---

*References 23, 32, 37, 38, 60, 75.

*References 16-19, 27, 35, 42, 43, 62, 79.

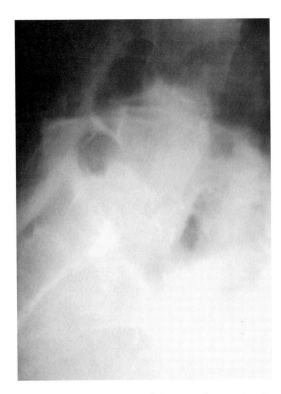

Figure 28-3. Ten-year followup of a two-level Cloward PLIF.

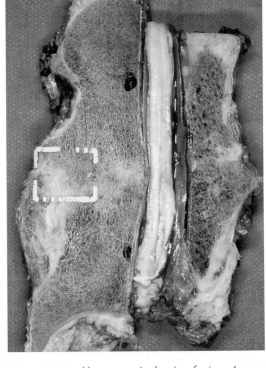

Figure 28-5. Horse cervical spine fusion, 6 years after Bagby's operation.

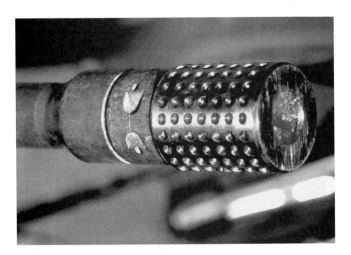

Figure 28-4. Bagby's basket: The original interbody fusion cage.

and developed the "Bagby basket." Using the horse cervical spine as his experimental model, he proved that the interbody zone could be permanently distracted and stabilized by means of this rigid, porous, hollow interbody spacer containing morselized bone graft[3,22,76] (Figure 28-4).

Bagby labeled this new fusion concept "distraction-compression fixation by means of a rigid housing containing bone graft." In a manner similar to that used by

Cloward, Bagby showed that if sufficient annular tension could be established, his bone graft–filled device would stabilize the motion segment, prevent collapse of the bone graft, and eventually fuse the interspace. By means of careful in vivo scientific studies involving radiographic, mechanical, and histologic methods, Bagby and his team proved that bony fusion did occur through the rigid basket. He attained an 88% fusion rate (proven by histologic examination), and many of the horses resolved their neurologic deficits. Some even went on to win races (Figure 28-5).

Bagby performed his pivotal work in this area in the late 1970s and early 1980s. Why was his great contribution to spinal surgery not immediately recognized and applied in humans? After pondering this very question for more than 10 years, I can conclude only that the oversight must be due to the following two factors. First, Bagby's original publications appeared only in veterinary journals. Most spinal surgeons do not read the veterinary literature. Second, many "experts" who were made aware of his work doubted that bone graft could grow in an area presumably "stress shielded" by rigid metal. They thought that Wolff's law would prevent bone growth and convert the graft into fibrous tissue. With fibrous tissue there would be no union. These opinions continue to be voiced today in spite of the overwhelming radiologic and histologic evidence to the contrary. When I encounter these antiquated objections, I am reminded of Galileo before the Inquisition, politely asking the bishops and cardinals, "Please, look beyond the Bible [conventional wisdom] and through the telescope [microscope]!"[73]

The BAK and Other Cages

Beginning in 1984, I collaborated with Bagby to modify his method and device for use in the human spine. We converted materials from the original stainless steel to titanium, beveled the leading edge of the implant, enlarged the cephalocaudal holes, and added threads to the device. Between 1983 and 1992, with the assistance of several other surgical and engineering colleagues, we developed tools and surgical techniques that made the method easier, safer, more precise, and more versatile. With the ideas of Gary Michelson, Douglas Kohrs, Thomas Oxland, and others, we added predistraction tools to the system that allowed surgeons to establish the correct degree of distraction and reestablish lordosis prior to device placement.[67] The resulting "BAK System" was extensively tested in vitro in several biomechanics laboratories prior to human use.[11,13,67] Remarkably, this testing established the fact that if the device were properly installed, the resultant annular tension would stabilize the motion segment in a manner nearly equivalent to that of pedicle fixation systems with interbody graft (i.e., circumferential fusions), but without the surgical trauma inherent to those massive surgical exposures (Figure 28-6).

Our team performed in vivo animal experiments using sheep, goats, and baboons. Radiographic and histologic results confirmed Bagby's concepts. During the years 1992 through 1996, all human use in the United States was restricted to a carefully constructed and executed FDA-approved, prospective, multicenter clinical trial involving 19 medical centers, 42 surgeons, and more than 1400 patients.

The U.S. Food and Drug Administration approved the BAK by expedited review on September 20, 1996.[25] The BAK is the only interbody fusion implant approved for human use in the United States by means of all surgical approaches (open posterior, open anterior, and laparoscopic). Studies involving cervical and thoracic versions of the BAK implant are nearly complete. The Ray device was approved shortly thereafter.[69,70]

THE PRESENT

Since 1996 several other "cages" have come into use. For the most part, these newly "invented" cages use the principles first suggested and proven by Bagby; Cloward; Lin; and Lin, Cutilli, and Joyce.[3,17,18,50,51] In an effort to limit surgical exposure, some surgeons prefer small-diameter cages that function more as spacers rather than the bone-hugging, deeply inserted baskets developed by Bagby, Kuslich, Michelson, and Ray.[69,70] As a result, there has been a recent increase in the popularity of ancillary fixation to augment the cages. This turn of events is unfortunate, in my view, because the added trauma and complications resulting from these 270- and 360-degree fusions is avoidable by proper use of the

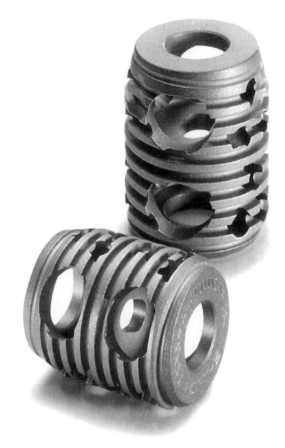

Figure 28-6. The BAK device.

original BAK design. MRI studies have proven that the extensive muscle retraction that is required for pedicle fixation injures paravertebral muscle tissue. It also leads to copious bleeding and increases the incidence of infection and postoperative pain.

Summary of BAK Human Clinical Studies

The aforementioned U.S. multicenter clinical trial proved that in appropriately selected patients, the BAK implant effectively stabilizes and fuses the interbody space with lower mortality and morbidity than previously available techniques. There were no instances of death, paralysis, or deep infection caused by or related to the implant in the U.S. clinical trial. Fusion success was comparable to or exceeded that reported for competitive procedures; specifically, it was greater than 90% at 3 years after the operation. The reoperation rate for device-related complications was less than 5%. A recent follow-up study of patients 4 and 6 years after surgery showed that pain relief, functional improvements, and fusion rates continue to improve at long term. Morbidity, in terms of blood loss, deep infection, hospital stay, and reoperation rates, was significantly less than that for posterolateral fixation systems.* The long-term follow-up study evaluated a 196 patient subset from the prospective Investigational Device

---

*References 40, 48, 53, 64, 80, 81.

Exemption (IDE) clinical trial using open surgical approaches. In addition to early postoperative examinations at 3, 6, 12, and 24 months, these patients were examined biannually with a minimum of 4-year follow-up. At each point, patient outcome was assessed by (1) a six-point scale evaluating pain relief and (2) functional improvement as determined by a functional impairment scale that assessed activities of daily living. Fusion rates were determined. The timing and ability to return to work was also determined. Complications and secondary operations were reported and categorized as non–device related or device related. The patient cohort (n = 196) with 4-year follow-up represented 25.6% of the original study population eligible at that time. Overall, the largest percentage of pain relief and functional improvements had occurred by 3 months, and these improvements were maintained at each follow-up (p < .05, comparing preoperative scores to subsequent follow-up scores). Overall fusion rate was 92.9% and 98.1% at 2 and 4 years, respectively. After 4 years, 62.7% of workers' compensation patients were gainfully employed. The complication rate in this cohort, defined as the number of postoperative patients experiencing one or more medical events *after* 2 years, was 13.8% (27 of 196 patients). Complications requiring a second operative procedure occurred in 8.7% (17 of 196 patients), and reoperations that were deemed device related were performed in 3.1% (6 of 196 patients). The results of this study suggest that the early positive benefits of interbody fusion cage procedures are maintained through 4 years with acceptably low morbidity.

The Current Status of Cage Technology

More than 100,000 patients have received the BAK and other BAK-like implants. Complications have of course occurred, and these complications have prompted a reaction in some quarters. Some surgeons have discontinued their use of the procedure. Other more vocal opponents have voiced the opinion that the threaded cage interbody fusion is fundamentally flawed and is therefore never indicated.

In an effort to determine the level of complications and general content or discontent with BAK and BAK-like procedures, a group of prominent spine surgeons recently formed a committee and performed a general survey of the membership of the North American Spine Society.

Carl, Kostuick, Abitbol, Huckell, Matsumoto, and Sieber reported the results of that survey to the North American Spine Society in 1999. Of the 655 responses obtained, 89% of surgeons reported using cage technology. This study reported the estimated results of 22,858 surgical cases[15] (Table 28-1).

The complication rates shown in Table 28-1 are very similar to the results of large multicenter studies of the BAK and Ray cages reported to the U.S. FDA in 1996.[48,69]

The Promise of Laparoscopic Spinal Fusion

At about the time when the author retired from his duties as medical director of the Spine-Tech company, the

Table 28-1	1999 North American Spine Society Survey of Surgeons' Use of Cage Technology (22,858 Cases, 655 Responses)
Percentage of surgeons rating cages results excellent or good	83.5%
Visceral injury rate	0.1%
Vascular injury	1.0%
Displacement-dislodgment	1.4%
Temporary neural injury	2.2%
Permanent neural injury	0.6%
Infection	0.3%
Retrograde ejaculation	1.2%
Revision surgery needed	2.7%

officers of that organization had become convinced that the future of interbody fusion lay in the application of the laparoscopic approach. Many prominent opinion leaders were convinced that the open approaches were either dead or dying. Most of the large-volume BAK surgeons were trained in the laparoscopic procedure and tried it out on patients. Follow-up reviews have found that very skilled specialty surgeons working in consort with very skilled access surgeons are able to accomplish L5 to S1 and even L4 to L5 fusions with about the same results but with somewhat higher complication rates and higher costs than mini-open approaches. Less than 10% of BAKs are being installed laparoscopically at present.

Probably stimulated by the success (clinical and financial) of BAK and Ray cages, other surgeons, engineers, and business executives have spent thousands of hours and millions of dollars developing newer cage designs. At least 30 designs currently exist. Each new cage design has its passionate defenders and detractors, all vying for the spine surgeon's ear. Biomechanical experiments are being carefully constructed to prove— or rather to suggest—that this or that design is mechanically or biologically superior.

Noncylindric Fusion Cages

Carbon fiber devices and other similarly constructed rectangular spacers, in combination with ancillary fixation (pedicle fixation for the most part), have resulted in very high fusion rates. Unfortunately, this has been accomplished at the price of fairly high complication rates and high reoperation rates. The clinical results are no better and the need for reoperation to remove fixation increases pain, cost, and disability.

Harms-type cages are being used with and without posterior fixation, apparently with good results. The technique appears to be gaining popularity. We must await definitive clinical studies comparable to the studies done on the threaded cages before direct comparisons can be made.

Lordosis

The current generation of new cage designs have focused on the preservation of lordosis in lower lumbar

> ## LORDOSIS
>
> - Normal lordosis is a result of a trapezoid-shaped vertebral body, a trapezoidal disc, or both.
> - Even though discs can degenerate and tilt forward as the nucleus deteriorates, fibers maintain their length and can be restored to correct lordotic position by simply distracting from the central portion of the disc before drilling and implanting cages.

fusions. Basing their logic on the known association of "flat back" in long scoliosis fusions and the premature degeneration of the one or two remaining mobile lower lumbar segments, several cage designers are emphasizing the importance of forcing the lumbar spine into "lordosis and balance." Several issues should be examined:

- "Normal lordosis" is the result of two mechanisms: a trapezoid-shaped vertebral body and/or a trapezoidal disc wherein the anterior annular fibers are longer than the posterior fibers.
- If the predistraction plugs are used correctly, they force the lumbar spine into the appropriate degree of lordosis that is proper for that segment. The cages then simply hold the motion segment at that position.
- Even though discs can degenerate and tilt forward as the nucleus deteriorates, the fibers maintain their length and can be restored to the correct lordotic position by simply distracting from the central portion of the disc before drilling and implanting cages.
- If, in a particular case, the mechanism of lordosis happens to be due to a trapezoid-shaped vertebral body with a parallel disc, forcing that segment into hyperlordosis by means of a trapezoidal distractor or "lordotic cage," the result may be the tearing of the annulus. That will cause loss of stability of the motion segment.
- When we studied a random subgroup of patients after BAK fusions, we did not find loss of lordosis.
- The original Ray cage tool designers recommended the use of lamina spreaders for their PLIF technique, without intradiscal distraction. This technique can and did cause a flattening of the normal lumbar curvature. The problem has since been remedied.
- Several recent unpublished studies were presented at the 1999 EuroSpine meeting indicating that minor degrees of "loss of lordosis" do not lead to clinical problems, provided that the remaining upper segments are mobile. Other reports failed to find any clinical improvement when lordotic cages were used.

Bony Cages

Cages constructed from bone allograft are also becoming popular. So far, the reported clinical studies involve small numbers of patients. These cages are used in a manner similar to metal cages, and made to look like threaded interbody cages.

Cage Fusion Failures and How to Prevent Them

Several complementary studies have confirmed the fact that cage interbody fusion has advantages over traditional methods.[6,40,54,66,80] A recent report by McAfee et al. identified the causes of failure in cage fusion procedures.[55] Of the 20 patients (their current experience is now up to 50) with failed cage fusions requiring revision surgery, all demonstrated some failure of surgical judgment or performance: improper diagnosis, insufficient distraction of the interspace, use of undersized cages, iatrogenic dural injury, inadequate bone graft, or inaccurate position of the cage. Three different unpublished studies have shown that the BAK Proximity version is less stable and less successful than the original BAK.

A recent review article presented several strategies to improve results and minimize problems.[46] The collective experience of many of the original BAK surgeons allows us to arrive at a general consensus regarding the general rules for ensuring success from cage fusion. By following these recommendations, the surgeon may expect a good to excellent outcome:

- The ideal case has the following characteristics:
  - A middle-aged laborer or a physically active nonlaborer whose activity demands heavy use of the back
  - One- or two-level degenerative disc disease with narrowing of the disc
  - MRI showing dehydration, annular tears, or both
  - An otherwise-healthy patient who is motivated to return to full activities following surgery
  - No contraindications (obesity, cancer, pregnancy, infection)
  - Spondylolisthesis not greater than Grade I
  - No compensation issues (issues are nonexistent or were being adjudicated prior to operation)
  - No osteoporotic patients
- The treating surgeon should make every effort to return the patient to light-duty employment *prior* to the operation.
- If the patient is taking narcotic drugs before the fusion operation, the patient should be weaned from these substances *prior* to the operation.
- The patient must understand the postoperative plan and agree to remain active and follow the plan in spite of remaining discomfort following the operation.
- Although cages can be installed from either the posterior or anterior route, the anterior, retroperitoneal route is best. It is easier and safer, it does not cause epidural scarring, and it results in a more stable construct. L5 to S1, especially in males, is approachable from either route.
- The cage should be installed deeply into the space using predistraction tools. The remaining one third of the disc space should be filled with cancellous bone (Figure 28-7).

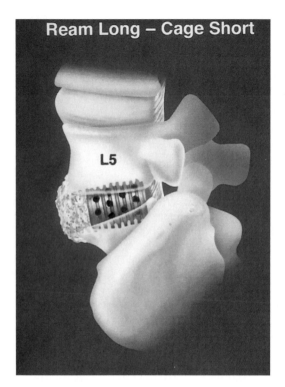

Figure 28-7. Proper installation of cages. *(Courtesy Dr. P. McAfee.)*

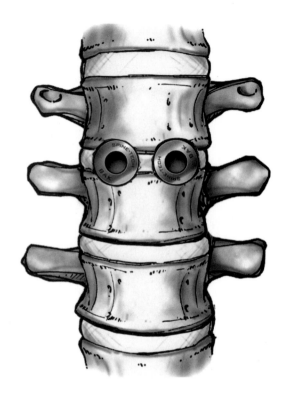

Figure 28-8. Threaded cage, designed for deep insertion into the vertebral end plates.

- Implant the cage deeply into the end plate bone using the largest-possible-diameter cage.
- Cages should not be removed unless they have migrated into dangerous positions—a very rare occurrence. Some cases require 12 to 18 months to become solid. Have patience. Keep the patient as active as possible. If nonunion is proven, simply add pedicle fixation without removing the cages.
- If pain continues in spite of apparent fusion, look for other causes of pain: adjacent level disease, sacroiliac disease, psychosocial factors, tumors, or other pelvic conditions.

The Present State of the Art

The state of the art in interbody fusion currently involves the use of autogenous bone graft–filled cylindric cages, metal and nonmetal, with and without ancillary fixation (depending on circumstances). In properly selected cases, and when done by careful and experienced surgeons, clinical results of surgery are good to excellent, fusion rates are high, and complications are acceptable in most series. Most failures, including the author's, are iatrogenic: poor surgical indications or poor surgical performance.

Stand-alone cages are proven effective in cases of advanced, uncomplicated one- and two-level degenerative disc disease. Ancillary fixation should be considered when segmental instability is moderate or severe.

Threaded fusion cages are proven technology: proven in the biomechanics laboratory, in animal pre-clinical studies, and in large multicenter studies. Other types of cages probably also work (Figures 28-8 and 28-9). After all, they nearly all utilize the basic principles of Cloward and Bagby. The other cage designs' efficacy and safety at this time are unproven. What they lack are the large, organized, multicenter clinical trials with long-term follow-up that characterize the threaded cage portfolio. Until these reports are complete and published in peer-reviewed journals, we must withhold our judgment.

Interbody Fusion: The Future

What is the future of interbody stabilization? Recent developments have raised hopes that soon, spinal fusion will be obsolete. These hopes hinge on the outcome of the following technologies:
- Thermal ablation of the disc
- Flexible posterior stabilization
- Artificial disc replacement
- Disc regeneration

Thermal ablation, or heat treatment of the damaged annulus, is currently being used in certain midstage degenerative disc patients. Advocates believe it works by cooking small nerve fibers near the outer annulus and by tightening and strengthening the collagen network. It appears that many patients obtain relief of pain.

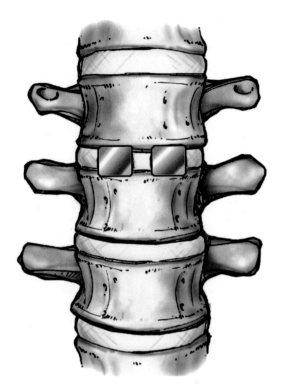

Figure 28-9.   "Spacer" design, which is more superficially implanted and may require additional hardware for stability.

Unfortunately, some patients have more pain for the first several weeks, and the procedure does not seem to work in advanced stages of disc degeneration. Early clinical trials did not contain a control group even though this type of procedure would seem ideal for that methodology. Long-term results (e.g., 4- to 6-year results) are unknown.

Flexible posterior stabilization, such as Graf tension band over pedicle screws and other nonrigid pedicle screw systems, are becoming somewhat popular, especially in certain areas of Europe. At this time, large clinical trials have not been done.

Artificial discs might be the "holy grail" for disc degeneration. Dozens of patents exist, but most have never been put into humans. The Link device has the longest history of use. It has been through three versions. The first two versions didn't work well, but proponents are very excited about version three. Multicenter trials are in progress in the United States, in a study using the BAK as the control device.

Hydrophilic artificial discs are undergoing clinical trials. The originators are claiming good results after some false starts during which a high percentage of patients experienced dislocation of the implant. A different implantation procedure is said to have solved the problem. Apparently, the device works best in early stage disc degeneration (e.g., at the time of the first disc protrusion).

Disc regeneration technology is in its infancy. The hope is that some day physicians may be able to use drugs, hormones, enzymes, or stem cells to force rejuvenation of damaged and aged disc tissue.

Summary and Opinions on Mobility Retention Strategies

At this time we need carefully performed multicenter clinical studies, in carefully selected patients, with long-term follow-up, before reasonable assessments can be made of the aforementioned technologies.

However, there are several reasons for suspecting that these mobility retention strategies may fail. Chronic mechanical low back pain occurs when the disc and the facet joints degenerate to a point where healing and reconstitution are probably no longer possible. Most of the pain is derived from the damaged and torn outer annulus. Some of the pain is derived from the inflamed facet capsule. Mobility retention strategies are unlikely to relieve pain derived from these structures. On the other hand, *if* these techniques can stop the chemical leakage from the disc, *and if* these techniques can reestablish and maintain disc height and annular distraction, *and if* degenerated disc tissue and facet degeneration can be regenerated back to normal, then these techniques may reduce or eliminate the discogenic pain. These techniques may then be almost as good as, or better than, a solid interbody fusion.

Proponents of these motion-retaining strategies assert that the "stiffness" imparted by one- or two-level lumbar fusion is a serious problem and an impediment to normal function.

Several facts contradict this assertion:

- About 90% of all middle-age back pain is derived from the two lowest discs: L4 to L5 and L5 to S1. When these levels are fused by interbody methods, the other discs remain (to the best of our knowledge) normal and mobile.
- Middle-age L4 to L5 and L5 to S1 discs have little mobility even when normal, perhaps contributing 6 to 20 degrees to the 90 to 120 degrees that are required to touch the floor with the hands, without bending the knees.
- Most people bend their hips and knees when attempting this maneuver.
- One- and two-level lumbar interbody fusion patients (unless harmed by destructive posterolateral fixation operations) do not complain about "stiffness." They simply bend a little more at the hips and knees in order to do the activities of daily living.
- One early artificial disc replacement device, and the one with the longest clinical experience, has an incidence of *fusion* of almost 50%! Might this not explain some of the good results?
- Presently, interbody (cage) fusion at one and two levels is clinically and radiographically successful (in skilled hands) in about 90% of appropriately selected cases, and the overall complication rate is low.

Advances in Osteoinduction

Starting with the pioneering research of Urist in the 1960s, the search for osteoinductive agents has accelerated over the past decade.[74] Several companies are poised to release products that promise to stimulate bone production at greater rates and reliability than ever before. Unfortunately, these agents cannot simply be injected into discs in order to generate fusion and stability.[7] Exact dosage and the proper milieu for bone formation appear to be essential for effectiveness.[8] Cost may also be a problem. The race is on, but the finish is probably a few years away.

The Story of the Optimesh

Is interbody cage fusion the final, definitive technology for treating degenerative disc disease? In spite of the admirable qualities already enumerated, the procedure remains a fairly large-scale operation, requiring great skill to perform properly and involving some significant risk. An example of a new spinal stabilization system is the Optimesh device.

The system involves removal of the diseased nucleus and inner annulus, and it distracts and fills the resulting cavity with bone or bone substitutes by an entirely new technology. The procedure can be performed through a 1- to 1.5-cm portal, through the most common posterior, posterolateral, anterolateral, and anterior or laparoscopic approaches. In the case of posterior approaches, the operation can be done using local or regional anesthesia, perhaps on an outpatient basis. Feasibility studies are complete, and biomechanical results are promising. Animal studies are under way.

The proprietary technologic features that make these advantageous characteristics possible include the following (Figures 28-10 and 28-11):

- Expandable reamers that can be placed through a 6- to 10-mm portal but expand inside to a diameter of 20 to 25 mm.
- A strong, porous, biocompatible surgical mesh that contains and retains the graft material (the BAG)
- Methods and devices for processing and injecting graft material into the Optimesh
- Osteoconductive bioceramic technology
- Osteoinductive technology

Experiments have been performed to determine whether injectable morselized bone graft (and other bioceramic compounds) could be sufficiently compressed within the interbody space, to produce the phase change from liquid to solid. Bonutti, Cremens, and Miller have described the drastic change in rigidity that results from compression of bone chips *outside* the body.[10] The resulting object, such as a bone-chip dowel, could then be inserted into an operative site. Optimesh technology gives the surgeon the ability to construct a rigid, compressed bolus of bone (and/or bioceramic) granules *within* a body cavity, through a portal opening that is significantly smaller than the cavity itself.

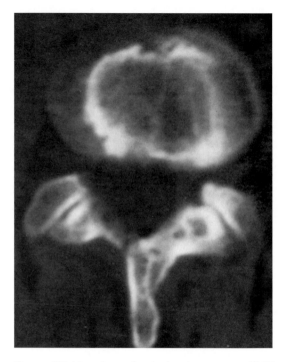

Figure 28-10. Bone formation in a mature PLIF. *(Courtesy Dr. P. Lin.)*

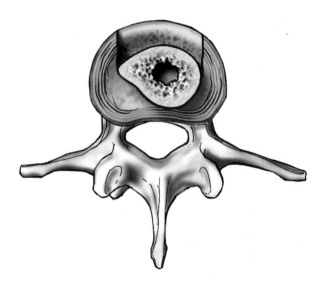

Figure 28-11. Dense cortical graft implants (and other flat, circular, inert spacers).

Several in vitro and in vivo experiments have been designed and completed to test the following hypotheses:

- That morselized bone graft (and/or other bioceramics) can be delivered easily, safely, and effectively into a body (or bony, or interbody) cavity (Figure 28-12)
- That the delivered morselized graft (and/or other bioceramics) can be compressed sufficiently within the body cavity to create a rigid structure

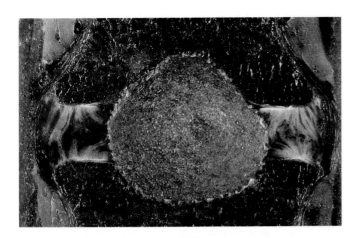

Figure 28-12. Coronal section of graft-filled Optimesh container in cadaver interbody space.

- That the rigid structure thus created will stabilize the target pathology as well as existing technology (e.g., cages or bone dowels)
- That the rigid structure thus created will maintain stability for a sufficient time and allow body tissues to grow through and around the rigid structure, eventually fusing the construct

CONCLUSIONS

These are interesting and rapidly changing times. For back pain sufferers, spinal research scientists, product developers, and practitioners, these are exciting and promising times. The diagnostic and therapeutic nihilism that characterized past centuries and decades is slowing fading. Although we remain unable to prevent degenerative disc disease and its attendant pain, or to cure the actual disease process, our ability to diagnose and treat the condition is advancing rapidly. Only time and extensive clinical experience will determine whether any of the new ideas listed in this chapter will prove to be better than conservative care or no care.

ACKNOWLEDGMENTS

The author respectfully dedicates this chapter to Ralph Cloward, MD, and George Bagby, MD. Dr. Cloward's achievements, dedication, courage, innovation, and service to humanity set the highest standards for those who follow. Dr. Bagby is the undisputed inventor and originator and father of the fusion cage concept. All others, including the author, were simply modifiers and facilitators of add-on features.

The author wishes to thank all of the dedicated, talented, and long-suffering individuals who worked tirelessly on the BAK projects, Optimesh projects, or both, especially Cynthia Ulstrom, Douglas Kohrs, John Dowdle, Ken Heithoff, John Sherman, Hansen Yuan, James Ahern, Matthew Garner, Richard Jansen, Thomas Oxland, Jane Garrett, Marilyn Wagner, David Stassen, Keith Eastman, David Shaw, Dan McPhillips, Paul Bottom, Scott Hook, Linda Golob, Duane Linnekugle, Douglas King, Pamela Snyder, Scott Raleigh, Karen Roche, Francis Peterson, Steven Wolfe, Cynthia Peck, and Joe Gleason.

Gary Michelson is acknowledged for his contributions to predistraction technology. Charles Ray is acknowledged for his Herculean efforts to teach and popularize cage fusion. John Brantigan is acknowledged for persistence in the face of adversity. Art Steffee is acknowledged for his pioneering spirit. Paul Lin is acknowledged for teaching the author the importance of the "Unipour" concept. Bob Cervenka and the Origin Group at Phillips Plastics are acknowledged for their foresight and courage in helping to accomplish the Optimesh project.

Additional credit is due to the artists and animators at Ghost Productions, Woodbury, Minnesota, who provided a majority of the artwork for this chapter: Stephan Kuslich, Jr., Nic Weiderhold, and Tony Meysenburg.

SELECTED REFERENCES

Fritzell P et al.: The Swedish spine study: lumbar fusion for chronic low back pain: a multicenter RCT comparing surgery with physiotherapy, *Eur Spine J* 9:300-301, 2000.

Kuslich SD et al.: The Bagby and Kuslich method of lumbar interbody fusion: history, techniques, and 2-year follow-up results of a United States prospective, multicenter trial, *Spine* 23:1267-1279, 1998.

McAfee PC et al.: Revision strategies for salvaging or improving failed cylindrical cages, *Spine* 24(20):2147-2153, 1999.

Ray CD: Threaded fusion cages for lumbar interbody fusions: an economic comparison with 360 degrees fusion, *Spine* 22:681-685, 1997.

REFERENCES

1. Andersson GBJ: The epidemiology of spinal disorders. In Frymoyer JW, ed: *The adult spine*, Philadephia, 1997, Lippincott-Raven.
2. Aprill C, Bogduk N: High-intensity zone: a diagnostic sign of painful lumbar disc on magnetic resonance imaging, *Br J Radiol* 65(773):361-369, 1992.
3. Bagby GW: Arthrodesis by the distraction-compression method using a stainless steel implant, *Orthopedics* 11:931-934, 1988.
4. Biering-Sorensen F: Low back trouble in a general population of 30-, 40-, 50-, and 60-year old men and women: study design, representatives and basic results, *Dan Med Bull* 29:289, 1989.
5. Blumenthal S, Baker J: The role of anterior lumbar fusion for internal disc disruption, *Spine* 13:566-569, 1988.
6. Blumenthal SL et al.: *Can threaded fusion cages be used effectively as stand-alone devices?* Annual Meeting of the North American Spine Society, 1999, Chicago, Ill.
7. Boden SD: Personal communication, 1998.
8. Boden SD, Stevenson S, eds: Bone grafting and bone graft substitutes, *Orthop Clin North Am* 30(4):635-645, 1999.
9. Bogduk N: Needle techniques in the diagnosis of low back pain. In Weinstein JN, Gordon SL, eds: *Low back pain: a scientific and clinical overview*, Rosemont, Ill, 1996, American Academy of Orthopaedic Surgeons, pp. 406-421.
10. Bonutti PM, Cremens MJ, Miller BG: Formation of structural grafts from cancellous bone fragments, *Am J Orthop*, July 1998, pp. 499-502.
11. Brodke DS et al.: Posterior lumbar interbody fusion: a biomechanical comparison including a new threaded cage, *Spine* 22(1):26-31, 1997.
12. Burns BH: An operation for spondylolisthesis, *Lancet* 1:1233, 1933.
13. Butts MK, Kuslich SD, Bechtold JE: *Biomechanical analysis of a new method for spinal interbody fusion*. Presented at the annual winter meeting of the American Society of Mechanical Engineers, Boston, Dec 1987.
14. Capner N: Spodylolisthesis, *Br J Surg* 19:374, 1932.

15. Carl AL et al.: *Interdiscal cage complications: a general consensus.* Presented at the annual meeting of the North American Spine Society, Chicago, Ill, 1999.

16. Christoferson LA, Selland B: Intervertebral bone implants following excision of protruded lumbar discs, *J Neurosurg* 42:401-405, 1975.

17. Cloward RB: Long-term result of PLIF. In Lin PM, ed: *Posterior lumbar interbody fusion*, Springfield, Ill, 1982, Charles C. Thomas.

18. Cloward RB: The treatment of ruptured intervertebral discs by vertebral body fusion, *Ann Surg* 136:987, 1952.

19. Crock HV: Observations on the management of failed spinal operations, *J Bone Joint Surg Br* 58(2):193-199, 1976.

20. Danforth M, Wilson P: The anatomy of the lumbosacral region in relation to sciatic pain, *J Bone Joint Surg* 7:109, 1925.

21. Davne AG, Meyers DL: Complications of lumbar spinal fusion with transpedicular instrumentation, *Spine* 17(Suppl):100-111, 1992.

22. DeBowes RM et al.: Cervical vertebral interbody fusion in the horse: a comparative study of bovine xenografts and autografts supported by stainless steel baskets, *Am J Vet Res* 45(1):191-199, 1984.

23. Deyo RA et al.: Cost, controversy, crisis: low back pain and the health of the public, *Annu Rev Public Health* 12:141-156, 1991.

24. Falconer MA, McGeorge M, Begg AC: Observations on the cause and mechanism of symptom production in sciatica and low back pain, *J Neurol Neurosurg Psychiatry* 11:13-26, 1948.

25. Food and Drug Administration (FDA): Summary of safety and effectiveness of the BAK interbody fusion system (PMA 950002), PMA Document Mail Center (HFZ-401), Center for Disease and Radiological Health, Washington DC, Sept 20, 1996.

26. Franklin GM et al.: Outcome of lumbar fusion in Washington State workers' compensation, *Spine* 19(17):1897-1903, 1994.

27. Freebody D: Anterior transperitoneal lumbar fusion, *J Bone Joint Surg Br* 53B(4):617-627, 1971.

28. Freemont AJ et al.: Nerve ingrowth into diseased intervertebral disc in chronic back pain, *Lancet* 350(9072):178-181, 1997.

29. Fritzell P et al.: The Swedish spine study: lumbar fusion for chronic low back pain: a multicenter RCT comparing surgery with physiotherapy, *Eur Spine J* 9:300-301, 2000.

30. Frymoyer JW: Magnitude of the problem. In Weisel SW et al., eds: *The lumbar spine*, ed 2, Philadelphia, 1996, WB Saunders.

31. Frymoyer JW, Nachemson A: Natural history of low back disorders. In Frymoyer JW, ed: *The adult spine: principles and practice.* New York, 1991, Raven Press, pp. 1537-1550.

32. Frymoyer JW et al.: Risk factors in low back pain, *J Bone Joint Surg Am* 65:213-218, 1983.

33. Fujimaki A, Crock HV, Bedbrook GM: The results of 150 anterior lumbar interbody fusion operations performed by two surgeons in Australia, *Clin Orthop* 165:164-167, 1982.

34. Gertzbein SD et al.: Semirigid instrumentation in the management of lumbar spinal conditions combined with circumferential fusion, *Spine* 21:1918-1926, 1996.

35. Goldner LJ, Urbaniak JR, McCollum DE: Anterior disc excision and interbody spinal fusions for chronic low back pain, *Orthop Clin North Am* 2:543-568, 1971.

36. Goldthwait JE: The lumbosacral articulation: an explanation of many cases of lumbago, sciatica, and paraplegia, *Boston Med Surg J* 164:365-372, 1911.

37. Greenough CG: Anterior lumbar fusion: a comparison of non-compensation patients with compensation patients, *Clin Orthop* 300:30-37, 1994.

38. Greenough CG, Fraser RD: The effects of compensation on recovery from low-back injury, *Spine* 14:947-955, 1989.

39. Grobler LJ et al.: BAK vertebral stabilization system: an experimental comparative investigation to evaluate this implant in a primate model. Presented at the 8th annual meeting of the North American Spine Society, San Diego, Calif, 1993.

40. Hacker RJ: Comparison of interbody fusion approaches for disabling low back pain, *Spine* 22:660-666, 1997.

41. Hirsch C: An attempt to diagnose the level of disc lesion clinically by disc puncture, *Acta Orthop Scand* 18:132-140, 1948.

42. Hodgson AR, Stack FE: Anterior spine fusion, *Br J Surg* 44:266, 1956.

43. Jaslow IA: Intercorporal bone graft in spinal fusion after disc removal, *Surg Gynecol Obstet* 82:215-220, 1946.

44. Knox BD, Chapman TM: Anterior lumbar interbody fusion for discogram concordant pain, *J Spinal Disord* 6(3):242-244, 1993.

45. Kuslich SD: Microsurgical lumbar nerve root decompression utilizing progressive local anesthesia, In Williams RW et al., eds: *Microsurgery of the lumbar spine*, Rockville, Md, 1990, Aspen, pp. 139-147.

46. Kuslich SD: Lumbar interbody cage fusion for back pain: an update on the BAK (Bagby and Kuslich) system, *Spine* 13(2):295-311, 1999.

47. Kuslich SD, Ulstrom CL: The tissue origin of low back pain and sciatica: a report of pain response to tissue stimulation during operations on the lumbar spine using local anesthesia, *Orthop Clin North Am* 22(2):181-187, 1991.

48. Kuslich SD et al.: The Bagby and Kuslich method of lumbar interbody fusion: history, techniques, and 2-year follow-up results of a United States prospective, multicenter trial, *Spine* 23:1267-1279, 1998.

49. Lee CK: Accelerated degeneration of the segment adjacent to a lumbar fusion, *Spine* 13(3):375-377, 1988.

50. Lin PM: Posterior lumbar interbody fusion technique: complications and pitfalls, *Clin Orthop* 193:16-19, 1985.

51. Lin PM, Cutilli RA, Joyce MF: Posterior lumbar interbody fusion, *Clin Orthop* 180:154-168, 1983.

52. Lindblom K: Diagnostic puncture of intervertebral discs in sciatica, *Acta Orthop Scand* 17:231-239, 1948.

53. Matsuzaki H et al.: Problems and solutions of pedicle screw plate fixation of lumbar spine, *Spine* 15(11):1159-1165, 1990.

54. McAfee PC: Interbody fusion cages in reconstructive operations on the spine, *J Bone Joint Surg Am* 81A(6):859-880, 1999.

55. McAfee PC et al.: Revision strategies for salvaging or improving failed cylindrical cages, *Spine* 24(20):2147-2153, 1999.

56. McCarron RF et al.: The inflammatory effect of nucleus pulposus, *Spine* 12:760-764, 1987.

57. Mixter WJ, Barr JS: Rupture of the intervertebral disc with involvement of the spinal canal, *N Engl J Med* 221:210-215, 1934.

58. Moore AT: The unstable spine: discogenic syndrome: treatment with a self-locking prop bone graft, *Intern Coll Surgeons* 8:64-72, 1945.

59. Murphy F: Experience with lumbar disc surgery, *Clin Neurosurg* 20:1-8, 1973.

60. Nachemson A: The lumbar spine: an orthopaedic challenge, *Spine* 1:59-71, 1976.

61. Nystrom B: *Open mechanical provocation under local anesthesia: a definitive method for locating the focus in painful mechanical disorder of the motion segment*, Falun, Sweden, Sept 9-11, 1992, Swedish Orthopaedic Society, abstract p. 73.

62. O'Brien JP et al.: Simultaneous combined anterior and posterior fusion, *Clin Orthop* 203:191-195, 1986.

63. O'Dowd JK et al.: BAK cage: Nottingham results. Annual meeting of the North American Spine Society. San Francisco, Calif, 1998.

64. Ohlin A et al.: Complications after transpedicular stabilization of the spine: a survivorship analysis of 163 cases, *Spine* 19(24):2774-2779, 1994.

65. Olmarker K, Rydevic B, Nordborg C: Autologous nucleus pulposus induces neurophysiologic and histologic changes in porcine cauda equina nerve roots, *Spine* 18:1425-1432, 1993.

66. Onesti ST, Ashkenazi E: The Ray threaded fusion cage for posterior lumbar interbody fusion, *Neurosurgery* 42(1):200-205, 1998.

67. Oxland TR: *Biomechanics of lumbar interbody fusion presentation.* International meeting of self-contained instrumented interbody fusion. Kuslich SD, ed: Oct 1994, Minneapolis, Minn.

68. Porter R: *The greatest benefit to mankind: a medical history of humanity,* New York, 1997, WW Norton.

69. Ray CD: Threaded fusion cages for lumbar interbody fusions: an economic comparison with 360 degrees fusion, *Spine* 22:681-685, 1997.

70. Ray CD: Threaded titanium cages for lumbar interbody fusions, *Spine* 22:667-680, 1997.

71. Rolander S: Motion of the lumbar spine with special reference to stabilizing effect of posterior fusion, *Acta Orthop Scand* 90:1, 1996.

72. Smyth MJ, Wright V: Sciatica and the intervertebral disc: an experimental study, *J Bone Joint Surg* 40:1401-1418, 1958.

73. Sobel D: *Galileo's daughter*, New York, 1999, Walker.

74. Urist MR: Bone formation by autoinduction, *Science* 150:893-899, 1965.

75. Waddell GW, Allan DB, Newton M: Clinical evaluation of disability in low back pain. In Frymoyer JW, ed: *The adult spine*, Philadelphia, 1997, Lippincott-Raven.

76. Wagner PC et al.: Evaluation of spine fusion as treatment in the equine wobbler syndrome, *J Vet Surg* 8:84-88, 1979.

77. Weinstein JW, Claverie W, Gibson S: The pain of discography, *Spine* 13:1344-1348, 1988.

78. Wiberg G: Back pain in relation to the nerve supply of the intervertebral disc, *Acta Orthop Scand* 19:211-221, 1950.

79. Wiltberger BR: Intervertebral body fusion by the use of posterior bone dowel, *Clin Orthop* 35:69-79, 1964.

80. Zdeblick TA, Ulschmidt S, Dick JC: *The surgical treatment of L5-S1 degenerative disc disease: a prospective randomized study.* Annual meeting of the North American Spine Society, Washington DC, 1995.

81. Zucherman J et al.: Clinical efficacy of spinal instrumentation in lumbar degenerative disc disease, *Spine* 13(5):570-579, 1988.

Prosthetic Vertebral Disc Replacement

Paul M. Arnold, David L. Kirschman,
Christopher Meredith

The intervertebral disc plays a key role in maintaining the stability and flexibility of the human spine. Its health is crucial in preserving the function of the surrounding bone, cartilage, and spinal cord. Abnormalities of the intervertebral disc are common, including herniation of the nucleus pulposus, degenerative disc disease, and segmental instability.[7] Techniques for diagnosing and treating these diseases have advanced rapidly in the past two decades. Diagnostic improvements include water-soluble myelography, magnetic resonance imaging, and provocative discography. Therapeutic advances include rigid, segmental pedicle screw fixation to enhance fusion rates; the use of allograft spacers and demineralized bone cement, as well as an increase in interest in interbody fusion; laparoscopic surgery to decrease operative time and complication rates; and intradiscal electrotherapy, a recently developed, minimally invasive procedure aimed at treating discogenic back pain by thermal coagulation of the painful disc.[22]

However, even with these recent advances, relief of back pain and/or solid fusion remains elusive in up to 30% of patients undergoing back surgeries. Some of the factors leading to this lack of successful outcome are not procedure-related per se and include patient selection, psychosocial factors, litigation, and so on. Nevertheless, several characteristics of spine surgery, including improper screw placement, inadequate decompression, postlaminectomy instability, pseudarthrosis, and graft site problems, can lead to patient dissatisfaction. Even when back pain is relieved and solid arthrodesis obtained, patients are at risk for adjacent disc degeneration, sometimes initiating a cascade of surgical procedures.[16]

Because of all these potential problems associated with interbody or transverse process fusion, interest has grown in artificial disc replacement as an alternative to rigid lumbar arthrodesis. Pioneered in Europe in the 1980s, the artificial disc has several advantages over rigid fusion in selected patients, according to its proponents.[1-6,8,10,23] The goal and potential advantage of the artificial disc is to replicate the biomechanics of the

> ### STATUS OF INTERVERTEBRAL DISC PROCEDURES
>
> - Abnormalities of the intervertebral disk
>   - Herniation of the nucleus pulposus
>   - Degenerative disc disease
>   - Segmental instability
> - Diagnostic improvements
>   - Water-soluble myelography
>   - Magnetic resonance imaging
>   - Provocative discography
> - Therapeutic advances
>   - Rigid, segmental pedicle screw fixation to enhance fusion rates
>   - The use of allograft spacers
>   - Demineralized bone cement
>   - Interbody fusion
>   - Laparoscopic surgery to decrease operative time and complication rates
>   - Intradiscal electrotherapy

normal disc at the treated level.* This serves to reduce mechanical forces that would be transmitted to adjacent segments in a rigid fusion, which ideally leads to a slowing or halting of the degeneration of adjacent discs and prevents spondylosis, disc herniation, stenosis, and instability. The artificial disc would also restore anatomic disc height, potentially avoiding compression of exiting lumbar nerve roots at the neuroforamen. Sagittal alignment would be achieved, restoring lordosis and the appropriate facet motion. Pseudarthrosis would also be eliminated as a cause of postoperative failure.

The design goals of an implantable disc should include endurance and mechanical strength, biocompatibility, long-term implant stability, normal disc geometry and kinematics, immediate fixation on implantation, and ease of use on implantation with low rates of failure.†

---

*References 1, 3, 7, 9, 12-14, 17, 18.
†References 1-3, 9, 13, 14, 17, 18, 21.

> ### ADVANTAGES OF THE ARTIFICIAL DISC
>
> - Potential advantage: Replicates the biomechanics of the normal disc at the treated level
> - Reduces mechanical forces transmitted to adjacent segments in rigid fusion
> - Leads to slowing or halting of degeneration of adjacent discs
> - Prevents spondylosis, disc herniation, stenosis, and instability
> - Restores anatomic disc height, potentially avoiding compression of exiting lumbar nerve roots at the neuroforamen

> ### REQUIREMENTS FOR SUCCESS OF THE ARTIFICIAL DISC
>
> - Mechanical strength and endurance
>   - Must last several decades
>   - Must endure up to 1 billion motion cycles over a 40-year life span
> - Biocompatibility
>   - Should not lead to excessive inflammatory reaction
>   - Should not be organotoxic or carcinogenic
> - Must closely replicate the stiffness of normal discs
>   - Stiffness maintained in all three planes of rotation, as well as axial compression
>   - Sagittal plane stiffness most important because flexion and extension are the most common movements in the lumbar spine
> - Implant geometry, dynamics, kinematics, and constraint of motion also crucial

Mechanical strength and endurance are key ingredients to the success of the artificial disc. These implants are considered permanent and thus need to last several decades* Kostuik[15] estimates that the implant will be required to endure up to 1 billion motion cycles over a 40-year life span. The advent of reliable prostheses in modern orthopedic joint replacement has bolstered the knowledge and confidence that such a construct is possible.

Biocompatibility is another important consideration in artificial disc design.† The implanted material should not lead to excessive inflammatory reaction, nor should it be organotoxic or carcinogenic. Materials should be chosen to maximize wear resistance of the implant-bone interface, which determines the ultimate success of the implant. Thus the ability to firmly interlock the implant to the bony surface is a key hurdle to overcome.

Kostuik[15] has summarized several other characteristics crucial to artificial disc success—namely, implant geometry, dynamics, kinematics, and constraint of motion. The shape of the implant should be maintained within the confines of the normal disc space, and long-

term restoration of disc heights must occur to restore loading of the facets.

The artificial disc should closely replicate the stiffness of the normal disc.[1,9,12-14,18] This stiffness will need to be maintained in all three planes of rotation, as well as axial compression. Sagittal plane stiffness is the most important of the three, because flexion and extension are the most common movements in the lumbar spine.

Since sagittal plane motion is the predominant movement of the lumbar spine, the artificial disc will have to allow for this bending, as well as bending in all other planes.[20] The axes of bending rotation will also have to conform to the healthy lumbar disc, allowing for precise sagittal plane movement and preventing movement that would harm the nerve roots or cauda equina.*

As previously mentioned, prosthetic discs have been available in Europe for several years and are currently undergoing initial and late clinical evaluation at selected centers in the United States.[4-8,10,23] The first reported series of artificial disc replacements was probably by Fernstrom in the 1960s.[10] His device was a spheric metal ball placed in the disc space. This device replaced the nucleus pulposus and not the entire disc. Fernstrom noted that the majority of his patients had migration of the ball into the vertebral body with subsequent disc space collapse.[10] There have been more recent attempts at nucleus pulposus replacement only. These efforts are predicated on normal annular anatomy. Intervertebral height and annular tension are restored to normal following nucleus pulposus replacements. Ray has developed a nucleus pulposus device, which consists of injecting a hydroscopic gel (hyaluronic acid) into the disc space.[21] The gel is contained in a semipermeable membrane (fluid-filled cylindric sacs), and two of these devices are replaced at each disc level via a posterior approach. The water content in the artificial discs increases over time, increasing the discal volume. Biomechanical studies following discectomy show normal segmental stability is achieved after hydroscopic gel injection, and failure rates are equivalent in intact discs compared with those replaced with the gel.[21] Clinical results of gel injection were quite promising, with 8 of 10 patients showing improvement in back pain.[21] Yuan has also recently reported his experience with a hydrogel disc in baboons.[23] These studies showed restoration of normal biomechanics and disc height.

Several strategies have been proposed for replacement of the entire disc. Enker et al. made one of the earliest attempts at total disc replacement.[8] Their device consisted of a polyethylene nucleus and cobalt-chromium end plates. The end plates were later modified to titanium, and the nucleus changed to rubber. Results in a small series of patients were reported in 1993, with relief of back pain in four out of six patients.[8] Kostuik[15] has developed an artificial disc made of titanium and cobalt chromium. The prosthesis was tested in sheep by being fixed to the adjacent vertebra after implantation. The artificial disc has a wedge

---

*References 1-3, 9, 13, 14, 17, 18.
†References 1-3, 9, 13, 14, 17, 18, 21.

---

*References 1-3, 9, 12-14, 17, 18.

REPORTED SERIES OF ARTIFICIAL DISC REPLACEMENT

- First by Fernstrom about 35 years ago
  - Used a spherical metal ball placed in the disc space
  - Replaced nucleus pulposus and not entire disc
  - For majority of patients, ball migrated into vertebral body with subsequent disc space collapse
- More recent attempts at replacing only the nucleus pulposus
  - Predicated on normal annular anatomy
  - Intervertebral height and annular tension restored to normal
  - May consist of injecting a hydroscopic gel (hyaluronic acid) into the disc space contained in a semipermeable membrane (fluid-filled cylindric sacs)
- Replacement of entire disc
  - Polyethylene or rubber nucleus with cobalt-chromium or titanium end plates
- Wedge elastic shape and a bony porous in-growth surface

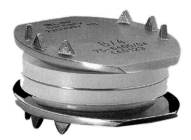

Figure 29-1. The SB Charité III artificial disc, completely assembled. The prosthesis consists of two cobalt-chromium alloy end plates and a central polyethylene core. It is the most commonly implanted artificial disc in Europe.

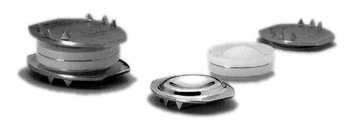

Figure 29-2. The SB Charité III artificial disc, unassembled.

elastic shape and a bony porous ingrowth surface. Results at 6 months after implantation showed significant bone ingrowth in two of the three sheep.

The prosthesis with the most extensive use worldwide is the SB Charité III artificial disc (Figures 29-1 and 29-2). The concept for this disc is 15 years old, and the disc itself has undergone several major design changes.[2-5] The SB Charité III artificial disc is currently available in Europe, and several series with long-term follow-up are monitoring its success.

A cogent description of the SB Charité III is given by Griffith et al.[11] The SB Charité III is made of two cobalt-chromium alloy end plates and a central ultra–high molecular weight polyethylene core. The three components are physically independent, allowing near-physiologic segmental mobility. A metal ring encircles the outside of the central polyethylene core to act as an x-ray marker. The end plates of the SB Charité III are produced in either an oblique or parallel dimension, allowing for versatility. The oblique-shaped artificial disc is usually employed at the L5 to S1 level; the parallel prosthesis is used at all other lumbar levels. The heights of the central polyethylene core range from 7.5 to 11.5 mm. The in situ flexion and extension angle is estimated to be 14 degrees. The end plates are attached to the vertebral body by means of anchoring teeth along the border of the prosthesis.

Indications for disc replacement generally mirror indications for interbody lumbar fusion; indeed, as previously noted, disc replacement evolved because of the complications and failure rates associated with lumbar fusion.* These indications include symptomatic disc disease at one or more levels; disc resorption with loss of disc height; postdiscectomy pain; and lateral recess stenosis secondary to decreased disc height with or

---

*References 2-5, 7, 8, 16, 23.

INDICATIONS AND CONTRAINDICATIONS FOR DISC REPLACEMENT

- Indications (generally mirror indications for interbody lumbar fusion)
  - Failed nonsurgical therapy
  - Symptomatic disc disease at one or more levels
  - Disc resorption with loss of disc height
  - Postdiscectomy pain
  - Lateral recess stenosis secondary to decreased disc height with or without osteophytes
  - Intact posterior elements, allowing artificial disc to serve in load-sharing capacity along with the facets
- Contraindications
  - Metabolic bone diseases, including osteoporosis, because of subsidence issues
  - Infection
  - Cancer
  - Exuberant scar formation from previous surgery
  - Spondylolisthesis
  - Central spinal stenosis
  - Instability secondary to loss of the posterior elements
- Laminectomy: Treatment of choice for symptomatic spinal stenosis
- Interbody or transverse process fusion: More stability and less wear and tear for spondylolisthesis and postlaminectomy instability

without osteophytes. This last syndrome may respond to restoration of normal disc height. Enker et al. add the caveat that the posterior elements should be intact, allowing the artificial disc to serve in a load-sharing capacity along with the facets.[8] All patients should have

failed nonsurgical therapy before artificial disc replacement is considered.

Contraindications to artificial disc replacement include metabolic bone diseases, including osteoporosis, because of subsidence issues; infection; cancer; exuberant scar formation from previous surgery; spondylolisthesis; central spinal stenosis; and instability secondary to loss of the posterior elements.[4-8,20,21] Laminectomy remains the treatment of choice for symptomatic spinal stenosis. An interbody or transverse process fusion will provide more stability and less wear and tear in cases of spondylolisthesis and postlaminectomy instability.

The technique for implanting the artificial disc is similar to that of an anterior lumbar interbody fusion[4-6] (Figure 29-3). An anterior retroperitoneal approach is used. After the appropriate disc level is exposed, a standard anteroposterior x-ray film is obtained to localize the center of the disc space. The annulus is opened and the disc is removed. As noted previously, the oblique-shaped artificial disc is used for the L5 to S1 interspace, and the parallel disc is used for the other lumbar levels. After the discectomy, the space is measured for implant trial sizing. The size of the artificial disc is determined by the diameter of the end plates of the vertebral body. The metallic artificial disc end plates are individually introduced into the disc space and tapped into place using an introducer. After the toothed superior and inferior end plates are affixed, distraction of the vertebral bodies is performed, allowing introduction of the central polyethylene sliding core. When distraction is released, the construct should be rigidly in place, with no sliding or motion between the bony end plates and the artificial disc. The ideal surgical construct is an appropriately sized prosthetic, placed centrally in the disc space, with no angulation of the construct relative to the adjacent vertebral bodies (Figures 29-4 and 29-5).

Several European studies have discussed the long-term results of patients undergoing implantation of the SB Charité III device.[2-8] Buttner-Janz et al.[4] reported their results in 1988. This initial series consisted of 62 patients, 83% of whom reported satisfactory or good results. David, in 1983, reported on 22 patients with a minimum 12-month follow-up.[6] In this study 65% of the patients had good or excellent results. Griffith et al.[11] reported their results using all three Charité devices. They followed 93 patients for an average of 11.5 months, and a statistically significant percentage of patients

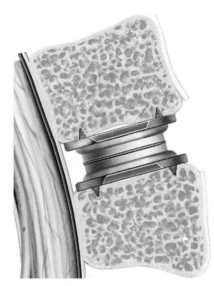

Figure 29-4. Schematic lateral diagram showing proper interbody placement of the artificial disc.

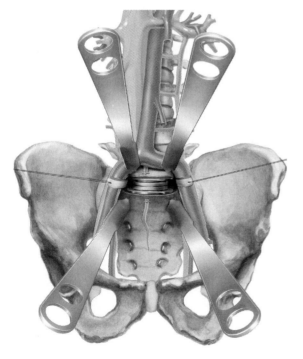

Figure 29-3. Schematic showing proper insertion technique of the artificial disc at the L5 to S1 interspace.

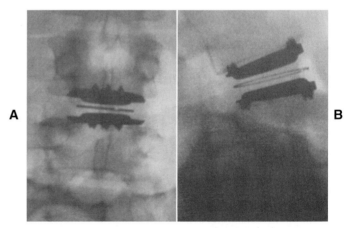

Figure 29-5. Anteroposterior **(A)** and lateral **(B)** postoperative x-ray films of a patient who had the SB Charité III disc placed at the L4 to L5 interspace. Note the central metal ring, which acts as an x-ray marker.

improved with respect to pain relief, lumbar motility, and distance walked. However, there was no difference in ability to return to work. Device failure occurred in six patients who received the Charité III prosthesis in this study.

Cinotti et al.[5] reported on 46 patients followed for a minimum of 2 years. In their study 63% had either good or excellent results overall, but only 40% of patients with multilevel disc replacement had satisfactory results. Of patients with no previous surgery, 77% were satisfied, as opposed to only 50% with previous surgery. There were no device-related complications rate. Lemaire et al.[19] have the largest and best followed series to date. They monitored 105 patients for an average of 4.25 years and noted that 79% of their patients had a good or excellent result, with an impressive 87% of patients returning to work. They had a 2.9% device-related complication rate. Zeegers et al.[24] followed 50 patients for an average of 2 years; 70% reported good or better results. Their device-related complication rate was 12%.

Surgical complications following disc replacement surgery can be classified as implant related or non–implant related.[2-6] Non–implant-related complications are generally the same as those associated with anterior lumbar spine surgery, including vascular injury (arterial or venous), ureteral injury, wound infection, hematuria, postoperative ileus, neurologic injury, dural tear with or without cerebrospinal fluid leak, deep venous thrombosis, and retrograde ejaculation. As expected, non–device-

related complication rates are similar to those of patients undergoing anterior lumbar interbody fusions.

Several potential complications are associated with the implantation of the artificial disc or the device itself. These include breakage of the end plates or failure of the central core, implant dislocation, migration of the implant, subsidence of the implant, malposition of the implant, and use of the wrong-sized implant (e.g., too small). Several of these complications might require reoperation, with subsequent replacement of the prosthesis or lumbar fusion. Technical failures will obviously be reduced as surgeons gain more experience with artificial disc replacement surgery. The overall complication rate in most of the aforementioned studies was 10% or less.

Optimal patient selection remains an elusive goal in lumbar spine surgery, and this remains true in disc replacement surgery. The most common cause of unsuccessful back surgery is poor patient selection. Cinotti, David, and Postacchini[5] note that 67% of patients involved in workers' compensation litigation reported unsatisfactory outcomes. This is a common problem confronting the spine surgeon. Despite excellent surgical technique and optimal implant placement, the previously cited series still had poor outcomes in 15% to 50% of patients.

What, then, is the future of the artificial disc in the United States? The long-term reliability, safety, and clinical efficacy are being intensively studied through several multicenter clinical trials in North America and Europe. The results may not be available for a few years.

Even then, the artificial disc will not replace lumbar fusion. It is contraindicated in areas such as spondylolisthesis, trauma, infection, stenosis, postlaminectomy syndromes, and osteoporosis, which are some of the most common problems facing the spine surgeon today. Artificial disc replacement may have a clinical role in one-level disc disease, but its efficacy goes down when

---

TECHNIQUE FOR IMPLANTING AN ARTIFICIAL DISC

- Technique is similar to an anterior lumbar interbody fusion.
- Use anterior retroperitoneal approach.
- After the appropriate disc level is exposed, localize the center of the disc space via standard anteroposterior radiograph.
- Open annulus and remove disc.
- After the discectomy, measure the space for implant trial sizing.
  - Use oblique-shaped artificial disc for L5 to S1 interspace.
  - Use parallel disc for other lumbar levels.
- Determine the size of the artificial disc by diameter of the end plates of the vertebral body.
- Individually introduce the metallic artificial disc end plates into the disc space and tap into place using an introducer.
- After the toothed superior and inferior end plates are affixed, perform distraction of the vertebral bodies, allowing introduction of the central polyethylene sliding core.
- When distraction is released, put the construct rigidly in place, with no sliding or motion between the bony end plates and the artificial disc.
- The ideal surgical construct is an appropriately sized prosthetic, placed centrally in the disc space, with no angulation of the construct relative to the adjacent vertebral bodies.

SURGICAL COMPLICATIONS

- Non–implant-related complications
  - Generally the same as those associated with anterior lumbar spine surgery
  - Vascular injury (arterial or venous)
  - Ureteral injury
  - Wound infection
  - Hematuria
  - Postoperative ileus
  - Neurologic injury
  - Dural tear with or without cerebrospinal fluid leak
  - Deep venous thrombosis
  - Retrograde ejaculation
- Implant-related complications
  - Breakage of the end plates or failure of the central core
  - Implant dislocation
  - Migration of the implant
  - Subsidence of the implant
  - Malposition of the implant
  - Use of the wrong-size implant (e.g., too small)

SUMMARY

- Long-term reliability, safety, and clinical efficacy are being intensively studied through several multicenter clinical trials in North America and Europe.
- The artificial disc will not replace lumbar fusion.
- Contraindications include spondylolisthesis, trauma, infection, stenosis, postlaminectomy syndromes, and osteoporosis.
- Disc prostheses will become another addition to the spine surgeon's armamentarium for a patient harboring degenerative lumbar disease.

two or more levels are treated. Yet one-level fusions are less common than multilevel fusion. It appears that, like interbody fusion devices, disc prostheses will become another addition to the armamentarium when a spine surgeon is faced with a patient harboring degenerative lumbar disease.

SELECTED REFERENCES

Griffith SL et al.: A multicenter retrospective study of the clinical results of the Link intervertebral prosthesis: the initial European experience, *Spine* 19:1842-1849, 1994.

Kostuik JP: Intervertebral disc replacement: experimental study, *Clin Orthop* 337:27-41, 1997.

Lemaire JP et al.: Intervertebral disc prosthesis: results and prospects for the year 2000, *Clin Orthop* 337:64-76, 1997.

Zeegers WS et al.: Artificial disc replacement with the modular type SB Charité III: 2-year results in 50 prospectively studied patients, *Eur Spine J* 8:210-217, 1999.

REFERENCES

1. Bao QB et al.: The artificial disc: theory, design, and materials, *Biomaterials* 17:1157-1167, 1996.
2. Buttner-Janz K: *The development of the artificial disc SB Charité*, Dallas, 1992, Hundley and Assoc.
3. Buttner-Janz K, Schellnack K, Zippel H: Biomechanics of the SB Charité lumbar intervertebral disc prosthesis, *Int Orthop* 13:173-176, 1989.
4. Buttner-Janz K et al.: Experience and results with the SB Charité lumbar intervertebral endoprosthesis, *Z Klin Med* 43:1785-1789, 1988.
5. Cinotti G, David T, Postacchini F: Results of disc prosthesis after a minimum follow-up of 2 years, *Spine* 21:995-1000, 1996.
6. David T: Lumbar disc prosthesis, *Eur Spine J* 1:254-259, 1983.
7. Diwan AD et al.: Current concepts in intervertebral disc restoration, *Orthop Clin North Am* 31:453-464, 2000.
8. Enker B et al.: Artificial disc replacement: preliminary report with a 3-year minimum follow-up, *Spine* 18:1061-1070, 1993.
9. Eysel B et al.: Biomechanical behavior of a prosthetic lumbar nucleus, *Acta Neurochir (Wien)* 141:1083-1087, 1999.
10. Fernstrom V: Arthroplasty with intercorporal endoprosthesis in herniated disc and in painful disc, *Acta Chir Scand (Suppl)* 357:154-159, 1966.
11. Griffith SL et al.: A multicenter retrospective study of the clinical results of the Link intervertebral prosthesis: the initial European experience, *Spine* 19:1842-1849, 1994.
12. Hedman TB et al.: Design of an intervertebral disc prosthesis, *Spine* 16:S256-260, 1991.
13. Heller, WG, Hedman TB, Kostuik JP: Wear studies for development of an intervertebral prosthesis, *Spine* 17:S86-S96, 1992.
14. Ingrana NA et al.: Materials and design concepts for an intervertebral disc spacer. I. Fiber-reinforced composite design, *J Appl Biomater* 5:125-132, 1994.
15. Kostuik JP: Intervertebral disc replacement: experimental study, *Clin Orthop* 337:27-41, 1997.
16. Lee CK: Accelerated degeneration of the segment adjacent to a lumbar fusion, *Spine* 13:375-377, 1988.
17. Lee CK et al.: Development of a prosthetic intervertebral disk, *Spine* 16:S253-S255, 1991.
18. Lee CK et al.: Prosthetic intervertebral disc. In Frymoyer JW, ed: *The adult spine: principles and practice*, ed 2, Lippincott-Raven, 1997, Philadelphia, pp. 2263-2276.
19. Lemaire JP et al.: Intervertebral disc prosthesis: results and prospects for the year 2000, *Clin Orthop* 337:64-76, 1997.
20. Pearcy MJ: Stereoradiography of lumbar spine motion, *Acta Ortho Scand (Suppl)* 212:1-41, 1985.
21. Ray CD: The artificial disk. In Weinstein JD, ed: *Clinical efficacy and treatment of low back pain*, New York, 1992, Raven, pp. 205-226.
22. Saal JS, Saal JA: Management of chronic discogenic low back pain with a thermal intradiscal catheter: a preliminary report, *Spine* 25:382-388, 2000.
23. Yuan HA: Nucleus replacement: a concept for functional replacement. *Proceedings of the 6th International Meeting on Advanced Spine Techniques*, Vancouver, 1999.
24. Zeegers WS et al.: Artificial disc replacement with the modular type SB Charité III: 2-year results in 50 prospectively studied patients, *Eur Spine J* 8:210-217, 1999.

Interbody Fusion Devices: Biomechanics and Clinical Outcomes

J. Kenneth Burkus

With fusion of the unstable spinal motion segment, the patient can gain significant relief from discogenic pain and segmental spinal instability. However, a posterior or posterolateral fusion does not always restore the structural integrity of a painful degenerative or unstable lumbar disc. In addition, injury to the spinal muscles during the traditional posterior approach can affect the ultimate rehabilitation potential of the lumbar spine. An interbody fusion provides intersegmental distraction, immediate stabilization, and facilitation of fusion without damaging the posterior soft tissues. Anterior lumbar interbody fusion has a high rate of fusion without interference with the posterior spinal muscles. With the addition of instrumentation, the posterior lumbar interbody fusion technique allows the surgeon to perform a circumferential fusion through the traditional posterior approach to the lumbar spine. With this procedure, the structural support of the spinal motion segment, as well as the rate of fusion, is enhanced. Combined anterior and posterior surgery enhances stability rates of fusion for revision and highly unstable lumbosacral conditions.

Both traumatic injuries and degenerative wear and tear of the intervertebral disc can lead to collapse of the disc space and segmental instability of the spine. The loss of the ability of the intervertebral disc to accommodate physiologic biomechanical stresses can cause pain. Fusion of the unstable spinal motion segment can provide significant relief from this progressive, disabling, painful condition.

Spinal fusions can be performed anteriorly, posteriorly, or posterolaterally. Instrumentation can also be used to stabilize the spinal motion segment and to promote fusion. Traditionally, fusions in the lumbar spine have been performed through a posterior approach. The posterior spinal elements are exposed, the facet joints are decorticated, and the bone grafts are placed laterally over the transverse processes. A posterolateral or intertransverse process fusion provides stability in the presence of rotational, translational, and iatrogenic instability patterns when the disc is intact.

A certain percentage of patients do not benefit from posterior or posterolateral fusion. Despite proper patient selection and technically well-performed surgery, some patient outcomes are compromised.[62] The posterolateral approach and the lateral exposure of the transverse processes of the lumbar spine may compromise the patient's functional outcome.[31] The paraspinal muscles must be detached from the posterior spinal elements and transverse processes during the surgical exposure for the lateral fusion. This injury to the spinal muscles limits the ultimate rehabilitation potential of the lumbar spine.[6] Several studies have demonstrated significant loss of paraspinal muscle strength and muscle atrophy after posterolateral lumbar spinal fusion in patients with persistent back pain.[29,48,56] After the paraspinal muscles are stripped from their anatomic attachments to the spine, they are reattached to the lateral fusion mass and retained spinal elements. Postoperative healing and scar tissue formation interfere with the normal, independent function of the paravertebral muscle groups. The loss of their normal anatomic attachment sites, formation of scar tissue, and loss of independent muscle function compromise the paravertebral muscles. Lumbar spine stabilization procedures that do not interfere with the posterior spinal muscles or that limit posterolateral dissection offer some significant advantages.

The development of a pseudarthrosis, or the lack of bridging bone at the site of surgery, remains one of the most common complications of spinal surgery. A failed fusion is associated with persistent pain after low back surgery. Spinal instrumentation has been developed to immobilize spinal segments and to promote bony healing. The use of posterior spinal implants to internally stabilize the spine has led to increased rates of fusion after lumbar surgery.[65]

Both biomechanical and clinical studies have shown that a posterior or posterolateral fusion does not always adequately stabilize a degenerative or painful lumbar disc. Motion occurs between vertebral bodies in the presence of a solid posterolateral fusion.[53] It may occur through the pedicle, through the normal elastic

---

EPIDEMIOLOGY

- Eighty percent of adults experience low back pain during adulthood.
- Workers younger than 45 years lose time from work and experience disability.
- Risk factors: Repetitive bending, stooping, and lifting.
- Factors predisposing to persistent pain: Trauma, sciatica, alcoholism, and job dissatisfaction.
- Prevention is difficult because the cause is elusive and variable.

---

properties of the spinal motion segment adjacent to the disc, or through the disc itself. To restore the structural integrity of a painful degenerative or unstable disc, an interbody fusion is required.[62]

EPIDEMIOLOGY

In the United States, low back pain is a common disorder that affects an estimated 80% of people at some time in their adult lives. Low back symptoms are the most common causes of time lost from work and of disability in persons younger than 45 years. The incidence of disabling low back pain among workers is approximately 2% per year. Male and female workers have a similar incidence of low back complaints, which peak in the fourth and fifth decades of life. Workers most at risk for the development of low back symptoms perform repetitive bending, stooping, and lifting tasks. Factors that predispose to recurrent and persistent low back complaints include trauma, sciatica, alcoholism, and job dissatisfaction.

The incidence of low back pain and the resulting disability has increased since the 1980s. Although some risk factors associated with the occurrence of low back pain have been identified, few preventative modalities have effectively decreased the number of low back injuries, in part because the exact cause of low back pain is difficult to identify and varies from patient to patient. A patient's disability from degenerative disc disease and segmental instability can be related to activity level, muscular control of the spinal segment, and psychologic factors.

PATHOPHYSIOLOGY

Degeneration of the intervertebral disc is a physiologic process that can be detected in some adults in their second decade of life. The pattern of degenerative changes varies and is in part dependent on hereditary factors, activity levels, and injury patterns. The hydrophilic proteins within the nucleus change over time, and the nucleus loses some of its water-binding capability, lowering the hydration of the nucleus from 88% to 60%.[43] With aging of the disc, the boundary between the nucleus pulposus and annulus fibrosus becomes poorly defined.

PATHOPHYSIOLOGY

- Low back pain is caused by degeneration of the intervertebral disc in part due to hereditary factors, activity levels, and injury patterns.
- Effects of aging: Change in hydrophilic proteins, loss of water-binding capacity of nucleus, and a poorly defined boundary between nucleus pulposus and annulus fibrosis.
- Radial fissure to the outer fibers of the annulus fibrosis leads to pain due to inflammatory biochemical degradation of the disc matrix that irritates nerve endings.
- Disc space narrowing due to long-term desiccation and cavitation causes abnormal motion, instability, and pain.

Tears in the annulus fibrosus occur as a part of the degenerative process of the disc.[45] An injury to the spinal motion segment can lead to fissuring of the annulus fibrosus and protrusion of the nucleus outside the confines of the disc space. The pathology of internal disc disruption is characterized by the disruption of the inner portion of the annulus fibrosus in the form of a radial fissure. Discogenic pain is not related to degenerative changes within the disc space; rather, it is related to annular disruption. The disc becomes painful as a result of an inflammatory biochemical degradation of the disc matrix that causes a chemical irritation of the nerve endings in the outer fibers of the annulus.[43,54] More than 70% of fissures reaching the outer third of the annulus are associated with pain.[55] A review of more than 800 discograms found that the outer annulus was the origin of pain reproduction.[40] In a clinical study, Kuslich et al.[35] documented that a similar painful response to stimulation of the annulus occurred at surgery.

The gradual desiccation and cavitation of the nucleus over time can lead to loss of disc space height. Disc space narrowing results in the overlapping of the facet joints and laxity of the intersegmental ligaments, in turn causing abnormal motion patterns, instability, and pain.

SIGNS AND SYMPTOMS

Internal disc disruption, discogenic back pain, and degenerative lumbar disc disease refer to a specific pain syndrome that originates from degenerative changes and instability patterns within the intervertebral disc.[7,19] These syndromes are characterized by chronic and, at times, incapacitating low back pain, which is often referred to the buttock and posterior aspect of the thigh. A vague, long history of intermittent episodes of pain interspersed with diminishing intervals of relief characterizes the onset of symptoms. Pain is usually related to vigorous activities and is somewhat relieved by rest. Prolonged sitting may also be painful, and patients often report difficulty finding a comfortable position. The pattern of referred leg pain rarely extends below the knees and radiates in a nondermatomal distribution into the lower extremities. Patients with these degenerative conditions do not usually exhibit

---

SYNDROMES

- Conditions treatable with interbody fusion
  - Internal disc disruption
  - Discogenic back pain
  - Degenerative lumbar disc disease
  - Postlaminectomy syndrome
  - Persistent low back pain after lumbar discectomy
- Symptoms
  - Chronic low back pain often referred to the buttock and posterior thigh
  - Intermittent pain with vigorous activity
  - Pain with prolonged sitting

IMAGING CHOICES

- Plain radiography
  - Signs of segmental spinal instability
  - Sagittal plane translation
- Magnetic resonance imaging
  - Preferred imaging technique
  - Spatial information
  - Characterization of tissues
    - Neurologic soft tissues
    - Bone marrow in vertebral body
    - Hydration of nucleus pulposus
    - Radial tears in annulus
- Discography
  - Most accurate for assessment of integrity of annulus fibrosus
  - Only technique for evaluation of characteristics and precise level of pain
  - Radial tears in annulus fibrosus
  - Early degenerative disc changes

---

objective neurologic deficits. Positive sciatic tension signs are also uncommon.

SPINAL IMAGING

Diagnostic imaging studies are only a part of the evaluation of patients reporting low back pain and must be interpreted in conjunction with physical findings and the medical history. Radiographic signs of disc degeneration are not statistically related to low back pain. Most clinical studies in which plain radiographs of the lumbar spine were examined found no association between low back pain and disc space narrowing, transitional vertebra, Schmorl's nodes, facet joint asymmetry, and radial traction spurs. Similarly, magnetic resonance imaging (MRI) studies performed on asymptomatic people have demonstrated that up to one third of the subjects have a substantial abnormality.[8]

Plain radiographs can show signs of segmental spinal instability such as disc space collapse, radial osteophyte formation, retrolisthesis, spondylolisthesis, or a combination of these. Obtaining supine flexion-extension lateral radiographs is sometimes necessary to demonstrate patterns of sagittal plane translation. These degenerative conditions must be differentiated from the lumbar instability patterns that characterize spondylolytic spondylolisthesis.

MRI is the preferred modality in the evaluation of lumbar degenerative disc disease. It is a noninvasive procedure that can display the spatial information in multiple planes and can characterize tissues more fully than can computerized axial tomography (CT). With optimal techniques, various aspects of the neurologic soft tissues can be emphasized, and the normal physiologic changes that occur with aging of the intervertebral discs can be studied. Bone marrow changes in the vertebral bodies, changes in hydration of the nucleus pulposus, and radial tears extending to the periphery of the annulus can be defined on an MRI scan.[3]

Discography can identify radial tears in the annulus fibrosus and early degenerative changes in the disc.[55,63] Discography is the most accurate method of assessing the integrity of the annulus and is the only direct means of evaluating pain characteristics and the precise level of pain production. The diagnosis of painful lumbar disc

---

NONOPERATIVE TREATMENT

- Limit nonoperative modalities to less than 4 weeks.
- Use for acute, not chronic, pain.
- Use modalities with exercise and strengthening program.

---

disease is confirmed with a positive provocative pain response to discography. To accurately identify the pain generator, discography must elicit a concordant reproduction of the patient's painful symptoms at the time of the injection. The radiographic findings and the provocative pain response seen with discography must be correlated with other neuroradiographic studies and clinical findings. Lumbar discs with outermost annular disruption on MRI are more likely to produce concordant pain on discography.[28] However, discography cannot be used alone to select patients for surgery.[22]

NONOPERATIVE TREATMENT

All patients who have symptoms consistent with degenerative lumbar disc disease or lumbar instability should undergo an intensive regimen of nonoperative treatment modalities. The use of modalities such as moist heat, massage, medication, mobilization, orthoses, and trigger-point injections should be limited to less than 4 weeks. Nonnarcotic analgesics can also be used for acute pain in the initial rehabilitation regimen. Modalities effectively treat the acute onset of pain but are not indicated for chronic pain. These modalities should be used in conjunction with an aerobic exercise and strengthening program. A physical therapy program that incorporates aerobic activity and trunk isometric strengthening exercises is initiated once the acute episode of pain has resolved.

BIOMECHANICS OF INTERBODY FUSION

Lumbar interbody fusions have several widely accepted clinical advantages over posterior or posterolateral lumbar fusions. Interbody fusion procedures place bone grafts within the disc space at the center of rotation of the vertebral motion segment. The intervertebral area is highly vascular, and the grafts have a wide contact area and are inserted in the weight-bearing axis of the spinal motion segment. Threaded interbody fusion devices and impacted spacers have been introduced and have been used to improve rates of fusion, to reestablish disc space height, and to restore normal sagittal contours. The structural characteristics of these implants provide significant advantages and benefits over traditional interbody fusion techniques, including intersegmental distraction, immediate stabilization, and facilitation of fusion. The intradiscal fusion devices provide mechanical support that promotes fusion and prevents subsidence and disc space collapse. These biomechanical considerations have been supported by clinical reports of back pain after solid posterolateral arthrodesis that was subsequently relieved after anterior discectomy and interbody fusion.[62]

The interbody fusion technique involves radical discectomy and restoration of normal disc space height. Distraction of the disc space places tension on the annulus fibrosis and compresses the implant.[5] Segmental stiffness significantly increases with increased distraction of the disc space and the use of larger cage sizes.[25] By providing an immediate reduction in motion, these devices promote fusion. Threaded constructs rely on end plate engagement, annular distraction, and proper positioning within the disc space to provide adequate fixation and promote interbody fusion. Impacted devices require supplemental spinal fixation.

Clinical studies have demonstrated that threaded interbody fusion cages and threaded cortical bone dowels provide sufficient stabilization of a lumbar spinal motion segment to promote fusion without supplemental stabilization.[4,14,34,51] The threaded fusion cages must withstand lumbar compressive loads while maximizing device porosity without fatigue failure and must promote load sharing between the device and the host bone. Threaded cages can be inserted either anteriorly or posteriorly, and these constructs have been evaluated in both static and dynamic testing (Figure 30-1). The implants must survive the normal loading of the spine. The compressive strength of the devices and graft materials in part determines the ability of the implants to maintain disc space height and annular tension.[30] Nachemson and Morris[42] performed pressure transducer studies to establish spinal loading patterns with specific activities. These ranged from 1000 to 3000 N. Other studies have shown that the maximum load to which the spine may be subjected in heavy lifting is greater. When Adams and Hutton[1,2] tested discs between adjacent vertebral bodies, they reported compressive failure values ranging from approximately 4000 to almost 13,000 N.

When used in isolated interbody grafting, certain bone grafts tend to collapse and fracture. Biomechanical analysis of the differing grafts identifies their weakness in static testing.[41,64] Cancellous autogenous bone fails at

---

> ### BIOMECHANICS
>
> - Threaded interbody cage
>   - Facilitates and improves fusion rates
>   - Provides immediate stabilization
>   - Reestablishes disc space height
>   - Restores normal sagittal contours
>   - Provides intersegmental distraction
>   - Provides mechanical support
>   - Promotes fusion
>   - Prevents subsidence and disc space collapse
> - Interbody fusion technique
>   - Involves radical discectomy and placement of bone graft at the center of rotation of the vertebral motion segment
>   - Restores normal disc space height, reduces motion, and promotes fusion

> ### BASICS OF FIXATION DEVICES
>
> - With less-than-physiologic compressive loads on the spine, some bone grafts fail
> - Interbody fixation devices provide stabilization, increased strength, reduced motion, and ease of insertion and incorporation of graft
> - Stabilization of a vertebral motion segment depends on the size of the implant, its position in the disc space, the size of the implant, and bone mineral density
> - Implants provide more stability in flexion and lateral bending than in extension and axial rotation

863 N, and tricortical wedges fail at 2257 N. Because the compressive strength of these grafts does not exceed the physiologic compressive loads on the spine, the loss of disc space height after insertion has been identified. Several clinical studies have documented loss of disc space height and deterioration in clinical outcome.[20,33,38] Cortical femoral rings have a very high compressive strength, failing at 65,000 N. Threaded cylindrical interbody devices offer increased strength to support cancellous graft material. These devices also allow for a controlled insertion, resistance to expulsion, and stabilization of the bone-implant interface, reducing micromotion and thus facilitating graft incorporation.

Cyclic or fatigue testing is also important in the performance of spinal constructs. Hedman et al.[26] proposed that 5 million cycles approximates 2.5 years of spinal loading. A Crock-type[19] unicortical graft survived 5 million cycles with a load of only 2000 N.

The stabilization of the spinal motion segment that the interbody fixation device provides is indicative of the biomechanical environment within the disc space (Figure 30-2). Reduction in motion within the spinal motion segment increases the potential for bony ingrowth and fusion. This has been studied in various animal and cadaver models by analyzing the immediate three-dimensional changes in flexibility of the spinal motion segment after insertion of the cage. The relationship

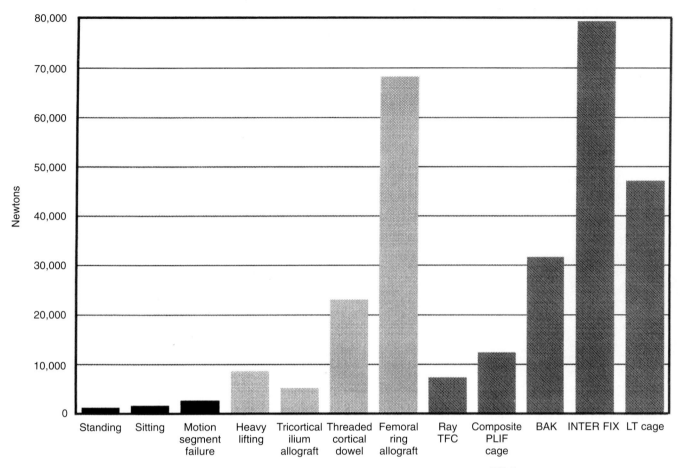

Figure 30-1. Static compression testing results of interbody constructs.[12,59,66]
TFC, threaded interbody cage; Ray TFC fusion (Surgical Dynamics, Norwalk, Conn.);
PLIF, posterior lumbar interbody fusion; *BAK* (Sulzer Spine-Tech, Minneapolis); *INTER FIX*
(Medtronic Sofamor Danek, Memphis); *LT*, lumbar tapered.

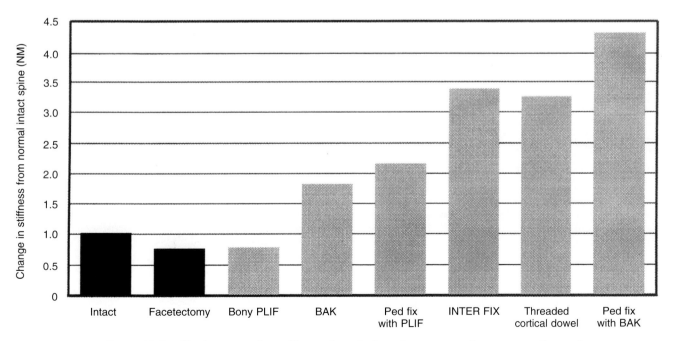

Figure 30-2. Flexion-extension stiffness of a spinal motion segment (instrumented/normal
spinal segment). *PLIF,* Posterior lumbar interbody fusion; *BAK* (Sulzer Spine-Tech,
Minneapolis); *Ped fix*, pedicle fixation; *INTER FIX* (Medtronic Sofamor Danek, Memphis).

between the implant and the vertebral motion segment is complex and is dependent on several factors, including the position of the implants within the disc space, the size of the implants, and the bone mineral density of the specimen. Two cylindrical implants are more stable than one in both calf and pig spines.[15] In the calf spine, Brodke et al.[12] found that the BAK interbody fusion system (Sulzer Spine-Tech, Minneapolis) provided stability comparable to the stability provided by pedicle screws with supplemental anterior interbody spacers.

In studies using human cadavers, Tencer et al.,[60] Lund et al.,[39] and Dimar et al.[21] did not find a significant increase in stiffness of the spinal motion segment when cages were inserted via the posterior lumbar interbody fusion (PLIF) technique. Tencer et al.[60] and Dimar et al.[21] identified motion reductions only in flexion and lateral bending. Reducing motion in extension and axial rotation was not achieved. Lund et al.[39] found no significant difference in the stabilizing effect of three different cage designs and found decreases in spinal motion segment in flexion and lateral bending. Further confirming these findings, Kettler et al.[32] tested the lumbar spinal motion segment after cyclic loading. Implants showed greater stability in flexion and lateral bending than in extension and axial rotation. Except for the study by Brodke et al.[12] that involved calf spines, all of these studies point to the potential inadequacy of the use of threaded interbody constructs from a posterior approach due to the inability to restore stability in both extension and axial rotation. This fact should be intuitive because, as larger cages are inserted to adequately restore the tension on the annulus and are sized correctly for the disc space, larger portions of the facet must be removed, thereby destabilizing the spinal motion segment. In addition, it is extremely difficult to quantitatively assess the differences in biomechanical findings not among tests but certainly among studies due to the varying morphometry and morphology of facet joints, end plates, and bone density from specimen to specimen. A good example is provided in the use of calf spines to test the biomechanical characteristics of cages. Calf spines contain a growth plate on both intervertebral end plates, a very small intradiscal space, cupped facets, and a significant increase in bone density at the end plate compared with the human intervertebral end plate, which make interpretation of the results to the human clinical practice a precarious activity.

Cylindrical Intervertebral Fixation Devices
BAK and Proximity Cages

The BAK threaded fusion cage is a hollow, fenestrated cylinder made of titanium. Its four large openings allow for graft contact with the host bone of the vertebral bodies and permits growth through the cage. These central openings have an area of 50 mm² (area of porosity for a 16- × 20-mm cage). A central internal ridge serves as the drive point for cage insertion and provides increased strength for the cage in axial loading. In fatigue testing, the BAK implant survived loads of 10,000 N at 5 million cycles.[46]

The Proximity device (Sulzer Spine-Tech) has similar design features to the BAK implant. The cylindrical

---

CYLINDRIC INTERVERTEBRAL FIXATION DEVICES

- BAK threaded fusion cage (Sulzer Spine-Tech, Minneapolis, Minn.): Survives loads of 10,000 N at 5 million cycles.
- Proximity implant: With stresses concentrated on its corners, it is more susceptible to subsidence.
- Ray (Surgical Dynamics, Norwalk, Conn) threaded fusion device: Only tested at a 1334-N load at 10 million cycles.
- INTER FIX cage (Medtronic Sofamor Danek, Memphis, Tenn.): Survives the equivalent of 2.5 years of physiologic compressive loading at the crush strength of vertebral bodies.
- Threaded cortical allografts: More static strength than traditionally used autograft and tricortical bone graft constructs; can survive a 7500-N load at 5 million cycles in fatigue strength testing.
- Impacted intervertebral fixation devices.
- Fail at less than 5300 N in compression testing.

---

contact areas between the cage and the host bone have been reduced to increase porosity and to reduce the center of rotation of two side-by-side implants. The porosity of the implant is 65 mm² (area of porosity for a 15.5- × 20-mm [13-mm BAK] cage). However, the loss of the cylindrical weight-bearing surface of the Proximity implant concentrates stresses on the corners of the implant and makes it more susceptible to subsidence.[13,14]

Ray Threaded Fusion Cage

The Ray TFC (Surgical Implants, Inc; Norwalk, Conn.) threaded fusion cage is a hollow, fenestrated, titanium cylinder. It has multiple small openings that allow bone graft to contact host bone and an 81-mm² area of porosity (for a 16- × 20-mm cage). The Ray cage was tested at only 1334 N at a 10-million–cycle run out.[52]

INTER FIX Cage

INTER FIX (Medtronic Sofamor Danek; Memphis) is a hollow, fenestrated cylinder made of a titanium alloy. This cage has thin walls compared with the BAK and Proximity devices. It also has self-tapping screw threads that eliminate the need for tapping and minimize the possibility of cross-threading. More important, the INTER FIX thread pattern increases the insertional torque of the implant and ensures a tight fit within the interspace. The close contact between the cage with the vertebral end plate enhances stability. It also allows direct apposition of the autogenous bone graft with the host trabecular bone on the vertebral body. Two implanted INTER FIX cages impart a stiffness of 3.2 times normal stiffness of the spinal motion segment.[49,66]

The INTER FIX cage is more porous (114 mm² area of porosity for a 16- × 20-mm cage) than the Ray, BAK, or Proximity implants. The design of the INTER FIX cage allows for increased porosity without sacrificing the strength of the implant, and it can withstand 9 tons of load.[49,66] The fatigue strength of the cage also far exceeds everyday in vivo loading of the spine because it can survive cyclic loading that is the equivalent of 2.5 years of physiologic loading at the crush strength of vertebral bodies.[2,26]

Threaded Cortical Allografts

Recent advances in bone allograft harvesting and bone preparation[17] have allowed for machining of a femoral allograft into threaded bone dowels that can be implanted into an intervertebral disc space like a metal cage is implanted. Cylindrical bone dowels are cut out of the diaphyseal portion of the intact femoral allograft specimen and consist of two intact cortical surfaces of the femoral allograft, the open intermedullary canal, and 2 to 3 mm of diaphyseal bone surrounding the medullary canal and linking the two cortical bony surfaces. Threads can be cut into the cortical portion of the cylindrical dowels. The natural hollow center (the intermedullary canal) of the allograft construct can be filled with autograft bone.

The static strength of cortical bone dowels provides for a substantial safety factor over maximum in vivo loads. Static testing of these implants shows that their strength is well above that of historically used bone graft constructs. Fatigue strength of the implants also provides a substantial safety factor over typically seen physiologic loads. In one study, the bone dowels survived a 7500-N run out to 5 million cycles.[9]

Impacted Intervertebral Fixation Devices

Brantigan, Steffee, and Geiger[11] reported on the biomechanical testing of a rectangular polymer polyetherketone ether ketone-ketone (PEKEKK) implant that is reinforced with randomly oriented, chopped carbon fiber. The implant is a hollow structure with struts to support weight bearing. The device failed at a load of 5288 N in compression testing.

Harms et al.[24] developed a vertically positioned titanium mesh cylinder that functions as an impacted spacer. This device provides anterior column load sharing support after radical discectomy and is always used in conjunction with posterior pedicle instrumentation. Although this device is strong enough to resist the compressive loading of the lumbar spine, the thin (1-mm) walls make it susceptible to subsidence into the end plates and vertebral bodies. Ideally, an interbody implant should have a balance between the support area and porosity for fusion.

ANTERIOR LUMBAR INTERBODY FUSION

One- or two-level degenerative lumbar disc disease is amenable to treatment by stand-alone anterior lumbar interbody fusion (ALIF).* Postlaminectomy syndrome, or persistent low back pain after lumbar discectomy, can also be successfully treated with interbody fusion.

---

*References 7, 14, 20, 33, 34, 38, 44, 50.

BASICS OF ANTERIOR LUMBAR INTERBODY FUSION

- Avoids injury to the posterior structures.
- Allows disc space expansion.
- Reestablishes the normal anatomic alignment and relationships of the spinal motion segments.
- Constantly compresses bone grafts in the intervertebral space.
- Complications occur with:
  - Osteoporosis and previous disc space infection
  - Spondylolytic spondylolisthesis
  - Two-level interbody fusion
- For solid arthrodesis: Use two interbody constructs placed completely within the disc space.

Procedures to stabilize the lumbar spine that do not interfere with the posterior spinal muscles offer some significant advantages.[6,29,31,48,56] The anterior approach to the spine completely avoids injury to the posterior paravertebral muscles. This approach also allows the surgeon to expand the disc space and to reestablish the normal anatomic alignment and relationships of the spinal motion segments in the lumbar spine. The anterior approach retains all posterior stabilizing structures and avoids epidural scarring and perineural fibrosis. ALIF procedures enable the surgeon to insert bone grafts into the intervertebral space and to place them in a biomechanically favorable position for fusion. These interbody grafts are under constant compression, which biomechanically encourages bone formation and fusion. Long-term follow-up studies have not shown significant rates of adjacent segment degeneration after ALIF.[47] Three-level lumbar disc disease can rarely be treated by anterior lumbar interbody fusion alone. Multilevel lumbar fusions (more than two disc space levels) are associated with high rates of pseudarthrosis, and these long lumbar fusions are also associated with significant restriction of lumbar motion and stress concentration within the sacroiliac joints.

Preoperative evaluation of plain radiographs and axial images on CT or MRI scans of the disc spaces is important in planning an anterior interbody fusion. Patients with a grade 2 spondylolisthesis or greater are not candidates for anterior lumbar interbody fusion alone. Spondylolytic spondylolisthesis is often associated with a high lumbosacral slip angle and a dysplastic or domed disc space. Patients with a high lumbosacral slip angle or osteoporosis of previous disc space infection are not candidates for anterior interbody fusion alone. These patients require a posterior segmental spinal fixation in addition to an interbody fusion. The intervertebral implants must stabilize the spinal motion segment by their attachment to the vertebral end plate. If the vertebral end plate and adjacent cancellous bone are inadequate to support the implants, the fusion will fail through subsidence of the implants and the development of segmental instability. Although spondylolytic spondylolisthesis is not a contraindication to stand-alone interbody fusion, this spinal deformity is associated with a higher risk for pseudarthrosis and loss of reduction after stand-alone interbody fusion.

Expansion of the collapsed disc space restores tenion to the soft tissues and ligamentous structures surrounding the disc space. Anterior distraction maneuvers often reduce any sagittal plane deformity (spondylolisthesis, retrolisthesis), reduce lateral plane deformity (scoliosis, lateral spondylolisthesis), and increase lumbar lordosis by tensioning these surrounding soft tissue elements (Figure 30-3). Establishing normal disc space height

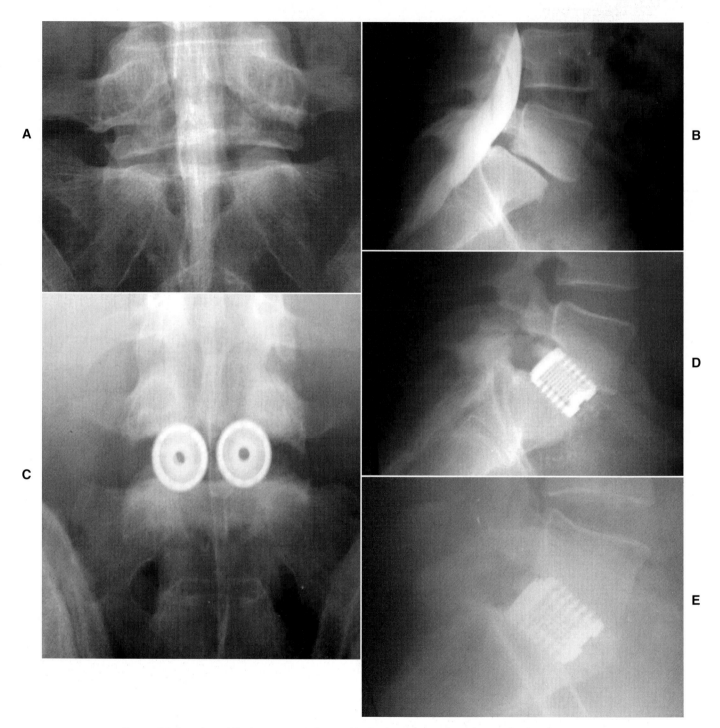

Figure 30-3.   **A** and **B,** Anteroposterior and lateral myelographic plain radiographs demonstrate grade I spondylolisthesis at L5 to S1 without nerve root impingement. There is disc space collapse without significant translational instability. **C** and **D,** Anteroposterior and lateral radiographs 4 weeks after surgery demonstrate central placement of the INTER FIX cages (Medtronic Sofamor Danek, Memphis), reduction in the spondylolisthesis, restoration of anatomic disc space height, and lumbar lordosis. **E,** Lateral radiograph at 1 year after surgery shows abundant anterior bone formation and no evidence of subsidence, loss of lordosis, or recurrence of sagittal plane deformity.

indirectly decompresses the neural foramina and enlarges the neuroforaminal opening.[16] Distraction of the soft tissue element of the motion segment also ensures that the interbody grafts are preloaded and compressed within the interspace. The use of preoperative templates helps ensure that the bone dowels will be properly seated within the disc space and will not extend outside the margins of the disc space. Axial images of the disc space from preoperative CT or MRI scans are helpful in determining the dimensions of the disc space. Constructs that are prominent anteriorly can impinge on and/or compress the adjacent vascular structures. Implants that are placed laterally or posterolaterally can narrow the neural foramina and impinge on the exiting nerve root or dorsal root ganglion.

Two interbody constructs are necessary to reliably and predictably achieve a solid arthrodesis. Single cage or dowel constructs used in interbody surgery are associated with subsidence and the development of a delayed union or pseudarthrosis. In most patients, placement of the single cage or dowel construct should be supplemented with a posterior stabilizing procedure. A single dowel does not provide adequate stabilization of the spinal motion to reliably promote fusion. Patients with osteoporosis are not good candidates for stand-alone ALIF because the vertebral end plates and the adjacent subchondral bone must support the implants.

A two-level interbody fusion has a higher rate of delayed union and nonunion after ALIF. Often, one of the two levels heals within 6 to 9 months after surgery. The adjacent level may take twice as long to fuse completely.

Subsidence of the implants affects approximately half of the patients. It occurs in the first 6 months after surgery and usually results in a loss of less than 15% of disc space height. Loss of reduction in sagittal contours rarely occurs in degenerative conditions; however, some loss of sagittal plane reduction is seen in patients with spondylolytic spondylolisthesis of more than 20%.

High fusion rates and improved clinical outcomes have been reported in single-level interbody fusion using threaded cortical allografts.[14] Kuslich et al.[34] reported on a large prospective, multicenter clinical series of patients treated with anterior stand-alone BAK devices.

POSTERIOR LUMBAR INTERBODY FUSION
Noninstrumented Technique

PLIF limits the extent of posterolateral soft tissue exposure, muscle stripping, and injury. For PLIF, the surgeon uses the traditional posterior approach to the lumbar spine, with dissection limited laterally to the facet joints. Through the PLIF approach, direct neural decompression can be completed, sagittal balance and disc space height can be restored, and intervertebral grafts can be placed in a biomechanically advantageous position.

Cloward[18] presented his technique for this demanding procedure in 1953. It involves wide exposure of the neural elements and a complete discectomy. The surgeon performs a wide laminectomy and facetectomies to place large structural bone grafts in the denuded and meticulously prepared disc space. With Cloward's technique, the posterior elements are sacrificed to achieve disc space

distraction, annular tension, and insertion of large structural grafts.

Lin et al.[37] modified Cloward's intervertebral grafting technique of structural grafts. This modified PLIF technique involves filling the disc space with strips of cancellous bone. It allows for preservation of the posterior elements and avoids the complication of inserting large structural grafts. Surgeons have made additional modifications to the bone graft technique and bone graft materials.

Instrumented Technique

PLIF procedures without supplemental posterior fixation are associated with graft retropulsion, graft collapse, and pseudarthrosis. Advances in spinal instrumentation have also been incorporated into modification of the PLIF technique. Steffee and Sitkowski[57] introduced segmental fixation using pedicle screws to stabilize the PLIF graft. Segmental fixation confers immediate stability, restores

---

POSTERIOR LUMBAR INTERBODY FUSION

ADVANTAGES
- Preservation of posterior elements
- No need to insert large structural grafts
- Direct neural decompression
- Restoration of sagittal balance and disc space height
- Placement of intervertebral grafts in a biomechanically advantageous position

RESULTS OF SUPPLEMENTAL POSTERIOR FIXATION
- Reduces graft retropulsion
- Reduces graft collapse
- Reduces pseudarthrosis

BASICS OF INSTRUMENTED TECHNIQUE

SEGMENTAL FIXATION
- Confers immediate stability.
- Restores normal sagittal contours.
- Enhances rate of fusion.
- Reduces graft extrusion and subsidence.
- Enhances stiffness of spinal motion after posterior lumbar interbody fusion in axial compression, axial torque, and flexion-extension torque.

IMPACTED INTERBODY SPACERS
- Always used with posterior segmental fixation; prevent subsidence.
- Improve fusion rates.

ANTERIORLY PLACED THREADED INTERBODY FUSION DEVICES
- Stand-alone devices that act as an instrumented posterior lumbar interbody fusion.
- Have high rates of fusion.
- Larger cages improve stiffness in rotation and lateral bending but necessitate increased mobilization and retraction of neural elements.

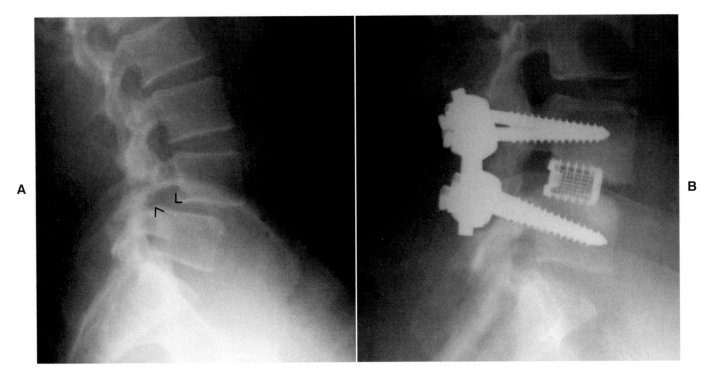

Figure 30-4. **A,** Standing lateral radiograph demonstrates degenerative spondylolisthesis and segmental kyphosis at the L4 to L5 interspace 9 months after a lumbar discectomy. **B,** Lateral radiograph 6 months after a posterior lumbar interbody fusion with cylindric interbody fusion cages and posterior segmental spinal fixation. The disc space height has been restored, and the segmental kyphosis has been reduced.

normal sagittal contours, and enhances the rate of fusion. It also reduces the complications of graft extrusion and subsidence (Figure 30-4). As previously discussed, Brodke et al.[12] demonstrated that segmental internal fixation greatly enhances the stiffness of the spinal motion after a PLIF procedure in axial compression, axial torque, and flexion-extension torque.

Impacted Interbody Spacers

Researchers have developed rectangular spacers that are impacted into prepared channels after complete discectomy. Carbon fiber implants and cortical allografts have been designed for insertion into the disc space in addition to morcellized autograft. These spacers provide structural support to the spinal motion segment. Their use has been shown to prevent subsidence and to improve rates of fusion. These impacted devices are always used in conjunction with posterior segmental fixation and are not used as stand-alone devices. Both the carbon fiber and allograft implants allow for radiographic visualization of the fusion mass and have similar modulus of elasticity to the host bone.

Brantigan et al.[10] reported successful fusion in all 26 patients treated with a carbon fiber–reinforced polymer impacted spacer and supplemental pedicle screw fixation. Tullberg et al.[61] found an 86% fusion rate in patients treated with this device montage. Agazzi et al.[4] reported a 90% rate of fusion but only a 66% rate of overall patient satisfaction.

The Harms cages have been widely used since 1991. Their use as impacted spacers in the treatment of spondylolisthesis was reported from a single group of investigators.[24] However, their use in a prospective, multicenter trial has not been completed.

Threaded Interbody Fusion Devices

Threaded cylindrical cages represent a new, distinct class of segmental spinal fixation devices. These devices were not designed as spacers that require segmental stabilization; rather, they were designed as stand-alone intervertebral devices that function as an "instrumented PLIF." Threaded interbody devices are biomechanically different from interbody spacers.

Initial clinical studies reported high rates of fusion and clinical success in certain centers; these results have not been widely reproduced. Biomechanical studies have shown that cage size is of some significance in stand-alone cage fusions and that stand-alone cages do not significantly increase spinal stiffness in studies using human cadavers. Larger cages improve stiffness in rotation and lateral bending. However, reduction of motion in flexion is not significantly improved with larger cages. Larger cages necessitate increased mobilization and retraction of the neural elements. A cylindrical device increases its medial-lateral dimensions equal to its increase in height, which necessitates a wide exposure and excessive retraction to place adequately sized implants. Excessive retraction of the nerve roots has

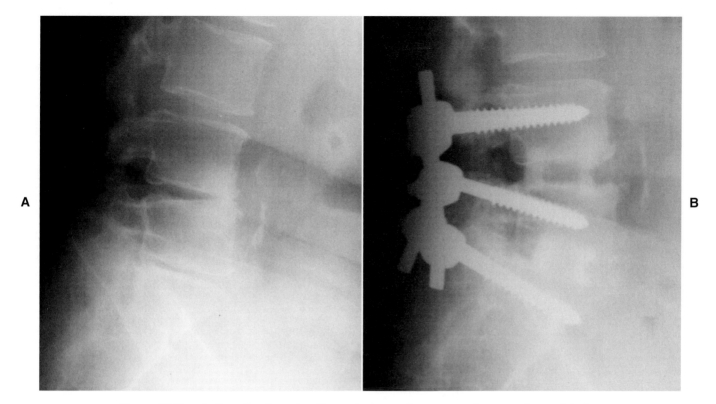

Figure 30-5. **A**, Standing lateral radiograph shows disc space collapse and spondylosis at both L4 to L5 and L5 to S1. There is a fixed kyphosis at L4 to L5. **B**, Standing lateral radiograph 6 months after anterior interbody fusion and posterior segmental stabilization. The disc space height and lordosis at both L4 to L5 and L5 to S1 has been restored.

been associated with neurologic deficits. As discussed, larger implants require more extensive facet joint resection or facetectomy, which further destabilizes the spinal motion segment.

Authors of clinical and radiographic studies on stand-alone interbody implants without supplemental fixation have reported fusion rates between 83% and 100%. Hacker[23] compared two groups of patients treated for disabling back pain: one group was treated with a stand-alone PLIF using BAK implants, and the other group was treated with combined anteroposterior fusion. He found equal patient satisfaction between the two groups. Ray[51] presented a prospective series of 236 patients treated with stand-alone interbody fusion and reported a 96% fusion rate at 2 years after surgery. These fusion criteria correlated with improved clinical outcomes. In this study group, only 65% had good to excellent clinical outcomes on the Prolo scale, and 14% had a poor result.

COMBINED ALIF WITH POSTERIOR STABILIZATION

Combined anterior and posterior spinal fusion was initially popularized in the treatment of traumatic spinal injuries and spinal deformity. The role of anterior and posterior fusion has been expanded to include use as a salvage procedure for failed lumbosacral fusions[63] and as a primary procedure for the treatment of discogenic back pain and lumbar instability.[27] This two-staged procedure

addresses both anterior and posterior sources of pain, has biomechanical advantages, and has a high rate of fusion.

High shear forces occur at the lumbosacral junction. The posterior elements, including the facets and ligaments, balance these forces. These forces undoubtedly contribute to the high incidence of degenerative changes at the lumbosacral junction. Posterior instrumentation can restore the integrity of the posterior spinal elements to resist these shear forces and can contribute to stabilization of the spinal motion segment. Pedicle fixation and facet screws have been used as a posterior tension band to stabilize anterior interbody fusion constructs.[27,58]

Circumferential fusions are best used in patients with significant patterns of instability, as demonstrated by high lumbosacral slip angles, angulation of more than 5 degrees on preoperative flexion-extension lateral radiographs, grade 2 spondylolisthesis or greater, and multilevel fusions (Figure 30-5).

Clinical studies have shown high rates of fusion with this technique. These two-staged procedures are associated with higher rates of complications, including postoperative infection. They also necessitate prolonged hospitalization and have increased costs.

CONCLUSIONS

The high rates of fusion associated with interbody techniques may be attributed in part to removal of the body end plates and exposure of bleeding cancellous bony surfaces, reestablishment of anatomic intradiscal height and tension of the annulus and ligamentous structure around the disc space, and use of autogenous grafts. Threaded interbody constructs provide adequate strength to ensure that no plastic deformation occurs within the maximum physiologic range. Dynamic testing of these implants has also shown that the fatigue performance of these implants occurs within normal daily physiologic loading. Stability testing has shown that when inserted anteriorly, these devices reduce intervertebral motion and increase spinal stiffness. Clinical outcomes using these interbody fusion devices can be improved by increasing rates of fusion and improving the sagittal contour of the lumbar spine.

SELECTED REFERENCES

Rolander SD: Motion of the lumbar spine with special reference to stabilizing effect of posterior fusion: an experimental study on autopsy specimens, *Acta Orthop Scand Suppl* 90:1-144, 1966.

Sutterlin CE et al.: Threaded cortical dowel: "construct stiffness testing," technical monograph, Gainesville, Fla, 1996, University of Florida Tissue Bank.

Weatherley CR, Prickett CE, O'Brien JP: Discogenic pain persisting despite solid posterior fusion, *J Bone Joint Surg Br* 68:142-143, 1986.

REFERENCES

1. Adams MA, Hutton WC: Mechanics of the intervertebral disc. In Ghosh P, ed: *Biology of the intervertebral disc*, Boca Raton, 1988, CRC Press, pp.39-71.
2. Adams MA, Hutton WC: Can the lumbar spine be crushed in heavy lifting? *Spine* 7:586-590, 1982.
3. Aprill C, Bogduk N: High-intensity zone: a diagnostic sign of painful lumbar disc on magnetic resonance imaging, *Br J Radiol* 65:361-369, 1992.
4. Agazzi S, Reverdin A, May D: Posterior lumbar interbody fusion with cages: an independent review of 71 cases, *J Neurosurg* 91:186-192, 1999.
5. Bagby GW: Arthrodesis by the distraction-compression method using a stainless steel implant, *Orthopedics* 11:931-934, 1988.
6. Beimborn DS, Morrissey MC: A review of the literature related to trunk muscle performance, *Spine* 13:655-660, 1988.
7. Blumenthal SL et al.: The role of anterior lumbar fusion for internal disc disruption, *Spine* 13:566-569, 1988.
8. Boden SD et al.: Abnormal magnetic-resonance scans of the lumbar spine in asymptomatic subjects: a prospective investigation, *J Bone Joint Surg* 72:403-408, 1990.
9. Boyd LM, Estes BT, Liu M: Biomechanics of lumbar interbody constructs: effect of design and materials [in French]. In Husson JL, LeHuec JC, eds: *Chirurgie Endoscopique et Mini-invasive du Rachis*, Montpelier, France, 1999, Sauramps Médical, pp. 181-192.
10. Brantigan JW, Steffee AD: A carbon fiber implant to aid interbody lumbar fusion: two-year clinical results in the first 26 patients, *Spine* 18:2106-2107, 1993.
11. Brantigan JW, Steffee AD, Geiger JM: A carbon fiber implant to aid interbody lumbar fusion: mechanical testing, *Spine* 16(6 Suppl):S277-S282, 1991.
12. Brodke DS et al.: Posterior lumbar interbody fusion: a biomechanical comparison, including a new threaded cage, *Spine* 22:26-31, 1997.
13. Burkus JK et al.: Subsidence evaluation of reduced lateral profile threaded constructs. Paper presented at the International Meeting on Advanced Spine Techniques, Barcelona, Spain, July 5-8, 2000.
14. Burkus JK et al.: Single-level anterior lumbar interbody fusion using threaded cortical bone allografts. Paper presented at the North American Spine Society Meeting of the Americas, Miami, 1991.

15. Butts M, Kuslich S, Bechold J: Biomechanical analysis of a new method for spinal interbody fixation. In Erdman A, ed: *1987 advances in bioengineering*, New York, 1987, The American Society of Mechanical Engineers, pp. 95-96.
16. Chen D et al.: Increasing neuroforaminal volume by anterior interbody distraction in degenerative lumbar spine, *Spine* 20:74-79, 1995.
17. Chen D, Kummer FJ, Spivak JM: Optimal selection and preparation of fresh frozen corticocancellous allografts for anterior interbody lumbar spinal fusion, *J Spinal Disord* 10:532-536, 1997.
18. Cloward RB: The treatment of ruptured intervertebral discs by vertebral body fusion. I. Indications, operative technique, after care, *J Neurosurg* 10:154-168, 1953.
19. Crock HV: Anterior lumbar interbody fusion: indications for its use and notes on surgical technique, *Clin Orthop* 165:157-163, 1982.
20. Dennis S et al.: Comparison of disc space heights after anterior lumbar interbody fusion, *Spine* 14:876-878, 1989.
21. Dimar JR et al.: Posterior lumbar interbody cages do not augment segmental biomechanical stability. Paper presented at the meeting of the Scoliosis Research Society, San Diego, 1999, pp. 22-25.
22. Gill K, Blumenthal SL: Functional results after anterior lumbar fusion at L5-S1 in patients with normal and abnormal MRI scans, *Spine* 17:940-942, 1992.
23. Hacker RJ: Comparison of interbody fusion approaches for disabling low back pain, *Spine* 22:660-665, 1997.
24. Harms J et al.: True spondylolisthesis reduction and monosegmental fusion in spondylolisthesis. In Bridwell KH, DeWald RL, eds: The textbook of spinal surgery, ed 2, Philadelphia, 1997, Lippincott-Raven, pp. 1337-1347.
25. Hasegawa K et al.: An experimental study of porcine lumbar segmental stiffness by the distraction-compression principle using a threaded interbody cage, *J Spinal Disord* 13:247-252, 2000.
26. Hedman TP et al.: Design of an intervertebral disc prosthesis, *Spine* 16:S256-S260, 1991.
27. Holte DC, O'Brien JP, Renton P: Anterior lumbar fusion using a hybrid interbody graft: a preliminary radiographic report, *Eur Spine J* 3:32-38, 1994.
28. Ito M et al.: Predictive signs of discogenic lumbar pain on magnetic resonance imagining with discography correlation, *Spine* 23:1252-1258, 1998.
29. Johnson B: The function of individual muscles in the lumbar part of the spinae muscle, *Electromyography* 10:5-21, 1970.
30. Jost B, Cripton P, Lund T: Compressive strength of interbody cages: the effect of cage shape and bone density. Proceedings of the ISSLS Annual Meeting, 1996, p. 151.
31. Kahanovitz N, Viola K, Gallagher M: Long-term strength assessment of postoperative diskectomy patients, *Spine* 14:402-403, 1989.
32. Kettler A et al.: Stabilizing effect of posterior lumbar interbody fusion cages before and after cyclic loading, *J Neurosurg* 92:87-92, 2000.
33. Kumar A et al.: Interspace distraction and graft subsidence after anterior lumbar fusion with femoral strut allograft, *Spine* 18:2393-2400, 1993.
34. Kuslich SD et al.: The Bagby and Kuslich method of lumbar interbody fusion. History, technique, and 2-year follow-up results of a United States prospective, multicenter trial, *Spine* 23:1267-1279, 1998.
35. Kuslich SD, Ulstrom CL, Michael CJ: The tissue origin of low back pain and sciatica: a report of pain response to tissue stimulation during operations on the lumbar spine using local anesthesia, *Orthop Clin North Am* 22:181-187, 1991.
36. Leong JC et al.: Long-term results of lumbar intervertebral disc prolapse, *Spine* 8:793-799, 1983.
37. Lin PM, Cautilli RA, Joyce MF: Posterior lumbar interbody fusion, *Clin Orthop* 180:154-168, 1983.
38. Loguidice VA et al.: Anterior lumbar interbody fusion, *Spine* 13:366-369, 1988.
39. Lund T et al.: Interbody cage stabilization in the lumbar spine: biomechanical evaluation of cage design, posterior instrumentation and bone density, *J Bone Joint Surg Br* 80:351-359, 1998.
40. Moneta GB et al.: Reported pain during lumbar discography as a function of annular ruptures and disc degeneration: a re-analysis of 833 discograms, *Spine* 19:1968-1974, 1994.

41. Morales RW, Pettine KA, Salib RM: A biomechanical study of bone allografts used in lumbar interbody fusions. Paper presented at the annual meeting of the North American Spine Society, Keystone, Colo, 1991.

42. Nachemson A, Morris JM: In vivo measurements of intradiscal pressure: discometry, a method for the determination of pressure in the lower lumbar discs, *J Bone Joint Surg Am* 46:1077-1092, 1964.

43. Naylor A: Intervertebral disc prolapse and degeneration: the biochemical and biophysical approach, *Spine* 1:108-114, 1976.

44. Newman MH, Grinstead GL: Anterior lumbar interbody fusion for internal disc disruption, *Spine* 17:831-833, 1992.

45. Osti OL et al.: Annular tears and disc degeneration in the lumbar spine: a post-mortem study of 135 discs, *J Bone Joint Surg Br* 74:678-682, 1992.

46. Oxland TR et al.: *The BAK Interbody Fusion System: an innovative solution*, Minneapolis, Spine-Tech, 1994, Form L1009 Rev A.

47. Penta M, Sandhu A, Fraser RD: Magnetic resonance imaging assessment of disc degeneration 10 years after anterior lumbar interbody fusion, *Spine* 20:743-747, 1995.

48. Rantanen J et al.: The lumbar multifidus muscle five years after surgery for a lumbar intervertebral disc herniation, *Spine* 18:568-574, 1993.

49. Rapoff AJ, Ghanayem AJ, Zdeblick TA: Biomechanical comparison of posterior lumbar interbody fusion cages, *Spine* 22:2375-2379, 1997.

50. Raugstad TS et al.: Anterior interbody fusion of the lumbar spine, *Acta Orthop Scand* 53:561-565, 1982.

51. Ray CD: Threaded titanium cages for lumbar interbody fusions, *Spine* 22:667-679, 1997.

52. *Ray Threaded Fusion Cage: a technical summary*, Norwalk, Conn, 1998, Surgical Dynamics.

53. Rolander SD: Motion of the lumbar spine with special reference to stabilizing effect of posterior fusion: an experimental study on autopsy specimens, *Acta Orthop Scand Suppl* 90:1-144, 1966.

54. Saal JS et al.: High levels of inflammatory phospholipase A2 activity in lumbar disc herniations, *Spine* 15:674-678, 1990.

55. Sachs BL, Vanharanta H, Spivey MA: Dallas discogram description: a new classification of CT/discography in low-back disorders, *Spine* 12:287-294, 1987.

56. Sihvonen T et al.: Local denervation atrophy of paraspinal muscles in postoperative failed back syndrome, *Spine* 18:575-581, 1993.

57. Steffee AD, Sitkowski DJ: Posterior lumbar interbody fusion and plates, *Clin Orthop* 227:99-102, 1988.

58. Stonecipher T, Wright S: Posterior lumbar interbody fusion with facet-screw fixation, *Spine* 14:468-471, 1989.

59. Sutterlin CE et al.: Threaded cortical dowel: "construct stiffness testing," technical monograph, Gainesville, Fla, University of Florida Tissue Bank, 1996.

60. Tencer AF, Hampton D, Eddy S: Biomechanical properties of threaded inserts for lumbar interbody spinal fusion, *Spine* 20:2408-2414, 1995.

61. Tullberg T et al.: Fusion rate after posterior lumbar interbody fusion with carbon fiber implant: 1-year follow-up of 51 patients, *Eur Spine J* 5:178-182, 1996.

62. Weatherley CR, Prickett CE, O'Brien JP: Discogenic pain persisting despite solid posterior fusion, *J Bone Joint Surg Br* 68:142-143, 1986.

63. Wetzel FT et al.: The treatment of lumbar spinal pain syndromes diagnosed by discography: lumbar arthrodesis, *Spine* 19:792-800, 1994.

64. Wittenberg RH et al.: Compressive strength of autologous and allogenous bone grafts for thoracolumbar and cervical spine fusion, *Spine* 15:1073-1078, 1990.

65. Zdeblick TA: A prospective, randomized study of lumbar fusion: preliminary results, *Spine* 18:983-991, 1993.

66. Zdeblick TA: Construct stiffness testing of the threaded interbody fusion device (TIBFD), IDE # G940127. Report prepared for Sofamor Danek Group, Inc, Aug 1994.

VI
Trauma

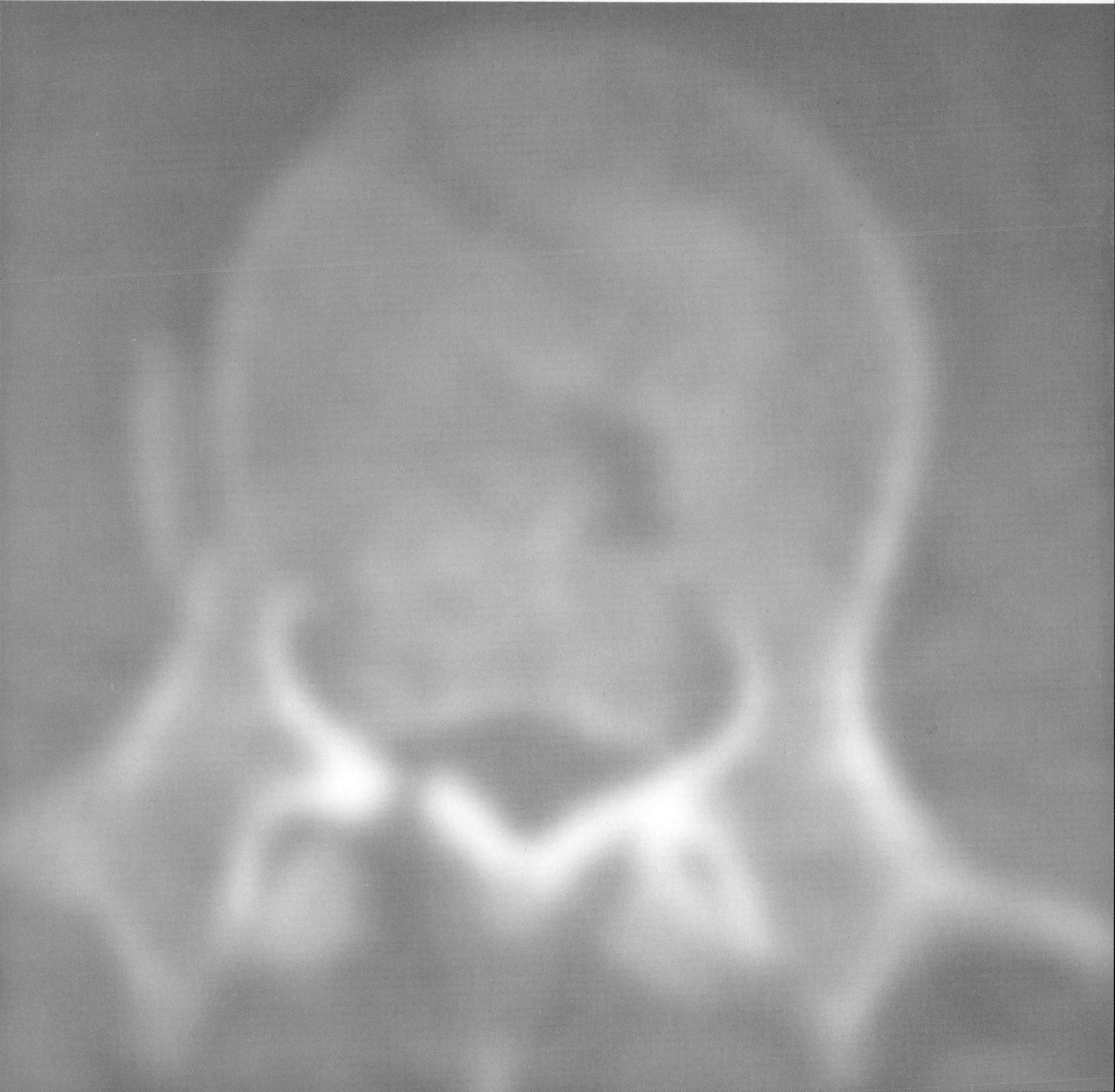

Pediatric Spinal Cord Injury

Randal R. Betz, Mary Jane Mulcahey

The initial evaluation and management (including determination of cause, diagnosis, initial treatment, and rehabilitation) of the child or adolescent with spinal cord injury differ from those of the adult because of the child's smaller size and the fact that children are still growing. Spinal cord injury without radiographic abnormality (SCIWORA) must be considered, as well as the possibility of delayed onset of neurologic deficits. Lap belt injuries frequently occur in children with spinal cord injury (SCI). Early evaluation must include the consideration of normal variance in radiographic evaluation, as well as the possibility of growth plate injuries. Key points of the initial management include head positioning during transport, halo traction, and indications for surgery.

EVALUATION

Roughly 200,000 people in the United States are presently living with some degree of SCI resulting from trauma,[12,21] and approximately 7800 to 11,000 new cases occur each year.[31] It is estimated that 4% to 14% of such injuries occur in children younger than age 15 years.[8,16,23,24] Causes for pediatric SCI parallel those in adults and include motor vehicle accidents in 40%, diving in 13%, other sports in 24%, gunshots in 8%, falls in 8%, transverse myelitis in 4%, and spinal cord tumors in 3% of cases.[35] Head injury concomitant with SCI occurs in 25% to 50% of patients,[11,30] and it is important

to recognize a potential head injury during the initial evaluation because its presence may significantly affect the rehabilitation process due to resulting perceptual, speech, and other associated deficits.

Thoracolumbar and lumbar spine injuries secondary to lap belt injuries demand particular attention. Retroperitoneal injuries have been reported in 30% to 50% of patients presenting with these spine fractures,[18,34] and neurologic deficits occur in 4% to 39%.* The variance in neurologic deficits in the reported series depends on whether the authors studied patients at a spinal cord injury rehabilitation center or in an emergency room.

The spine must be carefully evaluated in a patient with a known lap belt injury, preferably before the patient goes to the operating room (OR). If the spine cannot be evaluated because the patient is unstable hemodynamically, the patient should be treated as though he or she has the fracture until it is determined that he or she does not. Cases have been reported of children awakening paralyzed after an abdominal procedure when the child was previously neurologically intact, with paralysis probably occurring during manipulation on the OR table (Figure 31-1).

The flexion-distraction spine fracture secondary to a lap belt injury must be diagnosed on plain radiographs. It is extremely difficult to diagnose on CT scan because the plane of the distraction of the spine injury is the same as the axial CT cut.[37]

Long bone fractures occur in approximately 10% to 20% of patients, and internal fixation can help facilitate early rehabilitation of these patients.

The neurologic status of patients with SCI should be assessed using the current standards of the American Spinal Injury Association for motor, sensory, and impairment scores.[13] It should be remembered that children have different motor strengths, and what may be a motor strength of 5 in an adult may not be the same in a child.

During the radiographic assessment of the child, one must remember the normal radiographic variants seen. Pseudosubluxation of C2 on C3 is troublesome when seen on initial evaluation in an emergency room, especially in a child who may have sustained neck trauma.[9]

EVALUATION

- From 7800 to 11,000 new cases of SCI occur each year due to trauma (4% to 14% in children younger than age 15 years).
- Head injury is concomitant with SCI in 25% to 50% of cases.
- Flexion-distraction spine injury secondary to a lap belt injury requires careful evaluation on spinal radiographs.
- Remember normal radiographic variants in children.
- MRI is used for hard-to-see areas of the spine and can help delineate SCIWORA or injury to growth plates.

---

*References 14, 18, 19, 30, 34, 38.

401

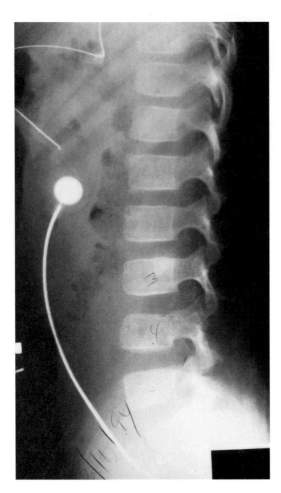

Figure 31-1. Lateral lumbar radiograph of a 4-year-old child who was involved in a motor vehicle accident. She was in a lap belt in the back seat at the time of impact. She was hemodynamically unstable and was rushed to the operating room for repair of retroperitoneal lacerations. The lateral radiograph shows some suggestion of injury at L3 to L4 disc and interspace.

If the posterior intralaminar line is not displaced, the pseudosubluxation seen is a normal variant (Figure 31-2, *A* and *B*).[36] If the line is disrupted, it is pathologic (Figure 31-3).

MRI following pediatric SCI can show problems not seen on plain radiographs. It can be beneficial in delineating spinal column injury in difficult-to-see areas such as C7 to T1[3] (Figure 31-4). SCIWORA has been reported in 10% to 20% of children with SCI.[2,20,33,39] In very young children, age 3 to 4 years, the association of SCIWORA with a Chiari malformation has been reported.[3] It is important to recognize the Chiari malformation because decompression of C1 and the foramen magnum has been reported to help with some recovery of function, especially when the lesion is incomplete. Growth plate injuries may be seen on MRI that may not be seen on radiograph, and the fragments can cause external dural compression that may be relieved by removing the fragment.[4,25,32]

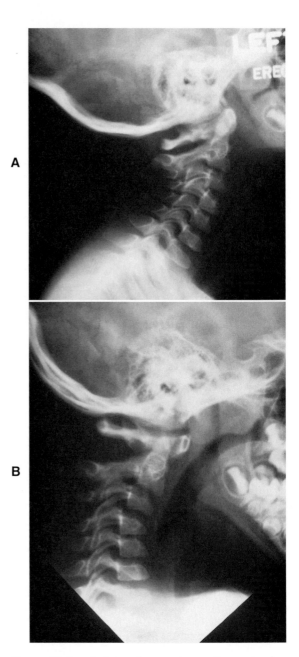

Figure 31-2. **A,** Lateral extension radiograph of the cervical spine. **B,** Lateral flexion radiograph shows pseudosubluxation of the anterior vertebral body of C2 on C3. The posterior intralaminar line (line of Swischuk) is intact. (*B, From Swischuk LE: Anterior displacement of C2 in children: physiologic or pathologic? A helpful differentiating line. Radiology, 122:759-763, 1977.*)

MANAGEMENT

The initial transport of the young child must allow for the head to be in extension. In children up to age 6 years, the head is disproportionately large in comparison to the torso, and lying flat on a spine board may cause flexion of the spine. Either cutting a hole in the spine board (allowing the head to recess) or elevating the torso on an additional pad (the preferred method)

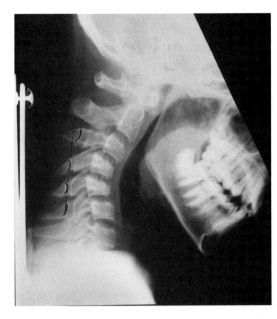

Figure 31-3. Lateral flexion cervical radiograph shows subluxation after C3 to C4. The posterior intralaminar line is disrupted to confirm that this is true instability.

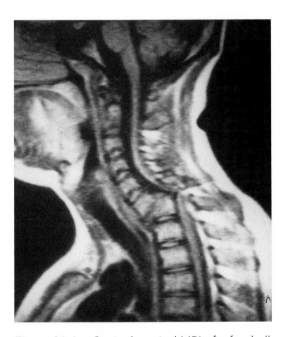

Figure 31-4. Sagittal cervical MRI of a football player with a fracture-dislocation of C6 on C7. Radiographs were indeterminate in defining the spinal column injury.

should allow the cervical spine to be in neutral position.[22]

Very little has been reported concerning injury modulation in children. Bracken et al. reported that methylprednisolone improves SCI recovery up to 5 motor points if administered within 8 hours of injury.[6] Although most treating physicians use methylprednisolone in cases of pediatric SCI, only 15% of the patients in the

MANAGEMENT

- Children's disproportionate head size requires careful positioning on a spine board during initial transport.
- Use of methylprednisolone, ganglioside, and hypothermia in children is not well supported.
- Halo traction is preferable to cervical traction in children under age 12 years.
- Decompression for incomplete neurologic deficits is appropriate for children.
- Type of surgical stabilization requires careful consideration secondary to implications on spinal growth.

study by Bracken et al. were age 13 to 19 years, and the study included no data on patients younger than age 13 years. One published study on the use of ganglioside (Sygen) in adult SCI showed some effectiveness in neural recovery,[16] but some recent evidence in animal studies show it may inhibit the effect of steroids administered simultaneously. The effects of hypothermia have been reported in animal studies but have not been documented in humans.[1]

Cervical traction in children under age 12 years is associated with increased risk compared with its use in adults, and primary halo traction may be preferred. Martinez-Lage et al.[27] reported dural leaks with Crutchfield tongs in patients under age 12 years. Halo fixators can safely be used in children.[14] The number of pins must be increased to 8 or 10 and the torques reduced, using 2 pounds/inch instead of 8. One may need to take standard halo rings and drill additional holes (Figure 31-5).[5,29] CT scans of the head for children younger than age 6 years have been recommended to help determine the best pin sites.[15,26] Should the halo become loose or for some reason not be able to be applied, a Minerva-type cervicothoracolumbosacral orthosis (CTLSO) would be an option and has been used successfully by the first author.

The indications for decompression in adults as defined by Bradford and McBride[7] for incomplete neurologic deficits are also appropriate for children. Alignment is another issue when considering surgery. In the pediatric population, residual deformity greater than 10 degrees secondary to fracture in complete SCI will enhance the chances of developing a spinal deformity.[28] When the posterior ligaments are disrupted (generally when there is greater than 25 degrees of kyphosis), surgery is usually recommended. The type of surgical stabilization must be carefully considered. Although the new multisegmented hook-screw-rod systems are attractive in that they minimize the need for postoperative immobilization, more spine levels must be instrumented and fused, and this may have an adverse effect on the overall growth of the spine. For the flexion-distraction lap belt injury, posterior wiring without fusion is an attractive alternative because it allows the spine to be stabilized, heal, and continue to grow. Wires can break from fatigue at what appears to be an appropriate time without losing spine stability, and the spine continues to grow.

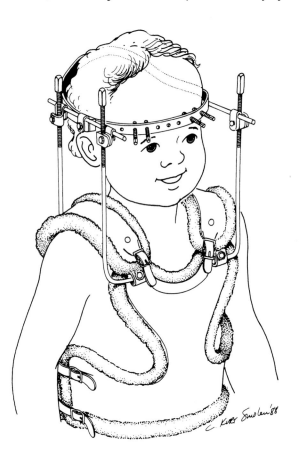

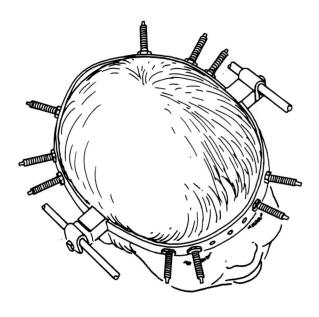

Figure 31-5. Schematic of halo placement in an infant. Note the increased number of pins from 8 to 10 or 10. Use 2 pounds per inch of torque instead of 8. *(From Mubarak SJ et al.: Halo application in the infant. J Pediatr Ortho, 9: 612-614, 1989.)*

CONCLUSIONS

The key unique areas in the evaluation of pediatric SCI include recognition of normal radiographic variants: SCIWORA is present in 10% to 20% of pediatric SCIs, and possible growth plate injury with retropulsion seen only on MRI can exist. Management issues include the use of a halo fixator for traction as opposed to Crutchfield or Gardner-Wells tongs in patients under age 12 years. Also, when stabilizing the spine with instrumentation, implications on future growth must be considered.

SELECTED REFERENCES

Betz RR et al.: Magnetic resonance imaging (MRI) in the evaluation of spinal cord injured children and adolescents, *Paraplegia* 25:92-99, 1987.

Cattell HS, Filtzer DL: Pseudosubluxation and other normal variations of the cervical spine in children, *J Bone Joint Surg Am* 47A:1295-1309, 1965.

Garfin SR et al.: Skull osteology as it affects halo pin placement in children, *J Pediatr Orthop* 6:434-436, 1986.

Glassman SD, Johnson JR, Holt RT: Seatbelt injuries in children, *J Trauma* 33:882-886, 1992.

Herzenberg JE et al.: Emergency transport and positioning of young children who have an injury to the cervical spine, *J Bone Joint Surg Am* 71A:15-22, 1989.

Mubarak SJ et al.: Halo application in the infant, *J Pediatr Orthop* 9:612-614, 1989.

Rumball K, Jarvis J: Seat-belt injuries of the spine in young children, *J Bone Joint Surg Br* 74B:571-574, 1992.

REFERENCES

1. Albin MS et al.: Study of functional recovery produced by delayed localized cooling after spinal cord injury in primates, *J Neurosurg* 29:113-120, 1968.
2. Anderson JM, Schutt AH: Spinal injury in children: a review of 156 cases seen from 1950 through 1978, *Mayo Clin Proc* 55:499-504, 1980.
3. Betz RR et al.: Magnetic resonance imaging (MRI) in the evaluation of spinal cord injured children and adolescents, *Paraplegia* 25:92-99, 1987.
4. Bondurant CP, Oró JJ: Spinal cord injury without radiographic abnormality and Chiari malformation, *J Neurosurg* 79:833-838, 1993.
5. Botte MJ, Byrne TP, Garfin SR: Application of the halo device for immobilization of the cervical spine utilizing an increased torque pressure, *J Bone Joint Surg Am* 69A:750-752, 1987.
6. Bracken MB et al.: A randomized, controlled trial of methyl-prednisolone or naloxone in the treatment of acute spinal-cord injury, *New Engl J Med* 322:1405-1411, 1990.
7. Bradford DS, McBride GG: Surgical management of thoracolumbar spine fractures with incomplete neurologic deficits, *Clin Orthop Rel Res* 218:201-216, 1987.
8. Burke DC: Injuries of the spinal cord in children. In Vinken PJ, Bruyn GW, eds: *Handbook of clinical neurology*, New York, 1976, Elsevier.
9. Cattell HS, Filtzer DL: Pseudosubluxation and other normal variations of the cervical spine in children, *J Bone Joint Surg Am* 47A:1295-1309, 1965.
10. Constantin S, Young W: The effects of methylprednisolone and the ganglioside GM1 on acute spinal cord injury in rats, *J Neurosurg* 80:97-111, 1994.
11. Desmond J: Paraplegia: problems confronting the anaesthesiologist, *Can Anaesth Soc J* 17:435-451, 1970.
12. Devivo MJ et al.: Prevalence of spinal cord injury: a reestimation employing life table techniques, *Arch Neurol* 37:707-708, 1980.

13. Ditunno JF Jr (ed): *International standards for neurological and functional classification of spinal cord injury*, Chicago, 1992, American Spinal Injury Association.
14. Garfin SR et al.: Complications in the use of the halo fixation device, *J Bone Joint Surg Am* 68A:320-325, 1986.
15. Garfin SR et al.: Skull osteology as it affects halo pin placement in children, *J Pediatr Orthop* 6:434-436, 1986.
16. Gehrig R, Michaelis LS: Statistics of acute paraplegia and tetraplegia on a national scale, *Paraplegia* 6:93-95, 1968.
17. Geisler FH, Dorsey FC, Coleman WP: Recovery of motor function after spinal-cord injury: a randomized, placebo-controlled trial with GM-1 ganglioside, *New Engl J Med* 324:1829-1838, 1991.
18. Glassman SD, Johnson JR, Holt RT: Seatbelt injuries in children, *J Trauma* 33:882-886, 1992.
19. Gumley G, Taylor TK, Ryan MD: Distraction fractures of the lumbar spine, *J Bone Joint Surg Br* 64B:520-525, 1982.
20. Hadley MN et al.: Pediatric spinal trauma: review of 122 cases of spinal cord and vertebral column injuries, *J Neurosurg* 68:18-24, 1988.
21. Harvey C et al.: New estimates of traumatic SCI prevalence: a survey-based approach, *Paraplegia* 28:537-544, 1990.
22. Herzenberg JE et al.: Emergency transport and positioning of young children who have an injury to the cervical spine, *J Bone Joint Surg Am* 71A:15-22, 1989.
23. Kewalramani LS: Autonomic dysreflexia in traumatic myelopathy, *Am J Phys Med* 59:1-21, 1980.
24. Kewalramani LS, Taylor RG: Multiple non-contiguous injuries to the spine, *Acta Orthop Scand* 47:52-58, 1976.
25. Lawson JP et al.: Physeal injuries of the cervical spine, *J Pediatr Orthop* 7:428-435, 1987.
26. Letts M, Kaylor D, Gouw G: A biomechanical analysis of halo fixation in children, *J Bone Joint Surg Br* 70:277-279, 1988.
27. Martinez-Lage JF et al.: Bilateral brain abscesses complicating the use of Crutchfield tongs, *Child Nerv Syst* 2:208-210, 1986.
28. Mayfield JK, Erkkila JC, Winter RB: Spine deformity subsequent to acquired childhood spinal cord injury, *J Bone Joint Surg Am* 63A:1401-1411, 1981.
29. Mubarak SJ et al.: Halo application in the infant, *J Pediatr Orthop* 9:612-614, 1989.
30. Nand S, Goldschmidt JM: Hypercalcemia and hyperuricemia in young patients with spinal cord injury, *Arch Phys Med Rehab* 57:553, 1976, [abstract].
31. National Spinal Cord Injury Association: *Fact sheet 2: spinal cord injury statistical information—spinal cord injury: the facts and figures*, Spinal Cord Injury Statistical Center at the University of Alabama at Birmingham, 1986.
32. Ogden JA: *Skeletal injury in the child*, Philadelphia, 1982, Lea & Febiger.
33. Pang D, Wilberger JE Jr: Spinal cord injury without radiographic abnormalities in children, *J Neurosurg* 57:114-129, 1982.
34. Rumball K, Jarvis J: Seat-belt injuries of the spine in young children, *J Bone Joint Surg Br* 74B:571-574, 1992.
35. Shriners Hospitals: *Shriners Hospitals annual statistical report for the Shrine units*, University of Alabama at Birmingham, 1991.
36. Swischuk LE: Anterior displacement of C2 in children: physiologic or pathologic? A helpful differentiating line, *Radiology* 122:759-763, 1977.
37. Taylor GA, Eggli KD: Lap-belt injuries of the lumbar spine in children: a pitfall in CT diagnosis, *Am J Roentgenol* 150:1355-1358, 1988.
38. Womack MS et al.: Pediatric spine injuries associated with lap seat belts. American Academy of Orthopaedic Surgeons Annual Meeting, San Francisco, Feb 1993.
39. Yngve DA et al.: Spinal cord injury without osseous spine fracture, *J Pediatr Orthoped* 8:153-159, 1988.

Pharmacology and Timing of Surgical Intervention for Spinal Cord Injury

Alexander R. Vaccaro, Basil M. Harris, Kush Singh

There is considerable debate as to the optimal acute treatment of spinal cord injuries. The main issues include the selection of efficacious pharmacologic agents designed to modify the secondary cascade of injury, as well as the value and timing of surgical decompression and stabilization. The direct clinical benefit of early surgery is a theoretical improvement in neurologic recovery over that of delayed surgery. The additional benefits may include the clinical advantages of a decreased length of hospitalization and its associated complications and a decreased time to rehabilitation and mobilization. Proper and timely surgical intervention may improve the physiologic environment so as to allow for maximum neurologic improvement.

Spinal cord trauma is a devastating injury to the unfortunate victim and a tremendous hardship to both family and societal support systems. Injury to the spinal cord is often irreversible, resulting in paralysis or even death. Although spinal cord injuries have been studied pervasively throughout history, a consensus regarding optimal medical and surgical treatments is yet to be reached. Controversy and confusion surround both the pharmacologic treatment regimen and the optimal timing of surgery that can maximally benefit a given patient. Successful therapies (pharmacologic and surgical) are thought to modify the primary and secondary cascades of neurologic injury. The natural history of the secondary injury cascade results in the inevitable, rapid deterioration of neural tissue (profound in the first 8 hours), defining a potential window of opportunity in which the effects of spinal cord injury could be reversed.[4,11,12,22]

Decompression and stabilization result in improved neurologic outcomes in cervical spine–injured patients with chronic long-term symptomatic spinal cord compression.[17] The debate remains on the optimal timing of acute surgical intervention in the setting of spinal cord or cauda equina injury. Prompt surgical intervention may minimize the secondary pathologic changes in neural tissue and allow for earlier advancement to rehabilitation. Delayed surgical intervention may forfeit the same benefits, but delayed surgery may allow a patient to be optimally medically stabilized before surgery. Review of a series of early studies tends to contraindicate prompt surgical intervention based on perioperative complications and increased mortality rates.[20] Conversely, more recent prospective and retrospective studies are inclined toward favoring early surgery, but cannot significantly discriminate between "early" (less than 72 hours) and "late" (more than 5 days) surgical treatment in terms of the degree of neurologic recovery.[14,17,22] In a recent study, Mirza et al.[14] concluded that surgery prior to 72 hours of injury is not associated with a higher complication rate, does not result in neurologic deterioration, and decreases hospitalization time.

EPIDEMIOLOGY

The annual incidence of acute spinal cord injuries for patients admitted to acute care hospitals in the United States has been estimated between 4 and 5.3 per 100,000 population, or between 7600 and 10,000 new spinal cord injuries per year.[21] An acute spinal cord injury is present in approximately 2.6% of all victims of major trauma, of which 43% to 46% result in complete loss of sensory and motor function below the level of the injury; approximately 55% occur in the cervical spine, 30% in the thoracic spine, and 15% in the lumbar spine.[13] Of the patients with injuries to the cervical spine, 40% present with a complete spinal cord injury, 40% with incomplete cord damage, and the remaining 20% with either no cord injury or only root lesions.[6]

The majority of spinal cord injuries are preventable, with the most common causes being motor vehicle collisions, falls, violence, and sports-related traumas. The patients are predominantly young men with an average age of 33 years.

EPIDEMIOLOGY

- 7600 to 10,000 spinal cord injuries per year in the United States.
- 55% cervical, 30% thoracic, 15% lumbar.
- 43% to 46% result in complete motor loss below the level of the injury.
- Cervical spinal injuries
  - 40% complete cord damage.
  - 40% incomplete cord damage.
  - 20% either no cord damage or only root lesions.
- Most spinal cord injuries are caused by motor vehicle collisions, falls, violence, and sports-related trauma.

PATHOPHYSIOLOGY

- Spinal cord injuries result in neurologic deterioration due to
  - Kinetic energy of traumatic event
  - Progressive secondary cascade of injury
- Primary traumatic event includes spinal cord compression and immediate neuronal and vascular injury.
- Secondary physiologic cascade involves both a vascular and a central nervous system response, including:
  - Hemorrhage
  - Inflammation
  - Membrane hydrolysis
  - Ischemia
- Initial pharmacologic treatment aims to counteract the mediators of inflammation.
- The inflammatory process is damaging at first but is vital for subsequent neural regeneration.

PHARMACOLOGIC TREATMENT

- National Acute Spinal Cord Injury Studies (NASCIS) I, II, and III
  - Study designs paralleled contemporary understanding of pathophysiology of spinal cord injury
  - Compared dosing and timing of glucocorticoid treatment (methylprednisolone) on neurologic recovery (motor and sensation)
- NASCIS I
  - Low-dose treatments with methylprednisolone ineffective
- NASCIS II
  - Validated that high doses of methylprednisolone improved neurologic recovery when administered within 8 hours of injury
- NASCIS III
  - Included initial bolus of high-dose methylprednisolone
  - If within 3 hours of injury, continued treatment for 24 hours
  - If within 3 hours to 8 hours of injury, recommended continued treatment for 48 hours

PATHOPHYSIOLOGY

The typical spinal cord injury includes compression of the spinal cord and immediate neuronal and vascular injury. Neurologic deterioration is due to the kinetic energy of the primary traumatic event and a progressive secondary biochemical cascade of injury. Since the extent of the injury is not determined solely at the moment of trauma, a potential window for surgical and pharmacologic therapies exists through which improved neurologic recovery could be attained. Delamarter, et al.[12] used a canine model to show the temporal relationship between the traumatic event and the extent of neurologic deterioration. Five groups of dogs were sequentially relieved of an experimental spinal cord compression (50% compression). The percent recovery of somatosensory evoked potentials (SEP) as measured at the posterior tibial nerve are shown in Figure 32-1. Only the animals whose spinal cords were either decompressed immediately or after 1 hour were able to attain a significant recovery, including walking, as well as bowel and bladder control. Animals whose spinal cords were compressed for 6, 24, or 168 hours remained paraplegic after decompression (immediately and at 6 weeks) and showed severe histologic damage (Figure 32-2).[12]

The complex secondary physiologic mechanisms resulting in spinal cord injury after trauma are still being elucidated. After an injury to the spinal cord, several phases of tissue repair occur. The acute phase involves both a vascular and a central nervous system (CNS) response, which includes membrane hydrolysis, or breakdown, resulting in the release of various neurotoxic and inflammatory mediators. These mediators damage the blood-brain barrier and consequently the spinal cord.[4,12,18] Pharmacologic treatment is aimed at counteracting these mediators in order to protect the cord from additional damage resulting from the initial traumatic event.

PHARMACOLOGIC TREATMENT

Studies of pharmacologic therapies have paralleled the contemporary understanding of the pathophysiology of spinal cord injury. The first National Acute Spinal Cord Injury Study (NASCIS I) compared 100-mg and 1000-mg doses of intravenous methylprednisolone sodium suc-

cinate given within 48 hours of injury. The study concluded that there was no difference in neurologic recovery (motor or sensation) at the 6-week or 6-month follow-up between either dosage group.[3] The second National Acute Spinal Cord Injury Study (NASCIS II) was used to validate the efficacy of very high doses of methylprednisolone on spinal cord recovery as witnessed in animal models on the human population. NASCIS II compared results between a placebo group, a group receiving methylprednisolone, and a group receiving naloxone. Groups were also split into those receiving the drug earlier or later than 8 hours after injury. Methylprednisolone was effective in modifying the deleterious effects of the secondary cascade of neural injury, with patients showing a significantly increased neuro-

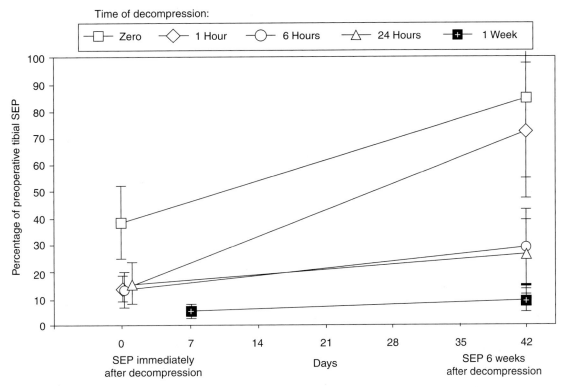

Figure 32-1. Recovery of posterior tibial somatosensory evoked potentials (SEP) after decompression of experimental spinal cord injury in five groups of six dogs each. All groups started at 100% SEP prior to compression. *(Redrawn from Delamarter RB, Sherman J, Carr JB: Pathophysiology of spinal cord injury: recovery after immediate and delayed compression, J Bone Joint Surg Am 77:1042-1049, 1995.)*

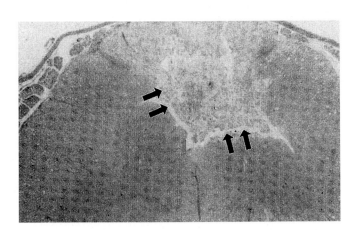

Figure 32-2. Hematoxylin-eosin stained section of spinal cord from experimental dog. Approximately 1 cm cephalad to induced 6-hour spinal cord compression. *Arrows* indicate degeneration in the central cord. *(Modified from Delamarter RB, Sherman J, Carr JB: Pathophysiology of spinal cord injury: recovery after immediate and delayed compression, J Bone Joint Surg Am 77:1042-1049, 1995.)*

logic recovery at 6 weeks, 6 months, and 1 year when given the steroid within 8 hours after injury.[4-6] Naloxone was less effective than methylprednisolone.

Promotion of endogenous mechanisms of neuronal regeneration is the goal of any medicinal treatment during the subacute postinjury period. Since neurons do not replicate, the focus instead is on regeneration and reconnection of various neural cell processes. The inflammatory process, damaging at first, is vital for subsequent neural regeneration. NASCIS II proved this by demonstrating a worsening in neural functional recovery if anti-inflammatory high-dose methylprednisolone was administered later than 8 hours after injury.[4] Thus, the difficult part of pharmacologic treatment is determining when to prohibit and when to promote the inflammatory process.

In a subsequent study (NASCIS III), Bracken et al.[7,8] compared the efficacy of high-dose methylprednisolone administered for 24 hours with methylprednisolone administered for 48 hours or tirilazad mesylate (a 21-aminosteroid) administered for 48 hours in patients with acute spinal cord injury. All patients received an initial bolus of methylprednisolone. The study involved 16 acute spinal cord injury centers in North America with a total of 499 patients. Compared with patients treated with methylprednisolone for 24 hours, those treated with methylprednisolone for 48 hours showed improved motor recovery at 6 weeks and 6 months after injury. The effect of the 48-hour methylprednisolone regimen was significant at 6 weeks and 6 months among patients whose therapy was initiated 4 to 8 hours after injury. Patients who received the 48-hour regimen and who started treatment at 4 to 8 hours were more likely to improve one full neurologic grade at 6 months, to show

ANIMAL STUDIES

- Surgical decompression with the addition of methylprednisolone resulted in maximum neurologic recovery.
- Surgical decompression (with or without methylprednisolone) was better than methylprednisolone alone.

SURGERY PLUS PHARMACOLOGIC AGENTS

- A significant difference between combined early surgery with any one of the following was clinically undetectable
  - Nimodipine (Ca^{2+} channel blocker)
  - Methylprednisolone
  - Nimodipine and methylprednisolone
  - No medical treatment

MODIFYING NEURAL REGENERATION

- Treatment with gangliosides (GM-1 sodium salt) possibly beneficial after initial treatment with high-dose methylprednisolone.
- Continuing elucidation of pathomechanics of spinal cord injury from animal models.
  - 5-HT: An important mediator in the early pathophysiologic responses of spinal cord injury (rat model).
  - Benzodiazepine receptors: May be involved in trauma-induced alterations in spinal cord evoked potentials, edema formation, and cell injury (rat model).
  - Prostacyclin: May offer beneficial neurologic effects by protecting myelinated axonal structures and limiting edema (rabbit model).
  - Others: With further study, additional neural recovery benefits may be derived from dihydropyridine member calcium channel blockers, axonal potassium channel blockers, or μ-opioid-receptor antagonists.

more improvement in 6-month FIM (functional improvement measures), and to have more severe sepsis and severe pneumonia than patients in the 24-hour methylprednisolone group and the tirilazad group. Other complications and mortality were similar among all groups. The authors concluded that patients with acute spinal cord injury who receive methylprednisolone within 4 hours of injury should be maintained on the treatment regimen for 24 hours. When methylprednisolone is initiated 4 to 8 hours after injury, patients should be maintained on steroid therapy for 48 hours. The response of several centers around North America to this study is an educated and informed decision-making process in selective patients in determining the duration of steroid administration for the 4- to 8-hour patient group.

Rabinowitz et al.[16] performed a study in which 18 dogs were prospectively split into three groups. In all dogs, the canal area at the L4 level (distal spinal cord) was constricted by 60% of its original value. Two groups received surgical decompression 6 hours after compression, with one of the groups also receiving methylprednisolone. The third group received methylprednisolone without surgery. The authors found that surgical decompression, with or without methylprednisolone, resulted in significantly better neurologic recovery than methylprednisolone alone. The authors also noted a better recovery in methylprednisolone-treated dogs undergoing surgery versus those without the drug, although this difference was not statistically significant. This study supports the secondary-injury theory of spinal cord injury, in which maximum neurologic injury is thought not to occur at the initial trauma, but to be due to pharmacologically controllable secondary mechanisms. Although the nylon compression method used may not accurately represent human spinal cord trauma, the study is significant for indicating that surgery in the setting of neural compression is needed in addition to pharmacologic treatment for maximal neurologic recovery. The authors note that more studies are required to further define the roles of surgical and pharmacologic treatment, as well as the appropriate timing of surgery.

Petitjean et al.[15] evaluated the effect of surgical intervention alone or in combination with nimodipine (a calcium channel blocker), methylprednisolone, or both on neurologic recovery during the acute phase of spinal cord injury. The study consisted of 106 spinal injured patients, including 48 with paraplegia and 58 with tetraplegia. Patients were randomly allocated into one of the four treatment groups described above. Early

spinal decompression was performed as soon as possible after injury. At 1-year follow-up, neurologic improvement based on America Spinal Injury Association (ASIA) score assessment was seen in each group; however, there was no advantage neurologically of one treatment over the others. Additionally, early surgery (49 patients), within the first 8 hours, did not influence ultimate neurologic outcome. The extent of the spinal injury (complete or incomplete lesion) was the only predictor of outcome. The authors concluded that at this time, due to the lack of supporting clinical studies, there was no evidence for the systematic use of specific medications or the timing of surgery in the spinal injury patient with a neurologic deficit.

The ability to modify neural regeneration was initially demonstrated histologically with the use of gangliosides in experimental neural injury.[7] These findings were supported clinically by the Maryland GM-1 Ganglioside Study. The study consisted of 44 patients, each receiving 100 mg of GM-1 sodium salt or a placebo once a day for 18 to 42 days. All patients received the first dose within 72 hours of injury. When compared with the placebo group, the GM-1 group had a statistically significant improvement in lower-extremity ASIA motor score at 1-year follow-up. This study formed the basis for a larger placebo-controlled multicenter study of 760 patients in which patients were randomized into three groups: (1)

Table 32-1	Pharmacologic Agents Beneficial in Neural Recovery	
Class	Drug Name	Mechanism of Action
Calcium channel blocker	Nimodipine	Dihydropyridine member calcium channel blocker
Potassium channel blocker	4-Aminopyridine	Axonal potassium channel blocker extends duration of action potentials
Opioid antagonist	Naloxone	μ-Opioid-receptor antagonist

high-dose methylprednisolone, (2) methylprednisolone followed by 100 mg GM-1 of sodium salt (Sygen), or (3) methylprednisolone followed by 200 mg of Sygen. The results of this study revealed a nonstatistical improvement in motor function in ASIA B treated patients (100 mg group) and an improved rate of recovery in ASIA C and D patients at 6 weeks with no statistical difference in ultimate recovery by 52 weeks. There was, however, no statistical improvement in neurologic recovery in the intent-to-treat group at follow-up.

Sharma et al.[19] examined the involvement of serotonin in early microvascular reactions and cell changes following trauma of the spinal cord. Serotonin antibodies were topically applied to the traumatized spinal cord in a rat model. Monoclonal 5-HT antibodies were applied 2 minutes after a focal trauma of the spinal cord was produced. The antibodies significantly reduced the breakdown of the blood-spinal cord barrier, edema formation, and cell changes in the traumatized rats that received 5-HT antiserum compared with the injured rats given saline. The results found 5-HT to be an important mediator involved in the early pathophysiologic responses of spinal cord injury.

In addition to serotonin, benzodiazepine receptor agonists appear to be involved in spinal cord injury pathomechanics. Winkler[24] investigated the influence of diazepam on spinal cord evoked potentials (SCEP), edema formation, and cell changes following spinal cord injury in a rat model. An injury was made at the T10 to T11 cord segments, with SCEPs recorded from the epidural space of the T9 level following stimulation of the right tibial and sural nerves. Spinal cord edema and cell changes were markedly pronounced 5 hours after injury. Pretreatment with diazepam attenuated the early SCEP changes induced by the trauma and reduced the later development of edema and cell injury. These results suggest that benzodiazepine receptors are involved in trauma-induced alterations in SCEP, edema formation, and cell injury.

Attar et al.[1] conducted a separate study on the early protective effects of Iloprost, a stable analog of prostacyclin, after spinal cord injury in rabbits. Sixteen adult male rabbits were injured by application of an epidural aneurysm clip. Half received an IV infusion of Iloprost, while the other half received an infusion of saline. Although no meaningful statistical difference between cortical somatosensory evoked potentials (CSEP) between the groups were found, light and electron microscopic studies showed that the Iloprost-treated group had moderate protection of myelin and axonal structures and limited edema. The authors concluded that intravenous Iloprost treatment after spinal cord

injury has a highly protective neurologic effect without any side effects.

Other pharmacologic agents have shown beneficial effects of neural recovery in basic science lab and animal spinal cord injury models (Table 32-1). Unfortunately, none of these agents has demonstrated any significant benefit in terms of functional neural recovery in well-designed controlled prospective human trials.

SURGICAL TIMING

Although not demonstrated by any human study, many researchers believe that a certain time period may exist (probably less than 2 to 3 hours) in which the removal of extrinsic pressure to the spinal cord may significantly benefit neural recovery. Previous studies by Levi and colleagues[2] as well as data from NASCIS II[4] have suggested clinically that the optimal timing of surgery is certainly less than 24 hours. However, a more precise time frame has yet to be elucidated.

Carlson et al.[10] conducted a study of the timing and efficacy of early decompression for spinal cord injury in a canine model. Twenty-one mature beagles were anesthetized and mechanically ventilated to maintain normal respiratory and acid-base balance. SEP from the upper and lower extremities were measured at regular intervals. The spinal cord was loaded dorsally at T14 under precision loading conditions until evoked potential amplitudes had been reduced by 50%. Spinal cord displacement was maintained for either 40 (n = 7), 60 (n = 8), or 180 minutes (n = 6), which was then followed by a 3-hour monitoring period. Regional spinal cord blood flow was measured with fluorescent microspheres at baseline (following laminectomy), immediately after stopping dynamic cord compression, and 5, 15, and 180 minutes after decompression. Within 5 minutes after stopping dynamic cord compression, evoked potentials were absent in all dogs. However, SEP recovery was observed in 6 of 7 dogs in the 40-minute compression group, 5 of 8 dogs in the 60-minute compression group, and 0 of 6 dogs in the 180-minute compression group. The authors concluded that the degree of early reperfusion hyperemia after decompression, important for potential neural recovery, was inversely proportional to the duration of spinal cord decompression and proportional to electrophysiologic recovery. After precise dynamic spinal cord loading to a point of functional conduction deficit (50% decline in evoked potential amplitude), a critical time period was found (1 to 3 hours) where intervention in the form of early spinal cord decompression led to effective recovery of electrophysiologic function.

OPTIMAL TIMING FOR SURGERY

- Neural recovery is enhanced by prompt removal of extrinsic pressure to spinal cord, although optimal time frame for surgery has not yet been clinically demonstrated.
- Clinical studies (NASCIS II and Levi et al.) suggest the optimal timing of surgery to be less than 24 hours.
- Experimentally, the degree of early reperfusion hyperemia after decompression is inversely proportional to the duration of spinal cord decompression and proportional to electrophysiologic recovery.
- After precise dynamic spinal cord loading to the functional conduction deficit (50% decline in evoked potential amplitude), critical time period of 1 to 3 hours identified when early spinal cord decompression leads to effective recovery of electrophysiologic function.

BENEFICIAL INTERVENTIONS

- Early surgical treatment: Reduces the length of hospital stay without increasing common medical complications.
- Aggressive adjunctive medical cardiopulmonary support: May enhance neural recovery in acute spinal cord injury patients.

ACUTE MANAGEMENT OF CERVICAL SPINAL CORD INJURY

- Maintenance of perfusion systolic blood pressure greater than 90 mm Hg
- Recognize neurogenic shock (differentiate from hypovolemic shock)
- 100% O_2 saturation via nasal cannula
- Early diagnosis by plain radiography
- Methylprednisolone therapy
- Loading dose of 30 mg/kg
- If within 3 hours of injury, follow by infusion at rate of 5.4 mg/kg per hour for 23 hours
- If within 3 to 8 hours of injury, follow by infusion at rate of 5.4 mg/kg per hour for 48 hours
- Early traction reduction for cervical fracture and dislocation
- Advanced spinal imaging (magnetic resonance imaging and/or computed tomography)
- Surgery if indicated for residual cord compression or fracture instability

© 1999 American Academy of Orthopaedic Surgeons. Modified from *J Am Acad Orthop Surgeons* 7(3):166-175, 1999. With permission.

In addition to the potential neurologic benefit of early surgical decompression, various investigators have also demonstrated improved function and medical recovery in this patient population. Campagnolo et al.[9] conducted a retrospective review of 64 patients with cervical, thoracolumbar spinal cord, or cauda equina injuries, evaluating the timing of surgical stabilization on length of hospital stay and medical complications following spinal cord injury. Patients were divided into two groups based on whether they underwent spinal stabilization less than or greater than 24 hours after injury. Although there was no statistical difference between the groups with respect to the occurrence of common medical complications, the length of stay between the two groups was statistically significant (less than 24-hour group: 47.5 days [SD ± 44.2] versus greater than 24-hour group: 54.7 days [SD ± 40.1]).

In addition to the potential benefits of early surgery of spinal cord patient recovery, it appears that aggressive adjunctive medical cardiopulmonary support may enhance the neural recovery in acute spinal cord injury patients. Vale et al.[23] conducted a prospective study in which they applied resuscitation principles of volume expansion and blood pressure maintenance in order to support adequate spinal cord blood flow to 77 patients who presented with acute traumatic neurologic deficit to the spinal cord between C1 and T12. According to the intensive care unit protocol, all patients were managed by using Swan-Ganz and arterial blood pressure catheters and underwent necessary fracture reduction and immobilization techniques as indicated. Intravenous fluids, colloids, and vasopressors were administered as necessary to maintain mean arterial blood pressure above 85 mm Hg. Surgery was performed in selected cases when neural decompression and stabilization was deemed necessary. Of the 77 patients involved in the study, 66 were followed at least 12 months postinjury using detailed neurologic assessments and functional ability evaluations. In those patients with complete cervical spinal cord injuries, 60% improved at least one

SUMMARY OF FINDINGS

- Early surgical decompression (less than 1 to 3 hours) combined with aggressive cardiopulmonary support and selected pharmacologic agents may significantly improve neurologic recovery after spinal cord injury or cauda equina injury.
- Appropriate combination of pharmacologic therapeutic agents or precise time period of when surgical intervention is most optimal in enhancing neural recovery remains to be demonstrated.

Frankel or ASIA grade, whereas 40% regained the ability to walk. In those patients with complete thoracic spinal cord injuries, 44% improved at least one Frankel or ASIA grade, whereas approximately 10% gained the ability to walk. At the 12-month follow-up review, 92% of patients with an incomplete cervical spinal cord injury demonstrated clinical improvement as compared to their initial neurologic status, whereas 88% of patients with an incomplete thoracic spinal cord injury demonstrated significant neurologic improvements at 1 year postinjury. The authors concluded that the improvement in neurologic outcome was in addition to and/or distinct from any potential benefit provided by surgery. It appears that early and aggressive medical management (volume resuscitation and blood pressure augmentation) of patients with acute spinal cord injuries optimizes the potential for neurologic recovery following an injury to the CNS.

CONCLUSIONS

Early surgical decompression (less than 1 to 3 hours) combined with aggressive cardiopulmonary support and selected pharmacologic agents may significantly improve neurologic recovery following spinal cord injury or cauda equina injury. What is not evident today is the appropriate combination of pharmacologic therapeutic agents or the precise time period of when surgical intervention is most optimal in enhancing neural recovery. It may turn out that surgical intervention is only useful if completed within 1 to 3 hours following injury, a time period that is often clinically impossible to accommodate. This places a greater emphasis on our arsenal of pharmaceutical agents in modifying neural repair and recovery. As the pathophysiologic mechanisms of spinal cord trauma are clarified, more advances will be made in our understanding of the value of surgical intervention and optimal pharmacologic treatment regimens in order to improve neurologic outcomes. As is always the case in difficult and challenging medical issues, more studies will need to be conducted in order to further refine our treatment approach for this unfortunate spinal disorder so that a recognized system of management may be developed to improve the lives of spinal cord injury patients.

SELECTED REFERENCES

Bracken MB et al.: A randomized, controlled trial of methylprednisolone or naloxone in the treatment of acute spinal-cord injury, *N Engl J Med* 322:1405-1411, 1990.

Delamarter RB, Coyle J: Acute management of spinal cord injury, *J Am Acad Orthop Surg* 7(3):166-175, 1999.

Delamarter RB, Sherman J, Carr JB: Pathophysiology of spinal cord injury: recovery after immediate and delayed decompression, *J Bone Joint Surg Am* 77:1042-1049, 1995.

Farmer J et al.: Neurologic deterioration after cervical spinal cord injury, *J Spinal Disord* 11(4):192-196, 1998.

Glaser JA et al.: Variation in surgical opinion regarding management of selected cervical spine injuries: a preliminary study, *Spine* 24(9):975-983, 1998.

Marion DW: Neurologic emergencies, head and spinal cord injury, *Neurol Clin* 16:485-502, 1998.

Mirza SK et al.: Early versus delayed surgery for acute cervical spinal cord injury, *Clin Orthop* 359:104-114, 1999.

Rosenfeld JF et al.: The benefits of early decompression in cervical spinal cord injury, *Am J Orthop* 1:23-28, 1998.

Salzman SK, Betz RR: Experimental treatment of spinal cord injuries. In Betz RR, Mulcaheny MJ, eds: *The child with a spinal cord injury*, Rosemont, Ill, 1996, American Association of Orthopaedic Surgeons, p. 63.

Sonntag VKH, Francis PM: Patient selection and timing of surgery. In Benzel EC, Tator CH, eds: *Contemporary management of spinal cord injury*, Park Ridge, Ill, 1995, American Association of Neurologic Surgeons, pp. 97-108.

Surkin J et al.: Spinal cord injury incidence in Mississippi: a capture-recapture approach, *J Trauma* 45(3):502-504, 1998.

Vaccaro AR et al.: Neurologic outcome of early versus late surgery for cervical spinal cord injury, *Spine* 22(22):2609-2613, 1997.

REFERENCES

1. Attar A et al.: Early protective effects of Iloprost after experimental spinal cord injury, *Neurol Res* 20(4):353-359, 1998.
2. Belanger E, Levi AD: The acute and chronic management of spinal cord injury, *J Am Coll Surg* 190(5):603-618, 2000.
3. Bracken MB et al.: Efficacy of methylprednisolone in acute spinal injury, *JAMA* 251:45-52, 1984.
4. Bracken MB et al.: A randomized, controlled trial of methylprednisolone or naloxone in the treatment of acute spinal-cord injury, *N Engl J Med* 322:1405:1411, 1990.
5. Bracken MB et al.: Methylprednisolone or naloxone treatment after acute spinal cord injury: 1-year follow-up date—results of the Second National Acute Spinal Cord Injury Study, *J Neurosurg* 76:23-31, 1992.
6. Bracken MB et al.: Effect of timing of methylprednisolone or naloxone administration on recovery of segmental and long-tract neurological function in NASCIS 2, *J Neurosurg* 79:500-507, 1993.
7. Bracken MB et al.: Administration of methylprednisolone for 24 or 48 hours or tirilazad mesylate for 48 hours in the treatment of acute spinal cord injury: results of the Third National Acute Spinal Cord Injury randomized controlled trial, *JAMA* 277:1597-1604, 1997.
8. Bracken MB et al.: Methylprednisolone or tirilazad mesylate administration after acute spinal cord injury: 1-year follow up, *J Neurosurg* 89:699-706, 1998.
9. Campagnolo DI, Esquieres RE, Kopacz KJ: Effect of timing of stabilization on length of stay and medical complications following spinal cord injury, *J Spinal Cord Med* 20(3):331-334, 1997.
10. Carlson GD et al.: Early time-dependent decompression for spinal cord injury: vascular mechanisms of recovery, *J Neurotrauma* 14(12):951-962, 1997.
11. Delamarter RB, Coyle J: Acute management of spinal cord injury, *J Am Acad Orthop Surg* 7(3):166-175, 1999.
12. Delamarter RB, Sherman J, Carr JB: Pathophysiology of spinal cord injury: recovery after immediate and delayed decompression, *J Bone Joint Surg Am* 77:1042-1049, 1995.
13. Marion DW: Neurologic emergencies: head and spinal cord injury, *Neurol Clin* 16:485-502, 1998.
14. Mirza SK et al.: Early versus delayed surgery for acute cervical spinal cord injury, *Clin Orthop* 359:104-114, 1999.
15. Petitjean ME et al.: Medical treatment of spinal cord injury in the acute stage (French), *Ann Francaises Anesth Reanimation* 17(2):114-122, 1998.
16. Rabinowitz RS et al.: Effect of urgent decompression, decompression and methylprednisolone, and methylprednisolone alone on the outcome of spinal cord injury: a blinded prospective, randomized trial in beagles. Presented at the annual meeting of the American Academy of Orthopaedic Surgeons, paper no. 514, Feb 26, 1996.
17. Rosenfeld JF et al.: The benefits of early decompression in cervical spinal cord injury, *Am J Orthop* 1:23-28, 1998.
18. Salzman SK, Betz RR: Experimental treatment of spinal cord injuries. In Betz RR, Mulcaheny MJ, eds: *The child with a spinal cord injury*, Rosemont, Ill, 1996, American Association of Orthopaedic Surgeons, p. 63.
19. Sharma HS, Westman J, Nyberg F: Topical application of 5-HT antibodies reduces edema and cell changes following trauma of the rat spinal cord, *Acta Neurochirurg Suppl* 70:155-158, 1997.
20. Sonntag VKH, Francis PM: Patient selection and timing of surgery. In Benzel EC, Tator CH, eds: *Contemporary management of spinal cord injury*, Park Ridge, Ill, 1995, American Association of Neurologic Surgeons, pp. 97-108.
21. Surkin J et al.: Spinal cord injury incidence in Mississippi: a capture-recapture approach, *J Trauma* 45(3):502-504, 1998.
22. Vaccaro AR et al.: Neurologic outcome of early versus late surgery for cervical spinal cord injury, *Spine* 22(22):2609-2613, 1997.
23. Vale FL et al.: Combined medical and surgical treatment after acute spinal cord injury: results of a prospective pilot study to assess the merits of aggressive medical resuscitation and blood pressure management, *J Neurosurg* 87(2):239-246, 1997.
24. Winkler T et al.: Benzodiazepine receptors influence spinal cord evoked potentials and edema following trauma to the rat spinal cord, *Acta Neurochirurg Suppl* 70:216-219, 1997.

Closed Treatment of Cervical Spine Injuries

Andrew Cree, Jens R. Chapman,
Carlo Bellabarba, Sohail K. Mirza

The instinctive impulse to protect the human neck after injury by collaring it with an external supportive device has been documented since the advent of civilization. The management of cervical spine trauma has evolved rapidly beyond this perspective during the past five decades. During the past two decades in particular, substantial advances in surgical instrumentation techniques have paralleled breakthroughs in neural imaging. Meanwhile, the designation of trauma treatment that avoids surgery has changed from "conservative" to "nonoperative," implying that it is the more cumbersome and in general less appealing treatment variant. Time-honored principles of nonoperative management are now sometimes being questioned, as surgical fracture treatment offers the hope of a "quick fix." Undoubtedly, however, there remains an ongoing role for nonoperative management of cervical spine fractures, be it in the form of a brace, a halo-vest assembly, a cranial skeletal traction, or combinations thereof. Such nonoperative interventions may have a role in the initial management phase, as an adjunct to surgical stabilization, or they may represent the definitive management of cervical spine trauma.

The aim of this chapter is to delineate the current role of closed management in cervical spine trauma. Controversies continue to exist regarding virtually every area of this topic, from the method, sequence, and timing of closed reduction to the indications for halo-vest management and the duration of brace wear. Although no consensus is likely to be found in the near future, the guidelines for the use of skeletal traction and the application of cervical spine orthoses, especially the halo vest, are reviewed.

ROLES OF TRACTION AND HALO MANAGEMENT

- Acute mode of treatment
- Adjunct to surgery
- Definitive treatment

ACUTE MANAGEMENT
Field Management

The management of cervical spinal trauma begins with treatment in the field. Well-established guidelines, such as those developed by the Advanced Trauma Life Support group of the American College of Surgeons[1] for the stabilization and extrication of patients at risk of neck injury, should be followed at all times. Although cervical spine trauma is most commonly associated with motor vehicle accidents and falls, the exposed nature of the cervical spine predisposes it to a wide variety of injuries and causes. A heightened degree of suspicion should be applied in the care of polytraumatized patients or patients presenting with cognitive impairment. Risk factors for cervical spine injuries based on large-scale epidemiologic data are becoming increasingly well defined.[8,32] Initial management should include a neurologic assessment and external neck and spine immobilization, extrication, and transport. Should emergent endotracheal intubation be necessary, external neck immobilization with manual in-line traction can limit potentially dangerous neck manipulation. Suitable treatment adjuncts for on-site external neck immobilization and patient transport consist of rigid neck collars and the use of a backboard or sandbags that surround the patient's head with the head taped to the backboard.

Cervical motion was most effectively limited with the use of sandbags and forehead tape compared with a range of commercially available rigid neck collars in studies conducted on normal volunteers and cadavers. The addition of a collar to the use of sandbags and tape alone helped reduce movement in extension only. In a comparison of various collars, the Philadelphia collar was comparable to all others but provided superior protection against extension[46,51] (Figure 33-1). Regardless of the choice of immobilization, routine patient transportation is preferably performed on a spine board, with a hard collar, possibly supplemented with sandbags and forehead tape.

Pediatric patients who are transported on a conventional backboard are prone to neck flexion due to their proportionally larger head size relative to their torso

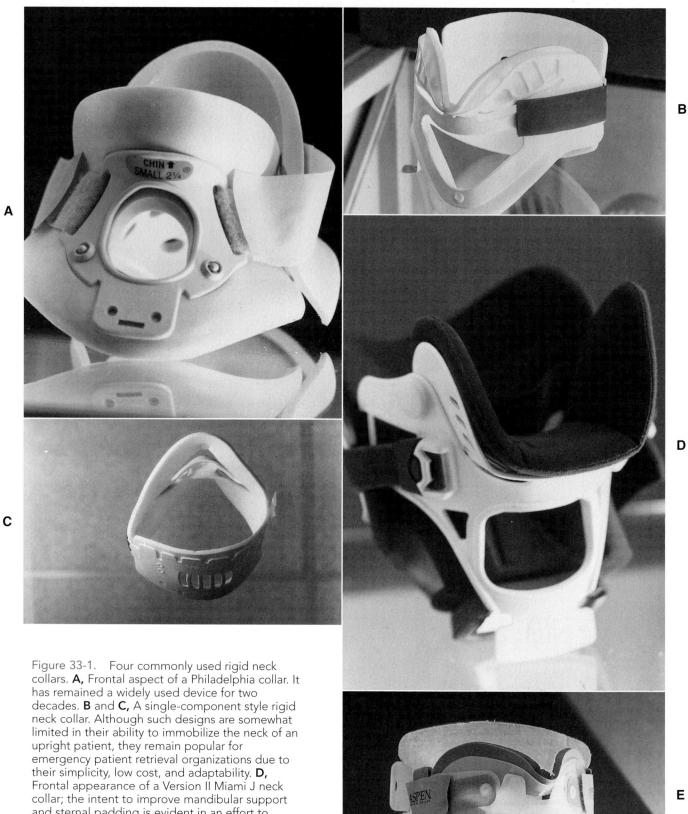

Figure 33-1. Four commonly used rigid neck collars. **A,** Frontal aspect of a Philadelphia collar. It has remained a widely used device for two decades. **B** and **C,** A single-component style rigid neck collar. Although such designs are somewhat limited in their ability to immobilize the neck of an upright patient, they remain popular for emergency patient retrieval organizations due to their simplicity, low cost, and adaptability. **D,** Frontal appearance of a Version II Miami J neck collar; the intent to improve mandibular support and sternal padding is evident in an effort to maximize external immobilization effects while minimizing focal soft tissue pressure points. **E,** Aspen collar, which has become popular for its comfort. Biomechanical studies that compared these devices offer sometimes conflicting data, depending on the individual setup.

PATIENT RETRIEVAL

- Field management
  - High degree of suspicion for cervical spine injury
  - Attention to advanced trauma life support guidelines for extrication
- Transport
  - Spine board
  - Head and neck immobilization with collar, sandbags, and tape superior to a hard collar alone
  - Occipital cutout in spine board for children to avoid excessive flexion

---

EMERGENCY DEPARTMENT MANAGEMENT

- Early recognition and treatment of cervical spine injury
- Serial neurologic examination
- Intravenous methylprednisolone for spinal cord injury
- Radiologic assessment
  - Initial lateral radiograph
  - Anteroposterior, open-mouth, swimmer's view
  - Computed tomography scan as helical screen, for poorly visualized regions, for injury determination
  - Beware of noncontiguous injury (40%)
- Prevention of further harm
  - Immobilization with collar, sandbags, or traction

---

diameter. Customized pediatric backboards, which feature an occipital recess or transport on a backboard with a folded sheet placed under the torso, can be used to avoid this phenomenon.[31]

Emergency Department Management

The emphasis at this stage of management should be the expeditious recognition, delineation, and emergency treatment of cervical spine injuries. The patient should be assessed and resuscitated using advanced trauma life support guidelines, and the appropriate sequence of investigations and treatment should be decided in conjunction with a multidisciplinary trauma team. Immobilization of the cervical spine should be continued throughout this phase. Clinical evaluation includes inspection and palpation of the entire back of the patient and neurologic assessment according to American Spinal Injury Association principles.[60] Patients with spinal cord injuries are commonly treated with high doses of intravenous methylprednisolone.[3] Determination of the radiographic needs of a patient can be made based on the specific clinical needs of a patient under sensible application of established diagnostic algorithms.[8] Increasingly, helical computed tomography (CT) scanning is used to either supplement or replace the conventional radiographic workup sequence of patients with suspected neck injuries. The role of urgent magnetic resonance imaging (MRI) for patients with neck trauma remains subject to debate. Well-accepted indications include patients with (1) a neurologic deficit unexplained with conventional radiographs and CT scans, (2) a progressive ascending neurologic deficit, or (3) an incongruous skeletal versus neurologic level of injury. Further diagnostic insights offered by MRI of the cervical spine include identification of soft tissue masses in the spinal canal, cord signal changes, and ligamentous disruption on specific images. Because MRI is commonly a time-consuming undertaking even in the most up-to-date trauma facilities, the perceived benefits of such a study obtained on an emergency basis should be weighed against possible disadvantages, such as delay of emergency treatment measures.

Skeletal Cranial Traction: Indications

In contrast to other regions of the spine, the cervical spine is amenable to realignment by nonsurgical techniques. This offers a clinician faced with a patient with a displaced cervical spine fracture and a manifest or potential spinal cord injury a chance at early and effective intervention. Manipulation of cervical spine fractures is rightly considered dangerous, but cranial traction as applied with tongs or a halo ring has a continuing role in the acute management of cervical spine trauma.

Although number of injury patterns are amenable to reduction with traction, this treatment measure is typically instituted in cases of facet joint subluxations or dislocations, as well as burst-type fractures. Certain upper cervical spine fractures, such as burst fractures of the atlas, traumatic spondylolisthesis of the axis, and odontoid fractures, are amenable to closed reduction with cranial traction as well.

Specific contraindications to cranial traction present with patients who have distractive neck injuries or certain types of skull fractures.[29,34] The presence of severe soft tissue injuries, such as scalping injuries, may preclude the safe application of cranial traction as well. The presence of any skull fracture as such does not necessarily rule out the safe application of skeletal traction. An understanding of the distribution of fracture lines and the avoidance of juxtaposition of pins and fracture regions are prerequisites if cranial tongs or a halo ring is considered for application. Lack of judicious application of cranial traction could, however, have devastating consequences, such as a depressed skull fracture or progressive dissociation of the cervical spine along with its neurovascular components (Figure 33-2).

We generally prefer spring-loaded tongs such as Gardner-Wells tongs because of their simplicity and ease of use. Under specific circumstances, primary halo application may be preferable, for example, for patients in whom a halo could be considered the definitive treatment. For pediatric patients, traction applied through multiple halo pins is usually safer and less prone to pullout than with a Gardner-Wells tong or a similar device.[40] For patients with distractive cervical spine injuries, such as atlanto-occipital dissociation, a halo ring and vest allow for a chance to maintain a closed reduction.

Skeletal Cranial Traction: Timing

Although not clearly proved, there is some evidence that rapid closed reduction may confer benefit in terms of neurologic recovery.[12,62] Because continued compression of the spinal cord can lead to further spinal cord injury

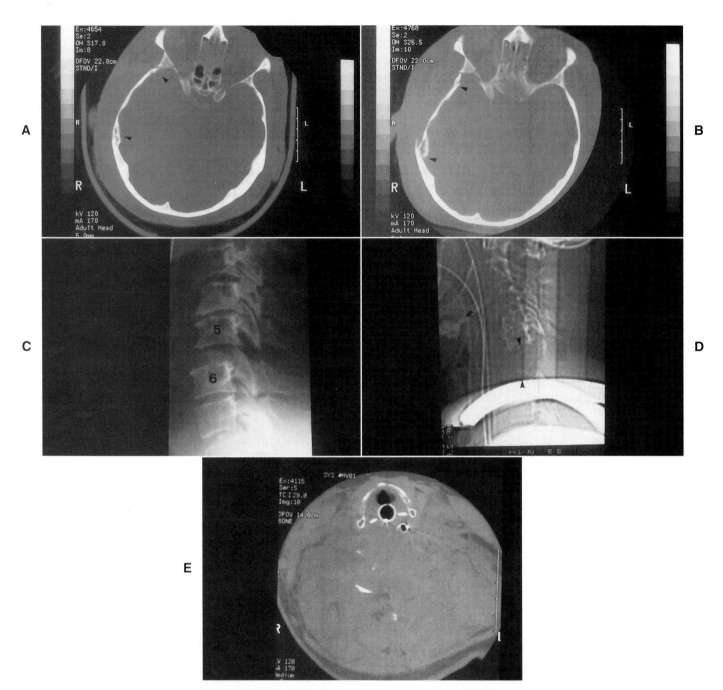

Figure 33-2. Contraindications to skeletal cranial traction. **A,** Nondisplaced parietal skull fracture on a head computed tomography scan of a polytraumatized patient with concurrent cervical spine fracture. **B,** Depression of the same skull fracture after Gardner-Wells tongs were applied to the patient's skull in an attempt to realign the cervical spine fracture. Due to seizures, the patient required a decompressive craniotomy and reconstructive surgery. It is crucial to establish or rule out the presence of skull fractures before the application of skeletal traction devices. **C,** Lateral cervical spine radiograph of a middle-aged woman who was brought to an emergency department unconscious after a high-speed motor vehicle crash. A distractive C5-on-C6 lesion can be seen on this study. The patient's neck was placed in 10 pounds of cranial traction despite the presence of this distractive lesion. **D,** On a scout film study of the head (computed tomography scan), a wide diastasis between the C5 and C6 segments can be identified. **E,** The axial view further shows the absence of any vertebrae, underscoring the presence of a profound ligamentous injury. To avoid overdistraction, before the placement of traction to the cervical spine, the presence of a distractive spine lesion should be ruled out by thoughtful analysis of the spine studies at hand and by review of sequential follow-up radiographs.

with irreversible changes manifest after 6 to 8 hours, reversal of such extrinsic cord compression by means of indirect spinal canal decompression through spinal realignment seems intuitively sensible. It is widely accepted that an early reduction effort should be undertaken in any patient with spinal cord injury in the presence of a fracture-dislocation. Controversy continues to surround the issue of timing of reduction efforts relative to obtaining diagnostic imaging tests in neurologically intact patients or patients who are cognitively impaired. Based on several case reports, the risk of neurologic deterioration after closed reduction attempts of cervical dislocations due to dislodgment of an intervertebral disc into the spinal canal became a focus of awareness. The incidence of postreduction spinal cord compromise caused by a disc herniation was estimated to range from 1.5% to 35%.[23,45,53] It therefore has been suggested that MRI be routinely obtained before attempts at reduction of a dislocated spine in patients who are neurologically intact and present in a cognitively impaired state. However, the time taken for imaging studies introduces a potentially critical delay in realigning, thereby indirectly decompressing the spinal cord.

Cotler et al. reported a series of 24 awake reductions of patients with lower cervical dislocations.[19] The procedure was found to be safe, and there were no instances of neurologic deterioration. Seventeen patients required in excess of 50 pounds of traction, up to a maximum of 140 pounds. Nine patients required manipulation as well. The same group reported on an additional series of 53 patients[61] who had a 68% incidence of neurologic improvement. There were no cases of neurologic deterioration, despite 39 patients requiring more than 50 pounds of traction.

In a prospective series of consecutive patients with lower cervical fracture dislocations, Grant et al. reported successful early closed reduction in 80 of 82 patients.[28] The average time until completion of reduction was 2.5 hours. Subsequent MRI showed an incidence of disc disruption in 24% of patients and an incidence of disc herniation in 22% of patients. In 23% of patients with unilateral facet dislocations and 13% of patients with bilateral facet dislocations, a disc herniation was found on postreduction MRI. Neurologic improvement, as assessed within 24 hours from injury, was found in 64% of patients with Frankel grade A neurologic deficits and 98% of patients with incomplete spinal cord injury. The motor score improved by 10.1 points for patients presenting with complete spinal cord injury. Patients with incomplete spinal cord injury patterns were found to have improved by 12 points. Neurologic deterioration of one motor level severity was encountered in 1 of the 82 patients several hours after successful reduction with traction. No causal connection to the reduction efforts or a mass effect could be established. Based on this experience, we therefore recommend closed reduction using an established traction protocol for all patients with lower cervical spine fracture-dislocations.

Vaccaro et al. prospectively studied 11 patients with cervical spine dislocation with MRI before and after closed reduction and identified no neurologic deteriora-

---

ROLE OF MAGNETIC RESONANCE IMAGING IN EARLY MANAGEMENT OF CERVICAL SPINE TRAUMA

- Advantages
  - Identification of spinal cord compression
  - Signal changes in spinal cord (prognosis)
  - Soft tissue injuries: ligaments/disc
- Disadvantages
  - Time consuming
  - Manipulation of unstable injured spinal column during transfers
  - Contraindicated if hemodynamically unstable
  - Decreased patient monitoring during scan
  - Delay of treatment of other life-threatening injuries
  - Difficult to have around-the-clock availability
- Common indications
  - Safely performed after urgent reduction of the dislocated cervical spine in neurologically impaired patients

---

tion in their series. They concluded that early reduction before MRI was safe and recommended it as the optimal early approach to cervical spine trauma.[65] Although these two recent studies concurrently identify the safety and efficacy of early cervical spine reduction in general, individual circumstances such as the specific hospital infrastructure and patient factors have to be taken into account. Unnecessary delays of reduction of lower cervical fracture dislocations due to the unavailability of MRI should be avoided, however (Figure 33-3).

Skeletal Cranial Traction: Technique

Essential prerequisites for closed cervical reduction are appropriate fluoroscopic facilities, equipment, and personnel skilled in the techniques of reduction. Ideally, anesthesiology and operating room services should also be available to deal with the potential complications of this procedure. In the event of neurologic deterioration, rapid transfer to an MRI machine and subsequent surgery should be within the capabilities of the institution. In the rural setting, decisions about timing of reduction should be made jointly between the referring and receiving physicians. The decision will depend on the nature of the injury, the presence of a neurologic deficit, the experience level of the referring physician, and logistic concerns in each case.

A patient has to be assessed for suitability of cranial traction reduction by a physician who is experienced in closed reduction of the cervical spine. After completion of the initial assessment and resuscitation, the patient is transported to the fluoroscopy suite in the emergency department. Preferably, the patient is awake and responsive and is positioned supine on a conventional trauma gurney fitted with a pulley and rack at its head-end. The patient should not be on a backboard, to avoid skin breakdown. An interscapular folded sheet or towel should be placed to allow for improved head positioning. Both shoulders should then be taped to the foot-end of

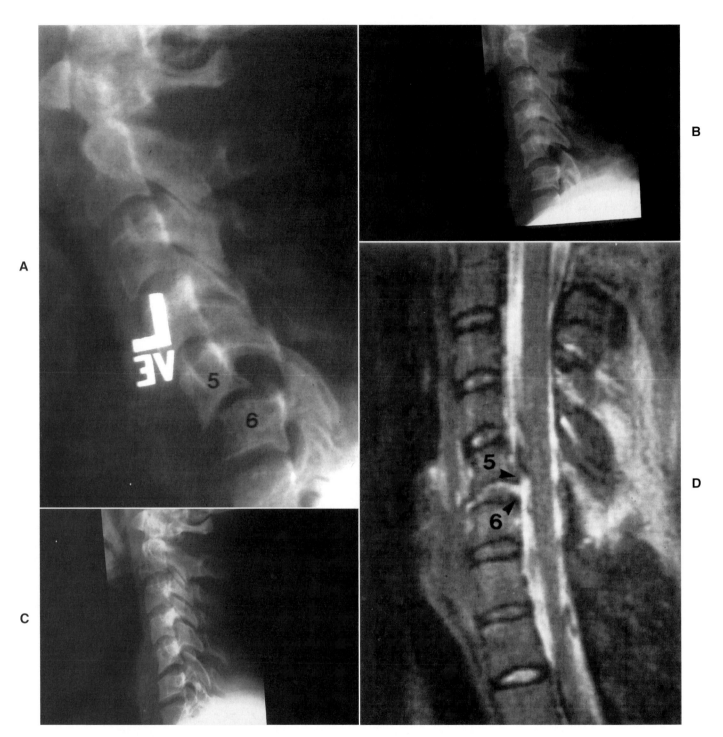

Figure 33-3. Closed reduction of facet dislocation. The lateral cervical spine radiograph of a 29-year-old man who presented after a motorcycle crash demonstrates a bilateral C5 to C6 facet dislocation. Aside from hyperreflexia in both upper and lower extremities, as well as elbow flexor weakness, the patient had no neurologic deficits. **A** and **B,** Successful reengagement of the facet joints at 80 pounds of traction, using the sequential cervical traction technique described by Grant et al.[28] At this point, the traction beam was lowered to a horizontal trajectory, and the weight was lowered to 20 pounds. **C,** The lateral cervical radiograph obtained after this correction shows nearly anatomic realignment and correction of kyphosis. **D,** A postreduction magnetic resonance image identified no mass effect on the spinal cord. Later, the patient received successful nonemergent cervical fusion.

the gurney under gentle traction to optimize radiographic spinal visualization and to prevent cranial migration of the patient during traction. The patient may also be temporarily placed in a reverse Trendelenburg position to prevent cranial sliding of the patient as larger weights are placed.

To make closed reduction as expedient as possible, the patient should receive intravenous analgesia and muscle relaxation with automated vital sign and oxygenation sensors that allow for continuous monitoring. Throughout the reduction efforts, the patient should preferably remain responsive and amenable to questioning and examination. The patient is asked to notify the physician immediately if any sensory or motor changes are noticed. Interval reexamination of both upper and lower extremities is performed between each increment of traction.

A baseline lateral fluoroscopic radiograph should be printed out for future comparison and to ensure adequate visualization of the lower cervical spine. For the short-term placement of Gardner-Wells tongs, shaving of the skull is not required. The intended pin placement site is then disinfected and anesthetized locally with subcutaneous and pericranial infiltration using a suitable local anesthetic. A sterile set of Gardner-Wells tongs is placed a fingerbreadth above the pinna of the ear, in line with the external auditory meatus. This point should be below the equator of the skull, which helps resist proximal migration of the pins. The pins are tightened simultaneously until resistance is felt and the spring indicator protrudes. Placement posterior to this position will provide a flexion moment, and anterior placement will provide an extension moment. This may be performed deliberately, to aid in the reduction of certain injury patterns or to assist in the maintenance of a reduction. However, neutral pin placement in an axial position is usually preferable. Flexion and extension of the head can then be varied by adjusting the height of the traction pulley and by placing pads under the patient's head.

It should be noted that stainless steel Gardner-Wells tongs have been found to pull out at 300 pounds in cadaver bone, whereas newer graphite/titanium materials failed at 75 pounds.[10] In addition, tongs show lower pullout strength after repeated use. Lerman et al. compared pullout strengths in a skull model with the use of a halo and new or used Gardner-Wells tongs. The pullout strength of the halo was 440 ± 37 pounds, and the pullout strengths of the tongs were 233 ± 49 pounds for new tongs, 185 ± 40 pounds for slightly used tongs, and 109 ± 10 pounds for heavily used tongs.[39] Lower pullout strength was attributed to spring or pin wear. If large reduction weights are anticipated, either a relatively new set of tongs, made from stainless steel, or a halo should be used.

At the commencement of the reduction, 10 pounds of traction weight is applied in an axial direction. Clinical reevaluation is then performed, followed by repeat fluoroscopic radiographs. It is crucial to rule out overdistraction of an occult cervical ligamentous injury on these early traction radiographs. In general, distraction efforts should be abandoned if widening of intervertebral interspace beyond 1.5 mm from baseline radiographs is encountered anywhere in the cervical spine. Weights are then increased in increments of 5 to 10 pounds, depending on the patient's size and injury type. After each weight change, fluoroscopic images are obtained and a neurologic

---

ACUTE CLOSED REDUCTION

- Indications
  - Facet fracture subluxation/dislocation
  - Burst fracture with canal compromise
- Contraindications
  - Most skull fractures
  - Severe local soft tissue trauma
  - Distractive ligamentous injury
- Timing
  - Within 2 hours of presentation
  - Reduction before magnetic resonance imaging in the awake, cooperative patient
  - Reduction in cognitively impaired patient before magnetic resonance imaging remains controversial
- Findings
  - Urgent reduction in emergency department with fluoroscopy safe and effective (98%)
  - Disc herniation
    - Bilateral facet dislocations: 13%
    - Unilateral facet dislocations: 23%

TECHNIQUE OF CLOSED REDUCTION WITH SKULL TRACTION

- Setup
  - Expert personnel
  - Fluoroscopy suite
  - Positioning with shoulder straps
  - Analgesia/sedation
  - Comprehensive monitoring
  - Local disinfectant, anesthetic
- Gardner-Wells tongs
  - 1 cm superior to pinna in line with external auditory meatus
  - Fingerbreadth above ear
  - Graphite tongs for routine care
  - Check for proper assembly
  - Use new stainless steel tongs if high weights anticipated (rare)
- Ten pounds of initial axial traction
  - Increase in 5- to 10-pound increments every 5 to 10 minutes
  - Neurologic and radiologic assessment at each step
  - Weights up to 140 pounds may be required
  - Flexion or extension moment by raising traction pulley, suboccipital or interscapular pad
- Cease if
  - Neurologic deficit; transfer to magnetic resonance imaging suite/operating room
  - Mechanical block
  - Greater than 1-cm distraction at injury level
- After reduction
  - Decrease weight to 20 pounds, and place towel in interscapular region to maintain neck in extension for most injury patterns

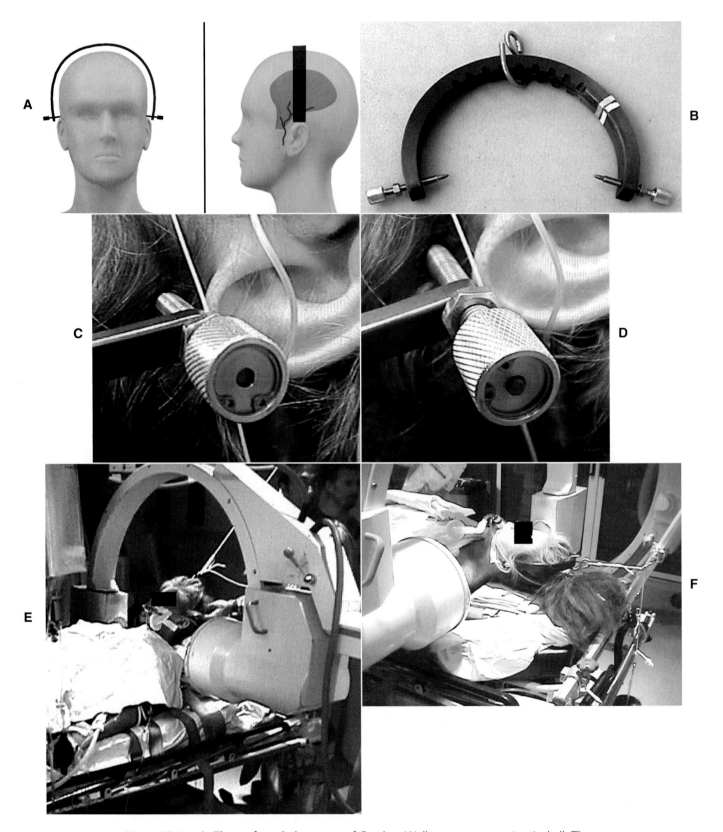

Figure 33-4. **A,** The preferred placement of Gardner-Wells tongs on a patient's skull. The presence of a skull fracture and distractive cervical spine lesion should be ruled out before the placement of such a device. **B,** Gardner-Wells tongs, showing the placement of a spring-loaded threaded bolt on one side *(X)* and, contralaterally, a conventional solid threaded bolt. **C,** Demonstrates the spring-loaded bolt with the indicator pin in retracted position. **D,** The pin has emerged by 2 mm, identifying correct loading pressure. **E,** Application of Gardner-Wells tongs in a patient using a flexion-type trajectory. **F,** The traction beam has been lowered after successful reduction of a cervical dislocation.

examination is performed. For patients with facet dislocation of the lower cervical spine, it is frequently helpful to raise the level of the pulley bar above the patient's head to disengage the facet joints (Figure 33-4, *C* and *D*).

On achieving reduction of the cervical spine, the head position is dropped into a neutral or slightly extended position. Hyperextension, however, should be avoided because it can lead to central spinal conal occlusion. The traction weight is reduced to 10 or 20 pounds. A repeat radiograph should now be obtained to confirm maintenance of the reduction. At this time, postreduction MRI and CT can be obtained to complete the diagnostic component of the cervical spine injury management. Should neurologic deterioration, overdistraction, or mechanical blockage of the reduction become apparent, closed reduction efforts should be abandoned in favor of emergency MRI and possibly CT as well as consideration for early open surgical reduction and internal fixation. In general, the medical literature does not support the use of manipulation for reducing fracture dislocations of the cervical spine (Figure 33-5).

Skeletal Cranial Traction: Limitations

In certain circumstances, it may not be appropriate to contemplate a closed reduction in the emergency department or, in fact, such a reduction may not be successful. If the goal of realigning the spinal canal and thus indirectly decompressing the spinal cord has not been met, urgent surgical intervention should be considered.

Manipulation of the dislocated cervical spine by means of gentle rotational force while cranial traction is applied has been occasionally reported. This technique should probably be left to very experienced spine surgeons and is not recommended for routine use.

Reasons for abandonment of closed reduction efforts also include an increasing neurologic deficit either before or during the reduction. Similarly, if the reduction is not successful with weights of 150 pounds or if excessive distraction at the injury site or elsewhere is identified, conversion to open reduction should be contemplated. Prolonged traction with large weights is not desirable due to a high likelihood of pin tract complications with either Gardner-Wells tongs or halo ring skeletal traction.

The issue of timing of reduction in cognitively impaired patients remains somewhat unresolved to date. Valuable real-time neurologic monitoring during closed reduction efforts as provided by serial examinations and patient feedback is limited or absent in such circumstances. A cautious approach with prereduction MRI therefore has been recommended.[23,45] Based on the more recent studies on this subject, it appears to be safe to proceed with closed reduction efforts even in cognitively impaired patients. Due to many variables among patients and hospital infrastructure, an individualized approach that maintains the basic treatment tents appears reasonable. Finally, if a neurologically impaired patient is shown to have residual spinal cord compression on postreduction MRI, early surgical decompression and stabilization should be considered (Figure 33-6).

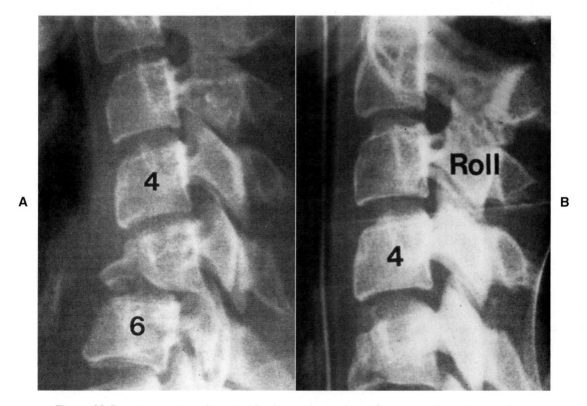

Figure 33-5. Restoration of cervical lordosis. The C5 burst fracture in this patient with incomplete spinal cord injury **(A)** was effectively realigned with 35 pounds of traction and placement of a folded towel under the neck **(B).** Care should, be taken, however, to avoid hyperextension of the cervical spine, because this has been shown to lead to a reduction in spinal canal volume.

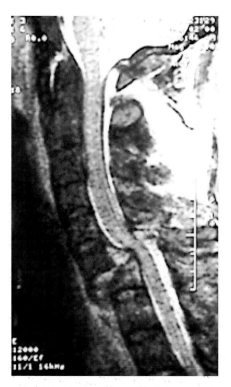

Figure 33-6. Magnetic resonance image showing a patient with complete cord injury at C4 level. The image was obtained before reduction due to the neurologic level of injury being higher than the injury, which consisted of a C5 to C6 bilateral facet dislocation. The image shows a large traumatic disc herniation protruding into the cervical spinal cord and cord signal changes extending rostrally well beyond the region of injury.

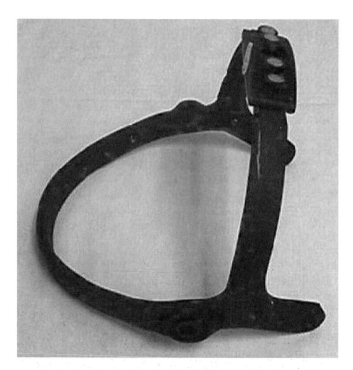

Figure 33-7. Halo ring with integrated transverse bar for traction. This device is suitable for patients with anticipated long-term traction. It easily can be converted for use with a conventional halo-vest assembly. Most manufacturers of halo rings provide a detachable traction bar that is secured to a halo ring with bolts.

INDICATIONS FOR URGENT SURGERY

- Increasing neurologic deficit due to mechanical compression
- Unsuccessful reduction
- Residual compression seen on magnetic resonance imaging in patient with neurologic deficit

---

RECUMBENT IMMOBILIZATION

- Cranial tong traction
  - Simple application
  - Long-term complication rate high
  - Roto Rest bed
  - Pulmonary toilet
  - Deep vein thrombosis prophylaxis
  - Decubitus prophylaxis
  - Repeat alignment assessment (radiographs)
- Halo traction
  - Easy conversion to halo vest
  - Controls head flexion and extension
  - Easily attachable to operating table
- Halo vest
  - "Portable traction"
  - Recumbent or partial mobilization options

DEFINITIVE MANAGEMENT
Skeletal Traction and Recumbent Treatment

Any form of nonoperative management of spinal trauma constitutes an attempt to counteract the forces of gravity as imposed on an upright skeleton while maintaining the best possible fracture alignment. In recognition of this fact, recumbent treatment has remained one of the oldest and simplest forms of spinal trauma management. In the cervical spine, the addition of judiciously applied skeletal traction adds the potential to correct traumatically induced malalignment by virtue of ligamentotaxis. Such traction may be applied with either a halo or tongs; although tongs are generally preferred in

the early stages of management, the halo confers advantages in its easy conversion to a halo vest. The halo also provides superior fixation to tongs, especially in the control of head flexion and extension (Figure 33-7). A desirable side effect of cranial traction is the very visible implied signal that the patient in question has an unstable spine injury, thereby minimizing the risk of inappropriate handling.[15]

Prolonged recumbent management for trauma indications has become increasingly unpopular due to a variety of issues. Medical concerns include thromboembolic events, pulmonary compromise such as pneumonia, decubital skin breakdown, pin tract infections, sepsis, and psychologic deterioration. Social issues are associated with the need for prolonged skilled nursing care, universally limited availability of suitable care sites, and usually significantly higher costs of care for cervical spine patients treated with this method. The benefits of rapid mobilization have become quite evident in the care of polytraumatized patients and are emerging as a desirable treatment element for elderly patients with cervical spine injuries.[2,47,56] For patients with certain isolated unstable cervical spine injuries, prolonged recumbence traction may, however, avoid the risks of potentially complex surgical procedures and loss of function due to lengthy fusion. In pediatric patients, nonoperative management can avoid growth arrest potentially caused by spinal surgery. Examples of unstable cervical injuries that can be effectively reduced with cranial traction are burst fractures, especially of the atlas; displaced forms of traumatic spondylolisthesis of the axis, such as the high-grade type II and IIa injuries; and odontoid fractures. Premature attempts at mobilization using brace or halo-vest immobilization of patients with such injuries is frequently accompanied by loss of reduction. Under such circumstances, prolonged recumbent traction is usually recommended for anywhere from 3 to 12 weeks. The end point in this phase of treatment is somewhat empiric but can be determined by reviewing upright radiographs at certain intervals, such as every 3 weeks. Stability concerns will then dictate the form of immobilization that is chosen after the conclusion of recumbent treatment[15] (Figure 33-8).

Principles of successful prolonged traction treatment involve rigorous attention to daily pin site care and the avoidance of pressure sores, especially about the sacrum and occiput, with skilled nursing care and the use of special traction beds such as the Roto Rest bed. Such an appliance can minimize the occurrence of dependent edema formation and pulmonary atelectasis. Vigilance for respiratory and urinary tract complications should be maintained throughout. Thromboembolism prophylaxis monitored by interval screening tests is a crucial component of this form of treatment to avoid potentially fatal complications. Adequate nutritional intake should similarly be monitored. Serial lateral cervical spine radiographs are required to assess the maintenance of an adequate reduction. Overdistraction as a function of progressive soft tissue relaxation effected by a continuous pulling force has to be taken into consideration, and adjustments to the traction force may have to be made.[29] It seems appropriate to involve any patient capable of decision making in the risks and implications of prolonged nonoperative treatment (see Figure 33-8).

Cervical Braces: Indications and Biomechanics

Various designs intended for external immobilization of the cervical spine are available. Johnson et al. described

---

LONG-TERM RECUMBENT CERVICAL TRACTION TREATMENT

- Advantages
  - Maintains fracture reduction via ligamentotaxis
  - Avoids fusions in complex fractures
  - Conversion to halo vest after initial fracture consolidation (range, 3 to 12 weeks; average, 4 to 6 weeks)
- Disadvantages
  - Lengthy high-intensity care (3 to 12 weeks)
  - Limited availability of qualified nursing care
  - Need for anticoagulation
  - Respiratory, urinary, and cutaneous complications frequent
  - High hospital cost
  - Uncertainty of treatment success after lengthy treatment course
  - Patient tolerance low

SKELETAL TRACTION: RELATIVE CONTRAINDICATIONS

- Patient factors
  - Elderly
  - Confused, intoxicated
  - Insensate
  - Comorbidity: Polytrauma, pulmonary compromise, cranial defects, dependent soft tissue lesions
- Injury pattern
  - Distractive injuries

CHOICE OF EXTERNAL IMMOBILIZATION

- Collars
  - Triage
  - Stable injuries
  - Stable postoperative spine
- Cervicothoracic orthosis
  - Relatively stable lower cervical spine injuries
  - Cervicothoracic injuries
  - Questionable fixation in postoperative patient
- Halo
  - Realignment of fracture
  - Unstable bony injuries
  - Best possible external immobilization required

---

four categories of such orthoses: (1) the collar, which can be made from various materials; (2) a poster brace, which includes mandibular and occipital pads connected to the torso by either two or four metal struts; (3) cervicothoracic orthoses, which differ from the poster braces by having metal connections between the anterior and posterior parts of the brace around the torso; and (4) the halo vest.[35]

In general, cervical orthoses such as the Necloc, Philadelphia, Miami J, and Stifneck collars are used either

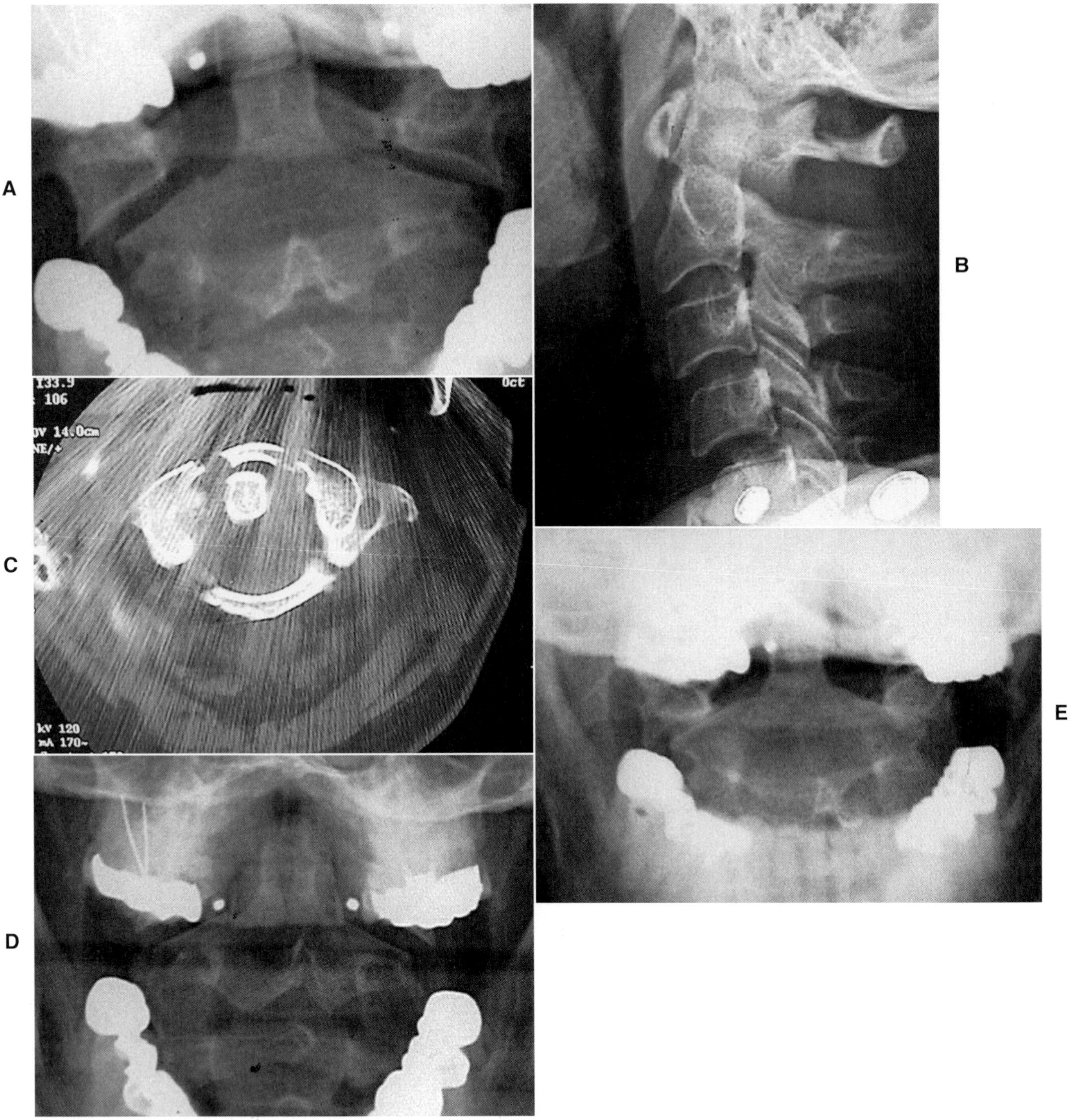

Figure 33-8. Treatment of unstable Jefferson fracture with prolonged traction. **A** to **C,** Open-mouth odontoid view, lateral cervical spine view, and axial computed tomography scan of a 54-year-old patient with unstable four-part atlas fracture. This neurologically intact patient had sustained this injury as a result of a fall from a balcony as an isolated injury. Based on the displacement of the open mouth odontoid view **(A)**, traumatic disruption of the transverse atlantal ligament was suspected. Initial reduction with Gardner-Wells tongs **(D)** could not be maintained with the patient placed in a halo-and-vest assembly despite multiple repeat manipulations **(E)**. The patient refused surgical treatment options, such as an atlantoaxial fusion. After returning into halo traction, the lateral masses of the atlas could be reduced successfully. The patient was mobilized after 2 weeks in a halo vest, with recurrent loss of reduction prompting return to cranial traction with the patient immobilized in a Roto Rest bed until week 8 of traction was completed. The patient remained in her halo vest for 8 additional weeks after recumbent traction. On completion of 4 months of immobilization from the time of injury, stable healing of the upper cervical spine was noted on flexion-extension radiographs **(F** and **G)**. The patient retained 45 degrees of lateral head rotation, despite having experienced partial loss of reduction on her final open-mouth odontoid radiograph, which was obtained 1 year after her injury **(H)**. The patient remains pain free and content with her choice of having avoided surgery.

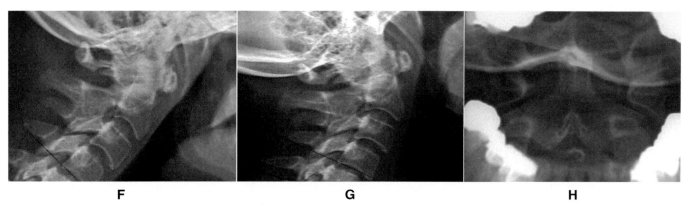

F
G
H

Figure 33-8, cont'd.

for the acute triage and resuscitation phase or in the postoperative period (see Figure 33-1). Some benign injuries, in which stability is not a concern, may be treated with simple cervical orthoses. They offer the patient comfort and proprioceptive feedback. Cervicothoracic orthoses offer more rigidity, especially in flexion and extension but less so in lateral bending and rotation. They are most useful in the management of injuries to the lower cervical spine. The halo vest remains the orthosis of choice when rigid immobilization of an unstable cervical spine injury is required. The phenomenon of "snaking" is an inherent limitation of all orthoses.[33] This pathologic motion is caused by the multisegmental and inherently mobile cervical spine being relatively fixed at either ends of an orthosis while allowing for flexion and adjacent level hyperextension to occur at its intercalary segments.

Results of biomechanical testing of the ability of external support devices to immobilize the cervical spine have been confusing and contradictory. There is little disagreement about the role of the soft neck collar. From a biomechanical perspective, it offers very little structural support to the cervical spine. Its use is mainly aimed at providing comfort from muscle spasms in the presence of an otherwise stable neck sprain or as an adjunct in a surgically stabilized patient. Johnson et al. compared the range of motion allowed by the four different device categories in 44 normal volunteers. They found the Philadelphia to be superior to the Necloc or Stifneck in preventing sagittal translation or rotation.[35] In contrast, Askins and Eismont and Eismont et al. performed a clinical study in normal volunteers and found the Necloc, followed by the Miami J, to be the most efficacious of five collars tested.[5,23] Hughes found that the Aspen collar reduced flexion to 31.5%, lateral bending to 51.1%, and rotation to 41% of normal levels in healthy volunteers.[33] Unfortunately, most studies have been in small groups of normal volunteers and may not reflect the pathologic situation.

Class 2 poster braces and class 3 cervicothoracic braces limit the amount of pivoting permitted by a conventional neck collar by incorporating the upper torso

into the brace construct. Overall, the cervicothoracic brace appears to be the most effective of these other orthoses. In the study of Johnson et al., the brace allowed 12.8% of flexion and extension, followed in order by the four-poster brace (20.6%), the Sterno-Occipito-Mandibular Immobilizer (SOMI) (27.7%), the Philadelphia collar (28.9%), and the soft collar (74.2%).[35] None of the conventional orthoses allowed less than half the normal range of lateral bending. Other points of note were that the cervicothoracic and SOMI braces were relatively effective in the lower cervical spine but that the SOMI was ineffective in limiting extension. The authors concluded that increasing the length and rigidity of an orthosis improved its efficacy (Figure 33-9). None of the conventional orthoses controlled lateral bending or rotation at any level or restricted flexion-extension in the upper cervical spine. More recently, Sharpe et al. assessed the use of a cervicothoracic brace and found that with or without an occipital flare and forehead strap, it did not control upper cervical spine motion well. However, such additions to the brace improved its rigidity in the lower cervical spine.[59] Benzel et al. assessed the use of a thermoplastic Minerva body jacket in a series of 155 patients and found good efficacy. In a motion segment unit study in 18 patients, superior immobilization was found with this device at the middle and lower cervical spine compared with published data for the halo. The authors advocated its use for most middle and lower cervical spine injuries.[7]

It appears reasonable to summarize from these data that orthotic devices have many inherent shortcomings and offer limited absolute immobilization of the cervical spine. For clinical purposes, however, complete stabilization of the cervical spine is frequently unnecessary. Awareness of the inherent limitations of braces and realistic expectations of their potential are essential for the treating physician. In principle, class 1 devices appear suitable for the treatment of soft tissue sprains; stable minor fractures, and most postoperative immobilization needs. Class 3 devices are suitable for the treatment of patients with relatively stable lower cervical or upper

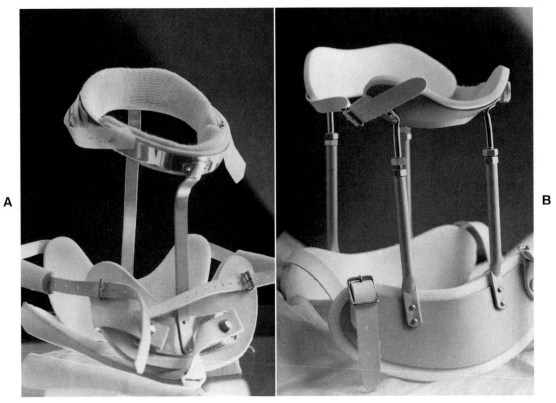

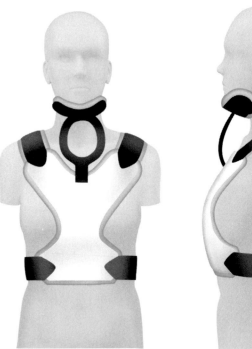

Figure 33-9.   Cervicothoracic braces. **A,** Variant of a SOMI-type brace, which predominantly relies on sternal contact with a shallow upper torso brace and close occipital and mandibular contact. **B,** An example of a four-poster brace. This type of brace offers some improvement of cervicothoracic stability by offering four upright bars, which do not obstruct radiographs. Both brace types are limited by poor torso purchase, which impairs immobilization, especially in larger patients. **C,** The Minerva brace has a more sizable torso plate while maintaining similar cranial attachments to the four-poster and SOMI-type braces.

thoracic fractures and for postoperative immobilization of patients with compromised bone quality. Important prerequisites of brace wear on the part of the patient are compliance, absence of major open wounds in the area covered by the brace, and an intact mandible as well as a pain-free temporomandibular joint. The most common complication associated with brace wear is the develop-

ment of occipital decubital ulcers, which is predominantly encountered in patients with head injuries and in the elderly population. Unfortunately, there are no simple answers to avoid this complication. Positional changes, regular inspection of soft tissues, and occasional substitution with other devices are helpful in the avoidance of skin breakdown.

HALO-VEST MANAGEMENT
Historical Background and Indications

Perry and Nickel described the use of a halo attached to a plaster body jacket for cervical immobilization for patients with poliomyelitis in 1959.[49] Before this, Bloom used a similar device during World War II to manage facial trauma in Air Force pilots. Blount attached the halo to a Milwaukee brace. Although this was unsuccessful, the halo vest rapidly evolved to be attached to a plastic vest with a sheepskin lining and has remained largely unchanged during the past 20 years.[9]

The halo continues to have a valuable role in the acute and definitive management of cervical spine trauma. In the acute phase, it allows ease of nursing and completion of the diagnostic workup of other injuries, whereas skeletal traction is often cumbersome. Beyond the immediate management, its benefits include superior immobilization over other forms of bracing, shorter hospitalization, fewer skin complications, and greater ease of access to wounds, and it leaves the mandible free for eating and chewing. It is also a useful adjunct to surgery, especially in the elderly or osteoporotic patient, in whom the quality of fixation may be suboptimal, or in the management of noncontiguous injuries. With the advent of polypropylene vests with a sheepskin or synthetic lining, patient wear comfort has been increased and the vest can be retightened easily. Variable position struts allow alteration of alignment and fracture reduction, while still allowing for the completion of adequate radiographs. The availability of newer materials such as aluminum, titanium, and graphite permit the use of MRI in such patients. Last, it confers some socioeconomic benefit in that it is a relatively cheap treatment modality and allows early discharge from the hospital. The psychologic impact of such treatment may be reduced by the availability of lower-profile halo design and is offset by the patient's ability to be mobilized early and to participate in a greater range of activities.

The benefits of the halo over the other orthoses include increased rigidity and more exact positioning of the injured cervical spine. Although cumbersome, they avoid direct pressure on the soft tissues of the chin and occiput, which are often injured in such patients; the halo also leaves the mandible free to allow for eating.

In general, halo-vest management is indicated in the unstable or potentially unstable cervical or upper thoracic spine in a patient who is not considered a surgical candidate. Although the halo vest confers superior stability compared with other braces, the morbidity associated with this device necessitates a clear understanding of indications and limitations of this device.

Components

The modern halo vest has evolved somewhat from the plaster of Paris and stainless steel version of Perry and Nickel.[49] The basic construct, however, has not changed significantly over time. In principle, a halo ring is attached with a number of pins to the skull. The ring is then attached to a body-conforming vest via connecting struts. Because many patients with cervical spine trauma require neuroimaging tests at various stages in their

---

HALO-VEST MANAGEMENT

- Role
  - Emergent reduction aid (distractive injuries)
  - Definitive treatment
  - Adjunct to surgery
- Benefits
  - Stiffest form of external immobilization
  - Short hospitalization period
  - Fewer skin complications
  - Ease of access to wounds
  - Leaves mandible free for eating
  - No temporomandibular joint impingement

---

management, MRI-compatible, nonferrous materials, which do not conduct electricity, should be used. To date, the most successful materials have been aluminum or carbon/graphite composites with plastic joints.

The halo vest should be lightweight, effective, and durable. It can be made of plaster of Paris, Fiberglas, or polyethylene. A more rigid fit is provided with the use of Fiberglas,[64] but it is labor intensive to apply, it cannot be removed quickly in the event of cardiopulmonary arrest, the underlying skin cannot be inspected, and the vest cannot be retightened. Because spine-injured patients typically lose considerable weight early, they would need at least one reapplication of the fiberglas vest. For this reason, the lightweight plastic vests are usually favored. They are more comfortable, durable, and adjustable. Most commercially available vests extend from the shoulders to the iliac crests, with cutouts for the arms and the breasts.[68] They are usually provided as detachable anterior and posterior halves. A range of sizes to accommodate extra large and pediatric patient dimensions should be available.

The uprights are typically four in number. It is preferable that they be low profile and be capable of multiplanar adjustment. They should be attached with interdigitating connectors, which provide for an increased stability. To avoid superimposition of radiographs, the uprights should be positioned away from the direct lateral or anteroposterior plane.

The halo ring is typically circular, but rings with an occipital cutout are easier to apply and help prevent inadvertent flexion through contact with the bed. The halo ring should be lightweight and should have multiple holes available to enable appropriate pin placement. The holes should be oval, with an independent locking mechanism, so that the pin placement is dictated by the patient's skull anatomy and not by the ring itself. This setup aids in placement of the pins perpendicular to the patient's skull. Ideally, the halo ring is placed in a distance of one to three fingerbreaths from the patient's skull. Hence, a variety of ring sizes should be available.

The pins are typically made of stainless steel or titanium. The pins should have a shoulder to help prevent skull penetration and should be placed with a torque screwdriver. Currently, a replacement for titanium pins, with low-electron-density materials, is being sought to increase CT and MRI compatibility[17] (Figure 33-10).

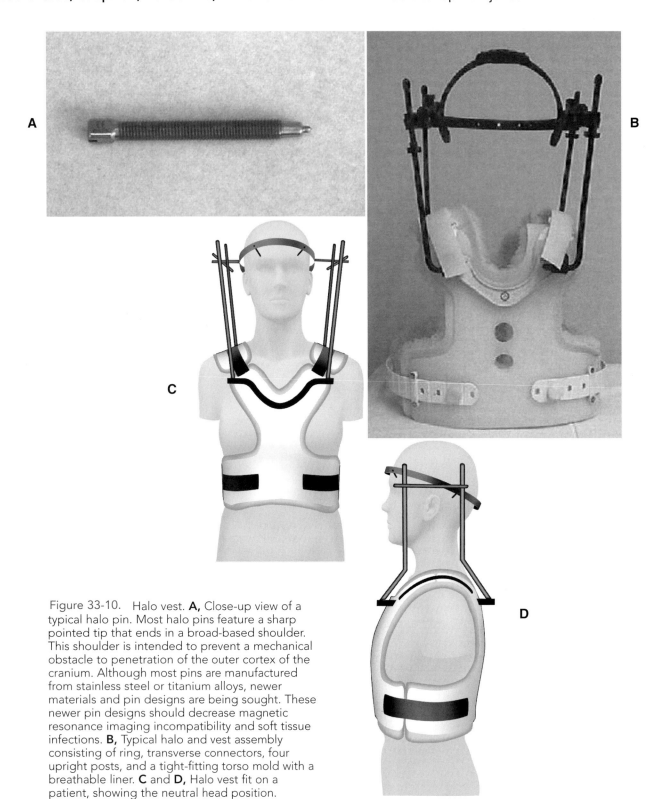

Figure 33-10.   Halo vest. **A,** Close-up view of a typical halo pin. Most halo pins feature a sharp pointed tip that ends in a broad-based shoulder. This shoulder is intended to prevent a mechanical obstacle to penetration of the outer cortex of the cranium. Although most pins are manufactured from stainless steel or titanium alloys, newer materials and pin designs are being sought. These newer pin designs should decrease magnetic resonance imaging incompatibility and soft tissue infections. **B,** Typical halo and vest assembly consisting of ring, transverse connectors, four upright posts, and a tight-fitting torso mold with a breathable liner. **C** and **D,** Halo vest fit on a patient, showing the neutral head position.

Biomechanical Aspects

The halo vest has been extensively investigated, but replication of the injury situation in experimental studies remains difficult. The halo vest provides remains, despite all of its limitations, the most effective form of external immobilization and is superior to other braces around the upper cervical spine.

Its efficacy is dependent on a firm fixation to the skull and to the torso. Independent of the snugness of fit at its cranial and caudal interfaces, "snaking" of the middle of the cervical spine still tends to occur.

Johnson et al. compared the halo vest with a Philadelphia, four-poster, cervicothoracic, and SOMI brace, using radiographs and photographs.[35] There was

HALO COMPONENTS

- Inventory
  - Availability of range of sizes
  - Range: Pediatric to extra large
- Vest
  - Adjustable, durable, and comfortable
  - Plastic with synthetic or sheepskin lining
  - Fiberglas more rigid, but cumbersome and usually requires reapplication
- Uprights
  - Low profile
  - Anodized coating
  - Multiplanar adjustability
  - Interdigitating connections
- Ring
  - Compatible with magnetic resonance imaging
  - Circular or occipital cutout
  - Lightweight
  - Multiple oval holes to allow placement of pins perpendicular to skull
- Pins
  - Magnetic resonance imaging compatibility preferable
  - Stainless steel or titanium
  - Sharp tip with broad shoulder to prevent dural penetration
  - Torque applicator or screwdriver available

HALO-VEST BIOMECHANICS IN COMPARISON

- More rigid, especially in upper cervical spine
- Restricts up to 75% flexion-extension motion at C1 to C2
- Superior control of lateral bending and rotation

75% restriction of atlantoaxial motion with the halo in a group of injured patients, but paradoxically, there was increased motion at the craniocervical junction. Although this study remains the most comprehensive comparison of external immobilization methods, the motion segment values in the halo group may have been altered by surgery, as five of the seven patients had a fusion performed.[35]

Lind et al. studied 31 patients with cervical spine injuries by using lateral radiographs in various positions. Strain gauges were attached to the uprights in the final 20 patients in the series. They found a mean motion of 51 degrees, which is 70% of normal.[43] The halo restricted motion best below C2 and poorly above it. There was a distraction force when the patient was supine. This was increased in shoulder shrug and arm exercises and decreased in sitting and standing. There was a positive correlation between supine distraction force and maximal cervical motion. This study was useful in showing the large variation in forces generated in the halo vest when the patient adopts different positions. It also contradicted the belief that distraction in a halo vest served to restrict cervical motion.

Relatively extensive cervical motion with everyday brace wear has been demonstrated in other studies as well. Depending on the experimental technique used, there is a large variation in the amount of cervical motion found in activities of daily living, ranging from 4%[35] to 31%[36] and up to 70%.[44] Walker et al. attached strain gauges to the apparatus and found that the forces were generated by the weight of the head and through distortion of the vest by the pushing effect of the abdomen,

arms, and shoulders. The largest forces were generated while seated or reaching sideways while lying. The amount of segmental motion decreases from the occipitocervical junction caudally.[67] Considerable distractive forces between the shoulders and halo are generated, especially with coughing, deep breathing, and shrugging of the shoulders.[36,44] It was hoped that the distractive forces between the shoulders and the halo would confer stability, but there is a positive correlation between the amount of distractive forces and the amount of cervical motion. Likewise, anteroposterior and mediolateral forces are similar in magnitude to the distractive-compressive forces, and this contributes to the loss of alignment in clinical series. Koch and Nickel and Lind et al. both documented that distractive forces were present in the supine position but became compressive forces in the erect position.[36,44]

There has been a general trend in recent years to make halo wear more attractive by decreasing the size of the body vests. Mirza et al. used a cadaver/plastic skull/Fiberglas composite model to assess nine different commercially available vests, after creation of a lesion at C5 to C6.[48] The nine vests demonstrated similar results. Segmental motion was related to vest tightness, deformability, and the amount of friction at the vest-thorax interface. Increasing the halo superstructure had no beneficial effect. It has been found that shortening a polyethylene vest leads to a loss of rigidity,[64] although Wang et al. concluded that a half-vest (nipple level) was effective for lesions above C5. A four-pad design, which generates lower forces in the halo struts, was associated with some decrease in midcervical segmental motion.[63]

These mechanical aspects of the halo-vest apparatus have clinical importance. Anderson et al. reported on a series of 42 patients with cervical spine injuries.[4] Lateral radiographs were performed in the supine and upright positions. There was greater than 3 degrees of angulation or 1 mm of translation in 77% of patients. Overall, there was an average of 7 degrees of angulation and 1.7 mm of translation between supine and sitting radiographs. The greatest motion occurred at the occipitocervical junction, where there was an average of 8 degrees of sagittal plane angulation. At noninjured sites, the average motion was 3.9 degrees.[4] Similar angular motion, ranging from 5 to 8.6 degrees, was reported for noninjured segments in studies by Koch and Nickel and Lind et al.[36,43] The surprising amount of motion found in the study by Anderson et al., however, did not translate into treatment failure.

Nevertheless, it remains important to check supine and upright radiographs for patients treated in a halo. The need to remain vigilant for loss of position was

HALO LIMITATIONS

- Subject to "snaking" phenomenon
- Distraction force generated by halo vest does not restrict cervical motion and is reversed to a compression force in sitting and standing
- From 4% to 70% of normal motion still occurs in activities of daily living
- Fracture reduction is altered on supine versus sitting radiographs
- 46% of patients have some loss of reduction during clinical course

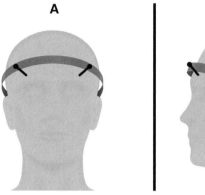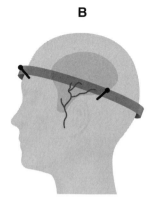

Figure 33-11. Halo ring placement. **A** and **B,** Schematical depictions of desirable pin locations for a typical four-pin halo ring placement. Incorrect placement can lead to increased pin tract complications, such as pin loosening, pullout, and infections.

highlighted by a report of five patients with facet subluxation and ligamentous injury who experienced recurrent dislocation in a halo.[69]

Application and Routine Care

The placement and care of a halo involve the combined skills of physicians, nursing staff, and orthotists. Complications are not infrequent, but appropriate care and supervision can minimize them.

Before the application of a halo, a checklist of necessary equipment should be recalled. It is imperative that the task be completed in an expeditious manner to minimize discomfort to the patient and to avoid early complications such as loss of fracture reduction.

The combined presence of a physician, who is skilled in halo application, and an orthotist, as well as an assistant, is helpful in expediting halo and vest application.

The patient should be positioned supine on a bed or gurney with adjustable height and a removable headboard. Fluoroscopy should also be readily available if a halo vest is applied in a patient with a highly unstable injury. Completeness of equipment and availability of ring and vest sizes appropriate for the patient should be checked before starting. Halo rings with an occipital cutout and temporary positioners greatly simplify the ring application.

The ring is secured to the patient's skull with three temporary positioning pins with blunt plastic suction caps. Ideally, the halo ring should lie in a plane perpendicular to the axis of the cervical spine and below the equator of the skull. This is usually about 1 cm above the orbital rim. There should be at least one fingerbreadth of clearance around the skull, and the halo should be clear of the pinnae of the ears.

In most adults, four pins provide adequate skeletal fixation. Six or even eight pins may be considered in pediatric patients and for patients with cranial defects, skull fracture, poor bone quality, or involuntary movement disorders. Anterior pins should be placed in the "safe zone" as described by Botte et al.[11] The ideal anterior pin location is approximately one fingerbreadth above the eyebrow in the lateral two thirds of the orbital rim. Medially, the frontal sinus and the supraorbital and supratrochlear nerves pose obstacles to safe pin place-

ment. The temporal fossa and the zygomaticotemporal nerve define the lateral boundary of the safe zone. The temporal fossa should be avoided because of its thin bone, risk of arterial bleeding, and possible interference with chewing[38] (Figure 33-11).

Before pin placement, the skin that is envisioned for pin placement is prepared with shaving, disinfection, and injected with a local anaesthetic agent such as 1% lidocaine with epinephrine. Care should be taken to infiltrate the pericranium with the anesthetic agent as well, to minimize patient discomfort. The pins are then advanced perpendicular to the skull with the patient's eyes closed and the forehead relaxed. After pin placement, adequate eye opening should be checked, and relaxing skin incisions should be placed if necessary. The posterior pins are placed directly diagonal to the anterior pins approximately two to four fingerbreadths above the mastoid process. In adults, the pins are then tightened to 6 pounds of torque in a diagonal sequence.

The anterior shell and uprights are then connected to the vest, and with continuing support to the head and cervical spine, the patient is log rolled to enable placement of the posterior shell and uprights. A check radiograph is completed and, the patient's condition permitting, the patient can then be sat up for a final tightening of the vest. A further radiograph should be obtained at this stage to ensure that there has been no loss of fracture reduction with elevation to the upright position.

Special care in the application of halo pins is necessary to prevent penetration, loosening, and infection. Penetration is best prevented by the use of a pin with a sharp point and a broad shoulder.[27] Some authors have proposed that loosening may be related to the amount of pin torque used at the time of insertion.

Some variation of opinion exists as to what is appropriate torque on the pins. Garfin et al. recommended the routine use of 8 pounds (1.12 Newton-meters) and single retightening at 48 hours based on a retrospectively controlled study compared with the use of 6 pounds of torque.[27] Rizzolo et al., however, conducted a randomized controlled study in 102 patients of complications with 6 versus 8 pounds of torque.[52] There was a trend, although not statistically significant, toward the occurrence of more complications with the use of 8 pounds of torque. Regardless of the torque used, a reduction in the compressive forces exerted by the posterior pin sites over the course of the treatment period may be expected.[25]

Retightening of pins may in part influence the rate of pin loosening and soft tissue infections. Botte et al. has recommended this as routine procedure at 48 hours.[11] Thereafter, a loose pin can be retightened if resistance is felt within one or two turns.[27] Otherwise, the pin should be removed and another inserted at a different location. Vertullo et al. similarly recommended routine retightening based on a comparison of 266 patients who received routine retightening at either 24 hours or 1 week.[66]

The common current practice is to insert pins with 6 pounds of torque and to retighten them once while the patient is still in the hospital. Pins are not routinely retightened beyond this, but a loose pin will be advanced if resistance is felt or replaced if grossly loose.

Patients and their care providers should be instructed in pin care. A ritual consisting of daily cleansing with cotton-tipped applicators and alcohol or hydrogen peroxide should be pursued fastidiously. Dressings or ointments of any sort should not occlude pin sites. Local disinfectants such as povidone-iodine may, however, be used around the pin insertion site several times a day.

Frequently asked questions surround the issue of personal hygiene. In principle, the halo vest should be kept dry during treatment. A regimen of rigorous daily skin care is important. Baths and showers are generally unsuitable for patients in a halo vest. Hair care is preferable performed with a dry shampoo. There is no need to routinely replace the lining of a halo vest. Should contamination of the lining necessitate an exchange, the possibility of a loss of fracture reduction should be considered.

Complications

Some degree of controversy surrounding the use of the halo is the perception of it being a cumbersome and complication-prone treatment modality. Fortunately, most complications are relatively minor and easily handled. Institution of an outpatient halo-care education and surveillance program can be helpful in reducing some of the more serious complications.

Patient selection can be another very significant contributing factor in avoiding complications. Cachectic elderly individuals or insensate patients who may not be able to complain of pressure points may experience a disproportionate incidence of skin breakdown. Patients with substantial preexistent deformities, such as found in ankylosing spondylitis or scoliosis, are prone to loss of fracture reduction. Pulmonary compromise may be present in patients with serial rib fractures, obese indi-

---

HALO-VEST APPLICATION

- Personnel
  - Physician, nurse, orthotist
- Equipment
  - Premeasured halo ring and vest, pins, wrenches, and screwdrivers
  - Fluoroscopy for realignment procedures
  - Sedation/local infiltration
- Halo placement
  - Temporary suction caps
  - Position halo 1 cm above orbital rim, below equator of skull, and leaving a fingerbreadth clearance above pinnae of ear and between skull and ring
- Tips
  - Recall "safe zone"
  - Check eyelid closure and swallowing
  - Apply torque to pins
    - Adults: 6 to 8 pounds
    - Children: 3 to 4 pounds
  - Retighten once at 24 to 48 pounds
  - Assess supine and erect radiographs

HALO: RELATIVE CONTRAINDICATIONS

- Elderly
- Severe cachexia
- Significant truncal deformity
  - Ankylosing spondylitis
  - Scoliosis
- Noncompliant patients
- Morbid obesity
- Tetraplegia
- Primarily ligamentous injury in adult with low chances of healing

---

viduals, patients with congestive pulmonary disease, and the elderly.[42]

The most common complications associated with halo-vest treatment are pin loosening, with an incidence of 5% to 36%, and pin tract infections, reported in 9% to 22% of patients.[27,43,52] Three basic types of infection may be differentiated: (1) superficial cellulitis, (2) deep soft tissue infection with purulence, and (3) osteomyelitis.[15] If any form of pin tract infection is noted, the patient should be examined for pin loosening and meningeal symptoms or drainage. In the absence of such, cellulitis can be treated with local wound care and oral antibiotics. In the presence of purulent drainage or abscess formation, local wound debridement and antibiotics are indicated. In the presence of spreading cellulitis, suspicion of dural penetration and gross pin loosening should be entertained, and pin removal, wound exploration and debridement, and institution of intravenous antibiotics are required (Figure 33-12). Pin retightening is contraindicated in a class 3 infection but can be considered for patients presenting with class 1 or 2 infections under the parameters discussed previously (Figure 33-12).

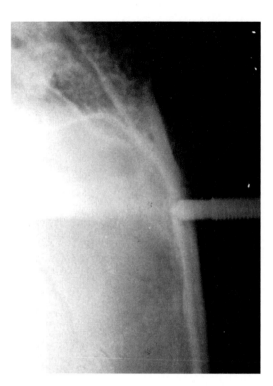

Figure 33-12. Pin tract complications. A pin loosening with osteolysis is shown on this tangential skull radiograph. This pin was clinically loose and infected. Surgical pin site debridement and hospitalization for intravenous antibiotics were required. Pin tract infections and loosening continue to pose considerable clinical challenges in the use of this device.

Pressure sores have been reported with an incidence of 0% to 11%.[27,63] Although vest design may contribute to this variability, more significant impact may be expected from the patient comorbidities. Patients with high levels of spinal cord injuries, severe head injuries, emaciation, and noncompliance are at a considerably elevated risk for skin breakdown. Skin care protocols and modified vests that use four pads with no pressure on the scapula can be of help in lowering the incidence of skin breakdown.[63]

Ring migration has been identified in 13% of patients.[27] This may be avoided in part by appropriate pin placement below the equator of the skull and the avoidance of the use of prolonged high-weight axial traction.

Unacceptable scars resulting from anterior pin sites may be anticipated in 4% to 11% of patients.[50] Pin migration and predisposition to keloid formation are some of the associated causes for this. Surgical revisions are rarely requested and usually should be delayed for approximately 1 year after halo removal.

The most common neurologic deficits associated with halo treatment are injuries to the supraorbital, supratrochlear, or facial nerve branches, with a reported incidence of 2% of patients being affected. Regard for the "safe zone" should minimize the rate of occurrence. If a

HALO: COMPLICATIONS

- Pin infection: 9% to 22%
- Pin loosening: 5% to 36%
- Pressure sores: 0% to 11%
- Ring migration: 13%
- Unacceptable scars: 4% to 11%
- Nerve injury: 2%
- Dysphagia: 2%
- Bleeding: 1%
- Dural puncture: 1%
- Loss of alignment: 7% to 15%

neural dysfunction in the area of pin placement is noted, the pin should be removed and placed at another site.

Dysphagia can occur in 2% of patients.[27] Difficulty in swallowing may be associated with excessive extension of the cervical spine and anterior bridging osteophyte formation. Manipulation of the cervical spine under fluoroscopy to achieve a more suitable head position while maintaining fracture alignment usually resolves this problem. A simple swallowing test with the patient drinking a cup of water in the upright position after realignment can be used to confirm the resolution of the problem. Problems with ingestion otherwise tend to be more frequently found with patients with cervicothoracic orthoses than with patients with halo vests. Lind et al. measured a diminution in pulmonary vital capacity with halo-vest wear in both neurologically intact and impaired patients.[42] Patients with pulmonary comorbidities may experience exacerbation of their underlying condition with halo-vest wear. Another cause of pulmonary deterioration is associated with aspiration during confinement to an external cervicothoracic immobilization. This problem is particularly common in geriatric patients and patients with cervical deformities.

Some patients have ongoing bleeding about the pin sites. This has been reported to occur in 1% of patients.[27] Although packing may be attempted, it is often unsuccessful, and a bleeding diathesis or the use of heparin or other anticoagulants needs to be excluded.

A rare, but feared, complication is dural injury with cerebrospinal fluid leakage, which is encountered in 1% of patients.[27,50] A patient with this complication should be closely monitored and treated with intravenous antibiotics. Pin removal and elevation of the head of the bed may be helpful. Fortunately, surgical repair to stop ongoing drainage is rarely necessary.

Any form of external fracture immobilization is associated with osteoporosis. In a study regarding the use of halo vests, Korovessis et al. found a 2.83% reduction in bone mineral density.[37] This was not related to age, gender, or injury level. The changes in bone density were reversible at 3 months after removal of the brace.

Loss of alignment is a relatively common occurrence that has been reported in 7% to 15% of patients.[4,13] Identification of loss of fracture reduction should prompt a reevaluation of the general treatment strategy. Patients with ligamentous injuries are usually more prone to experience recurrent loss of alignment (Figure 33-13).

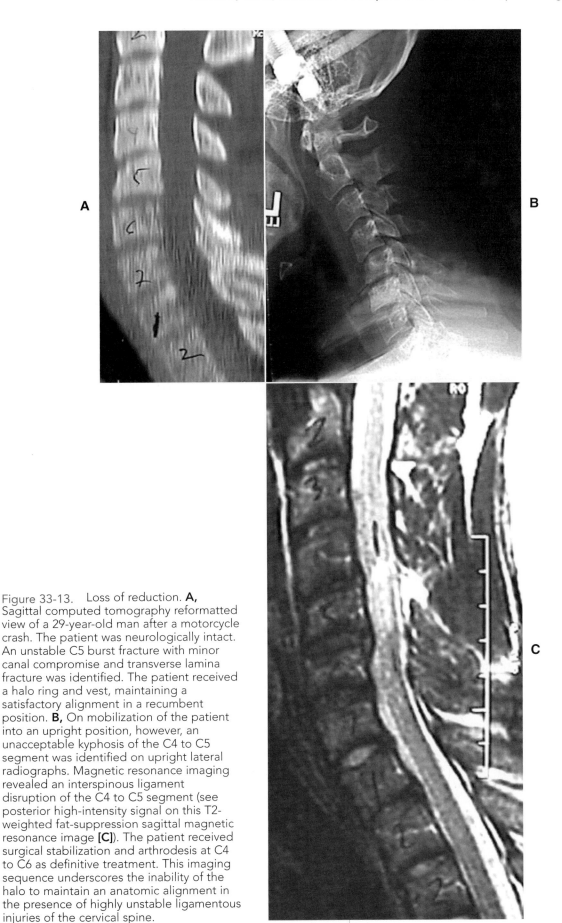

Figure 33-13. Loss of reduction. **A,** Sagittal computed tomography reformatted view of a 29-year-old man after a motorcycle crash. The patient was neurologically intact. An unstable C5 burst fracture with minor canal compromise and transverse lamina fracture was identified. The patient received a halo ring and vest, maintaining a satisfactory alignment in a recumbent position. **B,** On mobilization of the patient into an upright position, however, an unacceptable kyphosis of the C4 to C5 segment was identified on upright lateral radiographs. Magnetic resonance imaging revealed an interspinous ligament disruption of the C4 to C5 segment (see posterior high-intensity signal on this T2-weighted fat-suppression sagittal magnetic resonance image **[C]**). The patient received surgical stabilization and arthrodesis at C4 to C6 as definitive treatment. This imaging sequence underscores the inability of the halo to maintain an anatomic alignment in the presence of highly unstable ligamentous injuries of the cervical spine.

Continuation of nonoperative care may be a frustrating experience in such circumstances. Realignment efforts for patients with bony injuries may be more successful. Other options consist of returning the patient to recumbent cranial traction or converting to surgical care.

It is evident that the halo vest remains a useful tool in the management of cervical spine trauma. In a retrospective review, Rockswold et al. reported on 140 patients treated with a halo vest. Successful fracture healing was achieved in 78% of patients, with 25% of patients experiencing some form of complication, albeit usually of a minor nature.[54] In this study, a complication rate of 6% was identified with surgical care, with surgical complications being consistently more severe. Lind et al. clearly demonstrated limitations of the biomechanical aspects of fracture stabilization afforded by the halo.[43] Despite this, 90% of the 83 patients achieved uneventful healing. Range of motion was reduced overall, with an 18% decrease in rotation and side bending, whereas flexion and extension were preserved.[43]

Halo Use in Children

The halo vest perhaps has wider applicability in the management of cervical spine injuries in children than in adults. Spinal column injuries in the skeletally immature age groups, even if they involve ligamentous injuries, appear to have better chances of satisfactory healing results than do their adult counterparts. In addition, the effectiveness of braces may be limited by lack of compliance or mechanical stability. Cervicothoracic plaster of Paris molds, such as a Minerva cast, are frequently poorly tolerated and quite cumbersome.

The immaturity of the pediatric skull is, however, cause for some concern with the use of a halo. The principle of halo application in children is essentially similar to that in adults. It is helpful to review a CT scan of the skull to assess the bony thickness and appropriate sites for pin placement. To decrease the strain placed on each individual pin, the use of six to eight pins, positioned with respect to the "safe zone" anteriorly and into the thickest bone of the parietal and occipital cranium posteriorly, is recommended.

In a fetal calf skull model, Copley et al. assessed the angle of pin insertion and its influence on load to failure. As the insertion angle varied more from the perpendicular, there was a decreased load to failure.[18] Wherever possible, pins therefore should be inserted perpendicular to the skull, especially in children, to prevent pin loosening or pullout. Letts et al. compared a four-pin halo with an eight-pin halo in a human cadaver model and found significantly greater stiffness (24.2%) with the eight-pin halo.[40] Such a number of pins allow for a lower torque to be applied to each pin, and this in turn may help prevent dural penetration.

In a review of complications of halo-vest management in children, Dormans et al. reported on 37 patients, of whom one third were treated for traumatic injuries. The overall complication rate was 68%, mainly consisting of pin loosening and infection at the anterior sites. One patient experienced dural injury, one patient

---

HALO IN CHILDREN

- Immature skull
- High complication rate (68%)
- Review computed tomography scan of skull before pin placement
- Use six to eight pins, with low torque (3 to 4 pounds)
- Insert pins perpendicular to skull

---

experienced a supraorbital nerve injury, and in three patients, pin site scars were deemed objectionable by the patient or family. The authors postulated that a decrease in the size of the ring and an increase in the number of pins applied with lower amounts of torque would be helpful in diminishing these complications.[21]

MANAGEMENT OF COMMON FRACTURES
Basic Considerations

Any type of nonoperative treatment is limited by the nature of the skeletal injury. Mostly cancellous bone injuries with irregular large fracture surfaces and limited displacement have good chances to heal in a satisfactory fashion. In contrast, most structural ligamentous injuries in the adult spine have poor functional healing results if managed with any form of external immobilization.

The duration of brace wear is empiric but ranges from 6 weeks to 4 months. The end point for brace wear should be the demonstration of union on serial radiographs and stability on flexion-extension films. Chan et al. reported that radiologic union in 188 patients occurred at a mean of 11.5 weeks.[14] Vertullo et al. reported an average duration of brace wear of 9.5 weeks and a time to union of 12.2 weeks.[66] Some fracture patterns, such as a type 2 odontoid fracture, may require a full 12 weeks in the halo.[44]

By any standard of care, halo treatment should not be necessary for more than a minority of cervical spine injuries. As has been discussed, the halo is somewhat cumbersome and not without significant morbidity. It usually requires an extended period of use over a number of months, and it is not always well tolerated. Meanwhile, surgical techniques and implants have advanced to the point where many fractures that may previously have been treated with a halo are now being dealt with surgically.

Most inherently stable fractures or soft tissue injuries to the cervical spine can be treated with a collar or cervicothoracic orthosis[3]; these injuries include spinous process, laminar, and lateral mass fractures. Similarly, vertebral body compression fractures without retropulsion of fragments or a posterior ligamentous injury can be treated in this way. The main purpose of a brace in these circumstances is to enhance patient comfort, reduce the risk of further injury, and maintain alignment. The discomfort and morbidity of this device outweigh any theoretic advantages of the halo, such as improvement in fracture alignment.

The halo, however, has retained an important role of the management in certain fractures, especially in the

COMMON INDICATIONS FOR HALO MANAGEMENT

- Occipital condyle fractures
  - Type 2 (comminuted)
  - Type 3 (avulsion if no atlanto-occipital dissociation)
- Atlanto-occipital or atlantoaxial dissociation
  - Emergent reduction
  - Definitive management in pediatric patients
- Atlas fractures
  - Displaced
  - Unstable
  - Temporary recumbent traction
- Atlantoaxial injuries
  - Type 2 transverse atlantal ligament injuries
  - High-grade or old rotatory subluxation
- Odontoid fractures
  - Type 2
  - Type 3 displaced
- Traumatic spondylolisthesis of axis (Hangman's fracture)
  - Type 2 (high grade)
  - Type 2a (controversial)
- Subaxial cervical spine
  - "Stable" burst fracture
  - Unilateral facet fracture dislocation (controversial)
- Supplemental treatment
  - Compromised fixation in poor bone quality
  - Multilevel injury treatment

ATLAS FRACTURES AMENABLE TO HALO MANAGEMENT

- Anterior arch "blowout" fracture
- Displaced intraarticular lateral mass fracture
- "Jefferson"-type burst fracture
  - From 2- to 7-mm halo vest
  - Greater than 7 mm: Traction for 6 weeks and then vest[41]
  - Halo for transverse atlantal ligament bony avulsions (type 2 injuries)
  - 26% instability, nonunion at 3 months[20]

upper cervical spine. The basic principle behind halo management for such injuries consists of fracture reduction and realignment. Maintenance of satisfactory fracture reduction should then be assessed with supine and erect radiographs at the outset of management and serially over the next 3 months. This should be correlated with clinical review, especially neurologic examination. Depending on the radiologic assessment of union, a decision can be made about the duration of brace wear, but this will usually be in the region of 3 months. In some cases, fracture union itself may not be so much the end point for halo-vest management as the evaluation of stability parameters. These can be assessed on flexion-extension films after disconnection of the halo struts from the vest but before the removal of the halo ring. Commonly, patients receive a transitional period of bracing for 2 to 4 weeks on the completion of halo wear.

Craniocervical Junction Injuries

Most occipital fractures are suitable for nonoperative treatment, as long as they are not a manifestation of an occipitocervical dissociation. Surgical intervention for these injuries is rarely needed.

Occipitoatlantal dissociation injuries are receiving increasing attention due to an increased survival rate of these patients, who were previously believed to be non-survivable. The halo should be considered as an emergency reduction tool for patients presenting with an occipitoatlantal or atlantoaxial dissociation. Conventional traction usually leads to an unacceptable diastasis across the injury zone,[29] leaving the treating physician with a choice of attempting reduction and temporary stabilization with a halo or securing the patient with sandbags and tape until definitive treatment in the form of surgery can be contemplated. Halo treatment of an occipitoatlantal cervical dissociation beyond the initial stages is not advisable due to the poor craniocervical stabilization properties of this device.[44]

Atlas Fractures

Fractures of the atlas may be stable or unstable depending on the location of the fracture, displacement, and fracture comminution. In addition, its common association with other fractures in the cervical spine may predominate treatment decisions. Patients with isolated posterior arch fractures and minimally displaced fractures of the anterior ring usually do not require halo management due to the inherently stable nature of their fracture patterns. "Blowout" fractures of the anterior arch, intra-articular fractures of the lateral masses, and true burst or Jefferson fractures, however, are inherently unstable. Patients with such injuries usually are considered for halo treatment or surgical stabilization.

Burst fractures of the atlas are commonly referred to as Jefferson fractures. These injuries tend to be unstable and may require halo immobilization in absence of a predictably straightforward surgical treatment option for this injury. Lack of stabilizing properties of the halo becomes apparent when the halo is used for atlas fractures with disruption of the transverse atlantal ligament. Although acute fracture reduction with skeletal traction usually is readily possible, early mobilization of a patient with such an injury is not infrequently accompanied by recurrent splaying of the lateral masses. Levine and Edwards described temporary recumbent traction of 6 weeks' duration, followed by halo treatment, as successful management for 11 patients with such injuries.[41] Based on their experience, Levine and Edwards recommended immediate halo-vest treatment for patients with 2 to 7 mm of lateral mass spreading and several weeks of traction before conversion to halo treatment for patients with lateral mass splaying above 7 mm.

Dickman et al. differentiated transverse ligament disruptions into ligamentous type 1 injuries and bony type 2 avulsion lesions. Although patients with type 1 injuries were treated with primary atlantoaxial arthrodesis, those with type 2 injuries were treated with rigid external immobilization. A failure rate of 26% due to nonunion or persistent instability was noted.[20] These two more recent studies leave the treating physician somewhat in a quandary, because an ideal treatment for these injuries remains elusive. Prolonged recumbent traction followed by a halo vest has been reported to be successful but is frequently not well accepted due to secondary complications and cost.

Atlantoaxial Injuries

The classification of such injuries includes rotational, translational, and distractive patterns. Rotatory instability is commonly of nontraumatic origin and common in children. Most patients presenting with this problem acutely will resolve their deformity spontaneously. Skeletal traction has a role in the management of this condition for patients with pronounced displacement, delayed presentation for medical care, or unclear home care provisions. Weights in the region of 7 pounds in children, usually applied by halter traction, and of 15 pounds in adults, applied with cranial traction, are appropriate and gradually may be doubled as required. Fielding and Hawkins recommended maintaning traction for 1 week before deciding on the need for surgery or halo management for persistent subluxation.[24] In absence of atlantoaxial instability, surgery is rarely necessary.

Primary injuries to the transverse atlantal ligament can be treated nonsurgically if there is a bony avulsion present. Treatment decisions for these injuries were discussed earlier.

Distractive injuries at the atlantoaxial articulation are particularly unstable, and surgical management is appropriate.[34] Emergency halo-vest reduction with a compressive moment exerted and held through this orthosis is a temporizing measure until the patient can be treated surgically.

Odontoid Fractures

Halo-vest treatment continues to play a significant role in the management of patients with these fractures.[57] Successful healing of type 2 odontoid fractures remains a challenge with nonsurgical and surgical means. The multicenter Cervical Spine Research Society trial reported by Clarke and White concluded that all type 2 and type 3 fractures initially should be managed with skeletal traction. Those type 2 fractures with significant comminution, displacement (greater than 6 mm), and angulation (greater than 10 degrees), especially in elderly patients, may be considered for surgery; otherwise, the literature supports the use of halo immobilization for type 2 and type 3 fractures.[16] Dunn and Seljeskog reported on 128 patients with odontoid fractures, of whom 80 were treated in a halo. They concluded that

---

> ### ODONTOID FRACTURES AMENABLE TO HALO TREATMENT
>
> - Type 2 fractures without
>   - Segmental comminution
>   - Displacement of greater than 6 mm
>   - Angulation of greater than 10 degrees
>   - Elderly
>   - Delayed diagnosis
>   - Displacement or distraction in halo
> - Displaced type 3 fractures

> ### HANGMAN'S FRACTURES AMENABLE TO HALO TREATMENT
>
> - High-grade type 2 fractures (Francis criteria)
>   - Some displacement acceptable
> - Beware of distraction in type 2a injuries

---

type 2 or type 3 dens fractures should be treated in a halo if they were less than 1 week old, the patient was less than 65 years old, and the fracture was nondisplaced or displaced less than 2 mm posteriorly.[22]

These recommendations were similar to those of Hadley et al., who reported a series of 107 axis fractures, of which 59 were odontoid fractures. There was a 26% nonunion rate for the type 2 odontoid fractures. They noted that healing was quicker in a halo vest than with an SOMI and recommended the halo for external skeletal immobilization.[30]

Traumatic Spondylolisthesis of the Axis (Hangman's Fracture)

Patients with type 1 injuries as classified by Effendi and modified by Levine and Edwards have relatively stable fractures and usually can be treated successfully with a neck collar.[41] Type 2 injuries, which exhibit a greater than 3 mm displacement or angulation of greater than 10 degrees, may be considered for bracing or traction and reduction followed by a halo vest. Francis et al. found no difference in healing (overall, 94.5%) between immediate halo placement and the use of short- or long-term (6 weeks) traction.[26] Patients with type IIA fractures (distraction-hyperextension pattern) treated with traction will usually progressively malangulate with axial skeletal cranial traction. Levine and Edwards recommended immediate halo-vest placement with compression for patients presenting with this injury.[41] In their series of 15 patients with type 1 fractures, 29 patients with type 2 fractures, and 3 patients with type 2a fractures, there were no patients with nonunion. All patients with initially displaced fractures healed with significant residual deformity.[41] Type 3 injuries exhibit a displaced fracture through the pars interarticularis and a facet dislocation of the C2 to C3 joints. These injuries require open reduction and internal fixation and are not suitable for nonoperative treatment attempts.

Subaxial Injuries

Management of injuries that affect the subaxial spine has been less successful than that in the upper cervical spine. The exception to this has been the "stable" burst fracture, with the absence of a neurologic deficit and posterior ligament injury combined with a small vertebral body height loss, kyphosis, and neural canal compromise.[13,55,58] Surgical stabilization is widely considered to yield superior results for patients with significant posterior ligament injuries. An exception to this has been the management of unilateral facet dislocations, where treatment with closed reduction and a halo vest has been recommended.[6] Maintenance of anatomic alignment in a halo has been accepted as being essential for this treatment.[13] Neurologic deterioration and pain with persistent instability after conclusion of the halo treatment has been reported, however.[13,58]

SELECTED REFERENCES

Anderson PA et al.: Failure of halo vest to prevent in vivo motion in patients with injured cervical spines, *Spine* 16(10 Suppl):S501-S505, 1991.

Blackmore CC et al.: Cervical spine screening with CT in trauma patients: a cost-effectiveness analysis, *Radiology* 212(1):117-125, 1999.

Clark CR, White AA: Fractures of the dens: a multicenter study, *J Bone Joint Surg Am* 67(9):1340-1348, 1985.

Dormans JP et al.: Complications in children managed with immobilization in a halo vest, *J Bone Joint Surg Am* 77(9):1370-1373, 1995.

Fielding JW, Hawkins RJ: Atlanto-axial rotatory fixation (fixed rotatory subluxation of the atlanto-axial joint), *J Bone Joint Surg Am* 59(1):37-44, 1977.

Grant GA et al.: Risk of early closed reduction in cervical spine subluxation injuries, *J Neurosurg* 90(1 Suppl):13-18, 1999.

Johnson RM et al.: Cervical orthoses: a study comparing their effectiveness in restricting cervical motion in normal subjects, *J Bone Joint Surg Am* 59(3):332-339, 1977.

Letts M, Girouard L, Yeadon A: Mechanical evaluation of four- versus eight-pin halo fixation, *J Pediatr Orthop* 17(1):121-124, 1997.

Mirza SK et al.: Stabilizing properties of the halo apparatus, *Spine* 22(7):727-733, 1997.

Vertullo CJ, Duke PF, Askin GN: Pin-site complications of the halo thoracic brace with routine pin re-tightening, *Spine* 22(21):2514-16, 1997.

REFERENCES

1. American College of Surgeons: *Advanced trauma life support manual*, Chicago, 1992, The College.
2. Alander DH, Andreychik DA, Stauffer ES: Early outcome in cervical spinal cord injured patients older than 50 years of age, *Spine* 19(20):2299-2301, 1994.
3. An HS: Cervical spine trauma, *Spine* 23(24):2713-2729, 1998.
4. Anderson PA et al.: Failure of halo vest to prevent in vivo motion in patients with injured cervical spines, *Spine* 16(10 Suppl):5501-5505, 1991.
5. Askins V, Eismont FJ: Efficacy of five cervical orthoses in restricting cervical motion: a comparison study, *Spine* 22(11):1193-1198, 1997 (see comments).
6. Beatson TR: Fractures and dislocations of the cervical spine, *J Bone Joint Surg Br* 45:21-35, 1963.
7. Benzel EC et al.: The thermoplastic Minerva body jacket: a clinical comparison with other cervical spine splinting techniques, *J Spinal Disord* 5(3):311-319, 1992.
8. Blackmore CC et al.: Cervical spine screening with CT in trauma patients: a cost-effectiveness analysis, *Radiology* 212(1):117-125, 1999.
9. Blount WP: Use of the Milwaukee brace, *Orthop Clin North Am* 3(1):3-16, 1972.
10. Blumberg KD et al.: The pullout strength of titanium alloy MRI-compatible and stainless steel MRI-incompatible Gardner-Wells tongs, *Spine* 18(13):1895-1896, 1993.
11. Botte MJ et al.: The halo skeletal fixator: principles of application and maintenance, *Clin Orthop* 239:12-18, 1989.
12. Breig A, el-Nadi AF: Biomechanics of the cervical spinal cord: relief of contact pressure on and overstretching of the spinal cord, *Acta Radiol Diagn (Stockh)* 4(6):602-624, 1966.
13. Bucholz RD, Cheung KC: Halo vest versus spinal fusion for cervical injury: evidence from an outcome study, *J Neurosurg* 70(6):884-892, 1989 (see comments).
14. Chan RC, Schweigel JF, Thompson GB: Halo-thoracic brace immobilization in188 patients with acute cervical spine injuries, *J Neurosurg* 58(4):508-515, 1983.
15. Chapman JR, Anderson PA: Cervical spine trauma. In Frymoyer JW, ed: *The adult spine: principles and practice*: Philadelphia, 1997, Lippincott-Raven.
16. Clark CR, White AA: Fractures of the dens: a multicenter study, *J Bone Joint Surg Am* 67(9):1340-1348, 1985.
17. Clayman DA, Murakami ME, Vines FS: Compatibility of cervical spine braces with MR imaging: a study of nine nonferrous devices, *Am J Neuroradiol* 11(2):385-390, 1990.
18. Copley LA et al.: A comparison of various angles of halo pin insertion in an immature skull model, *Spine* 24(17):1777-1780, 1999 (published erratum appears in *Spine* 25(11):1460, 2000).
19. Cotler JM et al.: Closed reduction of traumatic cervical spine dislocation using traction weights up to 140 pounds, *Spine* 18(3):386-390, 1993.
20. Dickman CA, Greene KA, Sonntag VK: Injuries involving the transverse atlantal ligament: classification and treatment guidelines based upon experience with 39 injuries, *Neurosurgery* 38(1):44-50, 1996 (see comments).
21. Dormans JP: Complications in children managed with immobilization in a halo vest, *J Bone Joint Surg Am* 77(9):1370-1373, 1995.
22. Dunn ME, Seljeskog EL: Experience in the management of odontoid process injuries: an analysis of 128 cases, *Neurosurgery* 18(3):306-310, 1986.
23. Eismont FJ, Arena MJ, Green BA: Extrusion of an intervertebral disc associated with traumatic subluxation or dislocation of cervical facets: case report, *J Bone Joint Surg Am* 73(10):1555-1560, 1991.
24. Fielding JW, Hawkins RJ: Atlanto-axial rotatory fixation (fixed rotatory subluxation of the atlanto-axial joint), *J Bone Joint Surg Am* 59(1):37-44, 1977.
25. Fleming BC et al.: Pin force measurement in a halo-vest orthosis, in vivo, *J Biomech* 31(7):647-651, 1998.
26. Francis WR et al.: Traumatic spondylolisthesis of the axis, *J Bone Joint Surg Br* 63:313-318, 1981.
27. Garfin SR, Botte MJ, Nickel VL: Complications in the use of the halo fixation device, *J Bone Joint Surg Am* 69(6):954, 1987 (letter).
28. Grant GA et al.: Risk of early closed reduction in cervical spine subluxation injuries, *J Neurosurg* 90(1 Suppl):13-18, 1999.
29. Gruenberg MF et al.: Overdistraction of cervical spine injuries with the use of skull traction: a report of two cases, *J Trauma* 42(6):1152-1156, 1997.
30. Hadley MN, Browner C, Sonntag VK: Axis fractures: a comprehensive review of management and treatment in 107 cases, *Neurosurgery* 17(2):281-290, 1985.
31. Herzenberg JE et al.: Emergency transport and positioning of young children who have an injury of the cervical spine: the standard backboard may be hazardous, *J Bone Joint Surg Am* 71(1):15-22, 1989.
32. Hoffman JR et al.: Validity of a set of clinical criteria to rule out injury to the cervical spine in patients with blunt trauma, National Emergency X Radiography Utilization Study Group, *N Engl J Med* 343(2):94-99, 2000 (see comments).
33. Hughes SJ: How effective is the Newport/Aspen collar? A prospective radiographic evaluation in healthy adult volunteers, *J Trauma* 45(2):374-378, 1998.

34. Jeanneret B, Magerl F, Ward JC: Overdistraction: a hazard of skull traction in the management of acute injuries of the cervical spine, *Arch Orthop Trauma Surg* 110(5):242-245, 1991.

35. Johnson RM et al.: Cervical orthoses: a study comparing their effectiveness in restricting cervical motion in normal subjects, *J Bone Joint Surg Am* 59(3):332-339, 1977.

36. Koch RA, Nickel VL: The halo vest: an evaluation of motion and forces across the neck, *Spine* 3(2):103-107, 1978.

37. Korovessis P et al.: Spinal bone mineral density changes following halo vest immobilization for cervical trauma, *Eur Spine J* 3(4):206-208, 1994.

38. Krag MH, Byrt W, Pope M: Pull-off strength of Gardner-Wells tongs from cadaveric crania, *Spine* 14(3):247-250, 1989.

39. Lerman JA et al.: A biomechanical comparison of Gardner-Wells tongs and halo device used for cervical spine traction, *Spine* 19(21):2403-2406, 1994.

40. Letts M, Girouard L, Yeadon A: Mechanical evaluation of four-versus eight-pin halo fixation, *J Pediatr Orthop* 17(1):121-124, 1997.

41. Levine AM, Edwards CC: Fractures of the atlas, *J Bone Joint Surg Am* 73(5):680-691, 1991.

42. Lind B et al.: Influence of halo vest treatment on vital capacity, *Spine* 12(5):449-452, 1987.

43. Lind B, Sihlbom H, Nordwall A: Forces and motions across the neck in patients treated with halo-vest, *Spine* 13(2):162-167, 1988.

44. Lind B, Sihlbom H, Nordwall A: Halo-vest treatment of unstable traumatic cervical spine injuries, *Spine* 13(4):425-432, 1988.

45. Mahale YJ, Silver JR, Henderson NJ. Neurological complications of the reduction of cervical spine dislocations, *J Bone Joint Surg Br* 75(3):403-409, 1993.

46. McGuire RA, Degnan G, Amundson GM: Evaluation of current extrication orthoses in immobilization of the unstable cervical spine, *Spine* 15(10):1064-1067, 1990.

47. McLain RF, Benson DR: Urgent surgical stabilization of spinal fractures in polytrauma patients, *Spine* 24(16):1646-1654, 1999.

48. Mirza SK et al.: Stabilizing properties of the halo apparatus, *Spine* 22(7):727-733, 1997.

49. Perry JP, Nickel VL: Total cervical spine fusion for neck paralysis, *J Bone Joint Surg Am* 41:37-40, 1958.

50. Pierce DS: The halo orthosis in the treatment of cervical spine injury, *Instr Course Lect* 36:495-497, 1987.

51. Podolsky S et al.: Efficacy of cervical spine immobilization methods, *J Trauma* 23(6):461-465, 1983.

52. Rizzolo SJ et al.: The effect of torque pressure on halo pin complication rates: a randomized prospective study, *Spine* 18(15):2163-2166, 1993.

53. Rizzolo SJ, Vaccaro AR, Cotler JM: Cervical spine trauma, *Spine* 19(20):2288-2298, 1994.

54. Rockswold GL, Bergman TA, Ford SE: Halo immobilization and surgical fusion: relative indications and effectiveness in the treatment of 140 cervical spine injuries, *J Trauma* 30(7):893-898, 1990.

55. Romanelli DA et al.: Comparison of initial injury features in cervical spine trauma of C3-C7: predictive outcome with halo-vest management, *J Spinal Disord* 9(2):146-149, 1996.

56. Ryan MD, Taylor TK: Odontoid fractures in the elderly, *J Spinal Disord* 6(5):397-401, 1993.

57. Schweigel JF: Management of the fractured odontoid with halo-thoracic bracing, *Spine* 12(9):838-839, 1987.

58. Sears W, Fazl M: Prediction of stability of cervical spine fracture managed in the halo vest and indications for surgical intervention, *J Neurosurg* 72(3):426-432, 1990 (see comments).

59. Sharpe KP, Rao S, Ziogas A: Evaluation of the effectiveness of the Minerva cervicothoracic orthosis, *Spine* 20(13):1475-1479, 1995.

60. American Spinal Injury Association: *Standard for neurologic and functional classification of spinal cord injury*, revised, Atlanta, 1992, The Association.

61. Star AM et al.: Immediate closed reduction of cervical spine dislocations using traction, *Spine* 15(10):1068-1072, 1990.

62. Tarlov IM: Spinal cord compression studies: time limits for recovery after gradual compression in dogs, *Arch Neurol Neurosurg Psychol* 71:588-597, 1954.

63. Tomonaga T, Krag MH, Novotny JE: Clinical, radiographic, and kinematic results from an adjustable four-pad halovest, *Spine* 22(11):1199-1208, 1997.

64. Triggs KJ et al.: Length dependence of a halo orthosis on cervical immobilization, *J Spinal Disord* 6(1):34-37, 1993.

65. Vaccaro AR et al.: Magnetic resonance evaluation of the intervertebral disc, spinal ligaments, and spinal cord before and after closed traction reduction of cervical spine dislocations, *Spine* 24(12):1210-1217, 1999.

66. Vertullo CJ, Duke PF, Askin GN: Pin-site complications of the halo thoracic brace with routine pin re-tightening, *Spine* 22(21):2514-2516, 1997.

67. Walker PS et al.: Forces in the halo-vest apparatus, *Spine* 9(8):773-777, 1984.

68. Wang GJ et al.: The effect of halo-vest length on stability of the cervical spine: a study in normal subjects, *J Bone Joint Surg Am* 70(3):357-360, 1988.

69. Whitehull R et al.: Induction and characterization of an interface tissue by implantation of methylmethacrylate cement into the posterior part of the cervical spine of the dog, *J Bone Joint Surg Am* 70(1):51-59, 1988.

Cervical Spine Trauma: Upper and Lower

Gregg R. Klein, Alexander R. Vaccaro

It has been estimated that the annual incidence of spinal cord injury requiring hospitalization in North America is approximately 32 to 50 per million people.[35,80] The cervical spine accounts for about half of the 50,000 spinal cord injuries in the United States each year. Roughly 40% of these injuries are associated with a neurologic deficit.[50] Despite the advances in care and prevention of spinal cord trauma, the annual incidence is expected to increase from 11,500 in 1994 to approximately 13,400 in 2010.[79]

There is a bimodal age distribution in patients who sustain spinal injuries. The first peak is between 15 and 24 years of age, and the second peak occurs in patients older than 55.[48] The elderly population represent a unique subset of spinal trauma patients. One study reviewed 41 patients over 65 years of age who sustained cervical trauma and found that in 4 of the patients, cervical injuries were missed because of their innocuous (i.e., low-energy) injury mechanisms. In this age group 27% of patients died during their initial treatment. It was noted that those patients mobilized early had better outcomes than those patients treated with bed rest or traction.[59] Kannus et al.[46] reviewed the spinal cord admissions in Finland between 1970 and 1995 and found a 24% increase in the number of patients greater than 60 years of age admitted as a result of spinal trauma.

The introduction of well thought out and validated treatment protocols for spinal trauma has greatly improved the prognosis for the trauma patient. Treatment begins prior to arrival at the hospital in the initial "prehospital" management stage. This is divided up into (1) patient evaluation, (2) resuscitation, (3) immobilization, (4) extrication, and (5) transport.

It is important to assume that any patient who has incurred a traumatic event and is nonresponsive or intoxicated has a spinal injury until proven otherwise. Proper advanced trauma life support (ATLS) protocols should be instituted in the field. Additional trained personnel (i.e., emergency medical technicians, police officers, and firefighters) may be necessary if a complicated extrication is necessary. A cervical collar should be placed, and using in-line cervical traction, the patient should be transported to a rigid spine board. The head and neck should then be stabilized with head and side supports that attach to the spine board. The remainder of the patient's body should be secured to the board with straps. If the injury occurs during a sporting event, the helmet, if present, should be left in place until the patient reaches a secure setting. If a face mask is present, it may be removed to provide life support to the patient. The method of transport should be based on the distance the patient is from the hospital of destination.

Basic and advanced life measures are continued during patient arrival at the hospital. During the primary survey, the ABCs (airway, breathing, circulation) of life support are again reviewed. It is important to maintain optimal oxygenation to a patient with a spinal cord injury. Patients with high cervical injuries are often unable to maintain a sustainable airway, and if neurologic injury is present, early intubation is often required. Maintenance of adequate oxygenation will modify the adverse sequelae of the secondary cascade of neurologic dysfunction that occurs in the setting of a spinal cord injury. The patient's cardiovascular status should be evaluated for the presence of hypovolemic or neurogenic shock. In neurogenic shock the parasympathetic pathways are unregulated because of the disruption of the efferent sympathetic pathways. In both neurogenic and hypovolemic shock, hypotension is present. Neurogenic shock can be differentiated from hypovolemic shock by the presence of bradycardia in the setting of hypotension. Treatment of neurogenic shock involves placing the patient in Trendelenburg's position with judicious intravenous fluid administration. If necessary, pressors (e.g., atropine) may be given.

Appropriate pharmacologic therapy (methylprednisilone) for the treatment of spinal cord injury should be initiated if the patient comes to the hospital within 8 hours of injury.

CLASSIFICATION OF SPINAL CORD INJURY

Many different classification systems have been developed to define the nature of a spinal cord injury. In general a spinal cord injury can be described as complete, in which there is absence of motor or sensory function below the level of spinal injury, or incomplete, in which there is preservation of motor or sensory function

Box 34-1	ASIA Classification

- ASIA A—complete spinal cord injury
- ASIA B—sensation but no motor function below the level of injury
- ASIA C—motor function graded 3 or less distal to the level of injury
- ASIA D—motor function greater than 3 below the level of injury
- ASIA E—normal neurologic examination

Data from American Spinal Injury Association (ASIA): *Standards for neurological and functional classification of spinal cord injury—revised 1992,* Chicago, 1992, The Association.

below the level of injury. This may manifest as only preservation of sensation in the S4 to S5 distribution or contraction of the anal sphincter muscle group. The diagnosis of a complete injury cannot be made until the resolution of spinal shock. Spinal shock is defined as the transient loss of all motor function, sensation, and reflexes below the level of injury. In the majority of cases the duration of spinal shock is approximately 48 hours; however, it may be prolonged with certain medical comorbidities such as urinary tract infections or sepsis.[7] The return of sacral spinal reflexes such as the bulbocavernosus or anal wink signifies the end of spinal shock. An accurate assessment of the patient's neurologic status is imperative because it relates to the degree of anticipated neurologic recovery and the potential need for surgical intervention. In complete injuries significant neurologic recovery is less likely.

The American Spinal Injury Association (ASIA) scale (Box 34-1), which is a modification of the Frankel scale, is commonly used to grade spinal cord injury. It ranks injury from A through E. ASIA A is a complete spinal cord injury with absent sensory or motor function below the level of injury. ASIA B through D are incomplete spinal cord injuries. ASIA B represents the preservation of distal sensation but no motor function below the level of injury; ASIA C is defined as motor function of less than a grade 3 of 5 distal to the level of injury. ASIA D is an incomplete lesion with motor function of greater than or equal to 3 below the level of injury. Finally, ASIA E represents a normal spinal cord neurologic examination.[3]

SPINAL CORD SYNDROMES

Spinal cord injuries may also be classified based on the pattern of symptoms present, which is predicated on the anatomic location of the lesion within the spinal cord parenchyma. Four syndromes (Figure 34-1, *A* to *D*) have been described: central cord syndrome, anterior cord syndrome, posterior cord syndrome, and Brown-Séquard's syndrome.[69]

The central cord syndrome is most commonly seen in older patients who have preexisting cervical spondylosis. It is also the most common type of spinal cord syndrome. Patients present with motor deficits in the upper extremity with relative sparing of the lower extremity. The proposed mechanism is that of hyperextension with

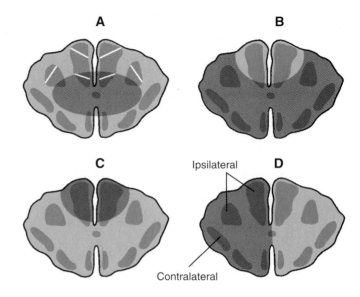

Figure 34-1. Spinal cord syndromes. **A,** Central cord syndrome. **B,** Anterior cord syndrome. **C,** Posterior cord syndrome. **D,** Brown-Séquard's syndrome.

resultant narrowing of the cervical canal diameter, resulting in anterior thecal sac compression by anterior vertebral body osteophytes and posterior thecal sac compression by inbuckling of the ligamentum flavum. Significant neurologic recovery in this syndrome is poor to fair.

Damage to the anterior two thirds of the spinal cord is seen in the anterior cord syndrome. This is clinically manifested as loss of motor function below the level of injury with variable changes in touch, pain, and temperature sensation. Functional recovery is dependent on the extent of injury (i.e., complete or incomplete).

The posterior cord syndrome is characterized by loss of vibrational sensation and proprioception. Gross touch may be spared because of the anterior location of the spinothalamic tracts. Functional outcome is fair.

Brown-Séquard's syndrome is due to damage of only one half of the spinal cord. There is ipsilateral motor weakness and loss of proprioception with contralateral loss of pain, temperature, and light touch. Functional prognosis is best in this type of spinal cord syndrome. Over 90% of patients with this syndrome will recover bowel and bladder function and will be able to ambulate.[12]

UPPER CERVICAL SPINE INJURIES
Occipital Condyle Fractures

Occipital condyle fractures are a relatively rarely reported injury. However, some studies show that occipital condyle fractures may occur in as many as 16% of patients with head or cervical injury.[55] An injury to the occipital condyle is usually due to axial compression associated with a lateral or anterior shear force. Many times a rotatory component may be involved. This injury may occur alone, with other noncontiguous injuries to the cervical

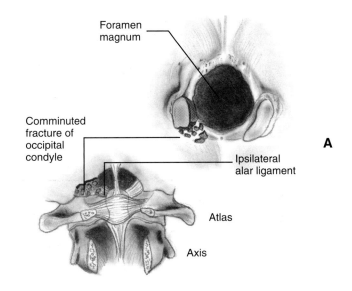

OCCIPITAL CONDYLE FRACTURES

- 33% incidence of associated atlanto-occipital injury
- Majority neurologically intact
- Beware of cranial nerve injuries
- Modality of choice: CT imaging
- Classification of Anderson and Montesano
  - I: Impacted, comminuted fracture—cervical orthosis
  - II: Extension of basilar skull fracture—cervical orthosis
  - III: Avulsion of alar ligament—halo, surgery

spine, or associated with subluxation or dislocation of the atlanto-occipital articulation. Goldstein et al.[36] found that as many as 33% of occipital condyle fractures were found to have evidence of atlanto-occipital injury.

Patient complaints and neurologic injury are variable. Many times the patient will have no neurologic deficit; however, occasionally significant impairment will exist, manifesting as complete quadriplegia with diaphragm paralysis. Patients may have suboccipital pain and head tilt. Cranial nerves IX, X, XI, and XII are particularly susceptible to injury, with rare injury occurring to cranial nerves VI and VII.[11,22,83]

Occipital condyle fractures are rarely diagnosed on cervical radiographs.[11,47] Bloom et al.[11] reported the presence of nine occipital condyle fractures in 55 (16.4%) patients who sustained high-energy blunt trauma to their head or upper neck. None of these fractures was diagnosed by plain radiography. It is therefore recommended that computed tomography (CT) be used as the imaging modality of choice if suspicion of an occipital condyle fracture is present.

The Anderson and Montesano classification of occipital condyle fractures[6] is a popular means of describing these injuries. It is divided into three types (Figure 34-2, *A* to *C*). Type I is a nondisplaced, impacted, comminuted fracture of the occipital condyle that is most commonly the result of an axial load. In a type I injury the ipsilateral alar ligament may be injured, but the tectorial membrane and contralateral alar ligament are intact. Type II injuries (Figure 34-3) are usually the result of a direct blow to the head. These injuries are considered extensions of a basilar skull fracture that may extend into the foramen magnum. The alar ligaments and tectorial membrane are intact. Type III injuries are displaced occipital condyle avulsion fractures of the alar and are potentially unstable if the tectorial membrane is disrupted.

Type I and II injuries are stable injuries and may be treated in a hard cervical collar for 2 to 3 months. Surgical intervention (i.e., arthrodesis) may be necessary for occipital condyle fractures with associated cervical spine injuries or persistent instability. Type III fractures are considered unstable and require halo-vest immobilization and possibly surgical stabilization.

Alternatively, Tuli et al.[82] developed a classification of occipital condyle fractures based on plain radiographs, CT and/or magnetic resonance imaging (MRI) studies.

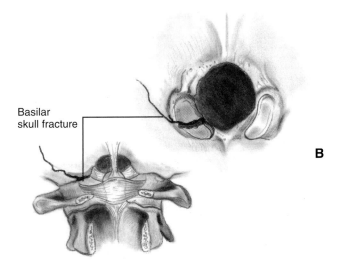

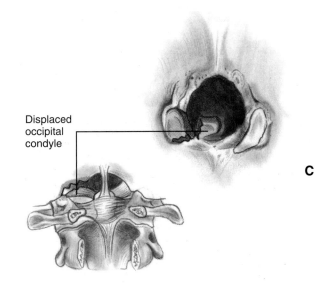

Figure 34-2. Anderson and Montesano classification of occipital condyle fractures. **A,** Type I. **B,** Type II. **C,** Type III.

Classification is based on fracture displacement and stability. Tuli type I (stable) occipital condyle fractures are nondisplaced. Type IIA (stable) fractures are displaced but without ligamentous instability, and Type IIB (unstable) fractures are displaced and have ligamentous instability.

Atlanto-Occipital Dislocations

The diagnosis of an atlanto-occipital dislocation, also referred to as craniocervical dissociation, is infrequently seen because of the high mortality associated with this injury subtype. The diagnosis of atlanto-occipital injuries has been increasing secondary to the improvement in prehospital stabilization and care of patients with spinal cord injuries. Its true incidence, however, cannot be adequately determined. These injuries tend to occur twice as commonly in children than adults because of the more horizontal orientation of the atlanto-occipital joint in children.[14]

In a postmortem review of 312 multitrauma victims, Alker et al.[2] found 19 atlanto-occipital dislocations. Likewise Bucholz and Burkhead[14] found 9 atlanto-occipital dislocations in 112 multitrauma fatalities.

The mechanism that leads to an atlanto-occipital dislocation is unclear. Alker et al.[2] proposed a hyperflexion force, whereas Bucholz and Burkhead[14] postulated that longitudinal traction combined with a hyperextension force is necessary to create this injury. Others attribute a rotatory component as the primary force involved.[64]

Stability at the atlanto-occipital articulations is composed of the anterior and posterior atlanto-occipital membranes, the apical alar and cruciate ligaments (occiput to axis), the tectorial membrane (occiput to axis), and the extensor musculature of the neck.

The clinical presentation of this injury is variable, but most patients have significant neurologic impairment. Submental lacerations, mandible fractures, and posterior pharyngeal wall disruption may indicate an atlanto-occipital injury. Injury to the brainstem, cranial nerves (VII to X most common), spinomedullary portion of the spinal cord, and/or cervical roots is common. Vascular insults such as vertebral or basilar artery injuries or subarachnoid hemorrhage at the craniocervical junction must be ruled out.[67]

Radiographic diagnosis is usually obvious as noted by a large gap at the atlanto-occipital junction. However, survivors of this injury may show only subtle radiographic evidence of an occipitocervical injury. Many radiographic indicators of atlanto-occipital injury exist. The degree of soft tissue injury may be a nonspecific indicator of injury at this level. At the C2 level a retropharyngeal space measuring greater than 7 mm may be a sign of injury. The Powers[66] ratio (BC/OA) (Figure 34-4) is the most common measurement used to evaluate the occipitocervical junction. It is measured on a lateral cervical radiograph, tomogram, or sagittal CT reconstruction. The Powers ratio is defined as the ratio of the distance from the basion (B) to the anterior edge of the posterior C1 arch (C) divided by the distance from the opisthion (O) to the posterior edge of the anterior C1 arch (A). A normal ratio is between 0.77 and 1.0; a value greater than 1.0 may suggest an injury to the atlanto-occipital junction or more specifically anterior displacement of the occiput in relation to the atlas.

Other radiographic markers[27,42,52] suggestive of atlanto-occipital dislocation include (1) displacement of Wackenheim's line, which is defined as a line that extends from the posterior tip of the clivus to the posterior tip of the odontoid; (2) a distance from the odontoid tip to the tip of the basion measuring greater than

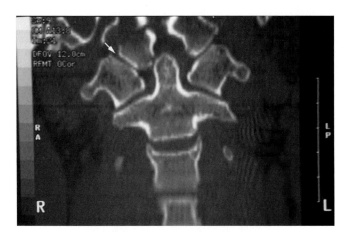

Figure 34-3. Coronal CT reconstruction demonstrating a type II occipital condyle fracture. The arrow shows the beginning of a linear fracture of the right occipital condyle at the level of the occipital to C1 articulation.

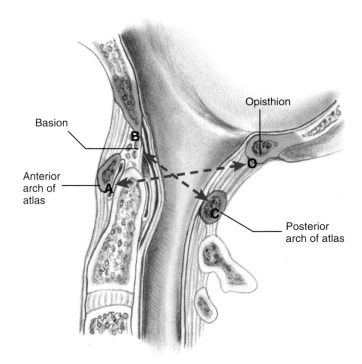

Figure 34-4. Powers ratio. A, Anterior arch of the atlas. B, Basion. C, Posterior arch of the atlas. O, Opisthion.

10 mm in children and 5 mm in adults; and (3) an incongruity in the relationship between the posterior margin of the foramen magnum and the spinolaminar line of C1, which should normally line up.

The most commonly used classification for atlanto-occipital injuries is described by Traynelis et al.[81] and is based on the direction of displacement of the occiput relative to the axis (Figure 34-5, *A* to *D*). Type I injuries are the most common and are described as anterior subluxation or dislocation of the occiput in relation to C1. Type II injuries are a distraction injury without evidence of dislocation, and type III injuries are posterior dislocations of the occiput in relationship to the atlas.

Treatment is aimed at obtaining immediate alignment and fracture stability. Type II injuries should be immobilized in a halo vest with slight axial compression applied to the skull. Type I and III injuries require closed reduction followed by halo-vest immobilization. Because of the degree and nature of ligamentous disruption associated with an atlanto-occipital dislocation, all three types should be treated with surgical stabilization of the occiput to the upper cervical spine followed by postoperative halo immobilization (Figure 34-6, *A* and *B*).

Atlas Fractures

Fractures of the atlas are relatively rare and account for only 2% of all spinal fractures and 10% of cervical spine fractures.[32,49] Common mechanisms include motor

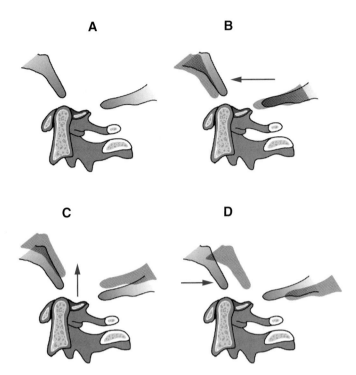

Figure 34-5. Traynelis classification for atlanto-occipital injuries. **A,** Normal atlanto-occipital relationship. **B,** Type I—anterior displacement. **C,** Type II—axial distraction injury. **D,** Type III—posterior displacement.

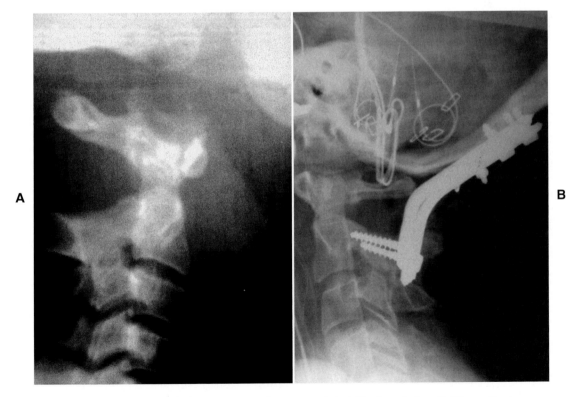

Figure 34-6. **A,** Lateral plain x-ray revealing an occipital C1 dissociation. **B,** The patient underwent a gentle closed reduction followed by a posterior occipital to C2 fusion with plates and screws to confer immediate stability.

ATLANTO-OCCIPITAL DISLOCATION

- High associated mortality
- More common in children
- Significant association with cranial nerve, vertebral artery, and cervical root injuries
- Normal Power's ratio (BC/OA) should be <1
- Traynelis classification
  - I: Distraction
  - II: Anterior subluxation/dislocation
  - III: Distraction
- All treated with closed reduction followed by posterior cervical fusion and halo immobilization

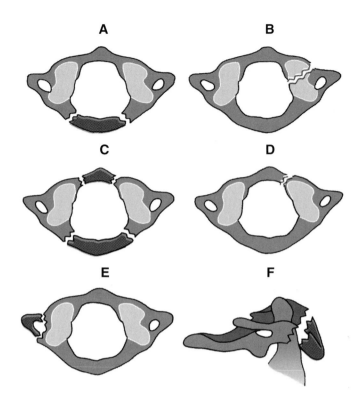

Figure 34-7. Patterns of atlas fractures. **A,** Levine and Edwards type I—posterior arch fracture. **B,** Levine and Edwards type II—lateral mass fracture. **C,** Levine and Edwards type III—classic Jefferson's or burst fracture. **D,** Unilateral anterior arch fracture. **E,** Transverse process fracture. **F,** Avulsion fracture of the anterior arch.

vehicle accidents, diving, falls from a height, or direct impact from objects falling overhead.[32] Over half of the documented atlas fractures are commonly associated with other cervical injuries.[57] Odontoid and axis fractures are the most frequent injuries associated with C1 injuries. Other concomitant injuries include occipital condyle fractures, rupture of the transverse ligament, and subaxial cervical fractures.[57]

Neurologic injuries are rare with C1 injuries because of the capacious size of the spinal canal at this level and the fact that many atlas fractures are space-expanding injuries (e.g., burst fractures). Patients usually complain of headaches and upper neck and suboccipital pain. However, because of the anatomic proximity of certain cranial nerves to the C1 ring, cranial nerve injuries may be observed. These may involve specifically cranial nerves IX, X, and XII. Connolly et al.[18] recently reported a case of Collet-Sicard syndrome (cranial nerves IX, X, XI, XII palsy without Horner's syndrome) after a Jefferson's burst fracture. The axial applied load causes the lateral masses to displace laterally and impinge on the cranial nerves. Associated injuries to the greater occipital nerves, suboccipital nerves, and vertebral arteries may also occur.

Atlas fractures are most commonly the result of an axial load applied to the head combined with either a flexion or an extension force. The mechanism for an anterior arch fracture is a flexion force associated with axial loading. Posterior arch fractures, which are the most common, are the result of an extension force combined with an axial load. The fact that posterior arch fractures are more common is consistent with findings of Doherty et al.[26] that the cortical bone of the posterior arch of C1 is the thinnest. Anatomic measurements performed found that the anterior-posterior and lateral dimensions of the atlas are generally constant between individuals. The sagittal canal diameter is approximately 32 mm, and the lateral dimension is approximately 29 mm. The thickness of the ring is approximately 6 mm anteriorly and 8 mm posteriorly. However, there is significant variability of lateral mass height and sagittal plane diameter.

Many classification systems have been proposed for atlas fractures (Figure 34-7, A-F). Levine and Edwards[58] classified atlas fractures into three types. In this classi-

fication system type I atlas fractures, which are fractures of the posterior arch of C1, were most common. If in isolation, these injuries are considered stable. Type II atlas fractures are fractures involving the lateral mass. These are the result of an axial load with a lateral bending moment. Type III atlas fractures are the classic burst or Jefferson type of fracture. These patients have either three (one in the anterior arch and two in the posterior arch) or four (two anterior and two posterior arch) fracture lines.

Occasionally low-energy forces such as a hyperextension moment may result in an avulsion fracture of the longus colli muscle at the anterior tubercle. A laterally applied axial load may also result in an isolated C1 transverse process fracture.

Fracture stability is based on the integrity of the transverse ligament. There is a high incidence of transverse ligament injuries associated with atlas burst fractures. If the transverse ligament is intact, the C1 injury is usually considered stable. Spence et al.[76] correlated the degree of lateral mass displacement to the integrity of the transverse ligament. They found a high incidence of transverse ligament disruptions with a combined lateral mass spread or overhang greater than 6.9 mm. If the lateral mass spread is less than 5.7 mm, there is high probability that the transverse ligament is intact.[76] This measurement can be made on an odontoid view or axial

CT scan. Because it is often difficult to visualize anterior or posterior arch fractures on plain radiography, CT is the recommended imaging modality for suspected C1 ring fractures. Heller et al.[44] reported that x-ray magnification must be accounted for in inferring injury to the transverse ligament. On an odontoid view, combined displacement of the lateral masses greater than 8.1 mm implies injury to the transverse ligament.[44] Injury to the transverse ligament may be inferred by the presence of an avulsion fracture of the medial tubercle of C1 at the insertion site of the transverse ligament. The integrity of the transverse ligament can also be evaluated by measuring the atlantodental interval (ADI) on a lateral cervical spine radiograph. Measurements of greater than 4 mm in the adult are highly suspicious for transverse ligament injury.[65] In addition, MRI may be used for direct visualization of the transverse ligament.[25]

Treatment of stable isolated atlas fractures is predominately nonoperative. Posterior ring, anterior tubercle, and transverse process fractures are treated successfully with a cervical hard collar. Traditionally many Jefferson's burst fractures and lateral mass fractures were treated with halo immobilization. However, in a retrospective review, Lee et al.[53] found that 12 patients with isolated burst fractures treated with 10 to 12 weeks of immobilization in a hard cervical collar achieved stable union without evidence of instability.

Unstable C1 injuries with an injury to the transverse ligament should be treated differently than isolated atlas fractures. Dickman et al.[24] have classified transverse ligament injuries into two types: type I involves disruption of the midsubstance of the ligament, and type II lesions are avulsions of the transverse ligament from the medial tubercle of C1. The authors found that no patient in a series of 15 with a type I ligament injury had healing of the ligament disruption with nonoperative treatment. Midsubstance ligament injuries in the adult have a poor propensity to heal and should be treated with an atlantoaxial fusion. Dickman et al.[21] found that 74% of patients with type II injuries healed without surgery. Type II injuries may be treated with a trial of halo immobilization, followed by close observation. Occasionally patients may be unable to tolerate halo immobilization, and surgical stabilization may become necessary. McGuire and Harkey[62] demonstrated an internal fixation method for unstable Jefferson's fractures using the Magerl C2 to C1 transarticular screw technique without postoperative halo immobilization. They obtained a successful solid fusion with maintenance of motion at the occipital cervical junction.

Atlantoaxial Subluxation

Traumatic atlantoaxial subluxation is most commonly the result of a motor vehicle accident. The mechanism is usually a combination of flexion, extension, and rotation. The C1 to C2 complex allows for significant rotation but is limited in anterior/posterior motion. The primary restraint to anterior subluxation of C1 on C2 is the transverse ligament, with the alar ligaments acting as a secondary restraint. These ligaments allow rotation of C1

ATLAS FRACTURES

- 10% of cervical spine fractures
- >50% have associated cervical injuries
- Neurologic injuries rare
- Posterior arch fractures most common
- Classification
  - I: Posterior arch fracture
  - II: Lateral mass fracture
  - III: Jefferson's (burst) fracture
- All stable fractures may be treated with a hard collar or halo-vest immobilization
- Transverse ligament conveys stability—evaluate for injury
  - Lateral mass overhang <5.7 mm—no transverse ligament injury
  - Lateral mass overhang >6.9 mm—high probability of transverse ligament injury
  - ADI >4 mm—possible transverse ligament injury
- Transverse ligament injury
  - Type I: Midsubstance tear/rupture—surgery
  - Type II: Avulsion fracture—no surgery

---

concentrically around the dens while limiting anterior subluxation. Through cadaveric studies Werne[86] has shown that dislocation of C1 to C2 occurs at 63 degrees of rotation, and further rotation will result in significant spinal canal compromise. Fielding et al.[31] similarly found that atlantoaxial dislocation will occur at 65 degrees of rotation if the transverse ligament is intact. At this degree of rotation the spinal canal is narrowed to 7 mm. If the transverse ligament is injured and there is 5 mm of displacement of C1 on C2, unilateral C1 to C2 facet dislocation will occur at 45 degrees of rotation with spinal canal narrowing approaching approximately 12 mm.

Clinically patients complain of limited cervical motion and suboccipital pain. The head may be in the "cock robin" position, in which the head is rotated 20 degrees in one direction and tilted 20 degrees in the opposite direction (Figure 34-8).

Radiographs are extremely useful in aiding the diagnosis of C1 to C2 instability. On the open-mouth anteroposterior (AP) "odontoid" view, C1 to C2 rotation may be observed. The lateral mass that is rotated forward appears wider and closer to the midline, whereas the contralateral lateral mass appears narrower and farther from the midline. The spinous processes may appear deviated from the midline. A CT scan or MRI may be helpful in providing more detail (Figure 34-9, *A* and *B*).

The atlanto-dens interval can be measured on the lateral radiograph to evaluate the integrity of the transverse atlantal ligament. Fielding et al.[31] classified fixed atlantoaxial subluxations into four types (Figure 34-10, *A* to *D*). Type I, which is the most common, is rotation without subluxation. There is less than 3 mm of displacement of C1 on C2, and this is within the normal range of physiologic motion. In type II injuries there is between 3 and 5 mm of anterior displacement of C1 on C2. This is the range that potentially signifies injury to the transverse ligament. In type III injuries there is more

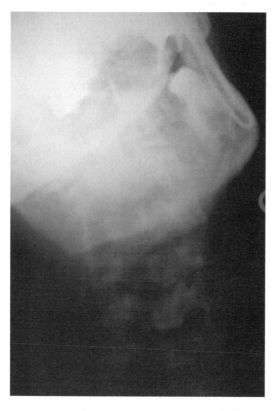

Figure 34-8. AP x-ray revealing the typical cock robin head position in a patient with a C1 to C2 rotatory dislocation.

than 5 mm of displacement of the atlanto-dens interval, signifying complete disruption of both the transverse ligament and supporting secondary ligamentous structures. Type IV subluxations are rare and are seen in patients with posterior displacement of the atlas on the axis. These are usually seen with odontoid injuries or in patients with rheumatoid arthritis who have erosion of the dens.

Treatment depends on the age of the patient, chronicity of the deformity, and the presence or absence of a neurologic deficit. Patients with type I acute traumatic atlantoaxial instability can be treated initially with head-halter traction (3 to 5 pounds) or a hard collar and sedation. If a reduction cannot be obtained within 1 to 2 weeks with collar immobilization or reduction does not occur with head-halter traction, skeletal traction is indicated. Once a reduction is obtained in a patient requiring traction, traction is maintained for 1 to 2 weeks followed by halo-vest immobilization. If reduction is not obtained, an open reduction and atlantoaxial arthrodesis followed by cervical orthosis or halo immobilization may be necessary. Type II and III injuries in children without a neurologic deficit may initially be treated with halo-vest immobilization. However, Type II and III atlantoaxial injuries are considered unstable, and C1 to C2 arthrodesis is recommended in the adult. Other indications for surgery include instability with neurologic symptoms, recurrence of deformity, prolonged nontreated deformity for greater than 3 months, or injuries resistant to nonoperative treatment.[4]

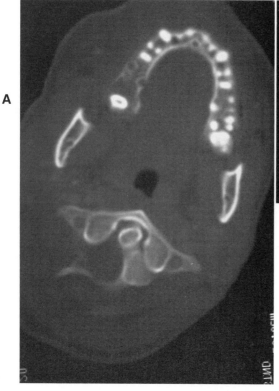

A

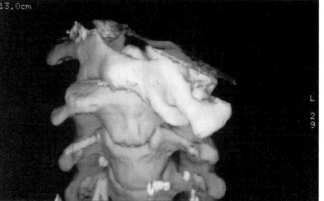

B

Figure 34-9. **A,** Transaxial CT scan revealing a dislocation of the right C1 to C2 articulation. **B,** Three- dimensional CT scan revealing a rotatory dislocation of the C1 to C2 articulation.

Odontoid Fractures

Odontoid fractures make up approximately 5% to 15% of cervical spine fractures, and approximately 25% are associated with a neurologic deficit. These injuries carry a 5% to 10% mortality rate. The mechanism of odontoid injuries is debated. It is felt that posteriorly displaced fractures are the result of a hyperextension force, whereas anteriorly displaced fractures are due to a hyperflexion force. Although many classification schemes exist for odontoid fractures, the most commonly used system is that of Anderson and D'Alonzo[5] (Figure 34-11, *A* to *D*). A type I fracture is an oblique fracture of the distal one third of the odontoid peg. It most likely represents an avulsion of the alar and apical ligaments. Some authors believe that this injury subtype is not an isolated injury and is a marker for serious injuries such as an atlanto-occipital dislocation.[15] Type II injuries are fractures involving the base of the dens where it meets the body of C2. Type III fractures extend into the cancellous portion of the body of C2 and usually involve one or both of the superior articular surfaces. Hadley et al.[39] have added a fourth type of fracture, type IIA, which is similar to type II injury but involves significant comminution of the odontoid base, making reduction difficult. They postulated that these injuries may involve injury to the ligamentous structure of the odontoid and may need more aggressive treatment. Puttlitz et al.[68] performed a finite element analysis based on cadaveric data to elucidate the mechanisms responsible for odontoid fractures. They found that hyperextension coupled with lateral shear or compression leads to type I fractures, and axial rotation and lateral shear can produce type II fractures. The authors were unable to find a model for type III fractures.

Treatment is guided by the type of odontoid fracture. Type I fractures that do not involve injury to the ligamentous structures supporting the atlanto-occipital articulation can be treated in a cervical orthosis for 3 months. There is debate about the ideal treatment for type II fractures due to the documented poor healing potential of the fracture in the elderly and the noted

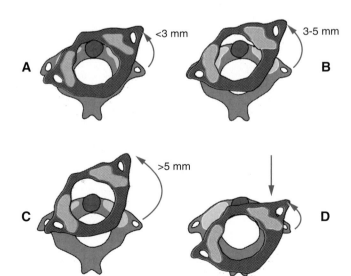

ATLANTOAXIAL SUBLUXATION

- Presentation often in the cock robin position with decreased range of motion (ROM)
- Lateral mass asymmetry visualized on AP open-mouth x-ray
- Fielding and Hawkins classification of atlantoaxial rotatory fixation
  - Type I: ADI <3 mm—transverse ligament intact
  - Type II: ADI 3 to 5 mm—transverse ligament insufficient
  - Type III: ADI >5 mm—complete disruption of transverse ligament
  - Type IV: Rare—posterior displacement of C1 on C2

Figure 34-10. Fielding and Hawkins classification of atlantoaxial rotatory fixation. **A,** Type I. **B,** Type II. **C,** Type III. **D,** Type IV.

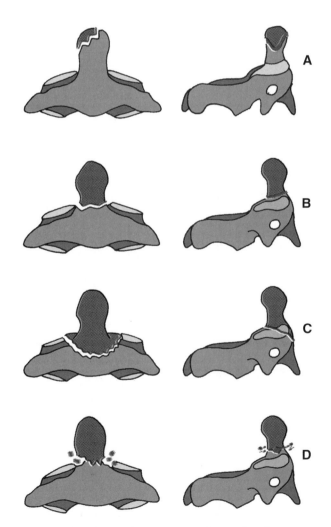

Figure 34-11. Anderson and D'Alonzo classification of odontoid fractures. **A,** Type I. **B,** Type II. **C,** Type III. **D,** Hadley type IIa odontoid fracture.

morbidity associated with prolonged halo treatment. In their review of 96 patients with type II odontoid fractures, Clark and White[17] found a 32% nonunion rate. They identified fracture displacement greater than 5 mm and angulation greater than 10 degrees as risk factors for nonunion or malunion in nonoperatively treated patients. In a review of 128 patients with an odontoid fracture, Dunn and Seljeskog[28] identified 65 years of age as a significant risk factor for nonunion of type II fractures. Currently it is recommended that displaced odontoid fractures undergo closed reduction with skeletal traction followed by collar or halo-vest immobilization. Relative indications for surgery include displacement greater than 5 mm, angulation greater than 10 degrees, age greater than 50 years, or failed attempted reductions or a history of fracture displacement or nonunion. Recently Lennarson et al.[54] found a 21 times higher risk of failure of halo immobilization for type II odontoid fractures in patients greater than 50 years of age. The authors recommended surgical intervention in this age group. Type IIA fractures with significant comminution may also be best treated with surgical stabilization.[40] Type III fractures are often successfully treated with halo-vest immobilization.[17]

Care must be taken when reducing odontoid fractures in skeletal traction. Harrop et al.[43] found that 40% of elderly patients with posteriorly displaced odontoid fractures experienced respiratory difficulty during acute flexion reduction of these fractures.

The gold standard for surgical treatment of type II odontoid fractures is C1 to C2 stabilization. More recently the use of anterior screw fixation has become more popular. A posterior C1 to C2 fusion theoretically decreases cervical rotation by as much as 50%. Odontoid screw fixation does not immobilize the C1 to C2 complex and thus theoretically preserves axial rotation.

Anterior odontoid screw fixation can be performed with either one or two screws (Figure 34-12). Studies comparing one- versus two-screw techniques show that there is no difference between the two in terms of load to failure. With either one- or two-screw fixation, fracture stability is only restored to one half of the native odontoid strength. In evaluating the cause of failure of odontoid screws, Doherty et al.[26] found that anterior odontoid screws fail secondary to screw bending in type II fractures and by screw cutout in type III fractures. Graziano et al.[37] compared screw fixation (one and two) versus C1 to C2 wiring and also found no differences between one and two screws with regard to bending and torsional stiffness. Screw fixation was stiffer than wiring in bending, but there was no difference in torsion. Chang et al.[16] reported 100% fusion with preservation of rotation in 12 patients undergoing single anterior odontoid screw fixation for type II odontoid fractures.

Many authors caution about the risk of anterior screw cutout in osteopenic bone in the elderly patient population. Berlemann and Schwarzenbach[10] reported on 19 patients over 65 years of age who were treated with anterior screw fixation. At an average follow-up of 4.5 years, the authors observed 16 cases of solid union at 3 to 6 months and 2 cases of pseudarthrosis that required no further treatment. Fifteen patients reported no symp-

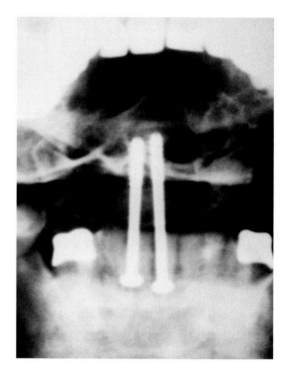

Figure 34-12. Open-mouth AP x-ray following anterior odontoid screw fixation for a type II odontoid fracture. Two 3.5-mm partially threaded screws were used to lag the fracture fragments together.

toms related to their fracture. The authors concluded that anterior screw fixation is successful in most elderly patients with type II odontoid fractures.

One should be vigilant about ruling out an associated transverse ligament injury in a patient for whom anterior odontoid screw fixation is considered. Greene et al.[38] reported on the treatment of three patients with an odontoid fracture and associated transverse ligament injury. They recommended posterior stabilization of these injuries because of the unpredictable nature of transverse ligament healing. Anterior screw fixation is contraindicated in this setting due to the potential for persistent transverse ligament nonhealing and late instability.

The method of management of an elderly patient with an odontoid fracture has evolved over the last two decades in terms of the recommendation for surgical intervention in the majority of patients. Many authors have reported a high rate of nonunion and morbidity and mortality in this patient population when treated nonoperatively and especially in a halo device. The majority of elderly patients are unable to tolerate prolonged immobilization, which is often a sequela of conservative treatment in this patient population.[8,41,73]

Traumatic Spondylolisthesis of the Axis

Traumatic spondylolisthesis of the axis is a fracture that extends through the C2 pars interarticularis bilaterally, resulting in an anterolisthesis of the C2 body on the C3 body. The term *hangman's fracture* is derived from the time

ODONTOID FRACTURES

- 5% to 15% of cervical spine fractures
- 25% incidence of associated neurologic deficit
- Anderson and D'Alonzo classification
  - Type I: Avulsion of the tip of dens—orthosis/rule out instability
  - Type II: Fracture through body of dens—halo versus surgery
  - Type III: Fracture extends into body of C2—halo
- Type II nonunion risk: >50 years of age, >5-mm displacement, redisplacement, angulation
- Posterior C1 to C2 fusion versus anterior odontoid screw fixation
- Must evaluate integrity of the transverse ligament

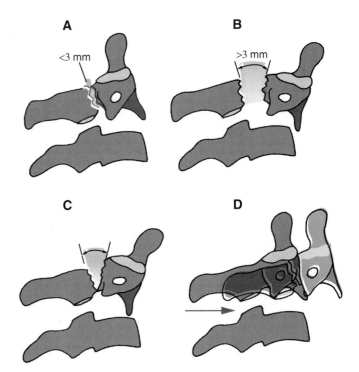

Figure 34-13. Levine and Edwards modification of classification of Effendi et al. of traumatic spondylolisthesis of the axis. **A,** Type I. **B,** Type II. **C,** Type IIa. **D,** Type III.

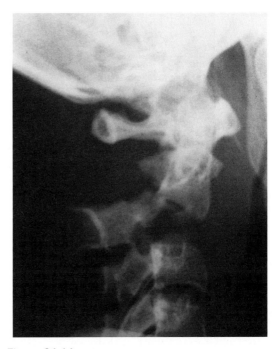

Figure 34-14. Lateral plain x-ray of a type IIA hangman's fracture. Note the significant degree of angulation with widening of the C2 to C3 disc space.

of judicial hangings, when the hangman's knot was placed under the victim's chin, resulting in a violent axial traction and hyperextension force at the time of hanging. Today as many as 75% of hangman's fractures are caused by motor vehicle accidents. These injuries make up approximately 12% to 18% of all cervical spine fractures, with a mortality occurring in as many as 25% to 40% of these injuries. Among the survivors of a traumatic hangman's fracture, there is a relatively low incidence of neurologic injury, primarily due to the large cross-sectional area of the spinal canal at the C2 to C3 level. In addition, when these fractures are bilateral, there is actually an increase in the size of the spinal canal during the fracturing process. The patients who do have a spinal cord injury are usually those with concomitant severe injuries such as a C2 to C3 facet dislocation.

Most patients present with nonspecific complaints of neck pain and report a sense of cervical instability. It is important to be aware of the possibility of other upper cervical spine (atlas, odontoid), cranial nerve, or vascular injuries.

The most commonly used classification is the Levine and Edwards[56] modification of the classification of Effendi et al.[29] (Figure 34-13, *A* to *D*). Type I fractures are bilateral fractures through the pars interarticularis (or adjacent superior and inferior articular processes) with less than 3-mm displacement of C2 on C3 and no angulation. By definition the C3 body is intact. Type II fractures have greater than 3-mm displacement of C2 on C3 with angulation. Commonly there is a wedge-compression fracture of the anterosuperior aspect of C3 or an avulsion fracture at the posteroinferior body of C2. Type IIa fractures (Figure 34-14) have severe angulation but little displacement. The fracture line in type IIa fractures is more oblique than the vertically oriented fractures seen in type I and II injuries. In type IIa fractures the anterior longitudinal ligament is intact, resulting in a secondary flexion deformity due to the disruption of the posterior longitudinal ligament. Type III fractures are fracture dislocations of C2 on C3 with either a unilateral or bilateral facet dislocation. Severe displacement and angulation may occur because there is disruption to both the anterior and posterior ligamentous structures.

Starr and Eismont[78] have identified an atypical variant of the hangman's fracture in which a fracture line extends through the posterior cortex of the C2 body. They noted a 33% incidence of neurologic injury in these patients because of narrowing of the spinal canal.

TRAUMATIC SPONDYLOLISTHESIS OF THE AXIS

- 12% to 18% of cervical fractures
- Mortality 25% to 40%
- Low incidence of mortality in type I and II fractures, increased in type III fractures
- Levine and Edwards classification
  - I: <3-mm fracture displacement—orthosis
  - II: >3-mm fracture displacement—traction reduction followed by halo
  - IIa: Angulation, minimal displacement—reduction with compression extension followed by halo
  - III: Fracture dislocation—open reduction if irreducible and surgical stabilization of the facet dislocation

Type I fractures are stable on flexion and extension radiographs and can be successfully immobilized with a cervical orthosis for 3 months. Coric et al.[19] treated 39 patients with hangman's fractures who had less than 6 mm of displacement in nonrigid immobilization (mostly Philadelphia collars) for 10 to 14 weeks and found that all patients healed in a stable manner.

Type II fractures can be successfully reduced via halo traction followed by halo-vest immobilization.[38] However, traction in a type IIa fracture may lead to significant fracture-fragment displacement. This fracture subtype is best treated with a compression-extension maneuver followed by halo-vest immobilization.

Muller et al.[63] have further subdivided type II fractures into three subgroups: flexion, extension, and listhesis. They recommended nonoperative (nonrigid) treatment for type II flexion and extension injuries. However, they found that type II spondylolisthesis type of injuries are unstable and have the potential for neurologic injury with nonoperative treatment.

Type III injuries are often difficult to reduce. If a successful reduction can be obtained with a unilateral facet dislocation, then halo immobilization is adequate for management of the C2 fracture, but surgical stabilization is recommended for the dislocated-facet injury. The majority of bilateral facet dislocations are difficult to reduce and usually require an open reduction and posterior C2 to C3 fusion followed by halo application to immobilize the pars fracture.

Axis Body Fractures

C2 body fractures have been classified by Benzel et al.[9] into three types. Type I are coronally oriented fractures, type II are sagittally oriented vertical fractures, and type III are horizontally oriented fractures and are equivalent to type III Anderson and D'Alonzo[5] odontoid fractures. Type II fractures appear as a C2 burst injury and may have retropulsion of bone into the spinal canal.

Fujimura et al.[33] reviewed 31 axis-body fractures and classified them into four types. Type I injuries are an avulsion fracture localized to the anteroinferior part of the axis body with anteroinferior displacement of the bony fragment. In type II injuries the fracture line runs transversely through the central region of the axis body. Type III injuries have an associated hangman's fracture with a comminuted burst fracture of the axis body, and a type IV injury is a fracture in the sagittal plane of the axis body. The authors recommend nonoperative management for type I and II fractures and surgical treatment (i.e., anterior C2 to C3 fusion) for type III and IV injuries.

SUBAXIAL CERVICAL SPINE

The subaxial cervical spine is biomechanically different from the upper cervical spine. The subaxial spine is responsible for 50% of cervical flexion, extension, and rotation. The posterior cervical facets are oriented 45 degrees in the coronal plane, which allows for significant motion. The three-column spine model divides the cervical spine into three distinct columns. The anterior column consists of the anterior half of the vertebral body, anterior annulus fibrosus, and anterior longitudinal ligament. The middle column includes the posterior longitudinal ligament, posterior annulus fibrosus, and posterior half of the vertebral body, and the posterior column is made up of the posterior ligamentous complex.[23]

The most commonly used classification system for subaxial cervical spine injuries is that described by Allen et al.[1] This classification is based on the mechanism of injury, including the direction of the injury force and the position of the neck at the time of injury. By knowing the probable mechanism of injury, one can predict the degree and type of bony and ligamentous injury. This classification is divided into six categories: compression flexion, vertical compression, distractive flexion, compression extension, distraction extension, and lateral flexion. Each category is then further subdivided into numbered stages, with the higher the number the more severe the injury.

Allen[1] found that common to all fracture patterns is the fact that compressive loads result in vertebral shortening whereas distraction results in spinal column lengthening. Although the majority of subaxial cervical spine fractures can be described by the Allen and Ferguson classification, some injuries are the result of combined forces and do not fit into any one category sufficiently. One study analyzed 10 cadaveric cervical spines by applying high-velocity flexion-compression loads to the head and demonstrated an array of injuries that were not adequately classified by existing systems due to multiple force vectors.[21]

Others describe subaxial cervical spine injuries based on their radiographic characteristics (i.e., compression fractures, burst fractures, teardrop fractures, posterior element fractures, avulsion fractures, and facet injuries).

Compression-Flexion Injuries

Compression-flexion (CF) injuries occur most commonly at the C4, C5, and C6 levels and make up approximately 20% of all subaxial spine fractures. The two most common mechanisms are motor vehicle accidents and

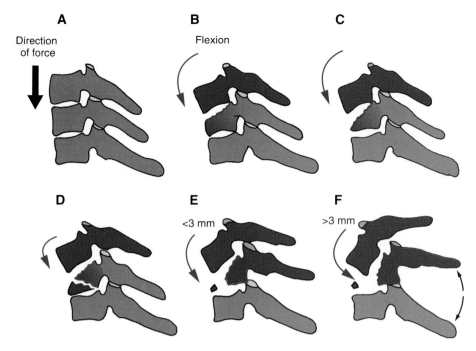

A Direction of force

B Flexion

C

D

E <3 mm

F >3 mm

Figure 34-15. Allen and Ferguson classification of compression-flexion injuries. **A,** Normal. **B,** Stage 1. **C,** Stage 2. **D,** Stage 3. **E,** Stage 4. **F,** Stage 5.

diving accidents. As the name describes, the anterior column fails in compression while the posterior column fails by distraction. Allen and Ferguson[1] divided CF injuries into five stages. The likelihood of spinal cord injury increases with the increasing stages of injury. They found evidence of a complete spinal cord injury in 25% of CF stage 3 (CFS3) injuries, 38% of CF stage 4 (CFS4) injuries, and 91% of CF stage 5 (CFS5) injuries.

In CF stage 1 (CFS1) (Figure 34-15, *B*) there is blunting and rounding of the anterosuperior margin of the vertebral body. As the force progresses to CF stage 2 (CFS2) (Figure 34-15, *C*) there is beaking of the antero-inferior vertebral body due to a loss of anterior vertebral body height. In CFS1 and CFS2 injuries the middle and posterior columns are spared, with some residual stability to the anterior column. Due to the relative stability of CFS1 and CFS2 injuries, they can be treated in a cervical orthosis or halo vest for approximately 10 to 12 weeks.

In a CFS3 injury (Figure 34-15, *D*), the CF force continues and causes an oblique fracture of the anterior vertebral beak from anterior superior to posterior inferior through the inferior subchondral plate. In a CFS4 injury (Figure 34-15, *E* and Figure 34-16) there is mild retrolisthesis of less than 3 mm of the vertebral body into the neural canal. These fractures, CFS3 and CFS4, may be treated in halo-vest immobilization if significant kyphosis or instability is not present. An MRI may be used to evaluate the degree of posterior ligamentous disruption present. Should instability in a CFS3 or CFS4 injury be a concern, either a posterior cervical fusion or an anterior corpectomy and fusion may be performed. If a neurologic deficit is present in the setting of anterior thecal sac

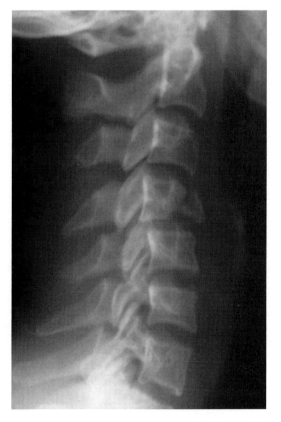

Figure 34-16. Lateral plain x-ray revealing a compression-flexion stage 4 injury involving the C4 vertebral body.

compression, an anterior procedure is recommended. If instability is still a concern after an anterior procedure, an additional posterior procedure may be necessary.

In a CFS5 injury (Figure 34-15, *F*) there is retrolisthesis or displacement of the fractured vertebral body into the neural canal of greater than 3 mm. By definition there is complete disruption of the posterior ligamentous complex resulting in a three-column injury. These injuries are often stabilized by an anterior decompression and stabilization procedure followed by a posterior fusion (Figure 34-17, *A* to *C*, and Figure 34-18, *A* and *B*).

Vertical Compression Injuries

Vertical compression (VC) injuries most commonly occur at the C6 and C7 levels as a result of a direct blow to the head or through blunt trauma from a motor vehicle or diving accident. This fracture subtype makes up approximately 15% of subaxial cervical injuries. In a VC stage 1 (VCS1) injury (Figure 34-19, *B*) there is a central "cupping" fracture of either the superior or inferior end plate. Ligamentous injury is uncommon. These injuries are usually treated with a cervical orthosis such as a hard collar.

In a VC stage 2 (VCS2) injury (Figure 34-19, *C*) the force progresses and causes a vertebral end plate fracture with minimal displacement of both the superior and inferior end plates. Again ligamentous injury is not common. Patients without neurologic injury may be treated with

---

COMPRESSION-FLEXION INJURIES

- 20% of subaxial cervical fractures
- Most common at C4, C5, C6 levels
- Treatment
  - CFS1 and CFS2—cervical orthosis or halo
  - CFS3 and CFS4
    - Halo if stable (posterior ligament intact)
    - Anterior or posterior surgery if instability present
    - Anterior decompression and fusion with neurologic injury and evidence of anterior thecal sac compression
  - CFS5—anterior and posterior procedure

VERTICAL COMPRESSION INJURIES

- Most common at C5 and C7
- 15% of subaxial cervical fractures
- Treatment
  - VCS1—cervical orthosis
  - VCS2—cervical orthosis or halo
  - VCS3—halo or anterior decompression and fusion in the presence of a neurologic deficit

---

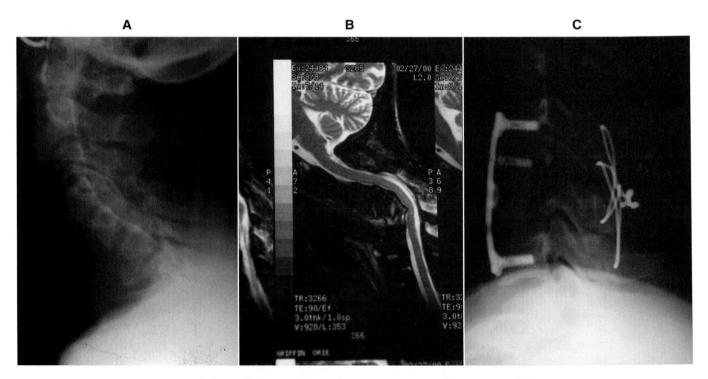

A   **B**   **C**

Figure 34-17.   **A,** Lateral plain x-ray revealing a compression-flexion stage 5 fracture to the C7 vertebral body. Note the significant degree of kyphosis. **B,** Sagittal plane MRI revealing an obvious cervical deformity in this advanced-stage compression-flexion injury. Note the tenting of the anterior thecal at the cervical thoracic junction. **C,** Lateral plain x-ray following a closed traction/reduction and anterior C7 corpectomy with fusion using iliac crest bone graft and anterior cervical plate followed by a posterior cervical wiring stabilization procedure.

either a cervical orthosis or halo-vest immobilization. VC stage 3 (VCS3) injuries (Figure 34-19, *D*) are similar to VCS2 injuries except there is displacement of the vertebral body into the spinal canal. Again these injuries may be treated with a halo vest. However, if neurologic injury is present, an anterior decompressive procedure followed by an instrumented fusion should be considered.

Distractive-Flexion Injuries

Distractive-flexion (DF) injuries account for approximately 10% of all subaxial cervical spine fractures. In a DF stage 1 (DFS1) injury (Figure 34-20, *B*) there is a divergence of the spinous processes (flexion sprain) with anterior facet subluxation of less than 25%. Often there is blunting of the anterosuperior vertebral margin of the

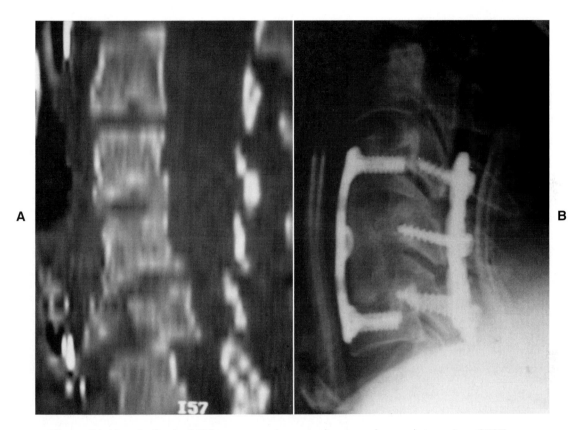

Figure 34-18. **A,** Sagittal CT reconstruction revealing an advanced stage (i.e., CFS5) injury to the C5 vertebral body. **B,** Lateral plain roentgenograph following an anterior C5 corpectomy and fusion with instrumentation followed by a posterior cervical stabilization with plates and screws.

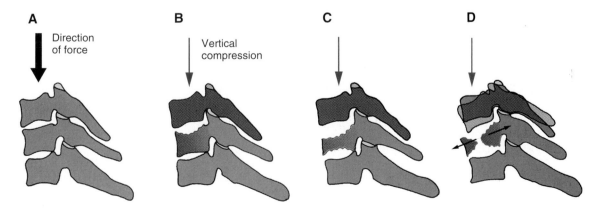

Figure 34-19. Allen and Ferguson classification of vertical compression injuries. **A,** Normal. **B,** Stage 1. **C,** Stage 2. **D,** Stage 3.

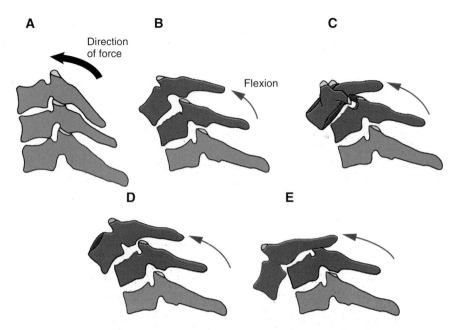

Figure 34-20.   Allen and Ferguson classification of distractive-flexion injuries. **A,** Normal. **B,** Stage 1. **C,** Stage 2. **D,** Stage 3. **E,** Stage 4.

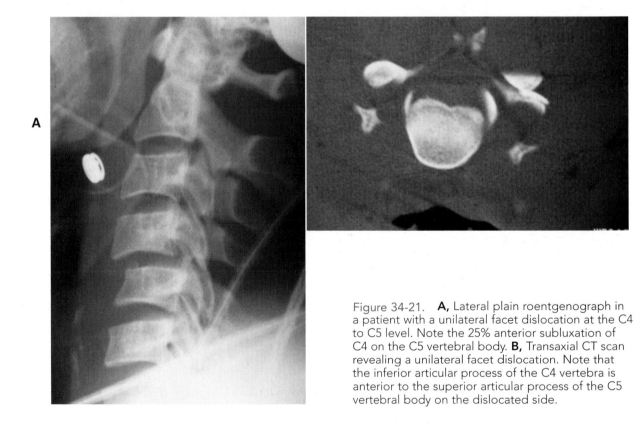

Figure 34-21.   **A,** Lateral plain roentgenograph in a patient with a unilateral facet dislocation at the C4 to C5 level. Note the 25% anterior subluxation of C4 on the C5 vertebral body. **B,** Transaxial CT scan revealing a unilateral facet dislocation. Note that the inferior articular process of the C4 vertebra is anterior to the superior articular process of the C5 vertebral body on the dislocated side.

caudad vertebral level. A DF stage 2 (DFS2) injury (Figure 34-20, *C*) is a unilateral facet dislocation (Figure 34-21, *A* and *B*) with 25% to 50% anterolisthesis of the cephalad vertebrae in relationship to the caudad vertebrae combined with a rotatory listhesis. DF stage 3 (DFS3) injuries (Figure 34-20, *D*) are bilateral facet dislocations (Figure 34-22, *A* and *B*) with greater than 50%

anterolisthesis of the cephalad vertebrae. DF stage 4 injuries (DFS4) (Figure 34-20, *E*) are a progression of DFS3 injuries with complete (100%) dislocation of the vertebral bodies with canal impingement.

The incidence of vertebral artery injury in cervical spine trauma has been documented to be around 19%.[34,85] This injury was seen more commonly following

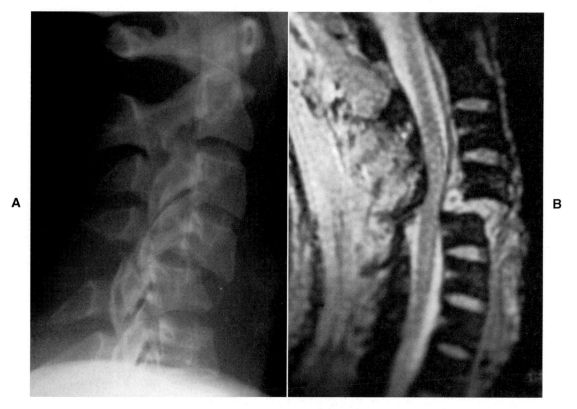

Figure 34-22. **A,** Lateral plain x-ray revealing a bilateral facet dislocation at the C4 to C5 level. **B,** Sagittal plain MRI of the same patient revealing a large extruded disc fragment at the C4 to C5 level. This patient required an initial anterior cervical discectomy to remove the disc herniation followed by an anterior open reduction and fusion procedure with anterior instrumentation.

DF and CF injuries to the cervical spine. In a cadaveric study Sime et al.[75] found that DF stage 2 through 4 injuries result in significant objective strain of the vertebral vasculature. DFS1 injuries did not demonstrate any significant stretch to the vertebral vasculature.

It is a recommendation of the authors that the vast majority of DF injuries undergo urgent closed-reduction skeletal traction during the initial evaluation in the trauma ward in a patient who is alert and awake and can cooperate with a neurologic exam. Closed reduction with Gardner-Wells stainless steel tongs is preferable to using carbon fiber MRI-compatible tongs when high weight reductions are anticipated. It is believed by the authors that an early successful closed reduction protects the neurologic elements from excessive motion during subsequent patient transfer and may potentially improve neurorecovery in compromised patients as compared with a delayed reduction. In a review of 210 patients with unilateral or bilateral facet dislocations, Lee et al.[51] found that those patients treated with early rapid reduction via traction had the best chance for neurologic recovery. Kahn et al.[45] have shown that delayed treatment (greater than 72 hours) of cervical facet dislocations had less successful outcomes than those reduced earlier than 72 hours. Again, closed cervical reduction of DF injuries should be performed only on awake, alert, nonintoxicated, and cooperative patients.

The documented incidence of herniated discs in this patient population may be as high as 54%.[71]

Cotler et al.[20] successfully reduced 24 patients with DF injuries (C4 to C7) using closed skeletal-tong traction with weights as high as 140 pounds. Occasionally, gentle manipulation by an experienced surgeon may be necessary to reduce a perched facet during the traction procedure.[77] Some authors argue that due to the high incidence of herniated nucleus pulposus at the time of cervical dislocation, an MRI should be obtained prior to reduction. However, in all documented permanent neurologic deterioration following a closed cervical reduction, patients were either under sedation or anesthesia during the reduction procedure.[30,71]

During a closed reduction a physician should monitor the neurologic status of the patient during each addition of weight or positional change. Should neurologic deterioration occur during awake reduction, the reduction procedure should be immediately stopped and the inciting event (i.e., weight addition) should be reversed. Ludwig et al.[61] reported a case of immediate quadriparesis during closed awake reduction. The mechanism was reversed, and an urgent MRI revealed a posterior epidural hematoma. The patient was taken to the operating room for an immediate posterior decompression. Postoperatively the patient had no evidence of a neurologic deficit.

An MRI should be performed following all successful closed reductions, all failed reductions, or in the presence of neurologic deterioration. The MRI will assist in guiding the approach to surgical treatment. The majority of DF injuries should be treated with surgical stabilization secondary to the ligamentous nature of the injury. Unilateral facet dislocations may be treated with an attempt at closed treatment with halo-vest immobilization. However, frequent follow-up is necessary and failure is common. Bucholz and Cheung[13] followed 20 patients with DF injuries treated with halo immobilization and found that 9 out of 20 (45%) ultimately required surgery. Shapiro et al.[74] found that 98% of patients treated with an open posterior reduction and stabilization went on to a successful result. They compared interspinous wiring and facet wiring using iliac crest bone graft to interspinous braided cable and lateral mass plating and found no significant difference between the two techniques.

Successfully reduced subluxations and dislocations without evidence of a herniated disc may be treated with a posterior stabilization procedure. A successful reduction in the presence of a herniated disc is best treated with an anterior decompression and fusion.

Unsuccessful closed reduction without the presence of a herniated disc requires an open posterior reduction and stabilization. This can be accomplished by using a posterior distraction maneuver to the dislocated vertebra using bony tenaculums or towel clips placed at the spinolaminar junction. A small nerve hook or Penfield is placed in the medial aspect of the dislocated facets while distraction is applied to the tenaculums. If necessary, a Kerrison punch may be used to remove a portion of the superior aspect of the superior articular processes to aid in the reduction.

An unsuccessful closed reduction with a documented herniated disc should first be treated with an anterior discectomy. Reduction may then be performed via an anterior reduction maneuver, or the wound can be closed and a posterior open reduction can be performed. This is all performed with the aid of spinal cord monitoring. With the use of Caspar distraction pins and a separate intervertebral spreader, an anterior reduction may be attempted with gentle distraction and a posterior rotatory force applied to the superior vertebrae. If successful, an anterior stabilization and fusion procedure should follow. Unfortunately, an open anterior reduction is not always successful. In this case the anterior wound is closed and a posterior reduction and stabilization is performed followed by returning to the anterior spine for an anterior fusion. Some surgeons may place an iliac crest bone graft in the anterior interspace following the anterior decompression in an exaggerated anterior position, with the expectation that a posterior reduction maneuver will pull the graft into an acceptable position. This may avoid the need to return to the anterior exposure. Another method of anterior grafting of an unreduced dislocation is the placement of a junction plate on the cephalad vertebral body in a position to hold in place a Smith-Robinson type of bone graft whose anterior surface is in line with the anterior cortex of the cephalad vertebral body. A small ridge or ledge is created in the inferior end plate of the cephalad vertebrae to prevent displacement of the graft into the canal during the posterior open reduction procedure.

DISTRACTIVE-FLEXION INJURIES

- 10% of all subaxial cervical spine fractures
- Allen and Ferguson classification
  - Stage 1—less than 25% subluxation
  - Stage 2—unilateral facet dislocation, 25% to 50% anterolisthesis
  - Stage 3—bilateral facet dislocation, > 50% anterolisthesis
  - Stage 4—bilateral facet dislocation, 100% anterolisthesis
- Urgent closed skeletal reduction in an awake, alert, cooperative patient
  - Gardner-Wells tongs preferred over carbon fiber or titanium pins due to failure of carbon fiber/titanium tong pin tips at weights exceeding 70 to 80 pounds
- Postreduction MRI necessary to evaluate presence of
  - Herniated nucleus pulposus (HNP)
  - Epidural hematoma
  - Significant soft tissue disruption
- Treatment
  - Successful closed reduction without HNP—posterior stabilization
  - Successful closed reduction with HNP—anterior decompression and fusion
  - Unsuccessful closed reduction without HNP—open posterior reduction and stabilization
  - Unsuccessful closed reduction with HNP—anterior decompression followed by either an anterior reduction and fusion stabilization procedure, or anterior grafting followed by a posterior open reduction and stabilization procedure or an anterior decompression followed by a posterior open reduction and stabilization procedure followed by an anterior fusion

---

Compression-Extension Injuries

Compression-extension injuries commonly result from motor vehicle or diving accidents. They are typically described as isolated posterior-element fractures but may involve the anterior bony elements, depending on the degree of force imparted to the spine. Compression-extension stage 1 injuries describe an injury to a unilateral vertebral arch. These are divided into three stages. Stage 1a (Figure 34-23, B1) is a fracture of the articular process. Stage 1b (Figure 34-23, B2) involves a fracture of the pedicle, and stage 1c (Figure 34-23, B3) involves a fracture of the lamina. Compression-extension stage 2 injuries describe the presence of bilateral vertebral arch fractures (Figure 34-23, C). If nondisplaced, these injuries are successfully treated with either a cervical orthosis or halo vest if necessary. Compression-extension stage 3 injury (Figure 34-23, D) consists of progressive injury to the posterior elements without vertebral body displacement. Compression-extension stage 4 injuries (Figure

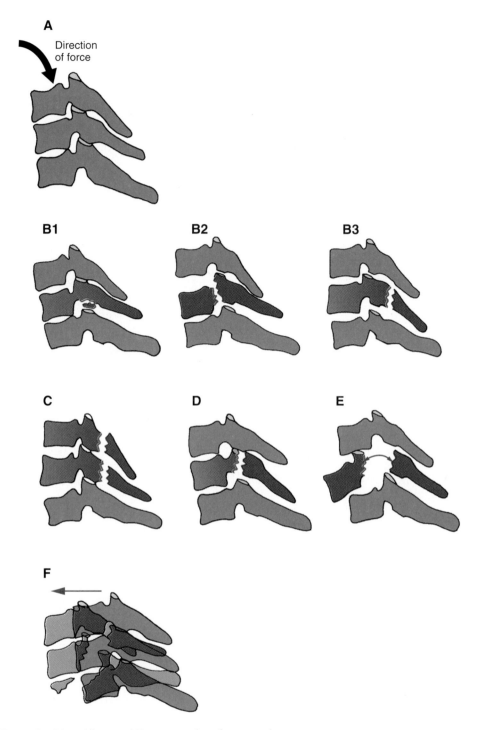

Figure 34-23.   Allen and Ferguson classification of compression-extension injuries.
A, Normal. **B1 to B3,** Stage 1a. **C,** Stage 2. **D,** Stage 3. **E,** Stage 4. **F,** Stage 5.

34-23, *E*) consist of bilateral posterior vertebral fractures with partial vertebral body displacement, and compression-extension stage 5 injuries (Figure 34-23, *F*) result in 100% anterior displacement of the injured vertebral body. Stage 3 injuries can be treated with a halo vest or with posterior surgical stabilization if necessary. Compression-extension stage 4 and 5 injuries are best treated with a posterior open reduction, decompression, and stabilization procedure. Should there be significant anterior

column injury, an adjunctive anterior stabilization procedure may be needed.[60]

Lifeso and Colluci[60] have described a rotationally unstable type of compression-extension stage 1 injury that involves a posterior unilateral lateral mass fracture of the pedicle, facet complex, or lamina along with a distractive injury to the anterior annulus and anterior longitudinal ligament that allows the vertebral body to rotate around the intact contralateral lateral mass. The

> ### COMPRESSION-EXTENSION INJURIES
>
> - Stages 1 and 2: Unilateral and bilateral neural arch fractures, respectively
> - Stage 3: Progressive posterior element injury without anterior body displacement
> - Stage 4: Posterior element injury with partial vertebral body displacement
> - Stage 5: Posterior element injury with complete body displacement
> - Treatment
>   - Stage 1 and 2—cervical orthosis or halo vest
>   - Stage 3—halo vest or posterior stabilization
>   - Stage 4 and 5—posterior open reduction, decompression, and stabilization

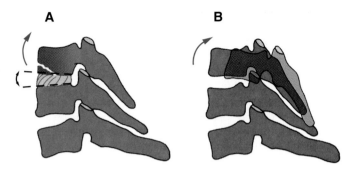

Figure 34-24. Allen and Ferguson classification of distraction-extension injuries. **A,** Stage 1. **B,** Stage 2.

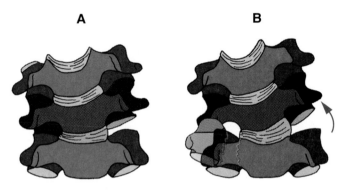

Figure 34-25. Allen and Ferguson classification of lateral flexion injuries. **A,** Stage 1. **B,** Stage 2.

authors compared traditional nonoperative and posterior surgical procedures to that of an anterior decompression and instrumented fusion and found better results in the group treated with anterior surgery.

Distraction-Extension Injuries

Distraction-extension injuries account for 22% of subaxial cervical spine injuries, with motor vehicle accidents and falls responsible for the majority of these injuries. Often these injuries appear benign, but if neglected they often result in significant neurologic morbidity. Many of these injuries are seen in elderly patients with either ankylosing spondylitis or diffuse idiopathic skeletal hyperostosis. In this patient population there is often a high degree of morbidity and mortality associated with this fracture subtype.[84] Allen classified these injuries into two stages. Distraction-extension stage 1 (DES1) injuries (Figure 34-24, *A*) consist of either failure of the anterior ligamentous complex or a transverse fracture through the vertebral body. Widening of the disc space is characteristically seen on plain radiographs. These injuries may be treated in a halo vest; however, due to the potential for vertebral displacement, many authors are recommending an anterior fusion procedure with anterior instrumentation acting as a tension band in injuries involving the disc space. Distraction-extension type 2 (DES2) (Figure 34-24, *B*) injuries involve a progression of the DES1 injury but with obvious disruption of the posterior ligamentous structures. These injuries are universally unstable and are best treated with an anterior cervical fusion with an anterior cervical plate acting as a tension band.[76] If closed reduction is necessary to improve alignment of this injury subtype, this is efficiently accomplished with bivector skeletal traction.[72] Injuries involving solely the bony skeleton are again extremely unstable but have a better prognosis for healing with rigid external immobilization than does an injury to the disc space.

Lateral Flexion Injuries

Lateral flexion injuries make up approximately 20% of subaxial cervical spine injuries. This type of injury is

> ### DISTRACTION-EXTENSION INJURIES
>
> - 22% of all subaxial cervical spine fractures
> - Commonly associated with ankylosing spondylitis or diffuse idiopathic skeletal hyperostosis—associated with a high morbidity and mortality
> - Stage 1: Anterior ligamentous injury or transverse body fracture—halo or anterior fusion and plating if involving the disc space
> - Stage 2: Anterior and posterior injury—anterior cervical fusion with plate acting as a tension band or a posterior open reduction and stabilization procedure followed by an anterior fusion if necessary

commonly seen after motor vehicle accidents and sports-related injuries such as football. Many injuries are missed on plain-film radiography, and a CT scan is recommended to detect occult injuries. Although spinal cord injury is rare with this injury subtype, brachial plexus and spinal nerve root injuries do occur. Lateral flexion stage 1 (LFS1) injuries (Figure 34-25, *A*) are nondisplaced vertebral arch fractures with asymmetric compression fractures. These injuries are best managed with a rigid cervical orthosis. In lateral flexion stage 2 (LFS2) injuries there is displacement of an ipsilateral arch fracture associated with a contralateral ligamentous tension

```
┌────────────────────────────────────────────┐
│                                              │
│          LATERAL FLEXION INJURIES            │
│          ─────────────────────────           │
│                                              │
│   • 20% of subaxial cervical spine injuries  │
│   • Stage 1—rigid cervical orthosis          │
│   • Stage 2—traction followed by posterior   │
│     stabilization                            │
│                                              │
└────────────────────────────────────────────┘
```

injury. LFS2 injuries (Figure 34-25, *B*) are best treated with reduction via skeletal traction followed by a posterior stabilization procedure. If spinal cord injury, nerve root injury, or anterior instability is present, an anterior decompressive procedure may be necessary.

CONCLUSIONS

Cervical spine trauma and spinal cord injury present the treating physician with a complex and challenging array of treatment decisions. Missed or incorrect diagnoses may lead to significant morbidity or prevent optimum return of neurologic function. Treatment begins long before the patient's arrival to the hospital, at the time of the injury recognition in the field. The advent of pre-hospital care protocols and emergency medical service (EMS) systems has significantly improved the quality of treatment and neurologic prognosis for the patient with a cervical spine injury.

The diagnosis of a cervical injury is based on a combination of clinical and radiographic (i.e., plain radiography, CT, and MRI) findings. Early diagnosis, pharmacologic intervention, and spinal stabilization are paramount to an optimal functional outcome. The timing of surgical intervention in this patient population with a neurologic deficit is still controversial, although many centers are urgently realigning the cervical elements to provide indirect relief of pressure on the neural elements.

The type of treatment of specific injuries is based on the mechanism of injury, anatomic location, severity of bony and ligamentous injury, and the medical status of the patient. It is imperative to be aware of other possible noncontiguous injuries that may affect treatment. Among the treatment options available, contemporary research and clinical trials are ongoing and are evaluating the most effective means of pharmacologic interventions and means of stabilization necessary to improve long-term functional outcome. Returning a patient to a functional and productive lifestyle is the ultimate treatment goal in the spinal-injury patient.

SELECTED REFERENCES

Allen BL et al.: A mechanistic classification of closed, indirect fractures and dislocations of the cervical spine, *Spine* 7:1-27, 1982.

An HS: Cervical spine trauma, *Spine* 23:2713-2729, 1998.

Anderson PA, Montesano PX: Morphology and treatment of occipital condyle fractures, *Spine* 13:731-736, 1988.

Benzel EC et al.: Fractures of the C-2 vertebral body, *J Neurosurg* 81:206-212, 1994.

Leone A et al.: Occipital condylar fractures: a review, *Radiology* 216:635-644, 2000.

Levine AM, Edwards CC: The management of traumatic spondylolisthesis of the axis, *J Bone Joint Surg Am* 67:217-226, 1985.

Levine AM, Edwards CC: Fractures of the atlas, *J Bone Joint Surg Am* 73:680-691, 1991.

Muller EJ, Wick M, Muhr G: Traumatic spondylolisthesis of the axis: treatment rationale based on the stability of different fracture types, *Eur Spine J* 9:123-128, 2000.

REFERENCES

1. Allen BL et al.: A mechanistic classification of closed, indirect fractures and dislocations of the cervical spine, *Spine* 7:1-27, 1982.
2. Alker GJ Jr, Oh YS, Leslie EV: Post mortem radiology of head and neck injuries in fatal traffic accidents, *J Neuroradiol* 114:611-616, 1975.
3. American Spinal Injury Association (ASIA): *Standards for neurological and functional classification of spinal cord injury—revised*, Chicago, 1992, The Association.
4. An HS: Cervical spine trauma, *Spine* 23:2713-2729, 1998.
5. Anderson LD, D'Alonzo RT: Fractures of the odontoid process of the axis, *J Bone Joint Surg Am* 56:1663-1674, 1974.
6. Anderson PA, Montesano PX: Morphology and treatment of occipital condyle fractures, *Spine* 13:731-736, 1988.
7. Atkinson PP, Atkinson JL: Spinal shock, *Mayo Clin Proc* 71:384-389, 1996.
8. Bednar DA, Prikh H, Hummel J: Management of type II odontoid process fractures in geriatric patients: a prospective study of sequential cohorts with attention to survivorship, *J Spinal Disord* 8:166-169, 1995.
9. Benzel EC et al.: Fractures of the C-2 vertebral body, *J Neurosurg* 81:206-212, 1994.
10. Berlemann U, Schwarzenbach O: Dens fractures in the elderly: results of anterior screw fixation in 19 elderly patients, *Acta Orthop Scand* 68:319-324, 1997.
11. Bloom AI et al.: Fracture of the occipital condyles and associated craniocervical ligament injury: incidence, CT imaging and implications, *Clin Radiol* 52:198-202, 1997.
12. Bosch A, Stauffer ES, Nickel VL: Incomplete traumatic quadriplegia: a ten-year review, *JAMA* 216:473-478, 1971.
13. Bucholz RD, Cheung KX: Halo vest versus spinal fusion for cervical injury: evidence from an outcome study, *J Neurosurg* 70:884-892, 1989.
14. Bucholz RW, Burkhead WZ: The pathologic anatomy of fatal atlanto-occipital dislocations, *J Bone Joint Surg Am* 60:279-284, 1979.
15. Burke JT, Harris JH: Acute injuries of the axis vertebrae, *Skeletal Radiol* 18:335-346, 1989.
16. Chang KW et al.: One Herbert double-threaded compression screw fixation of displaced type II odontoid fractures, *J Spinal Disord* 7:62-69, 1994.
17. Clark CR, White AA: Fractures of the dens: a multicenter study, *J Bone Joint Surg Am* 67:1340-1348, 1985.
18. Connolly B et al.: Jefferson fracture resulting in Collet-Sicard syndrome, *Spine* 25:395-398, 2000.
19. Coric D, Wilson JA, Kelly DL Jr: Treatment of traumatic spondylolisthesis of the axis with nonrigid immobilization: a review of 64 cases, *J Neurosurg* 85:550-554, 1996.
20. Cotler JM et al.: Closed reduction of traumatic cervical spine dislocation using traction weights up to 140 pounds, *Spine* 18:386-390, 1993.
21. Cusick JF et al.: Cervical spine injuries from high-velocity forces: a pathoanatomic and radiologic study, *J Spinal Disord* 9:1-7, 1996.
22. Demisch S et al.: The forgotten condyle: delayed hypoglossal nerve palsy caused by fracture of the occipital condyle, *Clin Neurol Neurosurg* 100:44-45, 1998.
23. Denis F: Spinal instability as defined by the three-column spine concept in acute spinal trauma, *Clin Orthop* 189:65-76, 1984.
24. Dickman CA, Greene KA, Sonntag VKH: Injuries involving the transverse atlantal ligament: classification and guidelines based on experience with 39 injuries, *Neurosurgery* 38:44-50, 1996.
25. Dickman CA et al.: Magnetic resonance imaging of the transverse atlantal ligament for the evaluation of atlantoaxial instability, *J Neurosurg* 75:221-227, 1991.
26. Doherty BJ, Heggeness MH, Esses SI: A biomechanical study of odontoid fractures and fracture fixation, *Spine* 18:178-184, 1993.
27. Dublin AB et al.: Traumatic dislocation of the atlanto-occipital articulation (AOA) with short term survival, with a radiographic method of measuring AOA, *J Neurosurg* 52:514-516, 1980.

28. Dunn ME, Seljeskog EL: Experience in the management of odontoid process injuries: an analysis of 128 cases, *Neurosurgery* 18:306-310, 1986.

29. Effendi B et al.: Fracture of the ring of the axis: a classification based on the analysis of 131 cases, *J Bone Joint Surg Br* 63:319-327, 1981.

30. Eismont GJ, Arena MJ, Green BA: Extrusion of an intervertebral disc associated with traumatic subluxation or dislocation of the cervical facets, *J Bone Joint Surg Am* 73:1555-1560, 1991.

31. Fielding JW, Hawkins RJ, Ratzan SA: Atlanto-axial rotatory fixation, *J Bone Joint Surg Am* 59:37-44, 1977.

32. Fowler JL, Sandhu A, Fraser RD: A review of fractures of the atlas vertebra, *J Spinal Disord* 3:19-24, 1990.

33. Fujimura Y, Nishi Y, Kobayashi K: Classification and treatment of axis body fractures, *J Orthop Trauma* 10:536-540, 1996.

34. Giacobetti FB et al.: Vertebral artery occlusion associated with cervical spine trauma: a prospective analysis, *Spine* 22:188-192, 1997.

35. Go BK, DeVivo MJ, Richards JS: The epidemiology of spinal cord injury. In Stover SL, DeLisa JA, Whiteneck GG, eds: *Spinal cord injury: clinical outcomes from the model systems*, Gaithersburg, Md, 1995, Aspen, pp. 21-55.

36. Goldstein SJ, Woodring JA, Young AB: Occipital condyle fracture associated with cervical spine injury, *Surg Neurol* 17:350-352, 1982.

37. Graziano G et al.: A comparative study of fixation techniques for type II fractures of the odontoid process, *Spine* 18:2383-2387, 1993.

38. Greene KA et al.: Acute axis fractures: analysis of management and outcome in 340 consecutive cases, *Spine* 22:1843-1852, 1997.

39. Hadley MN et al.: New subtype of acute odontoid fractures (type IIA), *Neurosurgery* 22:67-71, 1988.

40. Hadley MN et al.: Acute traumatic atlas fractures: management and long term outcome, *Neurosurgery* 23:31-35, 1988.

41. Hanigan WC et al.: Odontoid fractures in elderly patients, *J Neurosurg* 78:32-35, 1993.

42. Harris JH et al.: Radiologic diagnosis of traumatic occipito-vertebral dislocation. II. Comparison of three methods of detecting occipitovertebral relationships on lateral radiographs of the supine subject, *Am J Radiology* 162:887-892, 1994.

43. Harrop JS et al.: Acute respiratory compromise associated with flexed cervical traction after C2 fractures, *Spine* 26:E50-E54, 2001.

44. Heller JG, Viroslav S, Hudson T: Jefferson fractures: the role of magnification artifact in assessing transverse ligament integrity, *J Spinal Disord* 6:392-396, 1993.

45. Kahn A, Leggon R, Lindsey RW: Cervical facet dislocation: management following delayed diagnosis, *Orthopedics* 21:1089-1091, 1998.

46. Kannus P et al.: Continuously increasing number and incidence of fall-induced, fracture-associated, spinal cord injuries in elderly persons, *Arch Intern Med* 160:2145-2149, 2000.

47. Kelly A, Parrish R: Fracture of the occipital condyle: the forgotten part of the neck, *Emerg Med J* 17:220-221, 2000.

48. Kraus JF et al.: Incidence of traumatic spinal cord lesions, *J Chronic Dis* 28:471-492, 1975.

49. Landelis CD, Van Peteghem PK: Fractures of the atlas: classification, treatment and morbidity, *Spine* 13:450-452, 1988.

50. Lasfargues JE et al.: A model for estimating spinal cord injury prevalence in the United States, *Paraplegia* 33:62-68, 1995.

51. Lee AS, MacLean JC, Newton DA: Rapid traction for reduction of cervical spine dislocations, *J Bone Joint Surg Br* 76:352-356, 1994.

52. Lee C et al.: Evaluation of traumatic atlanto-occipital dislocations, *Am J Neuroradiol* 8:19-26, 1987.

53. Lee T, Green BA, Petrin DR: Treatment of stable burst fractures of the atlas (Jefferson fracture) with rigid cervical collar, *Spine* 23:1963-1967, 1988.

54. Lennarson PJ et al.: Management of type II dens fractures: a case-control study, *Spine* 25:1234-1237, 2000.

55. Leone A et al.: Occipital condylar fractures: a review, *Radiology* 216:635-644, 2000.

56. Levine AM, Edwards CC: The management of traumatic spondylolisthesis of the axis, *J Bone Joint Surg Am* 67:217-226, 1985.

57. Levine AM, Edwards CC: Treatment of injuries in the C1-C2 complex, *Orthop Clin North Am* 17:31-44, 1986.

58. Levine AM, Edwards CC: Fractures of the atlas, *J Bone Joint Surg Am* 73:680-691, 1991.

59. Lieberman IH, Webb JK: Cervical spine injuries in the elderly, *J Bone Joint Surg Br* 76:877-881, 1994.

60. Lifeso RM, Colucci MA: Anterior fusion for rotationally unstable cervical spine fractures, *Spine* 25:2028-2034, 2000.

61. Ludwig SC et al.: Immediate quadriparesis after manipulation for bilateral cervical facet subluxation: a case report, *J Bone Joint Surg Am* 79:587-590, 1997.

62. McGuire RA, Harkey HL: Primary treatment of unstable Jefferson's fractures, *J Spinal Disord* 8:233-236, 1995.

63. Muller EJ, Wick M, Muhr G: Traumatic spondylolisthesis of the axis: treatment rationale based on the stability of different fracture types, *Eur Spine J* 9:123-128, 2000.

64. Noboru H et al.: Traumatic anterior atlanto-occipital dislocation, *Spine* 18:786-790, 1993.

65. Oda T et al.: Experimental study of atlas injuries. II. Relevance to clinical diagnosis and treatment, *Spine* 16:S466-S473, 1991.

66. Powers B: Traumatic anterior-occipital dislocations, *Neurosurgery* 4:12-17, 1979.

67. Przybylski GJ, Clyde BL, Fitz CR: Craniocervical junction subarachnoid hemorrhage associated with atlanto-occipital dislocation, *Spine* 21:1761-1768, 1996.

68. Puttlitz CM et al.: Pathomechanisms of failures of the odontoid, *Spine* 25:2868-2876, 2000.

69. Reich SM, Cotler JM: Mechanism and patterns of spine and spinal cord injuries, *Trauma Q* 9:7-28, 1993.

70. Rizzolo SJ, Vaccaro AR, Cotler JM: Cervical spine trauma, *Spine* 19:2288-2298, 1997.

71. Robertson PA, Ryan MD: Neurologic deterioration after reduction of cervical subluxation, *J Bone Joint Surg Br* 74:224-227, 1992.

72. Rushton SA et al.: Bivector traction for unstable cervical spine fractures: a description of its application and preliminary results, *J Spinal Disord* 10:436-440, 1997.

73. Seybold EA, Bayley JC: Functional outcomes of surgically and conservatively managed dens fractures, *Spine* 23:1837-1845, 1998.

74. Shapiro S et al.: Outcome of 51 cases of unilateral locked cervical facets: interspinous braided cable for lateral mass plate fusion compared with interspinous wire and facet wiring with the iliac crest, *J Neurosurg* 91:19-24, 1999.

75. Sime E et al.: The effects of staged static cervical flexion-distraction deformities of the patency of the vertebral arterial vasculature, *Spine* 25:2180-2186, 2000.

76. Spence KF, Decker S, Sell KW: Bursting atlantal fracture associated with rupture of the transverse ligament, *J Bone Joint Surg Am* 52:534-539, 1970.

77. Starr AM et al.: Immediate closed reduction of cervical spine dislocations using traction, *Spine* 15:1068-1072, 1990.

78. Starr JK, Eismont FJ: Atypical hangman's fractures, *Spine* 18:1954-1957, 1993.

79. Stripling TE: The cost of economic consequences of traumatic spinal cord injury, *Paraplegia News*, 1990, pp. 50-54

80. Surkin J et al.: Spinal cord injury in Mississippi, *Spine* 25:716-721, 2000.

81. Traynelis VC et al.: Traumatic atlanto-occipital dislocation, *J Neurosurg* 65:863-870, 1986.

82. Tuli S et al.: Occipital condyle fractures, *Neurosurg* 41:368-377, 1992.

83. Urculo E et al.: Delayed glossopharyngeal and vagus nerve paralysis following occipital condyle fracture, *J Neurosurg* 84:522-525, 1996.

84. Vaccaro AR et al.: Distraction extension injuries of the cervical spine, *J Spinal Disord* 14:193-200, 2001.

85. Veras LM et al.: Vertebral artery occlusion after acute cervical spine trauma, *Spine* 25:1171-1177, 2000.

86. Werne S: Studies in spontaneous atlas dislocation, *Acta Orthop Scand Suppl* 23:1-28, 1957.

Cervical Spine Injuries in the Athlete: Return-to-Play Criteria

Alexander R. Vaccaro, Basil M. Harris, Robert Watkins

Fortunately, catastrophic cervical spine injuries during athletic participation are relatively uncommon. "Burner syndrome" and transient quadriparesis are more frequent injuries that have a wide spectrum of clinical severity and disabilities. The diagnosis of these injuries is not clinically difficult; however, the treatment after such an injury and decision on when or if the athlete may return to play are often unclear. Despite the frequency of cervical injuries among contact athletes, no consensus exists within the medical field on a standard guideline for return to the preinjury activity level. This chapter reviews the current literature to help determine reasonable return-to-play criteria after cervical spine injuries in the athlete.

Cervical spine injuries in the athlete account for 1 in 10 of the cervical spine injuries that occur in the United States.[8] Cervical spine injuries can happen to athletes at any level of participation ranging from unsupervised activities to organized contact sports. These injuries may occur during diving, surfing, skiing, football, boxing, lacrosse, wrestling, soccer, rugby, ice hockey, and gymnastics. The incidence of complete quadriplegia among high school and college football athletes has been reported to be as high as 2.5 per 100,000 in 1976 and as low as 0.5 per 100,000 in 1991.[4] The potentially catastrophic nature of this injury has prompted considerable effort by both the medical and athletic communities to determine risk factors and return-to-play criteria.

The decision to let an athlete participate in contact sports after a cervical spine injury is complicated and difficult. The decision should be based on the patient's medical history, physical examination, and the presence of imaging abnormalities. Several authors have set forth recommended guidelines for return to play.* Despite these recommendations, standardized return-to-play criteria have not been uniformly accepted by the medical community. Using 10 case histories, Morganti et al. surveyed 113 physicians in reference to their return-to-play recommendations.[10] The authors found no clear consensus on the postinjury management of cervical spine injuries, often due to each injury's uniqueness and individual presentation. In addition, in the majority of the cases there was no relationship between return-to-play recommendations and the medical consultant's years in practice, subspecialty training, or use of published guidelines.

TRANSIENT QUADRIPLEGIA

Cervical spinal cord neuropraxia with transient quadriplegia usually presents as temporary bilateral burning paresthesia and is associated with various degrees of bilateral extremity weakness. Its incidence in collegiate football players is approximately 7.3 per 10,000 athletes. The mechanism of injury is usually cervical axial compression with a component of either hyperflexion or hyperextension. Sensory and motor abnormalities are present bilaterally, usually for approximately 10 to 15 minutes; however, some patients may have residual symptoms for up to 48 hours or longer. Sensory disturbances vary from burning pain to loss of sensation. Motor abnormalities range from bilateral upper and lower extremity weakness to complete paralysis. Transient quadriplegia is associated with developmental cervical stenosis, kyphosis, the presence of a congenital fusion, cervical instability, and/or an intervertebral disc protrusion or herniation.[11]

Torg et al. developed the Torg ratio (defined as the anterior-posterior diameter of the spinal canal measured as the distance from the midpoint of the posterior aspect of the vertebral body to the nearest point on the corresponding spinolaminar line divided by the antero-posterior width of the vertebral body) to evaluate cervical stenosis of the cervical spine. They found that this radiographic sign was extremely sensitive in describing clinically significant cervical stenosis (93% sensitivity)

---

*References 1, 3, 5, 14, 15, 16, 18.

BACKGROUND

- Ten percent of 10,000 cervical spine injuries annually in the United States occur in athletes.
- Incidence of complete quadriplegia among high school and college football athletes varies.
  - As high as 2.5 per 100,000 in 1976
  - As low as 0.5 per 100,000 in 1991
- Medical and athletic communities seek risk factors and return-to-play criteria because of potentially catastrophic results.
- No clear consensus exists on postinjury management.
- Use of standardized return-to-play criteria is not uniformly accepted by medical community.

but had an extremely low positive predictive value for determining future injury (0.2%). This low positive predictive value precludes its use as a screening method for participation in contact sports. To date, there has been no proof that cervical spinal stenosis or a Torg ratio of 0.8 or less predisposes an athlete to permanent neurologic injury.[13]

Torg outlined a series of guidelines for the return to collision activities in patients with developmental stenosis of the cervical spinal canal following cervical cord neurapraxia. He categorized cervical congenital, developmental, and posttraumatic conditions as having no contraindication, relative contraindication, or absolute contraindication. Relative contraindication to play was defined as the possibility for recurrent injury despite the absence of any absolute contraindications to participate in contact sports. The patient had to understand that the degree of risk for reinjury was uncertain. For example, an asymptomatic athlete with a Torg ratio of less than 0.8 without any other cervical abnormality may return to sports without contraindication. However, a player with a Torg ratio of less than 0.8 and one previous episode of a spinal cord neurapraxia with or without intervertebral disc disease and/or degenerative changes represents a relative contraindication for return to play. A previously documented episode of neurapraxia with magnetic resonance imaging (MRI) findings of a cord abnormality (e.g., edema) in an athlete is an absolute contraindication for return to play. A documented episode of cervical cord neurapraxia associated with ligamentous instability, neurologic symptoms for more than 36 hours, and/or multiple episodes of neurapraxia is an absolute contraindication to the return to contact sports.[14]

Cantu et al. using case studies as examples, presented guidelines for return to contact sports after transient quadriplegia.[1,2] They proposed that an athlete may return to contact sports following the first episode of transient quadriplegia if there is complete resolution of symptoms, full range of motion, and a normal cervical spinal curvature without evidence of spinal stenosis on MRI, computed tomography (CT), or myelography. Relative contraindications to the return to sports include the presence of mild or minimal disc herniations and transient quadriplegia caused by minimal

contact. They believed that "functional" spinal stenosis (defined as a loss of the cerebrospinal fluid [CSF] around the cord or as deformation of the spinal cord as documented by MRI, CT with contrast, or myelography) was an absolute contraindication to the return to sports.

Using a newly developed computer technique for MRI, Torg et al.[14] measured the cord and canal diameters in 110 cases of cervical cord neurapraxia.[14] They found an overall recurrence rate of transient quadriplegia in 56% of players returning to contact sports; however, individuals with uncomplicated cervical cord neurapraxia did not present with a higher-than-normal risk for permanent neurologic injury. The risk of recurrence was increased with small Torg ratios (strongly predictive), smaller absolute disc level canal diameters, and less space available for the cord.[14]

BURNER SYNDROME

The burner syndrome, or "stinger," which is common in contact sports such as football and rugby, is described as a temporary episode of upper extremity unilateral burning dysesthesias with motor weakness. It has been reported that a stinger will occur in as many as 50% of athletes involved in contact or collision sports.[1,3] Patients usually describe a painful sensation that radiates from their neck to their fingertips after an impact load to the neck or shoulder. The deltoid (C5), biceps (C5 to C6), and spinatus muscles (C5 to C6) are the muscle groups most commonly involved. The pain usually lasts for a few seconds to minutes, but symptoms may persist for as long as a few weeks.[6,7,8] Three different mechanisms have been proposed for this syndrome: (1) stretch or traction injury to the brachial plexus; (2) extension of the cervical spine resulting in nerve root compression within the neural foramina; and (3) a direct blow resulting in injury to brachial plexus. This last mechanism in a football injury is thought to result from compression of the fixed brachial plexus between the player's shoulder pad and the superior medial scapula as the pad is pushed into the area of Erb's point (point of fixation of the upper trunk of the brachial plexus to the transverse process).[7] Chronic recurrent burners have been described as a recurrent neurapraxia or axonotmesis of the cervical nerve roots, often in the setting of cervical disc degeneration.[6,7,9] The C5 and C6 nerve root distribution is most commonly affected. The reported incidence of burner syndrome is between 49% and 65% in collegiate-level football players.

Meyer, et al. studied 266 collegiate football players and found that 40 of these players (15%) had reported a symptomatic stinger and that 31 of these athletes (11.6% of the 266) also complained of associated neck pain.[9] Thirty-four of these players (85%) reported an extension-compression mechanism, and six players (15%) noted a brachial plexus stretch etiology.[9] The mean Torg ratio was lower for the athletes with a history of a stinger (less than 0.8 in 47.5% of the players) than for the asymptomatic group (less than 0.8 in 25.1% of the players). Players with a Torg ratio of less than 0.8 had three times

CERVICAL SPINAL CORD NEURAPRAXIA WITH TRANSIENT QUADRIPLEGIA

- Incidence in collegiate football players approximately 7.3 per 10,000
- Usually cervical axial compression with a component of either hyperflexion or hyperextension
- Sensory disturbances from burning pain to loss of sensation
- Motor abnormalities from bilateral upper and lower extremity weakness to complete paralysis
- Present bilaterally usually for approximately 10 to 15 minutes, with residual symptoms that may last 48 hours or longer
- Transient quadriplegia associated with developmental cervical stenosis, kyphosis, congenital fusion, cervical instability, and/or an intervertebral disc protrusion or herniation

THE BURNER SYNDROME OR "STINGER"

- A temporary episode of upper extremity unilateral burning dysesthesias with motor weakness
- Occurs in up to 50% of athletes involved in contact collision sports
- Usually described as painful sensation radiating from neck to fingertips after impact load to neck or shoulder
- Deltoid (C5), biceps (C5 to C6), and spinatus muscles (C5 to C6) most commonly involved
- Pain lasts usually for a few seconds to minutes, but symptoms persist for up to a few weeks
- Mechanisms
  ○ Stretch or traction injury to brachial plexus
  ○ Extension of cervical spine resulting in nerve root compression within neural foramina
  ○ A direct blow causing injury to brachial plexus

the risk of incurring a stinger than did the players with ratios greater than 0.8. The authors noted that 45% of the athletes with a previous history of a stinger would suffer from recurrent episodes.

RETURN TO SPORTS

A difficult management scenario for the team's physician is deciding when an athlete may return to a competitive level of activity following a spinal injury. After reviewing the literature and clinical data, Torg and Ramsey-Emrheim set out to determine reasonable guidelines for the return to contact sports for an athlete who has suffered a cervical spine injury.[15] The following spinal conditions are considered to have no contraindications to participation in contact sports: (1) congenital conditions such as a type II Klippel-Feil anomaly (which involves only a one- or two-level cervical fusion with full range of motion and with no evidence of instability or the presence of cervical disc disease or other degenerative changes), (2) spina bifida occulta, (3) healed stable nondisplaced fractures without sagittal malalignment, and (4) asymptomatic disc herniations treated conservatively in the past. Asymptomatic patients who have had a one-level anterior or posterior cervical fusion for miscellaneous reasons who are neurologically intact, are pain free, and have a solid fusion are also able to return to sports.

For a patient with full cervical motion, no pain, and a normal neurologic examination, relative contraindications to the return to contact sports include (1) a previous upper cervical spine fracture such as a healed nondisplaced Jefferson fracture, a healed type I or type II odontoid fracture, and/or a healed lateral mass fracture of C2; (2) a healed, stable, minimally displaced vertebral body compression fracture without sagittal malalignment; (3) a healed, stable fracture of the posterior elements excluding spinous process fractures; (4) the presence of minimal residual facet instability after surgical or conservative treatment of cervical disc disease; and (5) a healed two- or three-level cervical fusion.

Absolute contraindications to the return to contact sports include (1) odontoid anomalies; (2) an atlanto-occipital fusion; (3) atlantoaxial instability; (4) atlanto-axial rotatory fixation; (5) certain Klippel-Feil anomalies (type I, defined as a mass fusion of the cervical and upper thoracic vertebrae, or a type II lesion with associated limited motion and/or associated occipitocervical anomalies or instability with or without disc disease and other degenerative changes); (6) the radiographic presence of a spear-tackler's spine, defined as a characteristic of a subset of football players who exhibit developmental stenosis of the cervical canal, persistent reversal of the normal lordotic cervical spine on neutral lateral x-rays, posttraumatic findings on roentgenograms and/or a documented history of using a spear-tackling technique[12]; (7) subaxial spinal instability defined by lateral roentgenograms that show 3.5 mm or more of horizontal displacement of one vertebrae on the other or greater than 11 degrees of rotation difference as compared with the adjacent vertebrae as measured on a lateral or flexion-extension radiograph[17]; (8) an acute fracture of either the body or posterior elements with or without ligamentous instability; (9) healed subaxial vertebral body fractures with sagittal malalignment; (10) an acute fracture of the vertebral body with associated posterior arch fractures and/or ligamentous laxity; (11) residual bony canal compromise from retropulsed bony fragments; (12) continued pain, abnormal neurologic findings or limited motion from a healed cervical fracture; (13) the presence of a symptomatic acute soft or chronic disc herniation with associated neurologic findings, pain, or limited motion; and (14) a successful one-level fusion in the presence of diffuse congenital narrowing of the cervical canal.

Maroon and Bailes have developed a three-stage classification system for the treatment of athletes with cervical spine injuries based on the neurologic deficit involved.[8] Type I injuries involve permanent spinal cord dysfunction. Type I patients include those with a complete spinal cord injury or incomplete lesions such as an anterior cord syndrome, the Brown-Séquard syndrome, the central cord syndrome, or a mixed incomplete syndrome. Type II injuries are transient spinal cord injuries, such as spinal concussion, neurapraxia, or "burning hands syndrome." Type III injuries consist of disorders involving radiologic abnormalities without a neurologic deficit, such as congenital and acquired spinal stenosis, herniated discs, unstable fractures and/or dislocations, stable spinal fractures (lamina, spinous process, and minor portion of vertebral body), unstable ligamentous injuries, and spear-tackler's spine.

Maroon and Bailes concluded that patients with type I injuries should not be allowed to return to sports.[8] Patients with type II transient injuries may be allowed to return to contact activities if a thorough workup is negative and neurologic symptoms do not recur. If the athlete experiences multiple episodes of these type II injuries, serious consideration for disallowing return to contact sports should be given. Type III injuries need to be evaluated on a case-by-case basis because some injuries that may be stable in the average person may not be stable under high-impact athletic activities. Athletes with a spear-tackler's spine, unstable fracture, and/or

dislocation as described by White et al., Panjabi, and Southwick and ligamentous instability requiring an orthosis or surgical treatment should be precluded from returning to contact sports.[17] Athletes with other type III injuries such as herniated intervertebral discs treated surgically, stable fractures of the cervical spine, congenital spinal stenosis and cases of congenital spinal fusion (except Klippel-Feil syndrome, a narrowed spinal canal, multilevel fusion, or instability on flexion and extension views) may safely return to contact sports.[8]

Weinstein has recommended that the decision for return to play after a "burner" syndrome be based on both clinical and electrodiagnostic studies.[16] After a "burner," those individuals who have demonstrable weakness are scheduled to undergo electromyographic evaluation. Players who demonstrate clinical weakness and moderate fibrillation potentials are withdrawn from play. Should sequential EMG studies reveal no spontaneous or mild or scattered positive waves with end motor recruitment, all suggestive of reinnervation, the athlete may return to the preinjury level of activity, if painless full range of motion with full strength has returned.

Box 35-1	Return-to-Play Criteria for Athletic Participation

NO CONTRAINDICATIONS TO RETURN TO PLAY
- Healed, stable C1 to C2 fracture with a normal cervical range of motion
- Single-level Klippel-Feil deformity (excluding the occipital to C1 articulation) with no evidence of instability or stenosis noted on MRI
- Spina bifida occulta
- Torg ratio less than 0.8 in an asymptomatic individual
- History of cervical degenerative disc disease, which has been treated successfully in the setting of occasional cervical neck stiffness with no change in baseline strength profile
- Healed, stable subaxial spine fracture with no sagittal plane kyphotic deformity
- Healed anterior single-level cervical fusion with or without instrumentation
- Previous history of two stingers or burners
- Asymptomatic clay-shoveler's fracture (C7 spinous process)
- Status after a single- or multiple-level posterior cervical microlaminoforaminotomy

RELATIVE CONTRAINDICATIONS TO RETURN TO PLAY
- The absence of any absolute contraindications to play; patient and family knowledge that there is a possibility of recurrent injury and an uncertain degree of risk
- Previous history of spinal cord neurapraxia for a patient with full return to baseline strength and cervical range of motion with no increase in baseline cervical neck discomfort
- A healed single-level posterior fusion with lateral mass segmental fixation
- Three or more previous stinger or burner injuries
- A healed, stable two-level anterior or posterior cervical fusion with or without instrumentation, excluding posterior segmental lateral mass screw fixation
- Symptomatic stinger or burner injuries or a history of cervical neurapraxia lasting more than 24 hours

ABSOLUTE CONTRAINDICATIONS TO PARTICIPATION
- Clinical history or physical examination findings of cervical myelopathy
- Presence of cervical spinal cord abnormality noted on MRI
- History of a C1 to C2 cervical fusion
- Asymptomatic ligamentous laxity (greater than 11 degrees of kyphotic deformity as compared with the cephalad or caudal vertebral functional spinal unit)
- Radiographic evidence of C1 to C2 hypermobility with an anterior dens interval of 4 mm or greater
- C1 to C2 rotatory fixation
- Evidence of spear-tackler's spine on radiographic analysis
- Radiographic evidence of a distraction/extension cervical spine injury
- A multiple level Klippel-Feil deformity
- An occipital C1 assimilation
- Radiographic evidence (MRI) of basilar invagination
- MRI evidence of Arnold-Chiari malformation
- Radiographic evidence of ankylosing spondylitis or diffuse idiopathic skeletal hyperostosis
- More than two previous episodes of a cervical cord neurapraxia
- Status after a cervical laminectomy
- A healed subaxial spine fracture with evidence of a kyphotic sagittal plane or coronal plane abnormality
- Radiographic evidence of significant residual cord encroachment following a healed, stable subaxial spine fracture
- Continued cervical neck discomfort or any evidence of a neurologic deficit or decreased range of motion from baseline following a cervical spine injury
- Symptomatic disc herniation
- Clinical or radiographic evidence of rheumatoid arthritis
- Three-level spine fusion

RECOMMENDATIONS

Following an episode of transient quadraparesis, the athlete should be removed from the sport for at least that particular event, even if a full recovery occurs during the sporting activity. If symptoms are momentary or resolve, a complete neurologic and radiographic examination should be performed on a timely basis and repeated as necessary if any persistent motor or sensory deficits are present. If the patient complains of significant neck stiffness, has worsening complaints of neck pain with axial head compression, or has persisting symptoms of neck pain, the player has a fracture until proven otherwise. If neurologic complaints are persistent at the time of injury, then a cervical orthosis should be applied. Special precautions should be taken in helmeted athletes (removal of shoulder pads and helmet at the same time) so inadvertent cervical manipulation is avoided. In the setting of a neurologic deficit, the patient should be expeditiously taken to a medical facility where steroid administration is possible and appropriate imaging studies may be obtained.

An athlete may return to play according to the criteria provided in Box 35-1. These are only guidelines, which should be modified appropriately, depending on the clinical scenario.

Recommended Clinical Pathway for an Athlete With Cervical Spine Injury

At the time of cervical injury, the athlete should be removed from the sport. A complete history and physical examination should be performed at the scene of the injury. In the setting of a stinger or burner injury, the patient is allowed to return to play at that sporting event if he or she has complete resolution of symptoms, returns to a baseline range of motion of the cervical spine, and returns to a baseline strength profile. Athletes who have a significant and sustained burner syndrome (other than brief or momentary) for the first time should not be allowed to participate in the current athletic contest until an MRI is performed to rule out a significant disc herniation or other structural abnormality. In the setting of persistent symptoms, cervical radiographs and a cervical MRI should be performed. If suspicion exists for an occult cervical spine fracture, a CT scan or SPECT scan may facilitate diagnosis.

CONCLUSIONS

The issue of return to play for an athlete after a cervical spine injury is controversial. Tremendous extrinsic pressures may be exerted upon the physician from noninvolved and involved parties. The decision to return an athlete to a particular sport should be based on the mechanism of injury, objective anatomic injury (as demonstrated by clinical examination and radiographic evaluation), and an athlete's recovery response. Due to the potential for significant catastrophic sequela from premature or inappropriate resumption of athletic participation, an understanding of the natural history of specific clinical syndromes and inherent risk factors should be familiar to the treating physician.

SELECTED REFERENCES

Cantu RC: Stingers, transient quadriplegia, and cervical spinal stenosis: return to play criteria, Med Sci Sports Exerc 29:S233-S235, 1997.

Cantu RC, Bailes JE, Wilberger JE: Guidelines for return to contact or collision sport after cervical spine injury, Clin Sports Med 17(1):137-146, 1998.

Torg JS, Ramsey-Emrhein JA: Suggested management guidelines for participation in collision activities with congenital, developmental, or postinjury lesions involving the cervical spine, Med Sci Sports Exerc 29:S256-S272, 1997.

Torg JS et al.: Neuropraxia of the cervical spinal cord with transient quadriplegia, J Bone Joint Surg Am 68:1354-1370, 1986.

Torg JS et al.: Cervical cord neurapraxia: classification, pathomechanics, morbidity, and management guidelines, J Neurosurg 87:843-850, 1997.

Weinstein SM: Assessment and rehabilitation of an athlete with a "stinger": a model for the management of noncatastrophic athletic cervical spine injury, Clin Sports Med 17(1):127-135, 1998.

Wilberger JE: Athletic spinal cord and spine injuries: guidelines for initial management, Clin Sports Med 17(1):111-120, 1998.

REFERENCES

1. Cantu RC: Stingers, transient quadriplegia, and cervical spinal stenosis: return to play criteria, Med Sci Sports Exerc 29:S233-S235, 1997.
2. Cantu RC, Bailes JE, Wilberger JE: Guidelines for return to contact or collision sport after cervical spine injury, Clin Sports Med 17(1):137-146, 1998.
3. Clancy WG, Brand RL, Bergfield JA: Upper trunk brachial plexus injuries in contact sports, Am J Sports Med 5:209-216, 1977.
4. Clarke KS: Epidemiology of athletic neck injury, Clin Sports Med 17(1):83-97, 1998.
5. Davis PM, McKelvey MK: Medicolegal aspects of athletic cervical spine injury, Clin Sports Med 17(1):147-154, 1998.
6. Levitz CL, Reilly PJ, Torg JS: The pathomechanics of chronic, recurrent cervical nerve root neuropraxia: the chronic burner syndrome, Am J Sports Med 25:73-76, 1997.
7. Markey KL, Di Benedetto M, Curl WW: Upper trunk brachial plexopathy: the stinger syndrome, Am J Sports Med 21:650-655, 1993.
8. Maroon JC, Bailes JE: Athletes with cervical spine injury, Spine 21:2294-2299, 1996.
9. Meyer SA et al.: Cervical spinal stenosis and stingers in collegiate football players, Am J Sports Med 22:158-166, 1994.
10. Morganti C et al.: Return to play after cervical spine injury, Spine 26(10):1131-1136, 2001.
11. Torg JS et al.: Neuropraxia of the cervical spinal cord with transient quadriplegia, J Bone Joint Surg Am 68A:1354-1370, 1986.
12. Torg JS et al.: Spear tackler's spine, Am J Sports Med 21:640-649, 1993.
13. Torg JS et al.: The relationship of developmental narrowing of the cervical spinal canal to reversible and irreversible injury of the cervical spinal cord in football players, J Bone Joint Surg Am 78A:1308-1314, 1996.
14. Torg JS et al.: Cervical cord neurapraxia: classification, pathomechanics, morbidity, and management guidelines, J Neurosurg 87:843-850, 1997.
15. Torg JS, Ramsey-Emrhein JA: Suggested management guidelines for participation in collision activities with congenital, developmental, or postinjury lesions involving the cervical spine, Med Sci Sports Exerc 29:S256-S272, 1997.
16. Weinstein SM: Assessment and rehabilitation of an athlete with a "stinger": a model for the management of noncatastrophic athletic cervical spine injury, Clin Sports Med 17(1):127-135, 1998.
17. White AA et al.: Biomechanical analysis of chemical stability in the cervical spine, Clin Orthop 109:85-96, 1975.
18. Wilberger JE: Athletic spinal cord and spine injuries: guidelines for initial management, Clin Sports Med 17(1):111-120, 1998.

Fractures and Dislocations of the Thoracolumbar Spine

Glenn R. Rechtine, II, Michael J. Bolesta

A spinal injury can be the most catastrophic event in a person's life. Fractures of the thoracolumbar spine are the most common spinal injuries. The vast majority of these do not involve any neurologic deficit. All patients sustaining multiple trauma should be evaluated for a spinal injury. Because of the common occurrence of multilevel spinal injuries, a patient with a single spinal injury should have the entire spine evaluated as well. It is common for the diagnosis of spinal injury to be delayed because of unconsciousness or alcohol or drug intoxication.[7,97,106] Motor vehicle crashes are by far the most common cause for spinal column injuries.* Men are more likely to sustain injury than are women. In elderly patients, falls are a much more common mechanism.[11,77,110]

PATIENT EVALUATION
History

Attention should be made to obtain a history from all patients. If the patient is conscious and can relate the mechanism of injury, this is important. The practitioner should also seek to elicit any history of paralysis,

---

> ### BASICS OF THORACOLUMBAR SPINAL FRACTURES AND DISLOCATIONS
>
> - Fractures of the thoracolumbar spine are the most common spinal injuries and typically do not involve any neurologic deficit.
> - All patients sustaining multiple trauma should be evaluated for a spinal injury.
> - Multi level spinal injuries are common; a patient with a single spinal injury should have the entire spine evaluated as well.
> - It is common to delay diagnosis because of unconsciousness or alcohol or drug intoxication.
> - Motor vehicle crashes are by far the most common cause for spinal column injuries.
> - Men are more likely to sustain injury than are women.
> - In elderly patients, falls are a much more common mechanism.

---

*References 2, 3, 7, 9, 14, 47, 77, 79, 110, 112.

sensory disturbance, or any other neurologic problem even if this was transient around the time of the injury. Reports from eyewitnesses and emergency medical technicians may also provide valuable information.

As with other injuries, an attempt should be made to obtain past medical history and information regarding other medical conditions that may influence treatment plans, such as heart condition, hypertension, anticoagulation, tobacco use, or corticosteroid treatment.

Physical Examination

The initial evaluation of the patient should include an overall assessment. This will follow the ABCs (Airway with cervical spine control, Breathing, and Circulation) as advocated by the advanced trauma life support course of the American College of Surgeons. Any deformity related to the spine should be noted. Palpation will identify areas of tenderness as well as gaps in the interspinous ligament. Any open wounds may indicate an open fracture.

Neurologic Examination

A detailed neurologic examination should encompass motor, sensory, rectal, and reflex examinations. The neurologic picture of a patient with a fracture of the thoracolumbar region can be very complex. Because of the anatomic arrangement of the conus medullaris and cauda equina, the possible neurologic deficits include complete cord injury, incomplete cord injury, mixed cord and root injury, and isolated root injury. It is very important to ascertain the level of any neurologic deficit and to document it over time through serial examination. A progressive neurologic deficit has a different prognosis and a different treatment plan.

Spinal shock occurs immediately after injury and is marked by absence of motor, sensory, or reflex activity below the level of the injury. Duration ranges from minutes to several days. In most circumstances, it resolves within 48 hours; return of the bulbocavernosus reflex heralds the end of spinal shock. In a fracture that occurs below the level of the conus, the bulbocavernosus reflex may be absent on the basis of a lower motor neuron injury. This lesion produces flaccid bladder and sphincter tone.

PATIENT EVALUATION

- Obtain complete history.
- Ask conscious patient to relate the mechanism of injury.
- Elicit any history of paralysis, sensory disturbance, or any other neurologic problem even if this was transient around the time of the injury.
- Seek reports from eyewitnesses and emergency medical technicians.
- Obtain past medical history and information regarding other medical conditions that may influence treatment plans.
- Note any deformity related to the spine.
- Use palpation to identify areas of tenderness as well as gaps in the interspinous ligament.
- Perform neurologic examination: Motor, sensory, rectal, and reflex.
- Possible neurologic deficits include the following:
  - Complete cord injury
  - Incomplete cord injury
  - Mixed cord and root injury
  - Isolated root injury
- Ascertain the level of any neurologic deficit; document it over time by serial examination.
- Be aware that a progressive neurologic deficit has a different prognosis and a different treatment plan.
- Assess for spinal shock
  - Occurs immediately after injury and is marked by lack of motor, sensory, or reflex activity below the level of the injury
  - Duration: Minutes to several days
  - Typically resolves within 48 hours
  - Return of the bulbocavernosus reflex heralded by the end of spinal shock
  - In a fracture that occurs below the level of the conus, the bulbocavernosus reflex may be absent on the basis of a lower motor neuron injury, producing a flaccid bladder and sphincter tone

TREATMENT

- Immobilize the patient before arrival in the emergency department.
- Be aware that corticosteroids, opiate receptor antagonists, gangliosides, and several other agents have been advocated for the acute treatment of spinal cord injuries.
- Methylprednisolone is the only drug in widespread clinical use at this time.
- Spinal radiographs
  - Obtain for all patients with a suspected spinal injury.
  - Anteroposterior and lateral views are required.
  - Standard chest and abdominal radiographs are inadequate for spinal evaluation.
- Obtain a computed tomography scan for all patients with a known thoracolumbar fracture.
- Magnetic resonance imaging (MRI).
  - Obtain MRI for thoracolumbar fractures, although this is not routine at most institutions.
  - Consider MRI in the following situations:
    - Patient has a neurologic deficit not explained by the bony injury.
    - Patient has a progressive deficit not explained by the previous studies.

TREATMENT
Patient Immobilization

The patient should be immobilized before arrival in the emergency department, usually on a backboard. It is necessary to rotate the patient to examine the skin and posterior ligamentous structures; this should be done while the patient is on a full-length backboard.[63,95] Once this procedure is carried out, the backboard should be removed to prevent decubitus ulceration.[34] It is at this point that we recommend using a kinetic bed such as a Roto Rest bed.

Pharmacologic Treatment

Corticosteroids, opiate receptor antagonists, gangliosides, and several other agents have all been advocated for the acute treatment of spinal cord injuries.* Methylprednisolone is the only drug in widespread clinical use

---

*References 11, 18-22, 53, 60, 61, 81, 96, 102.

at this time. The NASCIS studies (North American Spinal Cord Injury Study I, II, and III) involved a large number of patients receiving large doses of methylprednisolone within the first 8 hours after injury.[21] The statistical evaluation of these patients is somewhat troublesome but is currently thought to be the standard of care in most communities.[31] The factors to remember are that the study evaluated only spinal cord function and did not involve penetrating trauma. Therefore, there are no data to substantiate its use in patients with root level injuries, gunshot wounds, or other penetrating trauma.[62,89] The NASCIS III recommendations included a loading dose of 30 mg/kg of methylprednisolone given as an intravenous bolus, and if seen within 3 hours of injury, the patient is given 5.4 mg/kg per hour for 24 hours. If the patient presents 3 to 8 hours after the injury, the infusion is continued for 48 hours.[22] There is no reason to use steroids if not started in the first 8 hours, because the results were worse than no drug. Steroid therapy for cord injury associated with gunshot wounds was not studied by NASCIS and is associated with a higher complication rate.[62,89]

Radiographic Examination

Spinal radiographs should be obtained in all patients with a suspected spinal injury. As a minimum, anteroposterior and lateral views are required; standard chest and abdominal radiographs are inadequate for spinal evaluation.[15] Only patients with some clinical evidence or suspicion of thoracolumbar injury require radiographic assessment.[48,103,113]

Computed Tomography Scanning

A computed tomography scan should be obtained in all patients with a known thoracolumbar fracture.[8,91] This will better delineate any spinal canal compromise as well as fractures of the posterior elements.[29,76,92,114,117]

Myelography

Myelography is mentioned mainly for historical interest. At the present time, it is rarely used and has been replaced by magnetic resonance imaging (MRI). It is indicated when MRI is unavailable or contraindicated (e.g., patients with a pacemaker or ferromagnetic cerebral aneurysm clips).

Magnetic Resonance Imaging

MRI can be obtained for thoracolumbar fractures, although this is not routinely obtained at most institutions.[99,111] If the patient has a neurologic deficit that is unexplained by the bony injury or a progressive deficit that is not explained by the previous studies, MRI should be considered (Figure 36A-1).

CLASSIFICATION

At the present time there is no universally accepted classification for thoracolumbar injuries, although multiple attempts have been made. The original standard was that of Holdsworth; this considered the spine to consist of two columns.[65-67] The anterior column is loaded in compression. The posterior longitudinal ligament and all posterior structures are loaded in tension. This was the standard classification up until 1983, when Denis published his three-column theory.[40,41,43] This is based on analysis of computed tomography information. Images often showed the displacement of the posterior vertebral body into the spinal canal. The Denis scheme emphasized this component of the burst fracture, the most common injury in his series. This emphasis proved to be unwarranted. For a time, all burst fractures underwent surgical decompression and stabilization, but now it is known that the vast majority of burst fractures do not require surgical treatment. The retropulsed bone usually resorbs, and spinal stability returns with fracture healing.*

AO/ASIF (Magerl) Classification

Fritz Magerl spent more than 10 years studying thousands of radiographs to develop the AO/ASIF (Arbeitsgemeinschaft für Osteosynthesefragen/Association for the Study of Internal Fixation) classification system.[54,90] Type "A" injuries are the results of compression by axial loading (e.g., compression and burst fractures). Type "B" injuries are distraction injuries, and disruption may occur through the posterior or anterior structures (e.g., Chance injuries). Type "C" fractures are the result of a rotational force (e.g., fracture-dislocations with a rotary compo-

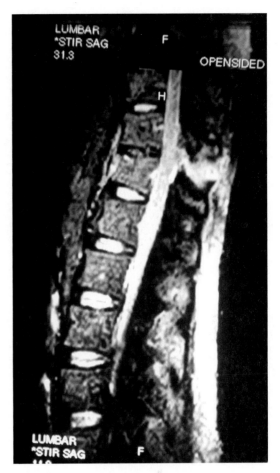

Figure 36A-1. Magnetic resonance image of the lumbar spine.

nent). Each type is divided into subgroups of increasing severity. The likelihood of neurologic deficit increases in the higher subgroups.

Spinal canal compromise and neurologic deficit do not correlate well.† The neurologic deficit may be the result of neural trauma that occurs at the time of injury rather than the residual canal compromise. Furthermore, spinal canal compromise is not permanent. Many studies have shown remodeling of the spinal canal after thoracolumbar fractures, both in patients who have been treated operatively and in those treated nonoperatively‡ (Figure 36A-2).

Fracture Biomechanics

Determining the degree of instability or potential instability is the key to appropriate treatment. There are mechanical and neurologic components. If we look just at the mechanical component, the burst fracture with posterior ligamentous disruption may not be able to withstand physiologic loads, and therefore the pattern is potentially unstable. This is temporary because if the bone is protected for a period of time and the spinal alignment is maintained, bone healing may occur and

---

*References 37, 59, 71, 74, 86, 100, 104, 118.

†References 12, 16, 23, 26, 28, 35, 44, 56, 70, 72, 75, 85, 87, 88.
‡References 37, 59, 71, 74, 86, 100, 114, 118.

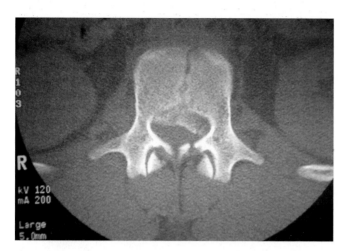

Figure 36A-2. Transverse section showing spinal canal compromise.

CLASSIFICATION AND NONOPERATIVE TREATMENT

- AO/ASIF (Arbeitsgemeinschaft für Osteosynthesefragen/Association for the Study of Internal Fixation) classification system
  - Type A injuries: Result of compression by axial loading (e.g., compression and burst fractures)
  - Type B injuries: Distraction injuries and disruption may occur through the posterior or anterior structures (e.g., Chance injuries)
  - Type C fractures: Result of a rotational force (e.g., fracture-dislocations with a rotary component)
- Spinal canal compromise and neurologic deficit do not correlate well.
- C7 vertebra should be centered over the sacrum in both sagittal and coronal planes when patient is standing or sitting.
- Nonsurgical treatment is indicated for most patients.
- Nonsurgical treatment is not appropriate in the following situations:
  - A complete dislocation with no bony contact: Healing cannot be expected to produce a stable spine
  - Significant soft tissue disruption such as a complete ligamentous disruption: Will not heal with stability
  - Documented neurologic deterioration: Mandates reassessment of management
  - Increasing pain or deformity despite appropriate nonoperative treatment: Signals failure of such treatment

---

the spinal column becomes stable. The neurologic instability is a neurologic injury that is worsening or failing to recover over time. These situations warrant work-up for correctable factors such as malalignment, uncontrolled mechanical instability, and neural compression.

Residual Kyphosis

Ideally, the C7 vertebra should be centered over the sacrum in both the sagittal and coronal planes when the patient is standing or sitting. The clinician should strive to achieve and maintain normal or near-normal sagittal curves. Both nonoperative and surgical management have a role in attaining a balanced stable spine.

TREATMENT OPTIONS

Nonsurgical treatment for thoracolumbar injuries is indicated in the vast majority of patients. This has been the mainstay for many years.* It is to be used for almost all compression fractures and most burst fractures. It is critical to distinguish acute and chronic mechanical instability. Just because the injury is mechanically unstable initially does not mean that it may not become stable after 4 to 6 weeks of immobilization in a cast or orthosis or with bedrest. It is difficult to justify decompression if the patient is neurologically intact. Increased deformity on upright radiographs, increased pain, and worsened neurologic symptoms or signs indicate failure of orthotic management and warrant modification of the treatment plan. The patient with a complete spinal cord injury may not be a good candidate for surgery and may be better treated nonoperatively as well.[101]

Nonsurgical treatment is not appropriate in the following situations. If there is a complete dislocation so that there is no bony contact, healing cannot be expected to produce a stable spine. Significant soft tissue disruption such as a complete ligamentous disruption will not heal with stability. Documented neurologic deterioration mandates reassessment of management. Increasing pain or deformity despite appropriate nonoperative treatment signals the failure of such treatment. If these conditions are not present, appropriate nonoperative treatment should be offered to all other patients.

Rechtine et al. reported a series of more than 100 patients treated using a kinetic bed.[101] It was shown to be a very effective treatment for both patients who are neurologically intact and those with neurologic deficits. When used properly, the Roto Rest bed can prevent decubitus ulceration, decrease atelectasis and pneumonia, reduce thromboembolism, and help protect the spinal column while it is healing. A vigorous exercise program is used to help decrease the deconditioning that comes with bedrest. Unless precluded by other injuries or diseases, all four extremities perform large repetition range-of-motion exercise against resistance. This exercise program may also diminish the likelihood of venous thrombosis and pulmonary emboli. The goal is for the patient to be as strong or stronger than before the injury. Deep venous thrombosis prophylaxis should include antiembolism stockings and sequential compression devices. Anticoagulation is not used for the first 72 hours after injury to avoid the risk of epidural hematoma; thereafter the clinician may deem anticoagulation appropriate.

After all injuries have been fully evaluated, it is appropriate to formulate a comprehensive treatment plan. The patient with an isolated stable spinal injury may be mobilized as tolerated. Nondisplaced posterior element

---

*References 4, 5, 18, 25, 36, 49, 51, 58, 73, 78, 80, 98, 100, 108.

fractures and many compression fractures can be mobilized without an orthosis. Upper thoracic compression fractures are not immobilized with standard off-the-shelf orthoses. An extension brace (e.g., CASH, Jewett) or a thoracolumbosacral orthosis (TLSO) may be used for thoracolumbar and lumbar compression fractures. Unlike the thoracic spine, which is stabilized by the rib cage, the thoracolumbar junction is subject to greater forces; most thoracolumbar compression fractures may benefit from a brace.

Patients who have a more severe injury that involves disruption of two or three of the spinal columns without disruption of the posterior ligamentous complex may be treated with a Roto Rest bed. Patients who are neurologically intact and those whose neurologic injury is stable or improving fall within this category. Patients with significant ligamentous disruption should be surgically stabilized. Individuals with deteriorating neurologic function would not be candidates for Roto Rest treatment if a surgically correctable cause can be identified. Nonoperative care may be appropriate for unrectifiable decline.

Severe compression fractures, burst fractures without severe comminution, and bony Chance fractures can be treated with a hyperextension cast.* Orthoses cannot provide the same reduction force as can well-molded hyperextension casts.

Patients with a neurologic deficit and insensate skin are not candidates for cast treatment. Braces used on insensate skin must be removed on a regular basis so the skin can be examined. Morbid obesity, burns, and other skin lesions may preclude bracing as well.

Surgical treatment provides options for those patients who are not candidates for nonoperative care. Instrumentation can restore sagittal and coronal plane alignment and indirectly decompress neural structures. However, surgery is attended by a higher complication rate. Certain complications, such as infection, are unique to surgery.[101] The patient should be given an accurate and balanced presentation of all treatment options. This facilitates informed consent.

Another controversy involving care of thoracolumbar fractures is the timing of surgical intervention. Intuitively it would make sense that a spinal canal decompression that is done immediately after the injury would provide a better neurologic recovery. This has been supported by animal studies, but this is not practical in clinical practice.[30,84] The work-up and stabilization take time. Immediate surgery is associated with greater hemorrhage. Surgical intervention should be performed as soon as the patient is ready and able to tolerate the surgery safely. The only proven advantage of surgical intervention is decreased hospital stay. The longer the patient is treated nonoperatively before surgery, the longer is the hospital stay.

Surgical Principles

The goals of surgical intervention are to provide immediate stability to the spine, decompress the neural ele-

---

SURGICAL INTERVENTION

- Goals
  - Provide immediate stability to the spine
  - Decompress the neural elements
  - Restore anatomic alignment
  - Reduce pain
- Absolute indications
  - Progressive neurologic deficit with a compressive lesion
  - Significant ligamentous injury
  - Dislocation
- Relative indications
  - Incomplete neurologic deficit that is not improving
  - Unacceptable deformity
  - Patient desire to avoid bed rest
  - Intractable pain

---

ments, restore anatomic alignment, and reduce pain. Ideally surgery would be limited to the injured vertebrae. This would produce minimal tissue disruption and optimize the transfer of forces and stresses around the injured area.

Indications

The absolute indications for surgical intervention are a progressive neurologic deficit with a compressive lesion, a significant ligamentous injury, and dislocation. Relative indications include an incomplete neurologic deficit that is not improving, an unacceptable deformity, patient's desire to avoid bedrest, and intractable pain.

Posterior Surgery

Historically, the first surgical approach for thoracolumbar trauma was a laminectomy, but now it is mentioned only for historical interest. Only rarely should laminectomy be performed in isolation for thoracolumbar injury. Harrington instrumentation provided the ability to stabilize the injured spine and allow earlier mobilization.[†] Before this, nonoperative treatment with plaster beds and prolonged bedrest was the only way to stabilize a spine. Disadvantages to Harrington instrumentation are lack of rotational rigidity, reliance on distraction, and limited ability to restore sagittal alignment. As the posterior rod systems became more rigid and added multiple points of fixation (e.g., CD [Cotrel Dubousset] and then TSRH [Texas Scottish Rite Hospital for Children] instrumentation), implant failure decreased.[‡] Luque championed the use of sublaminar wires, but it is not biomechanically suited for trauma.[68,109] The major disadvantage of these techniques was a requirement of extending two or three segments proximal and distal to the injury. Rae Jacobs described the rod-long/fuse-short technique.[1,39,69] This decreased the effects of the long segment fixation. Only the injured segments were actually grafted, and the

---

*References 4, 5, 49, 78, 80, 98, 100, 115.

†References 24, 26-28, 32, 42, 43, 45, 46, 50, 52, 56, 69, 70, 107.
‡References 10, 13, 33, 38, 57, 83, 93, 105, 109.

hardware extended two or three segments cranial and caudal to the injury. The rods and hooks are removed after approximately 1 year. The results in this technique appear to be reasonably good. Pedicle screw fixation provides the opportunity for short segment fixation. The problem with short segment fusions is that without anterior column support, implants are under a cantilever load, leading to significant screw failure. Another disadvantage of the posterior approach is that the neural elements lie between the surgeon and the displaced bone. Many techniques are available to restore the spinal canal from a posterolateral approach; these do not provide the degree of visualization that is possible with the anterior approach.

Anterior Surgery

Anterior approaches to the spine were initially developed for the treatment of tuberculosis. Eventually, this was modified to correct traumatic spinal canal compromise. Initially, a prolonged period of bedrest was necessary. The addition of posterior instrumentation to the anterior decompression and grafting allowed immediate patient mobilization. The next-generation spinal implants included anterolateral implants, which provide for immediate stability with only an anterior approach. The major advantages of the anterior approach are direct visualization for decompression of the spinal canal and reconstruction of the weight-bearing portion of the spine. The disadvantages are the extensive dissection of the retroperitoneal, transthoracic, transperitoneal, or thoracoabdominal approach and the biomechanical disadvantage of short segment anterior fixation.

Video-assisted thoracoscopic surgery has been applied to injuries of the thoracic spine to reduce the morbidity of the anterior approach.

ANTERIOR AND POSTERIOR APPROACHES

- Laminectomy is performed only rarely in isolation for thoracolumbar injury.
- Anterior approaches to the spine were initially developed for treatment of tuberculosis.
- Adding posterior instrumentation to anterior decompression and grafting allows immediate patient mobilization.
- Major advantages of anterior approach
  - Direct visualization for decompression of the spinal canal
  - Reconstruction of the weight-bearing portion of the spine
- Major disadvantages of anterior approach
  - Extensive dissection of the retroperitoneal, transthoracic, transperitoneal, or thoracoabdominal approach
  - Biomechanical disadvantage of short segment anterior fixation
- Complete dislocations may require combined anterior and posterior procedures.

Anterior and Posterior Surgery

Fracture-dislocations are often very unstable and may not be amenable to an isolated anterior or a posterior procedure. Complete dislocations may require combined anterior and posterior procedures. The majority of fracture-dislocations may be managed with posterior constructs using long segmental fixation extending several levels cranial and caudal to the dislocation. It will also require some sort of a rotational control with a linkage between the bilateral rod system. These unstable three-column injuries cannot be addressed by an anterior approach alone. The anterior instrumentation systems cannot withstand the forces that these injuries engender. McCormack and Gaines have a point system to predict short segment pedicle screw failure based on increasing comminution, fragment displacement, and kyphosis.[94] A high score is associated with failure of isolated posterior fixation due to excessive load on the screws. Anterior reconstruction is indicated in such severe injuries.

SPECIFIC INJURIES AND RECOMMENDED TREATMENTS
Nondisplaced Isolated Posterior Element Fractures

Transverse process fractures are avulsion injuries, and most are managed symptomatically and usually of no long-term consequence. The exception to this rule is the L5 transverse process, which is highly associated with pelvic and sacral fractures. The L5 transverse process fracture does not require specific treatment but should prompt a thorough examination of the sacrum and pelvis.

Gunshot Wounds

Most civilian gunshot wounds are low-energy wounds. Almost all in the thoracolumbar spine produce stable injuries. Most of the time, the bullet fragments need not be removed, and the fractures are treated nonoperatively. High-velocity gunshot wounds and shotgun wounds do require multiple debridements and may be associated with spinal instability. This spinal instability must be treated appropriately.

Compression Fractures

By definition, compression fracture involves only the anterior column. If the posterior ligamentous complex has been disrupted, this is a two-column injury and will require surgical intervention. As long as the anterior column is the only injured portion, this is generally stable and can be managed with early ambulation in an orthosis. Multilevel compression fractures indicate higher-energy injuries and must be assessed accordingly. Severe compression fractures may be a surgical indication, but this is rare.

Burst Fractures

Most of these patients will be neurologically intact. If there is a neurologic injury, most will be incomplete. One option would include nonoperative treatment on a kinetic bed. If the patient is neurologically intact with a stable burst injury, a hyperextension cast or a well-fit orthosis may be used. Proponents of operative management have stated that a neurologic injury, loss of vertebral body height greater than 50%, angulation of greater than 20 degrees, canal compromise of greater than 50%, lateral tilt greater than 10 degrees, or posterior ligament rupture is a surgical indication. Early surgical intervention with ligamentotaxis can restore spinal canal to an acceptable level. Care must be taken not to distract over a fixed kyphosis.

Another option for the isolated burst fracture would be in an anterior approach with decompression and anterolateral instrumentation. The association of a motor deficit and posterior element fracture has a high association with dural tear and entrapped nerve rootlets.

This injury pattern could be an argument for a posterior approach. In considering surgical treatment for burst fracture, arguably the most significant deciding factor is an associated complete posterior ligamentous disruption. This can usually be identified on physical examination by palpation of a gap between the spinous processes and marked posterior tenderness (Figure 36A-3).

Flexion Distraction Injuries

A seat belt injury (Chance or flexion distraction injury) can involve just bone, just ligaments, or a combination of both. With a bone-only injury, when anterior reduction can be obtained to an acceptable level, this fracture can be treated with either a rotating bed or hyperextension cast. Surgery is used if reduction fails, but when the

---

SPECIFIC INJURIES AND RECOMMENDED TREATMENTS

- Nondisplaced isolated posterior element fractures
  - Transverse process fractures: Avulsion injuries; most managed symptomatically; usually of no long-term consequence
- Gunshot wounds
  - Civilian gunshot wounds: Most low energy
  - Usually bullet fragments need not be removed; fractures treated nonoperatively
  - High-velocity gunshot wounds and shotgun wounds: Require multiple débridements; may be associated with spinal instability
- Compression fractures
  - If the posterior ligamentous complex disrupted: A two-column injury; requires surgical intervention

- Burst fractures
  - Most patients neurologically intact
- Flexion distraction injuries
  - Seat belt injury (Chance or flexion distraction injury): Can involve just bone, just ligaments, or a combination of both
- Fracture-dislocations
  - Tend to be high-energy injuries; carry a high likelihood of severe neurologic injury
  - Goals of treatment
    - Realign the spine
    - Provide stability
    - Allow for early mobilization of the patient
  - Usually require posterior or combined anterior and posterior stabilization

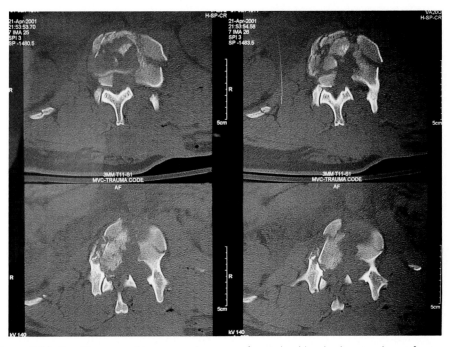

Figure 36A-3. Computed tomography scan of vertebral body showing burst fracture.

posterior column fails by ligamentous disruption, surgical intervention with segmental compression instrumentation system should be considered.

Fracture-Dislocations

Fracture-dislocations tend to be high-energy injuries and carry with them a high likelihood of severe neurologic injury. The goal of treatment is to realign the spine, provide stability, and allow for early mobilization of the patient. These will usually require posterior or combined anterior and posterior stabilization (Figures. 36A-4 and 36A-5).

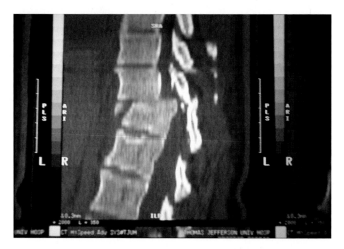

Figure 36A-4. Sagittal computed tomography scan showing fracture-dislocation of the spine.

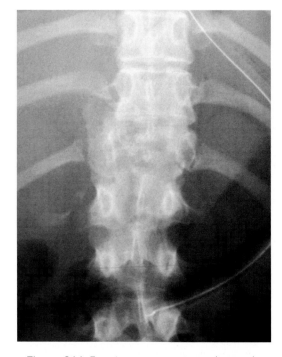

Figure 36A-5. Anteroposterior radiograph showing fracture of the lumbar spine.

POSTOPERATIVE MANAGEMENT

Many of the complications of surgical intervention are the same as those of nonoperative treatment. Measures to minimize pneumonia, atelectasis, and thromboembolism are high priorities for the postoperative patient. We have found that the Roto Rest or other kinetic bed is helpful in this regard. After 48 hours, the patient is ready to begin an active exercise and mobilization program. The patient is then placed in a regular hospital bed. Antiembolism stockings and sequential compression devices are used until the patient is fully mobile; this extends from arrival to the acute care hospital, through the surgery, and into the early postoperative period. The clinician may consider low-dose heparin or another form of anticoagulation after surgery in high-risk patients.

Nutrition has been shown to be very helpful in preventing infections and promoting fracture healing. As soon as possible, the patient should receive nutritional support after injury, resuming shortly after the operation. Steroidal and nonsteroidal antiinflammatory drugs (NSAIDs) and phenytoin (Dilantin) have an adverse effect on bone healing. If it is at all possible, NSAIDs are avoided for 3 months after surgery. There is experimental evidence that the cyclooxygenase-2 inhibitors may be less deleterious to bone healing than conventional NSAIDs. Smoking and tobacco abuse are strongly discouraged because of their detrimental effect on bone healing.

Orthoses are commonly used even with modern implants. Biomechanically, the orthosis does not provide much in the way of support in the face of a rod system. This orthosis is a reminder for the patient to limit their activity while the bone and soft tissues heal.

Exercise therapy, which is supervised by both physical therapy and occupational therapists, is part of our protocol for all spine trauma patients and continues from admission until discharge. Patients are instructed in what we hope becomes a lifelong home exercise program. While the patient is in the RotoRest bed, four extremity exercises with therapeutic rubber bands are used. If the patient has an extremity fracture, then exercise for that extremity is modified. If the patient has a neurologic deficit, then the muscle groups that are intact are exercised actively and the joints about paralyzed muscles are ranged passively and splinted to prevent unwanted contractures (e.g., heel equinus).

Complications of Nonoperative Treatment

The most dramatic complication is death. The most common cause of fatal outcomes with spinal injuries are thromboembolisms. The incidence is much higher in patients with complete neurologic deficits. It is important for the physician to recognize high-risk patients and to consider pharmacologic prophylaxis. This will not eliminate the problem, but it should minimize it. Antiembolic stockings and sequential compression devices are used unless lower extremity injuries preclude them. After the acute phase, low-dose anticoagulation may be added.

Decubitus ulceration will occur. Prevention should be preferable to treatment. It is important to remove the patient from the back-board as soon as possible.[34]

Urinary tract infections are an ongoing problem with any patient with a neurologic deficit. These can be minimized by removal of the indwelling catheter as soon as possible. If the patient has neurologic deficit, institute a program of intermittent catheterization. Atelectasis, pneumonia, and other pulmonary problems may be diminished by the use of respiratory therapy and kinetic beds.[64,101]

Late pain and neurologic deterioration are uncommon but can be addressed by surgical intervention if necessary.

Complications of Operative Treatment

All of the previously listed complications of nonoperative treatment can occur with operative treatment as well. One of the complications unique to surgical intervention is blood loss, which can require transfusion. Transfusion engenders an antigenic response, which may complicate future transfusion; can incite acute allergic response, which may be life threatening; and can transmit infectious disease, such as hepatitis and human immunodeficiency virus infection. Hypotensive anesthesia may help with blood loss, but when there is neurologic compromise, hypotensive anesthesia may not be the best choice.

An anterior approach can be associated with visceral and vascular injuries. Spinal fluid leakage can occur with any surgical approach and may require repair or grafting.

The chance of infection is higher in trauma patients than it is in the elective spine surgery population, by approximately 10%.[82,101] This may be related to the attendant soft tissue disruption and overall high energy involved in the injury.

Failure of fusion can occur even with modern instrumentation. Higher rates of nonunion will occur in patients with metabolic bone disorders, patients who are on drugs that alter bone healing, and those who persist in their tobacco abuse.

If the patient heals with an undesirable configuration, an osteotomy may be necessary. When instrumentation fails, there is loss of fixation and physiologic alignment; early surgical intervention is appropriate rather than waiting for bony healing as a malunion.

Bone grafting is intrinsically morbid. The most common patient complaint is donor site pain. This can sometimes be related to cluneal and lateral femoral cutaneous neuromas. Superior gluteal artery injuries can occur as well. Hematoma, pelvic fracture, and infection are also risks of graft harvest. In the future, it is hoped that technology will provide effective, safe, and cost-effective bone graft substitutes.

All surgical approaches have inherent morbidity. After an anterior approach, patients commonly note a muscular bulge and occasionally a hernia. A latissimus dorsi rupture is also possible. The dissection and the spinal instrumentation can injure visceral, vascular, or neural structures. The hardware may fatigue and bend or break. Instrumentation can loosen, resulting in loss of reduction, nonunion, and pain. Occasionally, it is necessary to revise or remove hardware just because it causes local soft tissue irritation.

Pain is an ongoing problem regardless of the method used for initial management. After the spine has been stabilized, decompressed, and anatomically restored, it is still possible for the patient to have ongoing pain. If reassessment shows no evidence of infection, nonunion, or persistent neural compression, a multidisciplinary pain program is probably the most appropriate treatment.

CONCLUSIONS

Fractures of the thoracolumbar area are the most common injuries associated with the spine. The spine

---

COMPLICATIONS

- To minimize complications of surgical intervention, such as:
  - Pneumonia
  - Atelectasis
  - Thromboembolism
- Kinetic beds are helpful.
  - After 48 hours, patient is ready to begin an active exercise and mobilization program, and then the patient is placed in a regular hospital bed.
- Antiembolism stockings and sequential compression devices are used until the patient is fully mobile.
- Consider low-dose heparin or another form of anticoagulation after surgery in high-risk patients.
- Nutrition is helpful in preventing infections and promoting fracture healing.
- Steroidal and nonsteroidal antiinflammatory medications (NSAIDs) and phenytoin (Dilantin) have an adverse effect on bone healing.
- If possible, NSAIDs are avoided for 3 months after surgery.
  - Selective cyclooxygenase-2 inhibitors may be less deleterious to bone healing than conventional NSAIDs.
  - Smoking is detrimental to bone healing.
- Thromboembolisms: Most common cause of fatal outcomes with spinal injuries
- Incidence: Much higher in patients with complete neurologic deficits
- Urinary tract infections: Ongoing problem with any patient who has a neurologic deficit; minimized by removal of the indwelling catheter as soon as possible
- Atelectasis, pneumonia, and other pulmonary problems: Diminished by the use of respiratory therapy and kinetic beds
- Blood loss: Complication unique to surgical intervention
- Spinal fluid leakage: Can occur with any surgical approach; may require repair or grafting
- Infection: Chance higher in trauma patients than in elective spine surgery population by approximately 10%
- Failure of fusion: Can occur even with modern instrumentation
- Higher rates of nonunion in
  - Patients with metabolic bone disorders
  - Patients on drugs that alter bone healing
  - Those who persist in their tobacco abuse

injury as well as the nonspinal injuries must be delineated to develop an appropriate treatment plan. This plan should provide the best opportunity for the patient to return to his or her preinjury status. The treatment of thoracolumbar spine injuries remains controversial at present. The treating physician should be adept at all aspects of nonoperative care as well as both anterior and posterior surgical approaches to the problem. If he or she does not possess all of these skills, the physician cannot adequately assess the most appropriate treatment for the patient. Nonoperative treatment will be appropriate for the vast majority of patients. Surgical intervention is indicated only when nonsurgical treatment will not produce an acceptably aligned and stable spine. If comparable results can be obtained with nonoperative treatment, this is preferable for most patients. Prospective multicenter studies with long-term follow-up will be needed to definitely address these issues, but the cost of such studies make them unlikely.

SELECTED REFERENCES

An HS et al.: Low lumbar burst fractures: comparison between conservative and surgical treatments, *Orthopedics* 15(3):367-373, 1992.

An HS et al.: Biomechanical evaluation of anterior thoracolumbar spinal instrumentation, *Spine* 20(18):1979-1983, 1995.

Anderson S, Biros MH, Reardon RF: Delayed diagnosis of thoracolumbar fractures in multiple-trauma patients, *Acad Emerg Med* 3(9):832-839, 1996.

Bradford DS, McBride GG: Surgical management of thoracolumbar spine fractures with incomplete neurologic deficits, *Clin Orthop* 218:201-216, 1987.

de Klerk LW et al.: Spontaneous remodeling of the spinal canal after conservative management of thoracolumbar burst fractures, *Spine* 23(9):1057-1060, 1998.

Holdsworth FW: Fractures, dislocations and fracture–dislocations of the spine, *J Bone Joint Surg Am* 52:1534-1551, 1970.

Lemons VR, Wagner FC Jr, Montesano PX: Management of thoracolumbar fractures with accompanying neurological injury, *Neurosurgery* 30(5):667-671, 1992.

Magerl F et al.: A comprehensive classification of thoracic and lumbar injuries, *Eur Spine J* 3(4):184-201, 1994.

Rechtine GR II, Cahill D, Chrin AM: Treatment of thoracolumbar trauma: comparison of complications of operative versus nonoperative treatment, *J Spinal Disord* 12(5):406-409, 1999.

Stanislas MJ et al.: A high risk group for thoracolumbar fractures, *Injury* 29(1):15-18, 1998.

Terregino CA et al.: Selective indications for thoracic and lumbar radiography in blunt trauma, *Ann Emerg Med* 26(2):126-129, 1995.

Weinstein JN, Colalto P, Lehmann TR: Thoracolumbar "burst" fractures treated conservatively: a long term follow-up, *Spine* 13:33-38, 1988.

REFERENCES

1. Akbarnia BA et al.: Use of long rods and a short arthrodesis for burst fractures of the thoracolumbar spine: a long-term follow-up study, *J Bone Joint Surg Am* 76(11):1629-1635, 1994.
2. American Academy of Orthopaedic Surgeons: *Emergency care and transportation of the sick and injured*, ed 4, Menashas, Wis, 1987, George Banta.
3. American College of Surgeons: *Advanced trauma life support manual*, Chicago, 1984, The College.
4. An HS et al.: Low lumbar burst fractures: comparison between conservative and surgical treatments, *Orthopedics* 15(3):367-373, 1992.
5. An HS et al.: Biomechanical evaluation of anterior thoracolumbar spinal instrumentation, *Spine* 20(18):1979-1983, 1995.
6. Anderson S, Biros MH, Reardon RF: Delayed diagnosis of thoracolumbar fractures in multiple-trauma patients, *Acad Emerg Med* 3(9):832-839, 1996.
7. Anderson PA et al.: Flexion distraction and Chance thoracolumbar spine fractures, *J Orthop Trauma* 3:160-161, 1989.
8. Ballock RT et al.: Can burst fractures be predicted from plain radiographs? *J Bone Joint Surg Br* 74(1):147-150, 1992.
9. Bedbrook GM: Stability of spinal fractures and fracture dislocations, *Paraplegia* 9:23-32, 1971.
10. Benli IT et al.: Cotrel-Dubousset instrumentation in the treatment of unstable thoracic and lumbar spine fractures, *Arch Orthop Trauma Surg* 113(2):86-92, 1994.
11. Benson DR et al.: Unstable thoracolumbar and lumbar burst fractures treated with the AO fixateur interne, *J Spinal Disord* 5(3):335-343, 1992.
12. Benzel EC: Short-segment compression instrumentation for selected thoracic and lumbar spine fractures: the short-rod/two-claw technique, *J Neurosurg* 79(3):335-340, 1993.
13. Benzel EC, Kesterson L, Marchand EP: Texas Scottish Rite Hospital rod instrumentation for thoracic and lumbar spine trauma, *J Neurosurg* 75(3):382-387, 1991.
14. Bohlman HH: Acute fractures and dislocations of the cervical spine: an analysis of three hundred hospitalized patients and review of the literature, *J Bone Joint Surg Am* 61(8):1119-1142, 1979.
15. Bolesta MJ, Bohlman HH: Mediastinal widening associated with fractures of the upper thoracic spine, *J Bone Joint Surg Am* 73(3):447-450, 1991.
16. Bosh A, Stauffer ES, Nickel VL: Incomplete traumatic quadriplegia: a ten year review, *JAMA* 216:473-478, 1971.
17. Braakman R et al.: Megadose steroids in severe head injury: Results of a prospective double-blind clinical trial, *J Neurosurg* 58(3):326-330, 1983.
18. Braakman R et al.: Neurological deficit in injuries of the thoracic and lumbar spine: a consecutive series of 70 patients, *Acta Neurochir* 111(1-2):11-17, 1991.
19. Bracken MB et al.: Efficiency of methyl prednisolone in acute spinal cord injury, *JAMA* 252:45-52, 1984.
20. Bracken MB et al.: Methylprednisolone and neurological function one year after spinal cord injury: results of the national spinal cord injury study, *J Neurosurg* 63:704-713, 1985.
21. Bracken MB et al.: A randomized, controlled trial of methylprednisolone or naloxone in the treatment of acute spinal-cord injury: results of the Second National Acute Spinal Cord Injury Study, *N Engl J Med* 322(20):1405-1411, 1990.
22. Bracken MB et al.: Administration of methylprednisolone for 24 or 48 hours or tirilazad mesylate for 48 hours in the treatment of acute spinal cord injury: results of the Third National Acute Spinal Cord Injury Randomized Controlled Trial National Acute Spinal Cord Injury Study, *JAMA* 277(20):1597-1604, 1997.
23. Bradford DS, McBride GG: Surgical management of thoracolumbar spine fractures with incomplete neurologic deficits, *Clin Orthop* 218:201-216, 1987.
24. Bradford DS et al.: Surgical stabilization of fracture and fracture–dislocation of the thoracic spine, *Spine* 2:185-196, 1977.
25. Bravo P et al.: Outcome after vertebral fractures with neurological lesion treated either surgically or conservatively in Spain, *Paraplegia* 31(6):358-366, 1993.
26. Broom MJ, Jacobs RR: Current status of internal fixation of thoracolumbar fractures, *J Orthop Trauma* 3:148-155, 1989.
27. Bryant CE, Sullivan JA: Management of thoracic and lumbar spine fractures with Harrington distraction rods supplemented with segmental wiring, *Spine* 8:532-537, 1983.
28. Burke DC, Murray DD: The management of thoracic and thoracolumbar injuries of the spine with neurological involvement, *J Bone Joint Surg Br* 58:72-78, 1976.
29. Campbell SE et al.: The value of CT in determining potential instability of simple wedge-compression fractures of the lumbar spine, *Am J Neuroradiol* 16(7):1385-1392, 1995.
30. Clohisy JC et al.: Neurologic recovery associated with anterior decompression of spine fractures at the thoracolumbar junction (T12-L1), *Spine* 17(8 Suppl):S325-S330, 1992.
31. Coleman W et al.: A critical appraisal of the reporting of the National Acute Spinal Cord Injury Studies (II and III) of methylprednisolone in acute spinal cord injury, *J Spinal Disord* 13(3):185-199, 2000.

32. Convery FR et al.: Fracture–dislocation of the dorsal-lumbar spine: acute operative stabilization by Harrington instrumentation, *Spine* 3:160-166, 1978.

33. Cotrel Y, Dubousset J, Guillaumat M: New universal instrumentation in spinal surgery, *Clin Orthop* 227:10-23, 1988.

34. Curry K, Casady L: The relationship between extended periods of immobility and decubitus ulcer formation in the acutely spinal cord-injured individual, *J Neurosci Nurs* 24(4):185-189, 1992.

35. Dall BE, Stauffer ES: Neurologic injury and recovery patterns in burst fractures at the T12 or L1 motion segment, *Clin Orthop* 233:171-176, 1988.

36. Davies WE, Morris JH, Hill V: An analysis of conservation (non-surgical) management of thoracolumbar fractures and fracture–dislocations with neural damage, *J Bone Joint Surg Am* 62:1324-1328, 1980.

37. de Klerk LW et al.: Spontaneous remodeling of the spinal canal after conservative management of thoracolumbar burst fractures, *Spine* 23(9):1057-1060, 1998.

38. de Peretti F et al.: Short device fixation and early mobilization for burst fractures of the thoracolumbar junction, *Eur Spine J* 5(2):112-120, 1996.

39. Dekutoski MB, Conlan ES, Salciccioli GG: Spinal mobility and deformity after Harrington rod stabilization and limited arthrodesis of thoracolumbar fractures, *J Bone Joint Surg Am* 75(2):168-176, 1993.

40. Denis F: The three-column spine and its significance in the classification of acute thoracolumbar spinal injuries, *Spine* 8:817-831, 1983.

41. Denis F: Spinal instability as defined by the three column spine concept in acute spinal trauma, *Clin Orthop* 189:65-76, 1984.

42. Denis F, Burkus JK: Diagnosis and treatment of cauda equina entrapment in the vertical lamina fracture of lumbar burst fractures, *Spine* 16(8 Suppl):S433-S439, 1991.

43. Denis F et al.: Acute thoracolumbar burst fractures in the absence of neurologic deficit, *Clin Orthop* 189:142-149, 1984.

44. DeWald RL: Burst fractures of the thoracic and lumbar spine, *Clin Orthop* 189:150-161, 1984.

45. Dickson JH, Harrington PR, Erwin WD: Harrington instrumentation in the fractured, unstable thoracic and lumbar spine, *Tex Med* 69:91-98, 1973.

46. Dickson JH, Harrington PR, Erwin WD: Results of reduction and stabilization of the severely fracture thoracic and lumbar spine, *J Bone Joint Surg Am* 60:799-805, 1978.

47. Dulchavsky SA, Geller ER, Iorio DA: Analysis of injuries following the crash of Avianca Flight 52, *J Trauma* 34(2):282-284, 1993.

48. Durham RM et al.: Evaluation of the thoracic and lumbar spine after blunt trauma, *Am J Surg* 170(6):681-684, 1995.

49. Finn CA, Stauffer ES: Burst fracture of the fifth lumbar vertebra, *J Bone Joint Surg Am* 74(3):398-403, 1992.

50. Flesch JR et al.: Harrington instrumentation and spine fusion for unstable fractures and fracture–dislocations of the thoracic and lumbar spine, *J Bone Joint Surg Am* 59:143-153, 1977.

51. Frankel HL et al.: The value of postural reduction in the initial management of closed injuries of the spine with paraplegia and tetraplegia. I, *Paraplegia* 7:179-192, 1969.

52. Gaines RW, Humphreys WG: A plea for judgment in management of thoracolumbar fractures and fracture–dislocations: a reassessment of surgical indications, *Clin Orthop* 189:36-42, 1984.

53. Geisler FH, Dorsey FC, Coleman WP: Recovery of motor function after spinal-cord injury: a randomized, placebo-controlled trial with GM-1 ganglioside, *N Engl J Med* 324(26):1829-1838, 1991.

54. Gertzbein SD: Scoliosis Research Society Multicenter spine fracture study, *Spine* 17(5):528-540, 1992.

55. Gertzbein SD: Neurologic deterioration in patients with thoracic and lumbar fractures after admission to the hospital, *Spine* 19(15):1723-1725, 1994.

56. Gertzbein SD: Spine update: classification of thoracic and lumbar fractures, *Spine* 19(5):626-628, 1994.

57. Graziano GP: Cotrel-Dubousset hook and screw combination for spine fractures, *J Spinal Disord* 6(5):380-385, 1993.

58. Guttmann L: Spinal deformities in traumatic paraplegics and tetraplegics following surgical procedures, *Paraplegia* 7:38-58, 1969.

59. Ha KI et al.: A clinical study of the natural remodeling of burst fractures of the lumbar spine, *Clin Orthop* (323):210-214, 1996.

60. Hall ED, Braughler NM: Non-surgical management of spinal cord injuries: a review of studies with glucocorticoid steroid methyl prednisolone, *Acta Anaesth Belg* 38:405-409, 1987.

61. Hamilton AJ, McBlack P, Carr D: Contrasting actions of naloxone in experimental spinal cord trauma and cerebral ischemia: a review, *Neurosurgery* 17:845-849, 1985.

62. Heary RF et al.: Steroids and gunshot wounds to the spine, *Neurosurgery* 41(3):576-583, 1997.

63. Herzenberg JE et al.: Emergency transport and positioning of young children who have an injury of the cervical spine: the standard backboard may be hazardous, *J Bone Joint Surg Am* 71(1):15-22, 1989.

64. Hodgson AR et al.: Anterior spinal fusion: the operative approach and pathological findings in 412 patients with Pott's disease of the spine, *Br J Surg* 48:172-178, 1960.

65. Holdsworth FW: Fractures, dislocations, and fracture–dislocations of the spine, *J Bone Joint Surg Br* 45:6-20, 1963.

66. Holdsworth FW: Fractures, dislocations and fracture–dislocations of the spine, *J Bone Joint Surg Am* 52:1534-1551, 1970.

67. Holdsworth FW, Hardy A: Early treatment of paraplegia from fractures of the thoracolumbar spine, *J Bone Joint Surg Br* 35:540-550, 1953.

68. Huckell CB et al.: A comparative analysis of distraction rods versus Luque rods in thoracic spine fractures, *Eur Spine J* 3(5):270-275, 1994.

69. Jacobs RR, Casey MP: Surgical management of thoracolumbar spinal injuries: general principles and controversial considerations, *Clin Orthop* 189:22-35, 1984.

70. Jacobs RR, Nordwall A, Nachemson A: Reduction, stability and strength provided by internal fixation systems for thoracolumbar spinal injuries, *Clin Orthop* 171:300-308, 1982.

71. Johnsson R et al.: Spinal canal remodeling after thoracolumbar fractures with intraspinal bone fragments: 17 cases followed 1-4 years, *Acta Orthop Scand* 62(2):125-127, 1991.

72. Kapandji IA: *Physiology of the joints*, vol 3, New York, 1974, Churchill Livingstone.

73. Karjalainen M, Aho AJ, Katevuo K: Painful spine after stable fractures of the thoracic and lumbar spine: what benefit from the use of extension brace? *Ann Chir Gynaecol* 80(1):45-48, 1991.

74. Karlsson MK et al.: Remodeling of the spinal canal deformed by trauma, *J Spinal Disord* 10(2):157-161, 1997.

75. Keene JS: Radiographic evaluation of thoracolumbar fractures, *Clin Orthop* 189:58-64, 1984.

76. Keene JS et al.: Significance of acute posttraumatic bony encroachment of the neural canal, *Spine* 14(8):799-802, 1989.

77. Keenen TL, Antony J, Benson DR: Dural tears associated with lumbar burst fractures, *J Orthop Trauma* 4(3):243-245, 1990.

78. Kinoshita H et al.: Conservative treatment of burst fractures of the thoracolumbar and lumbar spine, *Paraplegia* 31(1):58-67, 1993.

79. Kluger Y et al.: Diving injuries: a preventable catastrophe, *J Trauma* 36(3):349-351, 1994.

80. Knight RQ et al.: Comparison of operative versus nonoperative treatment of lumbar burst fractures, *Clin Orthop* 293:112-121, 1993.

81. Kobrine AI: The question of steroids in neurotrauma: to give or not to give, *JAMA* 251(1):68, 1984.

82. Kornberg M et al.: Surgical stabilization of thoracic and lumbar spine fractures: a retrospective study in a military population, *J Trauma* 24(2):140-146, 1984.

83. Korovessis PG, Baikousis A, Stamatakis M: Use of the Texas Scottish Rite Hospital instrumentation in the treatment of thoracolumbar injuries, *Spine* 22(8):882-888, 1997.

84. Krengel WF, Anderson PA, Henley MB: Early stabilization and decompression for incomplete paraplegia due to a thoracic-level spinal cord injury, *Spine* 18(14):2080-2087, 1993.

85. Kuner EH et al.: Ligamentotaxis with an internal spinal fixator for thoracolumbar fractures, *J Bone Joint Surg Br* 76(1):107-112, 1994.

86. Kuner EH et al.: Restoration of the spinal canal by the internal fixator and remodeling, *Eur Spine J* 6(6):417-422, 1997.

87. Lemons VR, Wagner FC Jr, Montesano PX: Treatment of patients with thoracolumbar fractures, *Contemp Neurosurg* 11:1, 1989.

88. Lemons VR, Wagner FC Jr, Montesano PX: Management of thoracolumbar fractures with accompanying neurological injury, *Neurosurgery* 30(5):667-671, 1992.

89. Levy ML et al.: Use of methylprednisolone as an adjunct in the management of patients with penetrating spinal cord injury: outcome analysis, *Neurosurgery* 39(6):1141-1148, 1996.

90. Magerl F et al.: A comprehensive classification of thoracic and lumbar injuries, *Eur Spine J* 3(4):184-201, 1994.

91. Martijn A, Veldhuis EF: The diagnostic value of interpediculate distance assessment on plain films in thoracic and lumbar spine injuries, *J Trauma* 31(10):1393-1395, 1991.

92. McAfee PC, Yuan HA, Lasda NA: The unstable burst fracture, *Spine* 7(4):365-373, 1982.

93. McBride GG: Cotrel-Dubousset rods in surgical stabilization of spinal fractures, *Spine* 18(4):466-473, 1993.

94. McCormack T, Karaikovic E, Gaines RW: The load sharing classification of spine fractures, *Spine* 19(15):1741-1744, 1994.

95. McGuire RA et al.: Spinal instability and the log rolling maneuver, *J Trauma* 27:525-531, 1987.

96. McIntosh TK, Faden AI: Opiate antagonists in traumatic shock, *Ann Emerg Med* 15:1462-1465, 1986.

97. Meldon SW, Moettus LN: Thoracolumbar spine fractures: clinical presentation and the effect of altered sensorium and major injury, *J Trauma* 39(6):1110-1114, 1995.

98. Mick CA et al.: Burst fractures of the fifth lumbar vertebra, *Spine* 18(13):1878-1884, 1993.

99. Mirvis SE, Borg U, Belzler H: MR imaging of ventilator-dependent patients: preliminary experience, *Am J Roentgenol* 149:845-846, 1987.

100. Mumford J et al.: Thoracolumbar burst fractures: the clinical efficacy and outcome of nonoperative management, *Spine* 18(8):955-970, 1993.

101. Rechtine GR II, Cahill D, Chrin AM: Treatment of thoracolumbar trauma: comparison of complications of operative versus nonoperative treatment, *J Spinal Disord* 12(5):406-409, 1999.

102. Sabel BA, Stein DG: Pharmacological treatment of central nervous system injury, *Nature* 323(6088):493, 1986.

103. Samuels LE, Kerstein MD: 'Routine' radiologic evaluation of the thoracolumbar spine in blunt trauma patients: a reappraisal, *J Trauma* 34(1):85-89, 1993.

104. Scapinelli R, Candiotto S: Spontaneous remodeling of the spinal canal after burst fractures of the low thoracic and lumbar region, *J Spinal Disord* 8(6):486-493, 1995.

105. Stambough JL: Cotrel-Dubousset instrumentation and thoracolumbar spine trauma: a review of 55 cases, *J Spinal Disord* 7(6):461-469, 1994.

106. Stanislas MJ et al.: A high risk group for thoracolumbar fractures, *Injury* 29(1):15-18, 1998.

107. Stauffer ES: Internal fixation of fractures of the thoracolumbar spine, *J Bone Joint Surg Am* 66:1136-1138, 1984.

108. Steindl A, Schuh G: Late results after lumbar vertebrae fracture with Lorenz Bohler conservative treatment, *Unfallchirurg* 95(9):439-444, 1992.

109. Stephens GC, Devito DP, McNamara MJ: Segmental fixation of lumbar burst fractures with Cotrel-Dubousset instrumentation, *J Spinal Disord* 5(3):344-348, 1992.

110. Stover SL, Fine PR: *Spinal cord injury: the facts and figures,* Birmingham, Ala, 1986, University of Alabama.

111. Tarr RW et al.: MR imaging of recent spinal trauma, *J Comput Assist Tomogr* 11:412-417, 1987.

112. Teifke A et al.: The safety belt: effects on injury patterns of automobile passengers, *Rofo Fortschr Geb Rontgenstr Neuen Bildgeb Verfahr* 159(3):278-283, 1993.

113. Terregino CA et al.: Selective indications for thoracic and lumbar radiography in blunt trauma, *Ann Emerg Med* 26(2):126-129, 1995.

114. Trafton PG, Boyd CA Jr: Computed tomography of thoracic and lumbar spine injuries, *J Trauma* 24:506-515, 1984.

115. Weinstein JN, Colalto P, Lehmann TR: Thoracolumbar "burst" fractures treated conservatively: a long term follow-up, *Spine* 13:33-38, 1988.

116. Willen J et al.: The natural history of burst fractures at the thoracolumbar junction, *J Spinal Disord* 3(1):39-46, 1990.

117. Yazici M et al.: Sagittal contour restoration and canal clearance in burst fractures of the thoracolumbar junction (T12-L1): the efficacy of timing of the surgery, *J Orthop Trauma* 9(6):491-498, 1995.

Thoracolumbar Trauma: Lower Lumbar Burst Fractures—L3 to L5

Dirk H. Alander

The treatment goals for lumbar burst fractures are stable healing with minimal residual deformity and freedom from pain. Nonoperative treatment takes advantage of the lumbar lordosis and the posteriorly shifting body axis to meet these goals. Hyperextension casting or bracing after limited bed rest allows a neurologically intact patient with a stable burst fracture to mobilize quickly. Decompression with internal fixation should be considered for the patient with a neurologic deficit and canal compromise, an unstable burst fracture pattern, or serious multiple injuries. Posterior decompression will suffice for most patients, whereas anterior decompression should be considered for patients with residual neurologic deficits and large canal compromise (30% to 50%). Posterior decompression is also indicated for patients with severe vertebral body comminution who also require reconstruction of the anterior and middle columns.

Biomechanical forces across the lower lumbar vertebral segments are reflected in the anatomic changes at each level. The treatment of burst fractures of the lower lumbar spine involves putting these forces to maximum use in either nonoperative or operative treatment modalities. Improvements in spinal instrumentation and operative techniques minimize the potential complications of older hook and rod systems and result in improved surgical outcomes. Relevant lumbar anatomy, considerations in the treatment decision-making process, and the pertinent treatment techniques for operative and nonoperative care of the lumbar burst fracture will be reviewed.

ANATOMY

From L3 to L5 the orientation of the facets continues to move toward the sagittal plane, the pedicles and the spinal canal increase in size, and the canal contents diminish at the caudal end of the spine. The anterior-to-posterior distance of the vertebral body gradually decreases in size, whereas the width of the body increases at progressively lower lumbar levels. The size

---

> ### ANATOMY
>
> - Orientation of lower lumbar pedicles increases their inclination of insertion in the transaxial plane about 2 degrees at each level.
> - Interpedicular distance increases caudally to the level of the sacrum.
> - Vertebral body height decreases and width increases approaching the sacrum.

---

of the pedicles increases toward the caudal end of the lumbar spine. The average diameter of the pedicle at L1 is 9 mm, progressing to 18 mm at the L5 level. The inclination of the facets becomes increasingly parallel to the axis of the sagittal plane of the spine so that rotation is limited, while allowing flexion at each level of approximately 6 degrees.

As the orientation of the facets changes, the axis of the pedicle also moves laterally about 2 degrees per level so that at L3 the pedicle axis is 15 degrees and at L5 approximately 20 degrees. This change in the pedicle axis is reflected in the increased interpedicular distance at the lower lumbar levels.

Several factors influence the type of fracture pattern that develops at the time of injury. These factors include the relative position of the vertebral body to the weight-bearing line of the body, the relative "fixed" ends of the thoracic spine superiorly and the pelvis inferiorly, and the mobility of the lumbar spine at the time injury.

The types of burst fracture described by Denis are related to the amount of deforming force, the relative position of the vertebral body to that force, and the axial load imparted to the vertebral body. Denis A and B are the most common types of lumbar fractures identified.[5] The Denis A fracture reflects a dominant axial load on a straightened lumbar spine. The pelvis tilts forward, causing the lumbar spine to lose its lordosis. The resulting load causes collapse of both vertebral end plates with the anterior and middle columns collapsing equally, resulting in a minimal degree of kyphosis. This fracture pattern is associated with widening of the pedicles, disruption of the pedicle–vertebral body junction, laminar fractures, and large retropulsed fragments of bone.

The Denis B burst fracture is caused by the addition of a flexion force as the axial load is applied.[5] The anterior column is more depressed than in the Denis A, and the retropulsed bone is directed posteriorly into the spinal canal at the level of the pedicles. Kyphosis of the vertebral body is greater than in the type A burst fractures due to the greater collapse of the anterior column. There is relative sparing of the posterior elements, leaving the pedicle–vertebral body junction intact.

TREATMENT DECISIONS

Burst fractures of the lumbar spine involve high energy and are frequently associated with injuries of the pelvis, sacrum, and spine (Figure 36B-1). The difficulties of nursing care, patient mobilization, and management of other orthopedic and nonorthopedic injuries must be taken into consideration when deciding how to treat the lower lumbar burst fracture. Patients need extremity exercises in bed, prophylactic treatment for deep venous thrombosis, and mobilization out of bed when a well-fitting orthosis or cast can be applied in a comfortable fashion.

Consideration for nonoperative treatment for the burst fracture involves the specific injury type, associated injuries, neurologic status, patient size, and compliance. Numerous studies support the treatment of neurologically intact patients with lumbar burst fractures nonoperatively.[1,4,8,11] The proponents of this approach note that there is little evidence that anatomic reconstruction relates strongly to clinical outcome. The chance of neurologic deterioration in nonoperatively treated patients is very small.[1] With the use of nonoperative care, those individuals with a neurologic deficit have been reported to have variable degrees of neurologic recovery,[3] most likely due to the peripheral nature of the nerve roots at the lumbar level. Hu et al.[7] have shown better improvement of neurologic status in patients who have undergone decompression than in those patients who have not. The criteria for choosing nonoperative treatment includes the following: a neurologically intact patient, an intact posterior column, no translational or rotational deformity, and intact facets. The patient must have a reasonable ability to wear a brace or cast and be willing to wear a brace/cast full time. The slender, neurologically intact patient with an isolated burst fracture is an ideal candidate for nonoperative treatment.

Consideration for operative treatment includes the overall status of the patient and associated injuries. Surgical treatment of the lower lumbar burst fracture is indicated for the following: patients with neurologic deficit and canal compromise or injury to the posterior column, including disruption of the facet joints; those with highly comminuted anterior and middle columns; and multiply-injured patients. Internal fixation and stabilization will facilitate patient care immediately

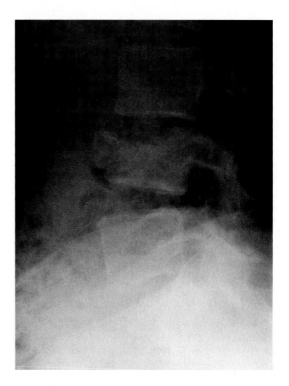

Figure 36B-1. Thirty-nine-year-old female suffered multiple extremity injuries and an L4 burst fracture with associated lower extremity radicular symptoms.

TREATMENT DECISIONS

- Burst fractures of the lumbar spine often involve high-energy injuries and associated injuries to the pelvis, sacrum, and spine.
- Use casting or a thoracolumbosacral orthosis (TLSO) in neurologically intact patients with stable burst patterns and an intact posterior column.
- Only a slight chance exists of neurologic deterioration in the neurologically intact patient.
- Stabilization and decompression improve the chance of neurologic recovery in the neurologically compromised patient.
- Consider operative intervention if:
  - There is a 50% or greater loss of the anterior column.
  - Kyphosis is greater than 20% to 30%.
  - There is a translational or rotatory malalignment with facet disruption.

after injury and in early phases of rehabilitation. Radiographic guidelines for operative treatment are not well defined. Most commonly accepted parameters for thoracolumbar fractures are loss of 50% or more of the anterior column, kyphosis at the fracture level of greater than 20 to 30 degrees, posterior column disruption (including those instances of translational or rotatory malalignment), or canal compromise of greater than 50% (Figure 36B-2). There is some concern that these guidelines are not stringent enough for the lumbar spine, with the recommendation that only 15 degrees of

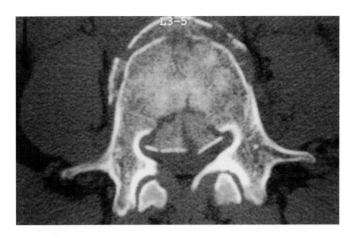

Figure 36B-2. Computed tomography (CT) scan at the level of injury shows approximately 70% canal compromise.

kyphosis be accepted.[10] The presence of a laminar fracture or spinous process fracture with a neurologic deficit should alert one to the possibility of root entrapment and dural tears; this can be an indication for surgery. Surgery should be considered for the patient with multiple trauma or a body profile that will not tolerate a full-time cast or brace.

NONOPERATIVE CARE OF LUMBAR BURST FRACTURES

The treatment of lower lumbar burst fractures in a nonoperative fashion has been recently delineated by Rechtine.[9] Initial bed rest is indicated until a well-fitting body cast or othosis is in place. Extremity range-of-motion and isometric exercises are initiated within the first several days of injury. Prophylaxis for deep venous thrombosis is started with pneumatic compression stockings and chemical prophylaxis (after confirmation that there is no active bleeding) and continued until the patient is freely mobile.

A well-molded cast is ideal in that it can be molded in hyperextension and conformed to each individual. There is a significant cost savings when using a cast compared with a clamshell thoracolumbosacral orthosis (TLSO). Fractures of the fifth lumbar vertebra require a pantaloon extension.[6] The cast is placed as soon as the patient can comfortably roll, usually within 2 to 3 days after injury. Once the cast is in place, mobilization should be initiated. Occasionally the use of a tilt table is helpful in making the first transition out of bed.

A clamshell TLSO is molded with lumbar hyperextension. A well-trained orthotist is a critical factor in brace management success. The orthotic must be worn at all times aside from daily hygiene until fracture consolidation and healing occurs. The brace should have an adequate relief of the anterior shell at the level of the hips to allow the hips to flex enough for sitting with minimal pressure to the femoral triangle. Discharge from the hospital is within 4 to 7 days, when independence in activities is demonstrated.

NONOPERATIVE CARE AND OPERATIVE CARE

- Initial bed rest followed by early casting or clamshell orthosis and mobilization
- Include pantaloon extension in cast or orthotic for L5 level fractures
- Goals
  - Anatomic realignment
  - Fracture stabilization
  - Short fusion
  - Neural decompression

OPERATIVE MANAGEMENT OF LOWER LUMBAR BURST FRACTURES

Anatomic realignment of the spine, stabilization of the fracture, and decompression of neural elements are the goals of operative management of lower lumbar burst fractures. Achieving a stable spine usually can be accomplished from the posterior approach with segmental instrumentation. The anterior approach allows for decompression at any level but is limited with regard to rigid fixation at the sacrum. In most cases the posterior approach allows for secure internal fixation of the fracture site and decompression of the neural elements. Anterior decompression, strut grafting, and stabilization are indicated for patients with severe vertebral body communication (with or without kyphosis) and neurologic deficits, those with continued neurologic deficit without improvement and a residual canal compromise, and for patients with nerve root compression.

Spinal instrumentation has evolved from the straight hook and rod systems into segmental systems that provide for stabilization, anatomic realignment, and limitation of motion segments. Short pedicle screw and rod constructs are used to avoid a "flat back" sagittal deformity and long arthrodesis of the lumbar spine and have increased the options for operative fixation of the lower lumbar spine. The principles of stabilization include limiting the number of lumbar segments fused, reestablishment of the sagittal lumbar contour, and reduction of the displaced bony fragments out of the spinal canal. Decompression of fracture fragments can usually be accomplished indirectly through distraction in the first 5 to 7 days after injury. Direct decompression is obtained by the transpedicular route or wide laminectomy in conjunction with vertebral distraction.

Improvement of spinal instrumentation systems and refinement of surgical techniques have made the option of operative care of the lower lumbar spine more attractive. The goals of operative treatment are decompression of the neurologic structures while providing initial stability to the injured vertebral segments, minimizing the number of vertebral segments of the fusion, and reconstructing the sagittal and coronal alignment of the lumbar spine (Figure 36B-3). The approach should be tailored to the greatest area of injury, anatomic limitations (such as limitation of anterior hardware at the L5 level when approached anteriorly), and technical expertise. In most cases a posterior approach will suffice.

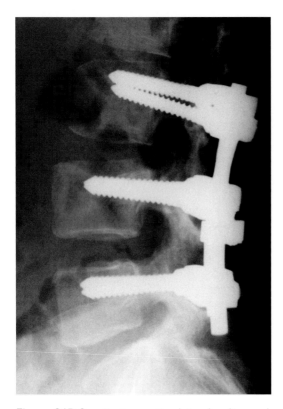

Figure 36B-3. Postoperative lateral radiograph shows elevation of the injured superior vertebral end plate and segmental fixation.

Systems utilizing hooks have the distinct disadvantage of needing a larger number of vertebral body segments for stable fixation. There is also limited ability to recreate the sagittal contour with these systems. Plates used with pedicle screws do not allow for easy distraction or manipulation of the involved segments.[2] The pedicle screw and rod construct allows for variable manipulation of distractive and compressive forces, and contouring of the rods allows for lumbar lordosis. Pedicle screw constructs also have the advantage of limiting the number of motion segments in an arthrodesis.

Short segment fixation of the lumbar spine meets the goals of stable fixation for the lumbar spine. There is the potential disadvantage of "settling" of the vertebral body if there is inadequate anterior and posterior support. The loss of sagittal correction may be the result of either bone or discal collapse.[3] The use of a well-fitting orthosis until a solid fusion is noted may help diminish settling.

Indirect decompression of the displaced fracture fragments is accomplished by distraction of the vertebral bodies above and below the level of injury. This is most easily done within the first several days after injury. Placing the largest-diameter pedicle screws to the depth of the midvertebral body helps secure the proximal and distal foundations for distraction. Distraction of the fracture followed by contoured rodding recreates the sagittal alignment. A transpedicular approach to the injured vertebral body should be considered if the pedicle and vertebral body are in contact. Preoperative computed

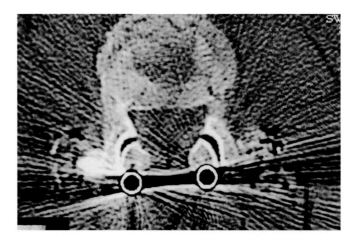

Figure 36B-4. Postoperative computed tomography (CT) scan shows reduction of the previously displaced posterior wall fragment.

tomography (CT) scans are necessary for planning the correct angle of entry into the pedicle and the vertebral body. A 4-mm round burr is used to create the entry site to the pedicle. The pedicle is entered with minimum effort to avoid uncontrolled plunging into bone. Manipulation of the vertebral body end plate can be accomplished with a pedicle probe or Akbarnia-designed instrument. Once the superior end plate of the vertebra is elevated, morselized bone is placed through the pedicle into the vertebral body. The pedicle screw is then placed into the pedicle and into the midportion of the vertebral body. The precontoured rod is attached to the screw. This maneuver supports the damaged end plate and aids in distraction ligamentotaxis of the fracture (Figure 36B-4). If there is a concern about the degree of indirect decompression after distraction, the screw on the left side can be left out to allow for an anterior retroperitoneal approach to the fractured vertebra.

The anterior approach to the lower lumbar spine is used when there will be inadequate middle and anterior column support after establishing the lumbar sagittal alignment. This includes wide displacement of the vertebral body fragments from the anterior and/or middle columns that leaves little structural support. At lumbar levels 3 and 4, anterior instrumentation is used to provide additional stability without a posterior procedure. Instrumentation for the fifth lumbar level is limited to the posterior side if one chooses to instrument after decompressive corpectomy and strut grafting. In either case, postoperative bracing is necessary.

CONCLUSIONS

Burst fractures of the lower lumbar spine in the neurologically intact patient can be treated with a cast or brace if the posterior column is intact. Operative treatment is reserved for kyphosis greater than 20 to 30 degrees, collapse of the anterior/middle column of greater than 50%, or an unstable fracture pattern resulting in translational or rotational instability. Contrary to the treatment of thoracic burst fractures, the decision to operate on the neurologically intact patient with a lumbar burst fracture should not be based solely on the degree of canal compromise. Short, posteriorly instrumented constructs implementing pedicle screws and contoured rods allow for stabilization and reconstruction of the lumbar sagittal alignment with a minimal number of levels fused.

SELECTED REFERENCES

An HS et al.: Low lumbar burst fractures: comparison among body cast, Harrington rod, Luque rod, and Steffee plate, *Spine* 16:S440-S444, 1991.

Andreychik DA et al.: Burst fractures of the second through fifth lumbar vertebrae, *J Bone Joint Surg Am* 78:1156-1166, 1996.

Chan DPK, Seng NK, Kaan KT: Nonoperative treatment in burst fractures of the lumbar spine(L2-L5) without neurologic deficits, *Spine* 18:320-325, 1993.

Hu SS et al.: The effect of surgical decompression on neurologic outcome after lumbar fractures, *Clin Orthop* 288:166-173, 1993.

Knight RQ et al.: Comparison of operative versus nonoperative treatment of lumbar burst fractures, *Clin Orthop* 293:112-121, 1993.

Rechtine GR: Non-surgical treatment of thoracic and lumbar fractures, *Instr Course Lect* 48:413-416,1999.

REFERENCES

1. An HS et al.: Low lumbar burst fractures: comparison between conservative and surgical treatment, *Orthopedics* 15:367-373, 1992.
2. An HS et al.: Low lumbar burst fractures: comparison among body cast, Harrington rod, Luque rod, and Steffee plate, *Spine* 16:S440-444, 1991.
3. Andreychik DA et al.: Burst fractures of the second through fifth lumbar vertebrae, *J Bone Joint Surg Am* 78-A:1156-1166, 1996.
4. Chan DPK, Seng NK, Kaan KT: Nonoperative treatment in burst fractures of the lumbar spine (L2-L5) without neurologic deficits, *Spine* 18:320-325, 1993.
5. Denis F: The three column spine and its significance in the classification of acute thoracolumbar spinal injuries, *Spine* 8:142, 1984.
6. Finn CA, Stauffer ES: Burst fracture of the fifth lumbar vertebra, *J Bone Joint Surg Am* 74:398-403, 1992.
7. Hu SS et al.: The effect of surgical decompression on neurologic outcome after lumbar fractures, *Clin Orthop* 288:166-173, 1993.
8. Knight RQ et al.: Comparison of operative versus nonoperative treatment of lumbar burst fractures, *Clin Orthop* 293:112-121, 1993.
9. Rechtine GR: Non-surgical treatment of thoracic and lumbar fractures, *Instr Course Lect* 48:413-416,1999.
10. Stauffer ES, ed: *Thoracolumbar spine fractures without neurological deficit*, American Academy of Orthopaedic Surgeons Monograph Series, 1993.
11. Weinstein JN, Collalto P, Lehmann TR. Thoracolumbar "burst" fractures treated conservatively: a long-term follow-up, *Spine* 13:33-38, 1998.

Sacral Fractures

Kirkham B. Wood, Francis Denis

The sacrum is the distal spinal segment, which is less commonly injured than the more cephalad spinal segments. However, injury to the sacrum may be a source of significant and complex disability. In this chapter, we present the spectrum of sacral and coccygeal trauma, classification schemes, radiologic diagnosis, surgical and nonsurgical, treatment, and any associated complications. The first section deals with higher-intensity sacral trauma that results in fracture, and the second section reviews sacral insufficiency fractures, a frequent cause of acute low back pain in the elderly, and sacral stress fractures, in which normal sacral bone fails under repetitive elevated stresses. In addition, fractures of the distal coccyx are described.

TRAUMATIC SACRAL FRACTURES

The stability of the sacrum is largely determined by its anatomic shape, with the more-caudal aspect shaped like a wedge and the anterior surface wider than the posterior aspect. The weight of the body imposes a vertical load that passes through the hips, such that the sacrum is the principal keystone that transfers loads from the spine to the pelvis.[26] When any deforming force is applied to the head or shoulders, the thoracolumbar spine typically receives the greatest impact, but when applied more distally, the lumbosacral region is affected, especially if the knees are extended. Nicoll[21] suggested that transverse fractures of the sacrum are thought to occur typically with the individual in a hip-flexed, knee-extended sitting position.

In 1937 Medelman[20] was the first to classify sacral trauma into three groups according to the direction of the fracture: longitudinal, horizontal, or oblique. In 1945 Bonnin[2] subsequently divided fractures into six different types: (1) juxtailiac marginal fractures, (2) fractures through the first or second sacral foramina, (3) compressed and comminuted body fractures, (4) traction fractures at the site of connecting ligaments, (5) transverse body fractures at the level of S2 or S3, and (6) fissure fractures that separate the lateral masses from the most proximal sacral foramina.

PATHOLOGIC ANATOMY

- Sacral stability largely determined by anatomic shape
  - Caudal aspect shaped like wedge
  - Anterior surface wider than posterior aspect
- Sacrum keystone in transfer of loads from spine to pelvis
- Transverse fractures of sacrum typically with individual in hip-flexed, knee-extended sitting position

---

CLASSIFICATION

- Sacral trauma classification: According to direction of fracture—longitudinal, horizontal, or oblique
- Fractures further divided
  - Juxtailiac marginal fractures
  - Fractures through first or second sacral foramen
  - Compressed and comminuted body fractures
  - Traction fractures at site of connecting ligaments
  - Transverse body fractures at level of S2 or S3
  - Fissure fractures separating lateral masses from most proximal sacral foramina
- One of the most readable and usable fracture schemes based on the medial or lateral location of the fracture relative to the sacral foramina
  - Zone I (alar zone): Fractures through the lateral ala
    - Most commonly associated with lateral compression pelvic injuries (e.g., pedestrian hit by a motor vehicle)
    - No damage to either foramina or central sacral canal
    - Superiorly displaced zone I fractures—trauma to the exiting L5 nerve root
  - Zone II (foraminal zone): Fracture line through one or more sacral foramina
    - Commonly extends over multiple levels
    - May also include the lateral ala, but does not extend into the central canal
  - Zone III (central canal): Central nerve root canal but frequently also zones I and II
    - Burst fractures of the sacrum or fracture dislocations (commonly seen in high-energy falls)
    - Transverse fractures of the sacrum
    - Rare in isolation, typically seen with other pelvic ring fractures; frequently associated with neurologic embarrassment
    - Usually occurs at S2 to S3 because this area encompasses the apical kyphotic angulation between the upper and lower aspects of the sacrum

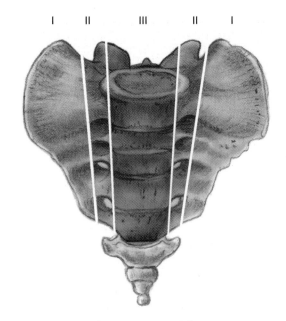

Figure 37-1. Schematic view of the sacrum divided into the three zones: alar *(I)*, foraminal *(II)*, and central *(III)*. (Redrawn from Denis F, Davis S, Comfort T: Sacral fractures: an important problem—a retrospective analysis of 236 cases, Clin Orthop Rel Res 227:67-81, 1988.)

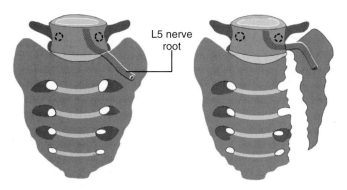

Figure 37-2. Anteroposterior view of the sacrum in which a displaced alar fracture impinges on the exiting L5 nerve root *(right)*.

Denis et al.[3] provided one of the most readable and usable fracture schemes based on the medial or lateral location of the fracture relative to the sacral foramina (Figure 37-1). They studied 236 sacral fractures in 776 pelvic injuries over a 10-year period and classified them into three principal zones. *Zone I* (alar zone) involves fractures through the lateral ala, which tend to be most commonly associated with lateral compression pelvic injuries (e.g., a pedestrian hit by a motor vehicle). There is no damage to either the foramina or the central sacral canal. Superiorly displaced zone I fractures can be associated with trauma to the exiting L5 nerve root[3,4] (Figure 37-2). *Zone II* (foraminal zone) involves a fracture line through one or more of the sacral foramina. These commonly extend over multiple levels. Fractures here

may also include the lateral ala but do not extend into the central canal. *Zone III* (central canal) fractures involve the central nerve root canal but frequently also include zones I and II. Burst fractures of the sacrum or fracture dislocations, commonly seen in high-energy falls, are examples of zone III injuries.

Transverse fractures of the sacrum are another type of zone III fracture. Rare in isolation and typically seen with other pelvic ring fractures, they are frequently associated with neurologic embarrassment.[3,4,22] They usually occur at S2 to S3 because this represents the apical kyphotic angulation between the upper and lower aspects of the sacrum. In addition, the superior aspect of the sacrum is stabilized by the sacroiliac joint, whereas the distal sacrum, the distal coccyx, and their ligamentous support may act as a lever arm on the superior body.[7]

Approximately one fourth of sacral fractures are complicated by neurologic injury.* These deficits can be either cauda equina–type radiculopathies of the sacral or lumbar nerve roots or whole plexopathies. They can occur either intradurally, extradurally within the canal, within the neural foramina, extraforaminally (plexus), or within the nerves beyond the sacrum itself. Injury to the L5 nerve root induces changes in sensation in the dorsum of the foot and lateral calf, as well as weakness of dorsiflexors of the foot. The S1 and S2 nerve roots are responsible mainly for hip extension, knee flexion, and plantar flexion with corresponding sensory dermatomes in the posterior aspect of the thigh, leg, sole and side of the foot, and genitalia (S2). The ankle jerk is typically diminished in lesions involving the S1 nerve root.

Injuries to the nerve roots S2 to S5 are commonly overlooked in trauma settings in large part due to the lack of obvious motor or sensory involvement in the lower extremities. The principal function of the S2 root is its role as a main contributor to the pudendal nerve. S2 innervates the musculature that forms the external urethral and anal sphincters, whereas S4 and S5 give sensation to the penis, labia, urethra, posterior scrotum, and anal canal.[7,31] S3 provides sensation to the uppermost medial thigh.

Coordinated voluntary control of the bladder and rectum is governed principally by the pelvic splanchnic autonomic nerves from S2 to S4. They are parasympathetic rami distributed to the bladder and rectum as the inferior hypogastric plexus. Their afferent fibers carry awareness of vesicle filling, whereas the efferent fibers initiate detrusor and rectal contraction. Sympathetic splanchnic nerves derive from the S2 and S3 ganglia. Their afferent fibers are responsible for pain and thermal information, whereas the efferent transmissions provide contraction of the urethral and anal sphincters and inhibit contraction of the muscular walls within their respected organ.

Neural injury to the roots S2 to S5 manifests principally by impairment of bowel and bladder continence and disturbances of sexual function. Often this aspect of the neurologic examination is overlooked or incomplete in the setting of urgent or multiple trauma.[7] The first

---

*References 2-4, 7, 22, 31, 34.

NEUROLOGIC CONNECTIONS

- Neurologic injury complicates about 25% of sacral fractures
  - Cauda equina–type radiculopathies of sacral or lumbar nerve roots
  - Whole plexopathies
- L5 nerve root injury
  - Changes in sensation in the dorsum of the foot and lateral calf
  - Weakness of foot dorsiflexors
- S1 and S2 nerve roots
  - Hip extension, knee flexion, and plantar flexion
  - Sensory dermatomes in posterior aspect of thigh, leg, sole, and lateral foot and genitalia (S2)
  - Ankle jerk typically diminished in lesions involving S1 nerve root
- S2: Musculature forming external urethral and anal sphincters
- S3: Sensation to uppermost medial thigh
- S4 and S5: Sensation to penis, labia, urethra, posterior scrotum, and anal canal
- Pelvic splanchnic autonomic nerves from S2 to S4
  - Coordinate voluntary control of bladder and rectum
  - Afferent fibers carry awareness of vesicle filling
  - Efferent fibers initiate detrusor and rectal contraction
  - Parasympathetic rami distributed to bladder and rectum as inferior hypogastric plexus
  - Sympathetic splanchnic nerves derive from S2 and S3 ganglia
    - Afferent fibers: Pain and thermal information
    - Efferent transmissions: Contraction of urethral and anal sphincters; inhibit contraction of muscular walls within respective organ
  - Often overlooked or incomplete in urgent or multiple trauma
  - First indication of lower sacral neuropathology comes days or weeks later when first complaints of perineal numbness or voiding difficulties are noted

ASSOCIATED INJURIES AND CONDITIONS

- Comminuted foraminal fractures may be highly associated with segment radiculopathy, especially at more cephalad levels of the sacrum (S1 to S2).
- Transverse fractures of the sacrum are nearly always associated with some neural injury; usually cauda equina and occasionally plexopathy.
- Vertical sacral fractures are much less commonly associated with neurologic injury, probably in part related to a proclivity for lateral alar zone I.
- From 80% to 90% of sacral fractures occur with pelvic fracture.
- Also associated with thoracolumbar fractures, varying degrees of pelvic disruption, bladder damage and bladder neck tearing, presacral hematoma from laceration of the middle sacral artery or presacral venous plexus, rectal lacerations, and cerebrospinal fluid leakage.

all patients complain of disturbance in bladder function consistent with the bilateral deficit within the canal. Vertical sacral fractures, on the other hand, are much less commonly associated with neurologic injury, probably due in part to their proclivity for the lateral alar zone I. However, when a neuropathy is found, it tends to be either radicular (L5) or plexopathic (L5 to S1) in nature ("far out syndrome").[3,31]

It has been noted that sacral fractures occur in conjunction with some form of pelvis fracture in 80% to 90% of cases. Other injuries associated with sacral fractures include thoracolumbar fractures, varying degrees of pelvic disruption, bladder damage and bladder neck tearing, presacral hematoma from laceration of the middle sacral artery or presacral venous plexus, rectal lacerations, and cerebrospinal fluid leakage.[7]

RADIOLOGY

Conventional radiographs of the pelvis can fail to adequately demonstrate trauma to the sacrum for a number of reasons: Anteroposterior radiographs are often obscured by overlying intestinal gas, and, because the sacrum is curved, the upper segments may be superimposed on each other, making fracture identification difficult. Adequate lateral images may also be difficult to obtain in the acute trauma setting and can be obscured in the obese patient by the overlying pelvis.[4,31] Often because of these radiologic difficulties, as well as the aforementioned lack of obvious neuropathology during the acute trauma admission, persons with sacral fractures often experience a significant delay in diagnosis.[22]

There are, however, certain radiographic signs that should heighten one's suspicion of a sacral injury[2,15]: (1) patterns of pelvic ring fractures known to be associated with a sacral fracture, such as bilateral rami fractures, and (2) fracture of the transverse process of L5[4,5] (e.g., detection of an apparently isolated lower lumbar transverse process fracture may actually be a warning signal for a sacral fracture), and additional imaging is recommended.

indication of lower sacral neuropathology sometimes comes days or weeks later, when the first complaints of perineal numbness or voiding difficulties are noted.

Neurologic injuries were seen in 51 of the 236 patients of Denis et al.[3] They were much more common in zones III (56.7%) and II (28.4%) than in zone I (5.9%). Within the central sacral canal, neurologic damage involved bowel, bladder, and sexual function in 16 of 21 patients. Ebraheim and Biyani[4] described eight persons with zone III fractures over a 7-year period of time, seven of whom had complete loss of bowel and bladder, and five also had sexual dysfunction.

The geometry and orientation of the sacral fracture play a strong role in the development of any neurologic sequelae. Foraminal fractures, when comminuted, can have a high association with segment radiculopathy, especially at the more cephalad levels of the sacrum (S1 to S2). Transverse fractures of the sacrum are nearly always associated with some degree of neural injury,[4,7,31] usually cauda equina, and occasionally plexopathy. Most

DIAGNOSTIC RADIOGRAPHIC PROCEDURES

- Can be a significant delay in diagnosis
  - Lack of obvious neuropathology during acute trauma admission
  - Conventional pelvic radiographs may not adequately demonstrate trauma to the sacrum
    - Anteroposterior radiographs often obscured by overlying intestinal gas
- Diagnostic yield increased by angling anteroposterior x-ray beam 50 degrees cephalad to the pelvis to show the sacral body and ventral foramina of zone II
  - With a curved sacrum, upper segments may be superimposed on each other
  - Adequate lateral images also difficult to obtain in acute trauma setting
    - Most useful in demonstrating sagittal angulation seen in transverse fractures or sacrolisthesis
  - Can be obscured in the obese patient by overlying pelvis
- Radiographic signs that should heighten suspicion of sacral injury
  - Patterns of pelvic ring fractures known to be associated with a sacral fracture, such as bilateral rami fractures
  - Fracture of transverse process of L5
    - For example, detection of apparently isolated lower lumbar transverse process fracture may warn of sacral fracture, and additional imaging is recommended
  - Significant anterior disruption of the pelvic ring even if the sacroiliac joint appears intact
- Computed tomography
  - Procedure of choice in evaluating complex sacral fractures, especially those of zone III or any fracture associated with a neurologic deficit
  - Sagittal reconstruction also advised to detect subtle transverse fractures
- Magnetic resonance imaging
  - Increasingly useful; primary ability to describe nerve roots within the canal and foramina
  - Also useful in highlighting areas of bony edema surrounding subtle fractures that may be missed on conventional radiography
  - Provides excellent sagittal images, including lumbar and sacral spine, on one view

A sacral fracture should also be suspected in cases of significant anterior disruption of the pelvic ring even if the sacroiliac joint appears intact.[4]

The diagnostic yield using plain radiography in more subtle cases can be increased by angling the anteroposterior x-ray beam 50 degrees cephalad to the pelvis to show the sacrum en face. This image not only provides an adequate view of the body of the sacrum but also clearly demonstrates the ventral foramina of zone II. Such fractures are commonly comminuted, and careful inspection allows identification of subtle fracture lines.[31]

Lateral radiography is most useful in demonstrating the sagittal angulation seen in cases of transverse fractures or sacrolisthesis.[4,22,26]

Computed tomography (CT) scanning offers superior resolution and probably is the radiographic procedure of choice in the evaluation of complex sacral fractures, especially those within zone III, or any fracture associated with a neurologic deficit. Sagittal reconstruction is also advised to detect subtle transverse fractures.[4]

Magnetic resonance imaging (MRI) is becoming increasingly useful, primarily in its ability to describe the nerve roots within the canal and foramina. It is also useful in highlighting areas of bony edema surrounding subtle fractures that may be missed on conventional radiography. Finally MRI provides excellent sagittal images that can include the lumbar and sacral spine on one view.

PHYSIOLOGIC TESTING

Electromyography can be useful at times in helping to localize an area of a sacral injury and even in suggesting a prognosis.[31] For example, injuries within the lumbar or sacral plexuses yield diffuse patchy electromyelographic changes: Because the paraspinal muscles derive their innervation proximally from the dorsal rami, plexus injuries therefore spare these muscles, whereas neuropathology from within the canal includes them in the injury pattern. The principal drawback to electromyography is that several weeks are needed to pass for real abnormalities to appear. It is also useful for only the lumbar and uppermost sacral roots because more-caudal levels below S2 have no real myotomal distribution.

A simple test in the clinical evaluation of bladder function is the measurement of postvoid residuals. Also, cystometrography can be used to elicit detrusor contraction through the active instillation of liquid into the bladder, as part of the examination of the mid to lower sacral roots. Structural lesions of the sacrum usually affect both sympathetic and parasympathetic control of the urinary system and manifest as detrusor areflexia and uninhibited sphincter relaxation. Cystometrography is most useful in confirming clinical impressions, but it can also be of some value in excluding a neurologic etiology for bowel or bladder dysfunction in the setting of local trauma to the lower urinary tract.[7,31]

TREATMENT

Because so many reports of sacral fractures have been anecdotal case reports or retrospective reviews that describe multiple treatment techniques, there actually has been very little experience in compiling a large series of similar injuries treated with various methods, surgical or nonsurgical.[3,31,34] The experience of Denis et al.[3] remains the most comprehensive to date and probably is the most useful in planning treatment.

The majority of adequately reduced and neurologically stable sacral fractures, such as those in zones I and II, can be easily managed by initial bed rest followed by progressive mobilization as comfort allows. If closed reduction is necessary, such as in vertically displaced alar fractures with L5 nerve root impingement, correction and maintenance of alignment can be accomplished through rest, skeletal traction if necessary, and/or hip spica casts.

Gunterberg's biomechanical data[11] suggest that much of the sacrum distal to the S1 to S2 level can be disrupted, including the lower half of the sacroiliac joint,

PHYSIOLOGIC TESTS

- Electromyography (EMG): Helps localize area of sacral injury and suggest prognosis; several weeks needed for real abnormalities to appear
- Structural sacral lesions: Usually affect sympathetic and parasympathetic control of urinary system and manifest as detrusor areflexia and uninhibited sphincter relaxation
- Clinical evaluation of bladder function: Measures postvoid residuals
- Cystometrography (CMG)
  - Elicits detrusor contraction through active instillation of liquid into the bladder, as part of the examination of mid to lower sacral roots
  - Most useful in confirming clinical impressions
  - Can exclude neurologic etiology for bowel or bladder dysfunction in local trauma to the lower urinary tract

MANAGEMENT OF SACRAL FRACTURES

- Sacral fractures as in zones I and II
  - Initially bed rest
  - Progressive mobilization as comfort allows if adequately reduced and neurologically stable
- Closed reduction necessary (in vertically displaced alar fractures with L5 nerve root impingement)
- Correction and maintenance of alignment through rest, skeletal traction if necessary, and/or hip spica casts
- Much of sacrum distal to S1 to S2 level can be disrupted (including the lower half of the sacroiliac joint) without significantly weakening the pelvic ring
- Sacral fractures associated with other pelvic ring fractures
- Anterior external fixation of the injured ring indirectly stabilizes the fractured sacrum
  - External fixation stabilizes an injured and bleeding pelvis
  - None of the "anterior" frames adequately stabilize major posterior injury to permit early weight bearing
  - Anterior approaches rare and ill advised; many have large presacral hematomas, risking massive hemorrhage
- Sacral laminectomy most common procedure: No comparison of results with those of nonoperative management available
- Posterior laminectomy and decompression of affected sacral neural structures: Best chance of nerve root recovery, especially with transverse fractures (varying degrees of angulation and fragment displacement often with kinking, tethering, or transection of nerve roots)
- Displaced and unstable longitudinal or vertical fractures
- Direct stabilization of the fractured sacrum
  - Can allow immediate mobilization of the patient out of bed
  - Pelvis unstable if more than 1 cm of posterior displacement exists
- Transforaminal zone II fractures with displacement
  - Realign with open reduction, decompression, and internal fixation
  - Direct internal fixation such as iliosacral screws or transsacral plating (can be supplemented with an anterior external frame)
- Overcompressing fragments when fixing longitudinal or foraminal fractures with screws risks trapping nerve roots
- Consider posterior plating for a significant foraminal fracture instead of lag screw fixation alone
- Closed reduction of displaced fractures with percutaneous fixation
  - Simplifies treatment and extensile exposure
  - Minimizes blood loss and potential infectious contamination
  - Concomitant anterior reduction and fixation without turning patient prone
- Caution
  - Depends on adequate fluoroscopic visualization
  - Thorough understanding of complex anatomic variations of the pelvis
  - Closed reductions are rarely perfect anatomically, and many prefer open reduction of sacral fractures associated with foraminal debris and neurologic injuries or with documented instability

without significantly weakening the pelvic ring. He concluded that in instances of subtotal destruction of the sacrum below S1, such as transverse fractures, gunshot wounds, and others, it probably was safe to allow full weight bearing at a relatively early stage. Higher transverse fractures (above S1 to S2) have been treated with bed rest and traction with moderate success.[22,31]

Because the majority of sacral fractures are associated with other pelvic ring fractures, anterior external fixation of the injured ring actually indirectly stabilizes the fractured sacrum.[4,31] It is important to remember, however, that although external fixation is a means of stabilizing the injured and bleeding pelvis, none of the "anterior" frames adequately stabilize a major posterior injury so as to permit early weight bearing.

When surgery is considered, anterior approaches to the injured sacrum are rare and ill advised because many of these injuries can have large presacral hematomas, and surgical violation may precipitate massive hemorrhage. Diastases of the pubic symphysis may render some alar fractures unstable yet be stabilized with anterior pubic plating.

Most neurologic deficits improve with time, although commonly it is not complete. Sacral laminectomy is the most common procedure, but a comparison of results with those of nonoperative management does not exist.[3,4] Posterior laminectomy and decompression of affected sacral neural structures provide the best chance of nerve root recovery, especially with transverse fractures, which show varying degrees of angulation and fragment displacement, often with kinking, tethering, or even occasional transection of nerve roots.[4,7,25,33]

On the other hand, Phelan et al.[22] described four patients with transverse fractures of the sacrum and neurologic deficits of bowel and bladder who recovered complete function with conservative treatment of bed rest and progressive ambulation. Even in instances of surgical decompression, perioperative bed rest with or without traction is indicated to effect osseous union.

In instances of displaced and unstable longitudinal or vertical fractures, direct stabilization of the fractured sacrum is occasionally possible.[4,27,33] A distinct advantage to this approach is that it can in many instances allow immediate mobilization of the patient out of bed.[27,34] Although the indications for internal fixation of isolated sacral fractures are variable, Templeman et al.[34] wrote that most authorities agree that the pelvis is unstable if more than 1 cm of posterior displacement exists.

Transforaminal zone II fractures with displacement should be realigned with open reduction, decompression, and internal fixation. If the sacroiliac joint is disrupted posteriorly and the alar region is intact or with minimal comminution, direct internal fixation such as with the use of iliosacral screws or transsacral plating is possible (and can be supplemented with an anterior external frame).[4,27] Care should be exercised when fixing longitudinal or foraminal fractures with screws by not overcompressing the fragments and risking entrapment of nerve roots. Lag screw fixation alone should not be performed in instances of significant foraminal fracture; that is, one should probably consider the use of posterior plating instead. Somatosensory evoked potential monitoring may be useful in avoiding this complication.[4,27]

Closed reduction of displaced fractures with percutaneous fixation has been advocated by some for several reasons: It simplifies the treatment and extensile exposure, and the attendant wound problems can be avoided.[27,34] Blood loss is minimized and potential infectious contamination in the polytrauma setting is lessened. In addition, concomitant anterior reduction and fixation can be accomplished without turning the patient prone. Their technique depends on adequate fluoroscopic visualization, however, and the surgeon must have a thorough understanding of the complex anatomic variations of the pelvis. Also, closed reductions are rarely perfectly anatomic. Many actually prefer open reduction of sacral fractures associated with foraminal debris and related neurologic injuries or with documented instability.[3,27,33]

INSUFFICIENCY FRACTURES

Insufficiency fractures of the sacrum can be an unsuspected cause of acute low back pain in the elderly, especially women, who have sustained unknown or relatively minimal trauma. They occur in abnormally fragile bone with reduced elastic resistance secondary to structural alterations as seen in osteopenia, involutional osteoporosis, or other metabolic bone disorders, including corticosteroid- or radiation-induced osteoporosis.[17,28,30,35]

The frequency of insufficiency fractures of the sacrum within the general population is not well known. A prospective study by Gaucher et al.[8] in a health clinic in Europe found an annual incidence of approximately 2% in women older than 60 years. Weber et al.[35] found 20 sacral insufficiency fractures in 2366 (0.9%) patients who presented with low back pain to the Department of Rheumatology at Stadtspital Triemli Zuerich during a 20-year period.

The demographics of sacral insufficiency fracture heavily favor postmenopausal women in their seventh, eighth, or ninth decade.[35] Most patients complain of dull low back pain, and many of these patients report exacerbation of the pain with direct pressure. Because the etiology is unclear, many patients complain of chronic pain for weeks, and the diagnosis is often quite delayed.[16] Although patients with insufficiency fractures of the sacrum almost universally have a normal neurologic examination,[9,30,35] neurologic findings have occasionally been reported, including paresthesias and urinary or bowel incontinence.[13,17,18,32] Finiels et al.[6] reviewed almost 500 cases of sacral insufficiency fractures and found an approximately 2% rate of neurologic compromise, with sphincter dysfunction being the most common. The true incidence may be somewhat underestimated, however, because many elderly individuals report "sphincter dysfunction," and concomitant symptoms of distal paresthesias and leg weaknesses may be overlooked.[13]

The imaging of insufficiency fractures of the sacrum can be difficult because in the elderly, the sacrum is frequently irregularly structured and has osteolytic and osteosclerotic areas. Plain radiography can be relatively insensitive, and often the fracture is missed completely, especially longitudinal fractures within the cancellous body of the lateral ala.[16,18,30,35] Bone scans, on the other hand, are remarkably reliable for pinpointing the diagnosis.[16,30,32] The most common anatomic presentation in insufficiency fractures is a longitudinal break parallel with the sacroiliac joint, which can be seen as an H or a butterfly shape when the fractures are bilateral. Commonly, due to both the patient's age and the rather insidious onset of the pain, many patients with insufficiency fractures have initially been presumed to have metastatic disease.[9] The increased uptake on bone scans confounded by the patchy osteoporosis has on many occasions resulted in such a diagnosis and the performance of unnecessary biopsies.[32]

CT is the definitive study,[16,32] and it reliably shows fracture lines within the anterior margin of the sacrum. Vacuumlike phenomena sometimes can be seen within the fractures, yet it lacks the destructive processes or soft tissue masses seen in metastatic disease. CT is best when combined with scintigraphy because longitudinal fractures can on occasion be misinterpreted as sacroiliitis on radionuclide imaging.

MRI has an increasing role in the examination and diagnosis of patients with subclinical insufficiency fractures due to its ability to image the reactive edema within the surrounding bone and to rule out metastatic pathology and with MRI the sagittal images of the entire spinal axis can be seen on one film.[32]

Fortunately, instability is not a problem with most sacral insufficiency fractures, and surgical intervention is almost never required. Bed rest with pain control, followed by gradual mobilization, is all that is typically needed. Even patients with clinical neuropathy or cauda equina–type syndromes often respond well with these measures.[13] Most patients become pain free and fully independent within 6 to 12 months.

INSUFFICIENCY FRACTURES, STRESS FRACTURES, AND COCCYGEAL FRACTURES

SACRAL INSUFFICIENCY FRACTURES
- Abnormally fragile bone with reduced elastic resistance secondary to osteopenia, involutional osteoporosis, or other metabolic bone disorders, corticosteroid- or radiation-induced osteoporosis
- Annual incidence approximately 2% in women older than 60 years
- Dull low back pain exacerbated with direct pressure
- Almost universally a normal neurologic examination
- Diagnosis frequently quite delayed
- Anatomic presentation
- Most common: Longitudinal break parallel with the sacroiliac joint
- Can be H- or butterfly-shaped appearance with bilateral fractures
- Plain radiography relatively insensitive, especially longitudinal fractures in cancellous body of lateral ala
- Bone scans remarkably accurate diagnostically
- Definitive study: Computed tomography
  - Reliably shows fracture lines in the anterior sacral margin
  - Best when combined with scintigraphy because longitudinal fractures can be misinterpreted as sacroiliitis on radionuclide imaging
- Magnetic resonance imaging
  - Useful in subclinical insufficiency fractures
  - Can image reactive edema within surrounding bone and can rule out metastatic pathology
- Instability not a problem—surgical intervention almost never required
- Require bed rest with pain control, followed by gradual mobilization

- Most patients become pain free and fully independent within 6 to 12 months

STRESS FRACTURES
- Mechanical or elastic resistance of bone normal but stressed beyond normal capacity
- Common finding in certain patient populations (military recruits, athletes, long-distance runners)
  - Typically of lower extremities but can affect lower lumbar spine and pelvis, including sacrum
- May be nutritionally based
  - Female long-distance runner: Amenorrhea common, leading to general weakening of bone in the sacrum
- Difficult to visualize with plain radiography; bone scintigraphy is the initial screening image of choice
- Most recover well with 4 to 6 weeks of rest; gradual resumption of activities, regulated by pain so as to prevent recurrent injury

COCCYGEAL FRACTURES
- Usually result from direct trauma to coccyx or fracture associated with childbirth
- Angulated sacrococcygeal or intercoccygeal segment on plain radiography
  - Normal variations of angulation of distal sacrococcyx described in asymptomatic populations
  - Bone scan imaging confirms diagnosis
  - Treatment
    - Symptomatic maneuvers (cushions and supports)
    - Injection therapy
- Coccygectomy in cases resistant to nonoperative care

STRESS FRACTURES

Stress fractures differ from insufficiency fractures in that they occur when the mechanical or elastic resistance of bone is normal but is stressed beyond its normal capacity. Stress fractures of the lower extremities are a common finding in certain patient populations, including military recruits, athletes, and long-distance runners,[19,29] and to a lesser degree, the lower lumbar spine and pelvis, including the sacrum, can be affected.[1,29] Stress fractures here may be nutritionally based as well: In the female long-distance runner, amenorrhea is common, which can lead to a general weakening of bone in the sacrum.[19]

The diagnosis of a sacral stem fracture is considered when low back and buttock or groin pain is found in susceptible individuals, such as long-distance runners, in whom osteoporosis and malignancy have been ruled out and there is no history of previous pelvic radiation. Many have localized tenderness over the sacrum and sacroiliac joint.

As in insufficiency fractures, stress fractures of the sacrum are extremely difficult to visualize with plain radiography, and bone scintigraphy remains the initial screening image of choice. CT scanning provides great bony detail, typically showing a sclerotic zone in the cancellous bone of the anterior aspect of the sacrum surrounding a faint linear lesion within the cortical bone.

Most individuals recover well with 4 to 6 weeks of rest and should be able to return to their normal activities by 2 months. The resumption of activities should be gradual, regulated by pain, however, so as to prevent recurrent injury.

COCCYGEAL FRACTURES

Coccygeal fractures can be a source of coccygodynia (tail bone pain) and are most commonly due to direct trauma to the coccyx[10,12,23,24] or fracture associated with childbirth.[14]

Plain radiography can often show an angulated sacrococcygeal or intercoccygeal segment, but some interpretive difficulty persists in that normal variations of the angulation of the distal sacrococcyx have been described in asymptomatic populations.[10,23] Bone scan imaging may help confirm the diagnosis.

Treatment includes symptomatic maneuvers such as the use of cushions and supports, injection therapy, and, in cases resistant to nonoperative care, coccygectomy. Wood et al.[36] studied 21 patients at a minimum follow-up of 2 years for total coccygectomy after painful traumatic coccygodynia and found that 86% had good or excellent results as reported on a patient questionnaire.

SELECTED REFERENCES

Denis F, Davis S, Comfort T: Sacral fractures: an important problem—a retrospective analysis of 236 cases, *Clin Orthop Rel Res* 227:67-81, 1988.

Routt ML, Simionian PT: Closed reduction and percutaneous skeletal fixation of sacral fractures, *Clin Orthop Rel Res* 329:121-128, 1996.

Taguchi T et al.: Operative management of displaced fractures of the sacrum, *J Orthop Sci* 4:347-352, 1999.

REFERENCES

1. Belkin SC: Stress fractures in athletes, *Orthop Clin North Am* 11:735-742, 1980.
2. Bonnin JG: Sacral fractures and injuries of the cauda equina, *J Bone Joint Surg Am* 27:113-127, 1945.
3. Denis F, Davis S, Comfort T: Sacral fractures: an important problem—a retrospective analysis of 236 cases, *Clin Orthop Rel Res* 227:67-81, 1988.
4. Ebraheim NA, Biyani A: Zone III fractures of the sacrum: a case report, *Spine* 21:2390-2396, 1996.
5. Fardon DF: Displaced fracture of the lumbosacral spine with delayed cauda equina deficit: report of a case and review of literature, *Clin Orthop* 120:155-158, 1976.
6. Finiels H et al.: Fractures du sacrum par insuffisance osseuse: meta-analyse de 508 cas, *Presse Med* 26:1568-1573, 1997.
7. Fountain SS, Hamilton RD, Jameson RM: Transverse fractures of the sacrum, *J Bone Joint Surg Am* 59:486-489, 1977.
8. Gaucher A et al.: Les fractures de contrainte de la ceinture pelvienne des sujets ages: fractures de insuffisance osseuse, *Semin Hop Paris* 62:2157-2161, 1986.
9. Gotis-Graham I et al.: Sacral insufficiency fractures in the elderly, *J Bone Joint Surg Br* 76:882-886, 1994.
10. Grosso NP, van Dam BE: Total coccygectomy for the relief of coccygodynia: a retrospective review, *J Spinal Disord* 8:328-330, 1995.
11. Gunterberg B: Effects of major resection of the sacrum, *Acta Orthop Scand Suppl* 162:1-38, 1976.
12. Gutierrez PR, Mas-Martinez JJ, Arenas J: Salter-Harris type I fracture of the sacro-coccygeal joint, *Pediatr Radiol* 1998, p. 28.
13. Jacquot JM et al.: Neurological complications in insufficiency fractures of the sacrum: three case reports, *Rev Rhumat EE* 66:109-113, 1999.
14. Jones ME, Shoaib A, Bircher MD: A case of coccygodynia due to coccygeal fracture secondary to parturition, *Injury* 28:549-550, 1997.
15. Laasonen EM: Missed sacral fractures, *Ann Clin Res* 9:84-87, 1977.
16. Leroux JL et al.: Sacral insufficiency fractures presenting as acute low-back pain: biomechanical aspects, *Spine* 18:2502-2506, 1993.
17. Lien HH et al.: Radiation-induced fracture of the sacrum: findings on MR, *Am J Radiol* 159:227, 1992.
18. Lock SH: Osteoporotic sacral fracture causing neurological deficit, *Br J Hosp Med* 49:210, 1993.
19. Major NM, Helms CA: Sacral stress fractures in long-distance runners, *Am J Radiol* 174:727-729, 2000.
20. Medelman JP: Fractures of the sacrum: their incidence in fractures of the pelvis, *Am J Radiol* 42:100-105, 1937.
21. Nicoll EA: Fractures of the dorsolumbar spine, *J Bone Joint Surg Br* 31:376, 1949.
22. Phelan ST, Jones DA, Bishay M: Conservative management of transverse fractures of the sacrum with neurological features: a report of four cases, *J Bone Joint Surg Br* 73:969-971, 1991.
23. Postacchini F, Massobrio M: Idiopathic coccygodynia, *J Bone Joint Surg Am* 1983, p. 65.
24. Raissaki MT, Williamson JB: Fracture dislocation of the sacro-coccygeal joint: MRI evaluation, *Pediatr Radiol* 29:642-643, 1999 (letter).
25. Rao SH, Laheri MR: Traumatic transverse fracture of sacrum with cauda equina injury: a case report and review of literature, *J Postgrad Med* 44:14-15, 1998.
26. Rodriguez-Fuentes AE: Traumatic sacrolisthesis S1-S2, *Spine* 18:768-771, 1993.
27. Routt ML, Simionian PT: Closed reduction and percutaneous skeletal fixation of sacral fractures, *Clin Orthop Rel Res* 329:121-128, 1996.
28. Saraux A et al.: Insufficiency fractures of the sacrum in elderly subjects, *Rev Rheum EE* 62:582-586, 1995.
29. Schils J, Hauzeur JP: Stress fracture of the sacrum, *Am J Sports Med* 20:769-770, 1992.
30. Schulman LL et al.: Insufficiency fractures of the sacrum: a cause of low back pain after lung transplantation, *J Heart Lung Transplant* 16:1081-1085, 1997.
31. Scmidek HH, Smith D, Kristiansen TK: Sacral fractures: issues of neural injury, spinal stability, and surgical management. In Dunsker SB et al., eds: *The unstable spine*, New Yorr, 1986, Harcourt.
32. Stabler A et al.: Vacuum phenomena in insufficiency fractures of the sacrum, *Skeletal Radiol* 24:31-35, 1995.
33. Taguchi T et al.: Operative management of displaced fractures of the sacrum, *J Orthop Sci* 4:347-352, 1999.
34. Templeman D et al.: Internal fixation of displaced fractures of the sacrum, *Clin Orthop Rel Res* 329:180-185, 1996.
35. Weber M, Hasler P, Gerber H: Insufficiency fractures of the sacrum: twenty cases and review of the literature, *Spine* 18:2507-2512, 1993.
36. Wood KB, Mehbod A, Goldsmith M: Coccygectomy for treatment of painful coccygodynia, *Spine* (in press).

Rehabilitation of the Spinal Cord Injury Patient

Mitchell K. Freedman, Guy W. Fried

Spinal cord injury (SCI) affects nearly every major organ system in the body. Following an injury, a thorough examination is performed to establish the neurologic baseline. Motor and sensory examination is performed according to the American Spinal Cord Injury Association (ASIA) neurologic classification system. This initial comprehensive examination allows multiple disciplines to monitor the patient and communicate with each other effectively. Functional rehabilitation begins in the perioperative period and is often a lifelong process. Treatment addresses not only neurologic recovery, but optimal use of residual function to achieve maximal functional status.

EPIDEMIOLOGY

The national prevalence of SCI is from 183,000 to 230,000.[24,48] Half of all injuries occur in patients between ages 16 and 30 years. However, there has been a steady increase in average age of injury from 28.5 years in 1973 to 1977 to 36 years from 1994 to 1998.[38] Males suffer 81% of spinal cord injuries. The most common causes of SCI are vehicular accidents (43%), violence (18.9%), sports accidents (11.1%), and falls (18.8%).[38] By age 30 years, more than 70% of violence-related injuries and 60% of vehicular injuries have occurred. SCI secondary to falls occurs more frequently in elderly populations.[24,38,48]

CLASSIFICATION OF SPINAL CORD INJURY

ASIA revised its classification system in 1996.[1] Tetraplegia refers to impairment of function in the arms, as well as to the trunk, legs, and pelvic organs secondary to impairment of motor and/or sensory function in the cervical segments of the spinal cord. Paraplegia refers to

damage to the spinal cord below the cervical segments and sparing the upper extremities. A complete injury occurs when there is no motor or sensory function preserved in the S4 to S5 sacral segments. An incomplete injury is characterized by the preservation of at least partial sensory and/or motor function below the neurologic level and including the S4 to S5 sacral segments (Box 38-1).

Motor examination is based on a six-point scale of muscle testing (Figure 38-1). The key muscles that are evaluated are listed in Figure 38-1. A motor level is derived for both sides. A muscle that is a 3 or 4 muscle grade is considered normal, provided that the next most rostral muscle is a 5/5 grade muscle. The presence or absence of tone and voluntary contraction of the anal sphincter is evaluated.

EPIDEMIOLOGY OF SPINAL CORD INJURY

- National prevalence: 183,000 to 230,000
- Average age: 36 years
- Etiology: Motor vehicle accidents, violence, sports, falls

Box 38-1	American Spinal Injury Association Impairment Scale

- **A = Complete:** No motor or sensory function is preserved in the S4 to S5 segments.
- **B = Incomplete:** Sensory but not motor function is preserved below the neurologic level and includes the S4 to S5 segments.
- **C = Incomplete:** Motor function is preserved below the neurologic level, and more than half of key muscles below the neurologic level have a muscle grade less than 3.
- **D = Incomplete:** Motor function is preserved below the neurologic level, and at least half of key muscles below the neurologic level have a muscle grade of 3 or more.
- **E = Normal:** Motor and sensory function is normal.

CLINICAL SYNDROMES
- Central cord
- Brown-Séquard
- Anterior cord
- Conus medullaris
- Cauda equina

Modified from the American Spinal Injury Association: *International standards for neurological and functional classification of spinal cord injury,* Chicago, revised 1996, American Spinal Injury Association.

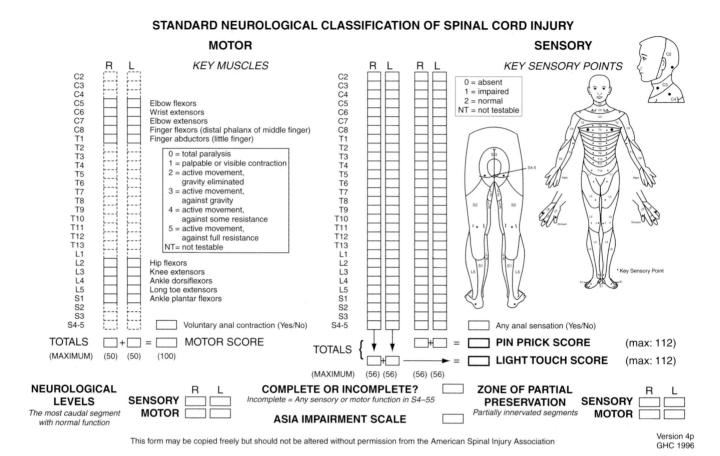

Figure 38-1. Standard neurologic classification of spinal cord injury. (*From the American Spinal Injury Association:* International standards for neurological functional classification of spinal cord injury, *Chicago, 1996, American Spinal Injury Association.*)

Sensory examination involves the evaluation of key sensory points (see Figure 38-1). Each dermatome is evaluated and graded for sharp and light touch sensation. Testing for sharp sensation is performed with a safety pin. Sensation is absent if the pin is not perceived as sharp. Sensation is impaired if there is diminished sensation or hyperesthesia. Sensation to touch is performed with cotton. The sensory level is defined bilaterally as the level above the most rostral abnormal segment.

Patients are generally evaluated in a supine position to allow for consistent monitoring from the initial evaluation, which is performed with the patient immobilized and in a supine position. The motor and sensory scales are documented and monitored for stability and progress throughout the rehabilitation course.

REHABILITATION

Rehabilitation of the SCI patient has several phases. Initially there is an evaluation and stabilization phase. The level and degree of neurologic injury is established. Medical and skeletal stability are evaluated and achieved. The second phase of treatment is the period immediately following the stabilization of the skeletal injury. Acute postoperative medical problems must be treated. The patient may be placed into an appropriate orthotic to stabilize the healing skeletal segment. The patient then moves into the subacute phase of rehabilitation. This may be limited by concurrent medical problems, including brain injury, extremity fractures, pressure ulcers, and autonomic dysfunction. Bracing may also limit progress.

There is close communication with the patient and family. Neurologic status and prognostication is reviewed on a regular basis. Interim and long-term discharge planning begins as early as possible. Therapy begins at bedside with splints and range of motion to prevent contractures. Muscle strength is maintained as much as possible. Positioning and nutrition are addressed to prevent pressure ulcers. Prophylaxis to prevent pulmonary emboli begins as rapidly as possible.[55] Patients are generally discharged to a rehabilitation center once they have achieved medical stability. However, there are times when patients may be discharged to an interim nursing home or subacute center if they are not able to participate in a full intensive rehabilitation program.

The average length of stay in inpatient rehabilitation was 144.8 days in the early 1970s. From 1990 to 1997, the

---

GOALS OF ACUTE REHABILITATION

- Neurologic/skeletal stability
- Medical stability
- Prevent pressure ulcers
- Maintain range of motion
- Patient and family teaching
- Initiate discharge planning

PROGNOSTICATION

- A complete injury at 72 hours after injury rarely becomes incomplete.
- At 72 hours after injury, preservation of pinprick sensation below the level of injury bodes well for progression to ASIA D and E levels.
- Patients with complete tetraplegia often gain one motor level in the first 1 to 2 years.
- Patients with 3/5 quadriceps strength by 2 months after injury may walk at 1 year.

---

average length of stay in acute rehabilitation changed from 74 days to 60 days. Discharge to nursing homes and rehospitalizations increased. High levels of functional ability, injuries that are less severe, and strong social support generally result in a shorter length of stay in the rehabilitation unit.[17]

The patient's ultimate function level depends on the degree of neurologic impairment. However, different levels of function may be achieved for a similar neurologic level depending on a given patient's motivation, age, body habitus, and general state of health. Typical levels of function for complete injuries are listed in Table 38-1.

PROGNOSTICATION

The prognosis may be more accurate 72 hours after the acute injury than in the emergency department.[6] Patients with ASIA A injury 72 hours after injury rarely become incomplete. If patients subsequently become incomplete, they rarely progress to an ASIA D or C classification.[12] Patients with ASIA B injuries who have preservation of pinprick sensation have an excellent chance to progress to ASIA D and E levels.[12] ASIA B patients without preservation of pinprick sensation are less likely to become ASIA C or ASIA D classifications.[26]

Patients with complete tetraplegia are likely to regain at least one motor level in the first 1 to 2 years. Recovery rates of one root level of function have been reported in 66% to 90% of patients.[49] The initial strength of the muscle is a predictor of achieving antigravity strength at the level caudal to the neurologic level of injury.[27] Thirty to forty percent of patients with 0/5 strength at the level caudal to the neurologic level of injury gain a level over the first 3 to 6 months. Patients with a grade 1 to 2 motor strength at the time of injury usually progress to the next neurologic level within 3 to 6 months of their injury.[15] The patient with a C4 injury may be less likely to progress by one motor level.[14,15]

AMBULATION

Tetraplegics who are motor and sensory incomplete at 72 hours after injury have a good chance to walk at 1 year. Maynard et al. reported that 47% of sensory-incomplete patients and 87% of motor-incomplete patients at 72 hours were walking at 1 year.[32] Patients who have a 3/5 quadriceps strength by 2 months have a good prognosis for ambulation at 1 year.[12]

MEDICAL COMPLICATIONS
Neurogenic Bowel

Bowel management after an SCI can be a lifetime balancing act between impaction and loose stool. There are several different methods of managing one's bowel with the goals of continence and timed regular evacuation. These goals can be accomplished by judicious use of laxatives and enemas/suppositories. Some patients prefer manual disimpaction. A frank discussion of bowel management includes the risks, benefits, and alternatives. A typical program would involve taking one Colace three times a day, two Senokot each noon, and one Fleet Bisacodyl Enema each night. It generally takes an oral laxative about 8 hours to be maximally effective. The stool moves down and gathers in the rectal vault, at which time an enema or suppository is used to complete evacuation. In the SCI population a colostomy is seldom indicated.

During initial hospitalization, gastrointestinal (GI) hemorrhage may develop in about 3% of patients. A GI hemorrhage and gastritis are believed to be secondary to the unopposed parasympathetic (vagal) action leading to acid secretion with the loss of sympathetic influence. The use of H$_2$ blockers and antacids is indicated.

Neurogenic Bladder

Fifty years ago renal complications were the leading cause of mortality in the SCI population. Over the years better diagnostics, management, and antibiotics have significantly improved renal disease.[50] Bacteriuria is the colonization of the bladder with bacteria; this will occur in about 80% of SCI patients. Asymptomatic colonization of the bladder alone does not warrant treatment. Patients with an SCI may not experience dysuria or urinary frequency; however, they may experience fatigue, autonomic dysreflexia (AD), or a change in their spasticity, which may herald a urinary tract infection and warrant treatment.

Neurogenic bladder function can be predicted by the level of neurologic injury. SCI patients do not have control over their autonomic nervous system and therefore tend to cocontract the bladder wall simultaneously with the bladder outlet; this is called detrusor-sphincter dyssynergia. Lesions below the spinal cord in the cauda equina tend to lead to a flaccid areflexic bladder.

Table 38-1	Typical Functional Outcomes for Patients With Complete SCIs

Location of Injury	Pressure Relief	Wheelchair Transfers	Wheelchair Propulsion	Ambulation	Orthotic Devices	Transportation
C3 to C4	Independent in power recliner wheelchair; dependent in bed or manual wheelchair	Total dependence	Independent in pneumatic or chin control–driven power wheelchair with power recliner	Not applicable	Upper extremity externally powered orthosis, dorsal cock-up splint, BFOs	Dependent on others in accessible van with lift; unable to drive
C5	Most require assistance	Assistance of one person with or without transfer board	Independent in power wheelchair indoors and outdoors; short distances in manual wheelchair with adapted handrims indoors	Not applicable	As above	Independent driving in specially adapted van
C6	Independent	Potentially independent with transfer board	Independent moderate distances with manual wheelchair with plastic rims or lugs indoors; assistance needed outdoors; independent in hand-driven wheelchair	Not applicable	Wrist-driven orthosis, universal cuff, writing devices, built-up handles	Independent in driving specially adapted van
C7	Independent	Independent with or without transfer board, including car, except to or from floor with assistance	Independent in manual wheelchair indoors and outdoors, except stairs	Not applicable	None	Independent driving car with hand controls or specially adapted van; independent placement of wheelchair into car
C8 to T1	Independent	Independent, including to and from floor and car	Independent in manual wheelchair indoors and outdoors; with curbs, escalators; assistance on stairs	Exercise only (not functional with orthoses); requires physical assistance or guarding	None	As above
T2 to T10	Independent	Independent	Independent	Exercise only (not functional with orthoses); may not require assistance	Knee-ankle-foot orthoses with forearm crutches or walker	As above
T11 to L2	Independent	Independent	Independent	Functional ambulation indoors with orthoses; stairs using railing	Knee-ankle-foot orthoses or ankle-foot orthoses with forearm crutches	As above
L3 to S3	Independent	Independent	Independent	Community ambulation; independent indoors and outdoors with orthoses	Ankle-foot orthoses with forearm crutches or canes	As above

From Delisa JA, Gans BM, eds: *Rehabilitation medicine: principles and practice*, ed 3, Philadelphia, 1998, Lippincott-Raven, pp. 1276-1277.
BFO, Balanced forearm orthosis.

Communication	Pulmonary Hygiene	Feeding	Grooming	Dressing	Bathing	Bowel and Bladder Routine	Bed Mobility
Independent with adapted equipment for phone or typing	Totally assisted cough	May be unable to feed self; use of BFOs with universal cuff and adapted utensils indicated; drinks with long straw after setup	Total dependence	Total dependence	Total dependence	Total dependence	Total dependence
As above	Assisted cough	Independent with specially adapted equipment for feeding after setup	Independent with adapted equipment	Assistance with upper extremity dressing; dependent for lower extremity dressing	Total dependence	Total dependence	Assisted by others and by equipment
Independent with adapted equipment for phone, typing, and writing; independent in turning pages	Some assistance required in supine position; independent in sitting position	Independent with equipment; drinks from glass	Independent with equipment	Independent with upper extremity dressing; assistance needed for lower extremity dressing	Independent in upper and lower extremity bathing with equipment	Independent for bowel routine; assistance needed with bladder routine	Independent with equipment
Independent with adapted equipment for phone, typing, and writing; independent in turning pages	As above	Independent	Independent	Potential for independence in upper and lower extremity dressing with equipment	Independent with equipment	Independent	Independent
Independent	As above	Independent	Independent	Independent	Independent	Independent	Independent
Independent	T2 to T6 as above; T6 to T10 independent	Independent	Independent	Independent	Independent	Independent	Independent
Independent	Not applicable	Independent	Independent	Independent	Independent	Independent	Independent
Independent	Not applicable	Independent	Independent	Independent	Independent	Independent	Independent

BLADDER MANAGEMENT

- Death from renal failure was previously the most common cause of mortality after spinal cord injury.
- Diagnostics, bladder management, and improved antibiotics have improved renal function.
- Urinary tract infection remains a frequent complication.
- Assessment of bladder management includes a detailed analysis of the patient, as well as the injury and personality characteristics such as reliability, hand function, and physiologic control of the bladder.

AUTONOMIC DYSREFLEXIA (AD)

- AD occurs in patients with injury at T6 level or above.
- Noxious stimulation below the level of injury leads to unopposed sympathetic release.
- Symptoms include severe hypertension and pounding headache.
- Primary treatment involves finding and removing the noxious stimulation.
- Raise head of bed to lower the blood pressure.
- Treatment may require antihypertensives such as nifedipine or nitroglycerin.

Options for treating a neurogenic bladder may include intermittent catheterization, an indwelling Foley catheter, condom catheterization, or spontaneous voiding. Urodynamics are important to evaluate the filling and voiding pressures associated with a neurogenic bladder. Discussion regarding the bladder management options needs to include the patient's functional strengths and weaknesses, including reliability, hand function, and physiologic control of the bladder.

Autonomic Dysreflexia

Autonomic dysreflexia (AD) is an uninhibited sympathetic nervous system response to noxious stimulation below the level of injury. It is manifested by a sudden onset of hypertension, pounding headache, flushing, perfuse sweating above the level of injury, piloerection, blurred vision, and nasal congestion. The hypertension, which may rise as high as 300 mm Hg, is dangerous. AD can cause strokes, seizures, and death.

AD generally affects patients who have a T6 level of injury or above; however, there have been reported cases as low as T10. AD occurs after the patient recovers from spinal shock. Spinal shock is a period of time after an injury during which reflexes cannot be elicited. It is typical that AD may begin to occur at least 2 months after injury. In general, AD will affect about half the patients with SCI above T6 at least once in their lifetime.

The pathophysiology involves an imbalance of the sympathetic and parasympathetic nervous systems. The splanchnic outflow is from T6 to L2.[10] Noxious sensory stimulation below T6 ascends in the sympathetic intermediolateral gray matter, leading to reflex sympathetic discharges. Inhibitory messages from the brain are blocked by the SCI. Thus the sympathetic discharges are unopposed with the release of norepinephrine and dopamine. Common noxious stimuli that cause AD include bladder distention, bowel impaction, kidney stones, epididymitis, pressure ulcers, and fractures.[19,40]

If AD is suspected, the blood pressure should be checked and monitored. If the blood pressure has increased, then the head of the bed should be elevated. The first line of treatment involves finding and correcting the source of noxious stimulation, for example, unkinking an indwelling Foley catheter and allowing the bladder to drain.

If no source of noxious stimulation is discovered and the blood pressure remains at a dangerous level, pharmacologic agents such as nifedipine or nitroglycerin may be used.

One must use caution in performing any procedure in an SCI patient whose injury level is above T6. Despite the fact that the patient may not feel pain during a procedure below the level of injury, anesthesia must be used to avoid AD. If no anesthesia is used, the body will respond with unopposed sympathetic reflex activity even though the patient does not subjectively perceive pain from the procedure.

Deep Vein Thrombosis and Pulmonary Embolism

Deep venous thrombosis (DVT) and pulmonary embolism are common and potentially lethal complications of acute SCI. Elements of Virchow's triad, which includes bed rest, hypercoagulability, and paralysis, predispose SCI individuals to DVT. Prospective studies indicate that 47% to 100% of acute SCI patients experience DVT.[35] The risk of DVT is highest within the first days after the acute injury, with 62% of patients demonstrating a positive venography by day 8.[43]

Pulmonary embolism occurs in close to 4% of all patients with SCI during their initial stay.[50] Pulmonary embolism is the most common cause of death in the SCI population. Studies indicate that 8% of the deaths in SCI individuals are caused by pulmonary embolism.[50] Death from a pulmonary embolism is 47 times as likely in the SCI person as in the uninjured person.[50]

Every effort should be made to prevent the occurrence of a DVT. It has been found that the combination of external pneumatic compression devices with subcutaneous heparin lowers the incidence of DVT. When possible, the pneumatic compression devices should be used during the high-risk period of the first 2 weeks after injury. It appears that the combination of the pneumatic compression devices and subcutaneous heparin works better than either modality alone. The current clinical practice guideline of the Consortium for Spinal Cord Medicine suggests that low–molecular weight heparin or adjusted-dose heparin begin at 72 hours after injury.[11,33] Inferior vena cava (IVC) filters are indicated for failed anticoagulation or if anticoagulation is contraindicated such as in an active bleed. IVC filters are not a substitute

---

DEEP VENOUS THROMBOSIS (DVT) PULMONARY EMBOLISM

- 47% to 100% of spinal cord injury (SCI) patients develop DVT.
- 62% of patients have a positive venogram by the eighth day of injury.
- 8% of SCI deaths are caused by pulmonary embolism.
- Low–molecular-weight heparin or adjusted-dose heparin should begin 72 hours after injury.
- Inferior vena cava (IVC) filters should be considered for anticoagulation failures or if anticoagulation is contraindicated.

PULMONARY COMPLICATIONS

- The higher the spinal cord injury, the more muscles of respiration are affected
  - Lowers the vital capacity
  - Raises risk of pulmonary complications, including pneumonia and atelectasis
- Innervation levels to the muscles of respiration
  - C3 to C5: Diaphragm
  - C5 to C8: Scalene muscles
  - T1 to T11: Intercostal muscles
  - T6 to T12: Abdominal muscles

---

for prophylaxis, which needs to be started as soon as possible. The consortium suggests that anticoagulation should continue in incomplete spinal cord patients until they are discharged home. The prophylaxis should continue for 8 weeks in an uncomplicated injury and for 12 weeks in a patient with other risk factors such as cancer, leg fractures, congestive heart failure, obesity, or age greater than 70 years.

Pulmonary Complications

Injury to the spinal cord can impair normal respiration. High tetraplegia can affect the phrenic innervation of C3 to C5 to the diaphragm. Because the diaphragm is a critical muscle of respiration, impairments in its innervation will lead to atelectasis, pneumonia, and ventilatory failure. The body stabilizes over time. The majority of patients admitted to a rehabilitation unit on ventilators, including 50% of the C3 tetraplegics, will be weaned off.[54]

Patients with acute SCI and intact diaphragmatic innervation will initially have vital capacities 25% to 30% of normal. This improves to 60% of normal over the next several months.[33] Serial vital capacities can be a useful bedside measure of pulmonary health. Changes in vital capacity may indicate pneumonia or ventilatory insufficiency. Consistent aggressive pulmonary toilet with chest physical therapy, assisted "quad" coughs, and bronchodilators is a useful adjunct.[30]

Lower tetraplegia affects the scalene accessory respiratory muscles innervated by the nerves C5 to C8. T1-T11 injuries affect the intercostal muscle functions. The intercostal muscles stabilize the chest wall during diaphragmatic excursion. The abdominal muscles are innervated between T6 and T12; they assist with coughing and forced expiration. In a tetraplegic patient, paradoxical breathing with retraction of the chest wall during inspiration can be seen because of the lack of chest stabilization by the intercostal muscles during diaphragmatic excursion.

Pressure Ulcers

Pressure ulcers are a major and preventable problem in the SCI population. Both acute and chronic SCI patients are at risk for ulcers. Studies indicate that there is at least a 25% incidence of pressure ulcers during the SCI patient's acute hospitalization.[7] Pressure is the most important characteristic leading to ulceration. The intensity and duration of tissue compression leads to ischemia. Laboratory evidence points to an inverse relationship between the length of time and the amount of pressure to cause tissue necrosis.[28]

Several characteristics of SCI patients put them at an increased risk, including immobility, diminished sensation, bowel and bladder incontinence, and changes in skin histology. Skin below the level of injury has lower concentrations of proline, lysine, and hydroxylysine compared with skin above the level of injury. These changes in histology have obvious implications with regard to skin integrity.[31] The economic cost of all pressure ulcers is well over a billion dollars a year. The human cost in losses is immeasurable.[36]

The key to healing pressure ulcers is to promptly identify the wound and minimize the contributing factors.

The U.S. Department of Health and Human Services clinical practice guideline on pressure ulcers identifies four stages of ulceration as determined by the degree of tissue damage observed.[4] Stage I is nonblanchable erythema of intact skin; the heralding lesion of skin ulceration. Stage II involves partial-thickness skin loss involving epidermis and/or dermis. The ulcer is superficial and presents clinically as an abrasion, blister, or shallow crater. Stage III involves a full-thickness skin loss involving damage or necrosis of the subcutaneous tissue that may extend down to, but not through, the underlying fascia. Stage IV involves full-thickness skin loss with extensive destruction, tissue necrosis, or damage to muscle, bone, or supporting structures. The presence of sinus tracts may also be associated with stage IV pressure ulcers.

The staging of ulcers recognizes some limitations. Identification of stage I pressure ulcers, for example, can be difficult in darkly pigmented skin. Also, when eschar is present, knowing the true depth of the wound is impossible until debridement.[9]

Every effort should be made to minimize contributing factors of the pressure ulcers. Early stabilization of the spine allows early mobilization of the patient out of bed and in shifting positions. It is key to maximize nutritional status. Serum albumin and lean body mass are good measures of nutritional status. With obesity it is important to

---

PRESSURE ULCER STAGING

- Stage I: Nonblanchable erythema of intact skin
- Stage II: Partial-thickness skin loss involving epidermis and/or dermis
- Stage III: Full-thickness skin loss involving damage or necrosis of subcutaneous tissue that may extend to underlying fascia
- Stage IV: Full-thickness skin loss with extensive destruction, tissue necrosis, or damage to muscle, bone, or supporting structures

---

CLASSIFICATION OF PAIN IN SCI

- Musculoskeletal
- Visceral
- Neuropathic pain at the level of injury
  - Central, radicular, or periperal pain below the level of injury
  - Central
- Other
  - Complex regional pain syndrome, posttraumatic syrinx, peripheral nerve lesion, headache

---

understand that adipose is poorly vascularized and should never be confused with a good nutritional status.[37]

Other factors contributing to pressure ulcers include bowel and bladder incontinence, which must be addressed and minimized.[41] Smoking diminishes tissue oxygenation and is associated with pressure ulcer formation.[29] Fevers increase tissue metabolism and oxygen demand, which also increase the risk of pressure ulceration.[20]

Pain

Pain occurs in 11% to 94% of patients with SCI and generally presents within 6 months of the injury. In the acute phase of rehabilitation, pain must be treated adequately so that patients can participate in their rehabilitation. On a chronic basis, 44% of patients with SCI claim that pain interferes with their daily activities. Pain can be so severe that a significant percentage of SCI patients would, if they had the chance, trade pain relief for loss of bladder, bowel, or sexual function.[2,5,38]

There are several classifications for types of pain in SCI patients.[16,47] Musculoskeletal pain is generally achy and confined to specific anatomic areas. Pain may occur from the overuse of upper extremities, abnormal gait patterns, and direct trauma or injury. Visceral pain is dull and vague. It is generally in the chest, abdominal, and/or pelvic area. Neuropathic pain is quite common. The pain is sharp, electric, and burning, etc. Segmental neuropathic pain at the level of injury may be secondary to radicular or central pain. A peripheral nerve lesion is also possible. Neuropathic pain that is caudal to the level of injury is most likely from a central etiology. In these cases, pain may be in the saddle distribution as well as into the extremities. Other reasons for pain include posttraumatic syrinx, headache associated with dysreflexia, peripheral nerve lesions, complex regional pain syndromes, and psychogenic pain.[5,47]

Treatment is challenging but critical so as to allow functional progress. Appropriate range of motion and strengthening is indicated. Proper positioning in the wheelchair must be achieved. Optimal body mechanics with ambulation and activities of daily living are critical. A transcutaneous electrical nerve stimulation unit may be helpful. Modalities that deliver ice or heat must be used with caution in the areas with sensory impairment. Biofeedback and relaxation techniques help patients manage their pain. Medication treatment includes topical ointments, nonsteroidal antiinflammatories, narcotic and nonnarcotic analgesics, tricyclic antidepressants, and membrane stabilizers.

Syrinx (Posttraumatic Cystic Myelopathy)

This condition is uncommon, occurring in 0.3% to 3.2% of SCI patients, although it can have potential devastating side effects. It usually occurs within the first few years of an injury. It is a cyst that develops in the center of the spinal cord around the level of injury. It can grow in a caudal or cephalad direction. It commonly presents with pain and numbness, which may be exacerbated by Valsalva maneuvers (coughing, sneezing, and straining). Weakness may occur with sensory loss. Magnetic resonance imaging is the most accurate means of diagnosis.[25] Once the syrinx is identified, it should be followed closely for changes. Primary treatment includes avoiding unnecessary Valsalva maneuvers. If the syrinx progresses, surgical shunting to the peritoneum can be helpful. Motor weakness and pain have a favorable prognosis with surgical intervention.[17]

Spasticity

Spasticity is a common side effect of SCI. Spasticity can be defined as a velocity-dependent increase in the resistance to passive range of motion caused by an upper motor neuron lesion. Deep tendon reflexes after acute SCI are initially depressed in the phase of spinal shock. Over several weeks to months the reflexes increase, sometimes to a severe level. Spasticity is usually treated if it interferes with function or hygiene or causes pain. Initial treatment starts with oral medication, including baclofen and tizanidine. If spasticity worsens, consideration can be given to dantrolene sodium and diazepam (Valium). If the patient does not have an adequate response to oral medications, consideration can be given to intramuscular botulinum toxin or phenol. If the intramuscular injections are not adequate to control spasticity, an intrathecal baclofen pump can be considered (Table 38-2).

Osteoporosis and Pathologic Fracture

SCI results in bone loss below the level of the lesion. The bone loss is greatest in the first 4 months after injury and levels off by 16 months.[23,42] Fractures occur in 4% of

---

SYRINX

- Incidence in the spinal cord injured population is 0.3% to 3.2%.
- Syrinx may occur years after injury.
- It commonly presents with pain and numbness.
- Treatment: Close observation and avoidance of Valsalva maneuvers; neurosurgical shunt indicated in a progressive syrinx.

SPASTICITY

- Upper motor neuron damage leading to velocity-dependent increase in resistance to a passive stretch
- Common side effect in spinal cord injury
- Treatment warranted if it causes a decrease in function or produces pain

---

OSTEOPOROSIS

- Bone loss below level of injury greatest in first 4 months after injury
- Bone loss levels off by 16 months after injury
- Fractures most common in distal femur and tibia
- Treatment in nonambulatory patients generally nonoperative

HETEROTOPIC OSSIFICATION

- New bone growth outside a joint
- Histologically similar to fracture callus
- May clinically present with a swollen leg, pain, and decreased range of motion
- Can ankylose joint, leading to decreased function
- Detected by serum alkaline phosphatase, x-rays, and bone scan
- Primary treatment: Range of motion
- Additional treatments: Etidronate and possibly radiation and indomethacin

---

Table 38-2	Treatment of Spasticity
ORAL MEDICATIONS	**POTENTIAL SIDE EFFECTS**
Baclofen	Fatigue
Tizanidine	Hypotension and increased liver function enzymes
Dantrolene	Hepatotoxicity
Diazepam	Fatigue, dependency
INJECTIONS	
Botulinum toxin	Localized weakness
Phenol	Localized pain/weakness
SURGERY	
Intrathecal baclofen	Refills necessary, pump malfunction

patients with SCI. The fractures are most common in the distal femur and tibia.[13]

Treatment of osteoporosis may include mobilization out of bed and standing.[8] Tiludrinate, a bisphosphonate, may be effective in reducing bone resorption.[21] Patients with lower extremity long bone fractures generally receive conservative treatment with the use of soft splints.[13] Shortening and angulation and even nonunion in the lower extremities of nonambulatory patients is acceptable.[34] Rotational deformity is not acceptable in patients who are ambulatory; these patients may require open reduction and internal fixation.[34]

Heterotopic Ossification

Heterotopic ossification is the development of new bone tissue around a joint. It occurs in 16% to 53% of the persons with SCI,[53] but only 3% develop severe limitation of joint range of motion. Heterotopic ossification occurs below the level of SCI.[22] The most common joint affected is the hip, and the second most common is the knee. Mature heterotopic ossification histologically resembles a fracture callus. It is similar to normal bone and has cortical and trabecular structures, as well as bone marrow.[51] Complications of heterotopic ossification may include nerve entrapment or pressure ulceration.

The clinical presentation may include a swollen leg, possibly pain, and decreased joint range of motion. The differential diagnosis must distinguish between DVT, cellulitis, and fracture.

Once the diagnosis is made, the treatment includes aggressive passive range of motion to maintain joint mobility. Etidronate disodium has been shown to be useful, especially if started early.[50,51] The optimal length of treatment may exceed the manufacturer's suggestion of 12 weeks. However, this has not been firmly established. Radiation and indomethacin have been found to be useful in treating heterotopic ossification in conditions other than SCI.[3,45,46]

Surgical resection of the heterotopic ossification is reserved for patients in whom the ankylosis causes significant loss of function or creates pressure ulceration. Caution must be taken to ensure that the bone has fully matured because of the vascular nature of the immature heterotopic ossification. Serial plain film x-rays, bone scans, and alkaline phosphatase can help determine maturity. Surgical complications include excessive bleeding, fractures, infection, and recurrence of heterotopic ossification.[52]

SELECTED REFERENCES

American Spinal Injury Association: *International standards for neurological and functional classification of spinal cord injury*, Chicago, 1996, The Association, 1996.

Consortium for Spinal Cord Medicine: *Acute management of autonomic dysreflexia: adults with spinal cord injury–presenting to health care facilities*, Washington, DC, 1997, Paralyzed Veterans of America.

McKinley WO et al.: Long-term medical complications after traumatic spinal cord injury: a regional model system analysis, *Arch Phys Med Rehabil* 80:1402-1409, 1999.

Nobunaga AI, Go BK, Karunas RB: Recent demographic and injury trends in people served by the model spinal cord injury care systems, *Arch Phys Med Rehabil* 80:1372-1382,1999.

Sidall PJ, Taylor DA, Cousins MJ: Classification of pain following spinal cord injury, *Spinal Cord* 35:69-75, 1997.

Stover SL, Delisa JA, Whiteneck GG: *Spinal cord injury: clinical outcomes from the model systems*, Gaithersburg, 1995, Aspen, pp. 302-305.

Yarkony GM, Formal CS, Cawley MF: Spinal cord injury rehabilitation: assessment and management during acute care, *Arch Phys Med Rehabil* 78:S48-S52, 1997.

REFERENCES

1. American Spinal Injury Association: *International standards for neurological and functional classification of spinal cord injury*, Chicago, 1996, American Spinal Injury Association.

2. Ankle AG, Stanghelle JK: Pain and life quality within two years of spinal cord injury, *Paraplegia* 33:555-559, 1995.

3. Ayers DG, Evart CM, Parkinson JR: The prevention of heterotopic ossification in high risk patients by low dose radiation therapy after total hip arthroplasty, *J Bone Joint Surg Am* 68:1423-1430, 1986.

4. Bergstrom N et al.: *Treatment of pressure ulcers*. Clinical Practice Guidelines, Public Health Service, Agency for Public Health Policy and Research, Rockville, Md, 1994, US Department of Health and Human Services.

5. Beric A, Dimitrijevic M, Lindblom V: Central dysesthesia syndrome in spinal cord injury patients, *Pain* 34:109-116, 1988.

6. Brown PJ et al.: The 72 hour examination as a predictor of recovery in motor complete quadriplegia, *Arch Phys Med Rehabil* 72:546-548, 1991.

7. Carlson CE et al.: Incidence and correlates of pressure ulcers development after spinal cord injury, *Rehabil Nurs Res* 1:34-40, 1992.

8. Chappard D et al.: Effects of tiludronate on bone loss in paraplegic patients, *J Bone Miner Res* 10:112-118, 1995.

9. Clinical Practice Guideline Number 3: *Pressure ulcers in adults: prediction & prevention*, Rockville MD, 1999, US Department of Health and Human Services, Public Health Service, Agency for Health Care Policy and Research, pp. 7-9.

10. Consortium for Spinal Cord Medicine: *Acute management of autonomic dysreflexia: adults with spinal cord injury presenting to healthcare facilities*, Washington, DC, Paralyzed Veterans of America.

11. Consortium for Spinal Cord Medicine: *Prevention of thromboembolism in spinal cord injury, clinical procedure guideline: spinal cord medicine*, Washington, DC, 1997, Paralyzed Veterans of America.

12. Crozier KS et al.: Spinal cord injury: prognosis for ambulation based on sensory examination in patients who are initially motor complete, *Arch Phys Med Rehabil* 72:119-121, 1991.

13. deBruin ED et al.: Changes of tibia bone properties after spinal cord injury: effects of early intervention, *Arch Phys Med Rehabil* 80:214-220, 1999.

14. Ditunno JF et al., eds: Spinal cord injury: clinical outcomes from the model systems, Gaithersburg, Md, 1995, Aspen, pp. 170-184.

15. Ditunno JF et al.: Motor recovery of the upper extremities in traumatic quadriplegia: a multicenter study, *Arch Phys Med Rehabil* 73:431-436, 1992.

16. Donovan WH, Dimitrijevic MR: Neurophysiologic approaches to chronic pain following spinal cord injury, *Paraplegia* 20:135-146, 1982.

17. Dworkin G, Staas WE: Post-traumatic syringomyelia, *Arch Phys Med Rehabil* 66:329-331, 1985.

18. Eastwood EA et al.: Medical rehabilitation length of stay and outcomes for persons with traumatic spinal cord injury: 1990-1997, *Arch Phys Med Rehabil* 80:1457-1463, 1999.

19. Erickson RP: Autonomic hyperreflexia: pathophysiology and medical management, *Arch Phys Med Rehabil* 61:431-440, 1980.

20. Fisher BH: Topical hyperbaric oxygen treatment of pressure sores and skin ulcers, *Lancet* 2:405-409, 1969.

21. Freehafer A: Limb fractures in patients with spinal cord injury, *Arch Phys Med Rehabil* 76: 823-827, 1995.

22. Garland DE: A clinical perspective on common forms of acquired heterotopic ossification, *Clin Orthop* 263:13-29, 1991.

23. Garland DE et al.: Osteoporosis after spinal cord injury, *J Orthop Res* 10:371-378, 1992.

24. Go BK, Devivo MJ, Richards JS: The epidemiology of spinal cord injury. In Stover SL, DeLisa JA, Whiteneck GG, eds: *Spinal cord injury*, Gaithersburg, Md, 1995, Aspen, pp. 170-184.

25. Hida K et al.: Post-traumatic syringomyelia: its characteristic magnetic resonance imaging findings and surgical management, *Neurosurgery* 35:886-891, 1994.

26. Katoh S, El Masry WS: Motor recovery of patients presenting with motor paralysis and sensory sparing following cervical spinal cord injury, *Paraplegia* 33:506-509, 1995.

27. Kirshblum SC, O'Connor KC: Predicting recovery in traumatic cervical spinal cord injury, *Arch Phys Med Rehabil* 79:1456-1466, 1998.

28. Koziak M: Etiology and pathology of ischemic ulcers, *Arch Phys Med Rehabil* 40:62-69, 1959.

29. Lamid S, Ghatit AZ: Smoking, spasticity and pressure sores in spinal cord injured patients, *Am J Phys Med Rehabil* 62:300-305, 1983.

30. Ledsome JR, Sharp JM: Pulmonary function in acute cervical cord injury, *Am Rev Respir Dis* 124:41-44, 1981.

31. Mawson AR et al.: Risk factors for early occurring pressure ulcers following spinal cord injury, *Am J Phys Med Rehabil* 67:123-127, 1988.

32. Maynard FM et al.: Neurological prognosis after traumatic quadriplegia: three-year experiences of California Regional Spinal Cord Injury Care System, *J Neurosurg* 50:611-616, 1979.

33. McKinley WO et al.: Long-term medical complications after traumatic spinal cord injury: a regional model system analysis, *Arch Phys Med Rehabil* 80:1402-1409, 1999.

34. McMaster W, Stauffer E: The management of long bone fracture in the spinal cord injury patient, *Clin Orthop* 112:44-52, 1975.

35. Merli GJ, Herbison GJ, Ditunno JF: Deep vein thrombosis in acute spinal cord injured patients, *Arch Phys Med Rehabil* 69:661-664, 1988.

36. Miller H, Delozier J: *Cost implications of the pressure ulcer treatment guideline*, Contract No. 282-91-0070, Columbia, Md, 1994, Center for Health Policy Studies, sponsored by the Agency for Health Care Policy and Research, p. 17.

37. Natow AB: Nutrition in prevention and treatment of decubitus ulcers, *Top Clin Nurs* 5:32-44, 1983.

38. Nepomuceno C et al.: Pain in patients with spinal cord injury, *Arch Phys Med Rehabil* 60:605-609, 1979.

39. Nobunaga AI, Go BK, Karunas RB: Recent demographic and injury trends in people served by the model spinal cord injury care systems, *Arch Phys Med Rehabil* 80:1372-1382, 1999.

40. Phillips WT et al.: Effect of spinal cord injury on the heart and cardiovascular fitness, *Curr Probl Cardiol* 23(11):657-663, 1998.

41. Powell JW: Increasing activity of nursing home patients and the prevalence of pressure ulcers: a ten year comparison, *Decubitus* 2:56-58, 1989.

42. Ragnarsson KT, Sell GH: Lower extremity fractures after spinal cord injury: a retrospective study, *Arch Phys Med Rehabil* 62:418-423, 1981.

43. Rossi E et al.: Sequential changes in factor VIII and platelets preceding deep vein thrombosis in patients with spinal cord injury, *Br J Haematol* 45:143-151, 1980.

44. Rossier AB, Bussat P, Infante F: Current facts on para-osteoarthropathy, *Paraplegia* 11:36-78, 1973.

45. Schaffer MA, Sosner J: Heterotopic ossification: treatment of established bone with radiation therapy, *Arch Phys Med Rehabil* 76:284-286, 1995.

46. Schmidt SA et al.: The use of indomethacin to prevent the formulation of heterotopic bone after total hip replacement, *J Bone Joint Surg Am* 70:834-838, 1988.

47. Sidall PJ, Taylor DA, Cousins MJ: Classification of pain following spinal cord injury, *Spinal Cord* 35:69-75, 1997.

48. Staas WE, Formal CS, Freedman MK, et al.: Spinal cord injury and spinal cord injury medicine. In DeLisa JA, Gans BM, eds: *Rehabilitation medicine: principles and practice*, ed 3, Philadelphia, 1998, Lipincott-Raven, pp. 1259-1291.

49. Stauffer ES: Neurologic recovery following injuries to the cervical spinal cord and nerve roots, *Spine* 9:532-534, 1984.

50. Stover SL, Delisa JA, Whiteneck GG: *Spinal cord injury: clinical outcomes from the model systems*, Gaithersburg, Md, 1995, Aspen, 92(127): 302-305.

51. Stover SL, Neimann KM, Miller JM: Disodium etidronate in the prevention of post-operative recurrence of heterotopic ossification in spinal cord injured patients, *J Bone Joint Surg Am* 58:683-688, 1976.

52. Stover SL, Neimann KM, Tulos JR: Experience with surgical resection of heterotopic ossification in spinal cord injured patients, *Clin Orthop* 263:71-77, 1991.

53. Venier LH, Ditunno JF: Heterotopic ossification in the paraplegic patient, *Arch Phys Med Rehabil* 52:475-479, 1971.

54. Wicks AB, Mentar RR: Long term outlook in quadriplegic patients with initial ventilator dependency, *Chest* 90:406-410, 1986.

55. Yarkony GM, Formal CS, Cawley MF: Spinal cord injury rehabilitation: assessment and management during acute care, *Arch Phys Med Rehabil* 78:S48-S52, 1997.

Soft Tissue Injuries of the Cervical Spine: Whiplash

Eeric Truumees

The Quebec Task Force on Whiplash-Associated Disorders defined whiplash as "an acceleration-deceleration mechanism of energy transferred to the neck." It may result from rear-end or side-impact motor vehicle collisions, but it can also occur during diving or other mishaps. The impact may result in bony or soft tissue injuries (whiplash injury), which in turn may lead to clinical manifestations (whiplash-associated disorders). In most cases, whiplash symptoms take a benign and self-limited course. In a small percentage of patients, a severe chronic pain syndrome may evolve. Social and medical costs related to chronic whiplash account for $4.5 billion per year in the United States alone.[119] A nonoperative regimen, including relative rest, antiinflammatory medications, and physical therapy, is recommended for the vast majority of cases. In longstanding cases, a multidisciplinary approach, including rehabilitation, work hardening, and counseling, may be appropriate.

Whiplash remains a contentious diagnosis with a "confusing and nonstandard"[104] terminology. A number of synonyms are used in the modern literature, including acceleration/deceleration injury, cervical sprain (strain) syndrome, and soft tissue neck injury. Much of the continuing controversy surrounding the legitimacy of whiplash stems from its poor representation in the literature. In the Quebec Task Force review, nearly all articles considered were rejected. Specifically, of the 10,382 articles reviewed, 62 were deemed acceptable (section 1, page 4), yielding a rejection rate of 99.4%.[38,104]

Whiplash was first described by Crowe in 1928[22] during a presentation on neck injuries at a meeting of the Western Orthopaedic Association. Present terminology differentiates whiplash injury, the mechanism, and whiplash-associated disorders, the clinical syndrome subsequently reported by some patients subjected to this mechanism. That is, whiplash injury occurs when force is indirectly applied to the neck by rapidly accelerating or decelerating the trunk. This mechanism is differentiated from a contact injury to the head, which may lead to a cervical spine fracture or dislocation.

Typically, rear-end injuries leading to cervical extension have been emphasized, but flexion injuries are also common. Ultimately, mixed-force vectors are seen in almost all cases, leading to a potentially complex pattern of injuries. Although people who complain of whiplash syndrome are typically involved in low-velocity collisions, potentially devastating injuries, including transverse atlantal ligament rupture, traumatic disc injury, and facet dislocations, may stem from similar mechanisms.

Whiplash syndrome refers to the wide variety of symptoms described by patients who sustain whiplash injury. These symptoms range from brief neck discomfort to severe neck pain in association with sympathetic and central nervous system dysfunction. The presence of chronic and bizarre symptoms after a seemingly minor trauma has led some authors to describe whiplash as a "type of psychoneurotic reaction."[37] However, although the relationship of suspected pathoanatomy to symptoms is not proved, most feel that whiplash has a physiologic cause, the recovery from which is complicated by psychosocial factors. [6,9,55,106]

No treatment, operative or nonoperative, has been convincingly shown to change the natural history of whiplash syndrome, but a number of complex treatment protocols have been developed by a variety of practitioners, including spine surgeons, physiatrists, psychiatrists, pain medicine specialists, and chiropractors.

EPIDEMIOLOGY

Ninety percent of whiplash cases stem from rear-end motor vehicle accidents (MVAs). In the United States, 4 million MVAs occur per year, and there are 1 million reported whiplash injuries. Deans et al.[26] found that 62% of patients taken to the emergency department after an MVA complained of neck pain. In Japan, approximately 50% of car-to-car traffic accidents result in neck injury.[79,90] A government mandate for head restraints in all cars manufactured after 1968 has reduced neck injuries by 18%.[78]

Internationally, whiplash epidemiology varies significantly. Differences are attributed to compensation systems and awareness of whiplash as a potential source of long-term difficulty. In Quebec, a no-fault system of injury reimbursement is used with a whiplash incidence of 70 per 100,000. Saskatchewan's confrontational tort system produces whiplash claims at a rate of 700 per 100,000. Similarly, a 13:100,000 incidence is recorded in the no-fault system of New Zealand, whereas Victoria, Australia, a tort state, reports an incidence of 106:100,000.[72]

Shrader et al.[99] found a remarkable absence of whiplash syndrome in Lithuania, where little expectation of disability or compensation exists relative to neck injuries. They hypothesized that chronic symptoms as a result of whiplash were not real and were primarily the result of avarice. This study was criticized for having "severe and fatal" selection bias.[13,25] In that no true population-based studies are available, all epidemiologic data are likely biased. For example, with alterations in compensation procedures, significant changes in reported incidence are noted.

Females account for up to 70% of the victims of whiplash.[39,55] A female's increased susceptibility may be due to the smaller neck muscle mass with its decreased ability to withstand acceleration forces. The lower incidence among physical laborers is attributed to their thicker neck muscle mass.[64] Women in their third and fourth decades are most commonly involved.[39,55]

PATHOMECHANICS

Our understanding of whiplash as an oscillatory injury stems from Gay and Abbott's description in 1953[39] of head and neck oscillation after rear-end MVAs. Since then, despite a number of animal, human volunteer, and cadaveric whiplash studies, the whiplash mechanism remains incompletely understood.[82,119] Numerous models have been proposed, often with conflicting data.[119]

BIOMECHANICALLY IMPLICATED FACTORS IN WHIPLASH

- Modality
  - Tension
  - Extension
  - Shear
  - Compression
  - Hyperextension
- Initial alignment: Native curvature of involved region
- Injury indices
  - Bending moment
  - Shear and axial forces
  - Head rotation
- Dynamic kinematics
  - Spinal segmental changes
  - Muscle activities—local curvature attenuation
  - Component motion during posteroanterior loading
- Vehicular
  - Effect of restraint system
  - Location and type of headrest
  - Seat design
  - Other interior components

Data from Yoganandan N, Pintar F, Kleinberger M: Whiplash injury: biomechanical experimentation, *Spine* 24(1):83-85, 1999.

Some authors find it useful to subcategorize whiplash into predominant flexion (deceleration) or extension (acceleration) injuries. In reality, the type of injury depends on the attitude of the head and neck at the time of impact, the point of impact, and the direction and amount of forces.[12] For example, if the head is in slight rotation at impact, the facet capsules, discs, and alar ligaments are prestressed, making them more susceptible to injury.

Severy et al.[102] used a motion picture technique to study extension injuries on anthropomorphic dummies and volunteers. With rear impact, the vehicle moves forward. The trunk and shoulders accelerate forward 100 msec later while the unsupported head lags behind. A higher peak acceleration is needed for the head to catch up (up to 11.4 g) (Figure 39-1). Even at low speed, this peak acceleration results in enormous forces (up to 45 kg). As the shoulders (moved by the car seat) travel under the head, the head recoils and the neck flexes. A kinematic response study in human test subjects[69] found that impacts of 6 to 8 km/hr directed 4.5 g of force axially through the cervical spine in a rapid compression-tension cycle. No extremes of hyperflexion or extension, such as those seen with similar extension moments in cadaveric models, were seen. Overall, a wide range of injuries are described, from mild muscular strain to decapitation. However, the more severe accident, the less likely that a whiplash injury is noted. Ultimately, low-velocity rear-end impacts (7 to 20 mph) are most often implicated.[102]

In a flexion injury, the driver of a car strikes a solid object head on. This collision causes flexion or elongation of the neck. Lateral flexion moments may also play a significant role in subsequent symptoms. In both forward and lateral flexion, neck excursion is limited by chin on chest or the shoulder, respectively.[102] Also, lateral flexion is strictly coupled with rotation, which leads to distraction of the ipsilateral facet and compression of the contralateral facet.[86] The effects of tension, axial load, and shear forces are difficult to separate, but,

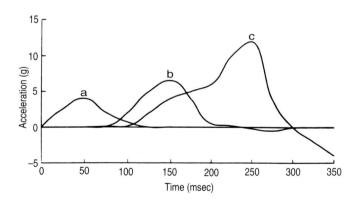

Figure 39-1. Idealized acceleration curves of the vehicle (*a*), shoulders (*b*), and head (*c*) after a rear-end impact. The peak acceleration of the head is significantly greater than that of the car and is followed by a significant deceleration. (*From Barnsley L, Lord S, Bogduk N: Whiplash injury: clinical review,* Pain *58:283-307, 1994.*)

clearly, some measure of shear parallel to the direction of impact will be seen. Because the muscles controlling direction and amplitude of movement respond after maximal deflection of the spine, movements are unlikely to occur around physiologic axes.

Vehicle factors should not be underestimated when calculating forces placed on the cervical spine during a whiplash injury. With decreasing vehicle mass, increased force is transmitted to the patient. With a harder seat back, decreased acceleration forces are seen and, ostensibly, less injurious loading. A well-positioned headrest or seat back that breaks away at the time at impact will lessen the injury to the cervical spine.[65,78,100] If the headrest is too low, the head will roll over the top into even more extension. Use of a seatbelt may increase the chance of whiplash. In one study, 73% of those wearing a seatbelt reported neck pain versus 53% of those who were not restrained.[26]

PATHOANATOMY

Because whiplash injury is rarely fatal, significant pathologic material is not available. The relationship between any demonstrated injury and symptom production remains circumstantial.[28] However, even a low-velocity MVA subjects the cervical spine to enormous forces that may injure various anatomic structures. One postmortem study of 16 MVA victims noted marked evidence of disc, facet, and soft tissue injury[110] (Figure 39-2).

With extension injuries, the posterior elements are compressed while the anterior elements are distracted. The facets, anterior soft tissues, anterior longitudinal ligament (ALL), and disc are thought to be at particular risk. The facet, as the first site of bone-to-bone contact, acts as a fulcrum to further flexion. Injuries may include capsule sprain or hematoma, cartilaginous shear with subsequent surface mismatch, and fracture. Some studies suggest an increase in the incidence of late facet joint degeneration in those sustaining whiplash injuries.[57,59] In one patient who died of unrelated causes 4 months after an MVA, postmortem examination revealed a healing facet fracture on the side of the patient's pain.[1] The postmortem examination of a patient whose suicide was attributed to severe neck pain found severe, unilateral facet arthrosis.[94]

Injury to the anterior soft tissues may include strain of the longus capitus and longus colli, strap muscles, and sternocleidomastoid muscle with significant hemorrhage and edema[48,65,115] (Figure 39-3). The sympathetic trunk, just medial, may also be injured. There have been reported cases of esophageal perforation after extension injuries over anterior osteophytes. MacNab[64] described acceleration-extension injuries sustained by monkeys strapped to a steel platform attached to two vertical guide rails. In this study, the platform was dropped from 2 to 40 feet. Altering the height produced various lesions from slight tears of the sternocleidomastoid muscle to ruptures of the longus colli and esophagus.

In the normal state, the ALL, which blends with the annulus, is effective in limiting neck extension.[24] With sufficient force, ALL and alar ligament sprains are seen.[29]

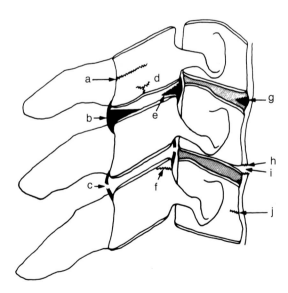

Figure 39-2. Commonly hypothesized injuries sustained via the whiplash mechanism. *a*, Articular pillar fracture; *b*, facet joint hemarthrosis; *c*, injury to the facet joint capsule; *d*, subchondral fracture of the facet; *e*, contusion to the meniscus of the facet joint; *f*, fracture of the articular process of the facet joint; *g*, tear of the annulus fibrosis; *h*, tear of the anterior longitudinal ligament; *i*, end-plate avulsion/fracture; *j*, compression fracture of the vertebral body. *(From Barnsley L, Lord S, Bogduk N: Whiplash injury: clinical review, Pain 58:283-307, 1994.)*

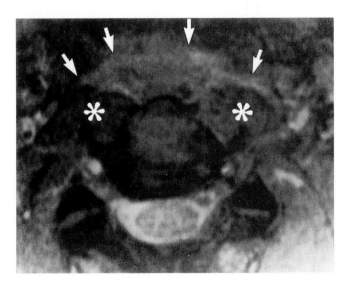

Figure 39-3. An axial T2 weighted magnetic resonance image of a patient sustaining a hyperextension mechanism. Mixed signal intensity of edema and hemorrhage are demonstrated in the retropharyngeal spaces *(arrows)* and the longus colli and capitus muscles *(asterisks)*. *(From Harris JH, Yeakley JW: Hyperextension-dislocation of the cervical spine: ligament injuries demonstrated by magnetic resonance imaging, J Bone Joint Surg Br 74:567-570, 1992.)*

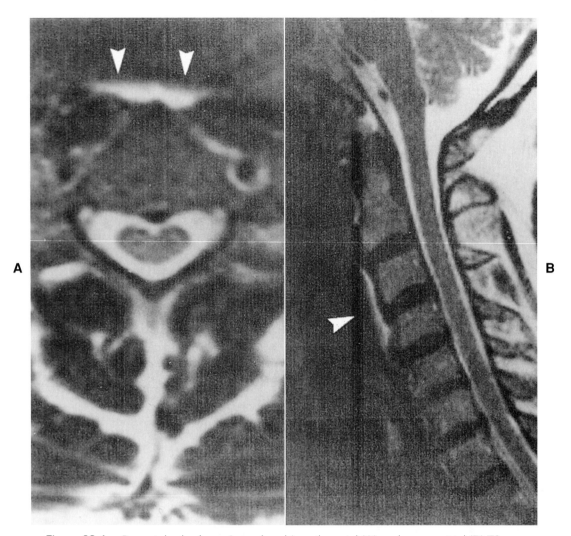

Figure 39-4.   Prevertebral edema *(arrowheads)* on the axial **(A)** and parasagittal **(B)** T2-weighted magnetic resonance images of a 66-year-old man with whiplash symptoms 7 days after the motor vehicle accident. *(From Ronnen HR et al.: Acute whiplash injury: is there a role for MR imaging? A prospective study of 100 patients, Radiology 201:93-96, 1996.)*

Although disc herniations occur, more frequently disc injury is thought to involve avulsion of the superior, anterior annulus. This avulsion may lead to loss of nutrition to the disc and early degeneration. Similarly, anterior end-plate fractures may occur. These fractures are typically radiographically occult but visible on magnetic resonance imaging (MRI). Harris and Yeakley[47] performed MRI evaluation on 8 patients whose hyperextension injuries were sufficiently severe to cause myelopathy. The authors found marked prevertebral edema, disruption of the ALL and annulus, separation of the posterior longitudinal ligament (PLL) from the subjacent vertebral body, posterior bulging or herniation of the nucleus pulposis, and tearing of the ligamentum flavum (Figure 39-4).

In 1926, Barre[11] described a complex of neurologic symptoms in patients with a history of cervical soft tissue injury. These symptoms include nervousness/irritability, cognitive and visual disturbances, headache, and vertigo and have come to be known as the Barre-Lieou syndrome. The anatomic substrate of this syndrome is still not well understood. One theory attributes these symptoms to cerebral injury such as concussion and hemorrhage.[32] Cranial nerve injuries (VI and IX through XII) and brainstem dysfunction have also been implicated.[52,53,80,81,111]

Wickstrom et al.[118] propelled primates on a cart and noted brain damage in 32%, cord damage in 57%, and nerve root damage in 0.7%. Ligamentous injury was noted in 11% and disc injuries in 2.3%. Unterharnscheidt[111] placed monkeys in acceleration sleds with their torsos restrained and head and neck unrestrained. These sleds produced hyperextension forces over 140 g and led to rupture of vertebral arteries, transection of the spinal cord, and massive atlanto-occipital separations. Ommaya et al.[76] demonstrated brain and spinal cord hemorrhage in monkeys subjected to acceleration/deceleration injuries. Ommaya and Yarnell[77] reported on two patients with subdural hematoma after whiplash injury. However, the rate of electroencephalographic abnormalities in patients with whiplash injuries is disputed.[41,60]

Barre[11] and Tamura[107] theorized that stretch or hemorrhage of cervical sympathetic chain or sympathetic fibers in cervical roots led to hypertonia of the sympathetic nervous system. Others attribute these changes to stimulation of peripheral sensory elements of C1 and C2 and compression of the vertebral artery and venous system. Raney et al.[93] were able to reproduce frontal headache, dizziness, and nausea after injection of saline subcutaneously in the upper cervical area. Tissington-Tatlow and Bammer[102] noted reversible headaches, dizziness, tinnitus, and partial loss of hearing and vision on one side by changing the position of the head and neck in cases of vertebral artery compression by spondylitic spurs. It is useful to note that the symptoms cited are common to postconcussion syndrome, chronic pain syndrome, and neurosis.

Some authors attribute ear complaints, tinnitus, and vertigo to inner ear injury.[19,40] Helliwell[46] described a case of bilateral vocal cord palsies with bilateral lateral rectus palsies after an acceleration injury. Amnesia, short-term memory loss, and loss of consciousness may be due to concussion or vertebral artery injury.[21,90,98] Finally, a central cord syndrome may be a rare complication in the elderly. Marar[67] reported 37 patients with varying degrees of central cord syndrome after hyperextension injury to the cervical spine. Some authors report that similar symptoms follow injury to the superficial branches of the cervical plexus adjacent to the sternocleidomastoid muscle. These fibers may be stretched concomitantly with the sternocleidomastoid muscle, and a positive Tinel's sign may be present for years after the injury.

Temporal mandibular joint (TMJ) problems may result from displacement of the articular disc anteriorly, where it may be caught and injured by the condyle.[46] In one study,[35] 15 of 40 patients had TMJ symptoms after hyperextension injury. These symptoms have been effectively treated with dental devices to restore bite and to place the mandibular condyle into a concentric relationship.[31]

With flexion-predominant moments, the anterior spinal elements are compressed while the posterior elements are distracted. This mechanism may lead to a spectrum of injury from mild strain to cord transection.[2,101,111] At low velocity, however, the chin strikes the chest and little soft tissue damage ensues.[102] On the other hand, if muscles are tensed in anticipation of the accident, collision could produce stretching with partial tearing of muscle leading to hemorrhage, inflammation, and muscle spasm. This injury mimics a flexion-sprain and may include traction injury to the greater occipital nerve or avulsion of a spinous process (clay shoveler's). At higher velocity, surviving patients usually incur bony injury.[3] In a series of 312 radiographic studies involving fatal accidents, Alker et al.[2] found a high proportion of flexion injuries involving the cranial-cervical junction and upper two cervical segments. Transverse atlantal ligament rupture may be seen with this mechanism in combination with a significant shear component.[33]

In cadavers, a whole range of intermediate lesions has been defined,[101] including rupture of the interspinous ligaments, capsular disruption, overriding facets, and

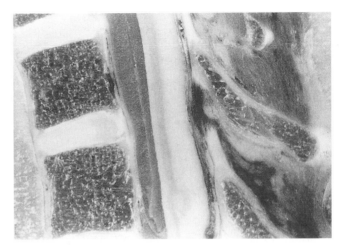

Figure 39-5. Anatomic specimen taken from a motor vehicle accident victim demonstrating rupture of the ligamentum flavum and overlying musculature. The disc is intact in this specimen. (From Jonnsson H, Cesarini K, Sahlstedt B, Rauschning W: Findings and outcome in whiplash-type neck distortions, Spine 19(24):2733-2743, 1994.)

stretch and rupture of the PLL and posterior annulus (Figure 39-5). Babcock[7] and Braakman and Penning[16] noted similar findings and added that a rotation vector led to unilateral facet dislocation, whereas more powerful flexion led to bilateral facet dislocation. The addition of axial loading, on the other hand, led to vertebral body fracture (wedge or teardrop).

SIGNS AND SYMPTOMS[17,43]

Clinical investigation into a given patient's complaints is limited by the lack of strict correlation of anatomic injury with symptom production.[28] The Quebec study was unable to find an acceptable scientific paper that confirmed the validity of any investigation into whiplash-associated disorder. However, when a patient presents with complaints of neck pain after an MVA, important steps include the following:

- Appropriate general trauma evaluation (ABCs)
- Musculoskeletal survey
- Cervical range of motion, tenderness, swelling, and deformity/step-off assessment
- Complete neurologic evaluation
- Exclusion of unstable spinal injury
- Specific investigation of symptomatic areas (e.g., cranial nerves)
- Exploration of the psychologic, social, and legal framework of the patient's complaints

Examination findings vary depending on the time from the accident. Within hours of the accident, evaluation is frequently negative. Later, however, tenderness, limited range of motion, and muscle spasm may develop. These findings may be affected by the predominant mechanism of injury. Evidence of hyperextension forces include face, forehead, and frontal scalp lacerations. Hyperflexion forces produce posterior occipital

TYPICAL WHIPLASH SYMPTOMS

- Neck pain
- Headaches
- Low back pain
- Shoulder and periscapular pain
- Arm pain
- Dizziness
- Paresthesias
- Tinnitus
- Visual symptoms
- Cognitive symptoms
- Emotional symptoms

CLASSIFICATION SYSTEM

- Norris and Watt classification
  - Group 1 (44%): Symptomatic but no physical examinition abnormalities
  - Group 2 (29%): Decreased range of motion, other possible physical findings, but no neurologic abnormalities
  - Group 3 (16%): Objective neurologic deficits
- Quebec classification
  - 0: No neck pain, no physical signs
  - 1: Neck pain, stiffness, tenderness; but no other physical signs
  - 2: Neck pain as above, but with other musculoskeletal symptoms (decreased range of motion, point tenderness)
  - 3: Neck pain with neurologic symptoms (decreased deep tendon reflexes, weakness, sensory deficits)
  - 4: Neck pain with known fracture or dislocation

scalp lacerations and posterior tenderness, particularly over the interspinous ligament.

Given the number and variety of symptoms that may be associated with whiplash, it is useful to subcategorize complaints. First, symptoms are described in terms of onset and persistence. It is useful when evaluating these patients to define acute, subacute, and chronic symptoms. Next, sites of pain origination and radiation are explored followed by assessment of neurologic and psychologic anomalies and work and litigation status.

Numerous classification systems have been devised that may be helpful both prognostically and in terms of treatment. The Norris and Watt Classification (N3), based on 61 patients who presented to the emergency department after an MVA, is similar to Quebec classification groups 1 through 3.[75] It is useful to keep a similar system in mind when evaluating a patient. Patients meeting high group criteria warrant a more intensive imaging and treatment approach.

Central neck pain is the most common complaint after whiplash and is seen in 88% to 100% of patients.[51,89] This pain is usually an aching in the back of the neck that increases with movement but may include occasionally sharp, lancinating pain with movement or may be associated with stiffness. Occasionally, difficulty lifting the head is noted, which could represent rupture of the strap muscles.[48,65,116]

Headache, the second most common complaint, is noted in 54% to 66% of patients.[50,55,66] These headaches are usually of the muscle contraction type and are suboccipital or occipital, radiating anteriorly to the temporal or orbital areas. Although such headaches may be related to concussion, they more likely represent muscle strain. The C1 to C3 dorsal primary rami, part of the trigeminocervical nucleus with the trigeminal nerve, have also been implicated. In one diagnostic block study, 27% of these headaches were attributed to the C2 and C3 facet joints.[62]

Radiating pain must be distinguished from paresthesias, which are also common. In one study, 33% of acutely symptomatic patients had radiating arm pain. Of those still symptomatic at 19.7 months, 37% noted radiating pain. Radiation has been attributed to myofascial injuries with trigger points, brachial plexopathies, thoracic outlet syndrome, peripheral entrapment neuropathies (e.g., carpal tunnel syndrome), radiculopathy, and

myelopathy. Often, this pain radiates along facet sclerotomes rather than dermatomes.[14] Most commonly, this pain extends to the shoulder, in particular to the interscapular area (40%)[50,89] (Figure 39-6). If facet injury is suspected, it may be localized to a specific facetal level.[5,30]

Commonly, pain may radiate along the ulnar nerve distribution. MacNab[64] believed this is due to scalenus spasm or hematoma pressing on the medial cord of the brachial plexus. Whiplash is also a common cause of thoracic outlet syndrome. In one study, a history of whiplash was reported in 56% of 491 patients undergoing surgical treatment for thoracic outlet syndrome.[96] Thoracic outlet syndrome is similar to whiplash in that, in general, findings are nonspecific and electrodiagnostic test results are often negative.[23] Rarely, patients with whiplash have radicular pain as the presenting problem. These patients should be evaluated for disc displacement.[48] Finally, radiation into the low back is seen in up to 35%.[55]

The *cervicoencephalic syndrome of Barre-Lieou* is one of many names given to the often bewildering array of central nervous system complaints seen in up to 20% of patients with whiplash syndrome.[20] These symptoms most commonly include fatigue, dizziness, irritability, depression, sleep disturbances, poor concentration, disturbed accommodation, and impaired adaptability to changes in light intensity. Vertigo and auditory and visual disturbances are common, especially *diplacucis*, which is the difference of sound perception in both ears, either in time or pitch, so that one sound is heard as two.[103] Intermittent aphonic hoarseness, temperature changes, and craniofacial complaints are reported and may be associated with pain, numbness, nausea, vomiting, and diarrhea.

These symptoms are often increased or provoked by *emotion, temperature, humidity,* or *noise*. Gay and Abbott[39] noted that significant soft tissue injury somehow resulted in an insult to the patient's personality structure, causing protracted symptoms. They could not

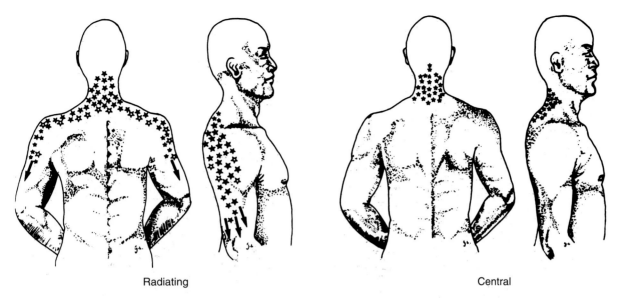

Radiating   Central

Figure 39-6.   Two typical patterns of pain are often described: central neck pain and pain with radiation to the shoulders and periscapular areas. *(From Squires B, Gargan MF, Bannister GC: Soft-tissue injuries of the cervical spine: 15 year follow-up, J Bone Joint Surg Br 78:955-957, 1996.)*

demonstrate whether this was an emotional reaction to the accident or revealed a predisposition to psychoneurotic behavior. Leopold and Dillon[62] noted that the emotional component to whiplash syndrome was integral and independent of litigation, concussion, or physical injury. They thought that injury to the head or neck carried strong, inherent, subconscious meaning. In one study, patients were found to be psychologically normal at the time of injury on the psychometric assessment portion of the General Health Questionnaire. Then increasing abnormalities were noted with increasing time from the injury.[38]

Other, miscellaneous complaints are reported by 8% to 20% of patients.[50,89] Early-onset *dysphagia*, often from retropharyngeal hematoma and pharyngeal edema, has prognostic significance. Later-onset dysphagia may be from psychologic factors. *TMJ syndrome*, including pain when opening the mouth, limited mouth opening, snapping of the jaw, and pain on chewing, is seen in 15% of patients.[31]

IMAGING

Cervical spine radiographs are indicated in any patient who comes to the office or emergency department with neck pain and a high energy of injury. In the trauma setting, this should include immobilization and lateral cervical spine radiographs. Neck pain, loss of consciousness, or neurologic change warrants a full cervical spine series: anteroposterior, lateral, oblique, and open-mouth odontoid views. In the elderly or those with suspected poor bone quality, radiographic evaluation should be routine.

The timing of dynamic radiographs remains controversial. Some obtain supervised flexion and extension radiographs (F/E) immediately.[26,73] Because mobilization

may be risky and muscle spasm may mask underlying pathology, I prefer a standing lateral radiograph in the acute period. F/E films are obtained on return to the office in 2 weeks. F/E films may be repeated at 6 to 12 weeks to rule out late instability.[26,49,68,73] Once obtained, F/E films should be carefully scrutinized for restricted motion at one interspace.[55]

Plain radiograph interpretation in whiplash is confounded by poor correlation with symptoms. Diagnostic difficulties include the variable significance of spondylotic findings in adult patients,[59] the lack of prior films for comparison, and the difficulty in detecting soft tissue injuries. Subluxation and angulation often spontaneously reduce before radiographic examination. Subtle changes on standing films and F/E should be sought.[115] Also, facet injuries are rarely detected with standard plain radiographic views.[61]

At least half of the radiographs obtained in patients with whiplash are unremarkable.[50] Spondylosis is seen in 8% to 31%[50] and may confer a worse prognosis. Often a loss of normal cervical lordosis is noted.[50] The significance of this finding is disputed. Cervical lordosis is lost on many supine lateral radiographs and may be seen in normal patients when they lower their chin. However, a sharp reversal of lordosis should be taken as a pertinent finding[55] (Figure 39-7).

An abnormal prevertebral contour also signals the possibility of significant injury (Figure 39-8). Penning[85] found a wide range of normal in prevertebral width. He recommended taking the upper limits of the normal values as a reference for abnormal width: 11 mm at C1, 6 mm at C2, 7 mm at C3, and 8 mm at C4. Such widening is greatest in early radiographs (0 to 3 days). It normalizes in 50% of cases after 2 weeks and in 90% of cases by 3 weeks. Prevertebral widening is especially pronounced in avulsion fractures and in hyperextension sprains (with

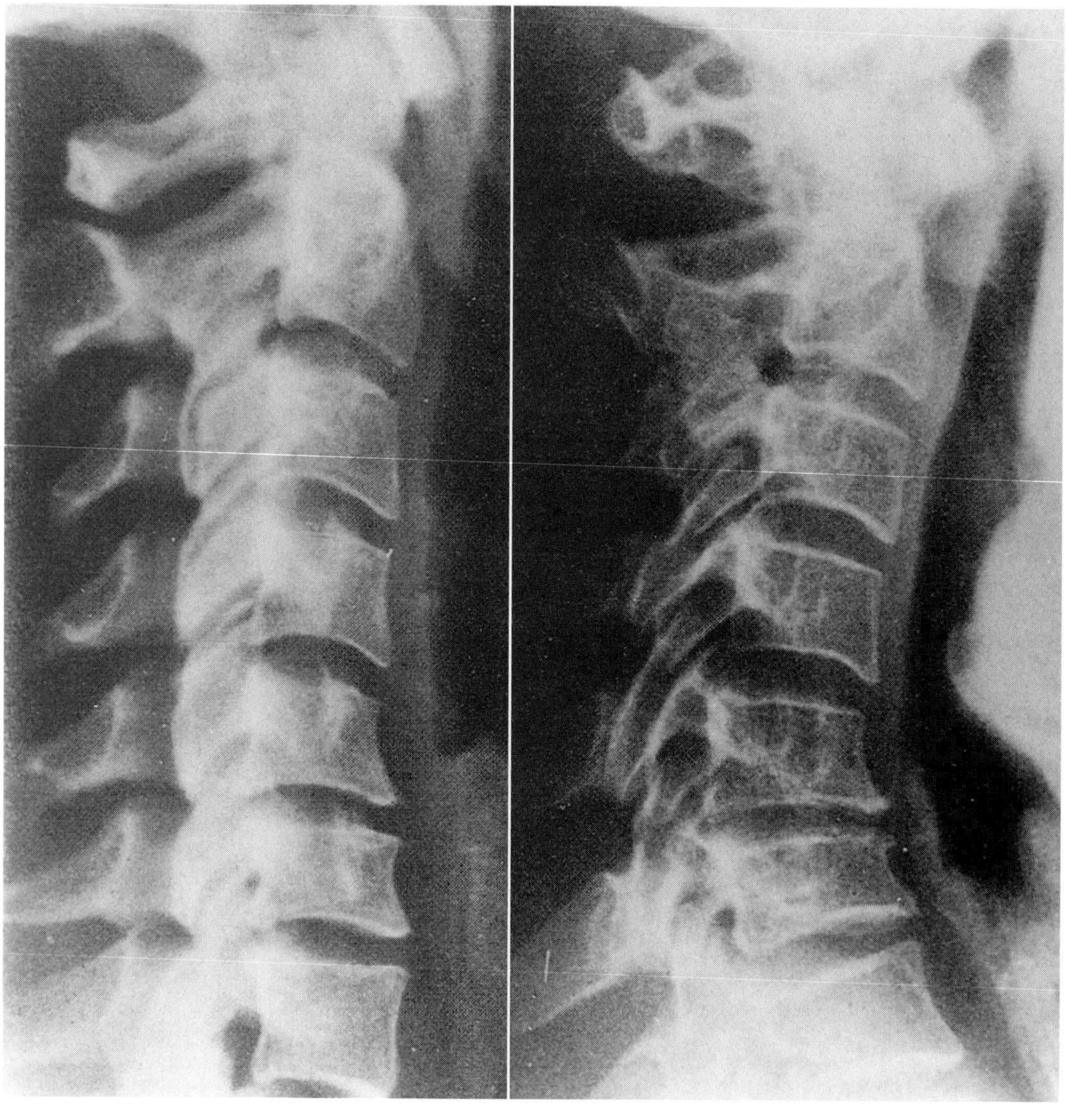

Figure 39-7.   Lateral cervical radiographs of two patients sustaining injuries via the whiplash mechanism. **A,** The cervical spine is straight. **B,** A kyphotic posture is noted. *(From Norris SH, Watt I: The prognosis of neck injuries resulting from rear-end vehicle collisions, J Bone Joint Surg Br 65:608-611, 1983.)*

SIX CHARACTERISTICS OF PATIENTS WITH A FLEXION PREDOMINANT MECHANISM

1. Localized kyphotic angulation at level of injury
2. Anterior rotation or displacement of affected vertebra
3. Anterior and superior displacement of superior facets with respect to inferior facets
4. Abnormal widening of involved interspinous space (fanning)
5. Anterior narrowing and posterior widening of involved disc space
6. Increase in distance between posterior cortex of subluxated vertebral body and anterior cortex of articular masses of subjacent vertebra

From Green JD, Hartle TS, Harris JH: Anterior subluxation of the cervical spine: hyperflexion sprain, *Am J Neuroradiol* 2:243-250, 1981.

disruption of the ALL and disc). Unless associated with fracture or dislocation of the bodies, widening should not be seen after pedicle, articular process, or spinous process fractures. On the other hand, if no prevertebral soft tissue swelling is noted, a disruptive hyperextension injury is very unlikely.

Absent true radicular pain, MRI is rarely indicated in this patient population.[48] One study of 100 patients found MRI had no role if radiographs were negative and the patient had no neurologic deficits.[95] The authors specifically looked for brainstem and posterior ligamentous abnormalities. If an MRI is ordered, short time inversion recovering (STIR) images, which are sensitive to edema, should be requested. Some authors recommend routine MRI, citing the need to exclude cord edema on T2 images or the possibility of important, occult lesions of the intervertebral discs.[24,87] Yet another

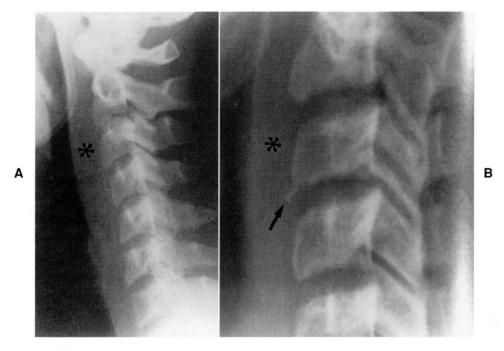

Figure 39-8. Lateral **(A)** and close-up spot **(B)** cervical radiographs of a hyperextension mechanism demonstrating diffuse prevertebral soft tissue swelling *(asterisks)*. A small avulsion fragment is noted *(arrow)*. The overall alignment is straight. *(From Harris JH, Yeakley JW: Hyperextension-dislocation of the cervical spine: ligament injuries demonstrated by magnetic resonance imaging, J Bone Joint Surg Br 74:567-570, 1992.)*

study reported, however, that significant disc tears may not be detected by MRI.[97]

Finally, discography as a provocative test and facet injections as a palliative test have been recommended. One double-blind study found facet injections to be an effective means of identifying the origin of pain.[8] Cervical discography, on the other hand, may have a high false-positive rate.[4] We do not routinely use either of these modalities.

NATURAL HISTORY

The natural history of whiplash syndrome has been variably described as favorable or guarded. In one report, 75% of patients recovered without treatment. The Quebec Task Force concluded that whiplash injuries result in "temporary discomfort," are "usually self-limited," and have a "favorable prognosis," and that the "pain [resulting from whiplash injuries] is not harmful." On the other hand, this report has been criticized for major methodologic flaws. Chronic, debilitating symptoms have elsewhere been reported in 12% to 44% of patients.[50,54,55,65]

Given the nature of whiplash, long-term outcomes assessment is problematic. For example, inclusion errors for prospective cohorts are likely, given delays in symptom onset and recurrence. In 22%, symptom onset was delayed to 48 hours.[26] In this group, outcome was not affected by late presentation. In another group of 93 patients with whiplash, 65 were symptomatic within 1 hour, 77 within 5 hours, and 85 within 15 hours.[50] Others

present weeks after the index trauma.[61] Moreover, in some patients, symptoms resolve only to recur later.

Once a patient is diagnosed with whiplash syndrome, the recovery curve is variable. For a large group of patients, the curve is best described as parabolic with an asymptote at 3 to 4 months from the accident date (Figure 39-9). That is, in most patients, recovery occurs in the early months. Then, a slower recovery rate is recorded for the remaining group over the next 3 months to 2 years. A small number of patients are left with essentially permanent symptoms. According to some reports, a given patient will reach a final state of recovery or continued, stable symptoms within 3 months.[66]

Various factors have been cited by different authors as adversely affecting outcome in patients with whiplash. One retrospective study grouped 102 patients into good (66%) and poor (34%) prognostic subgroups based on similar criteria. The good subgroup had an average time off work of 2 weeks (maximum, 16 weeks). One third of these patients took no time off. The poor group averaged 6 weeks off work. Although 20% of this group took no time off, 9% had not returned to work at 2 years.[66] One study found a decreased cervical range of motion to be the single best predictor of outcome.[38] In another study, if initial symptoms were severe enough to require bedrest, discomfort for 6 weeks was predicted. If, at the end of this period, neck discomfort was still noted all day, intermittent discomfort was noted for 6 months to 1 year.[65] The role of family size and marital status may be based on secondary gain issues outside of direct compensation.

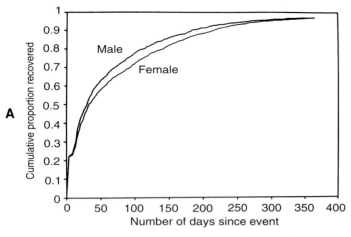
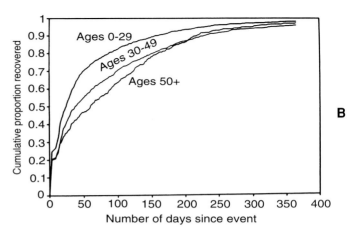

Figure 39-9. Recovery from whiplash over time as depicted by 1-year cumulative return to activity by gender **(A)** and age **(B)**. *(From Spitzer WO et al.: Scientific monograph of the Quebec Task Force on Whiplash-Associated Disorders: redefining "whiplash" and its management, Spine 20[Suppl]:S1-S73, 1995.)*

POOR PROGNOSTIC SIGNS IN WHIPLASH

- Female[55,57]
- Severity of initial symptoms[65]
- Degenerative changes[74]
- Radiating pain[44]
- Neurologic signs
- Muscle spasm[74,89]
- Significant neck stiffness[38]
- Thoracic and low back pain radiation[44]
- Age greater than 50
- Headache
- Married, large family unit
- Pending litigation

The role of these sociodemographic factors remains controversial, however. In one study, there was no difference between symptomatic and asymptomatic patients at 6 months in terms of: sex, education, mechanism of injury, collision fault, and time from injury to presentation.[89]

The presence of central, neurologic symptoms may not affect the outcome of neck pain in patients with whiplash. Patients with a Barre syndrome improve with the standard treatments as used for musculoskeletal complaints and at the same rate.[20] Radiation of pain may augur a worse prognosis, however. Greenfield and Ilfeld[44] studied short-term prognostic factors in 179 patients. They found that shoulder and arm pain were associated with slower progress to recovery. After 7 weeks, only 37% were asymptomatic.

Overall, a complete recovery is expected in 57% to 75% of patients. On the other hand, 8% to 12% continue to report severe pain and are unable to work or participate in preferred leisure activities.[42,79,87] The rest fall in between. Although the percentage with continuing, severe pain is small, given the large numbers of patients with whiplash, these failures compose a significant part of the chronic pain population.

In three succeeding studies, a single cohort of 61 patients with soft tissue injuries of the neck was followed up at 2, 10, and 15 years. Norris and Watt[73] found that 66% had neck pain at an average of 2 years after injury. Gargan et al.[38] reported on the same patients. After 10 years, 12% had severe symptoms and 28% had intrusive symptoms; 88% had some residual symptoms. At the 15-year mark, 40 patients were available for follow-up. In this group, 54% noted no change in their symptoms, 18% had improved in the 10- to 15-year term, and 28% deteriorated in that interval. Older patients and those with degenerative changes were more likely to have deteriorated. Of the 15-year cohort, 18% took early retirement due to problems they attributed to their whiplash. Interestingly, 60% of the symptomatic group had sought no further treatment in the interval; most stated that physicians were unable to help them. Thirty-three percent sought alternative remedies, including acupuncture and chiropractic, with no relief. Two patients subsequently underwent surgery; one had complete relief of symptoms and one had significant relief.

Radanov et al.[89,91,92] found that 27% of their cohort were symptomatic 6 months after their accident, and in a study published 2 years later, the authors reported that 27% of their cohort continued to have headaches 6 months after the accident. Hildingsson and Toolanen[50] found that 44% of their cohort were symptomatic an average of 2 years after the accident.

Litigation is a common element in whiplash syndrome. Even in 1956, 66% of patients were noted to have legal claims.[55] In a more recent study, 81% of cases involved litigation.[84] Hohl[55] found that patients who settled their litigation early (within 6 months versus after 18 months) had a much better prognosis (17% symptomatic versus 62% symptomatic). Some questioned whether this longer symptomatic duration reflected a "sick role" rather than a more serious injury. Gotten[42] studied 100 patients whose whiplash injuries prompted them to sue. Once settled, 88% were recovered and asymptomatic, and 12% needed further treatment. Of those satisfied with their settlement, 80% had no further or minimal discomfort. Only 25% of those who were not satisfied with their settlement experienced complete relief. The author noted a profound post-traumatic neurosis, including apprehension, nervous tension, and anxiety. Gotten thought that many patients were using the injury for psychosocial or financial gain.

Some authors note less resolution after litigation settlement than they originally expected. In one cohort, 39% noted symptomatic improvement after the settlement, but almost none had symptom resolution.[32] These symptoms were a continuing nuisance rather than significantly disabling. MacNab[65] reported that 45% of 266 patients had continued complaints even after settlement and did not believe that secondary gain was a major issue. He noted that in these same patients, wrist and ankle fractures healed, but the neck pain continued. Some studies have found similar rates of recovery independent of litigation.[55,74,84]

The role of whiplash injury in the acceleration of cervical spondylosis is debated.[108] In one study, radiographs taken 7 years after injury in a series of patients with no prior evidence of disc disease[53] revealed that spondylosis had developed in 9% at one or more levels. The expected incidence in this age group (mean, 30 years) was 6%. However, these radiographic changes did not correlate with symptoms. One 10-year follow-up study demonstrated increased rates of degenerative spondylosis compared with age- and gender-matched controls. In 30- to 40-year-old patients, spondylosis was seen in 33% of the patients with whiplash versus 10% in the control subjects. In another group, late degenerative changes were seen in 68% of patients at 10.8 years,[114] and these changes correlated with symptoms. On the other hand, other cohorts of 50 and 100 patients at a mean 5 and 8 years, respectively, from injury demonstrated no acceleration of degenerative changes.[61,83]

The social costs of chronic pain from whiplash syndrome should not be underestimated. For patients with whiplash in Quebec, 61.5% had less than a 2-month absence from work and accounted for 15.5% of the costs. Twenty-six percent missed 2 to 6 months and represented 38.5% of the costs, and 12.5% missed more than 6 months of work and accounted for 46% of the costs. In 1987, $18 million (Canadian dollars) were spent in Quebec alone on 4757 subjects. Of that expense, 70% was for income replacement.

MANAGEMENT
Nonsurgical Treatment

No treatment modality, surgical or nonsurgical, has been shown to alter the natural history of whiplash-associated disorder. Therefore, conservative measures are the most rational.

The cornerstone to this management is reassurance and education with "a supportive but optimistic approach."[89] Most patients should be placed in charge of their own recovery with encouragement to early motion and return to work.

TREATMENT OPTIONS FOR WHIPLASH SYNDROME

- Acute
  - Disease education and reassurance
  - Relative rest
  - Interval use of a soft collar
  - Analgesics: Nonsteroidal antiinflammatory drugs and acetaminophen
- Chronic
  - Exercise
  - Formal physical therapy
  - Continued analgesic agents
  - Other medications: Antidepressants
  - Behavioral and social intervention/counseling

The Quebec Task Force divided its treatment recommendations according to whiplash grade (Figure 39-10). Patients falling into Quebec groups 0 and 1 were immediately returned to work with no restrictions. Quebec group 2 patients were urged to return to work as soon as possible (usually 1 week). Quebec group 2 patients often required job restrictions for 3 weeks, and nonsteroidal medications were recommended for pain. The more severe pain noted in Quebec group 3 patients warranted short-term narcotics but an otherwise similar approach. Quebec group 4 patients were treated for their comorbid condition (e.g., herniated cervical disc).

Close follow-up is advised for all patients taken off work due to whiplash. This will allow graded but rapid return to normal duties. Disease education, including instruction in neck-sparing routines and reassurance, is critical.[40] Reassurance may be useful to stem the significant psychologic overlay in the whiplash syndrome.

Bracing and activity restriction, although not independently evaluated, are the only modalities that have undergone significant scientific study. There are two common philosophies: rest and early activity. MacNab[65] recommends bedrest in severe injuries to relieve the weight of the head and to more completely rest the neck. Many advise a short, initial period of rest, while splinting the neck with a soft cervical collar.[39,65,84] Others recommend an early, active mobilization program. Exercises often include short arc active motion for pain and spasm and passive range of motion to counteract stiffness. After 48 hours, active motion is added. Once the acute pain subsides, isometric strengthening to tolerance is added.

A prospective study of 201 patients compared immediate return to normal activities with a period of time in a cervical collar and off work. The return-to-work group did better in most categories, including pain localization, pain during daily activities, neck stiffness, memory, and concentration, and in terms of visual analog scale measurements of neck pain and headache.[15] Mealy et al.[71] reported on 61 patients selected at random to undergo 2 weeks of immobilization followed by gradual self-mobilization or local application of ice for 24 hours followed by daily therapy consisting of repetitive active and passive motion and heat. They found that over the

THE QUEBEC GUIDELINES FOR PATIENT CARE*

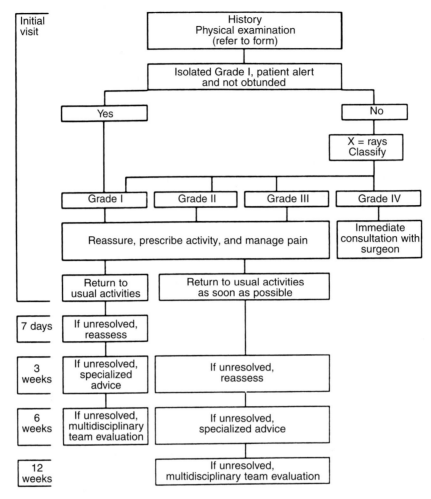

Figure 39-10.   The Quebec Task Force devised an algorithm for the care of patients with complaints related to a whiplash mechanism of injury. *(From Spitzer WO et al.: Scientific monograph of the Quebec Task Force on Whiplash-Associated Disorders: redefining "whiplash" and its management, Spine 20[suppl]:S1-S73, 1995.)*

short term (4 to 8 weeks), the active treatment group had significantly lower pain scores. Also, at 8 weeks, the active group had a significantly better range of motion.

McKinney[70] randomized 247 patients into three treatment groups: (1) rest for 10 to 14 days followed by self-mobilization, (2) physical therapy for 6 weeks consisting of both active and passive modalities, and (3) advice on self-mobilization, which consisted of 30 minutes of instruction given by a physiotherapist. At 2 years, no differences were found between the rest and intensive physical therapy groups. The early self-mobilization group recovered more quickly (mean, 3.4 months) and had significantly fewer symptoms 2 years after the injury.

Pennie and Agambar[84] randomized 135 patients to early physical therapy or rest in a soft collar for 2 weeks and then self-mobilization after the patients were taught a program of active exercises. Their conclusions were that given adequate instruction, a self-mobilization

program is equal to a more extensive physical therapy program.

A number of medications have been recommended for patients with whiplash. Most commonly nonsteroidal antiinflammatory drugs and other analgesics are prescribed. Although evidence documents the effectiveness of nonsteroidal antiinflammatory drugs for acute pain, no data supports its use for chronic pain. High-dose steroids have been recommended based on implied neurologic system injury. A prospective study in 40 patients found that methylprednisolone, given within 8 hours, decreased the number of sick days.[88] The authors cautioned that more studies are needed to determine which patients in particular would benefit.

Narcotics are often given for acute, severe pain. Efforts should be made to use lower-potency agents and to wean patients from these early. There is no role for chronic narcotic use in patients with whiplash. The use of muscle relaxants remains controversial.

Antidepressants may be especially useful to improve sleep and for depression that is commingled with chronic pain complaints.[112]

At 2 months from the onset, the success of these simple, nonoperative measures drops off, reflecting the natural history in chronic whiplash syndrome. At this time, a multidisciplinary evaluation, including psychosocial evaluation, is beneficial in exploring impediments to improvement and returning the patient to function.

Other unproved or controversial methods of whiplash care include injections. Cervical epidural injections have been recommended with no supportive data. A randomized clinical trial of sterile water versus saline triggerpoint injections in patients 4 to 6 years after whiplash injury was undertaken. Although this was not a blind study, it documented an increased pain relief and range of motion with sterile water injections.[17] Greater occipital nerve injections have been recommended in patients with flexion injuries. If these prove to be only temporarily beneficial, nerve resection is advocated.[28]

Perhaps more commonly supported are intra-articular injections in the cervical facets.[14,30] Injection studies have shown the facet joint to be a source of local neck pain and referred pain, transmitted by adjacent posterior primary rami. This pain may be relieved with steroid and anesthetic injections. However, the duration of relief has varied: some report no change versus the control group.[10]

Other techniques include pulsed electromagnetic treatments, which were yielded no better results than those when patients were placed in soft collars at 12 weeks.[34] Also, magnetic necklaces were used in patients with a 1-year history of neck and shoulder pain; no differences were noted between the magnetic or sham necklaces.[58] A number of other modalities have been recommended with no supportive evidence, including acupuncture, traction, manipulation, massage, heat, ice, cervical pillows, electrical stimulation, and ultrasound. Some of these methods may be used empirically.

Surgical Treatment

Surgical treatment for axial neck pain in whiplash syndrome is discouraged. However, some have reported acceptable results; these are usually in the context of another, discrete pathoanatomic entity, often frank disc displacement or ligamentous instability. In patients with persistent radicular pain confirmed by neuroimaging studies, an anterior cervical discectomy and fusion may be recommended.[27] As in any posttrauma patient, significant posterior ligamentous disruption must be excluded. Unstable patients may benefit from anterior plate fixation and/or anterior and posterior cervical fusion to achieve stability.

The use of an anterior cervical discectomy and fusion for patients with chronic axial complaints is more controversial. Some recommend selection for surgery based on MRI or discographic findings.[118] Jonnsson et al.[61] argued that the lack of adequate follow-up in previous series contributed to missed surgically treatable pathology. In their study, they monitored 50 patients over 5 years. Of these patients, 19 had radiating pain and normal F/E radiographs. An anterior cervical discectomy and fusion was undertaken for patients with neck or radiating pain that was severe and "in complete agreement with clinical and radiographic findings." At a mean of 5.5 months from surgery, complete relief of symptoms and no complications were reported.

Tamura[107] retrospectively investigated 40 patients with Barre-Lieou syndrome after whiplash injury. He noted a clear correlation between root sleeve defects at C3 to C4 on special oblique myelographic views and cranial symptoms. In 21 patients, anterior cervical discectomy and fusion was performed at the C3 to C4 level. Of the 20 patients available for review, 19 had complete resolution of the Barre-Lieou symptoms.[107]

Occasionally, posterior stabilization is recommended for patients demonstrating major instability by White and Panjabi's criteria[116] (Figure 39-11). In one report, attempted closed treatment resulted in dangerous long-term instability in more than one third of these patients.[113] In the report of Jonson et al.,[59] two patients presented with nonradiating neck pain and segmental instability on dynamic radiographs. A posterior cervical fusion was undertaken, with complete pain relief in both (Figure 39-12).

Finally, in patients reporting temporary relief with facet injections, open or radiofrequency rhizolysis is occasionally recommended. No data support this practice.

CONCLUSIONS

As understanding of the whiplash mechanism grows, the close delineation of anatomic injuries sustained remains elusive. More important, the relationship of the injury mechanism to resultant symptoms is poorly understood. Therefore, the diagnosis and treatment of patients with whiplash remain contentious. Ultimately, the whiplash syndrome probably represents a three-tier problem. First, the characteristic indirect injury exposes the neck to acceleration/deceleration cycles, imparting significant force to the tissues. A physiologic disturbance to anatomic structures of the cervical spine is likely. However, in most patients, the neck pain and stiffness engendered by this injury resolve quickly. In others, a second tier of abnormal pain response contributes to a protracted period of incapacitation. This second, or psychologic, tier may be magnified by a third, socioeconomic, tier. Here, recovery is further compromised by the secondary gains afforded patients through litigation, time off work, and a sick role within the family. The predominance of one or another of these tiers differs between individuals. Proper evaluation of a whiplash patient, therefore, includes not only a complete history and physical examination to fully define the extent of a patient's injuries but also an understanding of the context in which the injury and recovery will take place. In most patients, reassurance, education, and mild analgesics are all that are required for the patient to quickly return to normal activities. In

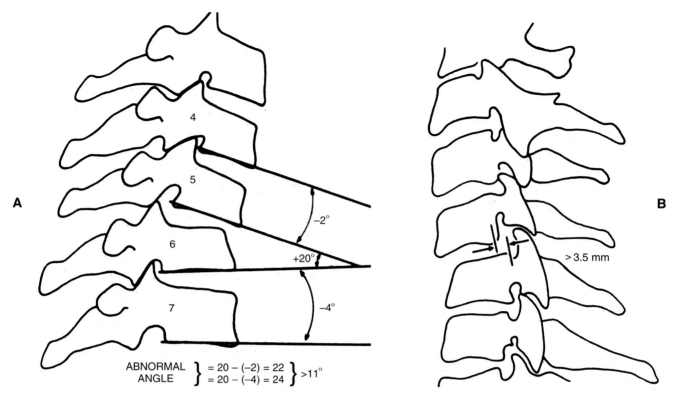

Figure 39-11.   White et al. defined cervical instability based on biomechanical tests of cadaveric preparations. They stated that increased angular motion greater than 11 degrees **(A)** and horizontal displacement greater than 3.5 mm **(B)** denote instability. *(From White AA et al.: Biomechanical analysis of clinical stability in the cervical spine, Clin Orthop 109:85-95, 1975.)*

certain, acutely distressed individuals, relative rest, a cervical collar, and a short course of narcotics may be helpful. In these more affected patients, aggressive follow-up with the introduction of formal physical therapy may be beneficial. Ultimately, a small percentage of chronically painful and dysfunctional patients will remain in this condition. These patients are best treated in the context of a multidisciplinary pain clinic with the appropriate psychologic, social, and rehabilitative support. Surgery is reserved for those patients with comorbid conditions such as disc displacement or ligamentous instability.

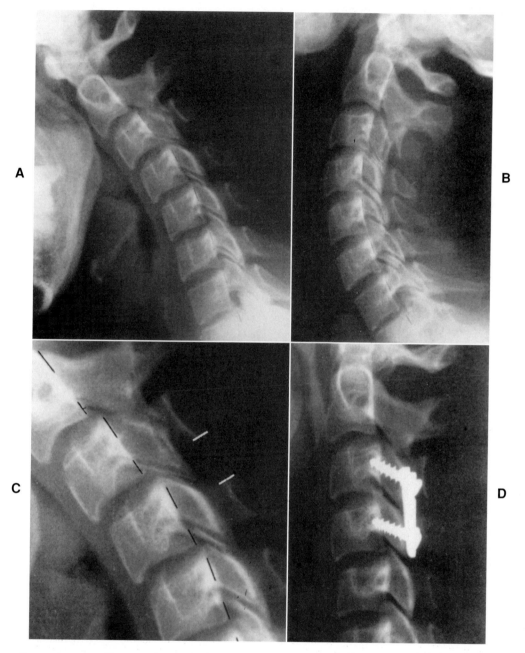

Figure 39-12. These radiographs depict a 23-year-old woman with continued neck pain after a rear-end motor vehicle accident. On flexion and extension, 5 mm of anterior translation and 13 degrees of sagittal angulation are noted (**A** to **C**). At surgery, the ligamentum flavum and facet joint capsules were found to be ruptured. A fusion with lateral mass plating was performed. Six months later, the segment remains stable and the patient is symptom free (**D**). *(From Jonsson H et al.: Findings and outcome in whiplash-type neck distortions, Spine 19(24):2733-2743, 1994.)*

SELECTED REFERENCES

Barnsley L, Lord S, Bogduk N: Whiplash injury: clinical review, *Pain* 58:283-307, 1994.

Freeman MD, Croft, AC, Rossignol AM: Whiplash associated disorders: redefining whiplash and its management by the Quebec Task Force: a critical evaluation, *Spine* 23:1043-1049, 1998.

Gargan MF, Bannister GC: Long-term prognosis of soft tissue injuries of the neck, *J Bone Joint Surg Br* 72:901-903, 1990.

Harris JH, Yeakley JW: Hyperextension-dislocation of the cervical spine: ligament injuries demonstrated by magnetic resonance imaging, *J Bone Joint Surg Br* 74:567-570, 1992.

Norris SH, Watt I: The prognosis of neck injuries resulting from rear-end vehicle collisions, *J Bone Joint Surg Br* 65:608-611, 1983.

Schrader H et al.: Natural evolution of late whiplash syndrome outside the medicolegal context, *Lancet* 347:1201-1211, 1996.

Spitzer WO et al.: Scientific monograph of the Quebec Task Force on Whiplash-Associated Disorders: redefining "whiplash" and its management, *Spine* 20(suppl):S1-S73, 1995.

Squires B, Gargan MF, Bannister GC: Soft-tissue injuries of the cervical spine: 15 year follow-up, *J Bone Joint Surg B* 78:955-957, 1996.

Whitecloud TS, Seago RA: Cervical discogenic syndrome: results of operative intervention in patients with positive discography, *Spine* 12:313-316, 1981.

REFERENCES

1. Abel MS: Occult traumatic lesions of the cervical vertebrae, *CRC Radiol Nucl Med* 6:469-553, 1975.
2. Alker GJ et al.: Post mortem radiology of head/neck injuries in fatal traffic accidents, *Radiology* 114:611-617, 1975.
3. Allen BL et al.: A mechanistic classification of closed, indirect fractures and dislocations of the lower cervical spine, *Spine* 7:1-27, 1982.
4. Aprill CR, Bogduk N: Prevalence of cervical zygoapophyseal pain, *Spine* 17:744-747, 1992.
5. Aprill CR, Dwyer A, Bogduk N: Cervical zygapophyseal joint pain patterns: a clinical evaluation, *Spine* 15:458-461, 1991.
6. Awerbuch M: Whiplash injury in Australia: illness or injury? *Med J Aust* 157:193-219, 1992.
7. Babcock JL: Cervical spine injuries, *Arch Surg* 3:646-651, 1976.
8. Barnsley C, Lord SM, Bogduk N: Comparative local anesthetic blocks in the diagnosis of cervical zygoapophyseal joint pain, *Pain* 55:99-106, 1993.
9. Barnsley L, Lord S, Bogduk N: Whiplash injury: clinical review, *Pain* 58:283-307, 1994.
10. Barnsley C et al.: Lack of effect of intraarticular corticosteroids for chronic pain of the zygoapophyseal joints, *N Engl J Med* 330:1047-1050, 1994.
11. Barre JA: Sur on syndrome sympathetique cervicale posterior, et cause frequent: l'artrite cervicale, *Rev Neurol* 45:1246, 1926.
12. Bauze RJ, Ardran GM: Experimental production of forward dislocation in the human cervical spine, *J Bone Joint Surg Br* 60:239-245, 1978.
13. Bjorgen IA: Late whiplash syndrome, *Lancet* 348:124, 1996.
14. Bogduk N, Marsland A: Cervical zygo-apophyseal joints as a cause of neck pain, *Spine* 13:610-617, 1988.
15. Borchgrevink GE et al.: Acute treatment of whiplash neck sprain injuries. a randomized trial of treatment during the first 14 days after a car accident, *Spine* 23:25-31, 1998.
16. Braakman R, Penning L: The hyperflexion sprain of the cervical spine, *Radiol Clin Biol* 3:309-320, 1968.
17. Bryn C et al.: Subcutaneous sterile water injections for chronic neck and shoulder pain following whiplash injuries, *Lancet* 341:449-452, 1993.
18. Carpenter S: Injury to the neck as cause of vertebral artery thrombosis, *J Neurosurg* 18:849, 1961.
19. Chester JB Jr: Whiplash, postural control, and the inner ear, *Spine* 16:716-720, 1991.
20. Chrisman OD, Gervais RF: Otologic manifestations of the cervical syndrome, *Clin Orthop* 24: 34-39, 1962.
21. Coburn DF: Cerebral artery involvement in cervical trauma, *Clin Orthop* 24:61-63, 1962.
22. Crowe HE: *Injuries to the cervical spine.* Presented at the annual meeting of the Western Orthopaedic Association, San Francisco, 1928.
23. Cuetter AC, Bartoszek DM: The thoracic outlet syndrome: controversies, overdiagnosis, overtreatment, and recommendations for management, *Muscle Nerve* 12:410-419, 1989.
24. Davis S et al.: Cervical spine hyperextension injuries: MR findings, *Radiology* 180:245-251, 1991.
25. de Mol BA, Heijer T: Late whiplash syndrome, *Lancet* 348:124-125, 1996.
26. Deans GT et al.: Neck sprain: a major cause of disability following car accidents, *Injury* 18:10-12, 1987.
27. DePalma AF, Subin DK: A study of the cervical syndrome, *Clin Orthop* 38:135, 1965.
28. Dunn EJ, Blazar S: Soft tissue injuries of the lower cervical spine, *ICL* 36:499-512, 1987.
29. Dvorjak J, Hayek J, Zehnder R: CT-functional diagnosis of the rotational instability of the upper cervical spine, *Spine* 12:197-205, 1987.
30. Dwyer A, Aprill C, Bogduk N: Cervical zygoapophyseal joint pain patterns: a study in normal volunteers, *Spine* 15:453- 457, 1990.
31. Ernest EA III: The orthopedic influence of the TMJ apparatus in whiplash: report of a case, *Gen Dentist* 27:62-64, 1979.
32. Evans RW: Some observations on whiplash injuries, *Neurol Clin* 10:975-997, 1992.
33. Fielding JW et al.: Tears of the transverse ligament of the atlas: a clinical and biomechanical study, *J Bone Joint Surg Am* 56:1683, 1974.
34. Foley-Nolan D et al.: Pulsed high frequency (27MHz) electromagnetic therapy for persistent neck pain: a double blind, placebo controlled study of 20 patients, *Orthopaedics* 13:445-451, 1990.
35. Frankel VH: Temporomandibular joint pain syndrome following deceleration injury to the cervial spine, *Bull Hosp Joint Dis* 26:47, 1969.
36. Freeman MD, Croft AC, Rossignol AM: Whiplash associated disorders: redefining whiplash and its management by the Quebec Task Force: a critical evaluation, *Spine* 23:1043-1049, 1998.
37. Gargan MF, Bannister GC: Long-term prognosis of soft tissue injuries of the neck, *J Bone Joint Surg Br* 72:901-903, 1990.
38. Gargan MF et al.: The behavioral response to whiplash injury, *J Bone Joint Surg Br* 79:523-526, 1997.
39. Gay JR, Abbott KH: Common whiplash injuries of the neck, *JAMA* 152:1678-1704, 1953.
40. Gebhard JS, Donaldson DH, Brown CW: Soft tissue injuries of the cervical spine, *Orthop Rev Trauma*, May 1994, pp. 9-17.
41. Gibbs FA: Objective evidence of brain disorder in cases of whiplash injury, *Clin Electroencephalogr* 2:107-110, 1971.
42. Gotten N: Survey of one hundred cases of whiplash injury after settlement of litigation, *JAMA* 162:865-867, 1956.
43. Green JD, Hartle TS, Harris JH: Anterior subluxation of the cervical spine: hyperflexion sprain, *Am J Neuroradiol* 2:243-250, 1981.
44. Greenfield J, Ilfeld FW: Acute cervical strain evaluation and short term prognostic factors, *Clin Orthop* 122:196-200, 1977.
45. Grimm RJ et al.: The perilymph fistula syndrome defined in mild head trauma, *Acta Otolaryngol Suppl* 464:1-40, 1989.
46. Hannheimer J et al.: Cervical strain and mandibular whiplash: effects upon the craniomandibular apparatus, *Clin Prev Dent* 11:29-32, 1989.
47. Harris JH, Yeakley JW: Hyperextension-dislocation of the cervical spine: ligament injuries demonstrated by magnetic resonance imaging, *J Bone Joint Surg Br* 74:567-570, 1992.
48. Harris WH, Hamblen DL, Ojemann RG: Traumatic disruption of cervical inter-vertebral disc from hyperextension injury, *Clin Orthop* 60:163-167, 1968.
49. Helliwell M: Bilateral vocal cord paralysis due to whiplash injury, *Br Med J* 288:1876-1877, 1984.
50. Herkowitz HN, Rothman RH: Subacute instability of the cervical spine, *Spine* 9:348-365, 1984.
51. Hildingsson C, Toolanen G: Outcome after soft-tissue injury of the cervical spine: a prospective study of 93 car-accident victims, *Acta Orthop Scand* 61:357-359, 1990.
52. Hildingsson C, Wenngren BI, Toolanen G: Eye motility dysfunction after soft-tissue injury of the cervical spine: a controlled, prospective study of 38 patients, *Acta Orthop Scand* 64:129-132, 1993.
53. Hildingsson C et al.: Oculomotor problems after cervical spine injury, *Acta Orthop Scand* 60:513-516, 1989.

54. Hodgson SP, Grundy M: Whiplash injuries: their long term prognosis and relationship to compensation, *Neuroorthopedics* 7:88-91, 1989.

55. Hohl M: Soft tissue injuries of the neck in automobile accidents, *J Bone Joint Surg Am* 56:1675-1682, 1974.

56. Hohl M: Soft tissue neck injuries. In *The cervical spine*, Philadelphia, 1983, JB Lippincott.

57. Hohl M, Hopp E: Soft tissue injuries of the neck: factors influencing prognosis, *Orthop Trans* 2:29, 1978.

58. Hong CZ et al.: Magnetic necklace: its therapeutic effectiveness on neck and shoulder pain, *Arch Phys Med Rehabil* 63:462-466, 1982.

59. Irvine DH et al.: Prevalence of cervical spondylosis in a general practice, *Lancet* 1:1089-1092, 1965.

60. Jacome DE: EEF in whiplash: a reapprasial, *Clin Electroencephalogr* 18:41-45, 1987.

61. Jonsson H et al.: Findings and outcome in whiplash-type neck distortions, *Spine* 19:2733-2743, 1994.

62. Leopold RL, Dillon H: Psychiatric considerations in whiplash injuries of the neck, *Pa Med J* 63:385-389, 1960.

63. Lord S et al.: Third occipital nerve headache: a prospective study, *J Neurol Neurosurg Psych* 57:1187-1190, 1994.

64. MacNab I: Acceleration injuries of the cervical spine, *J Bone Joint Surg Am* 46:1979-1999, 1964.

65. MacNab I: The "whiplash syndrome," *Orthop Clin North Am* 2:389-403, 1971.

66. Maimaris C, Barnes MR, Allen MJ: Whiplash injury of the neck: a retrospective study, *Injury* 19:393-396, 1988.

67. Marar BC: Hyperextension injuries of the cervical spine: the pathogenesis of damage to the spinal cord, *J Bone Joint Surg Am* 56:1655-1662, 1974.

68. Mazur JM, Stauffer ES: Unrecognized spinal instability associated with seemingly "simple" cervical compression fractures, *Spine* 8:687-692, 1983.

69. McConnell WE et al.: *Analysis of human test subject kinematic responses to low velocity rear end impacts: vehicle and occupant kinematics—simulation and modeling (SP-975).* International Congress and Exposition, Society for Automotive Engineers, 1993, pp. 21-30.

70. McKinney LA: Early mobilization and outcome in acute sprains of the neck, *Br Med J* 299:1006-1008, 1989.

71. Mealy K, Brenan H, Fenelon GCC: Early mobilization of acute whiplash injuries, *Br Med J* 292:656-657, 1986.

72. Mills H, Horn G: Whiplash: man-made disease? *N Z Med J* 99:373-374, 1986.

73. Nash CL: Acute cervical soft tissue injury and late deformity, *J Bone Joint Surg Am* 61:305-307, 1979.

74. Norris SH: The prognosis of neck injuries resulting from rear end vehicle collisions, *J Bone Joint Surg Br* 65:9, 1983.

75. Norris SH, Watt I: The prognosis of neck injuries resulting from rear-end vehicle collisions, *J Bone Joint Surg Br* 65:608-611, 1983.

76. Ommaya AK, Faas F, Yarnell P: Whiplash injury and brain damage: an experimental study, *JAMA* 204:295-299, 1968.

77. Ommaya AK, Yarnell P: Subdural hematoma after whiplash injury, *Lancet* 2:237-239, 1969.

78. O'Neill B et al.: Automobile head restraints: frequency of neck injury claims in relation to the presence of head restraints, *Am J Public Health* 62:399-406, 1972.

79. Ono K, Kanno ML: Influences of the physical parameters on the risk to neck injuries in low impact speed rear-end collisions. Presented at the International Conference on the Biomechanics of Impacts, Eindhoven, the Netherlands, Sept 8-10, 1993.

80. Oosterveld WJ et al.: Electronystagmographic findings following cervical whiplash injuries, *Acta Otolaryngol* 111:201-205, 1991.

81. Ortengren T et al.: Membrane leakage in spinal ganglion nerve cells induced by experimental whiplash extension motion: a study in pigs, *J Neurotrauma* 13:171-180, 1996.

82. Panjabi MM et al.: Simulation of whiplash trauma using whole cervical spine specimens, *Spine* 23:17-24, 1998.

83. Parmar HV, Raymaker R: Neck injury from rear impact road traffic accidents: prognosis in persons seeking compensation, *Injury* 24:75-78, 1993.

84. Pennie BH, Agambar LJ: Whiplash injuries: a trial of early management, *J Bone Joint Surg Br* 72:277-279, 1990.

85. Penning L: Prevertebral hematoma in cervical spine injury: incidence and etiologic significance, *Am J Roentgenol* 136:553-561, 1981.

86. Penning L: Changes in anatomy, motion, development, and aging in upper and lower cervical disk segments, *Clin Biomech* 3:37-47, 1991.

87. Pettersson K et al.: MRI and neurology in acute whiplash trauma: no correlation in prospective examination of 39 cases, *Acta Orthop Scand* 65:525-528, 1994.

88. Pettersson K, Toolanen G: High-dose methylprednisolone prevents extensive sick leave after whiplash injury: a prospective, randomized, double-blind study, *Spine* 23:984-989, 1998.

89. Radanov BP et al.: Role of psychosocial stress in recovery from common whiplash, *Lancet* 338: 712-715, 1991.

90. Radanov BP, Dvorak J, Valach L: Cognitive deficits in patients after soft tissue injury of the cervical spine, *Spine* 17:127-131, 1992.

91. Radanov BP et al.: Factors influencing recovery from headache after common whiplash, *Br Med J* 307:652-655, 1993.

92. Radanov BP, Sturzenegger M, Di Stefano G: Long-term outcome after whiplash injury: a 2-year follow-up considering features of injury mechanisms and somatic, radiologic, and psychosocial findings, *Medicine* 74:281-297, 1995.

93. Raney AA, Raney RB, Hunter CR: Chronic post traumatic headache and the syndrome of cervical disk lesion following head trauma, *J Neurosurg* 6:458, 1949.

94. Rauschning W, McAfee PC, Jonsson H Jr: Pathoanatomic and surgical findings in cervical spine injury, *J Spinal Disord* 2:227-230, 1989.

95. Ronnen HR et al.: Acute whiplash injury: is there a role for MR imaging? A prospective study of 100 patients, *Radiology* 201:93-96, 1996.

96. Sanders RJ, Pearce WH: The treatment of thoracic outlet syndrome: a comparison of different operations, *J Vasc Surg* 10:626-634, 1989.

97. Schellhas K et al.: Cervical discogenic pain: prospective correlation of magnetic resonance imaging and discography in asymptomatic subjects and pain sufferers, *Spine* 21:300-312, 1996.

98. Schneider R, Schemm G: Vertebral artery insufficiency in acute and chronic spinal trauma, *J Neurosurg* 18:348, 1961.

99. Schrader H et al.: Natural evolution of late whiplash syndrome outside the medicolegal context, *Lancet* 347:1201-1211, 1996.

100. Schutt CH, Dohan FC: Neck injury to women in auto accidents, *JAMA* 206:2689-2692, 1968.

101. Selecki BR, Williams HBL: *Injuries to the cervical spine and cord in man*, Australian Medical Association, Medical Monograph No 7., South Wales, Australian Medical, 1970.

102. Severy DM, Mathewson JH, Bechtol CO: Controlled automobile rear end collisions: an investigation of related engineering and medical phenomena, *Can Serv Med J* 11:727, 1955.

103. Shifrin LZ: Bilateral abducens nerve palsy after cervical spine extension injury: a case report, *Spine* 16:374-375, 1991.

104. Spitzer WO et al.: Scientific monograph of the Quebec Task Force on Whiplash-Associated Disorders: redefining "whiplash" and its management, *Spine* 20(suppl):S1-S73, 1995.

105. Squires B, Gargan MF, Bannister GC: Soft-tissue injuries of the cervical spine: 15 year follow-up, *J Bone Joint Surg Br* 78:955-957, 1996.

106. States JD, Korn MW, Massengill JB: The enigma of whiplash, *N Y State J Med* 70:2978-2980, 1970.

107. Tamura T: Cranial symptoms after cervical injury: etiology and treatment of the Barre-Lieou syndrome, *J Bone Joint Surg Br* 71:283-287, 1989.

108. Teasell RW, Shapiro AP, Mailis A: Medical management of whiplash injury, *Spine* 7:481-499, 1993.

109. Tissington-Tatlow WF, Bammer HG: Syndrome of vertebral artery compression, *Neurology* F:331, 1957.

110. Twomey LT, Taylor JR: Whiplash syndrome: pathoanatomy and physical treatment, *J Man Manip Ther* 1:26-29, 1993.

111. Unterharnscheidt F: Traumatic alterations in the Rhesus monkey undergoing −GX impact accelerations, *Neurotraumatology* 6:151-167, 1983.

112. Ward N: Tricyclic antidepressants for chronic low back pain, *Spine* 11:661-665, 1986.

113. Waters RL et al.: Cervical spinal cord trauma evaluation and non-operative treatment with Halo-vest immobilization, *Contemp Orthop* 14:35-45, 1987.

114. Watkinson A, Gargan MF, Bannister GC: Prognostic factors in soft tissue injuries of the cervical spine, *Injury* 22:307-309, 1991.

115. Webb JK et al.: Hidden flexion injury of the cervical spine, *J Bone Joint Surg Br* 58:332-337, 1976.

116. White AA et al.: Biomechanical analysis of clinical stability in the cervical spine, *Clin Orthop* 109:85-95, 1975.

117. Whitecloud TS, Seago RA: Cervical discogenic syndrome: results of operative intervention in patients with positive discography, *Spine* 12:313-316, 1981.

118. Wickstrom JK et al.: Hyperextension and hyperflexion injuries to the head and neck of primates. In Gurdjain ER, Thomas LM, eds: *Neckache and backache*, Springfield, Ill, 1970, Charles C Thomas, pp. 108-119.

119. Yoganandan N, Pintar F, Kleinberger M: Whiplash injury: biomechanical experimentation, *Spine* 24:83-85, 1999.

Degenerative and Isthmic Spondylolisthesis: Evaluation and Management

Richard A. Balderston, Russell S. Brummett, II

In 1772 Herbiniaux, a Belgian obstetrician, made the first observation of a spondylolisthesis in a woman with a difficult delivery secondary to narrowing of her pelvic outlet caused by a forward slip of the fifth lumbar vertebra on the sacrum. The actual term *spondylolisthesis* was coined in 1854 by Kilian.[33] Subsequent investigators demonstrated that sectioning of the pars interarticularis resulted in an olisthesis. Isthmic spondylolisthesis is defined as a translation of one vertebral body on the adjacent caudal vertebra in an anterior direction secondary to bilateral failure of the pars interarticularis occurring either from fracture or elongation of the pars.

Degenerative spondylolisthesis was described by Junghanns[18] in 1930 as a translation or pseudospondylolisthesis with no identifiable defect in the posterior neural arch. Macnab[24] reported this entity in the English literature in the early 1950s, and Newman[28] further defined the pathologic process by describing facet arthritis and hypertrophy at the level of the slippage. Neumann formally introduced the term *degenerative spondylolisthesis*.

EPIDEMIOLOGY

Valkenburg and Haanen[40] noted a 10% prevalence of degenerative spondylolisthesis in women in their seventh decade or older. Several studies have demonstrated that women are affected at a rate five times greater than men.[22] In addition, patients with diabetes mellitus have an increased prevalence of degenerative spondylolisthesis.

The prevalence of adult isthmic spondylolisthesis is approximately 6% across all demographic groups. Spondylolysis, or a defect in the pars without associated slippage, has been found to have an incidence of 6.4% in Caucasian men, 2.8% in African-American men, 2.3% in Caucasian women, and 1.1% in African-American women. It is interesting that although pars defects are nearly twice as common in boys as in girls, high-grade slippage is four times more common in girls.[23] The

> ### DEFINITIONS AND EPIDEMIOLOGY
>
> **DEGENERATIVE SPONDYLOLISTHESIS**
> - Women affected at rate five times greater than men
> - Increased prevalence in patients with diabetes mellitus
> - Associated with differential mobility between spinal segments
> - Limited motion and relatively fixed position usually of inferior vertebra—most commonly L5
>
> **ISTHMIC SPONDYLOLISTHESIS**
> - Etiology somewhat controversial
> - Cause multifactorial and related to developmental, genetic, and biomechanical factors
> - Prevalence in adults about 6% across all demographic groups
>   - 6.4% in Caucasian men
>   - 2.8% in African-American men
>   - 2.3% in Caucasian women
>   - 1.1% in African-American women
> - Pars defects nearly twice as common in boys as girls; high-grade slippage four times more common in girls
> - Highest known incidence in Alaskan Eskimos (as high as 50%)

highest known incidence of isthmic spondylolisthesis is in Alaskan Eskimos, being as high as 50%.

ETIOLOGY AND PATHOPHYSIOLOGY

Degenerative spondylolisthesis is associated with a differential mobility between spinal segments.[30] This differential mobility is related to two factors. First is a limited motion and relatively fixed position usually of the inferior vertebra. This vertebra is most commonly L5, which is physically more attached by ligaments to the sacrum and pelvis than is the L4 vertebra. An obvious cause of increased stability is hemisacralization of L5, which has been reported to be four times more frequent in patients with degenerative spondylolisthesis than in the normal population.[22] In addition, the relative position of L5 within the pelvis as determined by its relationship to an intercrestal line drawn between the superior aspect of the iliac crests may cause increased stress at the L4 to L5 disc level when this line intercedes the L5 vertebral body and the disc lies superior to this.

With aging and chronic stress to the lower lumbar spine, persistent translatory forces cause increased wear on the L4 to L5 joint complex compared with L5 to S1. With normal degenerative disc disease, the mechanics of the L4 to L5 joints are altered to produce an altered force on the facet joints, which in the long term increases facet hypertrophy.[11] With time, increased translation occurs.

The exact etiology of isthmic spondylolisthesis remains somewhat controversial. The cause is multifactorial and appears to be related to developmental, genetic, and biomechanical factors. It is generally agreed that the failure of the pars and subsequent development of an isthmic spondylolisthesis is the result of a combination of both mechanical and familial factors. Sagi et al.[33] in 1998 demonstrated that uneven distribution of isthmic ossification results in formation of a potential stress riser in the region of the pars in the lower lumbar vertebrae, which is then susceptible to fatigue fractures. Fredrickson et al.[8] noted an inherited predisposition for spondylolisthesis and hypothesized that first-degree relatives were more prone to develop a defect in the cartilaginous region of the developing pars. Wynne-Davies and Scott[44] observed an increased incidence of dysplastic lesions in affected relatives and suggested that the inheritance pattern was autosomal dominant with variable expressivity and reduced penetrance. As Fredrickson et al. had previously noted, Wynne-Davies and Scott also observed an increased incidence of spina bifida occulta and believe this is an important marker of a spondylolisthesis predisposition.

Wiltse et al.[43] theorized that spondylolysis is a stress fracture in the pars and that repetitive microtrauma or microstresses are a factor in its development. Repetitive hyperextension in which the caudal edge of the inferior articular facet of L4 makes contact with the pars of L5 is considered to play a causative role. This is supported by a higher incidence in participants in certain sports activities, such as gymnasts,[16] football linemen,[37] and weight lifters.[1] Thus the etiology is multifactorial with an inherited predisposition that possibly manifests as a weakening of the pars and a subsequent defect occurring after repeated microtrauma.

PATHOANATOMY

Degenerative and isthmic spondylolisthesis usually describes an anterior translation of one vertebra compared with the subjacent vertebra. The amount of translation required to define degenerative spondylolisthesis varies among different authors, but the lower limit is between 2 and 5 mm, with a maximum percentage of slippage rarely exceeding 40%.[13] Isthmic spondylolisthe-

sis may present with any degree of slippage, varying from very minimal anterior translation to complete spondyloptosis. Although it has been well documented that significant slip progression may occur in childhood and adolescence,[36] adult slip progression is rarely discussed and its clinical importance is even disputed.[11] However, Floman[6] recently demonstrated that adult slip progression was associated with disc degeneration at the olisthetic level. As the biomechanical integrity of the disc is lost, the previously stable lumbosacral slip may then progress and result in pain and nerve root compression, much like that which occurs during the development of a degenerative spondylolisthesis.

Slippage at L4 to L5 occurs approximately six times more frequently than at the L3 to L4 disc space; degenerative spondylolisthesis may be present at any level of the lumbar spine.[22] Isthmic spondylolisthesis occurs most often at the lumbosacral junction. This is a result of pars defects being most prevalent at L5 (7%) followed by L4 and L3.[32] Oblique x-rays as well as a CT scan demonstrate an intact neural arch, thus differentiating degenerative spondylolisthesis from isthmic spondylolisthesis, in which the defect is in the pars interarticularis.

With slippage comes a constellation of anatomic changes. Commonly there is expansion of the facet joints due to degeneration resulting in an increase in facet joint surface area.[31] In addition, disc space degeneration and narrowing of the disc that subsequently occurs cause infolding of the ligamentum flavum. Fibrocartilaginous scar tissue may also accumulate at the site of the isthmic pars defect. The combination of these and other factors can lead to thecal sac encroachment.

PATHOANATOMIC FACTORS

- Anterior translation of one vertebra compared with subjacent vertebra.
  - Amount of translation is from 2 to 5 mm, with maximum percentage of slippage rarely exceeding 40%.
  - Posterior elements of superior vertebra are closer to posterior vertebral body of inferior vertebra, thus narrowing spinal canal.
  - Isthmic spondylolisthesis may have any degree of slippage, varying from very minimal anterior translation to complete spondyloptosis.
  - Lateral translation of superior vertebra is possible, which may or may not be associated with rotatory deformity.
- As biomechanical integrity of disc is lost, previously stable lumbosacral slip may progress, causing pain and nerve root compression.
- Slippage at L4 to L5 occurs about six times more frequently than at L3 to L4 disc space.
  - Degenerative spondylolisthesis may be seen at any level of lumbar spine.
  - Isthmic spondylolisthesis occurs most often at lumbosacral junction.
    - This is a result of pars defects being most prevalent at L5 (7%), followed by L4 (10%) and L3 (3%).

In either type of spondylolisthesis, spinal nerve impingement may be caused by multiple factors. With anterior translation of one vertebra on another, the posterior elements of the superior vertebra are closer to the posterior vertebral body of the inferior vertebra, thus narrowing the spinal canal. Thus the inferior facet joints of L4, the most commonly affected level in degenerative slips, will translate anteriorly with respect to the posterior body of L5.[34] The second common anatomic change that contributes to spinal nerve impingement is facet joint expansion due to degeneration and hypertrophy of the superior facet of L5. As this process occurs, the aspect of the facet joint immediately adjacent to the pedicle of L5 expands anteriorly from its position immediately posterior to the L5 nerve at the level of the L5 pedicle.[31] This process is primarily degenerative in nature.

Within the foramen itself, this material may accumulate, which produces pressure on the nerve associated with the superior vertebra as this nerve exits below its pedicle.

In contrast, isthmic spondylolisthesis more often demonstrates impingement of the L5 root secondary to accumulation of tissue within the lateral recess at the site of the pars defect. S1 nerve root compression occurs with higher-grade slips and is caused by tension from stretch of the root over the posterior edge of the sacrum.

Additional deformities with respect to positioning of the two vertebrae may also occur simultaneously. There may be lateral translation of the superior vertebra, which may or may not be associated with rotatory deformity. This rotatory deformity usually has a common axis between the middle and posterior columns of the spine. This additional type of deformity, scoliosis in the frontal plane with a Cobb angle greater than 10 degrees, may also occur.[29] These types of deformities may be classified as those with idiopathic scoliosis that has occurred in adolescence or early adulthood or as a primary de novo scoliosis resulting primarily from differential severity of disc degeneration in the frontal plane, resulting in tilting of the L4 vertebra due to this asymmetric loss of disc height.[22]

CLINICAL SYMPTOMS AND PHYSICAL EXAMINATION

The clinical presentation and physical examination findings of both isthmic and degenerative spondylolisthesis have many similarities. The most common chief complaint in patients with degenerative spondylolisthesis is back pain. The clinical course of the back pain as described by the patient is highly variable and may or may not be related to a traumatic episode. The back pain is usually mechanical and is relieved by recumbency. During the course of any particular day, the pain usually worsens as the day progresses and with increasing activity.

Unfortunately, a great many spinal disorders may produce very similar symptoms. At this point, the clinician cannot really determine if the back pain is related to abnormal translation forces at the level of the spondy-

lolisthesis, disc degeneration at the level of the spondylolisthesis, or some other spinal ailment entirely. Strategies will be discussed later in this chapter to aid the clinician if it becomes important for the surgeon to know with a little more clarity what is causing the patient's pain.

Another common presenting symptom is neurogenic claudication. This symptom results from chronic spinal nerve compression as described in the section on pathoanatomy.[15] The pain is usually multinerve radicular pain that affects multiple dermatomes and muscle groups in the lower extremities, most commonly involving L4, L5, and S1 distributions. The patients may also describe a monoradicular nerve pattern, usually involving L4 or L5. The pain in the distribution of the L4 nerve will commonly radiate down the anterior thigh to the knee and anterior calf. The pain in the L5 distribution is most commonly described in the area of the posterolateral thigh, lateral calf, and dorsum of the foot, occasionally extending directly onto the dorsum of the great toe. Patients may also describe lumbar flexion positions that allow them to diminish pain and increase their endurance. For example, patients may describe leaning forward while walking. This leaning-forward posture may occur while the patient is using a shopping cart, and

---

CLINICAL PRESENTATION AND PHYSICAL EXAMINATION FINDINGS

- Most common chief complaint: Back pain
  - Usually mechanical and relieved by recumbency
  - Usually worsens as day progresses and with increasing activity
  - Similar to pain of many spinal disorders, possibly related to abnormal translation forces at level of spondylolisthesis, disc degeneration at level of spondylolisthesis, or other spinal ailment entirely
- Neurogenic claudication
  - Results from chronic spinal nerve compression
  - Usually multinerve radicular pain that affects multiple dermatomes and muscle groups in lower extremities, most commonly involving L4, L5, and S1 distributions
    - L4—radiates down anterior thigh to knee and anterior calf
    - L5—area of posterolateral thigh, lateral calf, and dorsum of foot, occasionally extending directly onto dorsum of great toe
- Specific lumbar flexion positions may diminish pain and increase endurance
  - Example: Leaning forward while walking
- Symptoms worsened by any maneuver producing lumbar spine extension
  - Increased pain while walking down flight of steps
  - Paradoxically, feel weaker walking downhill in an extended posture as compared with walking uphill
  - Frequently patients who sleep supine or prone produce hyperextended position that awakens them from sleep with severe pain radiating down one or both legs
- Cauda equina syndrome unlikely

indeed they may comment that they are able to walk much farther in a supermarket while utilizing a shopping cart than they can in a shopping mall without a similar supportive device. Similarly, symptoms may be worsened by any maneuver that produces extension of the lumbar spine. Patients may feel increased pain while walking down a flight of steps. Paradoxically they may describe feeling weaker while walking downhill in an extended posture as compared with walking uphill. Frequently patients who sleep supine or prone may produce a hyper-extended position that will wake them from sleep with severe pain radiating down one or both legs.[21,42]

Cauda equina syndrome is an unlikely symptom in this patient population. However, careful questioning with respect to subtle changes in bladder function may be indicated. The physical examination of patients with degenerative spondylolisthesis may not be that much different from a normal physical examination of an age-matched control patient. In the standing position, the patient may assume a more flexed position with anterior translation of the thorax upon the pelvis. With palpation of the lumbar spine, a palpable step-off may be noted at the level of the spondylolisthesis. The iliolumbar ligaments, sacroiliac joints, sciatic notches, other spinous processes, paraspinal muscles, and trochanteric bursae should all be palpated and the presence of tenderness noted.

Range of motion of the lumbar spine is usually some-what limited due to the age and normal degenerative changes associated with this patient population. Forward flexion usually does not produce radicular symptoms. At this point the examiner should attempt to extend the lumbar spine to ascertain whether neurologic symptoms are being reproduced. Range of motion of the hip joints is also checked because many patients in this population have degenerative arthritis of one or both hips.

The neurologic examination includes sensory reflex and motor evaluation of the lumbar and upper sacral spinal nerves. Generalized hyporeflexia is usually present in this age-group. Differential loss of the quadriceps tendon reflex may indicate a compromise of the L4 nerve. Quadriceps weakness and atrophy should be noted. Extensor hallusis weakness should also be tested, because weakness would indicate an L5 nerve abnormality.

RADIOGRAPHIC EVALUATION

The diagnosis of spondylolisthesis is made with the lateral lumbar x-ray film. Concomitant findings may include disc space narrowing, end-plate irregularities, sclerosis, osteophytes, and traction spurs anteriorly about the disc. Flexion-extension views may be obtained but rarely demonstrate significant additional transla-tional instability.[42] Oblique views may demonstrate a pars interarticularis defect, which may be the only differ-entiating factor between an isthmic and degenerative spondylolisthesis in this age-group.

For patients with predominantly mechanical low back pain that has responded to conservative modalities, further x-ray evaluation is not indicated. With persistent

---

DIAGNOSIS

- Lateral lumbar x-ray film
  - Disc space narrowing
  - End-plate irregularities
  - Sclerosis
  - Osteophytes
  - Traction spurs anteriorly about the disc
- Flexion-extension views: Rarely demonstrate significant additional translational instability
- Oblique views: Pars interarticularis defect, which may be the only differentiating factor between an isthmic and degenerative spondylolisthesis
- No further x-ray evaluation required for patients with predominantly mechanical low back pain responding to conservative modalities
- Magnetic resonance imaging: Persistent back or leg symptoms unresponsive to conservative means:
  - Typically diminished cross-sectional area of spinal canal at level of the spondylolisthesis
  - Compression of L5 nerve at level of superior facet just inferior to disc at pedicle level
  - May be abnormalities in thickening of ligamentum flavum and discal compressive pathology
- Myelography and postmyelogram computed tomography (CT) scan: Helpful in patients with severe compression for greater detail of the components of compression on each spinal nerve
- Technetium bone scanning: Especially in patients with suddenly increased back pain, where concomitant fracture must be ruled out

---

back or leg symptomatology that is unresponsive to con-servative means, magnetic resonance imaging (MRI) is the next study of choice. Typically there is a diminished cross-sectional area of the spinal canal at the level of the spondylolisthesis secondary to the anatomic changes previously discussed. The MRI scan may also demon-strate the compression of the L5 nerve at the level of the superior facet just inferior to the disc at the level of the pedicle. In addition, abnormalities with respect to thick-ening of the ligamentum flavum and discal compressive pathology may also be noted.

In patients for whom surgery is contemplated, mye-lography and a postmyelogram computed tomography (CT) scan may be helpful in those patients with severe compression where the surgeon would like to know in greater detail the components of the compression upon each of the spinal nerves.

Technetium bone scanning may be obtained, espe-cially in patients with a sudden increase in back pain, where a concomitant fracture needs to be ruled out. Finally, metastatic disease, which may occur at the level of the spondylolisthesis, is usually demonstrated nicely on the MRI scan.

DIFFERENTIAL DIAGNOSIS

Epidemiologic studies have demonstrated that many roentgenographic findings, including degenerative and isthmic spondylolisthesis, may be entirely asympto-

---

DIFFERENTIAL DIAGNOSIS

- Patients with degenerative scoliosis may have an increased risk of degenerative spondylolisthesis.
- Examine patient in standing position and then leaning forward to confirm diagnosis of concomitant scoliosis, requiring standing x-ray films in posteroanterior (PA) and lateral plane of entire spine.
- Among elderly, degenerative disease of cervical spine is extremely common and may produce symptoms that radiate to lower extremities.
  - Any patient with bilateral leg weakness, hyperreflexia, and positive Babinski's reflex requires thorough upper motor neuron evaluation.
  - Flexion-extension plain x-ray films and magnetic resonance imaging (MRI) scan of cervical spine are then performed to aid in diagnosis of cervical compression.
- Osteoarthritis of the hip is seen in 10% to 20% of patients with degenerative spondylolisthesis.
  - Pain from degenerated hip commonly radiates to anterior thigh and may mimic L4 radiculopathy.
  - Medial knee pain, caused by degenerative joint disease or meniscal pathology, may mimic L4 radiculopathy.
  - Peripheral vascular disease is common in this patient group, and symptoms may closely mimic neurogenic claudication.

---

matic. Patients with a degenerative scoliosis may have an increased risk of a degenerative spondylolisthesis.[28] Examination of the patient in a standing position and then leaning forward will usually confirm the diagnosis of concomitant scoliosis. Standing x-rays in the postero-anterior (PA) and lateral plane of the entire spine are then necessary.

In the elderly population, degenerative disease of the cervical spine is extremely common and may produce symptoms that radiate to the lower extremities. Certainly any patient with bilateral leg weakness, hyperreflexia, and a positive Babinski's reflex requires a thorough upper motor neuron evaluation. Flexion-extension plain x-ray films and an MRI scan of the cervical spine are then performed and should aid in the diagnosis of cervical compression.

Osteoarthritis of the hip is noted in 10% to 20% of patients with degenerative spondylolisthesis. Pain from a degenerated hip commonly radiates to the anterior thigh and may mimic an L4 radiculopathy. In addition, medial knee pain, which may be caused by degenerative joint disease or meniscal pathology, may also mimic an L4 radiculopathy. Skilled care must be taken in all of these patients to palpate and perform a range of motion of both the hip and knee. Peripheral vascular disease is common in this patient group, and symptoms from it may closely mimic neurogenic claudication. Pain with ambulation is a typical finding, but it is related to decreased perfusion and oxygen delivery to the lower extremities during activity. Thus patients will have more difficulty walking uphill than patients with degenerative spondylolisthesis due to spinal stenosis. One test that

may be helpful is to have the patient ride a stationary bicycle in the flexed forward position. Neurogenic claudication from spinal stenosis due to degenerative spondylolisthesis will usually not produce increased pain. However, peripheral vascular disease will produce cramping in both calves the longer the duration of exercise. Patients with peripheral vascular disease need only to stop their activity to alleviate their symptoms, whereas patients with degenerative spondylolisthesis often must sit and flex the lumbar spine to produce symptom relief. There is a subset of patients who have both diseases. Proper studies are usually necessary to quantify the diminution of blood flow to the lower extremities. With equal degrees of vascular and neurologic involvement, the vascular problem is usually addressed first with surgical management. Patients with diabetic neuropathy may rarely have a painful radiculopathy. In patients with degenerative spondylolisthesis who also have diabetes and pain of a radicular nature, electromyography (EMG) and nerve conduction studies should be performed. Those patients with a significant neuropathic involvement due to diabetes have a diminished chance of a good result from conservative or surgical management.

Patients with increasing, severe low back pain in whom conservative treatment does not alleviate symptoms should be treated as if their spondylolisthesis were asymptomatic. Then a complete evaluation for other causes of low back pain, including fracture, infection, metastatic disease, or retroperitoneal tumor, should be sought until proven otherwise.

PATIENT MANAGEMENT
Conservative Treatment

When discussing any spinal disorder, it is important for the clinician to separate patients into two groups: those who are back-pain predominant and those who are leg-pain predominant. As you will see with spondylolisthesis, management of these two patient groups is completely different. Many problems related to patient expectation and outcome are related to the physician's inability to separate patients into these two primary categories. Thus patients who are back-pain predominant, 90% low back pain with 10% radicular component, are usually not surgical candidates. Decompression of the spinal nerve compression in a patient who is only having minimal radicular symptoms would only cause frustration for both patient and surgeon. For patients who are back-pain predominant, nonsteroidal antiinflammatory medication, a supervised physical therapy program including paraspinal and abdominal strengthening, and aerobic conditioning are all appropriate treatment options. Aerobic conditioning may include swimming, as well as nonimpact loading exercises such as stair climbing, stationary bicycle, or Nordic Track type of activities. Weight reduction, where appropriate, is also a good topic to emphasize. These interventions may help the patient to avoid surgery, particularly when symptoms are back-pain predominant without neurologic deficit.

PATIENT MANAGEMENT

- Clinician views patients in two groups
  - Back-pain predominant
  - Leg-pain predominant
- Back-pain predominant
  - 90% low back pain with 10% radicular component; usually not surgical candidates
  - Nonsteroidal antiinflammatory medication, supervised physical therapy program including paraspinal and abdominal strengthening, and aerobic conditioning
- Leg-pain predominant
  - Typically 6 to 12 months of symptoms needed before proceeding with further testing to determine cause of back pain
  - Nonoperative management as for back-pain predominant
    - Epidural steroids added for patients with initial failure of conservative treatment
  - Surgery done if fail nonoperative care, after 6 to 12 weeks of relentless radiculopathy

---

Nonoperative management of patients who are leg-pain predominant begins in a similar fashion. In addition, epidural steroids are usually added for those patients who have had an initial failure of the above treatment.[17] Epidural steroids are appropriate for patients who have monoradicular and neurogenic claudication syndromes. We have found that utilization of selective spinal nerve blocks with steroid delivery performed under image-intensifier localization may be extremely beneficial. At this point it is impossible to predict whether patients may indeed have weeks, months, or years of relief from this modality. At our clinic we have utilized epidural steroids three times per year when indicated for patients whose radicular symptoms do not warrant a surgical approach.

Patients Who Do Not Improve With Nonoperative Management

At the stage where patients do not improve with a period of bed rest, antiinflammatory medications, physical therapy, or epidural steroids, the treating physician must separate the treatment plan with respect to two groups of patients: those who have predominantly radiculopathy and those with predominantly low back pain. At this point these two groups of patients must be treated in an entirely different manner because the surgical indications vary greatly. For those patients with leg-pain–predominant symptomatology who have failed nonoperative care, after 6 to 12 weeks of relentless radiculopathy, surgery may be entertained. For patients with back-pain–predominant symptomatology, a much more prolonged period of nonoperative care is indicated before surgery is discussed. Typically 6 to 12 months of symptoms would be necessary before proceeding with further testing to determine the cause of the patient's back pain. At this point, if an MRI scan has not already

been obtained, then it would be performed at this time to rule out infection, tumor, or occult fracture. In the appropriate patient who has back-pain–predominant symptomatology, discography may be indicated at this time.

The Role of Discography in the Management of Patients With Back-Pain–Predominant Symptomatology Related to Degenerative and Isthmic Spondylolistheses

In general, any patient with a back-pain–predominant disorder of the lumbar spine requires diagnostic discography before any surgical procedure. Discography's main purpose is to determine levels of concordant low back pain symptomatology with low-pressure mechanical stimulation of a particular disc. In our study of spondylolisthesis and back pain, 50% of patients had symptoms of concordant back pain symptomatology related to testing of another unsuspected disc level.[3] In back-pain–predominant patients for whom discography is negative, spinal fusion surgery has a much less predictable outcome. In patients with concordant pain at the level of the spondylolisthesis, anterior fusion with or without posterior fusion will give a more reliable result than posterior fusion alone. As Vaccaro et al.[39] reported, posterior fusion for back-pain–predominant patients, especially those patients with compensation or litigation factors, has a high likelihood of failure.

OPERATIVE TREATMENT OF LEG-PAIN–PREDOMINANT SYMPTOMATOLOGY ASSOCIATED WITH DEGENERATIVE AND ISTHMIC SPONDYLOLISTHESES

The primary indication for surgery in patients with degenerative and isthmic spondylolisthesis is radicular pain unresponsive to nonoperative management. Other operative indications include presentation with symptoms of stenosis or radiculopathy, neurologic deficits or cauda equina symptoms, or severe difficulty with standing or walking secondary to sagittal plane imbalance. Patients who have physical signs of neurologic dysfunction prior to surgery have a better outcome than patients with solely radicular pain.[11] Only 10% to 15% of patients treated nonoperatively for sciatica related to degenerative or isthmic spondylolisthesis eventually require surgical management.[11]

The principal goal of surgery for lower extremity symptoms related to spondylolisthesis is decompression of the neural elements at the level of the deformity.[20,27] Patients may be frail with concomitant medical problems, and a thorough preoperative medical evaluation is required.[42] The use of epidural anesthesia may decrease the likelihood of excessive blood loss. Careful attention to patient positioning should be carried out to avoid undue pressure on bony prominences.[11]

The surgical approach includes a midline muscle-splitting incision that divides the paraspinal muscles at the level of the spinous processes and the lamina of the two involved vertebral bodies. In addition, the facet joint at the level of the compression must be completely exposed along its medial posterior and lateral aspect. The spinous processes may then be removed, followed by a decompressive laminectomy usually beginning at the inferior level of L5 and proceeding superiorly. By the time the pedicular level at L5 is reached, there is usually increasing compression of the neural elements. At this point, care must be taken to free any adhesions at the level of the ligamentum flavum and bone before continuing in the cephalad direction. For an L4 to L5 decompression the laminectomy must be carried to the midpoint of the pedicle of L4.

At this point, lateral decompression is carried out by decompressing the medial aspect of the superior facet of L5. Care must be taken to expose the L4 and L5 spinal nerves bilaterally. When a probe is used, be sure that adequate space is available for the nerve to exit at the L4 and L5 foramen.[11,22] Also the L5 spinal nerve must be retracted medially to check for disc herniation and especially a superiorly migrated free fragment. With an intact annulus, routine discectomy is not performed.

At this point in the operation, in general a bilateral lateral spinal fusion is performed. Many investigators have reported satisfactory outcome with adequate surgical decompression without surgical fusion in 60% to 96% of patients.[4,46] However, residual back pain has been reported in as many as 73% of patients who have undergone decompression without fusion.[22] The presence of a postoperative slippage with resultant mechanical instability and recurrent spinal stenosis is thought to be in part responsible for progressive leg and low back symptoms.[12,19,35]

Lombardi et al.[22] retrospectively evaluated three different surgical approaches in 47 patients with symptomatic spondylolisthesis. In patients who had bilateral lateral spinal fusion, clinical results were greatly enhanced in contrast to procedures not incorporating a fusion.

The role of fusion in patients who have undergone decompression for degenerative and isthmic spondy-lolisthesis was definitively clarified by Herkowitz and Kurz[12] in a prospective concurrent series of well-matched patient groups who underwent decompression with or without fusion. For patients with fusion, 96% had a good to excellent result compared with only 46% who had a good to excellent result when posterior fusion was not performed.[12] These results are in agreement with the findings of other retrospective studies,[21,35] further demonstrating the importance of including a fusion (Figure 40-1).

The use of internal pedicle screw fixation has become much more widely accepted as an adjunct to spinal fusion in the surgical treatment of degenerative and isthmic spondylolisthesis. There is still some debate as to whether instrumentation truly improves fusion rates and clinical outcome. A recent study by Moller and Hedlund[26] failed to demonstrate a superior outcome with supplementary instrumentation over fusion alone in 77 patients. However, other authors have found improved fusion rates and continue to recommend the use of instrumentation to augment fusions.[9,41] In 1994 the largest retrospective historical cohort study of pedicle screw fixation in addition to bilateral lateral fusion was reported.[45] A total of 2684 patients with symptomatic spondylolisthesis were reviewed. This study demonstrated a statistically higher fusion rate in patients who underwent pedicle screw fixation to supplement their fusion than in noninstrumented patients (82.5% versus 74.5%). In patients with leg pain–predominant spondylolisthesis we currently perform bilateral lateral fusion with or without instrumentation (Figure 40-2). Factors related to the use of instrumentation include osteopenia, height of disc space, patient preference, and additional pathology, including rotatory scoliosis.

The question with regard to reduction of high-grade isthmic spondylolisthesis is a controversial one. Several authors have reported unacceptable pseudarthrosis rates following in situ fusion for high-grade spondylolisthesis. Causative factors are likely the increased stress on posterolateral bone graft, relatively small surface area for grafting, coexisting sagittal plane imbalance, and an incompetent lumbosacral disc. Therefore reconstruction must take into account the paramount importance of anterior column support. Rigid instrumentation and restoration of lumbosacral competence, either through anterior grafting or restoring spinal alignment, are essential. In addition, major neurologic complications with instrumented reduction procedures occur in as many as 30% of cases. Most complications have been temporary, but several studies reported the occurrence of permanent neurologic injury with reduction of high-grade spondylolisthesis even in the hands of accomplished deformity surgeons.[2,14,25] These studies have also demonstrated that the most important factor predicting patient success in function, pain, and satisfaction was the presence of a solid arthrodesis, which we believe can be accomplished with adequate anterior column support and rigid posterior stabilization. These reasons, as well as our inability to justify the risks of a reduction procedure, have led us to

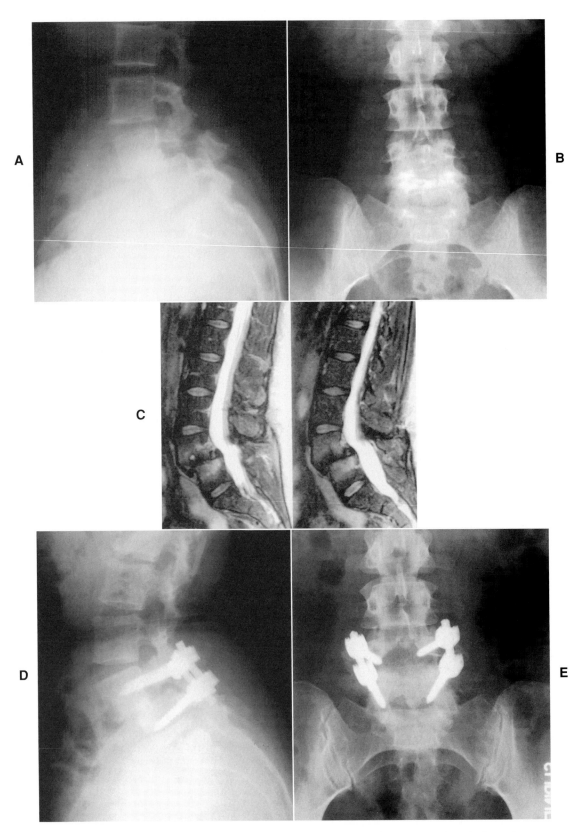

Figure 40-1.   A 50-year-old woman had a 5-year history of predominantly right lateral thigh and foot pain and associated lower back pain. Examination demonstrated a palpable step-off at L4 to L5. **A** and **B,** Films demonstrated an L4 to L5 grade II spondylolisthesis and associated disc space narrowing with an isthmic defect of the pars interarticularis. **C,** An MRI scan showed the spondylolisthesis and associated end-plate inflammatory changes. **D** and **E,** An L4 laminectomy and posterior spinal fusion with instrumentation and bilateral lateral fusion was performed at L4 to L5. Postoperatively the patient's symptoms resolved, and she resumed activities as tolerated without difficulty.

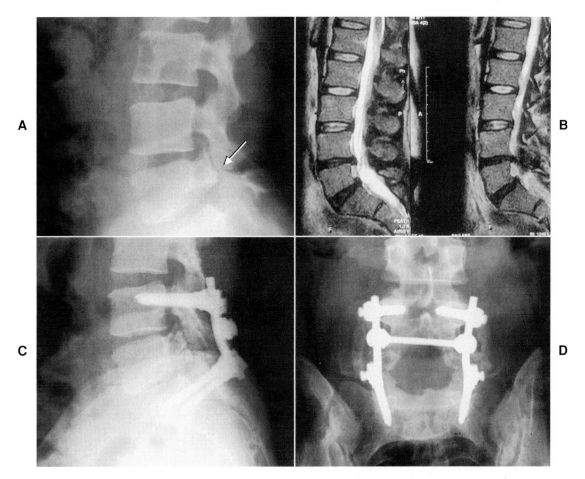

Figure 40-2. **A,** A 48-year-old man with a 10-year history of lower back pain and worsening right buttock, lateral leg, and dorsal foot pain initially responded to physical therapy and selective nerve root blocks. **B,** Symptoms recurred 1 year later, and an MRI scan demonstrated the L5 to S1 spondylolisthesis and degenerative disc disease of L4 to L5 and L5 to S1 with herniation of L4 to L5 and caudal migration of disc fragment. **C** and **D,** Operative management was elected and included posterior spinal fusion, L4 to L5 laminectomy and discectomy, and pedicle screw instrumentation. Films demonstrated incorporation of the graft and additional fusion mass formation. At follow-up all symptoms had resolved and the patient was tolerating all activities.

recommend the use of a postural reduction with circumferential arthrodesis without direct reduction of the spondylolisthesis.

OPERATIVE TREATMENT OF BACK-PAIN–PREDOMINANT SYMPTOMATOLOGY ASSOCIATED WITH DEGENERATIVE AND ISTHMIC SPONDYLOLISTHESES

Those rare patients with degenerative and isthmic spondylolisthesis who are candidates for surgery related to back-pain–predominant symptoms are evaluated by discography. Patients who demonstrate a positive discogram at the spondylolisthesis level then have a surgical fusion performed. Because of the pain reproduction factors inside the disc that are stimulated by the discography, anterior fusion is always performed. At this time we perform a retroperitoneal approach,

inserting a structural graft or prosthesis at the affected level (Figure 40-3). During anterior surgery, care must be taken to avoid the presacral sympathetic plexus because damage to this structure may result in retrograde ejaculation. The graft material may include femoral ring or bone dowels. One or two bone dowels may be used. A prosthetic choice would include the BAK or other titanium cage technology. At the time of the writing of this chapter, the issue of stand-alone fusion with respect to anterior fixation devices in patients with spondylolisthesis is highly questionable.[7,10] For this reason a posterior bilateral lateral fusion with decompression and instrumentation is also used. In patients who have discography positive for two levels of concordant pain, anterior fusion is performed at two levels followed by posterior decompression and instrumented fusion over the same levels posteriorly (Figure 40-4).

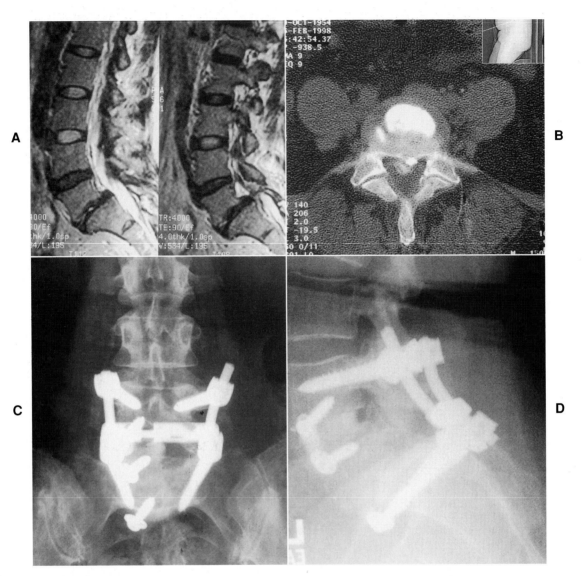

Figure 40-3.   A 43-year-old woman presented with a 1-year history of primarily lower back pain and less severe right lateral thigh and leg pain. Epidural injections alleviated the lower back pain somewhat; however, right lower extremity pain persisted. **A,** An MRI scan demonstrates L4 to L5 and L5 to S1 degenerative disc disease and an L5 to S1 spondylolisthesis with associated right L5 foraminal narrowing. **B,** A discogram was performed and was positive for concordant pain reproduction at L5 to S1 disc level, and a postdiscogram CT scan demonstrated disc fissuring of L4 to L5 as evidenced by extravasation of dye into the spinal canal. **C** and **D,** Operative management consisted of an anterior/posterior fusion with femoral ring allograft anteriorly and pedicle screw fixation posteriorly in conjunction with a bilateral lateral fusion and decompression of L5 neural foramen. At follow-up both the lower back pain and right lower extremity pain were essentially resolved, and the patient was tolerating all activities.

The results of surgical management of radiculopathy are 70% to 85% successful, whereas the relief of low back symptoms is slightly less predicable over the long term.[15,38] Increased age and associated morbidities are significant risk factors for diminished success of the outcome over a long-term follow-up. Deyo et al.[5] have demonstrated as many as 25% of elderly patients will have concomitant orthopedic and systemic complications that compromise long-term results. The importance of patient selection cannot be overly stressed when treating this pool of elderly, often frail, patients.

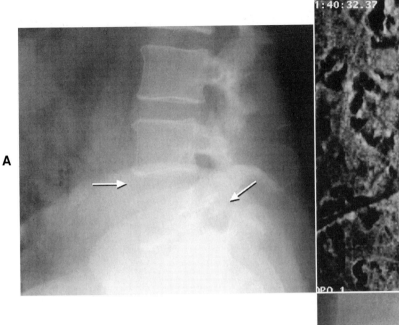

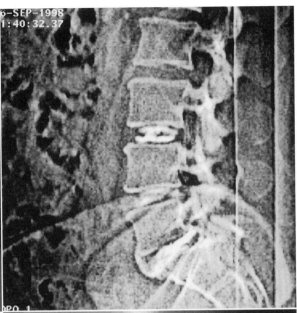

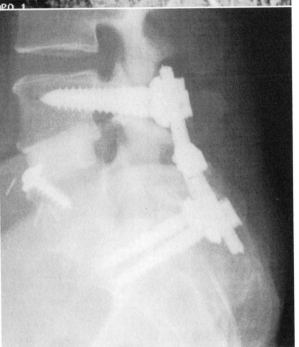

Figure 40-4. A 40-year-old man presented with the chief complaint of progressive lower back pain and associated left posterior thigh, calf, and dorsal foot pain that began after sustaining a fall 2 years prior to presentation. The pain was aggravated by flexion and extension of the lumbar spine, and the patient had received little relief with antiinflammatories, physical therapy, and epidural injections. **A,** X-ray films demonstrated the L5 to S1 spondylolisthesis with associated facet hypertrophy. An MRI scan also showed degenerative disc disease at the L4 to L5 and L5 to S1 intervertebral disc levels. **B,** A discogram revealed concordant pain at L4 to L5 and L5 to S1, and CT scan demonstrated a normal L3 to L4 disc but noted a degenerative disc at L4 to L5 and left lateral annular tear of L5 to S1. **C,** An L4 to S1 anterior fusion with femoral rings was performed and supplemented with posterior decompression and fusion with pedicle screw instrumentation. At follow-up, significant improvement of the patient's lower back pain and near total resolution of left lower extremity pain had been achieved.

OPERATIVE TREATMENT FOR BACK-PAIN–PREDOMINANT PATIENTS

- Associated with degenerative and isthmic spondylolistheses
- Anterior surgical fusion
- Perform on patients who demonstrate a positive discogram at the spondylolisthesis level only
  - Approach retroperitoneally with insertion of a structural graft or prosthesis at the affected level
  - Avoid presacral sympathetic plexus because damage to this structure may result in retrograde ejaculation
  - Graft material may include femoral ring or bone dowels
  - Prosthetic choice includes the BAK or other titanium cage technology

- Posterior bilateral lateral fusion with decompression and instrumentation
- Patients with discography positive for two levels of concordant pain: Perform anterior fusion at two levels followed by posterior decompression and instrumented fusion over the same levels posteriorly
- Results of surgical management of radiculopathy: 70% to 85% successful, whereas relief of low back symptoms is slightly less predicable over long term

SELECTED REFERENCES

Herkowitz AN, Kurz LT: Degenerative lumbar spondylolisthesis with spinal stenosis: a prospective study comparing decompression and decompression and intertransverse process arthrodesis, *J Bone Joint Surg Am* 73:802-808, 1991.

Kim SS et al.: Factors affecting fusion rate in adult spondylolisthesis, *Spine* 15:979-984, 1990.

Lombardi JS et al.: Treatment of degenerative spondylolisthesis, *Spine* 10:821-927, 1985.

Lonstein JE: Spondylolisthesis in children: cause, natural history and management, *Spine* 24(24):2640-2648, 1999.

Newman PH: The etiology of spondylolisthesis, *J Bone Joint Surg Br* 45:39-59, 1963.

Wiltse LL, Widell E Jr, Jackson DW: Fatigue fracture: the basic lesion in isthmic spondylolisthesis, *J Bone Joint Surg Am* 57:17-22, 1975.

REFERENCES

1. Bradford D: Management of spondylolysis and spondylolisthesis, *Instruct Course Lect* 32:151-162, 1983.
2. Bradford DS, Gotfried Y: Staged salvage reconstruction of grade IV and V spondylolisthesis, *J Bone Joint Surg Am* 69:191-202, 1987.
3. Cohen MW, Maurer PM, Balderston RA: *Pre-operative evaluation of adult isthmic spondylolisthesis with discography.* Presented at the annual meeting of International Society for the Study of the Lumbar Spine, Adelaide, Australia, April 19, 2000.
4. Dall BE, Rowe DE: Degenerative spondylolisthesis: its surgical management, *Spine* 10:668-672, 1985.
5. Deyo RA et al.: Morbidity and mortality in association with operations on the lumbar spine: the influence of age, diagnosis and procedure, *J Bone Joint Surg Am* 74:536-543, 1992.
6. Floman Y: Progression of lumbosacral isthmic spondylolisthesis in adults, *Spine* 25:342-347, 2000.
7. Flynn JC, Hogue MA: Anterior fusion of the lumbar spine, *J Bone Joint Surg Am* 61:1143-1150, 1979.
8. Fredrickson BE et al.: The natural history of spondylolysis and spondylolisthesis, *J Bone Joint Surg Am* 66:699-707, 1984.
9. Fueger P et al.: *Transpedicular fixation for the treatment of isthmic spondylolisthesis.* Presented at the eighth annual meeting of the North American Spine Society, San Diego, Calif, Oct 1993.
10. Grobler LJ et al.: Decompression for degenerative spondylolisthesis and spinal stenosis at L4-5: the effects on facet joint morphology, *Spine* 18:1475-1482, 1993.
11. Grobler LJ, Wiltse LL: Classification, nonoperative, and operative treatment of spondylolisthesis. In Frymoyer JW, ed: *The adult spine: principles and practice*, New York, 1991, Raven Press, pp. 1655-1704.
12. Herkowitz AN, Kurz LT: Degenerative lumbar spondylolisthesis with spinal stenosis: a prospective study comparing decompression and decompression and intertransverse process arthrodesis, *J Bone Joint Surg Am* 73:802-808, 1991.
13. Heron LD, Tripp AC: L4-5 degenerative spondylolisthesis: the results of treatment by decompressive laminectomy without fusion, *Spine* 14:534-538, 1989.
14. Hu SS, Bradford DS, Transfeldt EE, Cohen M: Reduction of high grade spondylolisthesis using Edward instrumentation, *Spine* 21:367-371, 1996.
15. Inoue S et al.: Degenerative spondylolisthesis pathophysiology and results of anterior interbody fusion, *Clin Orthop* 227:90-98, 1988.
16. Jackson DW, Wiltse LL, Cirincoine RJ: Spondylolysis in the female gymnast, *Clin Orthop* 117:68-73, 1976.
17. Johnsson KE, Rosen I, Uden A: The natural course of lumbar spinal stenosis, *Clin Orthop* 279:82-86, 1992.
18. Junghanns H: Spondylolisthesis. Ohne spalte im zwischenbelenkstu ("Pseudo-spondylolisthesen"), *Arch Orthop Unfall-Chir* 29:118-127, 1930.
19. Kabins MB et al.: Isolated L4-L5 floating fusions using the variable screw placement system: unilateral vs bilateral, *J Spinal Disord* 5:39-49, 1992.
20. Katz JN et al.: The outcome of decompressive laminectomy for degenerative lumbar stenosis, *J Bone Joint Surg Am* 73:809-816, 1991.
21. Kim SS et al.: Factors affecting fusion rate in adult spondylolisthesis, *Spine* 15:979-984, 1990.
22. Lombardi JS et al.: Treatment of degenerative spondylolisthesis, *Spine* 10:821-927, 1985.
23. Lonstein JE: Spondylolisthesis in children: cause, natural history and management, *Spine* 24(24):2640-2648, 1999.
24. Macnab I: Spondylolisthesis with an intact neural arch: the so-called pseudo-spondylolisthesis, *J Bone Joint Surg* 32:325-333, 1950.
25. Molinari RW et al.: Complications in the surgical treatment of pediatric high grade isthmic dysplastic spondylolisthesis: a comparison of three surgical approaches, *Spine* 24:1701-1711, 1999.
26. Moller H, Hedlund R: Instrumented and noninstrumented posterolateral fusion in adult spondylolisthesis, *Spine* 13:1716-1721, 2000.
27. Nakai O, Oookawa A, Yamaura I: Long-term roentgenographic and functional changes in patients who were treated with wide fenestration for central lumbar stenosis, *J Bone Joint Surg Am* 73:1184-1191, 1991.
28. Newman PH: The etiology of spondylisthesis, *J Bone Joint Surg Br* 45:39-59, 1963.
29. Pritchett JW, Bortel DT: Degenerative symptomatic lumbar scoliosis, *Spine* 18:700-703, 1993.
30. Rosenberg NJ: Degenerative spondylolisthesis: predisposing factors, *J Bone Joint Surg Am* 57:467-474, 1975.
31. Rosomoff HL: Lumbar spondylolisthesis: etiology of radiculopathy and role of the neurosurgeon, *Clin Neurosurg* 27:577-590, 1980.
32. Rowe G, Roache M: Etiology of the separate neural arch, *J Bone Joint Surg Am* 35:102, 1953.
33. Sagi HC, Jarvis JG, Uhthoff HK: Histomorphic analysis of the development of the pars interarticularis and its association with isthmic spondylolysis, *Spine* 23(15):1635-1640, 1998.
34. Satomi K et al.: A clinical study of degenerative spondylolisthesis: radiographic analysis and choice of treatment, *Spine* 17:1329-1336, 1992.
35. Sedgewick TA et al.: Surgical treatment of degenerative spondylolisthesis with associated spinal stenosis. Presented at the annual meeting of the Scoliosis Research Society, Minneapolis, Minn, Sept 27, 1991.
36. Seitsale S et al.: Progression of spondylolisthesis in children and adolescents: a long-term follow-up of 272 patients, *Spine* 16:417-421, 1991.
37. Semon RL, Spengler D: Significance of lumbar spondylolysis in college football players, *Spine* 6:172-174, 1981.
38. Takahaski K et al.: Long-term results of anterior interbody fusion for the treatment of degenerative spondylolisthesis, *Spine* 15:1211-1215, 1990.
39. Vaccaro AR et al.: Predictors of outcome in patient with chronic back pain and low-grade spondylolisthesis, *Spine* 22:2030-2040, 1997.
40. Valkenburg HA, Haanen HCM: The epidemiology of low back pain. In White AA III, Gordon SL, eds: *American Academy of Orthopaedic Surgeons symposium on idiopathic low back pain*, St Louis, 1982, Mosby, pp. 9-22.
41. West JL, Bradford DS, Ogilvie JW: *Steffee instrumentation: 2 year results.* Presented at the annual meeting of the Scoliosis Research Society, Baltimore, 1988.
42. Whiffen JR, Neuwirth MG: Degenerative spondylolisthesis. In Bridwell KH, Dewald RL, eds: *The textbook of spinal surgery*, vol 2, Philadelphia, 1991, JB Lippincott, pp. 657-674.
43. Wiltse LL, Widell E Jr, Jackson DW: Fatigue fracture: the basic lesion in isthmic spondylolisthesis, *J Bone Joint Surg Am* 57:17-22, 1975.
44. Wynne-Davies R, Scott JH: Inheritance and spondylolisthesis: a radiographic family survey, *J Bone Joint Surg Br* 61:301-305, 1979.
45. Yuan HA et al.: A historical cohort study of pedicle screw fixation in thoracic, lumbar, and sacral spinal fusions, *Spine* 19:2279S-2296S, 1994.
46. Zdeblick TA: A prospective, randomized study of lumbar fusion, *Spine* 18:983-991, 1993.

Adult Deformity: Scoliosis and Sagittal Plane Deformities

Keith H. Bridwell

The natural history of curves that are not treated in the skeletally mature patient is quite variable. Some large curves may progress at the rate of 1 degree per year.[17] De novo curves may progress as rapidly as 3.3 degrees per year.[10] Lumbar curves are more likely to progress than are thoracic curves. The curves do not necessarily progress at a constant rate. A substantial percentage of large scoliosis curves progress into adulthood.

INDICATIONS FOR SURGICAL INTERVENTION

The four main indications for surgical treatment of adult scoliosis[8,11,12] are (1) a large deformity based on Cobb measurement, rotational deformity, and balance in the coronal and sagittal plane; (2) progressive deformity; (3) back or leg pain; and (4) pulmonary or neurologic dysfunction related to the deformity. With significant lumbar curves, radicular leg pain may occur in conjunction with spinal stenosis and rotatory subluxations. Ideally, the patient should be relatively healthy and emotionally stable.

PRESURGICAL ASSESSMENT

Pulmonary function testing should be performed on any patient who has preexistent pulmonary disease or in whom an anterior approach or a thoracoplasty is being performed. Preoperative nutritional testing is of benefit as well. Some patients benefit from preoperative and perioperative enteral or parenteral hyperalimentation. Long-cassette standing coronal and sagittal plain radiographs show the erect deformity. Flexibility films should be performed to assess the correctability of curves. Appropriate flexibility films may include a long-cassette coronal supine film, long-cassette right and left side benders, a supine hyperextension lateral view, and a push-prone or fulcrum bending anteroposterior view. For patients who are having fusions down to L4, L5, or the sacrum, magnetic resonance imaging and/or provocative discography may play a role in deciding on the distal fusion level.

FUSION LEVELS

For the most part, patients between the ages of 20 and 35 who do not have substantial degenerative changes can be treated as one would a teenager. When the patients are older than age 35 and degenerative changes start to develop, it is important to assess the amount of disc degeneration at L3 to L4, L4 to L5, and L5 to S1, as well as whether stenosis/fixed tilt/listhesis coexist below.[4] Fusion levels for older patients (with superimposed degenerative changes) who require distal lumbar spine fusions are not clearly delineated.

THE SAGITTAL AND CORONAL PLANES

In the sagittal plane, the top and bottom of the fusion should extend into areas of lordosis to avoid junctional kyphosis. In the coronal plane, it is ideal for the fusion

---

INDICATIONS FOR SURGICAL TREATMENT

- Size of the deformity
- Evidence of the deformity's progression
- Patient symptoms (relative)
  - Back pain
  - Leg pain
  - Pulmonary compromise
  - Neurologic dysfunction

RADIOGRAPHIC ASSESSMENT

- Upright long cassette films
- Appropriate flexibility films

areas to be stable and neutral above to stable and neutral below and preferably horizontal if the fusion is below L2. Thus fusions should stop and start in stable and neutral zones. (*Stable* means centered on the middle of the sacrum, and *neutral* refers to rotation.)

SURGICAL APPROACHES

Factors that determine whether a posterior or circumferential fusion are needed include the magnitude of the curve, curve flexibility, and the patient's sagittal balance. Patients with lumbar curves are more likely to benefit from anterior surgery and structural grafting than are those with thoracic curves. Also, patients with kyphotic segments are more likely to benefit from anterior surgery and anterior structural grafting than those with lordotic segments. Severe rotatory subluxations are relative indications for anterior surgery because structural grafting opens up the disc space and creates a ligamentotaxis effect to reduce the subluxation (Figure 41-1).

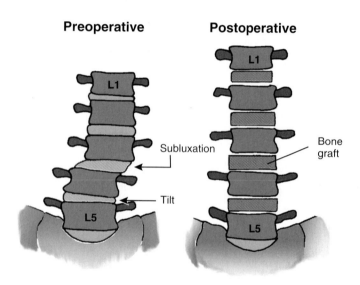

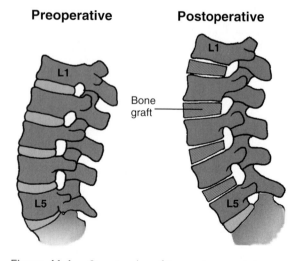

Figure 41-1.   Structural grafting reduces rotatory subluxation and lordoses of the spine and opens up the foramen.

Most thoracic curves can be treated with posterior-only surgery (Figure 41-2). Most long fusions to the sacrum require anterior and posterior surgery in the lumbar spine, structural grafting at L4 to L5 and L5 to S1, and four-point fixation of the sacrum and pelvis. It is also important to align the patient's spine in either neutral or negative sagittal balance with a long fusion.[3,7,16]

Patients with severe imbalance and stiff curves may benefit from either triplane osteotomies or vertebral column resection procedures. In most cases, if anterior and posterior surgeries are contemplated, the anterior surgery is performed before the posterior surgery. Decisions about whether to perform circumferential surgery on one day or separate days are based on the patient's preoperative nutritional status and comorbidities, physician and surgical team experience, and the anticipated length of the surgical procedure.

BONE GRAFTING

Allograft bone posteriorly in the adult spine seems to have little or no benefit.[1] However, anterior structural grafting in the form of mesh cages packed with autogenous bone or fresh frozen tricortical iliac grafts or fresh frozen femoral ring grafts packed with autogenous bone is a reasonable source of graft material.[5,9,15]

SPINAL FIXATION

Segmental fixation should always be used in surgery for adult deformity. In the young, very flexible, nonosteoporotic patient, an anterior-only surgery for a thoracic or a thoracolumbar curve may be considered, but this is the exception rather than the rule for the adult patient. With posterior constructs, either hooks or pedicle screws are reasonable choices in the thoracic spine. In the lumbar spine, pedicle screws are preferred by most.

DEGENERATIVE OR DE NOVO SCOLIOSIS

De novo scoliosis occurs in patients older than 40.[10] The deformity occurs as a result of disc degeneration with

---

ADULT DEFORMITIES

- Usually need posterior-only and circumferential operations
- Bilateral segmental fixation preferred
- Multilevel lumbar fusions and fusions for kyphosis generally require circumferential fusion

---

GRAFT CHOICES

- Posterior spine: Autogenous morselized bone graft preferred
- Anterior spine: Autogenous morselized bone combined with either allograft structural bone or cages

asymmetric collapse. Often the spine does not autostabilize, because of the lack of osteophytes and facet hypertrophy, so rotatory subluxations, vertebral tilt, and kyphosis occur. Although there are some reports in the literature that the male-to-female ratio is 1:1, it clinically appears that females are more likely to develop substantial problems than are males. These patients are more likely to have significant coexistent medical problems than are those with idiopathic scoliosis and superimposed degenerative changes.

The five potential treatments include (1) nonsurgical treatment, (2) decompression alone, (3) decompression with posterior fusion and instrumentation, (4) posterior decompression with anterior and posterior fusion, and (5) posterior decompression and posterior instrumentation with a vertebral column resection procedure. The indications for surgical treatment are coexistent spinal claudication symptoms or significant progressive deformity with progressive coronal or sagittal imbalance.

If such patients are out of balance in both the coronal and sagittal planes, then correctives include anterior structural grafting to create a ligamentoataxis effect or a posterior resection procedure such as a pedicle subtraction osteotomy to restore spinal alignment. Long fusions and instrumentations in this population of patients seem to carry a significant incidence of adjacent segment transition syndrome.

DE NOVO SCOLIOSIS

- Can occur in patients older than 40 years
- Such patients often have significant comorbidities
- Treatment produces more controversy than adult idiopathic scoliosis with superimposed degenerative changes

---

INDICATIONS FOR SURGICAL TREATMENT OF DE NOVO SCOLIOSIS

- Spinal imbalance
- Progressive deformity
- Substantial spinal claudication symptoms

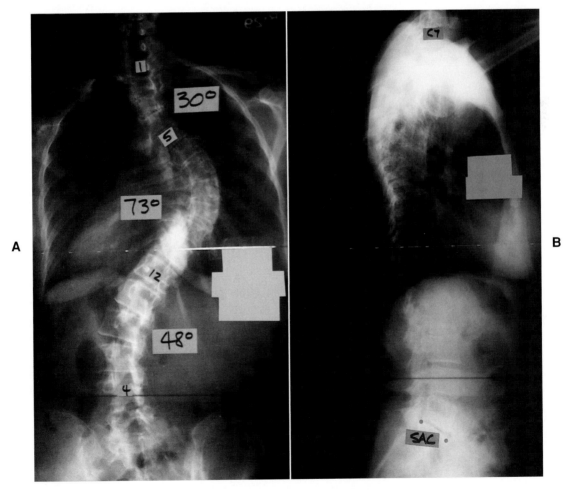

Figure 41-2. **A,** Upright coronal radiograph before surgery. **B,** Upright sagittal radiograph before surgery.

Continued

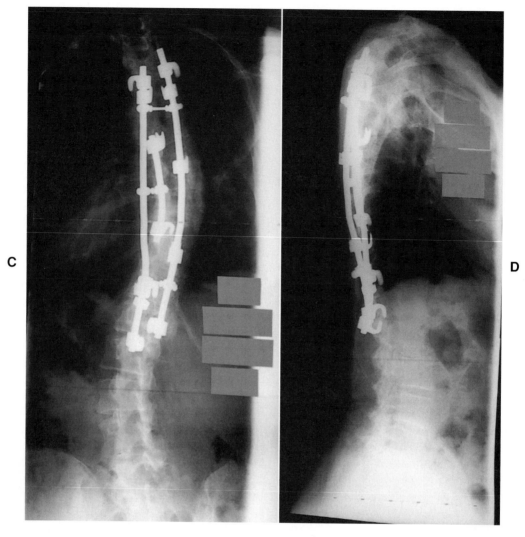

Figure 41-2, cont'd.   **C,** Upright coronal radiograph 7 years after surgery. **D,** Upright sagittal radiograph 7 years before surgery.

Continued

IATROGENIC FIXED KYPHOSIS

A plumb line dropped from C7 that falls anterior to the lumbosacral disc represents positive sagittal balance; through the disc neutral balance; and behind the disc negative balance. The most common causes of fixed sagittal imbalance are (1) posterior lumbar fusion with Harrington distraction instrumentation, (2) anterior spinal fusion with Zielke or Dwyer instrumentation without structural grafting, (3) uninstrumented fusion with pseudarthrosis, and (4) breakdown adjacent to degenerative fusion. Fixed sagittal imbalance syndrome is quite disabling. It causes fatigue pain and disabling functional problems because of the patient's inability to stand erect. These patients often have to hyperextend the neck, flex the knees, and maximally extend the hips to maintain a relatively erect posture (head over sacrum).

Surgical treatment of fixed sagittal imbalance syndrome includes either multiple Smith-Petersen oste-

---

FIXED SAGITTAL IMBALANCE

- Many causes and presentations
- An extremely disabling condition
- Treatments
  - Multiple Smith-Petersen osteotomies, usually with anterior and posterior surgery
  - A single pedicle subtraction osteotomy
  - Technically demanding with substantial risks

---

otomies or pedicle subtraction procedures.[2,13,14] The Smith-Petersen osteotomies are done posteriorly through the posterior column between pedicles above and below as a closing wedge (Figure 41-3). The Smith-Petersen osteotomies close the posterior and middle column, lengthen the anterior column, and often require anterior structural grafting (Figure 41-4). The pedicle subtraction procedure is V shaped in the sagittal plane

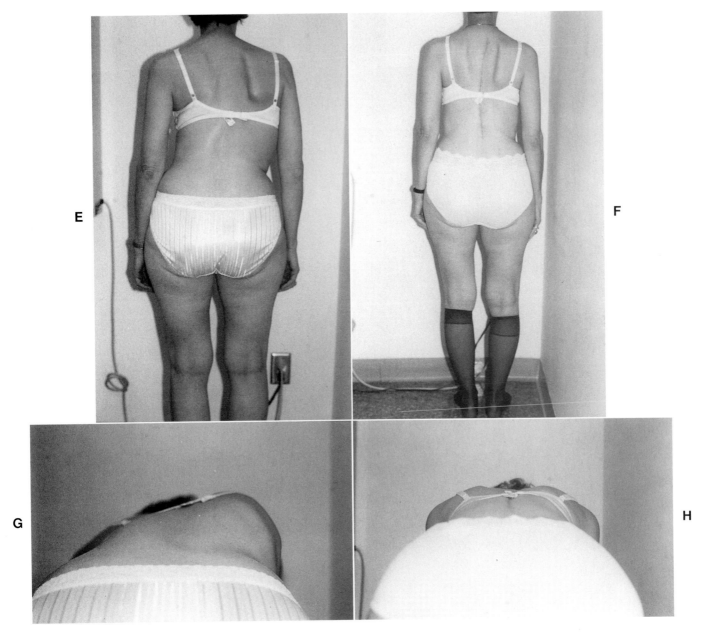

Figure 41-2, cont'd.   **E,** Clinical photograph before surgery showing trunk shift.
F, Clinical photograph after surgery. **G,** Rib hump before surgery. **H,** Rib hump after surgery.

and shortens the posterior and middle column without lengthening the anterior column (Figures 41-5 and 41-6). The goal of corrective surgery for fixed sagittal imbalance syndrome is to have a plumb line dropped from C7 on the sagittal standing radiograph fall through or behind the lumbosacral disc. It is safer to perform the osteotomies in the midlumbar spine. Smith-Petersen osteotomies, if performed through residual scoliotic deformities at the apex, have the potential to lengthen the convexity, shorten the concavity, and therein create a coronal imbalance problem that is less likely to occur with pedicle subtraction procedures.

CONCLUSIONS

Relief of back pain in a patient with adult deformity is somewhat unpredictable. Although "pain" is quoted in our literature as a major indication for the performance of adult deformity surgery, I do not consider it to be the major indication. Substantial deformity, progressive deformity, and progressive pain are better indicators. Rendering a patient with adult scoliosis totally pain free is not usually a reasonable goal. Most patients who undergo surgery for adult spinal deformity do have a significant improvement in pain, but not necessarily all, and most do not achieve complete pain relief.

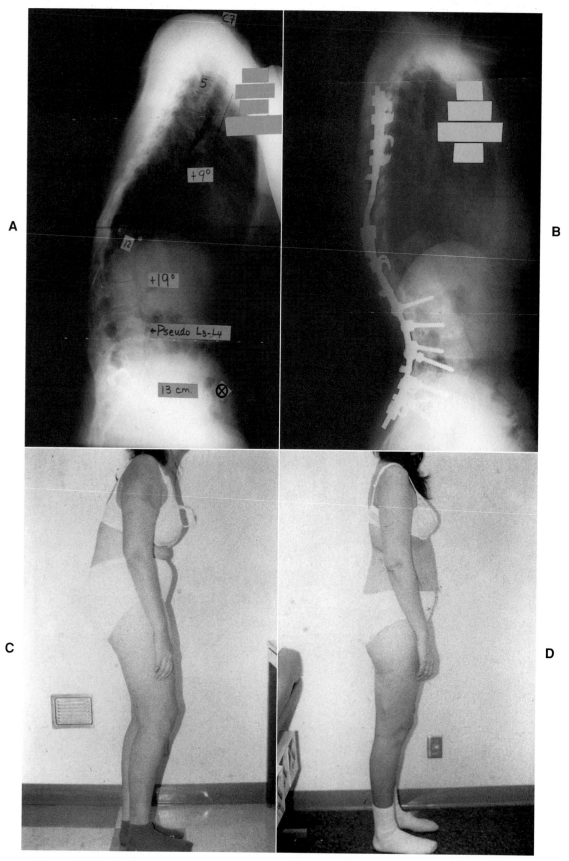

Figure 41-3. **A,** Upright sagittal radiograph before surgery, showing positive sagittal balance. **B,** Upright sagittal radiograph at 2 years and 8 months after several Smith-Petersen osteotomies, showing negative sagittal balance. **C,** Clinical photograph before surgery. **D,** Clinical photograph after surgery.

Before

After

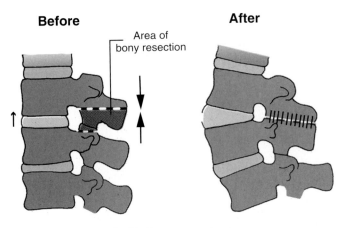

Area of
bony resection

Figure 41-4. Smith-Petersen osteotomy.

The assessment of fusion status in adult deformity is quite difficult. Multiple segments are assessed, and the segments are camouflaged by the instrumentation. My philosophy is that one can be reasonably confident of fusion only when a patient has no change in the implants or in the correction of the deformity at 3 to 5 years after surgery. Otherwise, assessments such as bone scans, oblique radiographs, flexion/extension films, and so on in a situation where the implants are still present are not terribly helpful modalities. On the other hand, if the implants are removed, flexibility radiographs and bone scans may be valid. However, the premature removal of implants in the adult patient with deformity is not wise and often reveals otherwise asymptomatic pseudarthroses.[6]

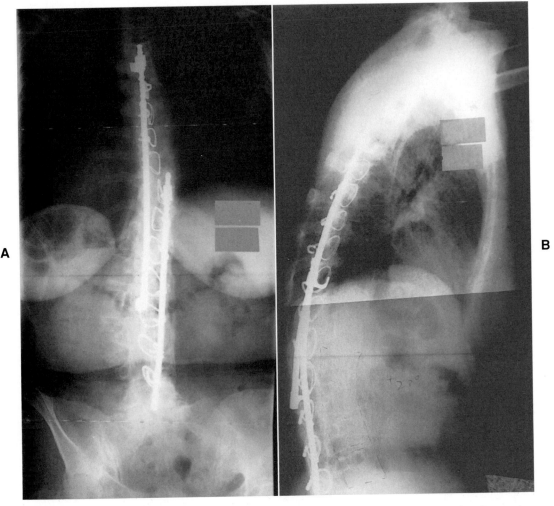

Figure 41-5. **A,** Upright coronal radiograph before surgery. **B,** Upright sagittal radiograph before surgery, showing positive sagittal balance.

Continued

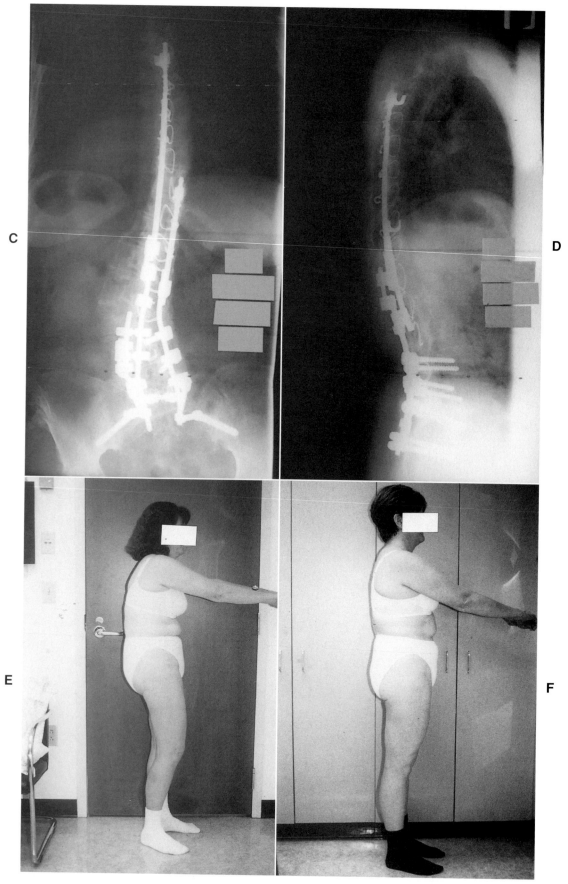

Figure 41-5, cont'd. **C,** Upright coronal radiograph after surgery. **D,** Upright sagittal radiograph 2 years after a pedicle subtraction osteotomy, showing neutral sagittal balance. **E,** Clinical photograph before surgery. **F,** Clinical photograph after surgery.

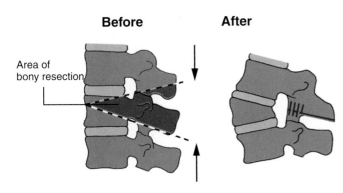

Before   **After**

Area of
bony resection

Figure 41-6.   Three-column pedicle subtraction osteotomy.

SELECTED REFERENCES

Booth KC et al.: Complications and predictive factors for the successful treatment of flatback deformity (fixed sagittal imbalance), *Spine* 24(16):1712-1720, 1999.

Bradford DS: Adult scoliosis: current concepts of treatment, *Clin Orthop* 229:70-87, 1988.

Dekutoski MB et al.: Fusion to the sacrum in adult idiopathic scoliosis: the role of sagittal balance, *Orthop Trans* 17(1):125, 1993.

Dickson JH et al.: Results of operative treatment of idiopathic scoliosis in adults, *J Bone Joint Surg Am* 77(4):513-523, 1995.

Grubb SA, Lipscomb HJ, Coonrad RW: Degenerative adult onset scoliosis, *Spine* 13(3):241-245, 1988.

Kostuik JP: Decision making in adult scoliosis, *Spine* 4(6):521-525, 1979.

Weinstein SL, Ponseti IV: Curve progression in idiopathic scoliosis, *J Bone Joint Surg Am* 65(4):447-455, 1983.

REFERENCES

1. An HS, Lynch K, Toth J: Prospective comparison of autograft vs. allograft for adult posterolateral lumbar spine fusion: differences among freeze-dried, frozen, and mixed grafts, *J Spinal Disord* 8(2):131-135, 1995.

2. Booth KC et al.: Complications and predictive factors for the successful treatment of flatback deformity (fixed sagittal imbalance), *Spine* 24(16):1712-1720, 1999.

3. Bradford DS: Adult scoliosis: current concepts of treatment, *Clin Orthop* 229:70-87, 1988.

4. Bridwell KH: Where to stop the fusion distally in adult scoliosis: L4, L5, or the sacrum? In Pritchard DJ, ed: *Instructional course lectures*, vol 45, Rosemont, Ill, 1996, American Academy of Orthopaedic Surgeons, pp.101-107.

5. Bridwell KH et al.: Anterior fresh frozen structural allografts in the thoracic and lumbar spine: do they work if combined with posterior fusion and instrumentation in adult patients with kyphosis or anterior column defects? *Spine* 20(12):1410-1418, 1995.

6. Deckey J, Court C, Bradford DS: Loss of sagittal plane correction after removal of spinal implants, *Spine* 25(19):2453-2460, 2000.

7. Dekutoski MB et al.: Fusion to the sacrum in adult idiopathic scoliosis: the role of sagittal balance, *Orthop Trans* 17(1):125, 1993.

8. Dickson JH et al.: Results of operative treatment of idiopathic scoliosis in adults, *J Bone Joint Surg Am* 77(4):513-523, 1995.

9. Eck KR et al.: Analysis of titanium mesh (Harms) cages in adults with minimum two-year follow-up, *Spine* 25(18):2407-2415, 1999.

10. Grubb SA, Lipscomb HJ, Coonrad RW: Degenerative adult onset scoliosis, *Spine* 13(3):241-245, 1988.

11. Kostuik JP: Decision making in adult scoliosis, *Spine* 4(6):521-525, 1979.

12. Kostuik JP: Adult scoliosis. In Bridwell KH, DeWald RL, eds: *The textbook of spinal surgery*, ed 1, Philadelphia, 1991, JB Lippincott, pp. 249-278.

13. Kostuik JP et al.: Combined single stage anterior and posterior osteotomy for correction of iatrogenic lumbar kyphosis, *Spine* 13(3):257-266, 1988.

14. LaGrone MO et al.: Treatment of symptomatic flatback after spinal fusion, *J Bone Joint Surg Am* 70(4):569-580, 1988.

15. Molinari RW et al.: Minimum 5 year follow-up of anterior column structural allografts in the thoracic and lumbar spine, *Spine* 24(10):967-972, 1999.

16. Saer EH III, Winter RB, Lonstein JE: Long scoliosis fusion to the sacrum in adults with nonparalytic scoliosis: an improved method, *Spine* 15(7):650-653, 1990.

17. Weinstein SL, Ponseti IV: Curve progression in idiopathic scoliosis, *J Bone Joint Surg Am* 65(4):447-455, 1983.

VIII

Pediatric Deformity

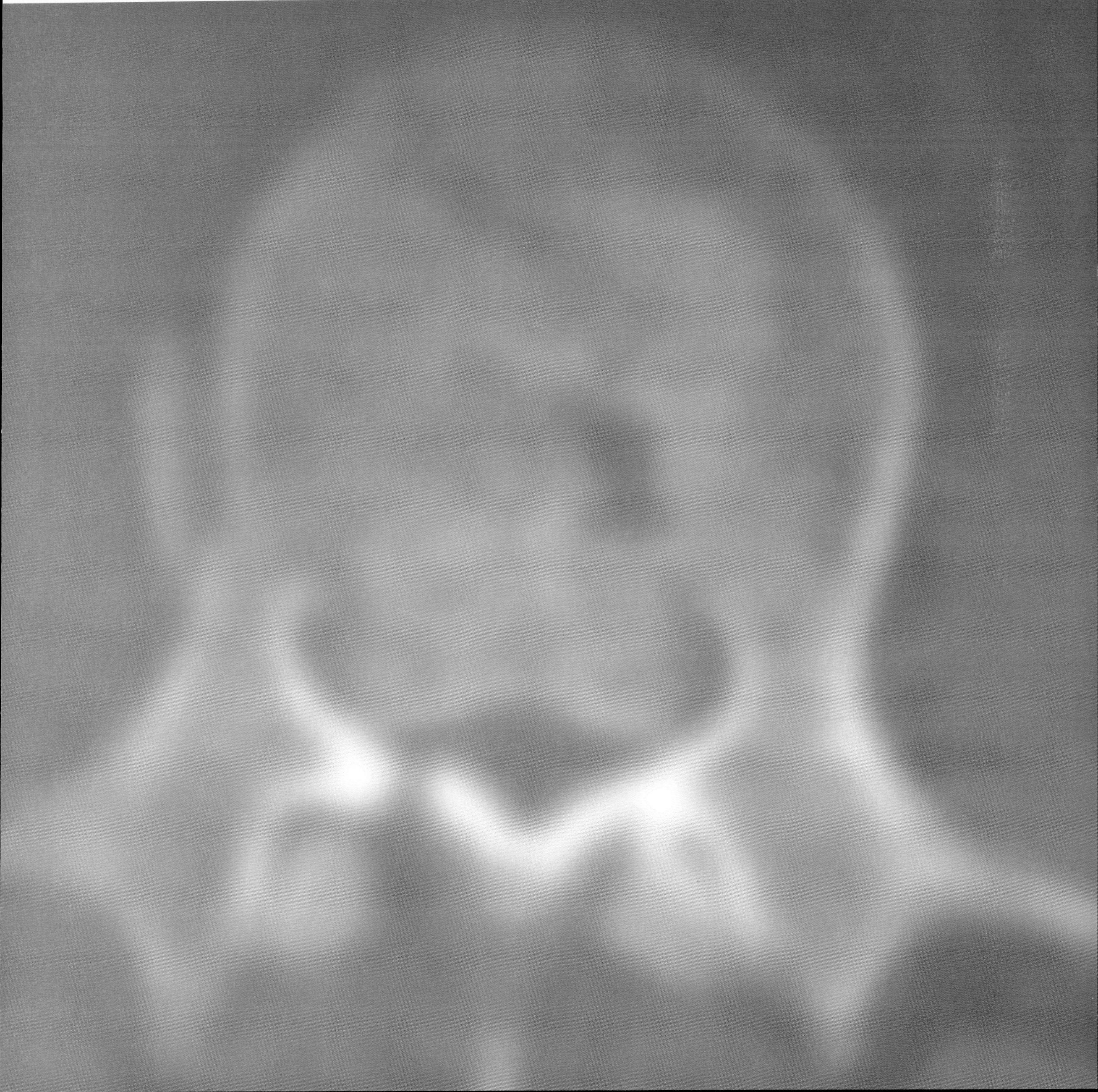

Pediatric Spondylolisthesis

Denis S. Drummond, Scott A. Rushton

There are few spinal conditions with management as controversial as spondylolisthesis. This controversy is the result of a lack of understanding of the biomechanical causes and sequelae of this disorder. It is difficult for the surgeon to develop a rational plan of treatment, in particular, for high-grade spondylolisthesis. Further, management of high-grade slips requires a plan that takes into account the delicate balance between the risks and benefits of surgical treatment.

Spondylolisthesis is defined as a translation of one vertebral body on the adjacent caudal vertebra in an anterior direction or, with more severe cases, in an anterior and caudal direction. When anterior translation is less than one half of the horizontal length of the adjacent vertebra, the condition is defined as low-grade spondylolisthesis. Translation greater than 50% is defined as high-grade spondylolisthesis. Generally, spondylolisthesis occurs as a result of dysplastic formation of the adjacent articular facets or a defect in the pars interarticularis, most commonly at L5 to S1.

CLASSIFICATION

Wiltse and colleagues[52] defined two similar, but, in their view, pathologically different types of spondylolisthesis.

DEFINITIONS AND CLASSIFICATION

- Translation of one vertebral body on adjacent caudal vertebra anteriorly
  - Low-grade: Anterior translation less than half the horizontal length of adjacent vertebra
  - High-grade: Translation greater than 50%
  - Severe: Vertebra translates both anteriorly and caudally
- Most common site: L5 to S1
- Developmental type (Marchetti and Bartolozzi)
  - Encompasses Wiltse types I and II
  - May result from
    - Dysplastic formation of adjacent articular facets (type I)
    - Defect in pars interarticularis from fatigue fracture (type IIA)
    - Elongation of pars interarticularis bilaterally (type IIB)
- Acquired type: All others

The dysplastic lesion (type I) is caused by a failure of the adjacent facets that allows anterior translation of the cephalad vertebral body on the caudal one, usually L5 on S1. The isthmic type (type II) was defined as a bilateral failure of the pars interarticularis, occurring either from a fatigue fracture (type IIA) or from an elongation of the pars interarticularis bilaterally (type IIB), a situation that appears radiographically like toffee being stretched. These varieties are defined as Wiltse type IIA and IIB spondylolisthesis, respectively.

Marchetti and Bartolozzi[24] have made a strong argument for their classification system, which combines the isthmic and dysplastic varieties described by Wiltse and classifies them as developmental spondylolisthesis. Marchetti and Bartolozzi classify all other types as acquired spondylolisthesis. Further, they believe that the pathology observed from the two developmental varieties arises as a result of the same developmental failure of the posterior elements. They describe two grades of dysplastic changes, each with differing prognosis. The high dysplastic posterior element dysplasia is at greater risk to progress to high-grade spondylolisthesis when compared with low-grade dysplasia.[24] Because the observational measurements, monitoring, and surgical treatment are conceptually similar for all of the developmental varieties of spondylolisthesis, Marchetti and Bartolozzi believe that their classification is more useful.[24]

In our experience, it is not always easy to distinguish the Wiltse type I and II lesions. His precise classification in these cases may, therefore, be irrelevant. Because the Marchetti and Bartolozzi classification system is simple and relevant to the experience of pediatric spine surgeons, we have chosen to embrace it (Table 42-1). Accordingly, this chapter will concentrate on developmental spondylolisthesis from the Marchetti and Bartolozzi classification. Whatever the classification system used, these patients require an understanding of the natural history of progressive spondylolisthesis.

INCIDENCE

Spondylolisthesis has rarely been diagnosed in the first year of life, but it is found in up to 5% of children age 5 to 7 years and in 6% at 18 years of age.[10,22,51] Rowe and Roche[41] reported that Caucasian males are more

551

Table 42-1	Spondylolisthesis Classifications	
Wiltse, Newman, Macnab	**Marchetti, Bartolozzi**	
Type 1: Dysplastic; due to dysplastic sacral facet	*Developmental:* Lysis or elongation	
Type 2: Isthmic; pars lesion	High dysplastic*	
Type 3: Degenerative; due to chronic instability	Low dysplastic	
Type 4: Traumatic; due to acute fracture	*Acquired:* Traumatic: Acute or stress	
Type 5: Pathologic; due to generalized bone disease	Post surgery Pathologic Degenerative	

*At risk for high-grade slip.

INCIDENCE

- Rarely diagnosed in first year of life, found in up to 5% of children 5 to 7 years old
- Incidence in males > females, Caucasians > African Americans; progression to high grade rare, but more likely in women
- Multifactorial etiology, related to genetic, developmental, and biomechanical factors
- Spina bifida occulta: Marker for posterior element dysplasia
  - Dysplasia in either superior sacral or inferior lumbar facets or both allows L5 vertebral body to slip forward on sacrum
  - Both dysplasia in posterior elements and changes in postural biomechanics are required to develop high-grade spondylolisthesis and spondyloptosis

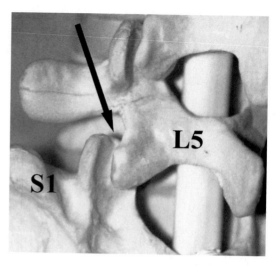

Figure 42-1.   Normal lumbosacral facet joint. The inferior facet of L5 and the superior facet of S1 are shown. Note the vertical orientation, which restrains translation. Wiltse has described the S1 facet as a buttress, and DeWald has likened the competent articulation to a bony hook.

frequently affected (6.4%) than African-American males (2.8%). Likewise, they observed spondylolisthesis in 2.3% of Caucasian women and in 1.1% of African-American women. Because this study was reported in 1953, it is possible that with the increased participation of girls and young women in more vigorous athletic pursuits, the gender difference for incidence may have decreased somewhat since then. The highest reported incidence for spondylolisthesis was in Alaskan Eskimos, where it was diagnosed in 13% of children and close to 50% of adults.[22]

The progression of a slip to high grade is relatively rare. Osterman[32] reported that close to 80% in his series were low grade and only 1% were high grade. Although spondylolisthesis appears more frequently in men, women are more likely to progress to a high-grade slip.[44]

ETIOLOGY

The cause of spondylolisthesis is multifactorial. It appears to be related to genetic, developmental, and biomechanical factors.

Fredrickson et al.[10] observed an inherited predisposition for spondylolisthesis. They hypothesized that kindred of affected patients were more prone to develop a defect in the cartilaginous anlage of the vertebral pos-

terior elements. Like others, they reported that spina bifida occulta is a marker for this.[2,8,26,46,54] Haukipuro et al.[13] reported a strong familial incidence for spondylolisthesis in Finish kindred with the same dysplastic vertebral pathology and markers. Haukipuro has traced two families and found developmental spondylolisthesis in three generations marked by posterior element dysplasia and spina bifida occulta. All of these patients had severe enough symptoms to require radiographic evaluation and treatment. In a separate study, Wynne-Davies and Scott[55] also observed a spina bifida occulta marker in relatives of patients affected with spondylolisthesis. Dysplastic lesions of the pars interarticularis, either a fracture or elongation, spina bifida occulta, a wide distal spinal canal, and dysplasia of both the inferior lumbar and sacral facets appear to be common components of spondylolisthesis, especially in high-grade slips.

Wiltse[51,52] has emphasized the importance of the buttress effect provided by the intact superior facet of S1. With dysplasia, this support effect is frequently lost, allowing the L5 vertebral body to slip forward on the sacrum. DeWald[8] has observed that the dysplasia can occur in either the superior sacral or inferior lumbar facets, or both of these, and that the competent relationship between the two can be likened to a bony hook that prevents translation (Figure 42-1). With facet dysplasia, the hook effect is lost to either a greater or lesser extent. In the presence of other conditions, including increased lumbar lordosis and an increased sacral inclination, the risk for anterior translation of one vertebral body on the other is increased. DeWald also believes that spina bifida occulta is an important marker for this dysplastic lesion. Recent observers of high-grade spondylolisthesis have also observed these same dysplastic features.[26,31,46]

Trauma appears to play a role in the development of the pars lesion, either as a stress fracture or as a dysplastic lengthening of the pars interarticularis. This hypothesis is based on the reports of spondylolysis in athletes, including gymnasts, football linemen, and weightlifters.[16,21,26,45] Despite these observations, one cannot help believe that those who developed spondylolisthesis had a predisposition, based in some degree on inheritance. It would appear that this genetic predisposition is responsible for the dysplastic lesion of the pars interarticularis and that postural biomechanics also play an important role, particularly for the larger and high-grade slips. It also appears that one of these features *alone* does not lead to a severe spondylolisthesis, which helps explain why most patients with developmental spondylolisthesis do not progress to high-grade slips. Both dysplasia in the posterior elements and changes in postural biomechanics are also required.[3,8,43,49] Although this question remains incompletely answered, it seems that a number of coexisting conditions are required to develop high-grade spondylolisthesis and spondyloptosis.

To our knowledge, spondylolisthesis has not been described in infants. The assumption is that one needs to obtain an upright posture to develop the necessary loads to affect a translation through the dysplastic posterior elements. DeWald's bony hook concept offers a particularly attractive hypothesis to explain how the slip occurs. He believes dysplastic posterior elements are incompetent to prevent vertebral translation when presented with increased lumbar lordosis and high postural loads.

Accordingly, the biomechanics of progressive high-grade spondylolisthesis are an important contributor to the development of the slip, the rate of translation, and the compensatory posturing and gait.

Anterior and caudal translation of the L5 vertebral body on the sacrum causes a relative kyphosis at the lumbosacral junction. This kyphosis and the associated instability have recently been appreciated as an important determinant of the extent and rate of translatory progression.[30,53] The kyphotic tilt of L5 on S1 has been described as the slip angle, which can be measured and followed to quantify progression (Figure 42-2).[53,54] Unfortunately, kyphosis and increasing slip angle occur late and are as much a result as a cause of progressive high-grade slips. Kyphosis and increasing slip angle, then, are both late results of high-grade spondylolisthesis and markers of the risk for spondyloptosis.

Increased lumbar lordosis is observed in virtually all cases of high-grade spondylolisthesis.[8,14,45,49] This occurs in response to abnormal morphology affecting the spine and pelvis and, further, as a compensatory response to an increasing translation and slip angle with a progressive unbalanced spine.[3,20,43,49,54] What begins as increased lumbar lordosis, a prerequisite for spondylolisthesis, is augmented by a secondary response to spinal imbalance, which causes further-increasing lordosis.[9,49] This augmentation can become an ongoing process with increasing loads that promote translation and create a further need for compensation to retain

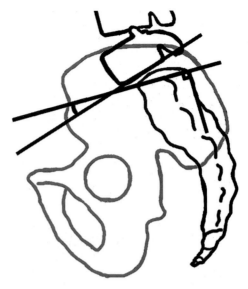

Figure 42-2. Measurement of the slip angle is shown. This measures the lumbosacral kyphosis that occurs when high-grade slips approach spondyloptosis. The kyphosis has great clinical significance to the biomechanics that influence progression and also may lead to failure of an arthrodesis.

ETIOLOGY

- Slip angle
  - Kyphotic tilt of L5 or S1
  - Can be measured and followed to quantify progression, but is late result of high-grade spondylolisthesis and marks risk for spondyloptosis
- Increased lumbar lordosis
  - Observed in virtually all cases of high-grade spondylolisthesis
  - Sagittal balance maintained by hyperlordosis and achieving more vertical inclination of sacrum
  - Compensation and spinal balance by sacral verticalization work only for short term
- Increased sacral inclination
  - Lends to shear loads at lumbosacral junction
  - Magnitude of forces varies directly with distance between sacrum on femoral heads
  - The more anterior the femoral heads are in relation to sacrum, the greater the tendency to spinal imbalance leading to increasing lumbar lordosis
  - Pelvic incidence
  - Combination of pelvic tilt and sacrococcygeal angle
    - Mean 53 degrees for adult males, 48 degrees for adult females
  - Biomechanics an important component of changes in posture and gait and shape adjacent lumbosacral vertebrae

sagittal balance. According to Dick and Elke,[9] sagittal balance can only be achieved by hyperlordosis, perhaps to anatomic extremes. When the need for further compensation to maintain sagittal balance occurs beyond the extremes of lumbar lordosis, a more vertical inclination of the sacrum is required.[9,19] Sacral verticalization

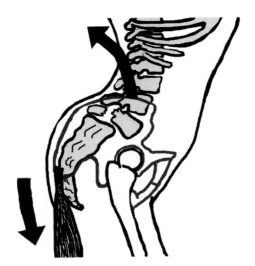

Figure 42-3. When the unbalanced spine can no longer be compensated by increasing lumbar lordosis, the sacrum is brought into a more vertical position by contracting the hamstrings. This effectively pulls the sacrum in a distal direction and, thus, also elevates the anterior pelvis into a more upright position.

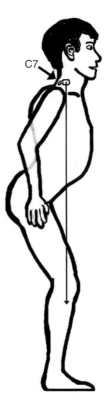

Figure 42-4. Demonstration of the postural change seen in high-grade spondylolisthesis. Gait changes typically accompany the postural change. Also, the plumb line from C7 depicts sacral overhang.

can only be accomplished by the contraction of the hamstrings, which rotates the ischium caudally and the anterior pelvis in a cephalad direction (Figure 42-3). This action, which occurs around the femoral heads, affects the posture and leads to functional disturbances. These disturbances include a crouched or waddling gait with a shortened stride length (Figure 42-4).

According to Roussouly compensation and spinal balance by sacral verticalization work only in the short term because, with time, the hamstrings and other extensors of the hips fatigue and become less effective in obtaining the upright posture and preserving spinal balance. With additional time, the muscles can atrophy and a state of decompensation ensues. Postural changes from poor spinal balance can, thus, become a functional problem associated with diminishing endurance and fatigue.[49] The relationship between lumbar lordosis and altered lumbosacral biomechanics due to spondylolisthesis clearly appears to be as important as the lack of a competent restraint from the dysplastic lumbosacral facets.

Because not all patients with dysplastic posterior elements develop a high-grade spondylolisthesis, the important question is what morphologic feature sets in motion the biomechanical cascade that leads to progressive translation and, in its most severe extreme, spondyloloptosis? Roussouly et al.[3,20,35,39,49] have described the sagittal morphology of the spine and pelvis, which appears to shed light on this question. They have defined measurements about the pelvis that provide insight to the development of increased lumbar lordosis, increased sacral inclination, and the risk for progressive slip. Their hypothesis is that the biomechanics, which dictate translation and progression, are related to the inclination of the sacrum and its distance from the femoral heads. Presumably, increased sacral inclination leads to shear loads at the lumbosacral junction and the magnitude of these forces varies directly with distance between the sacrum and the femoral heads. The more anterior the femoral heads are in relation to the sacrum, the greater the tendency to spinal imbalance. Balance, then, can only be achieved by further increasing lumbar lordosis.[3,9,12]

According to Roussouly et al.,[3,20,49] the critical biomechanical determinant is pelvic incidence, which relates the morphology of the pelvis and spine to postural biomechanics and the requirement for increasing lumbar lordosis to achieve spinal balance. The pelvic incidence is a combination of pelvic tilt and the sacral slope. Figure 42-5 shows that pelvic tilt is measured as an angle formed by a vertical line through the center of the femoral head and a line drawn from the center of the head to the midpoint of the superior sacral surface. The more anterior the femoral heads are placed in relation to the sacrum, the greater the pelvic tilt and pelvic incidence. A line extended from the superior sacral surface to the horizontal forms the sacrococcygeal angle. The greater the inclination of the sacrum, the greater the sacrococcygeal angle and pelvic incidence. Thus, pelvic incidence defines and measures the morphology that leads to lumbar lordosis and the biomechanical risk for progressive spondylolisthesis. The mean pelvic incidence is 53 degrees for adult males and 48 degrees for

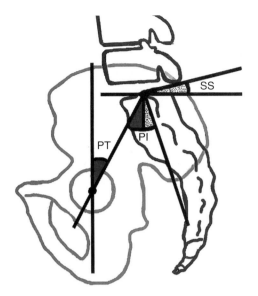

Figure 42-5. The pelvic incidence is shown. This is a result of primary changes in morphologic development of the spine and pelvis. Pelvic incidence is an angle *(PI)* that combines two others: pelvic tilt *(PT)* and sacral slope *(SS)*. It is an analysis of the combination of the slope of the sacrum and the distance of the femoral heads from the sacrum. It is considered to be responsible for increased lumbar lordosis, progression of translation, and spinal imbalance.

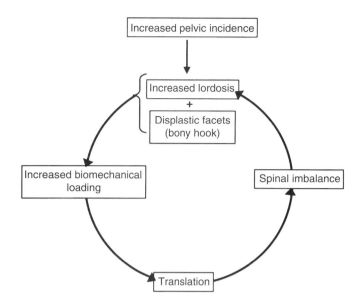

Figure 42-6. Vicious cycle of progression: The cycle that leads to spondylolisthesis and perpetual progression is depicted. The adverse biomechanics are initiated by the increased pelvic incidence and the slip permitted by the dysplasia of the L5 to S1 facets.

adult females.[20] Published mean values for children are unavailable.

Another biomechanical determinant is overhang, which measures the distance from the sacrum to the gravity line extending from C7 (see Figure 42-4).[32] This describes a moment arm, which determines the loads at the unstable lumbosacral junction. Normally, the plumb line extends through the body of S1.

There are, therefore, three biomechanical issues leading to the development of spondylolisthesis: First, the forces generated by an increased lumbar lordosis contribute to the development and progression of spondylolisthesis; second, biomechanics are an important component of changes in posture and gait, both of which are compensatory mechanisms to retain spinal balance; and, third, biomechanics shape the adjacent lumbosacral vertebrae.

Mechanical forces determine the shape of both the L5 vertebral body and the dome of the sacrum through the Heuter-Volkmann principle.[1,14,22] Because relatively greater loads are directed at the anterior part of L5 in chronic spondylolisthesis, the L5 vertebral body becomes trapezoidal with time, rather than rectangular. Similarly, the alteration to the body of the sacrum appears to be the result of instability at L5 to S1, where a teeter-totter effect associated with instability creates forces that lead to the dome shape.[14,22,26,34] These changes in vertebral shape are secondary and are, therefore, the result, not a cause, of high-grade slips. The conditions that lead to increased lumbar lordosis and high-grade spondylolisthesis are summarized in Figure 42-6.

CLINICAL FEATURES

Spondylolisthesis may develop silently and without apparent pain or other symptoms. Typically, this silent development occurs in patients presenting at younger than 10 years of age. The first alerting sign may be an exaggerated lumbar lordosis. With more extreme slips, tight hamstrings and changes of posture and gait may be observed, even in the absence of symptoms.[22] In symptomatic cases, mechanical back pain is the most common presenting complaint.[14,22,46] Typically, this pattern presents in the preadolescent and older age groups.

The severity of back pain may or may not correlate with the degree of slip. Radicular pain is less common, but is most often observed with progressive translation when instability is present. Impingement of the L5 root is seen more commonly than S1 radiculopathy and is caused by compression within the lateral recess by hypertrophic fibrocartilage at the site of the pars defect. In contrast, pain from the S1 root occurs with the higher grade slips and is caused by tension from stretch of the root over the posterior edge of the sacrum. This may lead to intense pain, muscle spasm, and sciatic scoliosis. As discussed earlier, hamstring contracture occurs from both pain and the attempt to achieve spinal balance.

The physical examination is marked by exacerbation of the pain on extending the spine and by maneuvers that expose the instability. Accordingly, pain is relieved by recumbence. Tight hamstrings are the rule and abnormal gait with flexed knees and hips and a short stride length are observed, particularly with the higher grade slips. Most patients exhibit an increased lumbar lordosis, which becomes extreme in more severe slips.

CLINICAL FEATURES

- May develop silently and without apparent pain or other symptoms
  - Particularly in patients younger than 10 years old
  - First alerting signs: Exaggerated lumbar lordosis, tight hamstrings, and changes in posture and gait
- Symptomatic cases: Mechanical back pain is most common presenting complaint
  - Typically in preadolescents and older
  - Degree of back pain may not correlate with degree of slip
  - Radicular pain less common
    - Impingement of L5 root more common than S1

RADIOGRAPHIC FEATURES

The standard radiographic examination is done to confirm the diagnosis, observe instability, measure the amount of translation, quantify lumbosacral kyphosis, and, when possible, estimate the state of spinal balance. The standard views include anteroposterior and lateral studies (both done standing), a spot or focused lateral, and the left and right obliques. The standing lateral allows accurate measurement of the amount of translation of the vertebral body along the surface of the next caudal one. The accuracy of diagnosis requires standard technique so that the radiographic view is perpendicular to the true lateral portion of the spine.[41,48,50]

The Meyerling measurement and classification systems, as well as the reported modifications to this system, divide the upper surface of S1 into quartiles, so that translation of L5 is expressed as a fraction or percent of the transverse dimension of S1 (Figure 42-7).[8,46] A high-grade slip is defined as one that has progressed to 50% or greater translation and is represented by grades III, IV, and V.

Another measurement, the slip angle, follows the progression of kyphosis at the lumbosacral junction.[53] Normally, the L5 to S1 disc space is wedged into lordosis with a mean of 14 degrees.[2,17] Therefore, a neutral or kyphotic angle is abnormal. A kyphotic slip angle, which increases with time, is worrisome because it points to a course that is progressing towards spondyloptosis.[30,42] The slip angle and its method of measurement are shown in Figure 42-2. Instability can be better shown on a standing lateral radiograph compared to one done supine. Further, one can appreciate the possibility for reduction of the slip angle with supine stress done over a bolster. Reduction can also be studied with views that extend the pelvis and lumbar spine. Roussouly et al. have developed views to study spinal balance and outline some normal spinal and pelvic morphology, which was discussed earlier.[3,20,49]

Unfortunately, in the United States we have not stressed these views enough and, in most centers, we are not accustomed to examining the whole spine from C7 to the sacrum, or to including the femoral heads in our sagittal radiographs. It is our belief that this will become a standard procedure. Only with appreciation of

RADIOGRAPHIC FEATURES

- Standard radiographic views
  - Standing anteroposterior and lateral
  - Spot or focused lateral
  - Left and right obliques
- Meyerling measurement and classification systems: Divide upper surface of S1 into quartiles
  - Translation of L5 is expressed as fraction or percent of transverse dimension of S1
- Slip angle: Follows progression of kyphosis at lumbosacral junction
  - Normally, L5 to S1 disc space is wedged into lordosis with mean of 14 degrees, therefore a neutral or kyphotic angle abnormal
  - Kyphotic slip angle, which increases with time, points to progressive course toward spondyloptosis
- Instability: Better shown on standing anteroposterior radiograph compared with supine
- Possible reduction of slip angle: Supine stress done over bolster
- Reduction: Studied with views that extend pelvis and lumbar spine
- Examining whole spine from C7 to sacrum (including femoral heads in sagittal radiographs) may become standard procedure in future
- Magnetic resonance imaging (MRI): Indicated when neurologic symptoms or signs coexist, particularly caudal equina syndrome
- Radiculopathy: Examine discs adjacent to slip and nerve roots before developing surgical plan
- Computed tomography (CT): Helpful for lateral recesses to localize root compression and may help visualize other abnormal anatomy

the spinal balance can we appropriately plan the surgical treatment.

Magnetic resonance imaging (MRI) is indicated when neurologic symptoms or signs coexist, particularly a caudal equina syndrome. Additionally, with radiculopathy, it is important to examine the discs adjacent to the slip and the nerve roots prior to developing a surgical plan. Computed tomography (CT) is helpful for examining the lateral recesses to localize root compression. Also, CT may help visualize other abnormal anatomy.

TREATMENT: GOALS AND PRINCIPLES

The majority of children with spondylolisthesis do well without surgical treatment.[22,30,46] Generally, the extent of slip the translation is not extreme, rapid progression is not observed, and the slip angle is near normal. Additionally, recalcitrant symptoms of pain and radiculopathy typically do not persist.

Invasive treatment for spondylolisthesis is, thus, not generally required and there is little need for prolonged activity restriction. When symptoms are a troublesome feature, temporary modification of activities, hamstring stretching, abdominal strengthening, and nonsteroidal antiinflammatory drugs (NSAIDs) are sufficient treatment.[22,46] Occasionally, brace treatment may be required,[22]

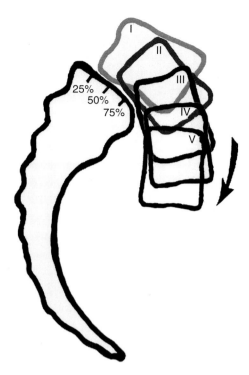

Figure 42-7. A modification of the Meyerling classification is depicted. Progression of translation or slip is related to the displacement of the body of one vertebra on another, in this case L5 on S1. Note the superior surface of the sacral body is divided into quartiles and each grade of translation is based on this. For example, grade I represents 25% translation and grade V describes spondyloptosis.

TREATMENT

- Children usually do well without surgical treatment
- For troublesome symptoms
  - Temporary modification of activities
  - Hamstring stretching and abdominal strengthening
  - Nonsteroidal antiinflammatory drugs (NSAIDs)
- Brace treatment occasionally required, followed by a gentle physical therapy program including abdominal strengthening, pelvic tilt, and hamstring stretching until asymptomatic
- Surgical treatment reserved for patients who have
  - Recalcitrant symptoms
  - Progressive horizontal translation that extends to 50% or more of length of adjacent vertebra (even if they are asymptomatic)
  - Failed nonoperative treatment
  - Young patients progressing to anticipated 50% translation considered operative candidates, particularly if younger than age 10 years (at risk to develop spondyloptosis)
- Surgical reduction has high risk for neurologic complications
- Surgical goal
  - Avoid high-grade spondylolisthesis
  - Fuse as few motion segments as possible
  - Restore or maintain spinal balance
  - Preserve neurologic status
  - Obtain solid arthrodesis
  - Treat clinical symptoms
- Approaches
  - Direct repair of pars defect
  - Posterior lateral fusion in situ (with or without decompression)
  - Instrumented posterior fusions (with or without decompression)
  - Anterior interbody fusions
  - Posterior interbody fusion
  - Posterior lateral fusion
  - Reduction or resection techniques

followed by a gentle physical therapy program including abdominal strengthening, pelvic tilt, and hamstring stretching.[33] This is done until the patient is asymptomatic. At this time, brace treatment is discontinued and physical therapy is increased to include back extension strengthening, exercises to increase spinal flexibility, and finally, an aggressive sports hardening therapy program to prepare the patient for a return to athletics. We have had many patients who successfully completed the outlined treatment program and resumed competitive athletics at a varsity level.

Surgical treatment is reserved for patients who have recalcitrant symptoms or a progressive horizontal translation that extends to 50% or more of the length of the adjacent vertebra, and those for whom nonoperative treatment has been unsuccessful. Even if they are asymptomatic, patients with translation of 50% or greater should also be considered as surgical candidates. Additionally, young patients who are progressing to an anticipated 50% translation should also be considered operative candidates, particularly if they are younger than 10 years of age.[14,30,42,46,52] These younger patients with progressive translation are at risk to develop spondyloptosis. The surgical goal is to avoid high-grade spondylolisthesis, but it must also be noted that surgical reduction has a high risk for neurologic complications.[29,42,43,46] If left untreated, however, the deformity leads to long-term problems that are disabling.[3,28,30,49] According to Roussouly and others, failure to avoid high-grade spondylolisthesis leads to extreme lordosis, spinal imbalance, and compensatory changes of posture and gait.[3,20,49] Eventually, the extensors of the hip fatigue and become unable to maintain spinal balance, which leads to failure to maintain an upright posture. At this point, surgically treating high-grade, kyphotic slips with posterior lateral arthrodesis is associated with a high rate of failure.[12,29,30] Accordingly, it would be prudent to treat spondylolisthesis prior to the development of a slip that measures 50% translation or greater and prior to the development of a significant slip angle.

Additional goals of surgical treatment in the management of spondylolisthesis are to fuse as few motion segments as possible, restore or maintain spinal balance, preserve neurologic status, obtain a solid arthrodesis, and treat the patient's clinical symptoms. A number of methods are available to aid the surgeon in accomplishing the above goals. These include direct repair of the pars defect, posterior lateral fusion in situ (with or without decompression), instrumented posterior fusions (with or without decompression), anterior interbody fusions, posterior interbody fusion, posterior lateral fusion, and reduction or resection techniques. Perhaps the least controversial approach is the use of a posterior in situ fusion for treatment of a low-grade spondylolisthesis. In contrast, the management of a high-grade spondylolisthesis (grade III to V) is controversial among surgical practices and within the literature. Segmental repair of the pars defect works well for spondylolysis, but, although conceptually attractive, it is not a viable option for significant spondylolisthesis.

Low-Grade Spondylolisthesis

Managing a low-grade (grade I to II) spondylolisthesis with a competent lumbosacral disc usually has a rewarding clinical outcome. Qualified candidates present with a low-grade slip, controlled lumbosacral lordosis, near normal slip angle and restoration of a bony hook through a solid posterolateral arthrodesis. We have also observed positive postsurgical outcomes in the majority of patients with a low degree of dysplasia and listhesis.

A high degree of success has been reported after posterolateral arthrodesis alone in patients with low-grade slips (Meyerling grades I and II) and in those with near normal slip angles.[14,30,42,52] Like others, we have been successful in the majority of these patients and have only observed pseudoarthrosis in 2 of approximately 100 patients, both of whom were varsity athletes. Both athletes, one, a 22-year-old college football player, and the other, a high school swimmer, required reexploration and fusion for pseudoarthrosis and persistent symptoms. A similar observation was reported by others.[30]

High-Grade Spondylolisthesis

High-grade spondylolisthesis is much more likely to develop pseudoarthrosis, persisting mechanical back pain and radicular symptoms.[14,29,30,42] The results of pseudoarthrosis are persisting pain, continued translation, progression, and ensuing increased slip angle. Pseudoarthrosis following a posterior lateral fusion performed in situ for high-grade spondylolisthesis has been reported by Grzegorzewski, Newton, Molinari, Seitsalo, and Schwab.[12,29,30,43,44] Grzegorzewski[12] noted pseudoarthrosis progression in 5 of 19 patients despite treatment with posterior lateral fusion followed by a pantaloon cast, non-weight-bearing for the first 4 months, and an additional 6 months in an orthosis. Newton[30] observed 3 of 39 patients treated for high-grade spondylolisthesis with in situ fusion who developed pseudoarthrosis, all of whom initially had a high kyphotic slip angle. Pseudoarthrosis was not detected in their patients with a neutral or lordotic slip angle. Molinari et al.[29] reported pseudoarthrosis in 5 of 11 patients with high-grade slips following posterior lateral fusion. They related the failure to dysplasia of the posterior elements and a small surface area of the transverse processes. They observed that circumferential

---

LOW-GRADE MANAGEMENT

- Low-grade (grade I to II) spondylolisthesis with competent lumbosacral disc
  - Presents with low-grade slip, controlled lumbosacral lordosis, near normal slip angle, and restoration of bony hook through solid posterolateral arthrodesis
- High degree of success after posterolateral arthrodesis alone for (Meyerling grades I and II) and near normal slip angles

---

HIGH-GRADE SPONDYLOLISTHESIS

- Much more likely to develop pseudoarthrosis, persisting mechanical back pain, and radicular symptoms
- Pseudoarthrosis results: Persisting pain, continued translation, progression, and ensuing increased slip angle
- Preoperative plan, consider role of instrumentation, need for reduction, resection techniques, and surgical approach—includes anterior, posterior, and combined approaches
- Must provide anterior column support through lumbosacral disc, using either anterior or posterior exposure
  - Importance in high-grade slips exemplified by low fusion rates after in situ posterior fusions not addressing importance of anterior column
- Surgical treatment options
  - Posterior fusion in situ without segmental spinal instrumentation or decompression followed by extension casting
  - Reduction with decompression, posterior instrumentation, and posterior column fusion
  - Reduction, decompression, and anterior/posterior fusion with posterior instrumentation
  - Postural reduction and circumferential fusion with transacral fibular interbody fusion providing anterior column support with decompression and instrumentation
  - Spondylectomy and instrumented fusion

---

arthrodesis without instrumentation appeared to be more successful. Similar observations have been made by others.[6,19,23,38,42]

The preoperative plan should consider the role of instrumentation, the need for reduction, resection techniques, and surgical approach, which includes the anterior, posterior, and combined approaches. When evaluating an approach, one must be able to provide anterior column support through the lumbosacral disc, using either an anterior or posterior exposure. The importance of anterior structural support in high-grade slips is exemplified by the low fusion rates following in situ posterior fusions that have failed to address the importance of the anterior column.[13]

Several authors have reported unacceptable pseudoarthrosis rates following in situ fusion for a high-grade spondylolisthesis. The nonunion rate ranges from 8% to 45% in some series, despite cast immobilization and activity restrictions. Causative factors are likely the increased stress on posterolateral bone graft, small surface area for grafting, coexisting spinal imbalance, and an incompetent lumbosacral disc. All of these factors contribute to an environment that jeopardizes bony fusion. Therefore, the reconstructive procedure chosen must resist the anterior shear and flexion forces that cause the deformity and generate tension across the graft to dissuade union. It seems intuitive, then, that rigid instrumentation and restoration of lumbosacral competence, either through anterior grafting or restoring spinal alignment, remain essential to the operative management of high-grade spondylolisthesis, especially those with a high kyphotic slip angle.

Anterior Column Support

We have experience treating 10 patients with high-grade spondylolisthesis with circumferential arthrodesis and structural graft to provide anterior column support without instrumentation. Treatment for all patients consisted of postural reduction, anterior fixation with an autograft or allograft fibula directed through L5 and into S1, and anterior arthrodesis at L4 to L5. This was followed by posterolateral arthrodesis from L4 to the sacrum without instrumentation. A pantaloon brace was worn for 6 months following surgery. Arthrodesis was achieved in all of the adolescent patients, but a loss of reduction was found in four of them. One 8-year-old patient developed a pseudoarthrosis with resorption of the fibular strut, lost reduction, and returned to the preoperative slip angle. The patient's condition was associated with mechanical back pain and left-sided radiculopathy, which required revision surgery. Because of this failed case, and because of the loss of correction in four others, we believe that we should have stabilized the arthrodesis with posterior instrumentation from L4 to S1. Others, including Bohlman and Cook, support this concept.[4,23,38]

The surgical treatment options for high-grade spondylolisthesis have been briefly discussed, and include posterior fusion in situ without segmental spinal instrumentation or decompression followed by extension casting; reduction with decompression, posterior instrumentation, and posterior column fusion; reduction, decompression, and anterior/posterior fusion with posterior instrumentation; postural reduction and circumferential fusion with transacral fibular interbody fusion providing anterior column support with decompression and instrumentation[4]; and spondylectomy and instrumented fusion.[11]

The published reports have indicated that surgery for high-grade spondylolisthesis has a higher risk of incurring major complications than surgery for low-grade spondylolisthesis. Postsurgical neurologic deficits ranging from radicular loss to cauda equina syndrome, loss of reduction, implant failure, pseudoarthrosis, and technical limitations have been frequently cited as sources of postsurgical morbidity.[5,15,25] These complica-

---

COMPLICATIONS WITH HIGH-GRADE SPONDYLOLISTHESIS SURGERY

- Higher risk of incurring major complications than surgery for low-grade spondylolisthesis
  - Postsurgical neurologic deficits ranging from radicular loss to cauda equina syndrome, loss of reduction, implant failure, pseudoarthrosis, and technical limitations; frequently cited as sources of postsurgical morbidity
- Major neurologic complications with instrumented reduction procedures: In as many as 15% to 30% of cases
  - Mechanism: Large increases in L5 nerve root tension with reduction greater than 50% of width of L5 vertebral body
  - With use of reduction techniques: Use spinal cord and spinal root monitoring
- Results of failure to achieve biomechanical harmony: Implant failure, loss of reduction, and eventual pseudoarthrosis
- Anterior structural support: Whether applied from anterior or posterior approach, provides mechanical advantages over posterior-only surgery
- Advantages of interbody structural grafting: Enhanced fusion rates, load-sharing capabilities, and no need for four-point pelvic fixation
- Whatever reconstructive approach is selected, ultimate goals of surgery: Prevention of slip progression, obtaining solid arthrodesis, preservation of neurologic function, and successful treatment of clinical symptoms
- Need for intraoperative reduction is controversial and possibly not justified
- Preference: Postural reduction followed by posterior-only circumferential arthrodesis using transsacral anterior column structural support

---

tions have been reported at varying rates for each of the above-mentioned procedures in separate series.

Major neurologic complications with instrumented reduction procedures occur in as many as 30% of cases. A review of the published literature regarding reduction shows that all of the existing series have at least one report in which a neurologic complication occurred. Fortunately, the majority of the neurologic sequelae were transient and resolution has been documented in long-term data. However, several studies have reported permanent neurologic loss following reduction of high-grade spondylolisthesis.[7,15] In a recent series, a 15% rate of neurologic injury occurred with reduction in the hands of accomplished deformity surgeons.[29] The mechanism appears to be large increases in L5 nerve root tension with reduction greater than 50% of the width of the L5 vertebral body.[36] Therefore, if reduction techniques are to be employed, we advocate the use of spinal cord and spinal root monitoring.

Failure to achieve biomechanical harmony in the surgical reconstruction of high-grade spondylolisthesis can result in implant failure, loss of reduction, and eventual pseudoarthrosis. The limitations of posterior-only instrumented reductions have been well documented in the literature, with hardware failure rates ranging from 25% to 83% in some series.[15,27] Furthermore, the biomechanical importance of anterior column interbody support has recently received attention in lumbar reconstructive surgery. Whether applied from an anterior or posterior approach, anterior structural support provides mechanical advantages over posterior-only surgery. The enhanced fusion rates, load-sharing capabilities, and obviating the need for four-point pelvic fixation are all reported advantages of interbody structural grafting.[27,29]

Whatever reconstructive approach is selected, the ultimate goals of surgery remain prevention of slip progression, obtaining a solid arthrodesis, preservation of neurologic function, and successful treatment of the clinical symptoms. Unfortunately, the literature is deficient in providing functional outcome data for the various surgical procedures available for the treatment of high-grade spondylolisthesis. Recently, Molinari et al.[29] reported patient-assessed function, pain, and satisfaction among three surgical procedures for high-grade isthmic dysplastic spondylolisthesis. The results suggest that the most important factor predicting patient success in function, pain, and satisfaction was the presence of a solid arthrodesis. Furthermore, the use of anterior column interbody structural support reduces the risk of implant failure and reduction loss and provides the highest fusion potential using a circumferential arthrodesis. There was no statistical difference in the above parameters, provided a solid posterior arthrodesis was achieved.

Therefore, the argument promoting reduction of a high-grade spondylolisthesis in order to optimize outcome and fusion potential is likely unjustified. In fact, the need for intraoperative reduction still remains controversial for reasons previously outlined. In all likelihood, it is our ability to obtain a solid arthrodesis and resist the abnormally high tensile stresses with sound constructs that optimize the clinical and radiographic outcomes. It is for these reasons, as well as our inability to justify the risks of a reduction procedure, that we prefer a postural reduction followed by a posterior-only circumferential arthrodesis using transsacral anterior column structural support.

TREATMENT TECHNIQUES
Posterolateral Arthrodesis

The Wiltse technique for posterolateral, or bilateral-lateral, arthrodesis is the authors' preferred method for low-grade spondylolisthesis because it is relatively easy to perform and has several advantages. First, the technique is extraarticular, which is appropriate because the arthrodesis is done anterior to the pathology and the instability. Second, when decompression and instrumentation are not required, as in the case of low-grade and stable slips, the muscle splitting approach rapidly and relatively nontraumatically leads to the desired fusion site. The site of entry is found approximately two finger breadths from the midline by incising the overlying fascia and palpating the facet joint (L5 for an arthrodesis at L5 to S1) and splitting the sacrospinalis muscle with a finger,

---

> ## POSTEROLATERAL ARTHRODESIS
>
> - Wiltse technique for posterolateral, or bilateral-lateral, arthrodesis
>   - Authors' preferred method for low-grade spondylolisthesis
>   - Extraarticular
>   - When decompression and instrumentation are not required (low-grade and stable slips), muscle splitting approach rapidly and relatively nontraumatically leads to desired fusion site
>   - Find site of entry: Approximately two fingerbreadths from midline by incising overlying fascia and palpatine in facet joint (L5 for an arthrodesis at L5 to S1) and splitting sacrospinalis with finger, elevator, or both
>   - Achieve hemostasis by electrocautery
>   - Expose lateral wall of the facets, transverse processes, and sacral alae and clean off all soft tissue
>   - Harvest cancellous bone graft from adjacent iliac crest, prepare fusion bed, and insert graft
>   - Can approach from midline, but skin and fascial incisions must be longer for same length of exposure; approach required when decompression or instrumentation planned
> - Use L5 facet to guide arthrodesis at L5 to S1; expose and meticulously clean transverse processes, sacral alae, and lateral wall facets to provide large bed for arthrodesis
> - Harvest cancellous bone graft from adjacent posterior iliac crest and then apply to bridge fusion site; to achieve successful arthrodesis, acquire large volume of bone graft
> - After insertion of graft, close two fascial incisions with running suture, effectively approximating sacrospinalis muscles
> - Close graft site and midline incision with drainage
> - Patient wears lumbosacral orthosis supporting one thigh for 3 months; orthosis worn for additional 3 months without thigh extension

an elevator, or both of these (Figure 42-8). Hemostasis is accomplished by electrocautery. The lateral wall of the facets, transverse processes, and the sacral alae are exposed and cleaned of all soft tissue. Cancellous bone graft is then harvested from the adjacent iliac crest, the fusion bed is prepared, and the graft is inserted.

The same area can be approached from the midline, but the skin and fascial incisions need to be longer to accomplish the same length of exposure. This approach is required when decompression or instrumentation is planned.

Either way, the L5 facet is the guide for arthrodesis at L5 to S1. It is important to expose and meticulously clean the transverse processes, sacral alae, and the lateral wall of the facets in order to provide a large bed for the arthrodesis. Cancellous bone graft can be harvested from the adjacent posterior iliac crest and then applied to bridge the fusion site. In order to achieve successful arthrodesis, it is important to acquire a large volume of bone graft.[18]

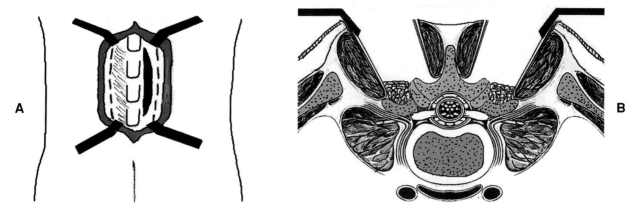

Figure 42-8.   The Wiltse posterolateral approach to arthrodesis. **A,** This is accomplished through a midline skin incision. The fascia is then incised as shown, approximately two finger breadths from the midline. For an L5 to S1 arthrodesis, the facets of L5 are the guides. They can be palpated through the paraspinal muscles. From there, the lateral wall of the facets, transverse processes, and the sacral alae can be identified and prepared for arthrodesis. **B,** The muscle splitting, which can largely be done with the index finger, easily leads to the facets and transverse processes. Note that the arthrodesis is extraarticular. It is important to meticulously clean the lateral wall of the facets, as well as the transverse processes and sacral alae. *(Data from Wiltse LL, Jackson DW: Treatment of spondylolisthesis and spondylolysis in children, Clin Orthop 117:92-100, 1976.)*

Following insertion of the graft, the two fascial incisions are closed with a running suture, effectively approximating the sacrospinalis muscles. The graft site and midline incision are then closed with drainage. A lumbosacral orthosis supporting one thigh is worn for 3 months and the orthosis is worn for an additional 3 months without the thigh extension. Figure 42-9 shows the radiographic and clinical pictures of an adolescent boy treated with postural reduction and posterolateral fusion using the Wiltse technique.

Postural Reduction With Posterior-Only Transsacral Arthrodesis

Our preferred technique for high-grade spondylolisthesis is similar to that previously described by Bohlman and others.[4,38,47] In contrast to his original description, several modifications have been added, including the use of rigid segmental instrumentation and fibular allograft strut grafting, thereby avoiding donor site morbidity (Figure 42-10). Despite the evolving enthusiasm for the restoration of a more normal sagittal plane contour, this technique permits adequate reduction of the slip angle while providing anterior interbody support through a posterior-only approach. This avoids any additional anterior surgery and the associated risks, including vessel injury and retrograde ejaculation, which is especially important in young males. In addition, our preferred technique provides an excellent opportunity for decompression of the lower lumbar and upper sacral nerve roots, which are commonly symptomatic. Furthermore, a more radical decompression is feasible through a sacroplasty in the setting of a sacral cauda equina syndrome. We consider the principal indications for this approach to include the presence of a high-grade

> ### PRINCIPLES OF POSTURAL REDUCTION WITH POSTERIOR-ONLY TRANSSACRAL ARTHRODESIS
>
> - Preferred technique for high-grade spondylolisthesis similar to that previously described by Bohlman and others with modifications.
>   - Include rigid segmental instrumentation.
>   - Use fibular allograft strut grafting (thereby avoiding donor site morbidity).
> - Despite evolving enthusiasm for restoring more normal sagittal plane contour, this technique permits adequate reduction of slip angle while providing anterior interbody support through a posterior-only approach.
> - Avoids additional anterior surgery and associated risks, including vessel injury and retrograde ejaculation, especially important in young males.
> - Preferred technique provides excellent opportunity for decompression of lower lumbar and upper sacral nerve roots, which are commonly symptomatic.
> - Principal indications include presence of high-grade spondylolisthesis (Meyerling grades III to V), severe mechanical low back pain, and neurologic dysfunction, including radicular pain, motor loss, or sacral cauda equina syndrome.

spondylolisthesis (Meyerling grades III to V), severe mechanical low back pain, and neurologic dysfunction, including radicular pain, motor loss, or a sacral cauda equina syndrome.

When performing our preferred approach, strict attention to detail is paramount in order to avoid complications and optimize surgical outcome. The patient is positioned prone on an operative frame or table that

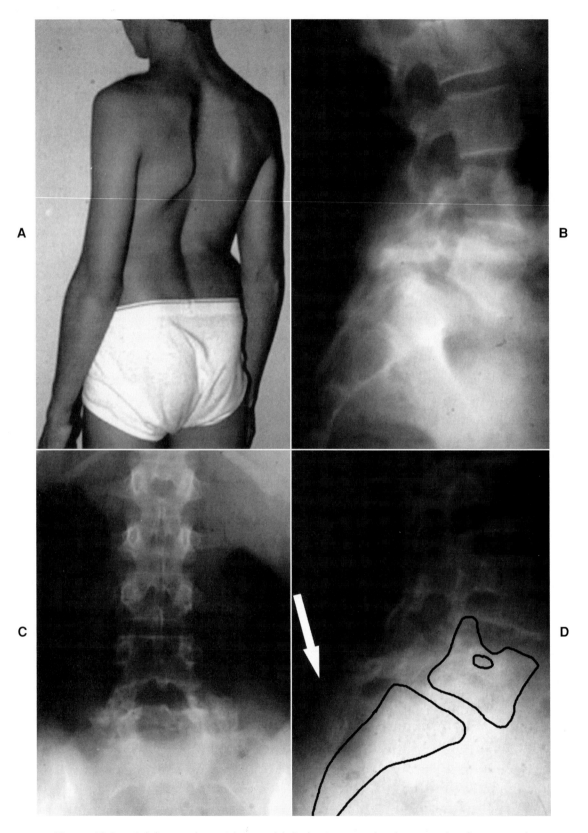

Figure 42-9.   Adolescent boy with spondylolisthesis treated with postural reduction and posterolateral fusion using the Wiltse technique. **A,** Preoperative picture. Note the sciatic postural lordosis. **B,** Preoperative lateral radiograph. He is developing a high-grade slip. **C,** Postoperative anteroposterior (AP) radiograph. Note the abundant lateral fusion mass. **D,** Postoperative lateral radiograph. *Arrow:* Note the abundant lateral fusion mass.

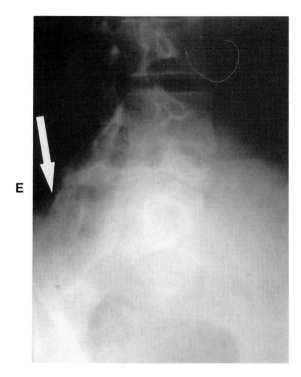

Figure 42-9, cont'd. **E,** Postoperative oblique radiograph. *Arrow:* Points to the posterolateral fusion.

permits hip extension and hyperextension of the lumbar spine. Historically, a well-padded four-poster frame had been used, but recent advances in spinal surgery tables allow for ease of positioning and visualization with fluoroscopy. Prior to initiating the procedure, intraoperative real-time images or static radiographs are obtained to ensure postural reduction of the slip angle and confirm visualization of the lumbosacral junction. Routine parenteral antibiotics are administered preoperatively and an intraoperative blood conservation system is used in concert with autologous donation.

A standard midline subperiosteal exposure of the lower lumbar spine and posterior aspect of the sacrum is carried out to the level of the second dorsal foramina. The lumbar transverse processes and sacral alae are widely exposed bilaterally to increase the lateral intertransverse area for grafting and decortication. Frequently, the autogenous iliac crest graft is harvested through a separate fascial incision after dorsal exposure to decrease the blood loss that occurs from a laminectomized spine. Furthermore, the graft can safely be harvested without the risk of inadvertent dural injury when working near exposed neural elements.

The spinal canal is entered at the L4 to L5 interlaminar space. A total bilateral laminectomy of L5, S1, and S2 is performed to adequately expose the dural sac and exiting nerve roots. An aggressive foraminotomy of the L5 and S1 nerve roots is carried out bilaterally to ensure decompression. Occasionally, the L5 pedicle is partially or completely excised to mobilize the exiting fifth lumbar root. All osseous fragments are retained for posterolateral grafting.

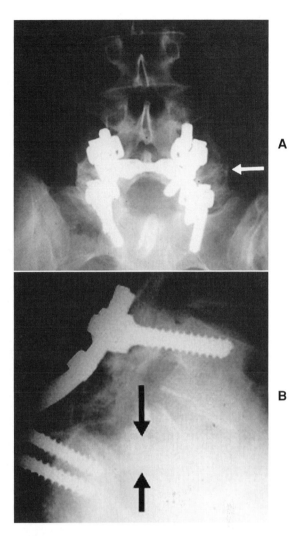

Figure 42-10. **A,** AP radiograph of a 17-year-old male 3 months following a posterior decompression and circumferential arthrodesis using Bohlman's technique. *Arrow:* Note graft position and signs of early consolidation in the intertransverse region. Our preference is the routine use of transpedicular segmental instrumentation with fibular allograft. **B,** Standing lateral radiograph of a 17-year-old male 3 months following a posterior decompression and circumferential arthrodesis using Bohlman's technique. *Arrow:* Note graft position in relation to L5 vertebral body and reduction of the slip angle with a postural reduction.

As reported and described by Smith and Bohlman,[47] a sacroplasty is indicated in those patients with a sacral cauda equina syndrome (Figure 42-11). This syndrome includes saddle anesthesia, proximal thigh dysesthesias, and bowel and bladder dysfunction. Although the myelogram and MRI show significant signs of compression, patients with preservation of distal sacral function do not require a sacroplasty.

When addressing the second-phase of the surgery an adequate exposure of the first and second sacral pedicle is mandatory. This will aid in localizing the starting point for transsacral interbody fixation. Our starting point is

TECHNIQUES OF POSTURAL REDUCTION WITH POSTERIOR-ONLY TRANSSACRAL ARTHRODESIS

- Position patient prone on operative frame or table that permits hip extension and hyperextension of lumbar spine.
- Prior to initiating the procedure, obtain intraoperative real-time images or static radiographs to ensure postural reduction of slip angle and confirm visualization of lumbosacral junction.
- Give routine parenteral antibiotics preoperatively.
- Use intraoperative blood conservation system in concert with autologous donation.
- Carry out standard midline subperiosteal exposure of lower lumbar spine and posterior aspect of sacrum to level of second dorsal foramina.
- Expose lumbar transverse processes and sacral alae widely bilaterally to increase lateral intertransverse area for grafting and decortication.
- Harvest autogenous iliac crest graft through separate fascial incision after dorsal exposure (often used to decrease blood loss that occurs from laminectomized spine).
- Safely harvest graft without risk of inadvertent dural injury when working near exposed neural elements.
- Enter spinal canal at L4 to L5 interlaminar space.
- Perform total bilateral laminectomy of L5, S1, and S2 to adequately expose dural sac and existing nerve roots.
- Carry out aggressive foraminotomy of L5 and S1 nerve roots bilaterally to ensure decompression; occasionally, L5 pedicle is partially or completely excised to mobilize exiting fifth lumbar root.

- Retain all osseous fragments for posterolateral grafting.
- When addressing second phase of surgery, obtain adequate exposure of first and second sacral pedicle to localize starting point for transsacral interbody fixation.
- Use angle of drilling approximately 15 degrees in cephalad toward midportion of L5 vertebral body; close fluoroscopic visualization of drill guide trajectory mandatory to avoid inadvertent anterior penetration and potential vascular injury.
- Ideally, locate guide pin directly below junction of anterior vertebral body and superior end plate of fifth lumbar vertebrae.
- Preferred technique: Use threaded guide pin and cannulated 10 to 15 mm ACL reamer for canal preparation (see Figure 42-14); once again, importance of continuous real-time image intensification cannot be overemphasized.
- Use of fresh-frozen fibula allograft to avoid the potential graft-site morbidity with autogenous harvest recommended.
- Postoperatively, immobilize patient in lumbosacral orthosis with articulated thigh extension for 3 months.
- For early postoperative rehabilitation include hamstring stretching, with more aggressive regimen after confirmation of union.
- External spinal stimulators recently added to postoperative protocol for adult patients.

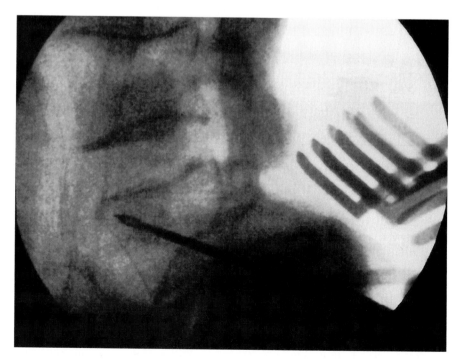

Figure 42-11. Intraoperative fluoroscopic lateral projection of ideal guide pin position. Position is just posterior to the junction of the anterior vertebral body line and superior implant.

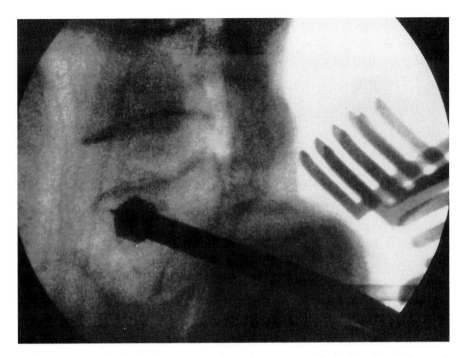

Figure 42-12.   Intraoperative fluoroscopic lateral projection of ideal position of cannulated ACL reamer. Note the position of the guide pin has remained unchanged. We routinely use a threaded guide pin and continued fluoroscopic visualization to prevent pin penetration.

similar to that described by Smith and Bohlman,[47] with careful retraction of the first and second sacral nerve roots. The angle of drilling is approximately 15 degrees in a cephalad direction toward the midportion of the L5 vertebral body (Figure 42-12). Close fluoroscopic visualization of the drill guide trajectory is mandatory to avoid inadvertent anterior penetration and potential vascular injury.[37] The ideal guide pin location is directly below the junction of the anterior vertebral body and superior end plate of the fifth lumbar vertebrae (Figure 42-13). We prefer a threaded guide pin and a cannulated 10- to 15-mm anterior curciate ligament (ACL) reamer for canal preparation (Figure 42-14). Once again, the importance of continuous real-time image intensification cannot be overemphasized.

We use fresh-frozen fibula allograft to avoid the potential graft site morbidity with autogenous harvest. The concerns regarding graft fracture or delayed incorporation with the use of allograft may be counterbalanced with segmental instrumentation. We routinely use monoaxial titanium transpedicular fixation by placing bilateral fixation points at the fourth lumbar and first sacral vertebra. The strong anterior column support permits leaving the S2 pedicles without instrumentation. Additionally, strict adherence to the principles of fusion biology should provide the ideal milieu for spinal union.

Postoperatively, the patient is immobilized in a lumbosacral orthosis with an articulated thigh extension for 3 months. Early postoperative rehabilitation consists of hamstring stretching, with a more aggressive regimen after confirmation of union. External spinal stimulators are a fairly recent addition to our postoperative protocol for adult patients.

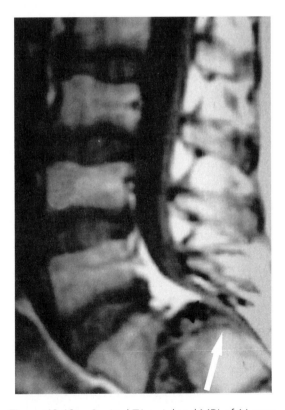

Figure 42-13.   Sagittal T1 weighted MRI of 16-year-old male with grade IV isthmic spondylolisthesis. Note incompetence of the lumbosacral disc, as well as the degree of lumbosacral kyphosis. *Arrow:* Projects to dorsal sacrum, which can require resection (sacroplasty) in the presence of a severe neurologic deficit.

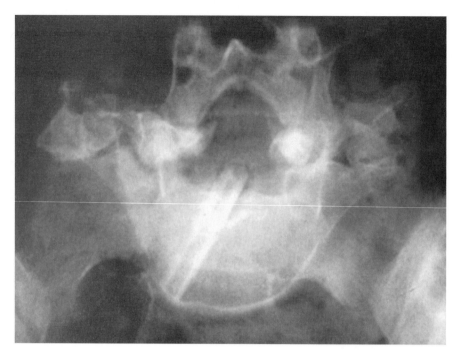

Figure 42-14. AP pelvic radiograph of 16-year-old male following an instrumented circumferential arthrodesis utilizing the Bohlman technique. Despite the lucency around the posterior graft, a solid arthrodesis was achieved.

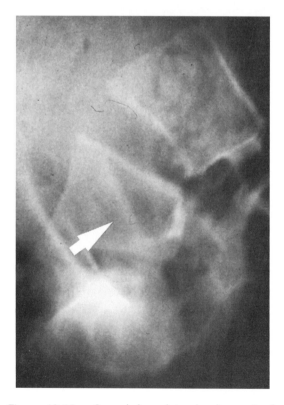

Figure 42-15. Coned-down lateral radiograph of the lumbosacral junction in a 15-year-old male 2 years following an uninstrumented arthrodesis. *Arrow:* Note the graft position in reference to the L5 vertebral body.

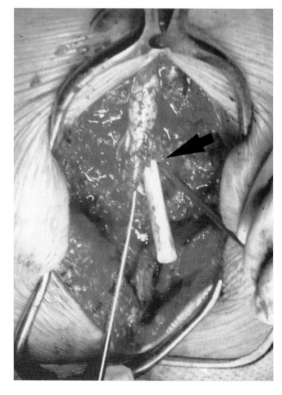

Figure 42-16. Intraoperative photograph identifying graft trajectory, as well as its position in reference to the first and second sacral nerve roots (arrow).

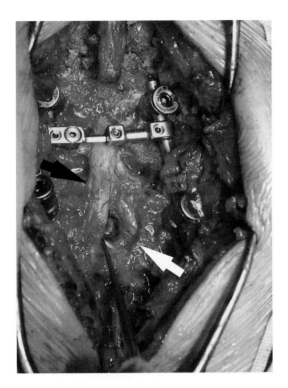

Figure 42-17. Intraoperative photograph illustrating the position of nerve roots following recession of fibular graft and position of segmental instrumentation. Note the wide decompression and the abundant bone graft in the posterolateral recess. Surgical instrument is pointing toward the posterior margin of the graft. *White arrow:* Points to the right sacral nerve roots. *Black arrow:* Points to the dorsal side of cauda equina.

The results published in the literature support our preference for a fibular allograft to provide anterior column support, posterolateral arthrodesis, and instrumentation from L4 to the sacrum as a viable option in the treatment of high-grade spondylolisthesis (Meyerling grades III to V). Smith and Bohlman's initial case series of 2 patients was the impetus for a later publication by Smith and Bohlman in which 11 patients were followed for an average of 64 months postoperatively.[4,47] All were treated with a posterior decompression and circumferential arthrodesis using a posterolateral noninstrumented fusion from L4 to S1 with transsacral fibula autograft interbody support (Figures 42-15 and 42-16). The majority of patients had a grade IV or V slip, neurologic deficit, and established nonunion after a previously failed reconstruction. At final follow-up, all 11 patients had a radiographic arthrodesis and all had complete neurologic return. In a more recent series, a group of 14 patients were treated with a decompression and circumferential arthrodesis using the technique of Bohlman.[38] Excellent results were observed in 13 patients, with one patient developing a nonunion and slip progression.

Despite the desire to "treat the radiograph" and restore the sagittal spinal alignment, we believe that the literature lacks convincing evidence supporting the reduction of a high-grade spondylolisthesis. In our opinion, the neurologic risks and associated postsurgical morbidity following reductions make postural reduction with posterior-only transsacral arthrodesis the most appealing technique. In our hands, this technique has provided a safe and effective means of stabilizing a high-grade lumbosacral spondylolisthesis. Furthermore, it avoids an additional anterior procedure while providing all of the benefits of anterior column support. From the few studies available, this technique, with the addition of segmental instrumentation, creates an excellent environment for arthrodesis (Figure 42-17).

SUGGESTED REFERENCES

Antoniades SB, Hammerberg KW, DeWald RL: Sagittal plane configuration of the sacrum in spondylolisthesis, *Spine* 25:1085-1091, 2000.

Berthonnaud E, Roussouly P, Dimnet J: The parameters describing the shape and the equilibrium of the set back pelvis and femurs in sagittal view, *Innov Techn Biol Med* 19:411-426, 1998.

Legaye J et al.: Pelvic incidence: a fundamental pelvic parameter for three-dimensional regulation of spinal sagittal curves, *Eur Spine J* 7:99-103, 1998.

Lonstein JE: Spondylolisthesis in children: cause, natural history, and management, *Spine* 24:2640-2648, 1999.

Molinari RW et al.: Complications in the surgical treatment of pediatric high-grade, isthmic dysplastic spondylolisthesis: a comparison of three surgical approaches, *Spine* 24:1701-1711, 1999.

Seitsalo S et al.: Progression of spondylolisthesis in children and adolescents: a long-term follow-up of 272 patients, *Spine* 16:417-421, 1991.

Smith JA, Hu SS: Management of spondylolysis and spondylolisthesis in the pediatric and adolescent population, *Orthop Clin North Am* 30:487-499, ix, 1999.

Vaz G et al.: Sagittal morphology and equilibrium of the spine and pelvis, *Spine J* 11:80-87, 2002.

Wiltse LL, Winter RB: Terminology and measurement of spondylolisthesis, *J Bone Joint Surg Am* 65:768-772, 1983.

REFERENCES

1. Antoniades SB, Hammerberg KW, DeWald RL: Sagittal plane configuration of the sacrum in spondylolisthesis, *Spine* 25:1085-1091, 2000.
2. Bernhardt M: Normal spinal anatomy: normal sagittal plane alignment. In Bridwell KH, ed: *Textbook of spinal surgery*, Philadelphia, 1997, Lippincott-Raven, 1997.
3. Berthonnaud E, Roussouly P, Dimnet J: The parameters describing the shape and the equilibrium of the set back pelvis and femurs in sagittal view, *Innov Techn Biol Med* 19:411-426, 1998.
4. Bohlman HH, Cook SS: One-stage decompression and posterolateral and interbody fusion for lumbosacral spondyloptosis through a posterior approach: report of two cases, *J Bone Joint Surg Am* 64:415-418, 1982.
5. Bradford DS: Treatment of severe spondylolisthesis: a combined approach for reduction and stabilization, *Spine* 4:423-429, 1979.
6. Bradford DS: Management of spondylolysis and spondylolisthesis, *Instr Course Lect* 32: 151-162, 1983.
7. Bradford DS, Gotfried Y: Staged salvage reconstruction of grade-IV and V spondylolisthesis, *J Bone Joint Surg Am* 69:191-202, 1987.
8. DeWald R: Spondylolisthesis. In Bridwell KH, ed: *Textbook of spinal surgery*, Philadelphia, 1997, Lippincott-Raven.
9. Dick W, Elke R: Significance of the sagittal profile and reposition of grade III-V spondylolisthesis, *Orthopade*, 26:774-780, 1997.
10. Fredrickson BE et al.: The natural history of spondylolysis and spondylolisthesis, *J Bone Joint Surg Am* 66:699-707, 1984.
11. Gaines RW, Nichols WK: Treatment of spondyloptosis by two stage L5 vertebrectomy and reduction of L4 onto S1, *Spine* 10:680-686, 1985.
12. Grzegorzewski A, Kumar SJ: In situ posterolateral spine arthrodesis for grades III, IV, and V spondylolisthesis in children and adolescents, *J Pediatr Orthop* 20:506-511, 2000.

13. Haukipuro K et al.: Familial occurrence of lumbar spondylolysis and spondylolisthesis, *Clin Genet* 13:471-476, 1978.
14. Hensinger RN: Spondylolysis and spondylolisthesis in children, *Instr Course Lect* 32:132-151, 1983.
15. Hu SS, Bradford et al.: Reduction of high-grade spondylolisthesis using Edwards instrumentation, *Spine* 21:367-371, 1996.
16. Jackson DW, Wiltse LL, Cirincoine RJ: Spondylolysis in the female gymnast, *Clin Orthop* 117:68-73, 1976.
17. Jackson RP et al.: Compensatory spinopelvic balance over the hip axis and better reliability in measuring lordosis to the pelvic radius on standing lateral radiographs of adult volunteers and patients, *Spine* 23:1750-1767, 1998.
18. Kim K et al.: Volumetric change of the graft bone after inter-transverse fusion, *Spine* 24:428-433, 1999.
19. Laursen M et al.: Functional outcome after partial reduction and 360 degree fusion in grade III-V spondylolisthesis in adolescent and adult patients, *J Spinal Disord* 12:300-306, 1999.
20. Legaye J et al.: Pelvic incidence: a fundamental pelvic parameter for three-dimensional regulation of spinal sagittal curves, *Eur Spine J* 7:99-103, 1998.
21. Letts M et al.: Fracture of the pars interarticularis in adolescent athletes: a clinical-biomechanical analysis, *J Pediatr Orthop* 6:40-46, 1986.
22. Lonstein JE: Spondylolisthesis in children: cause, natural history, and management, *Spine* 24:2640-2648, 1999.
23. Majd ME, Holt RT: Anterior fibular strut grafting for the treatment of pseudoarthrosis in spondylolisthesis, *Am J Orthop* 29:99-105, 2000.
24. Marchetti PG, Bartolozzi P: Classification of spondylolisthesis as a guideline for treatment. In Bridwell KH, ed: *Textbook of spinal surgery*, Philadelphia, 1997, Lippincott-Raven.
25. Maurice HD, Morley TR: Cauda equina lesions following fusion in situ and decompressive laminectomy for severe spondylolisthesis: four case reports, *Spine* 14:214-216, 1989.
26. McCarroll JR, Miller JM, Ritter MA: Lumbar spondylolysis and spondylolisthesis in college football players: a prospective study, *Am J Sports Med* 14:404-406, 1986.
27. McCord DH et al.: Biomechanical analysis of lumbosacral fixation, *Spine* 17:S235-243, 1992.
28. Meyers LL et al.: Mechanical instability as a cause of gait disturbance in high-grade spondylolisthesis: a pre- and postoperative three-dimensional gait analysis, *J Pediatr Orthop* 19:672-676, 1999.
29. Molinari RW et al.: Complications in the surgical treatment of pediatric high-grade, isthmic dysplastic spondylolisthesis: a comparison of three surgical approaches, *Spine* 24:1701-1711, 1999.
30. Newton PO, Johnston CE II: Analysis and treatment of poor outcomes following in situ arthrodesis in adolescent spondylolisthesis, *J Pediatr Orthop* 17:754-761, 1997.
31. Oakley RH, Carty H: Review of spondylolisthesis and spondylolysis in paediatric practice, *Br J Radiol* 57:877-885, 1984.
32. Osterman K, Lindholm TS, Laurent LE: Late results of removal of the loose posterior element (Gill's operation) in the treatment of lytic lumbar spondylolisthesis, *Clin Orthop* 117:121-128, 1976.
33. O'Sullivan PB et al.: Evaluation of specific stabilizing exercise in the treatment of chronic low back pain with radiologic diagnosis of spondylolysis or spondylolisthesis, *Spine* 22:2959-2967, 1997.
34. Penning L, Blickman JR: Instability in lumbar spondylolisthesis: a radiologic study of several concepts, *Am J Roentgenol* 134:293-301, 1980.
35. Peterson CK, Haas M, Harger BL: A radiographic study of sacral base, sacrovertebral, and lumbosacral disc angles in persons with and without defects in the pars interarticularis, *J Manipulative Physiol Ther* 13:491-497, 1990.
36. Petraco DM et al.: An anatomic evaluation of L5 nerve stretch in spondylolisthesis reduction, *Spine* 21:1133-1138; discussion 1139, 1996.
37. Rajaraman V et al.: Visceral and vascular complications resulting from anterior lumbar interbody fusion, *J Neurosurg* 91:60-64, 1999.
38. Roca J et al.: One-stage decompression and posterolateral and interbody fusion for severe spondylolisthesis: an analysis of 14 patients, *Spine* 24:709-714, 1999.
39. Rosok G, Peterson CK: Comparison of the sacral base angle in females with and without spondylolysis: *J Manipulative Physiol Ther* 16:447-452, 1993.
40. Rowe G, Roche M: The etiology of separate neutral arch, *J Bone Joint Surg Am* 35:102-109, 1953.
41. Saifuddin A et al.: Orientation of lumbar pars defects: implications for radiological detection and surgical management, *J Bone Joint Surg Br* 80:208-211, 1998.
42. Schlenzka D: Spondylolisthesis in childhood and adolescence, *Orthopade* 26:760-768, 1997.
43. Schwab FJ, Farcy JP, Roye DP Jr: The sagittal pelvic tilt index as a criterion in the evaluation of spondylolisthesis; preliminary observations, *Spine* 22:1661-1667, 1997.
44. Seitsalo S et al.: Progression of spondylolisthesis in children and adolescents: a long-term follow-up of 272 patients, *Spine* 16:417-421, 1991.
45. Shaffer B, Wiesel S, Lauerman W: Spondylolisthesis in the elite football player: an epidemiologic study in the NCAA and NFL, *J Spinal Disord* 10:365-370, 1997.
46. Smith JA, Hu SS: Management of spondylolysis and spondylolisthesis in the pediatric and adolescent population, *Orthop Clin North Am* 30:487-499, ix, 1999.
47. Smith MD, Bohlman HH: Spondylolisthesis treated by a single-stage operation combining decompression with in situ posterolateral and anterior fusion: an analysis of eleven patients who had long-term follow-up, *J Bone Joint Surg Am* 72:415-421, 1990.
48. Ulmer JL et al.: MR imaging of lumbar spondylolysis: the importance of ancillary observations, *Am J Roentgenol* 169:233-239, 1997.
49. Vaz G et al.: Sagittal morphology and equilibrium of the spine and pelvis, *Spine J* 11:80-87, 2002.
50. Wall MS, Oppenheim WL: Measurement error of spondylolisthesis as a function of radiographic beam angle, *J Pediatr Orthop* 15:193-198, 1995.
51. Wiltse LL, Jackson DW: Treatment of spondylolisthesis and spondylolysis in children, *Clin Orthop* 117:92-100, 1976.
52. Wiltse LL, Newman PH, Macnab I: Classification of spondylolisis and spondylolisthesis, *Clin Orthop* 117:23-29, 1976.
53. Wiltse LL, Winter RB: Terminology and measurement of spondylolisthesis, *J Bone Joint Surg Am* 65:768-772, 1983.
54. Wright JG, Bell D: Lumbosacral joint angles in children, *J Pediatr Orthop* 11:748-751, 1991 (comments).
55. Wynne-Davies R, Scott JH: Inheritance and spondylolisthesis: a radiographic family survey, *J Bone Joint Surg Br* 61:301-305, 1979.

Congenital Deformities of the Spine

John E. Lonstein

By definition congenital spinal deformities are due to abnormal vertebral development with the vertebral anomaly present at birth. Because of this, these children tend to have a curvature noted much earlier in life than the typical patient with idiopathic scoliosis.

This early development of the deformity has resulted in a tendency for the young child with congenital spinal deformities to receive less than optimum care. Congenital curves tend to be very rigid and resistant to correction. The curves are frequently allowed to progress, and because of all the years of growth, large deformities can result. These deformities must *not* be allowed to progress. In many cases early fusion is essential, being preferable to allowing severe curves to develop. Early fusion will *not* stunt the potential growth, because the area of the anomalies and the area that needs to be fused cannot grow in a normal vertical manner because of the abnormal growth potential.

CLASSIFICATION

Congenital deformities are classified a number of ways: (1) the type of anomaly, (2) the type of deformity (scoliosis, kyphosis, lordosis, or combinations—kyphoscoliosis and lordoscoliosis), and (3) the area of the spine involved (cervical, cervicothoracic, thoracic, thoracolumbar, lumbar, and lumbosacral).

CLASSIFICATION

- Basis of natural history
- Rationale for treatment
- Basis is growth imbalance
- Progression during growth spurts
  - Birth to 4 years of age
  - Adolescence
- Natural history/prognosis depend on
  - Type of anomaly
  - Area of anomaly
  - Deformity (scoliosis/kyphosis/lordosis)
  - Age
  - Sex

The vertebral anomaly is classified into abnormalities of segmentation, abnormalities of formation, or mixed problems, which can occur at any part in the vertebral ring (anterior, anterolateral, lateral, posterolateral, or posterior). It is important to remember that a hemivertebra is *not* an extra vertebra, but rather the remainder of the vertebra that did not form. In the area of the anomaly there is abnormal or absent growth potential due to an area of missing bone (formation defect) or missing growth plates (segmentation defect). Depending on where in the vertebral ring this occurs, the resulting deformity can be pure scoliosis, kyphosis, or lordosis, or a combination of scoliosis plus kyphosis or lordosis.

The difference in growth potential in the parts of the vertebral ring is the basis of the understanding of the natural history and the principles of treatment of congenital spine deformities. The magnitude of the deformity, its behavior, and rate of progression depend on the type of anomaly and the growth potential of the vertebrae in the area. The critical times of progression are during the periods of rapid growth in the growth spurts of infancy (birth to 4 years of age) and the adolescent growth spurt. In addition, the area of the anomaly and the deformity present (scoliosis/kyphosis/lordosis or combinations) also determine the natural history as discussed below.

PATIENT EVALUATION

Congenital spinal deformities occur during embryologic development, and thus the spinal anomalies are often accompanied by congenital anomalies involving other organs or systems, or the congenital spinal anomaly is part of a syndrome.[2] It is thus extremely important that

---

ASSOCIATED ANOMALIES

- Genitourinary 20% to 33%
- Cardiac 10% to 15%
- Intraspinal anomalies 20%
- Pulmonary
- Syndromes

---

these patients receive a complete evaluation, the evaluation not being restricted to the spine alone.

The most common associated congenital anomaly is found in the genitourinary tract. Studies of patients with congenital scoliosis by MacEwen et al.[11] revealed a 20% incidence of urinary tract anomalies on routine intravenous pyelography, whereas a study by Hensinger et al.[5] on cervical anomalies found a higher rate of 33%. Many of the anomalies noted are anatomic variations with normal renal function (e.g., unilateral kidney, cross-fused ectopia) that do not need urologic treatment, but significant obstructive uropathy can occur. Thus all patients diagnosed as having a congenital spine anomaly must have a renal tract evaluation. Renal ultrasound is the screening test, or a magnetic resonance imaging (MRI) scan is used as part of the spinal canal evaluation. An abnormal ultrasound or MRI is followed up with an intravenous pyelogram for definitive diagnosis. If an obstructive uropathy is found, appropriate urologic procedures should be performed before instituting orthopedic treatment of the spinal deformity.

A second area of concern is cardiac anomalies. As many as 10% to 15% of patients with congenital scoliosis have been noted to have congenital heart defects.[5,17] These may have previously been undetected. Murmurs should never be attributed to the scoliosis and must be thoroughly evaluated.

Examination of the back and extremities for evidence of a hidden neurologic disorder is very important. There is a high frequency of spinal dysraphism in patients with congenital scoliosis. These include Arnold-Chiari anomaly of the craniocervical junction, diastematomyelia, syringomyelia, and a tethered spinal cord. McMaster[14] reported that about 20% of his patients with congenital scoliosis had some form of dysraphism such as a tethered spinal cord, fibrous dural bands, diastematomyelia, or intradural lipoma. These neural canal abnormalities are frequently associated with cutaneous changes (hair patches, dimples, skin pigmentation, or hemangiomas), and various abnormalities on the examination of the lower extremities. These include flatfeet, cavus feet, vertical tali, clubfeet, and more subtle changes such as slight atrophy of one calf, a slightly smaller foot on one side, or asymmetric reflexes. On the other hand, it is possible for a patient to have one of these intraspinal anomalies and have no associated findings. The physician must evaluate the radiographs for any interpediculate widening or midline bony spicules. The use of MRI scans has greatly aided the evaluation of dysraphism. This imaging should be obtained in any patient having neurologic findings, foot deformities, bladder or bowel malfunction, cutaneous changes overlying the spine, or in whom a corrective spinal surgery is being planned[22] (Figure 43-1).

An accurate radiologic evaluation is essential. Supine radiographs should be obtained on all children unable to sit or stand unaided. A supine view is also obtained in older children to accurately visualize the area vertebral anatomy; the upright views shows the deformity. The convex growth is very important, and thus the quality of the bone and disc spaces on the convexity of the defor-

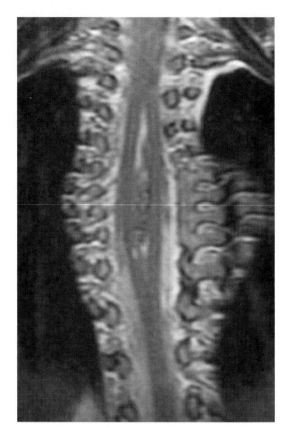

Figure 43-1. Coronal MRI scan of diastematomyelia in the thoracic spine showing interpediculate widening, midline bony spur with split spinal cord in this area.

mity must be clearly visualized and inspected. If the disc spaces are present and clearly defined, and the convex pedicles clearly formed, there is a possibility of convex growth, and the prognosis is poor. On the other hand, if the convex discs are not clearly formed, and the convex pedicles are poorly demarcated, there is less convex growth potential, and the prognosis is not as bad. It must be remembered that in the first 2 years of life cartilage forms a significant part of the vertebra, and therefore at this stage prognostication is not as accurate as in the older child.

Routine coronal and sagittal views are obtained initially to appreciate the deformity in both planes, with subsequent examinations or imaging modalities chosen depending on the deformity that exists. It is important to visualize the whole spine on both views because multiple anomalies are common, and they may be on opposite ends of the spine (e.g., one cervical and one lumbosacral). It is important to select accurate vertebral landmarks on the end vertebrae of the curves to be measured, with the same landmarks used for subsequent radiographs, ensuring the reliability of the evaluation. The accuracy of measurement in congenital scoliosis is less than in nonanomalous spines, the accuracy depending on choosing consistent end points for measurement and the clarity of these end points.[4]

SCOLIOSIS
Natural History

The natural history of congenital spinal deformities is the rationale for treatment of these deformities. The growth imbalance resulting from the congenital anomaly is the basis of this understanding. The growth potential in the area of the anomaly is best appreciated with high-quality radiographic evaluation.

Although one would theoretically like to associate a certain prognosis with a certain anomaly, this is not always possible. Careful documentation of the deformity and the magnitude of the curve by high-quality radiographs and photographs is necessary on the first examination. Subsequent serial photography and radiology are important. Children should be followed at 6-month intervals and must be followed until the end of their growth. Some patients have mild curves that are stable for many years and then suddenly become severe at the onset of the adolescent growth spurt. Some curves never progress at all and, after being followed for many years, do not result in any significant deformity. These patients of course do not require any treatment, and it is foolish to apply an orthosis or perform a fusion for a condition that is not progressive and not disabling.

In general, studies show that most curves are progressive, with 10% to 25% being nonprogressive.[8,23] The large study of McMaster and Ohtsuka[15] of 251 patients found that only 11% were nonprogressive, whereas 14% were slightly progressive, and the remaining 75% progressed significantly. The rate of curve increase depended on the area of the spine involved and the type of anomaly. Thoracic curves had the poorest prognosis, with the worst anomaly being a unilateral unsegmented bar (unilateral failure of segmentation) accompanied by single or multiple convex hemivertebrae.[13] The other anomalies with a poor prognosis were, in order, a unilateral unsegmented bar, double convex hemivertebrae, and a single free convex hemivertebra, with the bloc vertebra (bilateral failure of segmentation) having the best prognosis.

There are certain anomalies that are consistently associated with progression (the unilateral unsegmented bar) and so reliably malicious that the patient with this anomaly should have an immediate fusion, not waiting for progression. The unilateral unsegmented bar causes a total lack of growth on the concave side of the curve, and if growth continues on the convex side, a severe deformity will result. Once established, this deformity is extremely rigid and virtually impossible to correct except by complex and difficult surgery. Therefore it is far better to prevent the deformity from increasing than to correct it once it has become severe.

Hemivertebrae may be single or multiple and balanced or unbalanced.[20] In addition, they are classified on their relationship to the adjacent spine as being incarcerated or nonincarcerated, an incarcerated hemivertebra being "tucked into" the spine and not changing the contour of the spine. In addition, their relationship to the adjacent vertebrae is critical (segmented, semisegmented, or nonsegmented) because it gives an idea of the possible growth potential on the convexity of the

curve. Contralateral hemivertebrae (hemimetameric segmental displacement or hemimetameric shift) when balanced often may not progress and thus do not require treatment. When separated by several segments, a double curve is produced, and both curves may progress and require fusion. A single hemivertebra, which is the most common anomaly, may or may not cause a progressive deformity, this outcome being very difficult to predict.[15] The patient must be followed carefully, and with curve progression a fusion should be performed. A single hemivertebra at the lumbosacral level produces significant decompensation, because there is no room below the hemivertebra for natural compensation to occur. These patients may have a severe curve to one side, which is progressive with growth and is best seen clinically. A photograph of the back showing the balance in these patients is an essential part of the clinical evaluation.

Nonoperative Treatment
Observation

In cases where the natural history is unclear (isolated single or multiple hemivertebrae and mixed anomalies), the patient is followed for curve progression (Figures 43-2 and 43-3). Repeat x-rays are taken and carefully measured using consistent end vertebrae and consistent vertebral measurement points (pedicle or end plate). Because curve progression is slow, averaging 5 to 7 degrees a year,

---

SCOLIOSIS—NATURAL HISTORY

- 75% progressive
- 14% mildly progressive
- 11% nonprogressive
- Worst prognosis
  - Unsegmented bar with convex hemivertebra(e)
  - Unsegmented bar alone

SCOLIOSIS—NONOPERATIVE TREATMENT

- Observation
  - No role with unsegmented bar or if any kyphosis present
  - Used when natural history is unclear to document progression
  - Accurate measurement is essential
    - Same vertebrae
    - Same anatomic landmarks
    - Consistency is important
    - Compare current x-ray to initial and to last visit films
- Bracing
  - No role in congenital kyphosis, lordosis, short stiff scoliosis
  - Long flexible curves with anomaly part of the curve
  - Compensatory curve
  - Postoperative

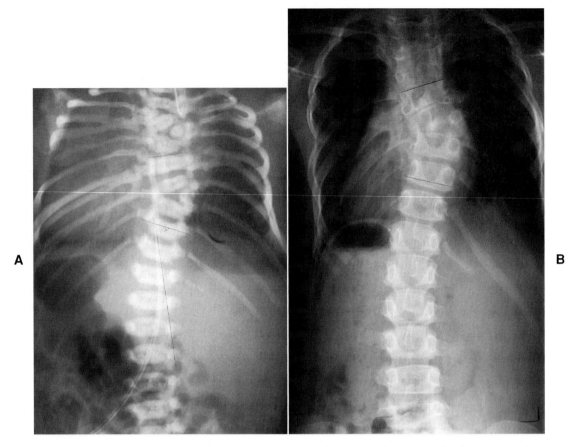

Figure 43-2.   **A,** Supine anteroposterior (AP) x-ray of newborn showing multiple congenital anomalies in the thoracic spine with areas of fused ribs in the upper thoracic and lower thoracic spine on the left and areas of fusion and additional vertebrae on the right—mixed anomaly, natural history is unclear. **B,** Age 5 years and 4 months. The areas of anomaly are now clearer with the upper thoracic spine showing bilateral failure of segmentation with no curve progression, but curve progression with a hemivertebra on the right side in the midthoracic area and fused ribs on the left with a resultant 37-degree curve.

if the current radiograph is only compared to the radiograph on the last visit, any slight difference may be ascribed to measurement error, and the progression will not be appreciated. The current film must always be compared to the film on the prior visit as well as to the original presenting x-ray. In cases that are difficult to measure, it is often useful to erase the marking on the three films and remeasure them using consistent landmarks. The timing of the repeat visits depends on the age of the child and the behavior of the scoliosis. In the period of rapid growth (the infantile and adolescent growth spurts) and where the curve is changing, return visits should be every 3 to 4 months. In stable curves in the time of steady growth in the juvenile years, yearly visits are possible.

Orthotic Treatment

Because the primary deformity in congenital scoliosis is in the bones rather than in the soft tissues, the curves tend to be rigid and thus they are *not* amenable to orthotic treatment. Nevertheless, there are definite indications for orthotic treatment of congenital scoliosis. The orthosis of choice is the Milwaukee brace, because

although underarm braces provide effective control, they do so at the expense of thoracic compression and a reduction of vital capacity—undesirable side effects.

Bracing is used in congenital scoliosis for curve control or to improve coronal imbalance. The curves that are responsive to bracing are compensatory curves, or where the anomalous area is part of a much longer curve that is flexible. It must be remembered that the anomalous area is not affected by the brace, and this area must be measured and followed separately. It is possible to control the whole curve but have an increase in the congenital scoliosis anomalous area. A study by Winter et al.[27] indicated that certain patients did well in the Milwaukee brace for many years, and a few could even be treated permanently in an orthosis, avoiding surgery. The best results were in patients with mixed anomalies that were flexible, or with a progressive secondary curve.

The other role for orthotic treatment in congenital scoliosis is for the treatment of coronal imbalance that may be decompensation or head tilt. With coronal decompensation with single or multiple anomalies, the Milwaukee brace can be effective in correcting the

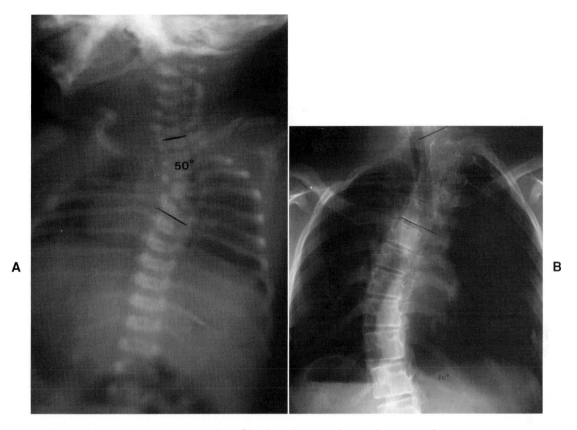

Figure 43-3.   **A,** A patient on day of birth with anomalies in the upper thoracic spine appearing to be a hemivertebra on the right with additional ribs on the right and a 50-degree curve. **B,** Age 8 years and 11 months. The upper thoracic curve is unchanged and has not progressed, and there is a compensatory curve below.

malalignment, allowing the spine to become balanced with growth. With head tilt in the young child with cervicothoracic or upper thoracic anomalies, the Milwaukee brace with an occipital pad can correct the head tilt.

The physician must recognize the role of the orthosis when it is used and must monitor this use to ensure that it accomplishes its goal—that is, it must control the curve with acceptable spine alignment. Careful monitoring both clinically and radiographically is necessary. If the patient's curve progresses or the coronal balance is not controlled despite the orthosis, fusion must be performed without further delay.

Surgical Treatment

Surgery is the most customary treatment of severe or progressive congenital scoliosis. Several types of operative procedures can be used. Two fundamental questions emerge: What is the best procedure? What is the best age for surgery?

In congenital scoliosis there is no simple answer to these questions. The operative treatment chosen must be tailored to that specific patient. It depends on the age of the patient, the type of deformity (scoliosis, kyphosis, lordosis, or a combination), the area of the deformity, the curve pattern, the natural history of the deformity, and the presence of other congenital anomalies.

The indications for surgery are first, an anomaly on presentation that has a guaranteed poor prognosis—a unilateral unsegmented bar with healthy convex growth, especially in the presence of a convex hemivertebra. In addition, double convex unsegmented hemivertebrae show severe progression. These anomalies should usually be treated fairly promptly without waiting for progression. The exception is the child under 9 to 12 months of age. In this case, surgery is planned for 12 to 18 months of age because surgery is easier at this age; the vertebrae are larger with less cartilage present.

In the majority of cases the anomaly is mixed in type, a combination of failure of segmentation and formation. A decision for surgery is made once progression occurs. This rule applies especially to the very young in whom the anomaly may be unclear because the vertebra is mainly cartilage. In these cases the crispness of the pedicle outlines gives an indication of the vertebral anatomy and growth potential. Any progressive curves should be treated surgically, irrespective of the age at which progression occurs. If a 25-degree curve in a 3-year-old child progresses to 35 degrees by 6 years of age, the curve requires surgical treatment. The tendency is to avoid surgery at this age for fear of "stunting the child's growth." In reality the child will grow taller if the curve is fused, rather than allowing the deformity to

SCOLIOSIS—SURGERY

- Indications
  - Unsegmented bar
  - Progressive deformity
- Procedures
  - Anterior hemiepiphysiodesis and posterior hemiarthrodesis (convex growth arrest)
  - Anterior/posterior fusion
  - Posterior fusion
  - Hemivertebra excision

progress, because the area of the anomaly is devoid of normal vertical growth potential.

There are four basic procedures for the surgical treatment of congenital scoliosis: posterior fusion, anterior and posterior fusion, convex growth arrest (anterior epiphysiodesis and posterior hemiarthrodesis), and hemivertebra excision. The fusion, posterior or combined, can be in situ or with correction by traction, casting, bracing, or instrumentation. The correction is maintained with casting, bracing, or instrumentation. Because fusion in congenital scoliosis is performed at a much earlier age than in other types of scoliosis, instrumentation becomes an adjunct to the procedure rather than an integral part of the fusion.

Convex Growth Arrest (Anterior Epiphysiodesis and Posterior Hemiarthrodesis)

Convex growth arrest was first described by MacLennan in 1922,[12] and subsequently by Roaf et al.[1,18,21] The convex growth arrest is achieved by anterior hemiepiphysiodesis and posterior hemiarthrodesis, and was designed to arrest excessive convex growth and allow the concave growth to occur and correct the deformity. It is thus indicated in cases with progressive scoliosis or marked scoliosis on presentation with single or adjacent convex hemivertebrae and a chance for concave growth with normal or near normal concave growth plates (i.e., there must not be an unsegmented bar on the concavity). To be successful the surgery must be performed when there are a sufficient number of years of growth remaining (i.e., under 5 years of age) and is contraindicated if there is any kyphosis in the area of the anomaly.

The anterior and posterior procedures are performed under the same anesthetic. It is essential to address the whole measured curve, sometimes adding a normal level to the convex fusion to increase the possibility of curve improvement by concave growth. The child is placed in a postoperative body cast extending to the legs, because correction can usually be obtained in the segments adjacent to the hemivertebra. The cast is appropriately trimmed so that the chest tube (inserted more anteriorly than normal) can be removed from under the cast. The child is kept nonambulatory for 3 to 4 months, the cast is removed, and the child is placed in a well-fitting Milwaukee brace that is worn full time for 12 to 18 months. This use of an orthosis after fusion in a young child is necessary because at 4 months postoperatively the fusion mass is immature, and continued support is necessary to achieve a strong, mature solid fusion. This protection is actually necessary in all cases of fusion in the young child. Convex growth arrest surgery can give two possible results. Gradual improvement of the curve over a number of years can result because of the concave growth. The surgery can give a fusion effect, which occurs where the concave growth potential is misjudged. Poor concave growth potential is actually present with no possibility of concave growth and curve improvement. The addition of an obviously healthy disc to the fusion area cranially and caudally increases the chance of a true epiphysiodesis effect. In some cases the curve may increase either immediately or years later. This is caused by residual convex growth and indicates a pseudarthrosis, which must be treated with repeat arthrodesis.

Combined Anterior and Posterior Fusion (Figure 43-4)

This has become an increasingly performed procedure for congenital scoliosis. It is used for thoracic, thoracolumbar, or lumbar curves with a poor prognosis (i.e., good convex growth potential). The multiple discectomies and fusion give an anterior growth arrest, which reduces or eliminates any bending of the fusion or "crankshaft" effect. In addition, improved correction usually results because of the multiple disc excisions, which are actually multiple convex wedge excisions. In addition, because of the combined approach, the pseudarthrosis rate is lower. This approach obviously adds the risks of an anterior procedure, even though these are small.

In the posterior procedure the correction can be obtained externally with traction or a cast or brace, or internally with instrumentation. The choice depends on the nature, magnitude, and flexibility of the deformity, the alignment of the spine (decompensation, head tilt), and the size and age of the child. In more severe deformities a combination of these methods is applicable (e.g., multiple discectomies to increase flexibility, traction to safely obtain correction with the patient awake and to achieve a balanced spine, and a cast to maintain this correction. The young child is kept nonambulatory for 3 to 4 months to eliminate the greatest deforming force on the spine: gravity. At this time the cast is removed, a Milwaukee brace is fitted, and the child is ambulatory, with brace wearing continuing for 12 to 18 months as mentioned earlier. In the older child, instrumentation is added with external support added for very active children or those with soft bone.

Posterior Fusion

Historically this procedure was the most common method of treatment of congenital scoliosis. The reported results are good[22,24] with curve stabilization; the failures are caused by curve increase, which in turn is caused by bending of the fusion mass (the "crankshaft effect") in 14% of cases, or by curve lengthening.

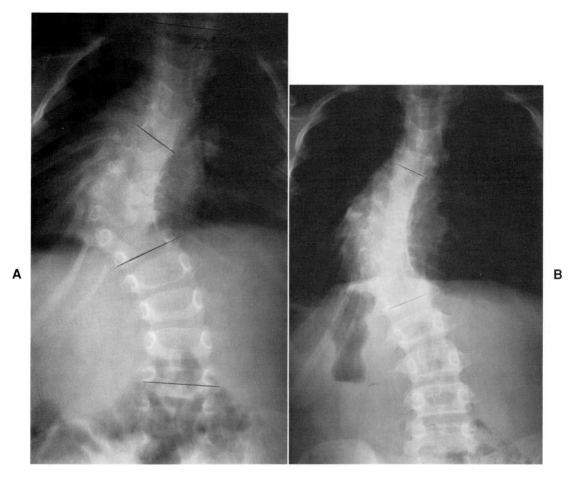

Figure 43-4. **A,** This patient was first seen at the age of 1 year and 11 months with a 60-degree left thoracic curve due to an unsegmented bar on the right side combined with a hemivertebra on the left as evidenced by the five ribs on the right and seven ribs on the left. **B,** She underwent an anterior/posterior arthrodesis with cast correction and immobilization postoperatively. At age 11 years and 0 months the curve is 43 degrees with a solid arthrodesis and excellent balance.

Currently, to prevent these side effects, a combined anterior and posterior fusion is used where the anterior fusion eliminates the anterior growth potential.

Today a posterior fusion alone is reserved for an older child with a moderate deformity that is still relatively flexible or is well balanced on presentation. The child must be old enough, usually over 10 years of age, so that the crankshaft effect is not a possibility. In these cases, correction is obtained and maintained with instrumentation, with external immobilization in a cast or brace being added when the fixation of the instrumentation is less than optimal. A posterior fusion alone is also used in cases of progressive mixed anomalies in which the anterior growth potential on the convexity of the curve is poor. A thick, wide posterior fusion stabilizes the curve and prevents subsequent anterior growth and bending of the fusion. In some of these cases a reinforcement of the fusion is performed at 6 months to increase the size of the fusion mass. If the convex anterior growth potential is good, especially in a younger child, it is better to stabilize the curve with the combined anterior and posterior approach.

The other role of a posterior fusion alone is in the case of progressive cervicothoracic anomalies, which are usually mixed in type and result in head tilt and shoulder elevation on the convexity of the curve. These anomalies tend to present in the young or during the adolescent growth spurt. In the young the deformity is still flexible, and the head tilt can be corrected as seen clinically by the use of gentle head traction in the supine child.

In these cases posterior fusion of the cervicothoracic curve is followed by immobilization in a Milwaukee brace with a head support behind the ear to correct the head tilt. The brace is worn until the head tilt corrects and the correction is stable—usually a number of years. In these children it is advantageous to fit the brace preoperatively and to allow the child and family to adapt to the brace before surgery, usually a period of 2 to 4 weeks. This makes the surgical procedure easier because the child is immediately placed in the brace to which he/she has already adapted. In the older child the head tilt may be rigid. In these cases the fusion is performed, with a halo being applied under the same anesthetic.

Postoperatively the halo is placed in traction with a lateral force to correct the head tilt. Once the head tilt is corrected, the head position is maintained with incorporation of the halo in a halo cast, which is used for 4 to 6 months until the fusion is solid.

It must be noted that instrumentation is an adjunct to the posterior fusion, being used to obtain or maintain correction. Correction with instrumentation is appropriate for curves in which it is safe to obtain correction in one procedure with the patient under anesthesia. There must be no evidence of spinal dysraphism, and the curve must be small enough and the child old enough that an anterior approach is not necessary to improve the correction or to ablate the anterior growth plates. Because there are many types of instrumentation available today, the surgeon should choose the system that best fits the child, the deformity, the safety factors, and the surgeon's experience.

A preoperative MRI scan is necessary when instrumentation is planned. This rules out any tethering problems, as well as any localized spinal stenosis.[23] In addition, spinal cord monitoring with the wake-up test is mandatory with the use of instrumentation in congenital spine deformities. Electronic monitoring can be used, but it augments rather than replaces the wake-up test.

Hemivertebra Excision (Figure 43-5)

Hemivertebra excision is essentially an anterior and posterior wedge osteotomy that is combined with correction and fusion. It is used for rigid angulated scoliosis in which compensation cannot be achieved with other methods.[9] It is usually applied in the lumbosacral area for a lumbosacral hemivertebra that causes decompensation, because there is no spine below the hemivertebra to allow compensation.[6,7,19] There is no way to achieve a balanced spine other than by a wedge excision, which is best performed before 5 years of age, before the secondary curve above has developed structural changes. The hemivertebra and the adjacent discs are excised using a lumbotomy approach, and a corresponding wedge of the hemivertebra and the pedicle are removed posteriorly with a fusion of the adjacent vertebrae. Depending on the age of the child and the size of the ver-

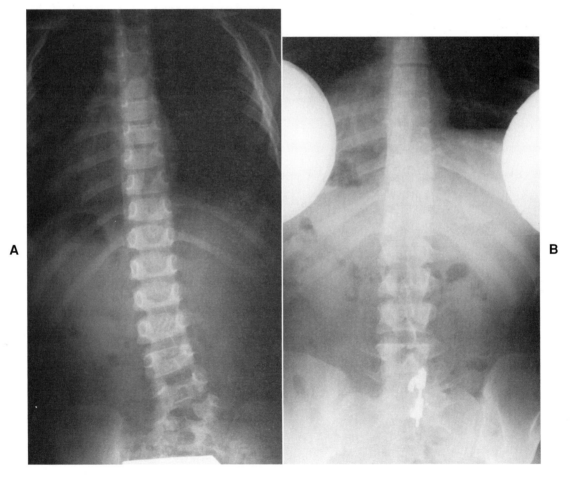

Figure 43-5. **A,** This patient presented at the age of 3 years and 0 months with a lumbosacral hemivertebra with decompensation to the left. **B,** An anterior/posterior hemivertebra excision was performed with fixation posteriorly with a short Harrington compression rod. Two years postoperatively the fusion is solid, and the coronal alignment is restored and maintained.

tebrae, the correction is maintained with a body cast with a leg extension or with the use of internal fixation.

KYPHOSIS
Natural History

Kyphotic deformities are less common than scoliosis, but they can have serious consequences if left untreated, causing paraplegia.

Congenital kyphosis can be caused by a failure of formation or a failure of segmentation, the former being more common. The failure of formation can be purely anterior, resulting in kyphosis, or more commonly anterolateral with a posterior corner hemivertebra, resulting in kyphoscoliosis. In general, kyphosis caused by failure of formation is universally progressive and can lead to paraplegia if untreated. The progression is caused by the growth imbalance and the mechanical effect of kyphosis.

Failure of formation gives a sharp angular kyphosis that tents the spinal cord, leading to cord compression and possible paraplegia. Paraplegia is more common in the upper thoracic area because in this area the spinal cord has the poorest collateral circulation—the so-called watershed area of the blood supply of the spinal cord. The paraplegia may occur early but is more common during the adolescent growth spurt with rapid increase in the untreated kyphosis, and it may occur after minor trauma.[3,10,16,25]

Kyphosis with any hemivertebra is thus important because it gives a different prognosis with progression and the danger of paralysis. This emphasizes the need to obtain coronal and sagittal views on all congenital deformities to appreciate the anomaly and deformity in three dimensions and to delineate whether the hemivertebra is lateral, posterior, or posterolateral.

Defects of anterior segmentation causing kyphosis are less common. They may involve single or multiple levels and may result in a rounded kyphosis with little risk of paraplegia. Kyphosis caused by a defect of segmentation commonly starts in the late juvenile years with progressive ossification of the disc space anteriorly. In the very early stages differentiation from Scheuermann's disease can be difficult, but with time the progressive anterior ossification becomes obvious. With the anterior bar and continued posterior growth, progressive kyphosis results. The rate of progression is less than that with a formation failure because the bar forms in the late juvenile years and the growth discrepancy is not as great.

KYPHOSIS

- Less common than scoliosis
- Types
  - Failure of formation (type I)
  - Failure of segmentation (type II)
  - Mixed
- Uniformly progressive
- Danger of paralysis with type I kyphosis

Nonoperative Treatment

There is no role for nonoperative treatment of congenital kyphosis. The natural history indicates a universally poor prognosis, and thus the treatment is surgical.

Surgical Treatment

In congenital kyphosis, the choices are between a posterior approach and a combined anterior and posterior approach. Because the defect is defined clearly, it is easier to discuss the treatment with respect to the vertebral anomaly.

Failure of Segmentation

The choice of treatment depends on the magnitude of the deformity and whether correction is desired.

Posterior fusion. If the defect is detected early with an acceptable kyphosis with no need for correction, a posterior fusion extending at least one vertebra cranial and one caudal to the segmentation defect is ideal. The fusion must include the whole of the abnormal sagittal curve. Abundant autologous iliac bone graft is added to achieve as thick a fusion as possible. Because the deformity is rigid, instrumentation is not used unless the congenital kyphosis is part of a longer kyphosis that requires treatment and fusion. This posterior fusion removes the deforming posterior growth forces.

Anterior and posterior approach. When the kyphosis presents later with a significant deformity that needs correction, the combined approach is best. Anteriorly the unsegmented areas are osteotomized with section of the anterior longitudinal ligament and removal of any residual disc posteriorly. The posterior annulus is left intact, and the spinal canal is not entered. An anterior fusion is now performed by packing the disc spaces with small chips of rib bone and extending the fusion to include any additional levels that need to be included in the fusion area. A sequential posterior fusion is now performed under the same anesthetic, fusing the whole extent of the kyphosis. Instrumentation and bone graft are added, the choice of instrumentation depending on the experience and preference of the surgeon.

Failure of Formation

The treatment plan depends on whether the kyphosis is detected early or late, and if late, whether neurologic loss, such as paraparesis or paraplegia, exists.

Posterior fusion (convex growth arrest). The best procedure is an early posterior fusion that extends one normal level cranial and caudal to the anomalous area. This is in effect a convex growth arrest that stops the posterior growth and allows the anterior growth to correct the deformity. This approach is best used on patients under 3 years of age and with kyphoses under 55 to 60 degrees. Postoperatively the child is placed in a hyperextension cast and is kept nonambulatory for 4 months. In the very young (under 18 months of age) it is generally recommended that routine exploration and graft augmentation be performed at 6 months to obtain a thick fusion. Following treatment in a cast nonambulatory, the child is immobilized in a brace and ambulated, the total time of immobilization being 18 months until the fusion is solid and mature.

The early posterior fusion allows anterior growth with a slow steady improvement in the angle of the kyphosis—a true epiphysiodesis effect. In their review of 17 cases of congenital kyphosis fused posteriorly alone before 5 years of age, Winter and Moe found improvement in the kyphosis in 12 patients (71%) with an average 9-year follow-up.[22]

In older children with less severe kyphosis (under 55 to 60 degrees) a posterior fusion alone can successfully control the kyphosis and stabilize the curve. Many of these cases are kyphoscoliosis, and instrumentation is added where possible to obtain any correction allowed by the flexibility of the deformity and to stabilize the curve during the fusion process.

Anterior and posterior fusion. For kyphosis greater than 55 to 60 degrees, an anterior and posterior fusion is necessary. It is important to include the whole extent of the kyphosis in the fusion, not limiting one's approach to the area of the anomaly. Anteriorly the tether is the abnormal cartilage in the area of the hemivertebra, the anterior longitudinal ligament, and the annulus fibrosis. These are all removed, and the discs are completely excised over the whole extent of the kyphosis back to the posterior annulus and to the opposite side.

Correction is obtained with manual pressure over the kyphosis and maintained with an anterior fusion with chips of bone inserted in the disc spaces. In addition, rib struts are added, bridging the kyphosis anteriorly and restoring the anterior support. In larger kyphoses with bone of adequate size, an anterior graft of allograft fibula is inserted to maintain the correction. The anterior strut is inserted in slots curetted in the vertebral bodies, with the anterior strut being inserted while correction is being obtained with pressure over the apex of the kyphosis. The principle is to build an anterior bridge, filling the concavity of the kyphosis with bone (rib struts).

A posterior fusion is now performed, usually sequentially under the same anesthetic. Instrumentation is added, which stabilizes the kyphosis and allows any possible correction at the ends of the curve. The third-generation multiple hook-rod systems are used today, with correction using cantilever correction. This is the safest force for the neural structures in these cases because it actually relaxes the spinal cord. The choice of instrumentation depends on the experience and choice of the surgeon.

With the use of instrumentation and secure fixation, the child is ambulatory without immobilization. If the fixation is not secure or is in question, additional external protection in a cast or brace is best. In the young patient in whom instrumentation is impossible or would not add sufficient stabilization, the child is placed in a hyperextension cast and kept nonambulatory for 3 to 4 months, at which time the child is mobilized in a brace that is worn for 12 to 18 months until the fusion is mature.

It is tempting in these cases to obtain correction in traction, either halo-gravity or halo-femoral. The use of traction with kyphosis carries a high incidence of paraplegia. The apex of the kyphosis is rigid with the spinal cord stretched over the apical vertebral bodies. Traction corrects the ends of the curve, pulling the cord against the apical bone with resultant neurologic loss. Traction thus plays no role in the treatment of congenital kyphosis.[10]

Treatment of Congenital Kyphosis and Neurologic Loss[10]

In patients who present with congenital kyphosis and *minor* neurologic deficits, the kyphosis is treated with a combined anterior and posterior fusion as described above. In these cases the straightening of the apex during the anterior procedure has the effect of releasing the compression of the apical bone against the spinal cord.

In cases of *mild* paraparesis with a flexible apex as shown on a hyperextension film, the patient is placed on bed rest. In some cases bed rest, which places the apex of the kyphosis in hyperextension, will result in improvement in the paraparesis. The bed rest is continued as long as there is neurologic improvement—usually a number of weeks. If the recovery is to normal or to a residual minor deficit, the improved position is stabilized with a combined anterior and posterior fusion as mentioned previously.

In cases presenting with more marked neurologic loss or in which the bed rest does not result in neurologic improvement in mild paraparesis, anterior spinal cord decompression is performed. The anterior approach and releases are performed as described above, followed by removal of the bone compressing the spinal cord over the whole area of compression identified on the preoperative imaging study. This allows the dural sac and cord to move anteriorly into decompressed area. An anterior fusion is now carried out with interbody fusion and the insertion of rib and fibula strut grafts as described previously.

The anterior decompression and fusion is followed by a posterior fusion with or without instrumentation. This can be under the same anesthetic, or in cases with excessive blood loss with the decompression, the posterior fusion is staged and performed 1 to 2 weeks later. The patient is kept nonambulatory for 2 to 4 weeks to allow maximal cord recovery and the postoperative edema in and around the cord to subside. Further treatment, as well as the need for external immobilization and following a period of nonambulation, depends on the use of posterior instrumentation and the security of its fixation as discussed above.

KYPHOSIS—TREATMENT

- No role for bracing
- Surgery
  - Early—posterior fusion (convex growth arrest)
  - Late—anterior/posterior fusion

LORDOSIS
Natural History

Congenital lordosis is the least common of the congenital spine deformities and is due to failure of posterior segmentation. The unsegmented bar can be only posterior, causing pure lordosis, but is more commonly posterolateral, causing lordoscoliosis The predominantly scoliosis cases have been discussed above, whereas those with lordosis as the major deformity are discussed here. The area of segmentation loss usually extends over multiple levels, and the deforming force is the anterior growth that usually results in a progressive deformity. With increasing lordosis there is reduction of the spine-sternal distance and alteration in the rib mechanics in respiration with resultant respiratory restriction, respiratory failure, and even early death.

Nonoperative Treatment

There is no role for any nonoperative treatment in congenital lordosis because the natural history is progression.

Surgical Treatment

The deforming force in these cases is anterior growth; therefore all cases need an anterior approach. The only method to correct the congenital lordosis is with an osteotomy of the unsegmented bar; thus any case requiring correction needs a combined anterior and posterior approach. Because these patients commonly have pulmonary restrictive disease, an anterior approach has greater risks. If there is already an element of pulmonary failure, these risks increase. If pulmonary artery hypertension is already present, surgery is probably contraindicated due to the high mortality in these cases.

Anterior Fusion (Convex Growth Arrest)

In early cases in which correction is not necessary, an anterior fusion is performed with disc excisions, removal of the cartilage end plates, and packing of the disc spaces with bone chips. This convex growth arrest removes the anterior growth potential and gives an anterior fusion opposite the unsegmented bar. This is the ideal procedure but is rarely performed because of the rarity of this anomaly, and because the child presents late with a larger lordosis.

LORDOSIS

- Posterior unsegmented bar
- Progressive
- Treatment
  - Early—anterior fusion (convex growth arrest)
  - Late—anterior/posterior procedure

Anterior and Posterior Procedure

Generally the cases present later where correction is necessary, involving anterior closing wedges and posterior osteotomy of the bar (Figure 43-6). Anteriorly the discs are excised over the whole area of the lordosis, and thin wedges of the adjacent vertebral end plates are excised, converting the disc excision into an osteotomy wider anteriorly. The disc spaces are not packed with bone chips because the wedges need to close.

Posteriorly multiple osteotomies of the unsegmented bar are performed, with exposure extending to all the vertebrae to be fused considering the coronal and sagittal curves. The best method for correction is with the passage of sublaminar wires and approximation of the spine to a kyphotically contoured rod. In addition, it may be necessary to perform bilateral rib resections to prevent the spine correction from being hampered by the ribs. This is performed in two stages: an internal thoracoplasty with rib resections performed during the anterior approach; and the opposite side resections performed during the posterior procedure. In some cases in which the lordosis is not too large, the same effect can be achieved with bilateral transverse process osteotomies during the posterior procedure. This process allows some spinal correction without the restriction imposed by the ribs.

CONCLUSIONS

All patients with a congenital spine deformity need a complete evaluation to exclude other congenital anomalies, especially those involving the spinal canal and its contents. Complete and accurate radiographic assessment in the coronal and sagittal planes is essential so that the type of vertebral anomaly and its anatomic position in the vertebral ring is established, as well as the associated deformity and its magnitude. What is important is the growth disturbance produced by the anomaly and the growth potential of the remainder of the vertebral ring; this imbalance results in the deformity and determines its rate of progression. Because the natural history of congenital deformities is well established, this assessment gives the prognosis and determines the treatment plan.

In general the treatment is fairly straightforward. Observation for curve progression is used for scoliosis anomalies in which the natural history and prognosis are not clear. Nonoperative treatment by bracing plays a limited role and is reserved for congenital scoliosis to improve spinal balance (including head tilt) and to control compensatory curves. There is no role for bracing in the treatment of rigid curves, congenital kyphosis, or congenital lordosis.

The principle of surgery is to balance growth, thus preventing curve progression. It is impossible to insert growth. Therefore the only thing that can be done is to remove the growth in the vertebral ring opposite the anomaly with an appropriate fusion. In some cases it is possible to perform a convex fusion where there is concave growth potential and sufficient growth remaining so that the concave growth corrects the curve (the

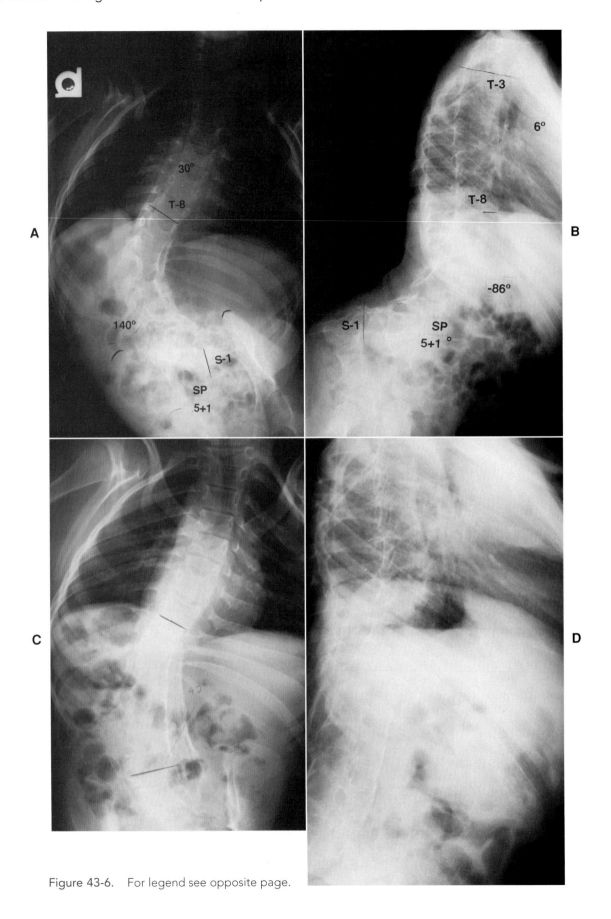

Figure 43-6. For legend see opposite page.

Figure 43-6. **A,** This patient presented at the age of 5 years and 1 month with a progressive lumbar deformity. She had severe hyperlordosis. Postero-anterior x-ray showed a severe 140-degree lumbar curve with unsegmented bars seen on the right side with fused pedicles from the low thoracic spine to the sacrum. **B,** Sagittal view showed the severe hyperlordosis with –86 degrees of lumbar lordosis due to the posterolateral bar. **C,** She underwent an anterior lumbar approach with multiple level discectomies, a posterior approach with transection of the fused bars where possible and bone grafting. The plan was to place her in 90-degree suspended halo-femoral traction postoperatively. As a result of the anterior procedure, she had severe spasm of the left iliac artery with a period of decreased circulation to the left leg, and thus the traction was not instituted. X-rays at this time showed correction of the scoliosis and lordosis, and therefore she was placed in a postoperative spica cast including both legs, which she wore for 4 months, followed by a thoracolumbosacral arthosis for 6 months. Three years later the scoliosis is corrected to 42 degrees with a solid arthrodesis visible. **D,** The lateral x-ray at this time shows correction of the lordosis with restoration of sagittal alignment.

epiphysiodesis effect). In other cases curve improvement is obtained with releases and correction, with the safest correction obtained in traction. It is also safer to shorten the convexity of a curve than to lengthen the concavity. Many surgical procedures are available—there is no ideal or correct procedure for a specific anomaly or deformity. The procedure and treatment plan chosen is tailored for the patient and depends on the anomaly, the deformity produced, its natural history, the patient's age, and the presence of other congenital anomalies, especially neurologic.

SELECTED REFERENCES

Holte D et al.: Hemivertebra excision and wedge resection in the surgical treatment of patients with congenital scoliosis, *J Bone Joint Surg Am* 77:159-171, 1995.

McMaster MJ, Ohtsuka K: The natural history of congenital scoliosis: a study of two hundred and fifty-one patients, *J Bone Joint Surg Am* 64(8):1128-1147, 1982.

McMaster MJ, Singh H: Natural history of congenital kyphosis and kyphoscoliosis, *J Bone Joint Surg Am* 81:1367-1383, 1999.

Winter RB: Convex anterior and posterior hemiarthrodesis and hemiepiphyseodesis in young children with progressive congenital scoliosis, *J Pediatr Orthopaed* 1(4):361-366, 1981.

REFERENCES

1. Andrew T, Piggott H: Growth arrest for progressive scoliosis: combined anterior and posterior fusion of the convexity, *J Bone Joint Surg Br* 67:193-197, 1985.
2. Beals RK, Robbins JR, Rolfe B: Anomalies associated with vertebral malformations *Spine* 18:1329-1332, 1993.
3. Dubousset J, Gonon EP: Cyphoses et cypho-scolioses angulaires, *Rev Chir Orthop Appar Mot* 69(Suppl II), 1983.
4. Facanha-Filho FAM et al.: Measurement accuracy in congenital scoliosis, *J Bone Joint Surg Am* 82:42-45, 2001.
5. Hensinger R, Lang JE, MacEwen GD: Klippel-Feil syndrome: a constellation of associated anomalies, *J Bone Joint Surg Am* 56:1246-1253, 1974.
6. Holte D et al.: Hemivertebra excision and wedge resection in the surgical treatment of patients with congenital scoliosis, *J Bone Joint Surg Am* 77:159-171, 1995.
7. King JD, Lowery GL: Results of lumbar hemivertebral excision for congenital scoliosis, *Spine* 16(7):778-782, 1991.
8. Kuhns JE, Hormell RS: Management of congenital scoliosis, *Arch Surg* 65:250-263, 1952.
9. Leatherman KD, Dickson RA: Two-stage corrective surgery for congenital deformities of the spine, *J Bone Joint Surg Br* 61:324-328, 1979.
10. Lonstein JE et al.: Neurological deficits secondary to spinal deformity: a review of the literature and report of 43 cases, *Spine* 5:331-355, 1980.
11. MacEwen GD, Winter RB, Hardy JH: Evaluation of kidney anomalies in congenital scoliosis, *J Bone Joint Surg Am* 54(7):1451-1454, 1972.
12. MacLennan GD: Scoliosis, *Br Med J* 2:864, 1922.
13. McMaster MJ: Congenital scoliosis caused by a unilateral failure of vertebral segmentation with contralateral hemivertebrae, *Spine* 23:998-1005, 1998.
14. McMaster M J: Occult intraspinal anomalies and congenital scoliosis. *J Bone Joint Surg Am* 66(4):588-601, 1984.
15. McMaster MJ, Ohtsuka K: The natural history of congenital scoliosis: a study of two hundred and fifty-one patients, *J Bone Joint Surg Am* 64(8):1128-1147, 1982.
16. McMaster MJ, Singh H: Natural history of congenital kyphosis and kyphoscoliosis, *J Bone Joint Surg* 81:1367-1383, 1999.
17. Reckles LH et al.: The association of scoliosis and congenital heart disease, *J Bone Joint Surg Am* 57:449-455, 1975.
18. Roaf R: The treatment of progressive scoliosis by unilateral growth arrest, *J Bone Joint Surg Br* 45:637-651, 1963.
19. Slabaugh PB et al.: Lumbosacral hemivertebrae: a review of twenty-four patients, with excision in eight, *Spine* 5:234-244, 1980.
20. Winter RB: *Congenital deformities of the spine,* New York, 1983, Thieme-Stratton.
21. Winter RB: Convex anterior and posterior hemiarthrodesis and hemiepiphyseodesis in young children with progressive congenital scoliosis, *J Pediatr Orthop* 1(4):361-366, 1981.
22. Winter RB, Moe JH: The results of spinal arthrodesis for congenital spine deformities in patients younger than 5 years old, *J Bone Joint Surg Am* 64:419-432, 1982.
23. Winter RB, Moe JH, Eilers VS: Congenital scoliosis: a study of 234 patients treated and untreated, *J Bone Joint Surg Am* 50:1-47, 1984.
24. Winter RB, Moe JH, Lonstein JE: Posterior spinal arthrodesis for congenital scoliosis, *J Bone Joint Surg Am* 66:1188-1197, 1984.
25. Winter RB, Moe JH, Wang JF: Congenital kyphosis, *J Bone Joint Surg Am* 55:223-256.
26. Winter RB et al.: Diastematomyelia and congenital spine deformities, *J Bone Joint Surg Am* 56:27-39, 1974.
27. Winter RB et al.: The Milwaukee brace in the nonoperative treatment of congenital scoliosis, *Spine* 1:85-96, 1976.
28. Winter RB et al.: The prevalence of spinal cord or cord anomalies in idiopathic, congenital and neuromuscular scoliosis, *Orthop Trans* 16:135, 1992.

Thoracoscopic Approach for Pediatric Deformity

Peter O. Newton

Thoracoscopy, also know as video-assisted thoracic surgery (VATS), has become a valuable tool in the treatment of pediatric spinal deformity. The thoracic region of the spine is an ideal location for minimally invasive endoscopic techniques, given the large, relatively open space of the chest cavity. Once the lung is deflated, using specialized endotracheal tubes, the spine is easily visualized and approached with endoscopic tools.

The goals of thoracoscopic anterior spinal surgery are the same as those of open surgery. The technique of exposure limits the incisions of the chest wall yet ideally allows comparable surgery on the spine itself. In general these goals in cases of pediatric spinal deformity include anterior release, fusion, crankshaft growth prevention, and in some cases deformity correction with instrumentation.

INDICATIONS FOR ANTERIOR RELEASE AND FUSION
Scoliosis

One of the most common indications for anterior thoracic procedures in scoliosis relates to the ability of the disc excision procedure to increase curve flexibility. Thoracic scoliosis has a variety of etiologies (idiopathic, neuromuscular, syndrome related) that are frequently not diagnosed or treated until the curve magnitude is relatively large and stiff. Strict guidelines on which curves are indicated for an anterior release are not established. In general those with a Cobb angle greater than 70 degrees to 75 degrees or bending to greater than 50 degrees are considered for release in order to increase flexibility, allowing greater correction with the subsequent posterior instrumentation procedure. The thoracoscopic approach is an alternative to open thoracotomy methods in all but the most severe cases.

Juvenile and young adolescent patients with progressive scoliosis are known to be at risk for continued crankshaft deformity when treated with a posterior fusion alone.[7] In these cases an anterior fusion limits anterior growth and prevents this late increasing deformity.[13] Thoracoscopic disc excision and fusion provides a minimally invasive option for such patients.[8,18]

Patients with spinal deformity associated with Marfan syndrome, neurofibromatosis (type I), or prior spinal irradiation are examples of those who may be associated with an increased risk of pseudarthrosis following an isolated posterior scoliosis correction. In cases such as these an anterior fusion procedure may improve the odds of successful arthrodesis.

Kyphosis

Controversy exists regarding the need for anterior procedures in cases of thoracic kyphosis,[4,21] although in many cases the release allows improved correction and the anterior fusion decreases the odds of later correction loss.[5] Kyphosis therefore is also a common indication for thoracoscopic release and fusion—followed by posterior instrumentation and fusion. Deformities related to both Scheuermann's disease and neuromuscular conditions, are amenable to this approach.

Congenital Deformity

Thoracoscopy has been applied to the treatment of congenital scoliosis as well.[18,23,25] The anterior portion of either a circumferential arthrodesis or growth-modifying hemiepiphysiodesis is theoretically possible via this endoscopic approach. The technical aspects of this surgery become more difficult, however, as the size of the child decreases. Although lower-thoracic–level hemivertebra may on occasion be indicated for excision, doing so thoracoscopically remains extremely challenging.

INDICATIONS: RELEASE AND FUSION

- Scoliosis
  - Large curve >70 degrees to 75 degrees
  - Stiff curve, bend >50 degrees
  - Crankshaft, triradiate cartilage open
  - Pseudarthrosis risk
- Kyphosis
- Congenital scoliosis
  - In situ fusion
  - Hemiarthrodesis

Many patients undergoing treatment for congenital scoliosis are less than 5 years of age and require anterior fusion over very few levels of the spine. The difference in the open (limited thoracotomy) and thoracoscopic (minimum of three to four portals) approaches decreases as the size of the child and chest decrease.

CONTRAINDICATIONS

As suggested above, small size of the patient is a relative contraindication to thoracoscopy. Lung deflation is more difficult in these cases, because standard-size double-lumen and bronchial-blocking endotracheal tubes are too large. Another contraindication is the presence of a markedly reduced working distance between the chest wall and the spine. This occurs in severe cases of scoliosis and limits both the field of vision (the endoscope is too close to the spine to obtain any perspective) and the maneuverability of the working instruments (e.g., rongeurs, curettes).

Visualization of the surgical field is mandatory in all surgical approaches and may be compromised in thoracoscopic surgery by incomplete deflation of the lung or pleural adhesions that prevent collapse away from the chest wall and spine. Pleural adhesions can be anticipated in patients with a history of prior ipsilateral thoracic surgery or significant pulmonary infection, both of which should lead the surgeon away from the thoracoscopic approach.

INDICATIONS FOR ANTERIOR SCOLIOSIS INSTRUMENTATION

Recently methods for thoracoscopic anterior scoliosis correction have been developed based on the principles of open thoracic anterior scoliosis instrumentation. Thoracic scoliosis correction is comparable with anterior and posterior methods, although the fusion is often shorter and kyphosis restoration greater with anterior instrumentation techniques.[3] Enthusiasm for this approach has been tempered by the extensive thoracotomy required and the high rate of rod fracture noted in the early reports. Adaptations to the instrumentation systems have made anterior scoliosis correction possible via entirely endoscopic methods.

The curve patterns amenable to this approach continue to be elucidated; however, in general, single thoracic curves and those double or triple curves in which only the thoracic component is structural may be considered for selective thoracic anterior instrumentation. The upper limits of curve magnitude and rigidity for which the thoracoscopic approach can effectively be applied is unknown, although it is the author's current practice to limit this procedure to those cases with a curve magnitude less than 70 degrees.

SURGICAL TECHNIQUE: DISC EXCISION AND FUSION

Much of the equipment required for spinal thoracoscopy is common to all endoscopic surgery. An endoscope

---

CONTRAINDICATIONS

- Pulmonary insufficiency
- Intrathoracic adhesions
  - Prior chest surgery
  - Prior infection
- Large curves > 100 degrees to 120 degrees—relative
- Reduced distance from chest wall to spine
- Small children < 4 to 5 years of age—relative

INDICATIONS: INSTRUMENTATION

IDIOPATHIC SCOLIOSIS
- Curves 40 degrees to 70 degrees
- Single thoracic curve
- Double curve with thoracic curve dominance

THORACOSCOPY EQUIPMENT

- Video monitor
- Video camera
- Light source
- Endoscopes—10 mm (0 degrees and 45 degrees)
- Ultrasonic dissector
- Thoracoports
- Rongeurs
- Endostitch
- Curettes

(10-mm diameter, 0-degree and 45-degree angle viewing), video camera, light source, and monitor have become standard in nearly all modern operating rooms. Access through the chest wall between the ribs is maintained with plastic tubular "ports." These ports provide a path to place the endoscope and working instruments into the chest cavity.

Patient positioning has traditionally been as for a thoracotomy in the lateral decubitus position (Figure 44-1). It has recently been suggested that in some cases prone positioning may be possible, avoiding the need to reposition the patient for the posterior procedure or even allowing simultaneous anterior release and posterior instrumentation. The ability to convert to an open approach may be restricted should that be necessary. The portal placement is necessarily more posterior, which may also be limited with the prone position; this may limit the anterior extent of spinal exposure and disc excision. As such, the author continues to prefer the lateral patient position for thoracoscopic spinal procedures.

The role of the anesthesiologist is critical to the success and safety of thoracoscopic surgery.[14] Complete ipsilateral lung deflation is essential to preventing lung parenchymal injury from passing instruments, as well as allowing visualization of the spine. Double-lumen endotracheal tubes are preferred in those patients large

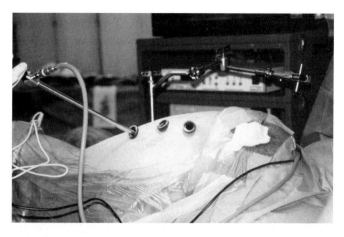

Figure 44-1. Portal placement for multilevel thoracic disc excision. The patient is positioned in the lateral decubitus position (head is to the right). The draping is wide to allow conversion to a thoracotomy should that be required.

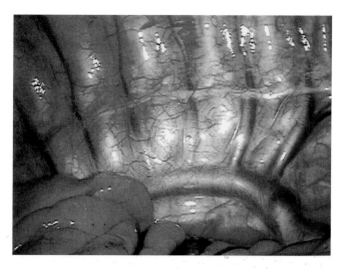

Figure 44-2. Thoracoscopic view of the spine, segmental vessels, and azygos vein. The lung is being displaced with an endoscopic fan retractor (proximal to the right, distal to the left).

SINGLE-LUNG VENTILATION

- Double-lumen endotracheal tube
- Bronchial-blocking Univent tube
- Main-stem bronchial intubation

---

enough to accept these devices. In juvenile patients a Univent bronchial-blocking tube provides an alternative. A small balloon advanced into the main-stem bronchus blocks ventilation to the lung on the side of the chest to be operated (convex side of scoliosis). In even smaller children a separate blocking balloon may be placed alongside a standard endotracheal tube or a main-stem intubation may be performed. In nearly all patients with normal preoperative pulmonary function, single-lung ventilation can be tolerated.

Following lung deflation, portals are established through the chest wall. The orientation of these portals may vary depending on the pathology, although in most cases of deformity release and fusion they are best placed in a linear relationship along the anterior axillary line. The inferior portals require a more slightly posterior placement to maintain an intrathoracic position due to the site of diaphragm insertion onto the anterior chest wall. Initial exposure of the spine often requires gentle retraction of the lung, at least until it becomes completely atalectatic (Figure 44-2). Division of the pleura overlying the spine may be either longitudinally over the length of the spine to be fused or transversely at each disc space. Treatment of the segmental vessels may be similarly individualized with either division or preservation, depending on the needs of the case or preference of the surgeon. In most cases the author prefers a longitudinal pleural exposure with division of the segmental vessels utilizing the Harmonic laparoscopic coagulating shears by Ethicon Endo-Surgery.

Division of the segmental vessels allows greater anterior spinal exposure for more complete annular release.

The levels of exposure possible thoracoscopically range from T2 to L1 with both the proximal and distal limits variable given the nature of the deformity. Exposure of the T12 to L1 disc and L1 vertebral body requires division of a small segment of the diaphragm insertion, which can be accomplished by extending the pleural incision distally into the diaphragm. The proximal thoracic spine in the right chest is often covered by the confluens of the segmental veins, which may appear daunting at the T3 and T4 levels. However, with slow, cautious use of the ultrasonic devices, these vessels can be sealed and divided safely, exposing the upper thoracic spine.

Disc excision techniques are similar to those utilized in open surgery. An annulotomy is performed with either the electrocautery or Harmonic scalpel. A rongeur is an excellent tool for the majority of the disc excision. These specially designed endoscopic rongeurs are available in extended lengths with a variety of angles (straight, up, right, left) to reach the depths of each disc space (Figure 44-3). An angled curette may also be used for removing residual end-plate cartilage and exposing the cancellous bony surface required for fusion. Although less critical from the standpoint of increasing flexibility, there is little doubt that if fusion is the goal, disc excision should be thorough. The method and type of bone grafting also appears important to the success of arthrodesis. This may be critical only in selected cases; however, all patients are at some risk for pseudarthrosis after posterior instrumentation and fusion procedures. Thus attention to bone grafting remains relevant. In those patients at greatest risk for pseudarthrosis, autogenous bone is best and the risk/benefit ratio must be analyzed on a case-by-case basis. Either cancellous allograft bone or autogenous bone (rib or iliac crest) can be delivered deeply into the disc space with a tubular plunger (Figure 44-4).

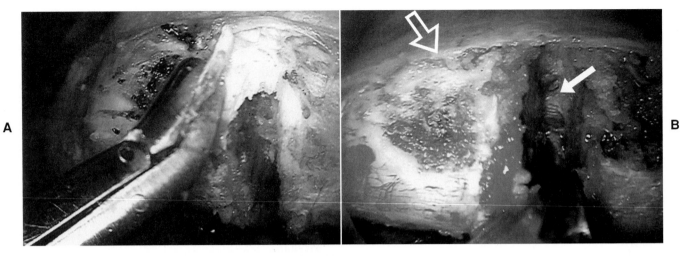

Figure 44-3.   **A,** Disc excision with removal of end-plate cartilage is performed with rongeurs and/or curettes. **B,** Complete disc removal exposing the posterior longitudinal ligament (PLL) is possible as seen. The cut edge of the pleura is marked with an *open arrow,* and the fibers of the PLL are marked with a *closed arrow.*

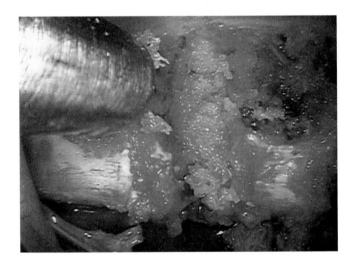

Figure 44-4.   The disc space can be seen to be filled with cancellous bone graft delivered with a tubular plunger that had been filled with graft material.

SURGICAL TECHNIQUE: ANTERIOR THORACOSCOPIC SCOLIOSIS CORRECTION

Although the long-term follow-up of this new technique does not yet exist, it is clear that thoracoscopic anterior instrumentation and fusion for the correction of thoracic scoliosis is technically possible (Figure 44-5). As with disc excision, the principles of the open surgical method remain. Segmental bicortical vertebral-body screw fixation is required of all vertebrae that are included in the fusion. In general the extent of the instrumentation is determined based on the standing posteroanterior (PA) preoperative radiograph and includes all the vertebrae that make up the measured Cobb angle.

Screw insertion endoscopically requires carefully planned portals directly lateral to the spine—approximately along the posterior axillary line. The image intensifier provides a means of determining the orientation of

SURGICAL TECHNIQUE

- Lateral position
- Three to four portals—linear relationship along anterior axillary line
    - Inferior portal—slight posterior placement to maintain intrathoracic position
- Complete ipsilateral lung deflation, gentle lung retraction
- Pleural incision—longitudinal
- Segmental vessels coagulated
- Sponge anterior to spine
- Annular incision
- Disc removal—rongeurs
- End-plate exposure—curette

THORACOSCOPIC INSTRUMENTATION

- Fuse/instrument entire curve based on standing posteroanterior (PA) preoperative radiograph
    - Includes all vertebrae that make up measured Cobb angle
- Segmental bicortical screw purchase—parallel to vertebral end plates
- Screw portals—directly lateral to spine as determined fluoroscopically along posterior axillary line
- Autogenous bone graft
- Contoured rod (4- to 4.75-mm diameter), prebent to desired degree of postoperative scoliosis and kyphosis
- Rod sequentially loaded into screws
- Segmental compression

the vertebrae and proper location of portal and screw position. Following thorough removal of disc material at each level to be fused, transverse vertebral body screws are inserted into each body parallel to the end plates. Penetration of the far cortex greatly enhances the fixation

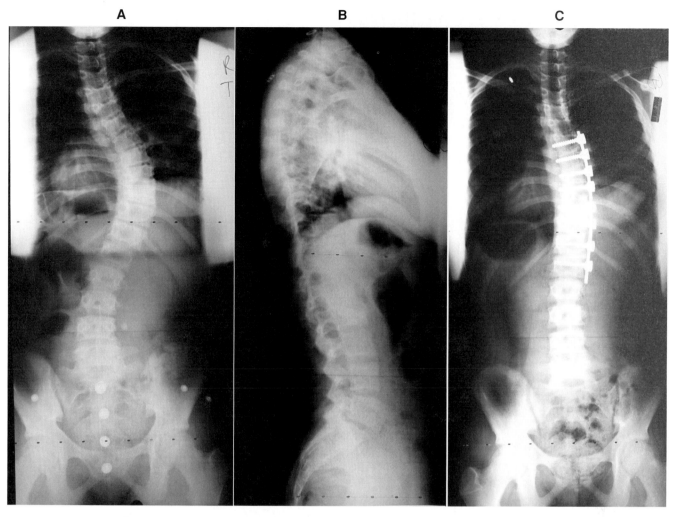

Figure 44-5. **A** and **B,** Preoperative posteroanterior (PA) and lateral radiographs of an adolescent female with idiopathic scoliosis. **C** and **D,** The deformity was corrected with anterior thoracoscopic instrumentation. The entire measured preoperative curve from T6 to L1 was fused with structural grafting performed at the inferior levels. **E,** The early postoperative clinical appearance demonstrates excellent trunk balance and shoulder symmetry.

Continued

and is mandatory at the proximal levels to reduce the risk of screw pullout. A contoured rod (4- to 4.75-mm diameter), prebent to the desired degree of postoperative scoliosis and kyphosis, is sequentially loaded into the screws and secured with locking nuts (Figure 44-6). Fully seating the rod into the screws may be accomplished with either a rod pusher or the use of reduction screws (with break-off extensions). Several styles of compressors have been developed to compress between levels. This is an important component to the anterior correction of scoliosis but must be performed in a cautious and controlled manner, particularly at the upper levels where screw fixation may be tenuous.

Bone grafting is critical to the success of this procedure, and autogenous graft (iliac crest or rib) is recommended. At the lower levels of the thoracic spine, distal to T11, structural anterior support may be required to aid in maintaining proper sagittal alignment.

OUTCOMES OF THORACOSCOPIC RELEASE AND FUSION

The thoracoscopic approach has obvious advantages associated with limited chest wall division compared with an open thoracotomy approach. These advantages (pulmonary function, reduced recovery period, less pain, improved cosmesis) will be realized only if the efficacy of the spinal procedure equals that of open surgery. Experimental animal and clinical studies suggest comparable efficacy in experienced hands.

Several experimental studies have been performed to analyze the extent of disc excision possible with thoracoscopic techniques. Biomechanical evaluations of the instability resulting from discectomy were equivalent between open and endoscopic approaches in a variety of animal models.[6,17,25] The extent of end-plate bony exposure has also been demonstrated to be similar with the two approaches experimentally.[11]

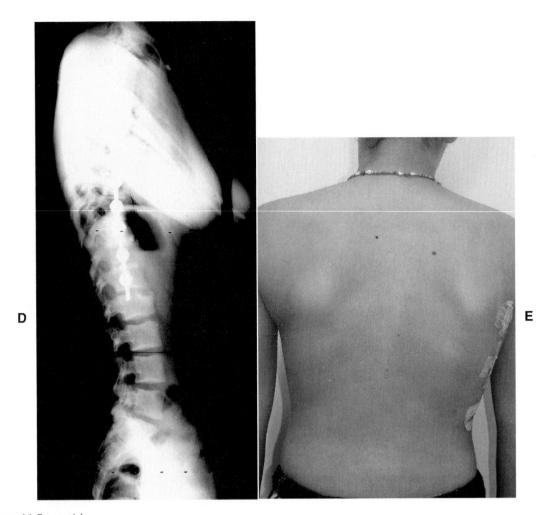

Figure 44-5, cont'd.

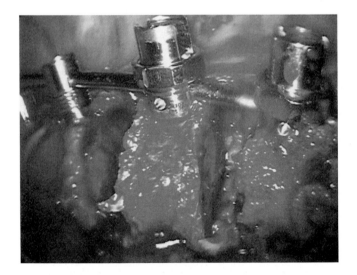

Figure 44-6. Vertebral-body screws and a rod have been placed endoscopically. This particular screw design incorporates extended "reduction" tabs that facilitate engaging of the locking nuts, as well as correcting the deformity. The extensions of the screws are broken off once the system is completely assembled.

The clinical results of thoracoscopic anterior release and fusion in patients with spinal deformity have been generally favorable though poorly controlled. A recent meta-analysis by Arlet[1] has nicely summarized the studies to date. There has clearly been an increase in the use of this method over the past decade, yet large controlled series with substantial follow-up are lacking.

The number of patients treated with release and fusion for spinal deformity reported in these series ranges from 3 to 65* and includes diagnoses of idiopathic scoliosis, neuromuscular deformity, Scheuermann's kyphosis, congenital scoliosis, and several miscellaneous conditions (Figure 44-7).

In the author's most recent experience, an average of 6.5 discs per patient were excised with the range 3 to 10 levels. The extent of release is difficult to define, but the percentage of curve correction has been comparable to results reported with open release. The results of kyphosis correction have also been satisfactory following thoracoscopic release, with the percentage of correction greater than 90% after posterior instrumentation.

---

*References 9, 10, 12, 15, 16, 18, 22-24.

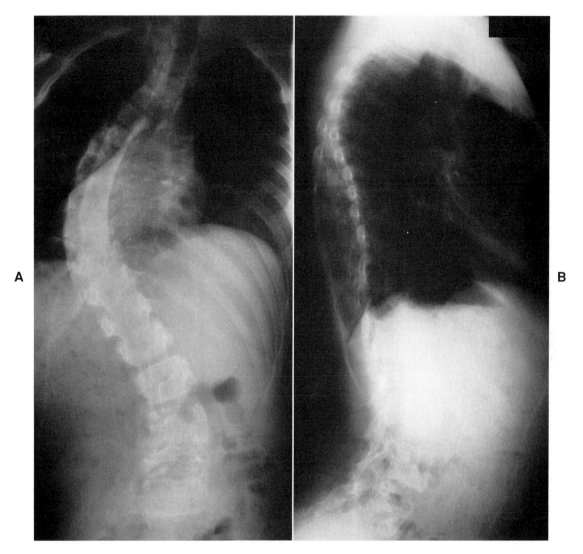

Figure 44-7.   **A** and **B,** Preoperative radiographs of a boy with neuromuscular scoliosis measuring 75 degrees. He was Risser grade 0, and the curve corrected just to 55 degrees on side bending.

Continued

The surgical time to perform thoracoscopic surgery in these cases has ranged from 90 minutes to 4 hours with a decrease in operative time as experience is gained. The total operative time per disc level excised averages 15 to 20 minutes (Figure 44-8). In the author's continued experience (greater than 120 cases), this trend has remained.

The blood loss and chest tube drainage reported has been comparable to open procedures with blood loss generally averaging less than 300 ml. Cases of excessive blood loss, however, have been reported[9,18,19] with at least two of these cases converted to open thoracotomy as a result.

There have not been cases of catastrophic complication resulting in either death or neurologic injury reported as a result of thoracoscopic release, although such cases have apparently occurred. As with all anterior spinal surgery, these risks exist and must be minimized. The training process necessary to perform thoracoscopy safely and effectively cannot be overemphasized. The approach is technically demanding, and the initial learning curve substantial. It is recommended that surgeons interested in initiating a thoracoscopic spinal surgery program begin by attending specially designed courses including hands-on human cadaveric and/or live-animal practical experiences. Visiting experienced surgeons and appropriate proctoring are required for the operating spinal thoracoscopy team (access surgeon and spinal surgeon).

OUTCOMES OF THORACOSCOPIC ANTERIOR SCOLIOSIS INSTRUMENTATION

Thoracoscopic anterior scoliosis correction has recently been introduced, and, as such, significant follow-up studies are lacking. In an experimental study utilizing a goat model, the author has demonstrated the feasibility and efficacy of multilevel anterior instrumentation with fusion performed thoracoscopically. The biomechanical

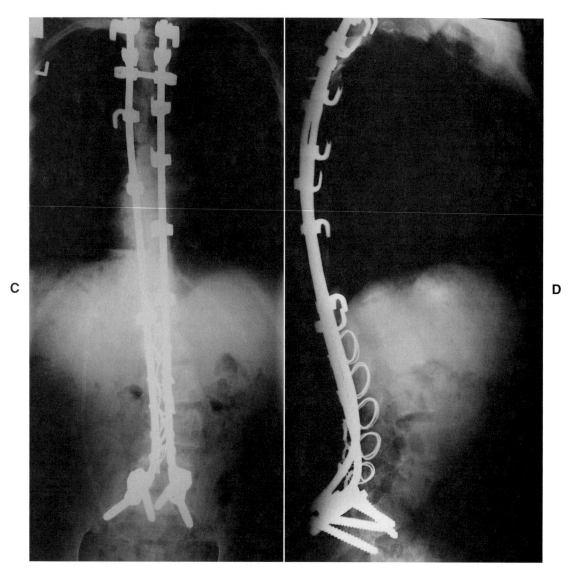

Figure 44-7, cont'd. **C** and **D,** He underwent a left thoracoscopic anterior release and fusion from T5 to L1, as well as a posterior instrumented fusion from T2 to the sacrum.

rigidity of the multilevel construct (four vertebral levels instrumented) was comparable for implants inserted endoscopically and under direct vision. In a comparison of fusion success, utilizing autogenous iliac crest and demineralized bone, there was significantly greater stiffness and radiographic consolidation after 4 months in the iliac-crest–grafted spines.

Picetti et al. reported in 1998 the first clinical case of multilevel anterior scoliosis correction performed thoracoscopically.[20] Since that time the experience has been increasing at several centers around the world. In the author's initial experience (first 30 cases), curve correction averaged greater than 60% with operative time ranging from 4½ hours to 7½ hours. The number of vertebrae instrumented ranged from six to eight, with the most cephalad vertebra instrumented T5 and the most distal level L1. No case has developed a loss of proximal screw fixation or rod fracture, although the follow-up period remains limited (all less than 2 years). Betz et al.

reported similar deformity correction comparing 30 open and 30 thoracoscopic anterior scoliosis corrections.[2] The postoperative recovery has been remarkably short compared to the open anterior and posterior procedures. Hospital discharge has been 1 to 2 days sooner. Quantification of shoulder and pulmonary function recovery is in progress, though anecdotally this appears more rapid as well.

The efficacy and exact role this operation will play in the treatment of idiopathic scoliosis remains to be defined, although many believe it will have a role with substantial benefit compared to open surgery.

THE FUTURE OF THORACOSCOPIC SPINE SURGERY

The role of thoracoscopy in the treatment of pediatric spinal deformity is clearly in evolution. Although early reports have suggested safety and efficacy, these results

Time/Disc vs. Case Number

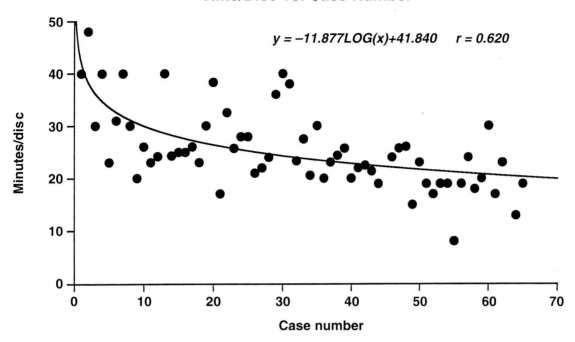

$$y = -11.877LOG(x)+41.840 \quad r = 0.620$$

Figure 44-8. In the author's initial thoracoscopic experience (65 cases) of anterior release and fusion for spinal deformity, the operative time per disc level treated decreased. This seemed to plateau after roughly 30 cases, with average anterior operative time for excision of 6 discs being 2 hours.

remain to be duplicated in large multicenter trials of the technique. Experience with the approach continues to grow as do the applications, most recently expanding into the area of anterior scoliosis instrumentation. A cautious optimism is prudent for all surgeons participating in the growth of this field. This approach, when done well in properly selected patients, has clear advantage over open thoracotomy, yet substantial experience and sound judgment are required to make this possible.

Further development will certainly continue in the techniques of discectomy, arthrodesis, and instrumentation. It is likely these advances will decrease the learning time required to perform these procedures.

SELECTED REFERENCES

Betz R et al.: Anterior instrumentation for thoracic adolescent idiopathic scoliosis: open and minimally invasive techniques. Presented at the 67th annual meeting of the American Association of Orthopaedic Surgeons, Orlando, Fla, 2000.

Betz R et al.: Comparison of anterior and posterior instrumentation for correction of adolescent thoracic idiopathic scoliosis, *Spine* 24(3):225-239, 1999.

Lischke V et al.: Thoracoscopic microsurgical technique for vertebral surgery: anesthetic considerations, *Acta Anaesthesiol Scand* 42(10):1199-1204, 1998.

Newton PO et al.: Anterior release and fusion in pediatric spinal deformity, a comparison of early outcome and cost of thoracoscopic and open thoracotomy approaches, *Spine* 22(12):1398-1406, 1997.

Newton PO, Shea KG, Granlund KF: Defining the pediatric spinal thoracoscopy learning curve: sixty-five consecutive cases, *Spine* 25:1028-1035, 2000.

Picetti GD III et al.: Anterior endoscopic correction and fusion of scoliosis, *Orthopedics* 21(12):1285-1287, 1998.

Regan JJ, Mack MJ, Picetti GD III: A technical report on video-assisted thoracoscopy in thoracic spinal surgery: preliminary description, *Spine* 20(7):831-837, 1995.

Rothenberg S et al.: Thoracoscopic anterior spinal procedures in children, *J Pediatr Surg* 33(7):1168-1170, 1998.

Waisman M, Saute M: Thoracoscopic spine release before posterior instrumentation in scoliosis, *Clin Orthop* 336:130-136, 1997.

REFERENCES

1. Arlet V: Anterior thoracoscopic spine release in deformity surgery: a meta-analysis and review, *Eur Spine J* 9:S17-S23, 2000.
2. Betz R et al.: Anterior instrumentation for thoracic adolescent idiopathic scoliosis: open and minimally invasive techniques. Presented at the 67th annual meeting of the American Association of Orthopaedic Surgeons, Orlando, Fla, 2000.
3. Betz RR et al.: Comparison of anterior and posterior instrumentation for correction of adolescent thoracic idiopathic scoliosis, *Spine* 24(3):225-239, 1999.
4. Bradford DS et al.: Scheuermann's kyphosis: results of surgical treatment by posterior spine arthrodesis in twenty-two patients, *J Bone Joint Surg Am* 57(4):439-448, 1975.
5. Bradford DS et al.: The surgical management of patients with Scheuermann's disease: a review of twenty-four cases managed by combined anterior and posterior spine fusion, *J Bone Joint Surg Am* 62(5):705-712, 1980.
6. Connolly PJ et al.: Video-assisted thoracic diskectomy and anterior release: a biomechanical analysis of an endoscopic technique, *Orthopedics* 22(10):923-926, 1999.
7. Dubousset J, Herring JA, Shufflebarger H: The crankshaft phenomenon, *J Pediatr Orthop* 9(5):541-550, 1989.
8. Gonzalez Barrios I, Fuentes Caparros S, Avila Jurado MM: Anterior thoracoscopic epiphysiodesis in the treatment of a crankshaft phenomenon, *Eur Spine J* 4(6):343-346, 1995.
9. Holcomb GW III, Mencio GA, Green NE: Video-assisted thoracoscopic diskectomy and fusion, *J Pediatr Surg* 32(7):1120-1122, 1997.

10. Huang T et al.: Complications in thoracoscopic spinal surgery. a study of 90 consecutive patients, *Surg Endosc* 13(4):346-350, 1999.

11. Huntington CF et al.: Comparison of thoracoscopic and open thoracic discectomy in a live ovine model for anterior spinal fusion, *Spine* 23(15):1699-1702, 1998.

12. Kokoska ER, Gabriel KR, Silen ML: Minimally invasive anterior spinal exposure and release in children with scoliosis, *J Soc Laparoendosc Surg* 2(3):255-258, 1998.

13. Lapinksy AS, Richards BS: Preventing the crankshaft phenomenon by combining anterior fusion with posterior instrumentation: does it work? *Spine* 20(12):1392-1398, 1995.

14. Lischke V et al.: Thoracoscopic microsurgical technique for vertebral surgery: anesthetic considerations, *Acta Anaesth Scand* 42(10):1199-1204, 1998.

15. McAfee PC et al.: The incidence of complications in endoscopic anterior thoracolumbar spinal reconstructive surgery: a prospective multicenter study comprising the first 100 consecutive cases, *Spine* 20(14):1624-1632, 1995.

16. Newton PO et al.: Anterior release and fusion in pediatric spinal deformity: a comparison of early outcome and cost of thoracoscopic and open thoracotomy approaches, *Spine* 22(12):1398-1406, 1997.

17. Newton PO et al.: A biomechanical comparison of open and thoracoscopic anterior spinal release in a goat model, *Spine* 23(5):530-535, 1998.

18. Newton PO, Shea KG, Granlund KF: Defining the pediatric spinal thoracoscopy learning curve. Sixty-five consecutive cases, *Spine* 25:1028-1035, 2000.

19. Papin P et al.: Treatment of scoliosis in the adolescent by anterior release and vertebral arthrodesis under thoracoscopy: preliminary results, *Rev Chir Orthop Reparatrice Appar Mot* 84(3):231-238, 1998.

20. Picetti GD III et al.: Anterior endoscopic correction and fusion of scoliosis, *Orthopedics* 21(12):1285-1287, 1998.

21. Ponte A, Siccardi G, Ligure P: *Scheuermann's kyphosis: posterior shortening procedure by segmental closing wedge resections.* Presented at the 29th annual meeting of the Scoliosis Research Society, Portland, Ore, 1994.

22. Regan JJ, Mack MJ, Picetti GD III: A technical report on video-assisted thoracoscopy in thoracic spinal surgery: preliminary description, *Spine* 20(7):831-837, 1995.

23. Rothenberg S et al.: Thoracoscopic anterior spinal procedures in children, *J Pediatr Surg* 33(7):1168-1170, 1998.

24. Waisman M, Saute M: Thoracoscopic spine release before posterior instrumentation in scoliosis, *Clin Orthop* 336:130-136, 1997.

25. Wall EJ et al.: Endoscopic discectomy increases thoracic spine flexibility as effectively as open discectomy: a mechanical study in a porcine model, *Spine* 23(1):9-15, 1998.

Adolescent Idiopathic Scoliosis

Randal R. Betz, Lawrence G. Lenke

The surgical treatment of adolescent idiopathic scoliosis (AIS) has advanced significantly during the past 25 years. This chapter provides an overview of treatment, concentrating specifically on the newer advances, including their advantages, results, and complications. Much of the problem in interpretation of the results of surgical treatment of AIS over the years has been due to the lack of a reliable classification system. Most surgical reviews are of treatments represented with different curve types with different degrees of flexibility and without regard to scoliosis being a three-dimensional deformity. In this chapter, we also present a new classification system that provides a mechanism to guide treatment as well as better comparison for evidence-based information in the future.

The goals of surgical treatment in AIS include correction and stabilization of the curve, reduction in the clinical deformity, and restoration or maintenance of a balanced spine. There are some clear indications for surgical treatment, and there are some gray areas. Factors other than the Cobb measurement of the curve often need to be considered, including the level of skeletal maturity, sagittal plane configuration, amount of vertebral rotation, clinical disfigurement, and knowledge of the natural history.

The indications for surgery in the adolescent generally are thought to include curves greater than 50 degrees. Weinstein et al.[81] studied curve progression after skeletal maturity and found that approximately 68% of thoracic curves progressed at least 5 degrees and 75 degrees progressed to the greatest extent over time. Lumbar curves in the adolescent generally need to be fused only for cosmetic disfigurement. Natural history studies during the past 20 years suggest that there is no increased risk of severe back pain.[19] Pregnancy is not an added risk factor for curve progression.[6] Curves between 35 degrees and 50 degrees without documented progression in adolescents need to be analyzed individually. In general, most should be observed for curve progression unless there is some concern with the cosmetic disfigurement. Skeletal maturity is an important factor in this analysis. For example, a 45-degree curve in a 14-year-old who is postmenarche and Risser stage 4 and is content with the cosmetic appearance should be observed. However, the same degree of curve in an 11-year-old girl who is premenarche and Risser stage 0 with open triradiates has an extremely high risk of progressing and should be considered for surgery, because bracing is ineffective for curves of this magnitude. The sagittal plane must be carefully analyzed when considering surgical treatment of AIS.[70] There is a group of patients with severe hypokyphosis or actual lordosis of the thoracic spine whom, because of the risk of adverse effects on pulmonary function, should be considered surgical candidates even if their Cobb angle measurement is not large enough to generally be considered for surgery.

Classification of Operative Adolescent Idiopathic Scoliosis

In the analysis of operative AIS, there lacks a universally agreed-on reliable classification system.[20,48] This makes comparisons of various surgical treatments difficult and does not allow for standardization of treatment.

A new, comprehensive, and surgical treatment–oriented classification system for AIS has been developed.[51] The classification consists of three components: specific curve types (1 to 6), lumbar spine modifier (A to C), and a sagittal thoracic plane modifier (−, N, and +).

GOALS OF SURGICAL TREATMENT IN ADOLESCENT IDIOPATHIC SCOLIOSIS

- Correction and stabilization of the curve
- Reduction in clinical deformity
- Restoration or maintenance of a balanced spine
- Factors (other than the Cobb measurement) to consider
  - Level of skeletal maturity
  - Sagittal plane configuration
  - Amount of vertebral rotation
  - Clinical disfigurement
  - Natural history

The six specific curve types (1 to 6) are based on the structural nature of each of the three regional spinal columns: proximal thoracic, main thoracic, and thoracolumbar/lumbar. Specific objective radiographic criteria in the coronal and sagittal planes separate structural from nonstructural curves (residual coronal curve ≥25 degrees on bending film or ≥20 degrees of kyphosis T2 to T5 or T10 to L2 on the erect lateral). A lumbar spine modifier (A to C) is added based on the relationship of the center sacral vertical line to the apex of the lumbar spine. Last, a sagittal thoracic modifier is added based on the T5 to T12 sagittal Cobb measurement (– for <+10 degrees; N for +10 degrees to +40 degrees; and + for ≥+40 degrees). Thus curve classification combines the specific curve type (1 to 6) with the lumbar spine modifier (A, B, or C) and sagittal thoracic modifier (–, N or +) to produce the specific curve classification (1A–, 1AN, 1A+, 1B–, 6CN, 6C+).

Classification reliability was tested by both the developers of the system and a randomly chosen independent group of Scoliosis Research Society members who were not involved in the formulation of this classification system. The interobserver and intraobserver reliabilities of the curve type by the developers of this system were $k = .83$ and $K = .92$, respectively, which equals good-to-excellent reliability for both.

A single-surgeon consecutive series[52] of 606 surgical cases found that adolescent idiopathic curves classified according to this new system had the following curve prevalence: type 1 (main thoracic), 51%; type 2 (double thoracic), 20%; type 3 (double), 11%; type 4 (triple major), 3%; type 5 (thoracolumbar/lumbar), 12%; and type 6 (thoracolumbar/lumbar-main thoracic), 3%. A retrospective review has shown this system to be 90% predictive of fusion of the appropriate structural curves.[52]

A schematic of the classification is shown in Figure 45-1.

POSTERIOR INSTRUMENTATION
General Posterior Spinal Fusion

Posterior spinal fusion with Harrington rod instrumentation was the mainstay of treatment for patients with idiopathic scoliosis. Excellent long-term results have been reported on selected thoracic fusions with the Harrington rod, with casting and bracing for postoperative care.[45] Long-term postoperative results show the patients doing well up to a 20-year follow-up, with

Curve Type

Type	Proximal thoracic	Main thoracic	Thoracolumbar/ lumbar	Curve type
1	Nonstructural	Structural (major*)	Nonstructural	Main thoracic (MT)
2	Structural	Structural (major*)	Nonstructural	Double thoracic DT)
3	Nonstructural	Structural (major*)	Structural	Double major (DM)
4	Structural	Structural (major*)	Structural	Triple major (TM)
5	Nonstructural	Nonstructural	Structural (Major*)	Thoracolumbar lumbar (TL/L)
6	Nonstructural	Structural	Structual (Major*)	Thoracolumbar/lumbar Main thoracic (TL/L-MT)

STRUCTURAL CRITERIA
(Minor Curves)

Proximal thoracic: + Side bending cobb ≥25°
+ T2–T5 kyphosis ≥+20°

Main Thoracic: + Side bending cobb ≥25°
+ T10–L2 kyphosis ≥20°

Thoracolumbar/lumbar: + Side bending cobb ≥25°
+ T10–L2 kyphosis ≥+20°

*Major = Largest Cobb Measurement, always structural
Minor = all other curves with structural criteria applied

LOCATION OF APEX
(SRS definition)

CURVE	APEX
THORACIC	T2–T11–12 DISC
THORACOLUMBAR	T12–L1
LUMBAR	L1–2 DISC–L4

Modifiers

Lumbar spine modifier	CSVL to lumbar apex		Thoracic sagittal profile T5–T12		
A	CSVL between pedicles		–	(Hypo)	<10°
B	CSVL Touches apical body(ies)		N	(Normal)	10°–40°
C	CSVL completely medial	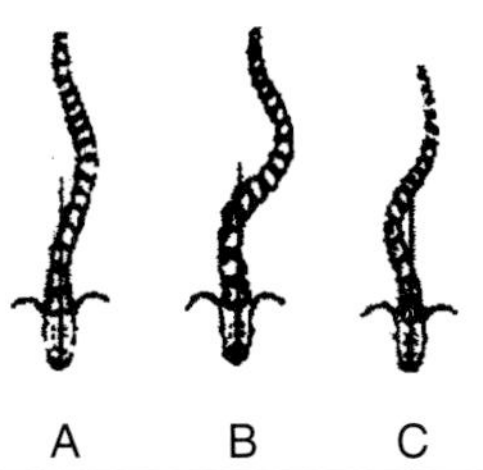 A B C	+	(Hyper)	>40°

Curve type (1-6)+ lumbar spine modifier (A, B, or C)+ thoracic sagittal modifier (–, N, or +)
Classification (e.g., 1B+): _____

Figure 45-1. Schematic of classification system of Lenke and colleagues. *(From Lenke LG, et al.: Adolescent idiopathic scoliosis: a new classification to determine the extent of spinal arthrodesis, J Bone Joint Surg Am 83:1169-1181, 2001.)*

conflicting reports on increasing back pain with fusion to the lower lumbar spine.[16,18,23,32]

In the mid-1980s, posterior spinal fusion with multi-segmented hook-rod systems became popular. Early and longer-term results have shown excellent results with regard to curve correction, maintenance of balance, and minimal complications.[2,37,47,68,72] Recently, pedicle screw fixation of both the lumbar spine and thoracic spine has become popular. Several reports show that screws are safe in the pediatric spine.[10,36,54] Studies of fixation of the lumbar spine of pedicle screws versus hooks show significant improvement in fixation and maintenance of curve correction.[3,17]

Pedicle Screws in the Thoracic Spine

During the past decade, the use of pedicle screw anchors in the treatment of AIS has expanded dramatically. Screws were used initially in the lumbar spine, then in the thoracolumbar junction, and now in the thoracic spine as well. This section discusses the rationale for use of pedicle screws in patients with AIS, specifically the feasibility, techniques for implantation, safety, and surgical results (Figures 45-2 and 45-3).

The use of pedicle screws in the pediatric population has been shown to be quite effective and safe in the lumbar spine.[1,10] These studies have shown improved coronal correction as well as lumbar lordosis in comparisons of pedicle screws versus hooks as lumbar anchors.[3,36] The correction of transverse plane rotation has been less optimal. Maintenance of correction over a minimum 2-year follow-up has been excellent, with minimal pseudarthrosis rates and subsequent requirements for revision.[10] Screws can be placed with or without image guidance (i.e., fluoroscopy), with most experienced scoliosis surgeons placing screws freehand using anatomic landmarks, a blunt pedicle seeker, careful palpation of intraosseous screw position before placement, and fluoroscopy and/or radiography in the coronal and sagittal planes to document accurate position.

As a surgeon gains experience, screws are often placed in the entire convexity of a lumbar curve up to the thoracolumbar junction. Interestingly, between T10 and S1, the smallest pedicles are usually L1 and L2*. The limiting factor for screw position is always the medial-lateral pedicle dimensions. The concave pedicle is always much more difficult to instrument than the convex pedicle, due to two factors: the concave pedicle tends to be slightly smaller in dimensions and more cortical, and the surgeon working on the concavity must drop his or her operative hand while probing the pedicle, often abutting the ipsilateral muscle mass in the process.

The use of screws in the proximal and mid-thoracic spine should be attempted only when the surgeon is extremely experienced and is comfortable placing screws in the lumbar spine and the thoracolumbar junction. Thoracic screws can be placed either with a freehand technique or using intraoperative fluoroscopy. Most, but not all, thoracic spines can accept intrapedicular screws at the apex of a scoliosis deformity.[64] In Dr. Lenke's experience, roughly 80% of thoracic vertebrae between T2 and T10 will accept intrapedicular screws at every level of the correcting rod (left-sided placement for a right convex idiopathic scoliosis). Again, the concave screws will be more difficult than the convex screws, with the pedicle being much more cortical on the concavity.[64]

The technique for thoracic pedicle screw placement involves freehand placement with careful, thorough dissection of the posterior elements. Two to three millimeters of the inferior facet should be osteotomized to clearly see the facet joint, for both decortication and screw placement. The starting point for screw placement varies as one proceeds from caudad to cephalad in the thoracic spine. In the lower thoracic regions (T10 to 12), the starting point is in line with the tip of the transverse process at its base at the junction to the lamina just at or lateral to the lateral aspect of the pars region. As one proceeds more cephalad in the thoracic spine (T5 to 9), the starting point is more medial and proximal. Thus, the most common starting point is the junction of the proximal edge of the transverse process where it meets both the superior facet and the lamina. The junction or groove between those three landmarks is the best spot to begin burring to locate the center of the pedicle. Often a pedicle "blush" is seen at the cancellous base of the pedicle. In smaller pedicles, this may not be seen, and the tip of the probe may be required to find this in a funnel-like technique. It is extremely helpful to use a small (approximately 2 mm) tip probe to locate the thoracic apical concave pedicles. Depending on the size of the pedicle, the probe will be quite snug going down the pedicle shaft, obviously with consideration of the previously placed screw direction. It is wise to err on the lateral side; plunging out laterally is safer than plunging out medially. Both the sagittal plane alignment and axial plane rotation must be kept in mind when placing thoracic screws. The pedicle seeker track is palpated to be absolutely sure that it is completely intraosseous. Normal screw diameters for the apical thoracic pedicles are between 4.5 and 5.5 mm. This is consistent with a study by O'Brien and colleagues,[64] which found the concave pedicle dimensions to be between 4 and 6 mm in patients with AIS. Again, the convex pedicles will be slightly larger and easier to find because of the increased amount of cancellous bone within the pedicle. Apical convex screws are somewhat safer to place (when paying attention to the amount of convex rotation present), because the spinal cord will be much closer to the apical concave pedicle than the convex pedicle.

Screw placement in the convex (left-sided) proximal thoracic region (T1 to T4) actually becomes easier because the pedicles are larger and one is working on the convexity. Screw placement starts slightly more distal at the proximal edge of the transverse process just medial to the lateral aspect of the pars. Concave proximal thoracic (T1 to T4) screws are more difficult to place because of small pedicle size.

Obviously, safe screw placement anywhere in the thoracic or lumbar spine is an absolute requirement for the

---

*David W. Polly, Jr., MD, Unpublished data.

A

B

C

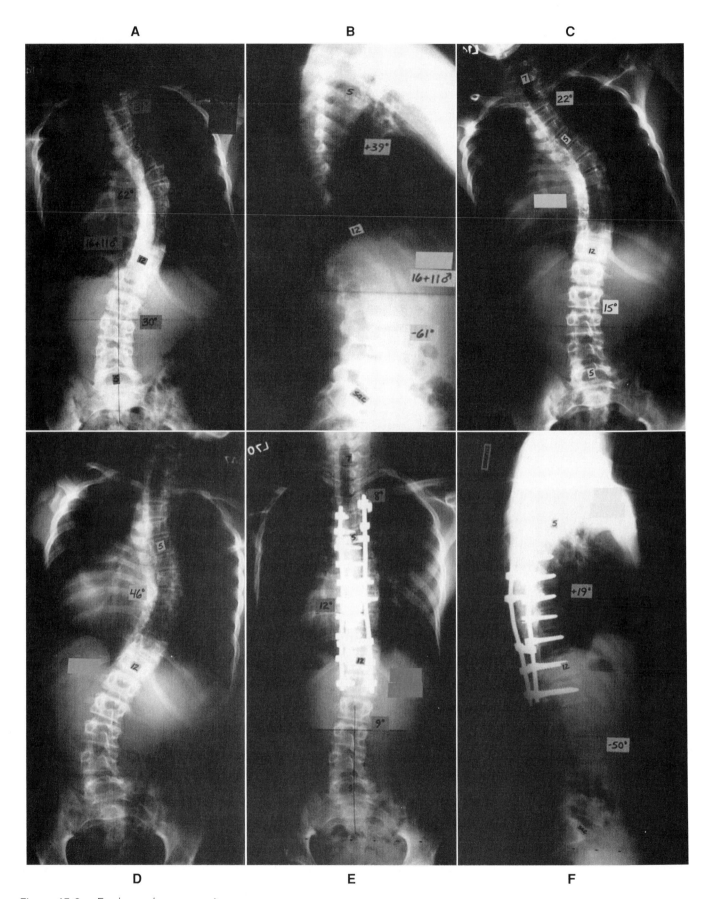

D

E

F

Figure 45-2. *For legend see opposite page.*

Figure 45-2. These views are from a 16-years and 11-month-old boy with adolescent idiopathic scoliosis. He is Risser stage 4 and nearly skeletally mature. **A,** Upright coronal long cassette radiograph shows a 31 degrees proximal thoracic, 62 degrees main thoracic, and 30 degrees thoracolumbar curve. **B,** His upright long cassette lateral radiograph shows 39 degrees of kyphosis between T5 and T12 and −61 degrees of lordosis between T12 and the sacrum. **C,** Side bending to the left demonstrates correction of the proximal thoracic curve to 22 degrees and the lumbar curve to 15 degrees. **D,** Side bending to the right shows correction of the right main thoracic curve to only 46 degrees. Thus this curve is classified 1AN by the Lenke et al. classification system. **E,** The patient underwent a posterior segmental instrumentation and fusion from T4 to L1 using thoracoplasty bone graft. His main thoracic curve was corrected to 12 degrees (81% correction) with spontaneous realignment in both the proximal thoracic and lumbar spine. L1 is appropriately centered on the sacrum and horizontal. **F,** Postoperative lateral radiograph shows sagittal alignment with 19 degrees of thoracic kyphosis between T5 and T12.

use of pedicle screws. One must be absolutely certain that the screw is completely intraosseous in all positions. This is done through several measures, including, most important, palpation of the screw track several times to confirm a bony floor and four intraosseous walls (medial, lateral, inferior, superior). Intraoperative fluoroscopy and/or radiography in both the coronal and sagittal planes before rod placement is imperative. Electrophysiologic techniques using electromyelographic stimulus can be quite helpful, similar to use in the lumbar spine (recording from the lumbar myotomes) as well as the mid and lower thoracic spine from T6 to T12 (recording from the rectus abdominus).[53] It cannot be overstressed how compulsive the surgeon must be to document accurate screw placement if one elects to use screws in patients with AIS.

There is a paucity of literature on the use of thoracic pedicle screws in patients with AIS. Suk et al.[74] followed 78 patients treated with different constructs: 31 patients treated with hooks alone, 23 patients treated with screws in a hook pattern, and 24 patients treated with segmental pedicle screws at every level of the correction rod. Postoperative Cobb correction was superior with the segmental screw constructs (72% versus 66% [screws in a hook pattern] versus 55% [all hooks]). They thought that 13 screws (3%) were malpositioned, but none produced any neurologic sequelae. Liljenqvist and colleagues[54] evaluated 120 screws in 32 consecutive patients and found that 25% of screws penetrated the pedicle wall or anterior vertebral cortex, with 1 screw revised due to proximity to the aorta. Their coronal curve corrections of 59% with screws were similar to 52% obtained with hooks.

There have been no published reports by North American authors on the use of thoracic pedicle screws for AIS. However, Dr. Lenke's experience includes the placement of more than 1000 thoracic pedicle screws in the past 3 years, with more than 500 of those used in patients with AIS. There have been no neurologic sequelae, no known pseudarthroses, and no revisions for any reason in these patients with AIS. Cobb correction has averaged nearly 70% (versus 50% with hooks).[52] Advantages to using thoracic pedicle screws instead of hooks have included the correction of thoracic hyperkyphosis by convex compression using segmental pedicle screws, treatment of skeletally immature

patients to minimize the risk of crankshaft via three-column screw fixations, maximization of apical translation without any intraspinal anchors (supralaminar hooks or sublaminar wires), the minimization of soft tissue striping above and below the lowest instrumented vertebrae that occurs with the use of hooks, and safe manipulation of the rod using firm cantilever forces without the risk of implant dislodgment or propulsion into the spinal canal (as can occur with supralaminar hooks, pedicle hooks, or sublaminar wires).

In conclusion, thoracic, thoracolumbar, and lumbar pedicle screws can be used safely for the surgical treatment of AIS. Strict attention to detail, confirmation of intraosseous placement, and surgical techniques that optimize segmental instrumentation are required for optimal success. Multicenter studies will be required to define the efficacy of this technique in individual surgeons' hands, as well as to provide justification for the routine use of thoracic pedicle screws in AIS.

Long-Term Effects of Posterior Spinal Instrumentation

Luk et al.[57] studied the effects of long spine fusions for scoliosis on the lumbosacral spine. They reviewed 22 patients with a minimum follow-up of 10 years. They found that most patients were pain free; only 1 of 22 (4.5%) had severe back pain. Radiographically, they noted the development of local kyphosis within the fused segment of the lumbar spine, although overall lordosis was maintained by hyperlordosis of the remaining segments. They proposed that this might predispose the patient to problems later and concluded that 10-year follow-up might not be adequate to evaluate the long-term effects of long scoliosis fusions on the unfused lumbosacral spine.

Two groups of independent investigators have reported results on the incidence of lower back pain after Harrington instrumentation and fusion into the lumbar spine. Cochran et al.[16] and Hayes et al.[40] have shown that the prevalence of back pain is related to the distal level of instrumentation. When compared with control groups, there was an increased risk of severe back pain when Harrington rod and fusion extended distally to the fourth or fifth lumbar vertebra. In contrast,

A

B

C

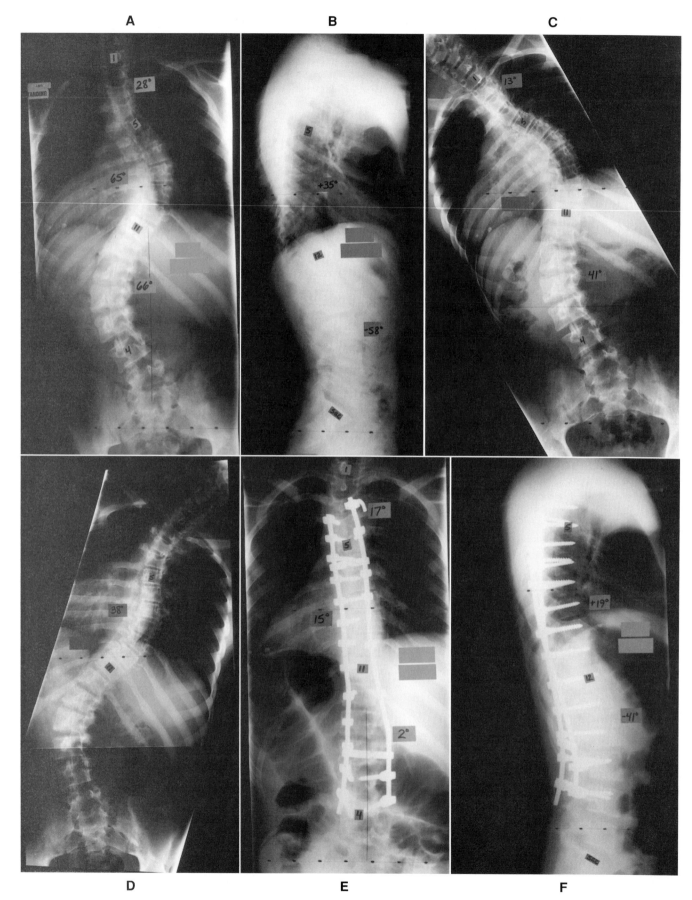

D

E

F

Figure 45-3. *For legend see opposite page.*

Figure 45-3. These views are from a 17-year 2-month-old skeletally mature boy with a double major adolescent idiopathic scoliosis curve pattern (Lenke 6CN). **A,** Upright long cassette radiograph demonstrates a 28 degrees proximal thoracic, 65 degrees thoracic, and 66 degrees lumbar curve. The lumbar modifier is "C." **B,** The long cassette lateral radiograph demonstrates +35 degrees of kyphosis between T5 and T12 and –58 degrees of lordosis between T12 and the sacrum. The sagittal modifier is "N." **C,** Side bending to the left demonstrates correction of the proximal thoracic curve to 13 degrees and the lumbar curve to only 41 degrees. **D,** Side bend correction of the main thoracic curve is to 38 degrees. The Lenke curve classification is 6CN. **E,** Posterior instrumentation and fusion was performed from T4 to L4 with transpedicular screw fixation at every level of the left side correcting rod in the thoracic concavity and lumbar convexity. The thoracic curve was corrected to 15 degrees (77% correction), whereas the lumbar curve was corrected to 2 degrees (97% correction). The L4 curve angle is improved horizontally with nice centralization of L4 and L5 postoperatively. **F,** The postoperative sagittal radiograph demonstrates normalized thoracic kyphosis and lumbar lordosis in a harmonious thoracolumbar junction.

Bartie et al.[4] reviewed the functional outcome of 172 patients followed an average of 19 years after posterior spinal fusion for idiopathic scoliosis (minimum follow-up was 10 years). The patients were treated with Harrington instrumentation to L2, L3, L4, or L5. The authors found no radiographic measurement or trend that could statistically predict a painful outcome. The patients and control subjects experienced similar back pain; however, control subjects functioned at a higher level. Based on available information, it seems prudent to avoid fusions into the lumbar spine if possible. When it is necessary to fuse into the lumbar spine, it is preferable that the distal extent of the fusion not be more caudad than L3. On the other hand, it is preferable to fuse to L4 and obtain a balanced spine than to stop the distal extent of the fusion more proximal and end up with trunk imbalance. It may well be that maintenance of normal sagittal contours in the lumbar spine is more important than the distal extent of fusion.

In a recent study, Gagnon et al.[31] reviewed a homogeneous Swedish population and found that, in the long term, surgery improves pulmonary function in patients with idiopathic scoliosis. They studied 42 women with thoracic curves averaging 59 degrees. Their preoperative vital capacities averaged 81% of predicted and were more likely to be diminished in patients with thoracic curves of greater than 50 degrees. Postoperatively, after an average 40% curve correction and at least 3 years of follow-up, there was an average 12% overall improvement in vital capacity. Lenke et al.[47] found that forced vital capacity was improved 21% in patients with idiopathic scoliosis treated with the Cotrel-Dubousset technique without thoracoplasty.

ANTERIOR INSTRUMENTATION
Thoracolumbar and Lumbar Scoliosis
Indications

The reported indications for anterior instrumentation in thoracolumbar and lumbar idiopathic scoliosis include the ability to save one or more distal fusion levels and to prevent crankshaft phenomenon in young patients.[60,65] Determining whether one can save distal fusion levels

---

INDICATIONS FOR ANTERIOR INSTRUMENTATION: THORACOLUMBAR

- The ability to save one or more distal fusion levels
- Prevention of the crankshaft phenomenon in young children

---

can be done by defining the lower instrumented vertebrae (LIV) anteriorly as the vertebrae in the Cobb angle having less than a 15-degree tilt to the pelvis on bending radiographs and less than 20% rotation.[61] The LIV can then be compared with a predicted level for posterior fusion.

A technique pioneered by Hall et al.[35] provides overcorrection of the instrumented apical three or four segments of thoracolumbar and lumbar curves and is performed to stop fusion at either L1 or L2, further saving additional fusion levels. They report a short segment overcorrection technique with derotation and overcorrection of the apical segment, fusing three or four segments. If the apex of the curve is a vertebral body, they fuse three segments, one body above and one below the apex. If the apex is a disc, they fuse two vertebral bodies above and two below, for a four-segment construct. They reported on 26 patients since 1983 with either Dwyer or VDS instrumentation (flexible threaded rods) and 18 patients with TSRH instrumentation (solid, rigid rods), with coronal correction averaging 100% and 108%, respectively. Development of kyphosis in the instrumented segment averaged 10 degrees in the Dwyer/VDS group and 9.9 degrees in the TSRH group. To date, no patient in their series has required extension of the fusion because of increased deformity distal to the LIV, nor have they had pain in any oblique segment below the fusion. Only long-term follow-up will determine if the oblique segment below the instrumentation becomes a clinical concern.

Approach

Thoracolumbar and lumbar approaches are well described in other textbooks. In general, one needs to enter the retroperitoneal space or the thorax through an interspace above the proposed upper instrumented level. Some surgeons prefer to take the rib; however, on closure, especially after the convexity has been corrected and straight, this leaves a defect in the chest wall. We prefer going through the intercostal space, which leaves less of a chest wall deformity. If one needs to harvest bone graft of the rib, one can take a longitudinal half of the rib.

One can shorten the length of the incision and extend the exposure by using a puncture approach to place the proximal or distal screw. Angled screwdrivers are available, but sometimes there is insufficient space between the rib and the vertebral body for them to work appropriately, and the puncture technique is helpful. It is strongly recommended that an intraoperative radiograph be obtained to confirm levels. If the level is too distal, the opportunity for saving a fusion level is lost. If it is too proximal, there is a high risk of decompensation.

Controversy still exists as to whether to remove the segmental vessels. Most surgeons still ligate the vessels, and in a large series reported by Winter et al.[85] of more than 1000 cases, there were no instances of intraoperative paralysis secondary to vessel ligation.

Creation of a periosteal sleeve is still controversial. It has been proposed to be very important in obtaining a solid fusion and facilitating clean disc and end plate excision. However, the disadvantages of this include increased blood loss and the tedious exposure required. It is essential for a thorough discectomy to use a disc spreader to spread the disc such that the end plate and posterior annulus can be removed all the way back to the posterior longitudinal ligament, maximizing the area of exposure for bone grafting. This exposure of the disc space then allows for structural graft placement for thoracolumbar and lumbar curve correction.

Variations of Instrumentation: Flexible

Examples of available flexible systems include the Zielke, Dwyer, and the Harms-MOSS system of 3.2-mm and 4-mm rods.* The derotation maneuver for derotating the lumbar spine and maintaining lordosis was popularized by Zielke and reported by Ogiela and Chan[65] and Moe et al.[60] The biggest problem with flexible rods has been the development of an average of 13 degrees to 20 degrees kyphosis in the instrumented segment.[56] This problem has been prevented by the use of solid, rigid rods[78] and the use of structural grafts for interbody spacers to provide anterior support.[39]

Variations of Instrumentation: Solid

A big advantage of the use of solid rods is that it eliminates postoperative bracing and casting. Examples of solid rod systems include TSRH (as reported by Turi et al.[78]), CD-Horizon, MOSS-Miami, Synergy, and ISOLA. Anterior structural support, as reported by Harms et al.,[39] appears to be most important with the use of

---

*References 28, 29, 46, 56, 60, 76.

> **INDICATIONS FOR ANTERIOR INSTRUMENTATION: THORACIC**
>
> • Potential to save two or more distal fusion levels
> • Ability to correct hypokyphosis (<20 degrees of kyphosis)
> • Skeletally immature patients

single solid rods to prevent kyphosis and obtain bone healing, although published reports of long-term studies are pending.

A dual–solid rod system (Kaneda Anterior Spinal System) has been reported to provide excellent coronal and sagittal results. The dual-rod system requires two screws in each vertebral body and may be beneficial for large patients to prevent nonunions and eliminate bracing.[44] In a study of 25 patients with thoracolumbar or lumbar scoliosis by Kaneda et al.,[43] the average correction rate was 83%. Preoperative kyphosis of the instrumented levels of 7 degrees was corrected to 9 degrees of lordosis. Sagittal lordosis of the lumbosacral area beneath the fused segments averaged 51 degrees before surgery and was reduced to 34 degrees after surgery. The trunk shift was improved from 25 mm before surgery to 4 mm at final follow-up evaluation. Apical vertebral rotation showed an average correction rate of 86%. At final follow-up evaluation, all patients demonstrated solid fusion without implant-related complications.

ANTERIOR INSTRUMENTATION
Thoracic Scoliosis
Indications

The indications for anterior instrumentation for correction of thoracic scoliosis include the potential to save two or more distal fusion levels (and/or the ability to correct hypokyphosis [less than 20 degrees of kyphosis]).[7] In addition, in skeletally immature patients an anterior release and fusion may be indicated to prevent the crankshaft phenomenon. In this situation, insertion of anterior instrumentation potentially involves less surgery than an anterior spinal arthrodesis followed by a posterior arthrodesis with instrumentation.[7]

In most cases where two or more distal levels can be saved, the curves are classified as King II, III, or IV or as type I according to the system of Lenke et al.[51] In those curves, there is a risk of the patient being unbalanced after posterior instrumentation of the thoracic curve alone.[9] The number of fusion levels to be saved must be predicted. The LIV that is instrumented with anterior thoracic instrumentation is the end vertebral body of the Cobb measurement, or, if there are two parallel vertebrae, the more distal vertebra is usually instrumented. This then can be compared with the predicted posterior LIV with either the stable vertebra or the Cotrel-Dubousset method.[14,71] In the Cotrel-Dubousset method, the disc below the proposed LIV on a bending radiograph must reverse 5 degrees and the LIV must have less than 20% rotation in the mature patient or be

PREDICTION OF FUSION LEVELS TO BE SAVED

- The lower instrumented vertebra addressed with anterior thoracic instrumentation is the end vertebral body of the Cobb measurement.
- With two parallel vertebrae, the more distal vertebra is used.
- This is comparable to the predicted posterior lower instrumented vertebrae by either the stable vertebra or the Cotrel-Dubousset method.
- In the Cotrel-Dubousset method, the disc below the proposed lower instrumented vertebrae on a bending radiograph must reverse 5 degrees and the lower instrumented vertebrae must have less than 20% rotation in a mature patient or be neutral in the immature patient.
- When there is evidence of thoracolumbar kyphosis on the preoperative radiographs, posterior instrumentation would need to be longer but not anterior.

SURGICAL TECHNIQUE FOR THORACIC CURVES: OPEN

- For more than seven levels, a double thoracotomy is necessary.
- Use a double-lumen tube.
- Make an incision in the intercostal space (at approximately T4 to T5).
- Make a second incision at T8 to T9.
- If a thoracoplasty is necessary, do it now.
- Obtain a radiograph to confirm the anatomic levels.
- Proximal screw stability is an issue with all anterior instrumentation. To overcome instability, place the screw in the superior third of the vertebra. Use a slightly longer proximal screw along with one or two washers to take up the space between the screw head and staple. The screw must penetrate at least 5 mm through the far cortex, producing bicortical purchase.
- Firmly pack the inferior discs between T10 and L2 with anterior structural support and bone graft to full anatomic height.
- Insert the rod and apply cantilever force.
- Obtain final correction by compressing each screw toward the apex.

neutral in the immature patient. When there is evidence of a thoracolumbar kyphosis on the preoperative radiographs, posterior instrumentation would have to be longer but not anterior instrumentation.[67] Residual hypokyphosis still occurs in up to 60% of cases after posterior multisegmented hook-rod systems,[7,47,67] and anterior instrumentation can consistently correct thoracic hypokyphosis and thoracic lordosis.

Surgical Technique: Approach

The usual approach to the thoracic spine involves a double thoracotomy through a single skin incision.[7,39] In general, for predicted anterior instrumentations of seven or fewer levels, a single incision through the interspace is all that may be required. For more than seven levels, in general a double thoracotomy is necessary to provide adequate exposure for disc clean out, anterior support, and instrumentation.

Surgical Technique: Open

The patient is intubated with a double-lumen tube for one-lung ventilation so that at the site of the thoracotomy, the lung can be kept deflated for the majority of the procedure to facilitate exposure of the anterior spine, as is done for thoracoscopy. The patient is then placed in a lateral decubitus position. A single skin incision is made approximately parallel to the eighth rib as is standard for a thoracotomy. The serratus anterior muscle is then mobilized and partially detached anteriorly. An incision is made in the intercostal space (at approximately T4 to T5 for instrumentation of the T5 vertebra). A second incision is made between the intercostal space of approximately three or four ribs distally (at T8 to T9 for instrumentation of T12). These intercostal space incisions can be adjusted proximally or distally, depending on the levels of the spine to be instrumented. For a short anterior instrumentation (seven or fewer levels), a single incision of the inter-

costal space may suffice. The most proximal level instrumented by the authors to date has been T3.

If the preoperative analysis of the patient suggests that a thoracoplasty is indicated for cosmesis, then it is easiest to perform it at this stage. Small pieces of rib are resected as posteriorly as possible in the intervening ribs between the two intercostal space entrances and above and below. For example, in the previous example, a piece of the ribs of T5 to T9 approximately 2 cm in length would be removed. If there is a very long rib deformity, additional pieces of ribs can be removed, such as from T4 or T10. It is best to do this at this stage, because the instrumentation will have minimal effect on correcting the rib deformity and the rib resections will facilitate retraction of the chest wall to make the discectomies and instrumentation easier to perform. The pieces of rib are used for bone grafting.

A radiograph should be obtained with a large needle in a disc space to confirm the anatomic levels. Because only selected fusion levels are performed using anterior instrumentation, it is absolutely critical to be correct in the levels. Next, the segmental vessels are ligated over each of the vertebral bodies to be instrumented. Some surgeons do not ligate the vessels but mobilize them and plan on slightly eccentric placement of the screw and staple or use no staple at all.* Staples are then inserted into the vertebral bodies. These are aligned so that they are in approximately the same anatomic position in each vertebral body, being as far posterior as possible while ensuring there is no possibility of penetration of the spinal canal with the staple prongs. Next, an awl is used to make the hole, and the screws are then inserted.

---

*T. Lowe, Personal communication.

It should be noted that proximal screw stability is an issue with all anterior thoracic instrumentation because of the risk for screws to pull out during correction. To overcome this problem, we now suggest the following precautions. In the most proximal vertebrae (e.g., T5), the screw is inserted eccentrically into the vertebral body. It is placed in the superior third of the vertebra but in the same position posteriorly as the other screws. This appears to add increased resistance to screw pull-out by abutting the screw threads against the superior end plate of the vertebral body and providing more bone between the screw and the apex of the curve to prevent ploughing. A slightly longer proximal screw is necessary so that the screw extends a bit out of the staple to align the rod with the other screws. In addition, we currently use one or two washers to take up this space between the screw head and staple, and the screw must penetrate at least 5 mm through the far cortex, producing bicortical purchase. Therefore, if the vertebral body measures 25 mm and one would normally put in a 30-mm screw to allow the threads to stick out 5 mm, we recommend a 35-mm screw with two washers. Because this technique has been used, no proximal screw pull-out has been observed as compared to a 10% prevalence before using this technique. It is important that all screw tips can be palpated on the concave side of the vertebral body. Before rod insertion, bone grafting should be placed in the disc spaces. Beginning distally, the disc spaces are wedged open and the interspaces are packed. It is important to pack the inferior discs between T10 and L2 firmly with anterior structural support and bone graft to full anatomic height. Structural anterior support, either autogenous or synthetic (e.g., titanium cage), should be used to help ensure maintenance of the sagittal profile. When grafting the apical vertebrae, the original sagittal contour must be considered. If the beginning sagittal profile is lordotic or hypokyphotic, only a small amount of graft should be inserted into the anterior disc space at the apex on the concave side of the curve. This allows the kyphosis to occur during compression with instrumentation. If, however, the patient starts with a normal kyphosis (greater than or equal to 20 degrees), the apical disc space should be wedged open to a normal height and bone graft applied solidly on the concave half of the disc space to provide a normal height as if the disc had been left intact. This still allows the convex side of the disc to compress. It is critical that the sagittal profile be controlled by the amount of bone graft, because the rod will be applied only in compression.

Once the bone grafting has been completed, the rod is inserted such that the sagittal alignment is established and the first two proximal nuts are tightened. It is important to remember to straighten out the operating table if it has been bent to facilitate the thoracotomy and disc exposure. In addition, it helps to have the anesthesiologist remove the axillary roll and pull on the lower arm at the axillary level on the concave side of the curve to facilitate correction of the curvature. With the rod inserted, a cantilever force is applied distally and the remaining nuts are inserted.

Final correction is obtained by compressing each screw toward the apex. Not all of the correction need be obtained in the first pass; it should be done slowly and incrementally.

VARIATIONS OF THORACIC INSTRUMENTATION
Flexible Rod Systems

The Zielke 3.2-mm rod and the Harms-MOSS 3.2- and 4-mm threaded rods have been used for correction of anterior scoliosis.[7,38] Harms et al.[39] reported that the flexible rod works well for controlled correction of the thoracic hypokyphosis and for more controlled correction with severe deformity of the thoracic spine. These flexible rods correct through controlled compression, in contrast to the single solid rods, which correct mainly through cantilever forces. The flexible rods theoretically have less chance to pull out than do the solid rods. However, the major problem with flexible rods is breakage, reported to occur at a rate of 31% in one series[7] and of 11% in another.[39] Despite these rates, the majority of the patients were asymptomatic with no loss of correction and no pain.

Various Rod Systems

Solid rod systems that are known to work in the thoracic spine include the 4- and 5-mm MOSS-Miami, CD Legacy, Horizon, the M-8 system, and ISOLA. Some of the systems are made from titanium alloy, and others are made from stainless steel. With regard to the 4- and 5-mm MOSS-Miami rods in stainless steel, rod breakage has been rare (2%) in the authors' experience with the Harms Study Group. There have been more broken rods with the 5-mm rods than with the 4-mm rods. It is theorized that there is settling of bone graft and that the 4-mm rod may allow the spine to collapse slightly and then go on to heal and that the 5-mm rod may be too stiff, preventing the spine from setting when the bone resorbs. The spine then develops a pseudarthrosis and the rod breaks. Longer-term results with titanium regarding optimal rod diameter and stiffness are not yet available.

Authors have reported on the use of dual-rod anterior instrumentation for thoracic scoliosis. Most recently, Kaneda et al.[44] reported excellent coronal and sagittal correction with their dual-rod system in 20 patients. They also demonstrated the value of rib head resection for axial plane correction. They reported 15% correction with compression alone and 58% correction with resection of the rib head followed by compression.

Thoracoscopic Technique

Once it has been decided that an anterior approach may be of benefit, a minimally invasive option for the approach may be considered. Dickman and Mican[22] compared costs of open versus thoracoscopic surgery and showed the length of stay in the intensive care unit with open procedures to be one third, the hospital stay to be one half, and the need for narcotic medication to be one half of that with thoracoscopy, but this study looked at one-level discectomy or corpectomy proce-

> ## THORACOSCOPIC TECHNIQUE
>
> When an anterior thoracic approach is deemed beneficial, consider a minimally invasive approach.

dures only. Newton et al.[62] compared open anterior release and fusion with thoracoscopic anterior release and fusion for deformity and showed no difference in length of stay but higher costs with the thoracoscopic procedure. Most surgeons still believe that the advantages of the thoracoscopic procedure include muscle sparing, less reduction in pulmonary function, and improved cosmesis, but these have yet to be proved.

A question that arises in use of the thoracoscopic approach for anterior release and fusion is whether adequate spine flexibility can be obtained. Wall et al.[80] looked at biomechanical flexibility obtained after thoracoscopic and open discectomy in swine and found it to be comparable; similar results were obtained in a goat model by Newton et al.[63] A clinical study that compared thoracoscopic release with open release was conducted by Newton et al.[62] in a small series of 10 patients in each group. This study showed no statistically significant difference in the amount of correction obtained via posterior instrumentation when the anterior release was done either open or thoracoscopically. A clinical study by Durrani et al.[27] showed no difference in humans.

The next question that arises is whether adequate disc annulus and end plate can be removed to create a good bed for fusion with thoracoscopic techniques. Bunnell[11] reported that more than 50% of the disc end plate had to be resected to obtain an adequate anterior spinal fusion (ASF). Huntington et al.[42] compared open versus thoracoscopic discectomies in a sheep model and found no statistically significant difference in the amount of end plate resected between the two approaches. In addition, they found no statistical difference in the number of discs that had 50% of their end plate resected. The Durrani study[27] again showed no difference in humans.

There are several variations of thoracoscopic instrument insertion. The Clements/Newton/Betz technique includes making two or three portals anterolaterally to perform annular release, disc removal, end plate obliteration, fusion, and thoracoplasty when needed. After this, additional portals are made in the posteroaxillary line perpendicular to the vertebral bodies for the placement of vertebral body screws. These screws are inserted for bicortical purchase and are visualized on the undersurface through the anterior portals. Intraoperative fluoroscopy use is minimal, and no cannulated guide pins are needed. After screw placement, the rod is inserted and correction is obtained through cantilever forces and through compression applied to the screws. The average operating room time for endoscopically instrumented cases is 5 to 7 hours, most of which is needed for meticulous discectomy, grafting, and thoracoplasty. The instrumentation component of the technique takes 1.5 to 2 hours.

In contrast, another method being developed for thoracoscopic technique is that of Picetti et al.,[66] who use only posterolateral portals for both the discectomy approach and insertion of the instrumentation. They also use a guide pin and cannulated screws and require intraoperative radiographic imaging. Extremely careful attention to the guide pin position is required. A case report of a tension pneumothorax on the contralateral chest secondary to guide pin migration has been reported.*

Results and Complications of Anterior Instrumentation for Thoracic Adolescent Idiopathic Scoliosis

Harms et al.[39] reported the results of 101 patients who underwent anterior instrumentation for thoracic scoliosis using the Harms-MOSS system. The average frontal correction was 73% (range, 32% to 100%), and the sagittal plane improved from an average of 10.9 degrees of hypokyphosis to a normal kyphosis averaging 27.9 degrees postoperatively. Spontaneous correction of the lumbar curve averaged 14.7 degrees (range, 0 to 47 degrees), and spontaneous correction of the upper thoracic curve averaged 16.2 degrees (range, 0 to 47 degrees). The rod fractured in 11 cases (11%), however, 4 of the 11 were associated with pseudarthrosis and only 3 of the 4 required revision surgery (3% of the total). They also reported a 22% incidence of proximal screw pull-out.

Betz et al.[7] reported the results of a comparison of 78 patients after anterior spinal arthrodesis with instrumentation with the Harms threaded rod versus 100 patients after posterior arthrodesis with multisegmented hook-rod systems. The average coronal correction of the main thoracic curve was 58% in the anterior group and 59% in the posterior group ($p = .92$). Analysis of sagittal contour showed that the posterior systems failed to correct a preoperative hypokyphosis (sagittal T5 to T12 <20 degrees) in 60% of cases, whereas 81% were normal postoperatively with anterior instrumentation. However, hyperkyphosis (sagittal T5 to T12 >40 degrees) occurred postoperatively in 40% of the anterior group when the preoperative kyphosis was greater than 20 degrees. Coronal balance was equal in both groups. An average of 2.5 (range, 0 to 6) distal fusion levels were saved using the anterior spinal instrumentation with variation depending on criteria used to determine posterior fusion levels. Selective fusion of the thoracic curve was performed in 76 of 78 patients (97%) of the anterior group compared with only 18 of 100 (18%) of the posterior group. Although these results were very supportive of the anterior instrumentation, there were problems with the 3.2-mm flexible rod that was used. With anterior instrumentation, a surgically confirmed pseudarthrosis occurred in 4 of 78 patients (5%), loss of correction greater than 10° occurred in 18 of 78 patients (23%), and breakage of the solid rod occurred in 24 of 78 patients (31%). Although the majority of patients with a broken rod were asymptomatic, the authors now advise the use of a 4.0-mm solid rod to eliminate this problem.

---

*A. Crawford, Personal communication.

Sweet et al.[77] recently reported a study of 89 patients who underwent a single solid rod ASF with a minimum 2-year follow-up (range, 2 to 6 years). The average coronal correction of thoracic curves was from 55 to 29 degrees (47%). The average correction of thoracolumbar/lumbar curves was from 50 to 15 degrees (70%). In the sagittal plane, kyphosis was improved in thoracic fusions from 24 to 30 degrees (T5 to T12) and lordosis maintained in thoracolumbar/lumbar fusions at −63 degrees (T12 to sacrum). Five patients (5.5%) developed a pseudarthrosis, four with implant failure. Three of the five required a posterior fusion, for a reoperation rate of 3.3%. The fourth and fifth patients were asymptomatic and appeared fused at 2-year follow-up with minimal loss of correction. Common risk factors for pseudarthrosis were smoking (four of five), weight greater than 70 kg (four of five), and, for thoracic pseudarthrosis, hyperkyphosis greater than 40 degrees T5 to T12 (two of three).

Commonly asked questions concerning selected fusion of the thoracic curve with anterior instrumentation include whether the spontaneous correction of the lumbar curve will continue to hold up over time and whether it is any better than selected posterior instrumentation. In a study by Lenke et al.,[50] not only did the lumbar curve spontaneously reduce predictably, but this correction either stayed improved or, on occasion, continued to improve during a 2-year follow-up. Although this similar pattern occurred in the posterior (control) group, the amounts of correction obtained were dramatically different. Overall, for thoracic curvatures instrumented selectively with ASF, they obtained 58% correction and the lumbar curve spontaneously corrected 56% at 2-year follow-up. In the posterior group, only 38% correction was obtained in the thoracic curve and, likewise, spontaneous correction of the lumbar curve was only 37%. This was found to be even more significant in the King II double major curves (Lenke et al. type 1C), where the mean thoracic curves were 65 degrees in the anterior group and 67 degrees in the posterior group. The mean residual curve was 27 degrees in the anterior group and 49 degrees in the posterior group, with percent corrections of 59% and 27%, respectively. Similarly, the residual lumbar curves at 2-year follow-up were only 21 degrees in the anterior group versus 37 degrees in the posterior group (50% and 30% correction, respectively).

Skeletal immaturity is an indication for anterior instrumentation to prevent crankshaft. The Harms Study Group noted a very large degree of hyperkyphosis in these immature patients at 2-year follow-up, with more than 70% of the patients having kyphosis greater than 40 degrees from T5 to T12. Recently, D'Andrea et al.[21] reported the phenomenon of progressive sagittal kyphosis after ASF in an immature patient. They showed that in patients at Risser stage 0 who underwent ASF, 60% developed kyphosis greater than 40 degrees compared with only 27% of patients operated on at Risser stages 1 to 4. The patients who progressed after the ASF did so an average of 15 degrees. Therefore, when performing ASF on immature patients, several members of the Harms Study Group currently advise reducing the residual kyphosis at the time of surgery through the use of structural interbody grafts, anticipating a 15-degree progression of sagittal deformity as the patient matures. The exact etiology of this progressive sagittal kyphosis is unclear. D'Andrea et al.[21] speculate that it may be due to overgrowth of the posterior elements with a solid ASF.

Graham et al.[34] observed 44 patients with thoracic AIS (average age 15 years) who had pulmonary function tests to evaluate volume (forced vital capacity), flow (forced expiratory volume in 1 second), and total lung capacity evaluated after thoracic anterior instrumentation. The results show a significant decline in pulmonary function test absolute values at 3 months postoperatively with continued improvement to baseline, with no statistical difference between preoperative values and those measured at 2 years postoperatively. These results are identical to those of posterior spinal fusion with thoracoplasty and raise the question of whether the temporary effect is secondary to the thoracoplasty associated with the ASF.

Results of Thoracoscopic Approach Versus Open Thoracotomy

In a study by Betz et al.,[8] 30 patients had anterior instrumentation inserted thoracoscopically. The average age at surgery was 14 years, and the average preoperative curve was 50 degrees. Follow-up ranged from 2 to 30 months. These patients were randomly matched with 30 patients who underwent open thoracotomy for insertion of anterior instrumentation by age, curve degree, and curve types according to Lenke et al.[51] Average age at surgery in this group was 14 years, and average preoperative curve was 48 degrees. Follow-up ranged from 11 to 26 months. Both thoracoscopic and open techniques included partial rib resection for thoracoplasty. All patients, whether the spine was exposed through open thoracotomy or by thoracoscopic technique, were similarly treated with rib resection for thoracoplasty and with a MOSS-Miami 4-mm solid rod. In the thoracoscopic versus open groups, results were as follows: coronal correction was 67% versus 65%. One patient's plumb line was out of balance (>2 cm) in both groups, and one patient in each group had more than 10 degrees of shoulder asymmetry. Sagittal measurement (T5 to T12) was 24 degrees preoperatively to 22 degrees postoperatively in the thoracoscopic group versus 21 degrees preoperatively to 27 degrees postoperatively in the open group. Estimated blood loss was 1028 ± 363 versus 484 ± 170 ml. Average operative time was 7 versus 4.5 hours. One patient in the thoracoscopic group had residual pleural effusion, and two patients in the open group had recurrent pneumothorax after the chest tube was discontinued. Two patients in the thoracoscopic group had a delayed peroneal palsy that was not detected until 24 hours postoperatively and completely resolved within 4 weeks. This was thought to be secondary to the prolonged operative time with the weight of the upper leg on the lower leg, which sustained the peroneal palsy. Rod breakage occurred early in the series, before better support of the anterior spinal column was achieved with better bone graft techniques and before the development of custom cages for thoracoscopic use.

Neuromuscular Scoliosis: Surgical Treatment

Lawrence G. Lenke, Randal R. Betz

A vast array of disorders fall into the category of neuromuscular.[2,7] However, they consist primarily of two main types of disorders: neurologic and muscular, which refer to their primary etiology (Box 46-1). They all result in disturbances in the musculoskeletal system, because of either altered innervation to the muscular system or lack of appropriate muscle tone and mass. Because of the importance of the musculoskeletal system in controlling the alignment and function of the spinal column, these disorders inherently alter the spinal column that has diminished supportive properties. Patients with neuromuscular disorders are commonly afflicted with spinal deformities such as scoliosis and kyphosis. They also can have global, coronal, and/or sagittal imbalance of the spinal column and pelvis that renders ambulation and/or sitting balance problematic.

Primary neurologic disorders that fall under the category of neuromuscular disease states include cerebral palsy, spina bifida, postpolio syndrome, and spinocerebellar syndromes, among others.[6,12] They can be categorized into upper versus lower motor neuron lesions. The prototypical upper motor neuron neurologic disorder is cerebral palsy, which is a static encephalopathy. Most commonly, it is caused by anoxic brain injury perinatally. It also can be caused by other disease entities in infants and children, such as various forms of asphyxiation and severe allergic reactions. These entities can produce a broad spectrum of disability ranging from a slight heel contracture that produces mild toe walking to a severely

---

Box 46-1 Neuromuscular Scoliosis

A. Neuropathic
  1. Upper motor neuron lesion
     a. Cerebral palsy
     b. Spinocerebellar degeneration
        i. Friedreich's
        ii. Charcot-Marie-Tooth
        iii. Roussy-Lévy
     c. Syringomyelia
     d. Spinal cord tumor
     e. Spinal cord trauma
     f. Other
  2. Lower motor neuron lesion
     a. Poliomyelitis
     b. Other viral myelitides
     c. Traumatic
     d. Spinal muscular atrophy
        i. Werdnig-Hoffmann
        ii. Kugelberg-Welander
        iii. Letterer-Siwe
  3. Dysautonomia (Riley-Day)
  4. Other
B. Myopathic
  1. Arthrogryposis
  2. Muscular dystrophy
     a. Duchenne's (pseudohypertrophic)
     b. Limb-girdle
     c. Facioscapulohumeral
  3. Fiber-type disproportion
  4. Congenital hypotonia
  5. Myotonia dystrophica
  6. Other

NEUROMUSCULAR DISORDERS

- Neurologic
  - Upper motor neuron
    - Cerebral palsy resulting in broad range of disability (spastic)
    - Spine cerebellar degeneration, including Friedreich's ataxia, Charcot-Marie-Tooth syndrome, and Roussy-Lévy
    - Pediatric spinal cord injury
    - Syringomyelia and spinal cord tumors
  - Lower motor neuron
    - Postpolio syndrome
    - Spina bifida
    - Spinal muscular atrophy
      - Type 1: Werdnig-Hoffmann
      - Type 2: Kugelberg-Welander
      - Type 3: Letterer-Siwe
  - Muscular
    - Duchenne's muscular dystrophy (flaccid)
    - Limb-girdle dystrophy
    - Facioscapulohumeral dystrophy
    - Arthropyosis, congenital myopathy, myotonic dystrophy, and Pierre-Robin syndrome

involved pentaplegic patient who has involvement not only of all four extremities but also of the cerebral cortex.

A group of syndromes called *spinocerebellar degeneration* also produces spinal deformities due to the altered muscular control of the spinal column. Three of the more common types of spinocerebellar degeneration are Friedreich's ataxia, Charcot-Marie-Tooth syndrome, and Roussy-Lévy. Friedreich's ataxia drastically alters balance and equilibrium of the entire body, including the spinal column. Charcot-Marie-Tooth is a debilitating disorder in which peripheral nerves do not function properly, producing musculoskeletal abnormalities such as cavus feet and scoliosis.

Pediatric spinal cord injury is another common cause of upper motor neuron neuromuscular scoliosis disorders. It is known that each child who becomes acutely paraplegic or quadriplegic before skeletal maturity develops a neuromuscular scoliosis that may interfere with wheelchair ambulation. Entities such a syringomyelia and spinal cord tumors can obviously cause upper motor neuron pathology, leading to neuromuscular scoliosis.

There are a variety of lower motor neuron lesions that produce neuromuscular scoliosis. Postpolio syndrome is an infrequently seen cause of neuromuscular spinal deformity, with its incidence decreasing drastically since the preventive polio vaccine. Spina bifida has many different forms, from quite benign incomplete posterior S1 arch formation to full-blown myelomeningocele with a thoracic level paraplegia. Certainly the degree of spinal bifida involvement correlates with the anatomic location and the propensity to develop spinal deformities. Various forms of spinal muscular atrophy also produce neuromuscular spinal deformities in patients, with forms that survive into childhood and young adulthood.[5] Type 1 is called Werding-Hoffman, which is usually severe and may be lethal at a young age. Type 2 is called Kugelberg-Wellander and are more benign, with patients living into the teenage years. Type 3 is called Letterer-Siwe and is noted in patients who can live into adult life with less severe involvement.

The prototypical muscular disorders are the muscular dystrophies; these include Duchenne's muscular dystrophy, limb-girdle, and facioscapulohumeral dystrophy.[15-17] All of these cause global weakness to the trunk and extremities, with Duchenne's being progressive, ultimately resulting in death as a teenager or young adult.

Other rare causes of muscular disorders that present with neuromuscular spinal deformities include entities such as arthropyosis, congenital myopathy, myotonic dystrophy, and Pierre-Robin syndrome.

In addition, most neuromuscular disorders can be categorized into those that have spastic versus flaccid spinal deformities. A classic spastic type of neuromuscular disorder is cerebral palsy, whereas the classic flaccid neuromuscular disorder is Duchenne's muscular dystrophy. Surgical treatment of spinal deformities associated with neuromuscular disorders are tailored to the amount of spasticity versus flaccidity displayed by the patient. Another important distinction of these neuromuscular

patients are whether they are ambulatory or nonambulatory. In general, ambulatory patients will not require instrumentation and fusion to the pelvis for their spinal deformities, whereas the nonambulatory patients will require this.[14,21] It is also important in these patients to ascertain their level of mental functioning. Many of these patients have normal mentation and cognitive abilities, such as those with spina bifida and postpolio syndrome. Others, however, have their mental capacities altered by their diseased state, including the most severe forms of pentaplegic cerebral palsy, in which patients may be completely unaware of their surroundings and incapable of interacting with their environment. All of these issues are extremely important to determine before entertaining corrective spinal deformity surgery if indicated for these neuromuscular patients.

INDICATIONS FOR SURGERY

Neuromuscular patients present to the spinal deformity surgeon because of increasing pain, standing or sitting imbalance, or body distortion due to their spinal deformity.[3,4] A history must be obtained from the patient and/or parent/caregiver with regard to the limitations and/or problems encountered by the patient. It is important to try to elucidate any pain symptoms, because this is, in our experience, a frequent but underemphasized area of concern for these patients. Any history regarding gait abnormalities in ambulatory patients and/or sitting problems for those who are nonambulatory is important to investigate. It is quite common for nonambulatory patients to have to prop themselves up with their upper extremities as their spinal deformity progresses. This limits the functional freedom that they have because all four of their extremities become useless for activities of daily living in this scenario. The use of orthotics in neuromuscular patients may help delay the progression of deformity but does not alter the natural history of those patients destined to progress in their deformity.[7,13]

SURGICAL OPTIONS FOR AMBULATORY PATIENTS

- Fusion rate is inherently lower for neuromuscular patients.
  - There is increased stress on the instrumentation, especially in patients with spasticity.
- Do not stop instrumentation constructs short, because neuromuscular patients are less able than are idiopathic patients to accommodate scoliosis correction in the unfused spine above and below.
- Consider anterior spinal fusion before posterior instrumentation.
  - The curve magnitude is large (>80 degrees measurement).
  - After anterior release fusion, definitive posterior instrumentation and fusion can be performed on the same day, after 1 week, or later.
- Intervening halo gravity traction may be indicated in severe kyphotic or scoliotic deformities.

SURGICAL OPTIONS FOR AMBULATORY PATIENTS

Certainly a variety of patients with neuromuscular disorders are fully ambulatory with an associated progressive spinal deformity. These patients usually have a level pelvis, so the goal is to seek correction and fusion of the spinal deformity while stopping short of the pelvis. In a scoliosis deformity, the goals are to provide secure segmental fixation from neutral vertebrae proximally to a true stable vertebral distally. Secure implants should be placed with a combination of screws, hooks, and/or wires to provide not only correction but also a stable construct[9] (Figure 46-1). The fusion rate for neuromuscular patients is inherently lower than for idiopathic patients, because increased stress will be placed on the instrumentation until the fusion becomes solid, especially in patients with spasticity.

The use of pedicle screws in the lumbar spine has been commonplace for quite some time, with hooks and/or wires used in the thoracic spine. More recently, the use of screws extending up into the thoracic spine has been more commonly performed. This has usually resulted in less bracing postoperatively because of the extremely secure fixation provided by these multiscrew constructs (Figure 46-2). It is extremely important not to "cheat" short on the fusion levels, especially distally. Neuromuscular patients do not have the same balance, spatial perception, and connective tissues to allow the unfused spine above and below to accommodate the type of scoliosis correction used for idiopathic patients. This is also true proximally, where junctional kyphosis is a common problem if the instrumentation construct is stopped too short (below T3 or T4) posteriorly.[23]

Often anterior and posterior fusions are required in neuromuscular patients who undergo fusion short of the pelvis. Indications for considering an anterior spinal fusion before posterior instrumentation and fusion include the following:

- Large curve magnitude (greater than 80 degrees Cobb measurement)
- Regional hyperkyphosis in the thoracic (≥+50 degrees), thoracolumbar, or lumbar (≥20 degrees) spine

Certainly coronal and sagittal flexibility radiographs can be used to assess the mobility of these large coronal and/or sagittal malalignments. If an anterior procedure is considered, it can be performed either endoscopically or open.[1,19] With either approach, thorough annulectomies and discectomies should be performed with autogenous rib autograft used for fusion. It is quite common not to have enough autograft rib bone to fill every disc space being fused in these patients. Thus a combination of structural versus nonstructural allograft can be quite helpful for anterior fusions as well. Because of the common pulmonary restrictive disease found in neuromuscular patients, the open thoracotomy approach has been more commonly performed, because the lung will not necessarily need to be deflated, just packed off in the working areas. After the anterior release and fusion, the definitive posterior instrumentation and fusion can be performed on the same day or 1 week later or even at a more distant time point. Occasionally, intervening halo gravity traction may be indicated, especially in patients with severe kyphotic deformities or scoliotic deformities. In this case, the definitive instrumentation and fusion can be performed after maximum correction with the halo gravity traction. Definitive posterior instrumentation and fusion are performed in a manner similar to that listed earlier, with the distal fusion level being the true stable vertebra (Figure 46-3).

Rarely, an anterior-only instrumentation and fusion may be performed for a neuromuscular disorder. The patient will obviously have a single curve amenable to anterior-only instrumentation and fusion and vertebral bodies large and strong enough to hold anterior implants. Pulmonary function tests should be checked preoperatively for this approach to be considered. By and large, the vast majority of ambulatory neuromuscular patients will be treated for their spinal deformity by posterior instrumentation and fusion with or without an anterior fusion.[2,22]

SURGICAL OPTIONS FOR NONAMBULATORY PATIENTS

The vast majority of neuromuscular patients who require spinal deformity correction are nonambulatory.[7] These patients invariably have neuromuscular scoliosis with pelvic obliquity with or without sagittal plane malalignment. Regardless of the etiology, the most common surgery performed includes a posterior instrumentation and fusion from the upper thoracic spine into the sacropelvic unit (Figure 46-4). If the posterior instrumentation and fusion are begun at the thoracolumbar junction and extended to the sacrum, invariably a junctional kyphosis will develop in the thoracic spine that requires revision

Text continued on page 616

SURGICAL OPTIONS FOR NONAMBULATORY PATIENTS

- Most neuromuscular patients are nonambulatory.
  - Extend posterior instrumentation and fusion from the upper thoracic spine (T2 or T3) into the sacropelvic unit.
  - Combined anterior and posterior fusion is often required for severely spastic deformities (e.g., cerebral palsy).
  - Stopping short of the pelvis is not advocated in patients with spastic disorders but may be possible in patients with flaccid disorders who also have a limited life expectancy.
  - For flaccid deformities (e.g., Duchenne's muscular dystrophy), treatment may be a posterior-only procedure, even for severe scoliotic deformities.
    - Luque-Galveston technique with proximal hooks (vs wires) can avoid proximal midline ligament disruption, which may lend to a junctional kyphosis.
    - In smaller patients, consider sublaminar wires (even a Drummond button wire), avoiding disruption of the midline ligaments supraadjacent to the upper instrumented vertebra.

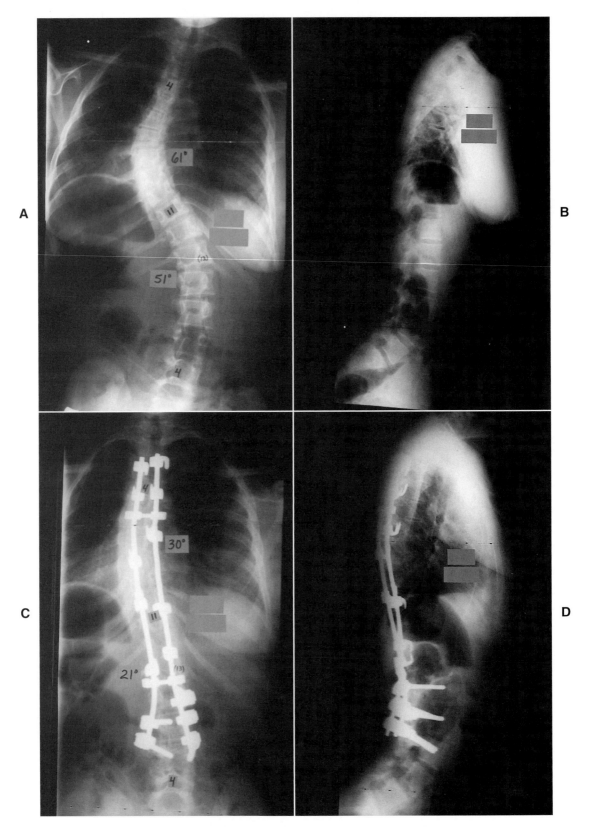

Figure 46-1. **A,** A 15-year and 1-month-old girl with diplegic cerebral palsy and a progressive double major scoliosis. **B,** The sagittal plane was unremarkable except for flattening of lower thoracic kyphosis and upper lumbar lordosis. **C,** The patient underwent a posterior instrumentation and fusion at T3 to L3 with segmental spinal instrumentation consisting of multiple hooks and distal pedicle screws. At 2 years after surgery, she has excellent coronal balance and curve correction is maintained. **D,** The sagittal plane shows slightly increased upper lumbar lordosis and overall good alignment.

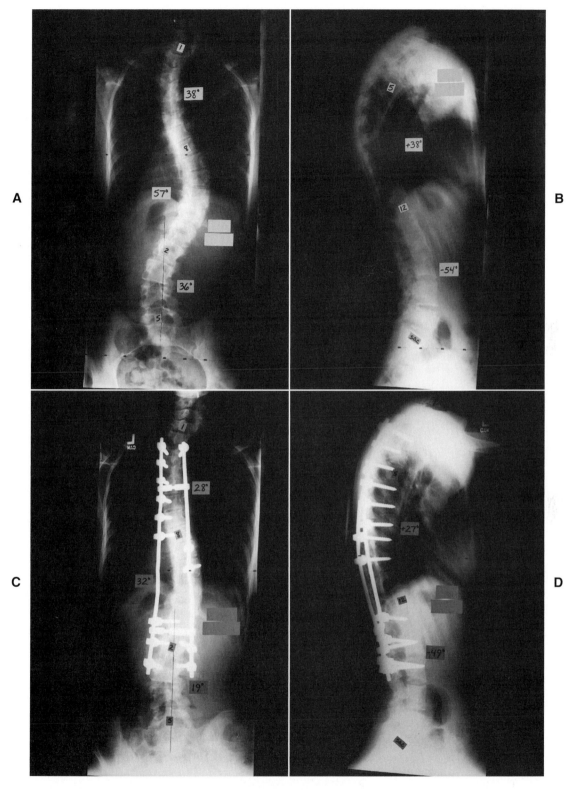

Figure 46-2.   **A,** A 16-year and 5-month-old girl with Friedreich's ataxia and a progressive double thoracic scoliosis. **B,** The sagittal plane showed 38 degrees of kyphosis at T5 to T12 and 54 degrees of lordosis from T12 to the sacrum. **C,** The patient underwent a posterior instrumentation and fusion at T3 to L3 with multilevel pedicle screw fixation. Her coronal alignment is shown with good positioning of the lowest instrumented vertebral L3. **D,** The lateral radiograph shows physiologic thoracic kyphosis and lumbar lordosis being maintained. No postoperative mobilization was used due to the strong fixation of multilevel screw placement.

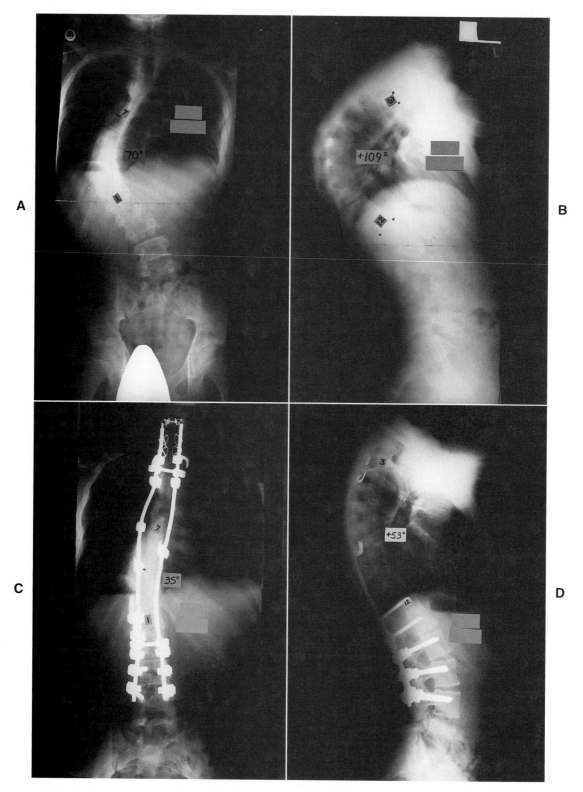

Figure 46-3.   A, A 15-year and 10-month-old boy who underwent surgical treatment for a low-grade astrocytoma in his mid and lower thoracic spine by a multilevel laminectomy. He presented to the scoliosis clinic with a 70-degree left thoracic curve. **B,** In the sagittal plane, the patient had a 109-degree postlaminectomy thoracic kyphosis at T3 to T12. He underwent a staged anterior open thoracotomy release and fusion, followed by halo gravity traction, and a posterior instrumentation and fusion several weeks later. **C,** The 3-year postoperative frontal radiograph shows 50% correction of the coronal scoliosis with good alignment of the spine. **D,** The 3-year postoperative lateral radiograph shows approximately 50-degree correction of the thoracic kyphosis with a solid anterior spinal fusion noted at T3 to T12.

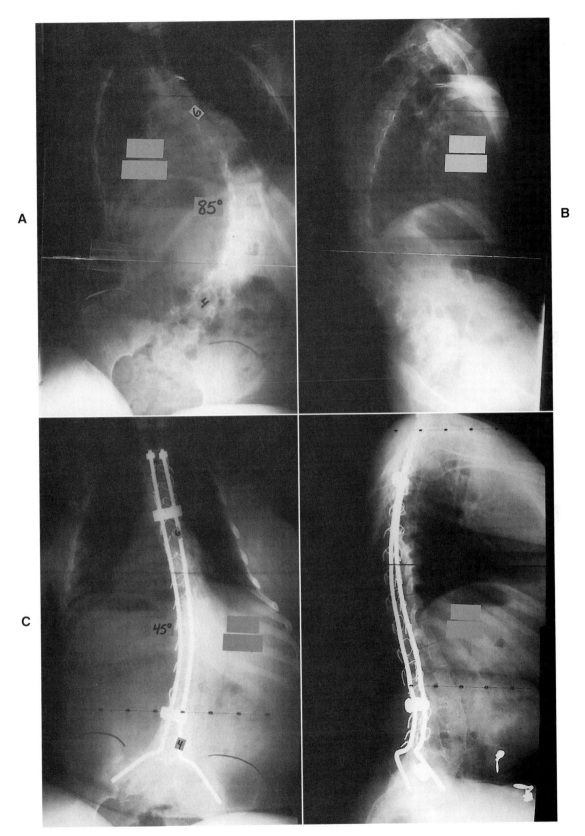

Figure 46-4.   An 8-year and 4-month-old girl with a spinal muscular atrophy. **A,** The patient presented with an 85-degree neuromuscular scoliosis and difficulty with sitting balance. **B,** The sagittal plane view showed a global kyphosis due to the poor muscle tone and posture. The patient underwent a posterior-only instrumentation and fusion from T2 to the sacrum with sublaminar wires and Galveston technique in her ilium. **C,** At 5 years after surgery, the patient has a stable spine over the pelvis with minimal pelvic obliquity. **D,** The 5-year postoperative lateral radiograph is unremarkable, showing good sitting sagittal alignment.

Continued

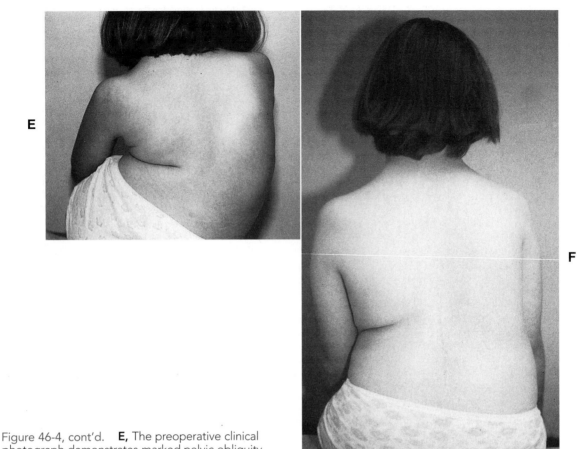

Figure 46-4, cont'd. **E,** The preoperative clinical photograph demonstrates marked pelvic obliquity and sitting imbalance. **F,** The 5-year postoperative clinical view demonstrates adequate sitting balance with ability to use the hands freely in space while sitting.

of the instrumentation up to the more proximal thoracic spine. Thus it is critical, even in the absence of a significant coronal and/or sagittal thoracic deformity, that the posterior instrumentation and fusion extend to the T2 or T3 level.

There is some thought that occasionally one can stop at L5 instead of fusing to the sacrum in nonambulatory patients with progressive neuromuscular scoliosis. We believe that this is not an appropriate option for patients with any type of spasticity because they may look well balanced soon after surgery but they will develop a progressive pelvic obliquity over time because of their spasticity. However, it may be possible to stop at L5 in some patients, especially in those with flaccid neuromuscular disorders such as Duchenne's muscular dystrophy, who also have a limited life expectancy.[7,10,16] However, we have limited experience with this and still recommend instrumentation and fusion posteriorly to the sacropelvic unit. Performance of the Galveston technique to the sacropelvic unit takes approximately 30 to 45 minutes of additional surgery time, with minimal additional blood loss. In addition, patients are at risk for the development of a significant pelvic obliquity at L5 that may interfere with appropriate sitting balance.

There are many other decisions to make in a non-ambulatory neuromuscular patient with significant neuromuscular scoliosis with pelvic obliquity that requires surgical treatment. Obviously, the type of neuromuscular disorder is important to assess. Specifically, patients who have a more spastic disorder (e.g., cerebral palsy) have a much more difficult deformity to treat than does a patient who has a more flaccid (e.g., Duchenne's muscular dystrophy) deformity. Thus, even with severe deformities, patients with a Duchenne's muscular dystrophy scoliosis are treated with a posterior-only procedure to avoid any diminution of their altered pulmonary function. Conversely, a severely spastic quadriplegic cerebral palsy patient often requires a combined anterior and posterior fusion with secure posterior instrumentation.[8] For the patient with a sagittal plane hyperlordosis, minimal bone should be packed into the disc spaces or, even occasionally, vertebral body osteotomies will have to be performed to effectively shorten the anterior column and to correct the hyperlordosis.

The simplest posterior construct for neuromuscular disorders is Luque's instrumentation with the Galveston technique of iliac fixation. The placement of sublaminar wires is a very inexpensive and secure way of segmental fixation. It certainly has stood the test of time.[13,14]

PLACEMENT OF GALVESTON ROD BENT INTO ILIUM

- Contour the proximal portion of rod to fit the spine before any implants are placed.
- Bend the concave rod somewhat straighter in the coronal plane.
- Next, place the concave rod (normally).
- Distract the two rods distally to fit the Galveston portion snugly into the ilium.
- Crosslink the rods both proximal and distal.
- Next, tighten the sublaminar wires on the concave side of the rod to translate the apex over to the midline.
- Firmly distract the rods apart so that on tightening of the apical wires, the spine is displaced to the rod (rather than the rod to the spine).

ANTERIOR PROCEDURES

- Anterior release and fusion
  - Beneficial for large structural deformities in the lumbar spine with severe pelvic obliquity
  - Secure fusion of all the lumbar levels; an anterior fusion of L5 to S1 has the best chance of fusing the lumbosacral junction
- Anterior instrumentation
  - Of possible benefit with single thoracolumbar/lumbar defect
  - May be of benefit where posterior spine is likely bifid, as in thoracolumbar/lumbar myelomeningocele scoliosis

In a similar fashion, creating Galveston bends in the distal rods and inserting them into the ilium at the posterior iliac spine, either intracortical or bicortical, is a tried and true method of providing sacropelvic fixation in long neuromuscular instrumentations to the pelvis. For flaccid neuromuscular disorders, the Luque-Galveston technique has been our main treatment construct. However, we have tended to use proximal hooks instead of wires to avoid proximal midline ligament disruption, which can produce a junctional kyphosis to the supraadjacent noninstrumented level (Figure 46-5). Some smaller patients will have excessively downsized posterior elements that will not allow hook fixation, and thus sublaminar wires with consideration even for a Drummond button wire at the very proximal level may be used. Again, this avoids disruption of the midline ligaments supraadjacent to the upper instrumented vertebra.[7] Another option is to place a unilateral sublaminar wire at the proximal level to avoid disruption of the contralateral facet capsule and ligaments.

The technical aspects of placing Galveston rod bends into the ilium is extremely important. We prefer to bend the Galveston portion to the rod first after preparation of the ilium bilaterally. The proximal portion of the rod is also contoured to fit the spine before the placement of any implants. This avoids retropulsing any sublaminar wires into the spinal canal when rods are being bent to fit directly onto the spine. Usually, the concave rod is bent somewhat straighter in the coronal plane to allow translational forces at the apex, which is better able to correct the deformity in the coronal plane. This involves the attachment of sublaminar wires and the placement of many proximal hooks. The concave rod is normally placed first into the ilium and then into the proximal implants. The contralateral rod is placed next. Before applying any apical translational forces, the two rods are distracted distally to fit the Galveston portion snugly into the ilium and cross-linked both proximal and distal. Next, the sublaminar wires are tightened on the concave rod to translate the apex over the midline. If the rods are not firmly distracted apart, the translational tightening of the apical wires tend to bring the rod to the spine

instead of bringing the spine to the rod. This also loosens the iliac fixation by pulling the Galveston bend of the rod out of the ilium medially, and it should be avoided. Another option is the use of a unit rod that connects two Luque rods simultaneously on the top. Although it may be difficult to insert the Galveston portion of the rods into both iliac crests simultaneously, it does provide the best control of pelvic obliquity, providing a stable platform to minimize imbalance.

For larger, more structural deformities in the lumbar spine with severe pelvic obliquity, especially in a skeletally immature patient, an anterior release and fusion can be extremely beneficial to mobilize the spine and provide an expeditious and solid circumferential fusion[8,11] (Figure 46-6). Normally, all convex levels in the lumbar spine down to the sacrum are fused. It is important to also attempt fusion for L5 to S1 anteriorly if at all possible. This provides the best chance of fusing the lumbosacral junction, which is inherently difficult to do with a posterior-only operation, especially in a spastic patient. Anteriorly, autogenous rib is normally placed within the disc for fusion. If more than four or five levels are being fused, one rib will not provide sufficient bone graft for these levels. Thus, a combination of allograft bone, structural and nonstructural, may be required. Demineralized bone matrix putty may also be used as a graft extender in these cases. The definitive posterior instrumentation and fusion procedure is usually performed on the same day as long as the blood loss has not been excessive, the patient is hemodynamically stable, and a motivated operating team is available.

Occasionally, the use of anterior instrumentation is beneficial. We find this to be most helpful in two situations: (1) with a single thoracolumbar/lumbar overhang curve where anterior instrumentation and fusion may be used as a sole correcting technique (Figure 46-7) and (2) in the face of thoracolumbar/lumbar myelomeningocele scoliosis deformities where the posterior spine is likely bifid and, thus, the best fixation of the spine will occur anteriorly in the vertebral bodies (Figure 46-8). In both of these situations, often smaller rod diameter instrumentation should be used because the vertebral bodies will be quite osteoporotic in these nonambulators. In patients with a high-level myelomeningocele who are instrumented and fused posteriorly, a flexible threaded

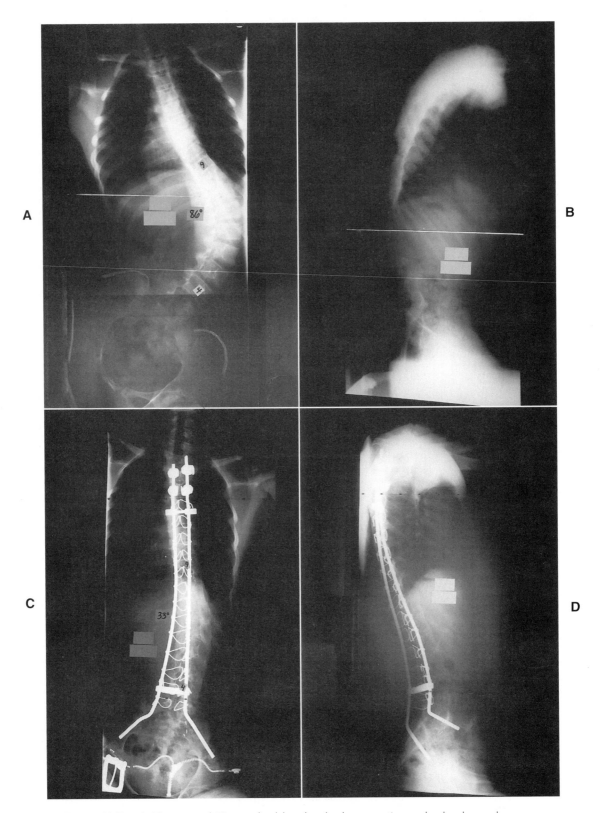

Figure 46-5. A 12-year and 10-month-old male who has spastic cerebral palsy and a neuromuscular scoliosis with pelvic obliquity. **A,** The frontal view shows an 86-degree thoracolumbar scoliosis with marked pelvic obliquity. **B,** The sagittal plane shows mild thoracolumbar kyphosis. The patient underwent a staged anterior and posterior fusion. The anterior fusion was from T10 to the sacrum, and the posterior fusion was from T3 to the sacrum. **C,** The 1-year postoperative frontal radiograph demonstrates excellent coronal balance with minimal pelvic obliquity. **D,** The 1-year postoperative lateral radiograph demonstrates excellent sagittal sitting alignment.

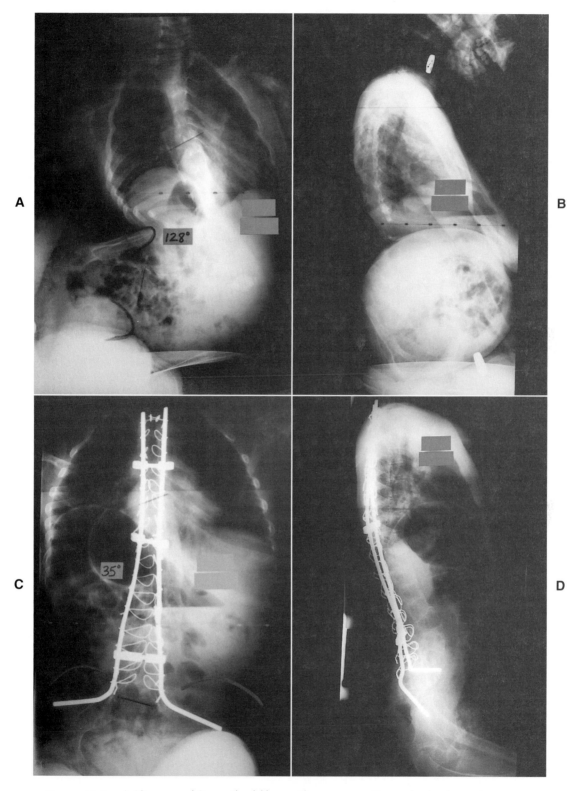

Figure 46-6.   A 13-year and 2-month-old boy with severe spastic cerebral palsy and a horrendous neuromuscular scoliosis. **A,** The frontal radiograph demonstrates a 128-degree scoliosis with a vertical pelvis. **B,** The sagittal plane is difficult to interpret because of marked three-dimensional deformity. The patient underwent a same-day anterior and posterior spinal fusion. He was anteriorly fused from T10 to the sacrum and posteriorly from T2 to the sacrum. He underwent intraoperative halo femoral traction in an attempt to balance the spine over the pelvis during the posterior procedure. **C,** The 2-year postoperative frontal radiograph demonstrates correction of the scoliosis to 35 degrees with a horizontal pelvis. **D,** The 2-year postoperative lateral radiograph demonstrates a solid thoracolumbar and lumbar spine fusion and good sagittal alignment.

Continued

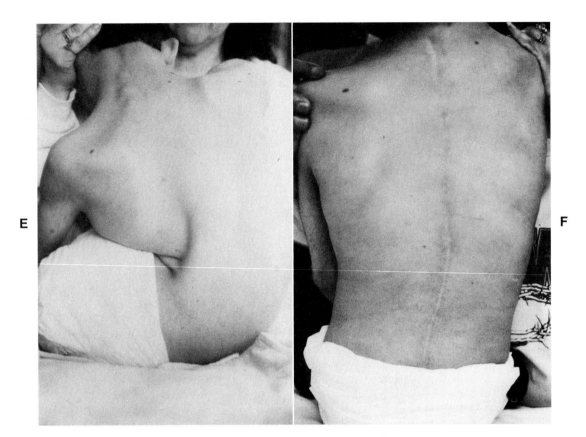

Figure 46-6, cont'd. **E,** The preoperative clinical photograph demonstrates marked sitting imbalance with body weight resting on the lower rib cage and right trochanteric region. **F,** The 2-year postoperative clinical photograph demonstrates the marked improvement in sitting balance.

rod is often quite beneficial when performing a careful anterior instrumented correction of the patient's thoracolumbar/lumbar scoliosis deformity. In patients with intact posterior columns, such as patients with cerebral palsy, we do not normally instrument the spine anteriorly, but we do recommend bilateral segmental fixation posteriorly in the thoracolumbar/lumbar spine with secure fixation to the sacropelvic unit.

Although sublaminar wires with Luque instrumentation and Galveston technique into the pelvis has traditionally been the gold standard for neuromuscular scoliosis, various modifications have been performed in the 1990s. First, as mentioned previously, the use of proximal hooks to avoid junctional kyphosis is now commonplace. The next alternative has been the use of iliac wing screws instead of Galveston rods for superior iliac wing fixation.[18] Iliac wing screws are all placed intracortical, with a diameter and length that the ilium will accommodate. Often, the ilium is quite dysplastic and fragile, and one must be very careful when placing screws and keeping them intracortical. A blunt gearshift and/or K wire can be placed down the pathway of the distal ilium, just proximal to the sciatic notch. Normally, this is where the cortical pathway provides the greatest diameter for screw placement. Usually a screw with a length of 50 to 70 mm and a diameter of 5.5 to 7.5 mm is placed. The advantage of the screws is that with the

appropriate multiaxial head or lateral connector, the more distal portion of the rod will not require a complex three-dimensional Galveston bend. It can also be kept quite vertical in the coronal plane, and just a sagittal plane bend can be performed to accommodate the lumbosacral junction into the ilium. This has been our preferred method of sacropelvic fixation for neuromuscular disorders during the past several years (Figure 46-9).

A very useful technique for obtaining a level pelvis with a balanced deformity is the use of intraoperative halo unilateral femoral traction. Halo and unilateral femoral traction pins are placed before the patient is positioned prone. A traction pin is placed in the femur unilateral to the high side iliac crest. Thus, with halo unilateral femoral traction, sufficient weight is placed on the femur to level the pelvis. The traction weight on the halo provides countertraction to resist the patient being pulled distally during the course of the operation. Approximately 10 to 20 pounds is placed on the halo and between 15 to 30 pounds is placed on the femur for correction of the pelvic obliquity (Figure 46-10). The goal is to have the pelvis level before the skin incision is made. Thus all of the implants are placed with the pelvis level, and less manipulation of the pelvis has to be performed because it is instrumented "in situ."

If the traction seems to be excessive, it can be temporarily removed during the exposure and replaced

Text continued on page 625

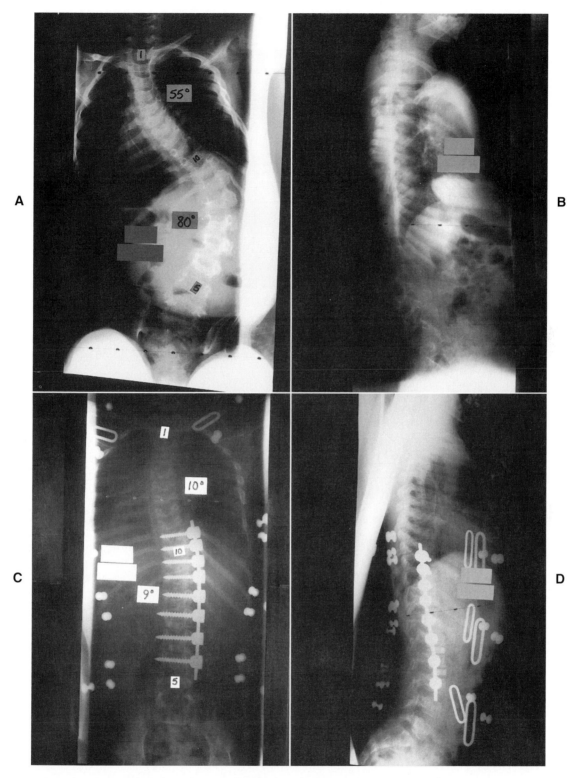

Figure 46-7.   A 10-year and 2-month-old boy with neuromuscular scoliosis from a high thoracic paralysis. **A,** The upright frontal radiograph demonstrates a 55-degree main thoracic scoliosis, which is compensatory to an 80-degree main lumbar scoliosis. The patient has mild pelvic obliquity and is nonambulatory. **B,** The sagittal plane is unremarkable and fairly straight. The patient underwent an anterior instrumentation and fusion with correction of the main curve in an attempt to allow the main thoracic curve above to compensate and to avoid fusion to the pelvis. **C,** Postoperative radiograph demonstrates marked correction of both the instrumented lumbar curve and spontaneous correction of the main thoracic curve. **D,** The sagittal plane gained in neutral alignment across the thoracolumbar and lumbar spine.

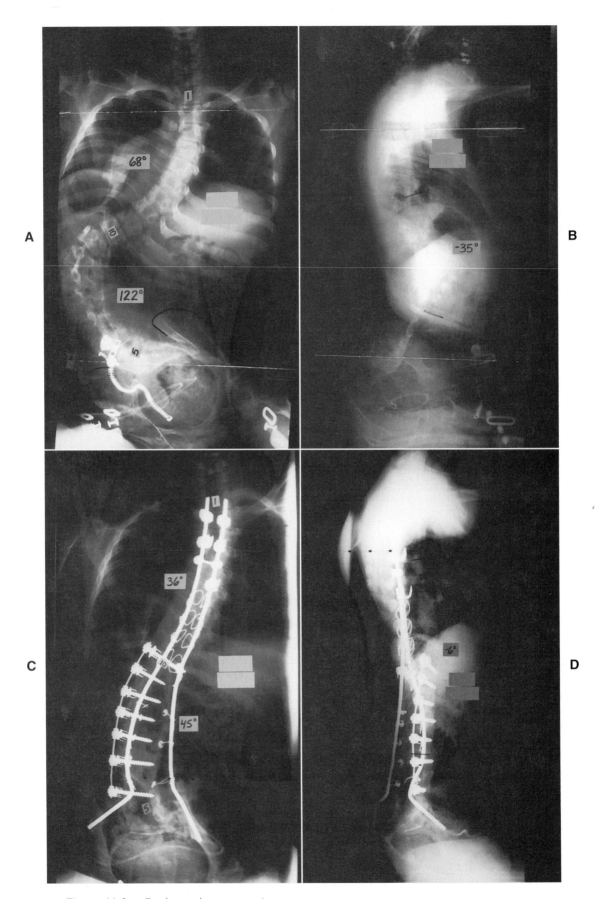

Figure 46-8. *For legend see opposite page.*

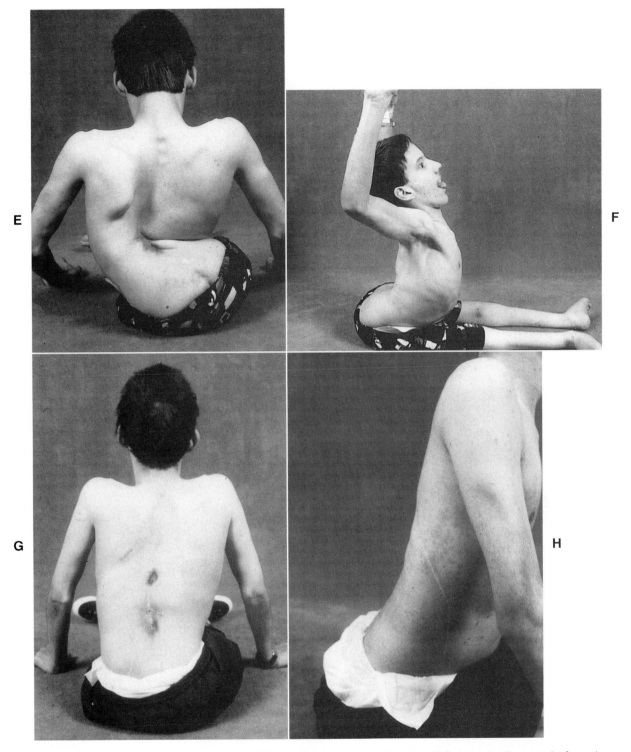

Figure 46-8.   A 16-year and 2-month-old male with a high-level myelomeningocele spinal deformity. **A,** The upright frontal radiograph demonstrates a 122-degree lumbar scoliosis with marked pelvis obliquity. The spine is bifid up to the T10 level. **B,** The sagittal plane shows a collapsing thoracolumbar lordotic deformity, which is difficult to visualize because of the three-dimensional malalignment. The patient underwent a staged anterior and posterior spinal fusion. First, through a left thoracoabdominal approach, he had anterior instrumentation and fusion at T10 to L4 and fusion alone from L4 to the sacrum. One week later, he underwent a posterior instrumentation from T2 to the sacrum with segmental fixation proximal and Galveston technique into the ilium bilaterally. **C,** The 2-year postoperative coronal radiograph demonstrates marked correction of the deformity with overall good balance and a fairly level pelvis. **D,** The 2-year postoperative lateral radiograph demonstrates a fairly straight spine with improved sitting balance. **E,** The preoperative clinical photograph demonstrates marked trunk shift and pelvic obliquity. **F,** The preoperative lateral photograph demonstrates marked collapsing spinal deformity of the spine onto the pelvis in a flexed position. **G,** The postoperative coronal clinical photograph demonstrates marked improvement in sitting balance. **H,** The postoperative lateral clinical photograph demonstrates improved trunk position on the pelvis.

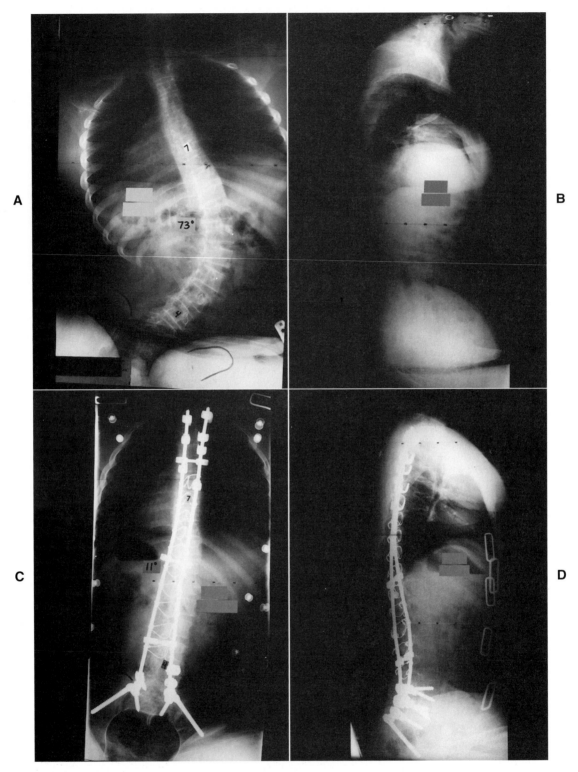

Figure 46-9.   A 15-year and 8-month-old boy with limb girdle muscular dystrophy who presented with a progressive thoracolumbar neuromuscular scoliosis. **A,** The upright frontal radiograph sitting demonstrates 73 degrees of scoliosis with marked pelvic obliquity. **B,** The sagittal plane radiograph shows a slight thoracolumbar kyphosis; otherwise, it is unremarkable. The patient underwent a single-staged posterior instrumentation and fusion from T2 to the sacrum using segmental fixation with hooks proximal, apical sublaminar wires, and pedicle screws distally. He had bilateral iliac wing screws used for sacral pelvic fixation. **C,** The postoperative frontal radiograph demonstrates marked correction of the patient's scoliosis and a level pelvis. **D,** The postoperative sagittal plane radiograph shows unremarkable sagittal alignment and good sitting balance.

MODIFICATIONS

- Iliac wing screws are an alternative to Galveston rods for superior iliac wing fixation: Intercortical screw placement 50 to 70 mm in length and 5.5 to 7.5 mm in diameter.
- Intraoperative halo and unilateral femoral traction can be used to obtain a level pelvis.
  - Place halo and pins before the patient is positioned prone.
  - Use traction pin in femur unilateral to the high-side iliac crest.
  - With approximately 10 to 20 pounds on the halo and 15 to 30 pounds on the femur, the pelvis can be made level before skin incision.
  - Spinal cord monitoring can be helpful to determine whether traction is excessive.
  - Remove halo and femoral pins at the end of the procedure.
- Halo gravity traction is used for coronal and/or sagittal plane deformities.
  - Use six- to eight-pin halo traction weight starting with 1 to 2 pounds and increase by 2 to 3 pounds per day up to 30% to 40% of body weight.
  - Perform frequent neurologic examinations with particular focus on cranial nerves VI, VII, and XII.
  - Obtain weekly lateral cervical spine radiographs to assess excessive distraction.

during the actual placement of the instrumentation. Spinal cord monitoring can be very helpful in this regard.[20] As soon as the instrumentation is complete, the traction weight is removed completely from the femur with approximately 5 pounds left on the halo to keep the head balanced. Another great advantage is that no pressure is placed on the prone face because all of the pressure rests on the halo pins (Figure 46-11). The halo and femoral traction pins are removed at the end of the procedure. Because the halo has been on for only a very short time, the pin tracks are not a long-term visible problem. In addition, because the patient is nonambulatory, in our experience, femur fractures have not developed from the temporary placement of the femoral traction pin. Obviously, this will not completely correct scoliotic curvatures normally, but the spine invariably assumes an acceptable coronal balance with a level pelvis that is the ultimate goal of neuromuscular scoliosis surgery. We have experience with this technique in more than 50 patients and have been quite pleased with the ability to obtain a level pelvis postoperatively.

We have also used halo gravity traction for neuromuscular patients with severe coronal and/or sagittal plane deformities (Figure 46-12). For the most part, patients who are candidates for preoperative halo gravity traction have a reasonably intact mental status so they can cooperate with the regimen. A six- to eight-pin halo is placed, and a graduated traction weight program is added, usually beginning with 1 to 2 pounds and increasing by 2 to 3 pounds per day up to 30% to 40% of body weight. Neurologic examinations, including a thorough cranial nerve examination (checking specifically for lateral rectus cranial nerve 6, hypoglossal cranial nerve 12, and facial cranial nerve 7 palsies), as well as weekly lateral cervical spine radiographs to assess for any excessive occipito-cervical or midcervical distraction are performed. The use of halo gravity traction is beneficial for several reasons. First, gradual correction of spinal deformity in either the coronal and/or sagittal planes may be performed. Because these patients are often quite osteoporotic, the use of correction with halo gravity traction is highly beneficial before the placement of posterior instrumentation. Second, patients benefit from improvement in their respiratory status. Increasing their chest wall diameter by optimizing their position allows for improved air movement and secretion mobilization. Simultaneous with the traction is the performance of daily respiratory therapy using intermittent positive pressure breathing, chest physiotherapy, and incentive spirometry if the patient is capable, as well as anteroposterior and lateral long cassette radiographs of the spine. The indications for the preoperative correction of spinal deformity with halo gravity traction include thoracic hyperkyphosis deformities and more proximally based severe scoliotic deformities rather than for those based more distal in the thoracic and lumbar spine, where vertical traction is less effective. Another alternative is halo-dependent traction with a CircOlectric bed.

The results of treatment of flaccid neuromuscular disorders are quite good. Most patients tend to heal readily even if only allograft bone is used.[4] In addition, their quality of life seems to be dramatically improved. Results for patients with spastic neuromuscular disorders are slightly inferior. Many of these patients have concomitant mental insufficiencies. In addition, their spasticity works against the instrumentation and subsequently makes fusion more difficult. Many of these patients need concomitant anterior as well as posterior procedures, which are usually performed on the same day. It is often helpful to consider perioperative hyperalimentation in these patients to decrease the wound and pulmonary complications that may occur. Although similar to the flaccid patients, successful clinical outcomes can be obtained with appropriate patient selection, meticulous surgical techniques, and preoperative and postoperative care.

Even though the same goals remain for the treatment of neuromuscular scoliosis patients, that being a solid arthrodesis with the head centered over the pelvis in both the coronal and sagittal planes, new techniques have provided much more rigid fixation to the spine to allow for rapid mobilization of the patient and improved patient outcomes.[4] Additional techniques such as those of halo gravity or halo-intraoperative traction can also be quite beneficial. Instrumentation constructs using secure posterior implants with strong fixation to the pelvis will decrease the pseudarthrosis rate. In addition, anterior fusions improve the fusion rate, especially in spastic neuromuscular patients and in those with fusion to the pelvis. Strict attention to detail and meticulous and efficient surgical techniques are necessary for the safe performance and ultimate success of neuromuscular scoliosis surgery.

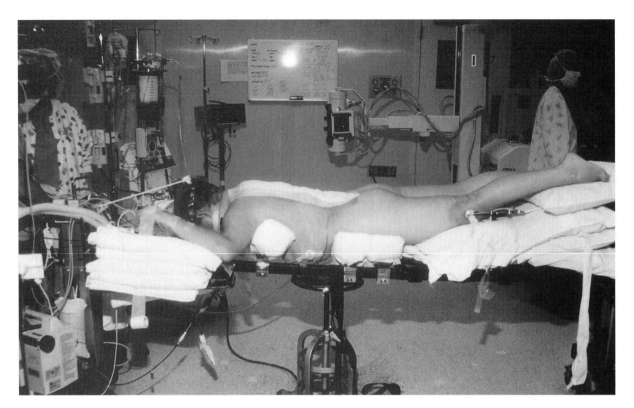

Figure 46-10.   The patient is in halo ipsilateral left femoral traction after staged anterior and posterior spinal fusion for neuromuscular scoliosis.

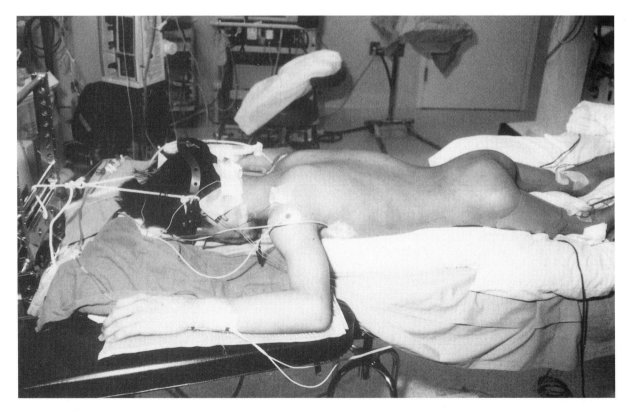

Figure 46-11.   A close-up view depicting halo femoral traction showing the free position of the face intraoperatively with all of the patient's weight of the skull resting on the halo pins.

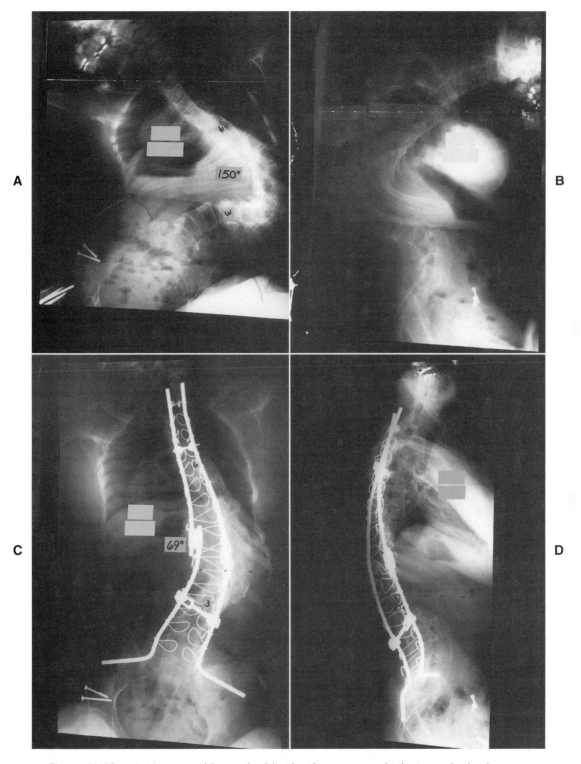

Figure 46-12.   A 14-year and 3-month-old girl with severe quadriplegic cerebral palsy and a severe spinal deformity. **A,** The upright frontal sitting radiograph demonstrates a 150-degree scoliosis with the apical spine abutting against the lateral chest wall. **B,** The lateral radiograph is difficult to interpret due to marked distortion from the spinal deformity. The patient underwent a staged anterior release, fusion, and posterior instrumentation and fusion separated by 6 weeks of halo gravity traction. Anteriorly, she was fused from T6 to the sacrum. Posteriorly, she had a fusion from T2 to the sacrum. **C,** At 3 years after surgery, the patient has marked correction of the deformity with good coronal balance and minimal pelvic obliquity. **D,** The 3-year-postoperative lateral radiograph demonstrates adequate sitting balance and a solid spinal fusion.

SELECTED REFERENCES

Bridwell KH et al.: Process measures and patient/parent evaluation of surgical management of spinal deformities in patients with progressive flaccid neuromuscular scoliosis (Duchenne's muscular dystrophy and spinal muscular atrophy), *Spine* 24:1300-1309, 1999.

Drummond DS: Neuromuscular scoliosis: recent concepts, *J Pediatr Orthop* 16:281-283, 1996.

Ferguson RL et al.: Same-day versus staged anterior posterior spinal surgery in a neuromuscular scoliosis population: the evaluation of medical complications, *J Pediatr Orthop* 16:293-303, 1996.

Granata C et al.: Long-term results of spine surgery in Duchenne muscular dystrophy, *Neuromusc Disord* 6:61-68, 1996.

REFERENCES

1. Arlet V: Anterior thorascopic spine release in deformity surgery: a meta-analysis and review, *Eur Spine J* 9(suppl)1:517-523, 2000.
2. Banta JV, Drummond DS, Ferguson RL: The treatment of neuromuscular scoliosis, *Instr Course Lect* 48:551-562, 1999.
3. Benson ER et al.: Results and morbidity in a consecutive series of patients undergoing spinal fusion for neuromuscular scoliosis, *Spine* 23:2308-2317, 1998.
4. Bridwell KH et al.: Process measures and patient/parent evaluation of surgical management of spinal deformities in patients with progressive flaccid neuromuscular scoliosis (Duchenne's muscular dystrophy and spinal muscular atrophy), *Spine* 24:1300-1309, 1999.
5. Carter GT et al.: Profiles of neuromuscular diseases. Spinal muscular atrophy, *Am J Phys Med Rehabil* 74(suppl 5):S150-S159, 1995.
6. Dias RC et al.: Surgical correction of spinal deformity using a unit rod in children with cerebral palsy, *J Pediatr Orthop* 16:734-740, 1996.
7. Drummond DS: Neuromuscular scoliosis: recent concepts, *J Pediatr Orthop* 16:281-283, 1996.
8. Ferguson RL et al.: Same-day versus staged anterior-posterior spinal surgery in a neuromuscular scoliosis population: the evaluation of medical complications, *J Pediatr Orthop* 16:293-303, 1996.
9. Girardi FP, Boachie-Adjei O, Rawlins BA: Safety of sublaminar wires with Isola instrumentation for the treatment of idiopathic scoliosis, *Spine* 25:691-695, 2000.
10. Granata C et al.: Long-term results of spine surgery in Duchenne muscular dystrophy, *Neuromusc Disord* 6:61-68, 1996.
11. Hamill CL et al.: Posterior arthrodesis in the skeletally immature patient: assessing the risk for crankshaft: is an open triradiate cartilage the answer? *Spine* 22:1343-1351, 1997.
12. Hart DA, McDonald CM: Spinal deformity in progressive neuromuscular disease: natural history and management, *Phys Med Rehabil Clin North Am* 9:213-232, 1998.
13. McCarthy RE: Management of neuromuscular scoliosis, *Orthop Clin North Am* 30:435-449, 1999.
14. McCarthy RE, Bruffett WL, McCullough FL: S rod fixation to the sacrum in patients with neuromuscular spinal deformities, *Clin Orthop* 364:26-31, 1999.
15. McDonald CM et al.: Profiles of neuromuscular diseases: Becker's muscular dystrophy, *Am J Phys Med Rehabil* 74(suppl 5):893-903, 1995.
16. McDonald CM et al.: Profiles of neuromuscular diseases: Duchenne muscular dystrophy, *Am J Phys Med Rehabil* 74(suppl 5):S70-S92, 1995.
17. McDonald CM et al.: Profiles of neuromuscular diseases: Limb-girdle syndromes, *Am J Phys Med Rehabil* 74(suppl 5):S117-S130, 1995.
18. Miladi LT et al.: Iliosacral screw fixation for pelvic obliquity in neuromuscular scoliosis: a long-term follow-up study, *Spine* 22:1722-1729, 1997.
19. Newton PO, Shea KG, Granlund KF: Defining the pediatric spinal thoracoscopy learning curve: sixty-five consecutive cases, *Spine* 25:1028-1035, 2000.
20. Owen JH et al.: Efficacy of multimodality spinal cord monitoring during surgery for neuromuscular scoliosis, *Spine* 20:1480-1488, 1995.
21. Widmann RF, Hresko MT, Hall JE: Lumbosacral fusion in children and adolescents using the modified sacral bar technique, *Clin Orthop* 364:85-91, 1999.
22. Yazici M, Asher MA: Freeze-dried allograft for posterior spinal fusion in patients with neuromuscular spinal deformities, *Spine* 22:1467-1471, 1997.
23. Yazici M, Asher MA, Hardacker JW: The safety and efficacy of Isola-Galveston instrumentation and arthrodesis in the treatment of neuromuscular spinal deformities, *J Bone Joint Surg Am* 82:524-543, 2000.

Congenital Intraspinal Abnormalities of the Cervical, Thoracic, Lumbar, and Sacral Spine

Lee M. Buono, Suken A. Shah,
Walter W. Frueh, Arjun Saxena,
Alexander R. Vaccaro

In this chapter, we review the most common congenital spinal dysraphisms, their presentation, and their treatment. Through an understanding of embryology and epidemiology, the treating physician can gain an understanding of the etiologic factors and approach to the treatment of these anomalies.

A wide range of congenital spine and spinal cord defects exist, but common to them all is an aberration in the embryogenesis of the neuropore and secondary effects on the adjacent mesenchymal structures. Although the lesion itself is localized to the spine, it may have far-reaching effects on the brain, appendicular skeleton, bowel, and bladder. Consequently, the approach to the care of the patient with a spinal dysraphism involves the expertise of the neurosurgeon, orthopedic surgeon, urologist, and rehabilitation medicine specialist.

CLASSIFICATION

The term *spinal dysraphism* is used to refer to the overall group of defects related to the abnormal development of the embryonic ectoderm, mesoderm, and neuroectoderm of the spine. *Myeloschisis* is a cleft that occurs in the spinal cord due to failure of the neural plate to form a neural tube. This term may also be used to describe rupture of the neural tube after closure. *Rachischisis* refers to a congenital fissure of the spinal column that may be limited (rachischisis partialis or merorachischisis), involve only the posterior elements (spina bifida), or may fatally involve the entire axis of the spine (rachischisis totalis or holorachischisis).

Spina bifida, which is a term that is often misused, is a developmental anomaly characterized by defective closure of the bony encasement of the spinal cord. This bony defect may involve protrusion of the meninges and/or neural elements and then is termed *spina bifida cystica*. Isolated bony defects without prolapse of such elements is termed *spina bifida occulta*. Clinical recognition of spina bifida occulta is often limited to incidental radiographic findings with or without cutaneous manifestations such as a tuft of coarse hair on a patient's posterior

CLASSIFICATION

- Spinal dysraphism: Abnormal embryonic development of the ectoderm, mesoderm, and neurectoderm
  - Myeloschisis: Spinal cord cleft secondary to failure of neural tube formation from neural plate
  - Rachischisis: Fissure of bony spinal column that may be limited or complete
  - Spina bifida cystica: Developmental defect characterized by incomplete closure of bony encasement of the spinal cord (pedicles, lamina, and spinous process) *with* protrusion of the meninges and/or neural elements
  - Spina bifida occulta: Developmental defect characterized by incomplete closure of the bony encasement of the spinal cord *without* protrusion of the meninges and/or neural elements
  - Occult spinal dysraphisms: Include other pathologic entities such as diastematomyelia, spinal lipoma, and neurenteric cysts
- Open versus closed neural tissue
  - Open lesions: Lack skin and soft tissue coverage
  - Closed lesions: Have skin and/or soft tissue coverage

trunk. Additional pathologic findings in spinal dys-raphism such as diastematomyelia, spinal lipomas, and neuroenteric cysts may be termed *occult spinal dysraphism.*

It is useful to divide these conditions based on whether the neural tissue is open or closed. The open lesions lack skin coverage of the defect and may have a component of myeloschisis, spina bifida, and exposure of the neural elements; the best example is a myelo-meningocele. Closed lesions may also have myelo-schisis or spina bifida but have no exposed elements. Conditions such as diastematomyelia, spinal lipoma, tight filum terminale, and dorsal dermal sinus can be classified as closed lesions.

EPIDEMIOLOGY

The incidence of myelomeningocele in North America has been reported to be approximately 1 to 1.5 per 1000 live births.[34] Geographic and ethnic variations have been reported; black and Asian populations have a lower inci-dence than do white ethnic groups. Overall, the inci-dence has been decreasing for the past 18 years.[71] In 1992, the Centers for Disease Control and Prevention studied the incidence of spina bifida in the United States and found the overall incidence to be 4.6 cases per 10,000 births. Furthermore, they reported the inci-dence was decreasing for the period of 1990 to 1993, and geographic and ethnic variations could not be found.[22]

Extensive searches for etiologic factors have only borne out that spina bifida has multifactorial causes. For the most part, attempts to implicate the maternal age, parity, infections, or the use of drugs have been incon-clusive.[37,65,67] However, maternal use of the anticonvul-sant valproic acid has been associated with neural tube defects.[15]

States of nutritional deficiency have been suspected as a cause for decades, but it was not verified until a large, randomized, controlled study by the British Medical Research Council showed that folic acid dietary supplements resulted in a 72% reduction in neural tube defects.[36] The U.S. Public Health Service now recom-mends that all women of childbearing age should consume 0.4 mg of folic acid per day to reduce the risk of a pregnancy with a neural tube defect.[14]

There is a tendency for spina bifida to recur in fami-lies, so genetics seems to play a role. The estimated risk of having a child with a neural tube defect is 0.1% to 0.2%. With one affected sibling, the risk of a second affected child increases to 2% to 5%, and the risk of a third affected child increases again to 10% to 15%.[23] The pattern of inheritance is unknown.

The occurrence of spina bifida occulta is much more common than the open neural tube defects. Reviews of spinal radiographs of patients without back complaints have shown 17% to 30% of asymptomatic individuals have spina bifida occulta, most commonly in the lum-bosacral region.[21] These defects have no clinical significance, but when associated with subtle neurologic findings or cutaneous malformations such as dimples, hairy patches, or hemangiomas, a thorough investiga-tion for a spinal dysraphism should be performed.

NORMAL EMBRYOLOGY

Spinal dysraphisms result from a malformation during the embryonic process, and a review of the normal process can aid in understanding the defects and the surgical anatomy that is important in treatment.

By day 17, the embryo is *trilaminar*, composed of an endoderm (adjacent to the yolk sac), ectoderm (adjacent to the amnion), and mesoderm (in-between). The endo-derm develops into the gut structures, the mesoderm into the skeleton and muscles, and the ectoderm into the skin and nervous system. As the mesoderm prolifer-ates, cells in the midline condense; this is called the *notochordal process.* The primitive pit deepens and extends through the notochordal process, forming a hollow tube. Along its ventral surface, the notochordal tube fuses with the endoderm, and portions of the endoderm undergo programmed cell death, causing a temporary communication of the yolk sac and amnion through the neurenteric canal. This is called *intercalation of the noto-chordal plate.* Then the notochordal plate re-forms into a cylinder, the notochord, and the endoderm reconsti-tutes. This is called *excalation of the notochord.*

Neurulation or neural tube, formation (Figure 47-1) begins with the development of the notochord. The ectoderm differentiates into the neural plate and enlarges and expands on each side of the developing neural groove. Simultaneously, the notochord induces paraxial mesoderm to condense and segregate into 42 to 44 paired segments called *somites* (Figure 47-2), which will ultimately form the vertebral bodies. The neural folds continue to grow and meet (fuse) in the midline. Closure of the neural tube progresses caudad and ros-trally as additional somites form. The final closure is at the level of the future L1 or L2 vertebral body. The lowest portion of the spinal cord forms via a separate process called canalization.

The superficial ectoderm separates from the neural tube and reconstitutes to form the future skin. The lateral mesenchyme migrates between the neural tube and ectoderm to form the meninges, neural arches, and paraspinal muscles.

The distal spinal cord forms after neurulation is com-plete. The caudal end of the neural tube and the rem-nants of the notochord form the caudal cell mass. Vacuoles form and coalesce in the caudal cell mass and then connect with the formed spinal cord rostrally. The most rostral end becomes the conus medullaris, and the

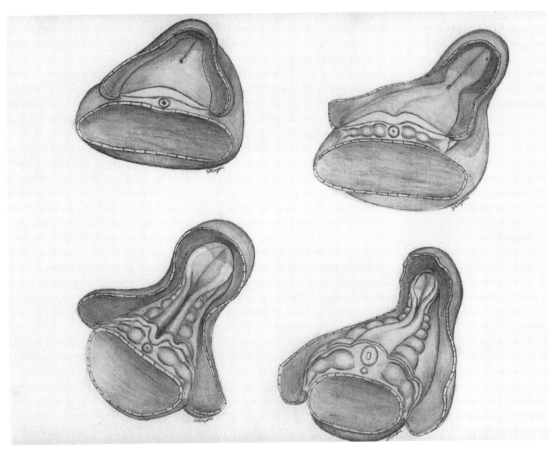

Figure 47-1. Neurulation with development of neural groove, notochord, and somites. *(Courtesy Dr. John Cooper.)*

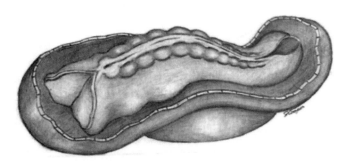

Figure 47-2. Closed neural tube displaying somites. *(Courtesy Dr. John Cooper.)*

remainder involutes to form the filum terminale (retrogressive differentiation). As the conus medullaris forms, it is located at the third coccygeal level.[49] Because the spinal column grows at a faster rate than the spinal cord, the conus apparently "ascends." This ascension occurs rapidly between 8 and 25 weeks, then comes to reside at L2 to L3 at birth, and then reaches the adult level of L1 to L2 in several months after birth.

SPINA BIFIDA CYSTICA

Most neurulation defects occur between 18 and 21 days' gestation.[38,44] Failure of fusion produces a variety of open defects through failure of disjunction of the neural and cutaneous ectoderm. Neurulation defects can be of three types: failure of neural tube closure, abnormal disjunction of the neural plate and ectoderm, or defective mesenchymal migration. The resulting anomalies have in common the absence of intact overlying skin. The risk is increased with a neural tube defect in a sibling or maternal folate deficiency.[18,64] Maternal serum alpha-1-fetoprotein (AFP) is commonly increased. This group of anomalies includes spina bifida aperta, meningocele, meningomyelocele, anencephaly, and cranioschisis. The most common type of neurulation defect is a myelomeningocele.

Meningocele

Spinal meningoceles are protrusions of dura and arachnoid though a bony defect in the spine (Figure 47-3). Although there may be other associated abnormalities, by definition, the neural elements do not permeate bony borders. As discussed earlier, the embryology and pathogenesis derive from a defective primary neurulation process. Accordingly, epithelialization of the overlying sac may vary from denuded dura to dysplastic or mature epithelium. Moreover, meningoceles may be located in a variety of locations depending on the site of the embryonic bony fusion defect. Most common in the posterior lumbosacral region, meningoceles may also

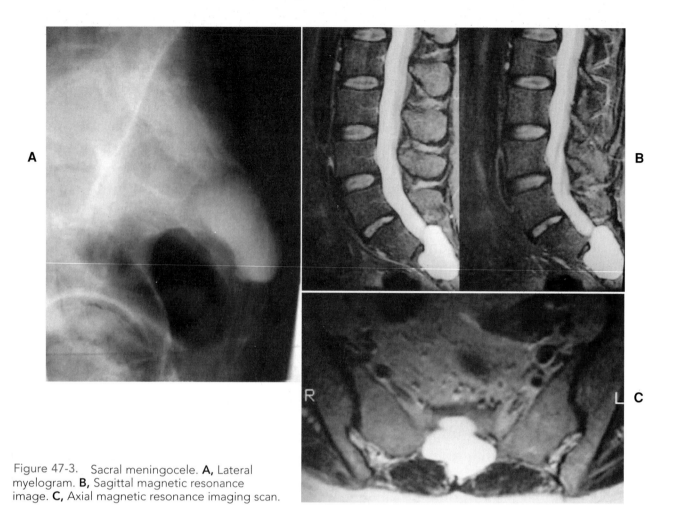

Figure 47-3. Sacral meningocele. **A,** Lateral myelogram. **B,** Sagittal magnetic resonance image. **C,** Axial magnetic resonance imaging scan.

OPEN DYSRAPHIC CONDITIONS: GENERAL

- Neurulation defects: Generally occur at 18 to 21 days' gestation
- Three types of neurulation defects
  - Incomplete neural tube closure
  - Abnormal dysjunction of neural plate and ectoderm
  - Defective mesenchymal migration
- All patients with open dysraphic conditions lack skin overlying the defect
- Maternal alpha-1-fetoprotein (AFP) typically increased

MENINGOCELE

- Defective primary neurulation process
- Protrusion of dura and arachnoid through bony spine defect
- Most commonly found in posterior lumbosacral region
- Often pedunculated with some epithelial covering (sometimes dysplastic)
- Normal neurologic examination without lower extremity deformity
- Surgical repair must include meticulous attention to goal of untethering cord

---

occur posterior at the cervical and thoracic level.[35,53] Anterior sacral, anterolateral cervical, lumbar, and thoracic locations have also been described.[44]

Epidemiology

Truly accurate epidemiologic data are lacking for meningoceles, in part due to their grouping with meningomyeloceles. However, estimates project the incidence to be less than one twentieth as frequent as meningomyeloceles.[71]

First described by Brock and Sutcliffe in 1972,[9] the use of routine maternal screening of AFP levels and fetal ultrasonography coupled with the U.S. Public Health Service advisory for recommended maternal consumption of folate has significantly reduced the incidence of spina bifida in North America.[31,71]

Although meningoceles have not yet been isolated for inheritance studies, evidence suggests that a mother with an affected child or the progeny of an affected female has a 3% to 5% risk of incurring any form of spinal dysraphism.[69]

Signs and Symptoms

Meningoceles are most commonly located in the lumbosacral region. They may be pedunculated and of varying sizes and are usually covered by some degree of epithelium whether dysplastic or not. Easily compressible, these lesions transilluminate and rarely leak cerebrospinal fluid (CSF).

Neurologic examination is normal without deformity of the lower extremities. Bowel and bladder function remains unaffected. Head circumference reflects the absence of hydrocephalus with a soft anterior fontanel.

This disorder is characterized only by the physical findings and invariably remains so in the postoperative period unless the spinal cord becomes tethered.

Surgery

Due to the rarity of CSF leak, operative intervention may be performed on a semielective basis. The sac is opened dorsally, and great care is taken to free normal nerve roots on entering the peduncle of the meningocele. The dura must be freed sufficiently to examine the contents of the spinal canal with the goal of untethering, and meticulous dissection must be followed to avoid later iatrogenic scarring. It may be necessary to perform a one- or two-level laminectomy to visualize the entire lesion. Once the neural elements are free, the dura is closed primarily with absorbable suture. The subcutaneous and skin layers are easily closed due to their redundancy. Concerns regarding long-term follow-up relate to retethering or de novo tethering later in life.

Meningomyelocele

Meningomyeloceles occur in 0.07% of live births in the United States and are more common in females[19] (Figure 47-4). It is now becoming increasingly clear that a variety of environmental and genetic factors play a role in the development of meningomyeloceles. Specifically, as previously mentioned, genetic risk factors include consanguinity and affected siblings.[19] Environmental factors include decreased maternal folate or vitamin A and use of valproate or carbemazepine.[39,40,54,63,70] The increased awareness of these risk factors has had a major impact on prevalence throughout the world.

Ten times more common than meningoceles, meningomyeloceles are also most often located in the lumbar spine.

Embryology

The myelomeningocele is the result of failure of neural tube closure. When the tube fails to close, the superficial ectoderm remains attached and lateral to the flat neurectoderm. The mesenchyme cannot migrate and, consequently, forms the bony, cartilaginous, and muscular elements laterally.[32] At the level of the defect, several contiguous vertebrae are affected: the pedicles and laminae have developed laterally and appear everted.[52] The transverse processes are directed anteriorly, and these deformities decrease the anteroposterior dimen-

---

MYELOMENINGOCELE: GENERAL

- Incidence in United States 0.04% of live births (more common in females)
- Genetic risk factors: Consanguinity and affected siblings
- Environmental risk factors: Decreased serum folate or vitamin A and uses of certain anticonvulsants (valproate and carbemazepime)
- Embryologic failure of neural tube closure
- Associated clinical findings
  - Hydrocephalus
  - Decreased intelligence quotient (IQ) scores
  - Bowel and bladder incontinence
  - Lower extremity deformities
  - Progressive scoliosis

---

sion of the canal. If the outward pedicle rotation is severe enough, the paraspinal muscles can develop anterior to the midcoronal plane of the spine and become flexors of the spine, creating or aggravating a kyphosis.[32]

Presentation

A multitude of associated anomalies may be found with meningomyeloceles. Their presence and severity play key roles not only in survival but also in ultimate level of function of the developing child. These key factors are hydrocephalus, intelligence, bowel and bladder continence, orthopedic problems, and ambulation. Their impact on outcome is paramount and therefore is discussed here.

The incidence of hydrocephalus ranges from 83% to 92%.[2,29] The etiology of hydrocephalus in this population stems from outflow obstruction of the fourth ventricle and/or impaired CSF absorption. Surprisingly, an autopsy study of 100 children revealed patency of the aqueduct of Sylvius in all.[20]

Most patients become symptomatic within the first 6 weeks after birth.[29] The development of delayed hydrocephalus plays an important role in surgical planning for the meningomyelocele. Most authors recommend concomitant shunting for patients with the slightest evidence of hydrocephalus on clinical or radiographic examination.[2,29,41] However, one may be reluctant to perform a shunting procedure for fear of assigning a child to the lifelong drawbacks of shunt dependence.

In the United States, 73% of patients with meningomyeloceles score greater than 80 on the intelligence quotient.[4,30] Lowered intelligence quotient scores are more closely related to central nervous system infections than to hydrocephalus if treated.[43] Although many variables in patient development, including the presence of congenital and related brain anomalies, may contribute to a lowered intelligence quotient, research suggests that the predominance of mental disability is due to concomitant meningitis or cerebritis.[48]

More than 80% of myelodysplastic patients incur bladder incontinence.[13] Fortunately, various methods of

A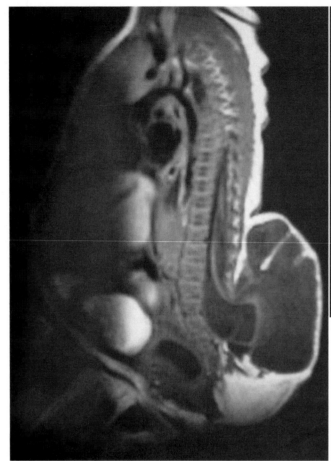

B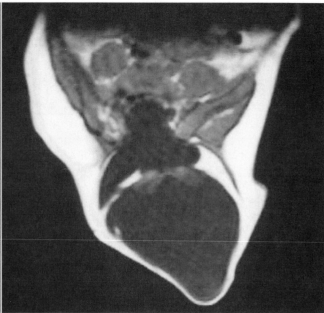

Figure 47-4. **A,** Sagittal magnetic resonance image. **B,** Axial magnetic resonance imaging scan.

urinary diversion procedures combined with sterile intermittent catheterization procedures exist to help manage these disabilities. Bladder incontinence remains a major issue in the chronic care of this patient population. This problem has proved to be more manageable with adequate patient training.

Lower limb deformities, progressive scoliosis, and other orthopedic conditions remain additional obstacles. It is imperative that patients receive adequate and continuous rehabilitation and monitoring throughout their lives. Early recognition of other associated vertebral anomalies, such as widened pedicles and anterior or posterior fusion defects, must be identified as potentially hazardous later in development. These defects may be distant to the location of the meningomyelocele. However infrequent, gastrointestinal, pulmonary, and cardiac abnormalities have also been associated with myelodysraphism.

The ability to ambulate at a functional level inside or outside of the household is an important goal of the patient and the caregiver. Data reveal that 23% to 59% of myelodysplastic individuals are able to ambulate without personal assistance.[66] The level of neurologic disability determines the strength of hip flexors, hip adductors, and quadriceps and hence the degree of functional ambulation.

Myelomeningoceles are frequently diagnosed prenatally through routine screening tests such as AFP, amnio-centesis, and ultrasound examinations.[50,60] This prenatal diagnosis allows education for the expectant parents and preparation for proper care at delivery. Rupture of the overlying membrane could result in central nervous system infection with the potentially devastating results previously mentioned. Even if not diagnosed prenatally, the keys to evaluation and treatment of the neonate with a myelomeningocele are to assess the general health of the infant and to identify associated problems that would preclude a surgical intervention. Prenatal diagnosis will become more critical in the future as surgical intervention in utero develops into common practice. The early goals are surgical closure of the defect, preservation of neurologic function, and prevention of infection. The defect is initially protected from trauma and drying through the application of a sterile, saline-soaked, nonadherent dressing.

The presence of associated anomalies of the genitourinary, cardiac, and gastrointestinal systems is evaluated. Ultrasound examinations of the head and urinary system and plain radiographs of the entire spine are obtained portably in the neonatal intensive care unit. Critical to preoperative planning is the presence of hydrocephalus, hydronephrosis, or occult dysraphisms. A thorough neurologic evaluation is undertaken to determine the functional level of the lesion and is preferable when the infant is quiet or sleeping. The sensory level is assessed, watching for a facial grimace or crying, proceeding distal to proximal. Voluntary motor function of the lower extremities is determined by stimulating the upper extremities (if unaffected) and watching for spontaneous contraction of lower extremity musculature. Various orthopedic anomalies such as clubfeet, hyperextended knees, or hip flexion contractures can give clues to the neurologic level as well.

The flat red neural plate may be visualized through the membrane. The surface of the neural plate represents the interior of the spinal cord, and therefore the central canal is located at the top of the plate and is continuous with the CSF beneath the sac. Skin, arachnoid remnants, and dura surround the neural pate and form the fluid-filled membrane of the sac. The sac varies in size and is often fragile, thereby demanding meticulous care in the preoperative period. The ventral surface of the neural plate is made up of the elements that would normally make up the outside of the spinal cord. The ventral nerve roots lie lateral to the midline, and the dorsal nerve roots lie lateral to them; both cross through the subarachnoid space and exit through the neural foramina. The neural placode is the structure formed by the flattened neural plate and nerve roots. The sac is lined by arachnoid, and the dura, displaced laterally, blends together with the surrounding skin at the margins. The spinal canal is tethered by its attachment to the skin, and its end is marked at this level most commonly in lumbosacral myelomeningoceles. In myelomeningoceles, which occur at higher levels, the spinal cord may have a normal configuration above and below the defect.[32]

Surgery

Although several techniques of myelomeningocele repair have been reported, anatomic reconstruction of the defect is most preferred by current surgeons.[32] The neural tube can be reconstituted, but the dural sac should be reconstructed to allow the tube to lie in a CSF-filled space. This attempts to provide the best environment for neural function of the placode and to decrease the risk of retethering at the repair site.[32] The fact that neural function persists in the placode is substantiated by the presence of function below the level of a myelomeningocele, the recovery of motor function postoperatively, and electrophysiologic studies on the neural placode.[42]

Closure of the myelomeningocele should be performed early. The incidence of infection and ventriculitis increases with delay in closure, and this can manifest in mental retardation and impaired function.[72] If the sac is not leaking, closure within 24 to 48 hours should be performed.[17]

The surgery is performed under general anesthesia with preoperative antibiotics and the infant positioned prone on chest rolls. Loupe magnification or an operating microscope is required to avoid injury to the neural structures. The initial step is to isolate the neural placode by incising the surrounding skin and arachnoid junction circumferentially. When the subarachnoid space is entered, the nerve roots are identified and pro-

> ### MYELOMENINGOCELE: SURGICAL CONSIDERATIONS
>
> - Goals
>   - Closure of defect
>   - Preservation of neurologic function
>   - Prevention of infection
> - Include both anatomic neural tube reconstitution and dural sac reconstruction
> - Infection rates directly correlate with delays in closure, so a 24- to 48-hour window is recommended for surgical reconstruction (assuming no cerebrospinal fluid leakage)
> - Monitor all patients postoperatively for signs of hydrocephalus with shunt placement if such condition arises
> - Infection and wound breakdown: Possibly as high as 12%

tected. Small fragments of skin, fat, or dura must be trimmed from the placode to avoid formation of delayed epidermoid tumors or inflammatory reactions.[75] Then the placode may be reconstituted into a tube by suturing the lateral arachnoid edges together, involuting the raw surface, and attempting to prevent adhesions to the dural repair.

The edges of the dura are then sharply dissected and mobilized, and closed in the midline to recreate a closed dural sac and subarachnoid space. Dural substitutes and grafts should be avoided to decrease the risk of wound breakdown and late inflammatory and fibrotic reactive tissue.[33] Provided sufficient dorsal fascia exists to close over the midline dural repair, an attempt should be made to add another layer of closure. The skin and underlying subcutaneous fat are carefully mobilized to close over the defect in the midline in two layers.

Significant hydrocephalus is present in 15% of neonates but develops subsequently in more than 90%; most require a procedure to divert CSF.[52] A ventriculoperitoneal shunt may be placed during the same procedure in those patients with enlarged ventricles.[7] Thoracolumbar kyphosis is present in about 15% of patients with myelomeningoceles at birth and may make closure difficult and increase wound complications at the site of the bony prominence. Some authors advocate a simultaneous kyphectomy by vertebrectomy and return of the paraspinal muscles to a position more consistent with extensor function. This may reduce the incidence of late spinal deformity.[68]

Postoperatively, the patient should be monitored for signs of hydrocephalus, and serial ultrasound examination of the ventricles is helpful. If hydrocephalus develops, a shunt is placed when infection has been ruled out. Direct pressure over the closed defect should be avoided, and the wound is monitored for CSF leak, infection, or breakdown. CSF leaks are usually self-limited or treated by shunting the underlying hydrocephalus. Infection and wound breakdown are problematic, occurring up to 12% in one study.[43]

OCCULT SPINAL DYSRAPHISM

Occult dysraphic conditions are those in which skin covers the neural elements and include spinal lipomas, diastematomyelia, dermal sinuses, tight filum terminale, and tethered cord. Although they arise from different embryologic errors, they have in common the presenting symptomatology of tethering of the spinal cord.

Cutaneous malformations such as a hairy patch, nevus, skin appendage (Figure 47-5 and Plate 47-1), or dimple with a pinhole can be a clinical clue for an occult spinal dysraphism. Diastematomyelia is associated with hypertrichosis, and spinal lipomas are associated with subcutaneous fat collections.

The term *tethered cord syndrome* represents a constellation of signs and symptoms that are associated with occult spinal dysraphisms. The syndrome can be present in the child on initial presentation or as a result of retethering in a previously treated lesion such as myelomeningocele. Symptoms include weakness of the lower extremities, deterioration of gait, spasticity, urinary incontinence, scoliosis, and pain. Nondermatomal sensory disturbances, which are asymmetric, may herald early changes, especially in the perineal area. Several pathophysiologic mechanisms exist to explain the syndrome complex, and most center around the decreased capacity of the tethered cord to stretch and dissipate energy with normal movement of the spinal canal. The focal traction on the cord leads to neural tissue injury. This mechanism also explains the onset of symptoms with physical exertion and growth. The treatment has evolved to aggressive surgical management and untethering of the spinal cord to arrest symptom progression.

SPINAL LIPOMA

With the exception of Chiari II malformations, spinal lipomas are associated with most forms of occult spinal dysraphism.[46] They may occur at any location in the spine and may be found within the canal with adhesions to the dura, spinal cord, or nerve roots.[46,47] Spinal lipomas are usually found in one of three circumstances: lipomyelomeningocele, fibrolipoma of the filum terminale, or intradural lipomas. Six forms of spinal dysraphism with lipoma have been described[11,16]; here, we limit the discussion to the most clinically relevant.

Lipomyelomeningocele

Approximately 84% of spinal lipomas are lipomeningomyeloceles[16] (Figure 47-6). The lipoma traverses a midline defect in the lumbar fascia, vertebral arch, and dura, finally merging with the spinal cord. There are three subtypes: terminal, dorsal, and transitional.[16] Each type is commonly associated with a tethered cord (Figure 47-7). This anomaly accounts for 20% to 56% of all occult spinal dysraphism and is responsible for roughly 20% of skin-covered lumbosacral masses.[11]

> **CLOSED DYSRAPHIC CONDITIONS: GENERAL**
>
> - Common clinical findings: Skin covering the neural elements
> - Symptomatic tethering of spinal cord common, with
>   - Lower extremity weakness
>   - Gait abnormalities
>   - Spasticity
>   - Urinary incontinence
>   - Pain and sensory disturbances
> - Types of closed or occult dysraphic anomalies
>   - Spinal lipomas
>   - Diastematomyelia
>   - Dermal sinuses
>   - Tight filum terminale
> - Cutaneous malformations
>   - Hairy patch and hypertrichosis
>   - Nevus
>   - Skin appendages
>   - Dimple with central pinhole

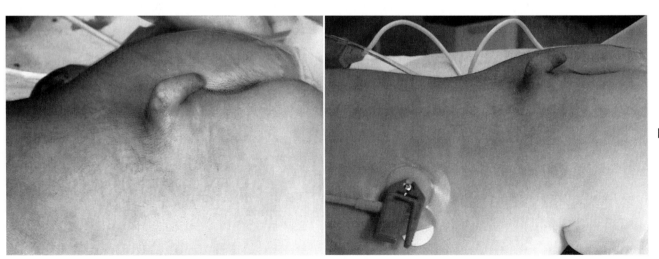

A **B**

Figure 47-5.   (See Plate 47-1) **A** and **B**, Posterior lumbar skin appendage in an infant with type I split cord malformation.

Embryology

Several theories have been proposed to account for the defect and its attachment of fat. McLone et al.[47] suggest that a single error of neurulation, a premature ectodermal disjunction, can allow mesenchyme to migrate to contact the inside of the forming neural tube and results in myeloschisis from the mesenchymal tissue, preventing neural tube closure. The mesenchyme differentiates into fat and adheres to the neural plate. The ectoderm dorsally fuses to create intact skin over the lesion.[47]

The dorsal aspect of the low-lying conus is often split at the level of the bifid spine. A fibrovascular band constricts the sac and neural tissue superiorly. The lipoma may pass through the dehiscent dura to become attached to the dorsal surface of the placode. Its extent may reach beneath the arches of intact cephalad vertebrae.

SPINAL LIPOMA

- Associated with most forms of occult spinal dysraphisms
- Can be cervical, thoracic, lumbar, or sacral and often found with adhesions to meninges and or neural elements
- Three most common types
  - Lipomyelomeningocele
    - Neurulation error characterized by premature ectodermal disjunction
    - Clinically: Usually normal at birth, but plegias and urinary incontinence develop by age 2 years
    - Magnetic resonance imaging definitive study to diagnose
    - Surgical correction elective, with main goal of untethering spinal cord
  - Fibrolipoma of filum terminale
    - Faulty retrogressive differentiation
    - Present with symptoms of spinal cord tethering
    - Surgical treatment involves filum division with careful resection of lipoma
  - Intradural lipomas
    - Most commonly cervical or thoracic
    - Usually present in second to fifth decades with monoparesis or paraparesis and pain

---

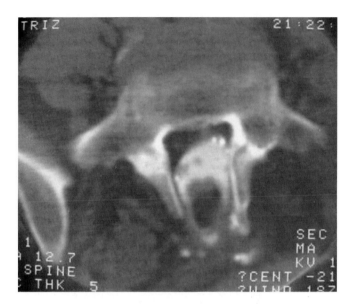

Figure 47-6.   Axial computed tomography myelogram of lipomyelomeningocele.

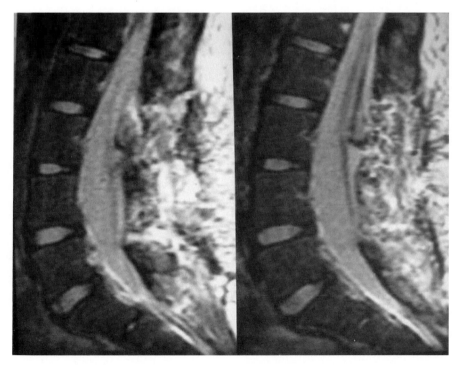

Figure 47-7.   Sagittal magnetic resonance imaging scan of a lumbar dorsal lipoma with tethered cord.

Presentation

The natural history of lipomyelomeningoceles is not well described in the literature, but in most reports, most patients are normal at birth and subtle neurologic deficits such as monoplegia or dribbling urine appear by age 2.[11] In a 1979 pediatric series,[11] 56% of patients presented with back masses, 32% with bladder dysfunction, and 10% with lower extremity deformities, weakness, or leg pain. The infants may be referred because of cosmetic concerns about the lumbosacral fat collection or cutaneous markings, which are present in half of the affected patients. The lipoma is typically located above the gluteal cleft, but it may extend into one buttock. Cutaneous stigmata such as hypertrichosis, a dimple, or aberrant pigmentation often provide clues to the pathology beneath the sac. It is the rule that these children are born without neurologic deficit. The incidence of neurologic deficit begins to unfold after the second year of life.

In neonates, ultrasound examination of the spine can often delineate the lipoma and spinal dysraphism. Plain radiographs of the spine may illustrate increased lumbar lordosis, segmentation defects of the distal vertebrae, and sacral deformities. Magnetic resonance imaging (MRI) is the definitive study and allows visualization of the neural plate, its orientation in the canal, and its relationship to the lipoma.

Surgery

Provided the neural elements are covered with intact skin, surgical intervention is performed on an elective basis. The goal of the surgery is to release or untether the cord to prevent neurologic deficits or to curtail them (Figure 47-8 and Plate 47-2). Because the lipomatous tissue extends into the cord, aggressive attempts at total removal of the lipoma from the cord should not be attempted. The safe untethering of spinal cords from lipomas and intradural debulking of the lipoma has been documented in several reports.[16,27] After subcutaneous flaps are mobilized, the dura is opened from the normal area superiorly and then carried down the lateral side of the neural plate in the area of the larger subarachnoid space (identified with MRI or ultrasound). If the incision is made too close to the cord-lipoma junction, the dorsal roots could be cut. After the subcutaneous mass is mobilized, the last intact vertebral arch is opened to work from normal dura. The fibrovascular band is identified and carefully sectioned to free the dural tube. After the neural plate is untethered, the lipoma can be debulked with a laser. The placode is reformed into a closed neural tube with absorbable suture. The pial margins are then closed, followed by the dura. A tension-free, watertight dural closure is accomplished by either primary apposition or placement of a fascia lata graft. Postoperatively, the patient is kept flat for several days after the operation to minimize CSF leakage into the subcutaneous dead space and to prevent tension on the wound.

Fibrolipoma of the Filum Terminale ("Fatty Filum")

Approximately 1% to 5% of autopsies and MRI examinations of the lumbar spine reveal a small lipoma of the filum terminale.[55,73] Most likely due to faulty retrogressive differentiation, the symptomatic variety is much larger in size and often located at the lower dorsal dural attachment.[51] Although nerve root irritation has been described, the most likely presentation clinically (the vast majority are asymptomatic) is due to spinal cord tethering.

Treatment for symptomatic individuals involves division of the filum terminale with removal of the interposed lipoma. Complete excision of the lipoma should be performed only in the absence of adhesion to nerve roots or the conus medullaris.

Intradural Lipoma

Completely intradural lipomas compose less than 5% of all spinal lipomas. They are more frequent in the cervical or thoracic spinal cord, and the canal is usually normal.[47] In cases in which the spinal cord is normal, the lipoma is most often in a dorsal, subpial, and juxtamedullary location.[5] The peak occurrence is between

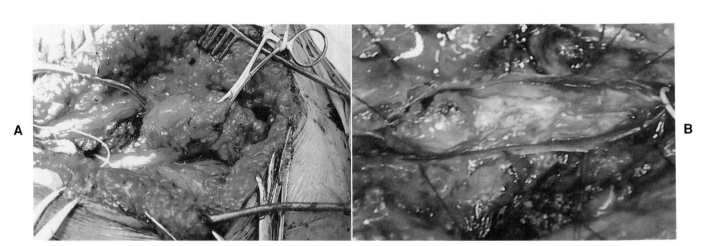

Figure 47-8. (See Plate 47-2) **A** and **B,** Intraoperative photographs of lumbar lipomyelomeningocele.

the second to fifth decades without sex predilection. Due to their location, the presenting symptom is most frequently monoparesis or paraparesis and pain.

Split Notochord Syndromes

This rare group of anomalies occurs during splitting of the notochord when connections persist between the gut and neuroectoderm. These anomalies include diastematomyelia, dorsal enteric communications, and enteric cysts. The most severe form of split notochord syndrome is the dorsal enteric fistula. Here we review the most common types and their treatments.

The nomenclature for the various phenotypes that arise from the split notochord syndrome has been misleading and misused and continue to be under some debate. We use the system proposed by Pang and colleagues[57,58]

The term *split cord malformation* (SCM) is used to describe all duplicate spinal cords. First proposed by Pang and colleagues[57,58] in 1992 as a unified theory, SCMs can be divided into two types. *Type I*, also referred to as a *diastematomyelia*, is defined as two separate hemicords with each enclosed in a dural tube (Figure 47-9). The hemicords are separated by an osseocartilaginous septum. *Type II* SCMs involve two hemicords enclosed by a single dural sheath. An intervening fibrous band separates the hemicords. This type may also be referred to as *diplomyelia* in the literature.

SPLIT NOTOCHORD SYNDROMES

- Diastematomyelia
- Diplomyelia
- Dorsal enteric communications
- Enteric cysts

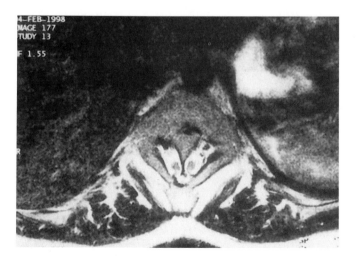

Figure 47-9. T2 axial magnetic resonance imaging scan of diastematomyelia (type I split cord malformation).

Embryology

According to the "unified theory" put forth by Pang and colleagues,[57,58] an ectodermal-to-endodermal adhesion forms into an accessory neurenteric canal. The resulting endomesenchymal tract bisects the notochord and neural plate. The result is two hemicords, each with a dural sac separated by a rigid osteocartilaginous septum or both contained in a single dural sac divided by a fibrous band. Each separate neural tube may vary in size.

Type I Split Cord Malformation (Diastematomyelia)

This type represents half of SCMs. At the level of the split cord, various abnormalities of the bony spine may exist.[26] Findings may include a septated vertebral body, agenesis of the intervertebral disc, and dorsal hypertrophic bone at the site of septal attachment.[24,28] Cutaneous abnormalities such as hypertrichosis (50% to 75%), lipoma, or nevi, as well as orthopedic foot deformities (i.e., clubfoot, neurogenic high arches), may be present. Approximately 85% are located from T9 to S1.[28] There is a female predominance (3.5:1), and roughly 20% of Chiari II malformations have diastematomyelia.[24]

Treatment of symptomatic individuals involved removal of the osseocartilaginous spike to untether the cord. Due to the possibility of additional tethering of the spinal cord at the filum level, one must perform the untethering portion at the level of the diastematomyelia before the filum to prevent spinal cord retraction against the caudal region of the spike. Before closure, the dura is reconstituted into a single tube.

Type II Split Cord Malformation (Diplomyelia)

Unlike type I, there are usually no spine abnormalities at the level of the split cord. However, type II SCM is associated with lumbosacral spina bifida occulta. The embryologic origins of types I and II SCM are similar, and therefore many of the findings of type I (cutaneous and orthopedic features) also appear in type II.

DIASTEMATOMYELIA

- Type I split cord malformation in Pang classification
- Two hemicords separated by an osseocartilaginous septum, each enclosed within a dural tube
- Often have bony spine abnormalities at level of split cord
  - Septated vertebral body
  - Disk agenesis
  - Dorsal hypertrophic bone
- Often have cutaneous anomalies such as hypertrichosis, lipoma, or nevi
- Female-to-male ratio of 3.5:1
- Often seen in association with Chiari II malformations
- Treatment
  - Untethering the cord by resection of osseocartilagenous spike
  - Reconstruction of dura into single tube

DIPLOMYELIA

- Type II split cord malformation
- Two hemicords separated by fibrous band enclosed in single dural sheath
- No spine abnormalities at level of split
- Associated with lumbosacral spina bifida occulta
- Treatment involves untethering cord

Treatment of symptomatic type II SCM involves primarily untethering the cord at the level of the lumbar spina bifida occulta. Subsequent lysis of the fibrous septum at the level of the SCM may not be required. Careful review of the preoperative and postoperative images as well as the neurologic examination is paramount in unveiling a symptomatic fibrous septum.

Presentation

This condition is reported to be three times more common in females than in males, and cutaneous manifestations are present in most patients (50% to 90%), most commonly a hairy patch or nevus.[26] Up to 25% of patients with diastematomyelia also have meningomyelocele, but the SCM is often not discovered until long after the closure of the myelomeningocele.

Some patients are asymptomatic for many years, but all will develop some neurologic sequelae; some adults may suddenly deteriorate. Adults typically have pain and urologic dysfunction, and their symptoms may be exacerbated by activity.[57] Children have pain less frequently and a more insidious progression.

Scoliosis is present in patients with SCM, and the curves are usually progressive. Congenital anomalies of the vertebral bodies are found along with the SCM, and the corollary is also true: 5% of patients with congenital scoliosis also have a diastematomyelia.[24] In addition to scoliosis, other orthopedic lower extremity abnormalities such as a cavovarus, planovalgus, clubfoot deformity, or limb length discrepancy, can be found with an otherwise normal neurologic examination.[28] In some patients, neurologic symptoms such as hyperreflexia, upper or lower motor neuron signs, or weakness can be ascertained, with or without limb deformities.

Plain radiographs of the spine reveal scoliosis, vertebral anomalies of the bodies, canal, or laminae in 90% of patients. A bony cleavage spur may be localized, usually in the area of the widest interpedicular distance. MRI allows evaluation of the entire spine and spinal cord and assessment of tethering, thickened filum terminale, lipomas, or syrinx cavities.[57] Computed tomography with myelography is useful to show bony abnormalities, the cleaving spur on the vertebral body, and its ossification status.[32]

The pathophysiology of symptoms in SCM is thought to involve traction on the spinal cord by the dividing septum, local ischemia of the cord, or the development of syringomyelia.[32]

Surgery

The goals of surgery in SCM, like other spinal dysraphisms, is to halt neurologic deficits, prevent further deterioration, and attempt to reverse any neurologic symptoms. Surgery is indicated in asymptomatic patients as well, due to the natural history of neurologic deterioration of patients with untreated SCM.[57]

SCM lesions are best approached posteriorly, with laminectomies to expose the normal dura above and below the septum, avoiding dissection in the midline of any bifid laminae. The dura is then dissected under magnification from the septum, with control of bleeding from the venous plexus in the area. The septum, if ossified, is then burred down to the level of the posterior aspect of the vertebral body. The dura is then opened longitudinally down both hemicords, the cleft portion is excised, and the dorsal opening is closed in the standard fashion. Any tethering is treated concomitantly.[32]

Most patients will have stabilization or improvement of neurologic symptoms and/or pain postoperatively.[26] The correlation of shorter symptom duration and better outcome after surgery is clear. Because the scoliosis can be expected to stabilize, consideration for spinal fusion should be delayed for many months to monitor progression of the spinal deformity.[26,28]

Enterogenous (Neurenteric) Cyst

Arising from failure of notochord and foregut separation, neurenteric cysts appear as thin-walled, fluid-filled masses.[8,58] The walls are lined by columnar and cuboidal epithelium with occasional mucin-secreting goblet cells. Peak age of presentation is 0 to 20 years, with a slight male predominance.[8,10] They are most commonly located in the thoracic (42%) and cervical (32%) spine.[10] The vast majority of these lesions (90%) occur ventral to the spinal cord and in the midline.[10] Vertebral anomalies may be found in 43% of cases.[8]

Embryology

By the eighteenth day of normal development, the floor of the notochord and endoderm disintegrates. Failure of separation of the notochord with the developing foregut results in retained endodermal material, which is then incorporated within the developing notochord.[64]

Presentation

An enlarging cyst may present with myelopathy and worsening neurologic deficit. Ruptured cysts present with a potentially severe chemical meningitis. The ventral location of the cyst may result in presentation of pain, which may be radiculopathic. Once confirmed by diagnostic imaging, a search for other signs of spinal dysraphism and tethering should follow.

Treatment

Incidental or asymptomatic neurenteric cysts may be followed with serial MRI examinations. Some authors

ENTERIC CYSTS

- Failure of notochord and foregut separation, resulting in gut epithelium–lined cyst
- Thin-walled, fluid-filled mass most common in thoracic and cervical spine
- Present clinically within first 20 years of life with myelopathy and potentially severe meningitis if cyst has ruptured
- Male predominance
- Asymptomatic cysts followed with serial magnetic resonance images
- High morbidity associated with surgical removal secondary to potential for chemical meningitis

Table 47-1	Chiari Malformations

Chiari I
   Cerebellar tonsils extend below the foramen magnum
Chiari II
   Abnormal corpus callosum
   Beaked tectum
   Small posterior fossa
   Large thalamic massa intermedia
   Low-lying torcula
   Hindbrain extends into cervical canal
   Kinked cervicomedullary junction
Chiari III
   Occiptocervical encephalocele
Chiari IV
   Cerebellar hypoplasia

contend that an enlarging cyst should be removed surgically due to the risk of meningitis or neurologic disability. However, the ventral location of these lesions often requires an anterior or a posterolateral approach. Therefore surgical removal is subject to a higher morbidity, and the risks and benefits in asymptomatic patients should be carefully weighed.

Once exposed, the lesion is carefully dissected without rupture of the membrane if possible. Should the contents of the sac leak, copious irrigation is used to blunt the possibility of postoperative meningitis. Complete removal of the sac is not always possible due to adhesion to the spinal cord. Care is taken to ensure the spinal cord is not tethered at the site of the lesion.

Dermal Sinus

Forming a tract beginning at the skin surface, a dermal sinus is lined with epithelium. It is most commonly found in the lumbosacral region (57%) and likely results from failure of the cutaneous ectoderm to cleave from the neuroectoderm during closure of the neural groove.[76] The incidence is approximately 1 in 2500 live births.[62]

The tract is 1 to 2 mm in diameter and often has a cephalic trajectory due to the migration of the spinal cord. The surrounding skin may have "port wine" pigmentation. The sinus may terminate superficially, connect to the coccyx, or extend to the dural tube (60%).[76] Along its course, the tract may dilate to form an epidermoid cyst containing keratin debris and lined with stratified squamous epithelium. It may also harbor a dermoid cyst containing skin appendages, hair follicles, and sebaceous glands. Up to 60% of dermal sinuses contain epidermoid or dermoid tumors.[62]

If the tract extends intradurally and remains patent, the potential for recurrent meningitis may be a presenting sign. Moreover, intrathecal extension may result in a tethered spinal cord. Therefore, due to its location, bladder dysfunction is often the initial presentation.

Treatment

Patency and extension into the thecal sac necessitate surgical repair. An ellipse is cut around the opening of

CHIARI MALFORMATION DESCRIPTIONS

- Hindbrain herniation first characterized by Chiari in 1891
- Four types
  - Chiari I: Cerebellar tonsils extend below foramen magnum
  - Chiari II
    - Abnormal corpus callosum
    - Beaked tectum
    - Small posterior fossa
    - Large thalamic massa intermedia
    - Low-lying torcula
    - Hindbrain extends into cervical canal
    - Kinked cervicomedullary junction
  - Chiari III: Occipitocervical encephalocele
  - Chiari IV: Cerebellar hypoplasia

the tract. Careful dissection to free the margins of the tract is performed without spilling the contents of the cyst. If the tract is found to be penetrating the spine, laminectomy is needed for full visualization. Extension through the dura occurs in the midline and requires careful subdural inspection of neural elements and eventual watertight dural closure.

CHIARI MALFORMATIONS

In 1891, Chiari described and categorized various types of hindbrain herniation[12] (Table 47-1). Although type IV is actually due to cerebellar hypoplasia, these categories have become the mainstay of today's descriptions. Types I and II are the most common of these abnormalities. Multiple theories regarding the pathogenesis of Chiari I and II malformations abound. Currently, the most widely accepted of these theories describes faulty equilibration of the CSF pressure wave after Valsalva maneuver.[45] Accurate or not, the theory aligns various data that have revealed that pressure differentials within the posterior fossa and craniovertebral junction play an important role in the symptomatology and pathogenesis of this disease process.

Chiari I Malformation

The Chiari I malformation exhibits no brainstem abnormality, but the cerebellar tonsils extend below the foramen magnum (Figure 47-10). Because about 15% of asymptomatic patients undergoing MRI for other reasons have some herniation of the tonsils below the foramen magnum, it is generally considered that 2 to 3 mm of extension is insignificant and can be considered normal.[1] Patients with symptoms of a Chiari malformation have herniation of more than 3 mm below the foramen magnum. Radiographic criteria (Table 47-2) for

tonsillar extension below the foramen magnum may be used as a guide for possible surgical intervention in symptomatic patients.

All patients with tonsillar herniation below the level of the foramen magnum greater than 12 mm are symptomatic.[6] Approximately 70% of patients with 5- to 10-mm tonsillar protrusion become symptomatic.[6] Occasionally, Chiari I malformations have been described to appear after frequent lumbar puncture or placement of a lumboperitoneal shut. There are no other associated brain malformations with type I Chiari malformations. However, skeletal abnormalities have been found in 25% of cases[59] (Table 47-3). Approximately 40% to 65% of patients

---

CHIARI MALFORMATION TYPE I:

- Greater than 2- to 3-mm extension below foramen magnum (15% of asymptomatic patients undergoing magnetic resonance imaging have 1 to 3 mm of herniation)
- Twenty-five percent of cases have skeletal abnormalities (basilar invagination, Klippel-Feil, atlanto-occipital fusion, cervical spina bifida occulta)
- Most accepted etiologic theory supports abnormal cerebrospinal fluid (CSF) flow dynamics
- Presenting symptoms
  ○ Pain
  ○ Occipital headache
  ○ Lhermitte's sign
  ○ Long tract signs
- Associated with syringomyelia and hydrocephalus
- Treatment: Observation in asymptomatic patients who have radiographic evidence of a syrinx
- Surgical treatment for symptomatic patients involves supratentorial decompression

---

Table 47-2	Radiographic Criteria for Chiari I
Age (yr)	Distance Below Formen Magnum (mm)
<10	6
<30	5
<80	4
<90	3

Table 47-3	Skeletal Abnormalities Associated With Chiari I
Finding	Incidence (%)
Basilar invagination	25-50
Klippel-Feil syndrome	5-10
Atlanto-occipital fusion	5
Cervical spina bifida occulta	5

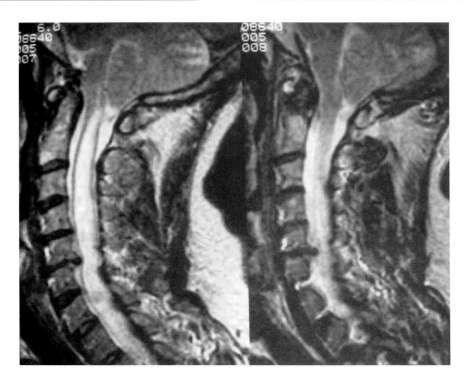

Figure 47-10. T2 sagittal magnetic resonance imaging scan of Chiari I malformation with syrinx.

develop hydrosyringomyelia.[59] The hydrodynamic theory proposed by Gardner[25] in 1965 continues to be widely accepted. According to Gardner, faulty CSF egress from the fourth ventricle transmits a force vector creating the syrinx during periods of Valsalva maneuver. Symptoms such as long tract signs and a suspended sensory loss are a direct affect of the damage the syrinx infers on the nearby pain and temperature fibers and corticospinal tracts.

Embryology

Perhaps the most widely accepted theory for the development of the Chiari I malformation involved CSF flow dynamics. Delayed or atretic opening of the foramina of Lushka and Magendie would create a larger and more sustained pressure gradient intracranially on Valsalva maneuver.[25] Any such maneuver, such as through coughing, would engorge epidural veins, increasing intracranial pressure. This increased pressure would further alter CSF flow equilibration should CSF outflow be partially obstructed while leaving the fourth ventricle. This continued stress to the posterior fossa contents throughout life would slowly prolapse the cerebellar tonsils out of the foramen magnum.

Presentation

Symptoms usually present in early adulthood and include pain, occipital headache, Lhermitte's sign, and long tract signs. Syringomyelia is present in 20% to 40% of asymptomatic individuals and 60% to 90% of symptomatic patients.[56] Hydrocephalus may be present in 25% of cases.[61] Presentation varies with age and may range from the aforementioned to signs of brainstem compression, including changes in phonation, dysphagia,

and hiccoughs. It is this metamorphosis of symptoms that may confuse the clinician and sends the patient "doctor shopping."

In adolescence, typical findings may include lower extremity weakness and spasticity, suspended sensory loss, upper extremity atrophy, truncal ataxia, scoliosis, neck pain on Valsalva, and cervical dysesthesias (Figure 47-11 and Plate 47-3). Presentation in adulthood adds nystagmus, vertigo, scoliosis, and the aforementioned bulbar symptoms.

Treatment

The decision to undergo craniocervical decompression is based on a number of factors. First, in the presence of symptomatic or radiographic hydrocephalus, a ventriculoperitoneal shunt should be placed first, despite the presence of any Chiari-related findings. Decompression of the supratentorial compartment may provide resolution of the Chiari malformation. Moreover, in the presence of elevated supratentorial pressures, decompression of the posterior fossa may induce further downward herniation, cerebellar prolapse, or even death.

The asymptomatic patient with incidental radiographic evidence of a Chiari I malformation should be observed. The exception, however, is the presence of a syrinx. Hydrosyringomyelia is likely to progress to neural insult, and the risk of permanent injury far outweighs the risk of surgical intervention.

The symptomatic patient without hydrocephalus should undergo craniocervical decompression. The patient is placed prone, and a midline incision is created in the avascular plane of the posterior soft tissues. Once muscle dissection is complete, careful identification of landmarks for the torcula and transverse sinus are marked for avoidance. After craniectomy, the dura is incised into a Y shape. Removal of the laminae of the atlas and axis may be performed depending on the level of tonsillar descent. A duroplasty is performed by placement of a triangle-shaped patch of Gore-Tex or other dural substitute. This dural closure must be water tight to prevent delayed CSF leakage. The muscle, fascia, and subcutaneous tissues are then closed in three layers.

Chiari II Malformation

The Chiari II malformation constitutes a variety of anomalies that affect the brain, skull, and spinal cord (Figure 47-12). Typically, the posterior fossa is small, and the cerebellum, pons, and medulla are displaced into the cervical canal to varying degrees, which results in compression of the brainstem. The most common associated findings are meningomyelocele (100%), hydrocephalus (90%), and medullary kinking (70%).[74] Other abnormalities are evident above the tentorium (Table 47-4).

Embryology

McLone et al.[46] proposed an embryologic theory to account for the pathoanatomy seen in a type II Chiari

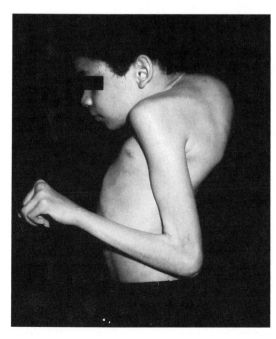

Figure 47-11. (See Plate 47-3) Photograph of adolescent patient with Chiari I malformation.

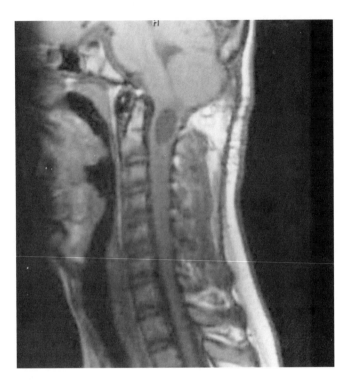

Figure 47-12. T1 sagittal magnetic resonance imaging scan of Chiari II malformation with syrinx.

Table 47-4	Chiari II: Associated Abnormalities
Skull and dura	Lacunar skull "lukenschadel"
	Low-lying torcula and transverse sinus
	Small posterior fossa
	Large foramen magnum
	Concave petrous temporal bone
	Shortened concave clivus
	Thin fenestrated falx cerebri
Hindbrain	Herniation of vermis, nodulus, uvula, and pyramis through foramen magnum
	Medullary kinking
	Tectal beaking
	Ectopic choroids
	Upward cerebellar herniation
Cerebrospinal fluid spaces	Hydrocephalus
	Elongated fourth ventricle
	Enlarged third ventricle
	Enlarged massa intermedia
	Colpocephaly
	Aqueductal stenosis
	Enlarged cisterna magna
Cerebral hemispheres	Heterotopias
	Polymicrogyria
	Callosal dysgenesis
Spine	Meningomyelocele
	Syrinx
	Diastematomyelia
	Incomplete atlas arch

CHIARI MALFORMATION TYPE II

- Most common associated findings
  - Myelomeningocele (100%)
  - Hydrocephalus (90%)
  - Medullary kinking (70%)
- Embryologic etiology most likely a failure of neuroectoderm to appose and adhere
- Presenting signs/symptoms
  - Dysphagia
  - Aspirations
  - Stridor
  - Spasticity
  - Scoliosis
- Surgical treatment: Decompression of hindbrain displacement
  - Multiple cervical laminectomies from C1 to caudal end of cerebellum with durotomy and patching to expand luminal volume

malformation due to failure of the neurectoderm to appose and adhere.[20] During normal embryogenesis, there is occlusion of the neurocele that accounts for ventricular dilatation, and in the absence of apposition, the inductive pressures on the surrounding mesenchyme can cause changes in the skull, posterior fossa, and hindbrain. Secondary changes in the cerebrum result from a lack of distention in the telencephalic ventricles.

Presentation

One fifth of patients with myelomeningocele and a Chiari II malformation will have symptoms of hindbrain compression.[74] Symptoms vary with age but are most significant before the age of 20 years. Infants have swallowing difficulties, presenting with poor feeding, repeated aspirations, apnea, or stridor from vocal cord paresis. Older children may have swallowing difficulties as well as extremity weakness. Adolescents typically have patterns of spasticity, sensory changes, and scoliosis, but this may be due to the development of syringomyelia.[74]

Because hydrocephalus can mimic hindbrain compression, shunt dysfunction or hydrocephalus must be ruled out. MRI has become the study of choice for evaluation of the craniocervical junction, the anatomy of the Chiari malformation, and cervical canal compression. Plain radiography and computed tomography may be used to determine the presence of associated occipitocervical anomalies, such as basilar invagination, atlantoaxial instability, or Klippel-Feil abnormalities.

The primary cause of death in myelodysplastic patients is respiratory embarrassment. Whether this is due to brainstem compression or primary hypoplasia of the medullary respiratory center remains a debate.

Surgery

The treatment of Chiari II malformations involves decompression of the hindbrain displacement into the cervical canal. The operation is often referred to as "posterior fossa decompression," but this is actually a misnomer, because the exposure is limited to the cervical spine. Multiple cervical laminectomies are performed from C1 to the caudal extent of the cerebellum, and frequently a tight dural band is found below the arch of C1.[32] The dura is opened in the midline and covered with a patch to create an expanded space. Any syrinx found during the exposure can be shunted.

The outcome after surgery is related to symptomatology at presentation. The outcome is poor in infants with severe brainstem dysfunction, particularly those with stridor or vocal cord paralysis. This may be due to irreversible ischemia of the brainstem or structural abnormalities that do not respond to decompression. Older patients with long tract signs do well after decompressive surgery.[61]

SYRINGOMYELIA

Syringomyelia is a pathologic fluid-filled cavity in the spinal cord that is lined by astrocytes. Hydromyelia, on the other hand, is an enlarged central canal of the spinal cord lined by ependymal cells. Hydromyelia is most commonly seen in Chiari II malformations and meningomyeloceles. Both are not the primary manifestation of a disease process but rather a result of a variety of mechanisms for fluid accumulation. Moreover, the fluid within hydromyelia may dissect through the ependymal layer, becoming a syringomyelia. Therefore the term *hydrosyringomyelia* is preferred while discussing pathogenesis. Patients with spinal dysraphism, tethered cord, and Chiari malformations are at risk of syrinx development (Figure 47-13). Small cavities that remain stable may continue to be asymptomatic to the patient.

As previously reviewed, the origin of syringomyelia is theorized to be due to obstruction of CSF across the foramen magnum.[56] Altered hydrodynamic forces in the spinal subarachnoid space force fluid into and down the spinal cord because the space cannot accommodate pressure changes from CSF pulse flows at systole with each heartbeat. However, other well known causes of hydrosyringomyelia include trauma, arachnoiditis, and neoplasm.

Presentation

Clinically, a developing or expanding hydrosyringomyelia mimics the lesion of a central spinal cord injury unless in a steady state. Dynamic syrinx will create a rather reliable constellation of symptoms and signs that, when revealed on examination, should alert the practitioner to pursue radiographic evidence.

Interruption of the crossing spinothalamic fibers is usually the first affected modality. Loss of pain and temperature with a dissociated and suspended sensory loss will create Charcot joints and evidence of chronic dissociated neglect with ulcers and lesions on the extremity. As the lesion enlarges, long tract signs begin to develop through compression of the neighboring corticospinal tracts. Loss of fine motor control in the upper extremities with spastic weakness of the lower extremities follows. Dysesthesias develop commonly in a C2 distribution and are exacerbated by cough or Valsalva maneuver. Disturbance of the descending sympathetic fibers may result in a Horner's syndrome. Lhermitte's sign is a

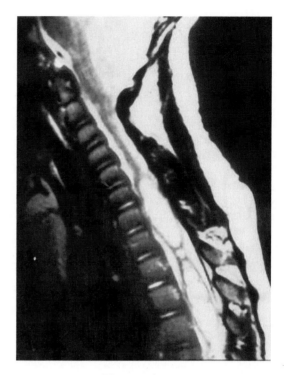

Figure 47-13. T2 sagittal magnetic resonance imaging scan of loculated cervical syrinx.

common entity and forewarns traction of the dorsal columns under the constraints of the enlarging diameter of the cord. Dynamic interference with spinal cord function can cause symptoms. Scoliosis due to disruption of the neural axis is a frequent presenting symptom. The use of MRI is paramount in the diagnosis and follow-up of these lesions.

Treatment

Treatment is indicated in those patients who are symptomatic or in those with large or extensive syringomyelia, even without symptoms. Data on the natural history of syringomyelia reveal that 35% of patients who received no treatment had no progression, and most of these were only mildly involved. Continuous neurologic progression occurs in 55%, and 10% of patients develop intermittent progression.[3]

Due to the unpredictability of the clinical course, surgical intervention is reserved for patients with symptomatic lesions or large dynamic lesions. Patients who are asymptomatic with small lesions can be followed with serial MRI. The current recommendation for patients with CSF occlusion at the foramen magnum is to undergo posterior fossa decompression with craniectomy and dural incision above the foramen magnum to allow adequate decompression. If the syrinx is at the same level of decompression, fenestration and shunting into the subarachnoid space can be performed, but the results of decompression alone appear to be similar. The size of the syrinx will decrease in 40% to 60% of cases.[32] Alternatively, without compression at the foramen magnum, the syrinx can be fenestrated locally and shunted. With resolution of the syringomyelia, patients will experience an improvement in their symptoms, even if a small syrinx remains on follow-up MRI.

CONCLUSIONS

Patients with congenital spinal anomalies represent a heterogeneous group of patients with individual conditions that can challenge the clinician involved in spinal care. Advances in embryologic research and medical imaging have improved the care of these patients. In most cases, surgical intervention has improved the natural history of spinal dysraphism, and continued follow-up is necessary to detect problems after surgery. A multidisciplinary clinic is essential to the management of these patients and their associated needs.

SELECTED REFERENCES

Ames MD, Schut L: Results of treatment of 171 consecutive myelomeningoceles: 1963-1968, *Pediatrics* 50:466-470, 1972.

Brock DJH, Sutcliffe RG: Alpha fetoprotein in the antenatal diagnosis of anencephaly and spina bifida, *Lancet* 2:197-199, 1972.

Cass AS, Spence BR: Urinary incontinence in myelomeningocele, *J Urol* 110:136-137, 1973.

Czeizel AE, Dudas I. Prevention of the first occurrence of neural-tube defects by periconceptional vitamin supplementation, *N Engl J Med* 327:1832-1835, 1992.

Emery JL: Deformity of the aqueduct of Sylvius in children with hydrocephalus and meningomyelocele, *Dev Med Child Neurol* 16:40-48, 1974.

Jorde LB, Fineman RM, Martin RA: Epidemiology of neural tube defects in Utah, *Am J Epidemiol* 119:487, 1984.

Lorber J: Results of treatment of meningomyelocele: an analysis of 524 unselected cases, with special reference to possible selection for treatment, *Dev Med Child Neurol* 13:279-303, 1971.

Okumra R et al.: Fatty filum terminale: assessment with MR imaging, *J Comput Assist Tomogr* 14:571-573, 1990.

Paul KS et al.: Arnold-Chiari malformation: review of 71 cases, *J Neurosurg* 58:183-187, 1983.

Pollack IF et al.: Outcome following hindbrain decompression of symptomatic Chiari malformations in children previously treated with myelomeningocele closure and shunts, *J Neurosurg* 77:881, 1992.

Powell KR et al.: A prospective search for congenital dermal abnormalities of the craniospinal axis, *J Pediatr* 87:744, 1975.

Samuelsson L, Skoog M: Ambulation in patients with myelomeningocele: a multivariate statistical analysis, *J Pediatr Orthop* 8:569-575, 1988.

Shurtleff DB, Lemire RJ, Warkany J: Embriology, etiology, and epidemiology. In Shurtleff DB, ed: *Myelodysplasias and extrophies: significance prevention and treatment*, New York, 1986, Grune & Stratton, p. 39.

Wright RL: Congenital dermal sinuses, *Progr Neurol Surg* 4:175, 1971.

REFERENCES

1. Aboulezz AO et al.: Position of cerebellar tonsils in the normal population and in patients with Chiari malformations: a quantitative approach with MR imaging, *J Comput Assist Tomogr* 9:1033, 1985.
2. Ames MD, Schut L: Results of treatment of 171 consecutive myelomeningoceles: 1963-1968, *Pediatrics* 50:466-470, 1972.
3. Anderson NE, Willoughby EW, Wrightston P: The natural history and influence of surgical treatment in syringomyelia, *Acta Neurol Scand* 71:472, 1985.
4. Badell-Ribera A, Shulman K, Paddock N: The relationship of nonprogressive hydrocephalus to intellectual functioning in children with spina bifida cystica, *Pediatrics* 37:787-793, 1966.
5. Barkovich AJ, Naidich TP: Congenital anomalies of the spine. In Barkovich AJ: *Pediatric neuroimaging*, New York, 1990, Raven, pp. 227-271.
6. Barkovich AJ et al.: Significance of cerebellar tonsillar position on MR, *AJNR* 7:795-799, 1986.
7. Bell WO, Arbit E, Fraser RA: One stage myelomeningocele closure and ventriculoperitoneal shunt placement, *Surg Neurol* 27:233, 1987.
8. Bentley JFR, Smith JR: Developmental posterior enteric remnants and spinal malformation: the split notochord syndrome, *Arch Dis Child* 35:76-86, 1960.
9. Brock DJH, Sutcliffe RG: Alpha fetoprotein in the antenatal diagnosis of anencephaly and spina bifida, *Lancet* 2:197-199, 1972.
10. Brooks BS et al.: Neuroimaging features of neurenteric cysts: analysis of nine cases and review of the literature, *AJNR* 14:735-746, 1993.
11. Bruce DA, Schut L: Spinal lipomas in infancy and childhood, *Child Brain* 5:192, 1979.
12. Carmel PW, Markesberry WR: Early descriptions of Arnold-Chiari malformation: the contribution of John Cleland, *J Neurosurg* 37:543, 1972.
13. Cass AS, Spence BR: Urinary incontinence in myelomeningocele, *J Urol* 110:136-137, 1973.
14. Centers for Disease Control: Recommendations for the use of folic acid to reduce the number of spina bifida cases and other neural tube defects, *JAMA* 269:1233, 1993.
15. Centers for Disease Control: Valproic acid and spina bifida: a preliminary report: France, *Morb Mortal Rep CDC* 32:565, 1982.
16. Chapman, PH: Congenital intraspinal lipomas: anatomic considerations and surgical treatment, *Child Brain* 9:37, 1982.
17. Charney EB et al.: Management of the newborn with myelomeningocele, *Pediatrics* 75:58, 1985.
18. Czeizel AE, Dudas I: Prevention of the first occurrence of neural-tube defects by periconceptional vitamin supplementation, *N Engl J Med* 327:1832-1835, 1992.
19. Elwood JM, Elwood JH: Genetic models. In Elwood JM, Elwood JH, eds: *Epidemiology of anencephalus and spina bifida*, New York, 1980, Oxford University Press, pp. 236-247.
20. Emery JL: Deformity of the aqueduct of Sylvius in children with hydrocephalus and meningomyelocele, *Dev Med Child Neurol* 16:40-48, 1974.
21. Fidas A et al.: Prevalence and patterns of spina bifida occulta in 2407 normal adults, *Clin Radiol* 38:587, 1987.
22. Flood T et al.: Spina bifida incidence at birth: United States: 1983-1990, *Morb Mortal Rep CDC* 41:497, 1992.
23. Fraser F: Genetic counseling in some common pediatric diseases, *Am J Hum Genet* 26:636, 1974.
24. French BM: Midline fusion defects and defects of formation. In Youmans JR, ed: *Neurological surgery*, ed 2, Philadelphia, 1982, p. 1236.
25. Gardner WJ: Hydrodynamic mechanism of syringomyelia: its relation to myelocele, *J Neurol Neurosurg Psychiatry* 28:247, 1965.
26. Gower DJ et al.: Diastematomyelia: a 40 year experience, *Pediatr Neurosci* 14:90, 1988.
27. Hoffman HJ et al.: Management of lipomyelomeningoceles: experience at the Hospital for Sick Children, Toronto, *J Neurosurg* 62:1, 1985.
28. Humphreys RP, Hendrick EB, Hoffman HJ: Diastematomyelia, *Clin Neurosurg* 30:436, 1983.
29. Hunt GM: Open spina bifida: outcome for a complete cohort treated unselectively and followed into adulthood, *Dev Med Child Neurol* 32:108-118, 1990.
30. Hunt GM, Holmes AE: Factors related to intelligence in treated cases of spina bifida cystica, *Am J Dis Child* 130:823-827, 1976.
31. Jorde LB, Fineman RM, Martin RA: Epidemiology of neural tube defects in Utah, *Am J Epidemiol* 119:487, 1984.
32. Kaufman BA: Congenital intraspinal anomalies: spinal dysraphism: embryology, pathology, and treatment. In Bridwell KH, DeWald RL, eds: *The textbook of spinal surgery*, ed 2, Philadelphia, 1997, Lippincott-Raven, p. 365.
33. Keller JT et al.: Repair of spinal defects: an experimental study, *J Neurosurg* 60:1022, 1984.
34. Khoury MJ, Erickson JD, James LM: Etiologic heterogeneity of neural tube defects: clues from epidemiology, *Am J Epidemiol* 115:538, 1982.
35. Langman J: Medical embryology: human development: normal and abnormal, Baltimore, 1995, Williams & Wilkins.

36. Laurence KM et al.: Double-blind randomised controlled trial of folate treatment before conception to prevent occurrence of neural tube defects, *Br Med J* 282:1509, 1981.

37. Layde PM, Edmonds LD, Erickson JD: Maternal fever and neural tube defect, *Teratology* 21:105, 1980.

38. Lemire RJ et al.: *Normal and abnormal development of the human nervous system*, Hagerstown, Md, 1975, Harper & Row.

39. Lindhout D, Omtzigt JG: Teratogenic effects of antiepileptic drugs: implications for the management of epilepsy in women of childbearing age, *Epilepsia* 35:19-28, 1994.

40. Little BB et al.: Megadose carbamazepine during the period of neural tube closure, *Obst Gynecol* 82:705-708, 1993.

41. Lorber J: Results of treatment of meningomyelocele: an analysis of 524 unselected cases, with special reference to possible selection for treatment, *Dev Med Child Neurol* 13:279-303, 1971.

42. McLone DG: Results of treatment of children born with a myelomeningocele, *Clin Neurosurg* 30:407, 1983.

43. McLone DG, Dias LS: Complications of myelomeningocele closure, *Pediatr Neurosurg* 17:267, 1991.

44. McLone DG, Dias MS: Normal and abnormal early development of the nervous system. In Cheek WR et al., eds: *Pediatric neurosurgery: surgery of the developing nervous system*, Philadelphia, 1994, WB Saunders, pp. 1-39.

45. McLone DG, Knepper PA: The cause of Chiari II malformation: a unified theory, *Pediatr Neurosci* 15:1, 1989.

46. McLone DG, Mutluer S, Naidich TP: Lipomeningoceles of the conus medullaris, *Concepts Pediatr Neurosurg* 3:170, 1983.

47. McLone DG, Naidich TP: Laser resection of fifty spinal lipomas, *Neurosurgery* 18:611, 1986.

48. McLone DG et al.: Central nervous system infections as a limiting factor in the intelligence of children with myelomeningocele, *Pediatrics* 70:338-342, 1982.

49. Moore KL: *The developing human: clinically oriented embryology*, Philadelphia, 1970, WB Saunders.

50. Morrow RJ, McNay MB, Whittle MJ: Ultrasound detection of neural tube defects in patients with elevated maternal serum alpha fetoprotein, *Obstet Gynecol* 78:1055-1057, 1991.

51. Moufarrij NA et al.: Correlation between magnetic resonance imaging and surgical findings in the tethered spinal cord, *Neurosurgery* 25:341-346, 1989.

52. Naidich TP, McLone DG: Congenital pathology of the spine and spinal cord. In Taveras JM, Ferucci JT, eds: *Radiology: diagnosis, imaging, intervention*, Philadelphia, 1989, JB Lippincott.

53. Naidich TP et al.: Congenital anomalies of the spine and spinal cord embryology and malformations. In Atlas SW, ed: *Magnetic resonance imaging of the brain and spine*, ed 2, Philadelphia, 1996, Lippincott-Raven, pp. 1265-1337.

54. Nau H: Transfer of valproic acid and its main active unsaturated metabolite to the gestational tissue: correlation with neural tube defect formation in the mouse, *Teratology* 33:21-27, 1986.

55. Okumra R et al.: Fatty filum terminale: assessment with MR imaging, *J Comput Assist Tomogr* 14:571-573, 1990.

56. Oldfield EH et al.: Pathophysiology of syringomyelia associated with Chiari I malformation of the cerebellar tonsils: implications for diagnosis and treatment, *J Neurosurg* 80:3, 1994.

57. Pang D: Split cord malformation. II: Clinical syndrome, *Neurosurgery* 31:481, 1992.

58. Pang D, Dias MS, Ahab-Barmada M: Split cord malformation. I: A unified theory of embryogenesis for double spinal cord malformations, *Neurosurgery* 31:451-480, 1992.

59. Paul KS et al.: Arnold-Chiari malformation: review of 71 cases, *J Neurosurg* 58:183-187, 1983.

60. Platt LD et al.: The California Maternal Serum Alpha Fetoprotein Screening Program: the role of ultrasonography in the detection of spina bifida, *Am J Obstet Gynecol* 166:1328-1329, 1992.

61. Pollack IF et al.: Outcome following hindbrain decompression of symptomatic Chiari malformations in children previously treated with myelomeningocele closure and shunts, *J Neurosurg* 77:881, 1992.

62. Powell KR et al.: A prospective search for congenital dermal abnormalities of the craniospinal axis, *J Pediatr* 87:744, 1975.

63. Rosa FW: Spina bifida in infants of women treated with carbamazepine during pregnancy, *N Engl J Med* 324:674-677, 1991.

64. Rosenberg IH: Folic acid and neural tube defects: time for action? *N Engl J Med* 327:1875-1877, 1992.

65. Rudd LN: *Genetics: disorders of the developing nervous system: diagnosis and treatment*, Boston, 1986, Blackwell Scientific, p. 47.

66. Samuelsson L, Skoog M: Ambulation in patients with myelomeningocele: a multivariate statistical analysis, *J Pediatr Orthop* 8:569-575, 1988.

67. Seller MJ: The cause of neural tube defects: some experiments and a hypothesis, *J Med Genet* 20:164, 1983.

68. Sharrad WJW: Spinal osteotomy for congenital kyphosis in myelomeningocele, *J Bone Joint Surg Am* 50:466, 1968.

69. Shurtleff DB, Lemire RJ, Warkany J: Embryology, etiology, and epidemiology. In Shurtleff DB, ed: *Myelodysplasias and extrophies: significance prevention and treatment*, New York, 1986, Grune & Stratton, p. 39.

70. Smithells RW, Sheppard S, Scorah CJ: Vitamin deficiencies and neural tube defects, *Arch Dis Child* 51:944-950, 1976.

71. Stone DH et al.: Declining prevalence of hydrocephalus, *Eur J Epidemiol* 53:398, 1989.

72. Tachdjian MO: *Pediatric orthopaedics*, Philadelphia, 1990, WB Saunders.

73. Uchino A, Mori T, Ohno M: Thickened fatty filum terminale: MR imaging, *Neuroradiology* 33:331-333, 1991.

74. Vandertop WP et al.: Surgical decompression of the symptomatic Chiari II malformation in neonates with myelomeningocele, *J Neurosurg* 77:541, 1992.

75. Venes JL, Stevens EA: Surgical pathology in tethered cord secondary to myelomeningocele repair: implications for initial closure technique, *Concepts Pediatr Neurosurg* 4:165, 1983.

76. Wright RL: Congenital dermal sinuses, *Progr Neurol Surg* 4:175, 1971.

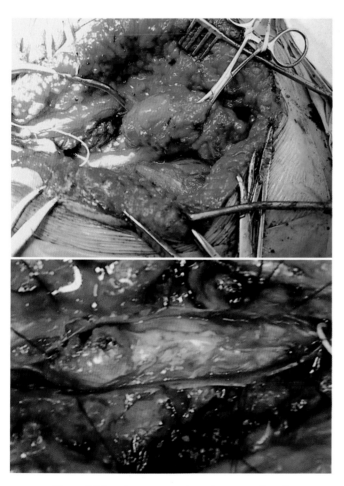

Plate 47-1.　**A** and **B,** Posterior lumbar skin appendage in an infant with type I split cord malformation.

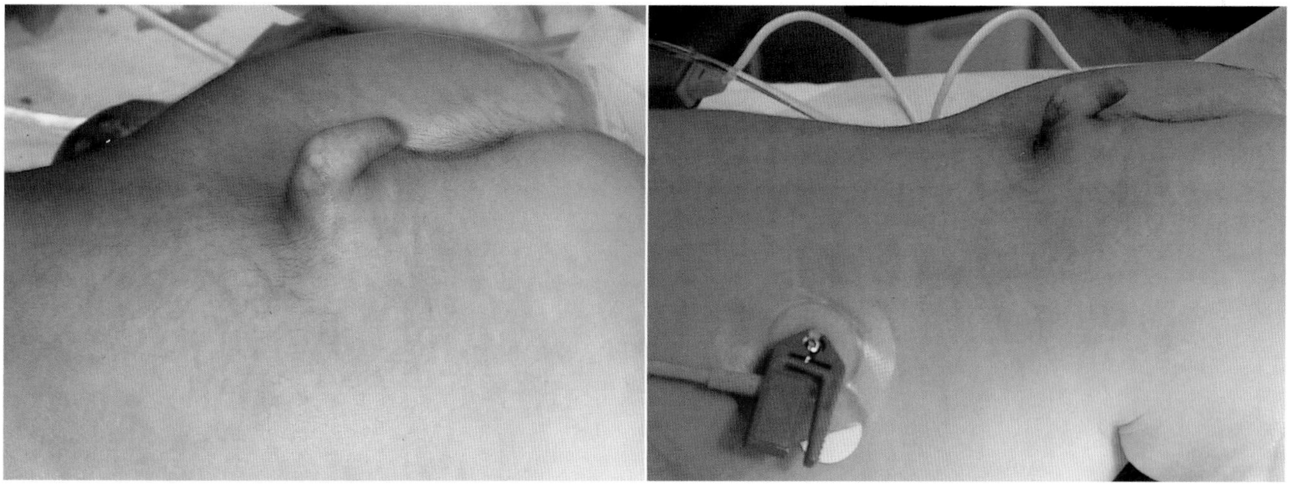

Plate 47-2.　Intraoperative photographs of lumbar lipomyelomeningocele.

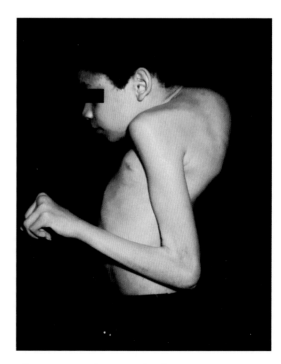

Plate 47-3.　Photograph of adolescent patient with Chiari type I.

Skeletal Dysplasia

Peter G. Gabos

Management of spinal deformity in a patient with a skeletal dysplasia is a challenging undertaking. Recognition that a skeletal dysplasia is not a localized skeletal abnormality but rather a generalized *systemic* abnormality is critical to avoid potentially disastrous outcomes. The timing and selection of surgical procedures for spinal deformity will vary according to each patient's underlying diagnosis and clinical manifestations. Underlying medical fragility can complicate surgical treatment, such as an underlying cardiovascular abnormality in Marfan syndrome, or thrombotic tendencies in homocystinuria. Often, attention may be directed to an area of obvious deformity, such as a severe thoracic kyphoscoliosis, leaving a less obvious but no less important anomaly, such as odontoid hypoplasia, unnoticed. A full understanding of the patient's underlying disorder that extends beyond the musculoskeletal system, often with the help of a multidisciplinary team approach, is a prerequisite for the safe and effective management of spinal deformity in the various skeletal dysplasias.

MARFAN SYNDROME

Introduction

Marfan syndrome represents one of the more common generalized disorders of connective tissue, characterized by abnormalities of the ocular, cardiovascular, and musculoskeletal systems. Management of spinal deformity in this disorder may pose several treatment challenges due to the potential for abnormalities at virtually every level of the axial skeleton.

Epidemiology

The prevalence of Marfan syndrome has been estimated to be 1 in 10,000 in the United States,[12] without racial or ethnic predilection. Marfan syndrome is inherited as an autosomal dominant disorder, with a wide range of pleiotropism and clinical variability. Males and females appear to be affected equally, and as many as 25% of cases arise as new mutations.

Etiology

The genetic basis for Marfan syndrome has recently been elucidated, and involves a mutation in the fibrillin-1 gene (FBN1) located on the long arm of chromosome 15 (15q21.1).[11,17,23] Fibrillin is a large glycoprotein that is an element of the microfibrillar system of elastic tissues that are commonly affected in Marfan syndrome, including the suspensory ligament of the ocular lens, aorta, and periosteum.

Clinical Features

The diagnostic criteria for Marfan syndrome include a positive family history and characteristic abnormalities of the ocular, cardiovascular, and musculoskeletal systems. Although genetic analysis may establish the diagnosis, a combination of any two of these features is considered diagnostic. The major criteria include, but are not limited to, ectopia lentis (superolateral subluxation of the lens), aortic dilatation, scoliosis, and chest wall deformity (pectus excavatum or carinatum). Minor criteria include arachnodactyly, increased metacarpal index, positive thumb sign, positive wrist sign, dolichostenomelia, crossed knee sign, generalized ligamentous laxity, tall stature, dolichocephaly, long narrow facies, high-arched palate, myopia, retinal detachment, and mitral valve prolapse. The application of the term

---

DIAGNOSTIC CRITERIA
FOR MARFAN SYNDROME

Two or more of the following major criteria
- Positive family history (may now include presence of a detected mutation in FBNI known to cause Marfan syndrome)
- Ectopia lentis
- Aortic dilation
- Scoliosis
- Pectus excavatum or carinatum

For the index case
- If family/genetic history not contributory: Major criteria in at least two organ systems plus involvement of a third organ system
- If a mutation known to cause Marfan syndrome in other family members is detected: One major criterion in an organ system and involvement in a second organ system

From *Pediatrics* 98(5):978-982, 1996.

forme fruste to individuals who manifest only few or minor features of the Marfan phenotype has been criticized, and should likely be abandoned.

Radiographic Features

Radiographic survey of a patient with Marfan syndrome, as expected, may reveal many of the skeletal manifestations of the disorder. When considering operative treatment of spinal deformities in these patients, one must pay particular attention to identifying the presence of any of the myriad of spinal abnormalities, alone or in combination, that have been described in Marfan syndrome, and that are elucidated below.

Spinal Deformities

Spinal involvement is seen in up to 75% of patients with Marfan syndrome, and includes coronal and sagittal plane deformities such as scoliosis; thoracic lordosis and thoracic, thoracolumbar, and lumbar kyphosis; spondylolisthesis; dural ectasia; meningocele formation; and cervical spine abnormalities, either alone or in combination. Back pain may be a common associated complaint. Evaluation of the spine in Marfan syndrome therefore requires careful scrutiny from the occiput to the sacrum to assess for these abnormalities. As well, these patients require thorough evaluation by an ophthalmologist and cardiologist due to associated ocular, cardiovascular, and pulmonary anomalies. Such scrutiny is critical if surgical intervention is contemplated; however, most surgeons agree that surgery is not contraindicated in cases of such associated anomalies.

Scoliosis

Scoliosis represents the most common spinal disorder in Marfan syndrome, characteristically presenting in the first decade. The various patterns of curvature are similar to those seen in idiopathic scoliosis, with a somewhat higher incidence of double major thoracolumbar curves. Progression of curvature appears to be more rapid and stiffer curves may be seen. Accordingly, bracing may be indicated for relatively smaller curves in young patients, although most authors have contended that bracing is largely ineffective in halting the progression of curvature. Curves greater than 45 degrees should be treated with a brace only if surgery is being delayed for some reason.

Surgical treatment of scoliosis in Marfan syndrome is recommended for curves measuring greater than 45 to 50 degrees, or for lesser degrees of curvature demonstrating rapid progression despite bracing. Some authors have identified a high rate of pseudarthrosis and mechanical problems with instrumentation in Marfan patients.[4,27,28] Robins et al.[27] reviewed 64 patients with Marfan syndrome and scoliosis, 14 of whom underwent surgical treatment for curves averaging 75 degrees. Using a combination of meticulous facet fusion of all structural curves, autogenous bone grafting, Harrington instrumentation in 11 of the 14 patients, and postoperative

---

> ### SPINAL ABNORMALITIES IN MARFAN SYNDROME
>
> - Scoliosis
> - Thoracic lordosis
> - Thoracic and thoracolumbar kyphosis
> - Spondylolisthesis
> - Dural ectasia
> - Meningocele
> - Cervical anomalies

> ### SCOLIOSIS IN MARFAN SYNDROME
>
> - Most common spinal deformity
> - Infantile/juvenile presentation common
> - Typical patterns of curvature; double major thoracolumbar curves most frequent
> - All curve components may be structural
> - Rapidly progressive, stiffer curves
> - May be painful

---

immobilization, correction comparable to the average correction seen on preoperative supine bending radiographs was achieved. Five pseudarthroses occurred. Of these, two underwent repair and subsequently fused, two lost correction and one was lost to follow-up. The authors state that the pseudarthrosis rate was no higher in this series than for fusions done for idiopathic scoliosis during the same time period. One additional patient required a two-stage procedure due to excessive intraoperative blood loss, and one deep wound infection occurred. There were no cases of paralysis or death. Savini et al.[28] reported on 17 patients with Marfan syndrome who underwent posterior spinal fusion for severe curves using the Harrington method. Failure of fixation in the form of hook rotation or dislodgement occurred in seven patients. Two cases of pseudarthrosis are described, one in a patient with 180 degrees of scoliosis and 180 degrees of kyphosis who later went on to fuse after multiple procedures. She subsequently died secondary to a cardiac complication. The other pseudarthrosis occurred following "fracture of arthrodesis callus" following a fall, with subsequent rupture of the lamina and hardware failure. Two cases of superficial infection occurred. Birch and Herring[4] described their operative experience in nine patients with Marfan syndrome and spinal deformity. Four patients required revision for multiple pseudarthroses. In these four cases, instrumentation included two patients with Luque-type segmental fixation, and one patient with Harrington instrumentation and segmental wiring. The remaining patients underwent Harrington instrumentation only, with one case of an infected pseudarthrosis. Although the authors proceeded to recommend segmental internal fixation in every patient with Marfan syndrome, their best results were obtained in cases where nonsegmental instrumentation was employed.

A   B   C

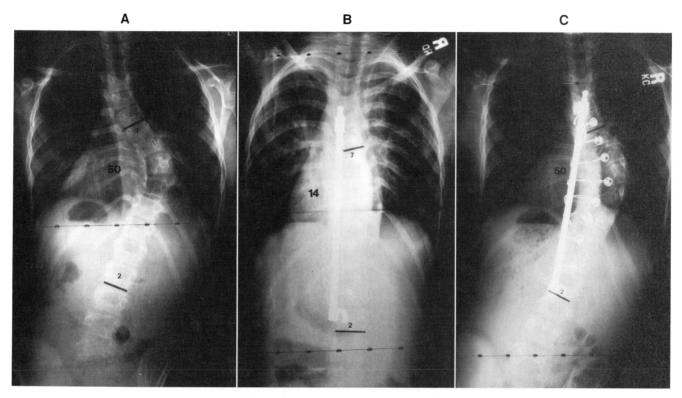

Figure 48-1.   Pseudarthrosis and failure of instrumentation after posterior spinal fusion in a 14-year-old patient with Marfan syndrome. **A,** Preoperative curve measures 50 degrees from T7 to L2. **B,** Postoperatively, correction to 14 degrees is achieved using Harrington instrumentation and spinous process wires. **C,** Pseudarthrosis and subsequent hardware failure ensued with return to previous deformity.

TREATMENT OF SCOLIOSIS IN MARFAN SYNDROME

Nonoperative
- Bracing has limited role/success
- May be indicated for smaller curves (20 degrees) in young patients
- Not indicated for curves greater than 40 to 45 degrees

Operative
- Spinal fusion indicated for curves greater than 45 to 50 degrees
- Pseudarthrosis and instrument failure may be increased
- Include structural curves in the fusion
- Pay meticulous attention to detail
- Consider postoperative immobilization

Postoperative
- Perform frequent radiographic evaluation for pseudarthrosis

In general, it would appear that scoliosis in Marfan syndrome can be successfully treated surgically with a fairly low complication rate. Frequent radiographic surveillance of the spine is required in every patient with Marfan syndrome in whom scoliosis has been detected to allow for surgical treatment before severe deformity ensues. All associated spinal abnormalities must be recognized and addressed where appropriate, especially when surgical correction of scoliosis is planned. Due to the progressive and rigid structural nature of the curves, fusion levels should include all areas of spinal involvement. Secure instrumentation should be employed, and, even in cases where more modern hook and/or pedicle screw and rod segmental spinal fixation are employed, consideration should be given to postoperative immobilization. Frequent radiographic assessment of the fusion mass is required and any areas of pseudarthrosis identified should be addressed (Figures 48-1 to 48-4).

Thoracic Lordosis

Patients with Marfan syndrome may exhibit a reversal of the normal sagittal alignment of the spine, with thoracic lordosis and lumbar kyphosis (Figure 48-5). Thoracic lordosis can be severe, and can lead to cardiopulmonary compromise, especially in cases where concomitant pectus excavatum is present. It is the second most commonly encountered spinal deformity in Marfan syndrome. Winter[36] reported on the use of Harrington distraction rods and sublaminar wires in two patients with severe thoracic lordoscoliosis in Marfan syndrome, with good results. More modern instrumentation systems could likely produce similar results if careful attention to detail is maintained.

Text continued on page 656

Figure 48-2. *For legend, see opposite page.*

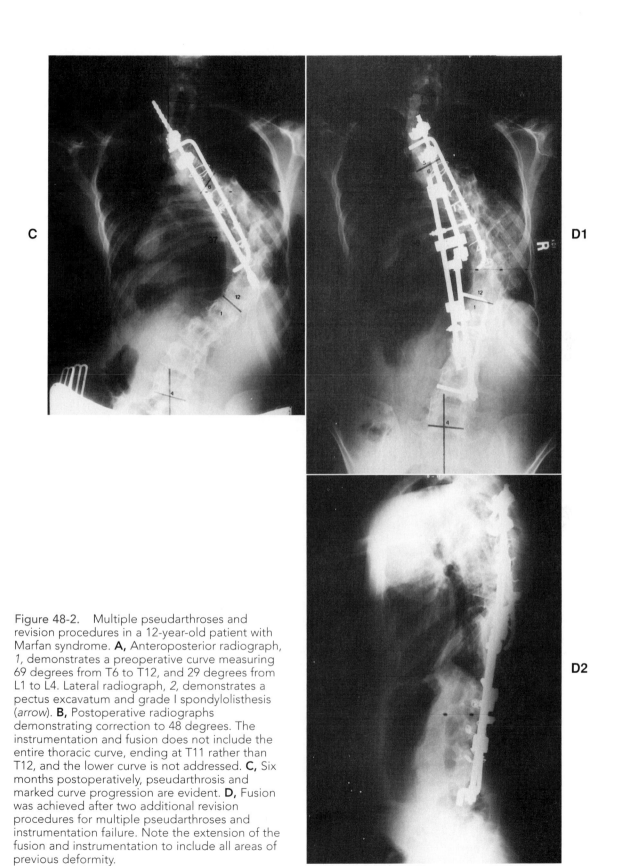

Figure 48-2.   Multiple pseudarthroses and revision procedures in a 12-year-old patient with Marfan syndrome. **A,** Anteroposterior radiograph, *1,* demonstrates a preoperative curve measuring 69 degrees from T6 to T12, and 29 degrees from L1 to L4. Lateral radiograph, *2,* demonstrates a pectus excavatum and grade I spondylolisthesis (*arrow*). **B,** Postoperative radiographs demonstrating correction to 48 degrees. The instrumentation and fusion does not include the entire thoracic curve, ending at T11 rather than T12, and the lower curve is not addressed. **C,** Six months postoperatively, pseudarthrosis and marked curve progression are evident. **D,** Fusion was achieved after two additional revision procedures for multiple pseudarthroses and instrumentation failure. Note the extension of the fusion and instrumentation to include all areas of previous deformity.

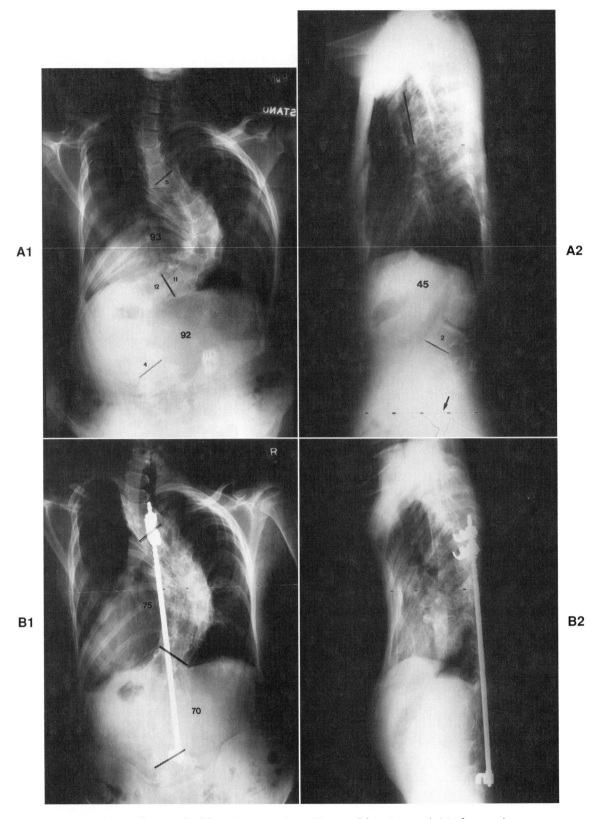

Figure 48-3.   Severe double major curve in a 15-year-old patient with Marfan syndrome.
A, Anteroposterior radiograph, *1,* demonstrates a preoperative curve measuring 93
degrees from T5 to T11, and a 92-degree curve from T12 to L4. Lateral radiograph, *2,*
demonstrates reversal of the normal sagittal contour, with narrowed anteroposterior chest
diameter and a 45-degree thoracolumbar kyphosis. A grade III spondylolisthesis is
present at L5 to S1 *(arrow).* **B,** Although residual deformity remains, solid fusion was
achieved using meticulous fusion technique and nonsegmental Harrington
instrumentation followed by 6 months of postoperative casting.

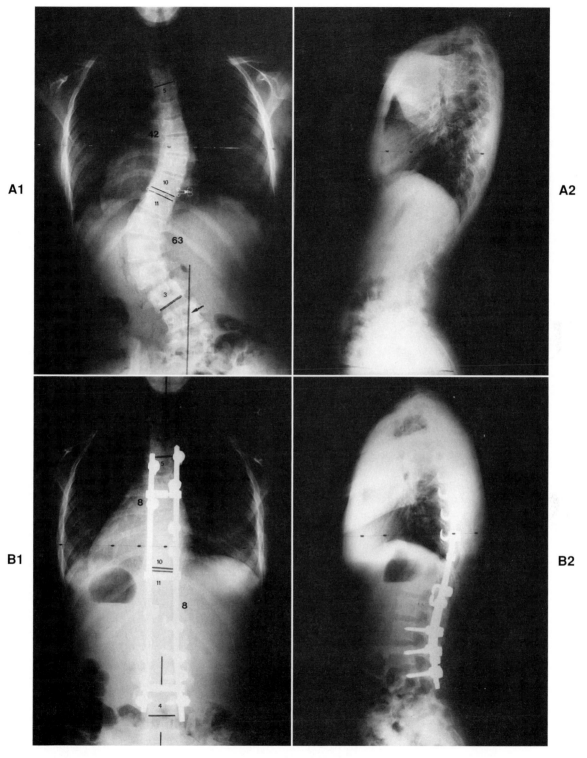

Figure 48-4.   Double major curve in an 11-year-old patient with Marfan syndrome. **A,** Preoperative radiographs demonstrate a 42-degree curve from T5 to T10 and a 63-degree curve from T11 to L3. The center sacral line (arrow) most nearly bisects L4, and there is marked translation of the thorax to the left. **B,** Postoperative radiographs following posterior spinal fusion with segmental instrumentation from T5 to L4. Solid fusion with restored coronal and sagittal balance was achieved. More modern instrumentation constructs do not, however, replace meticulous attention to fusion technique.

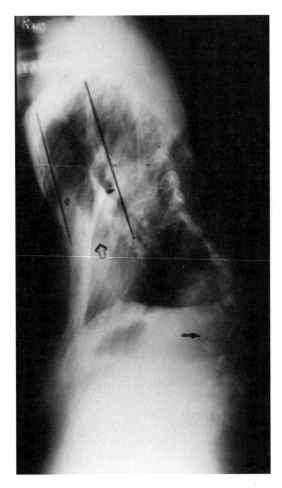

Figure 48-5. Lateral radiograph demonstrating reversal of the normal sagittal spinal alignment, with thoracic lordosis (*small solid arrow*) and pectus excavatum (*small open arrow*), resulting in a narrowed anteroposterior chest diameter (*large open arrow*). Thoracolumbar kyphosis is evident (*large solid arrow*).

Thoracic and Thoracolumbar Kyphosis

Kyphosis in the thoracic and thoracolumbar spine has also been reported in Marfan syndrome. End-plate irregularities may mimic those seen in Scheuermann's disease. When severe kyphosis is present in conjunction with scoliosis, the addition of anterior procedures may be necessary when surgical correction of scoliosis is planned. In the report by Birch and Herring,[4] one patient with a primary thoracolumbar kyphosis required reoperation for a pseudarthrosis that occurred after posterior spinal fusion using Luque segmental fixation. Amis and Herring[2] reported a case of iatrogenic kyphosis in a patient with Marfan syndrome who underwent distraction by Harrington instrumentation. The authors attributed the facet dislocation and disc-space disruption to reduced tensile strength of the tissues.

Spondylolisthesis

Spondylolisthesis has been infrequently reported in Marfan syndrome. Although uncommon, the reported cases have been severe. Savini et al.[28] reported one case of spondyloptosis in a 7-year-old girl with Marfan syndrome who subsequently underwent reduction of the slip and posterior spinal fusion using Harrington instrumentation from T3 to the sacrum for progression of scoliosis to 80 degrees. Winter[34] reported two cases of spondyloptosis. Both were treated successfully with the Gill procedure and posterolateral fusion, although the indication for the decompression was unclear. One of the patients was noted to have a 27-degree right thoracic scoliosis that improved on the supine preoperative radiograph. This olisthetic scoliosis resolved after the treatment of the spondyloptosis. Taylor[33] reported on an 11-year-old girl with Marfan syndrome who had a 70-degree scoliosis and a grade IV spondylolisthesis. The patient's spondylolisthesis was treated by posterior fusion and the Gill procedure, followed by a two-stage anterior and posterior spinal fusion using Harrington instrumentation 1 year later.

Dural Ectasia and Meningocele

Several authors have described the presence of dural ectasia as a common finding in Marfan syndrome. Pyeritz et al.[26] found widening of the lumbosacral canal in 63% of 57 patients with Marfan syndrome who underwent computed tomography (CT) scanning for some other clinical indication. They described bony abnormalities ranging from mild thinning of the pedicles and foraminal erosion to near total erosion of the pedicle and meningocele formation. Several other reports have verified meningocele formation in the sacral, lumbar, and thoracic spine. The etiology is thought to involve abnormal dural structure, with subsequent dilatation from cerebrospinal fluid pressure.

Cervical Anomalies

There are scant reports of cervical spine abnormalities in Marfan syndrome. Yajnik et al.[37] reported a case of basilar impression in a 16-year-old male with Marfan syndrome, manifested as persistent occipital headaches and visual disturbance. Levander et al.[19] reported atlantoaxial instability in a 24-year-old female with Marfan syndrome with progressive neurologic involvement that resolved after posterior occipitocervical fusion. Hobbs et al.[15] noted that 54% of 104 patients with Marfan syndrome who underwent lateral neutral and flexion-extension cervical spine radiographs had increased atlantoaxial translation. Sixteen percent of patients had cervical kyphosis and 36% had basilar impression. However, complaints of neck pain did not differ significantly from that of age-matched controls. In spite of these abnormalities, the frequency of neurologic compromise in Marfan syndrome is rare, but the risk of neurologic damage from trauma may be theoretically increased.

Conclusions

Spinal abnormalities are frequently encountered in Marfan syndrome. Although attention is often given to the scoliosis due to its rapid progression and rigidity, careful scrutiny for the myriad of spinal abnormalities described is critical when surgical intervention is planned. Preoperative evaluation for any ocular, cardiovascular, or pulmonary abnormality is required. Although a high rate of pseudarthrosis and instrumentation failure has been noted by some authors in patients undergoing spinal fusion for scoliosis in Marfan syndrome, good results should be attainable with attention to meticulous fusion technique, selection of proper fusion levels, and secure instrumentation.

NEUROFIBROMATOSIS
Introduction

Neurofibromatosis is a multisystemic, hereditary disease involving components of the neuroectoderm, mesoderm, and endoderm. Accordingly, various manifestations of the disorder can include abnormalities of the skin, nervous system, skeleton, and soft tissue. Neurofibromatosis has recently been classified into two clinical forms. Neurofibromatosis-1 (NF-1), so-called peripheral neurofibromatosis, is the more common type, and is characterized by café-au-lait macules, neurofibromas, optic gliomas, iris hamartomas, and musculoskeletal abnormalities. Neurofibromatosis-2 (NF-2), so-called central neurofibromatosis, is characterized by bilateral schwannomas of the vestibular portion of cranial nerve VIII, although schwannomas of other peripheral nerves may occur, as well as meningiomas and ependymomas. NF-2 does not appear to have any spinal or other orthopedic manifestations, and dermal lesions are unusual. None of the eighth cranial nerve tumors are found in NF-1.

Epidemiology

Neurofibromatosis is the most common single-gene disorder of humans, affecting nearly 1 million people worldwide. NF-1 has been found to affect approximately 1 in 4000 individuals. It is inherited as an autosomal dominant disorder, with variable penetrance and a reportedly high rate of spontaneous mutation. NF-2 is the less common form, affecting approximately 1 in 100,000 individuals.

Etiology

The gene locus of NF-1 has been linked to the long arm of chromosome 17. NF-2 has been localized on the long arm of chromosome 22.

Clinical Features

NF-1 can be easily distinguished from NF-2 by the absence of cranial nerve tumors, and characteristic abnormalities of the skin, nervous system, and musculoskeletal system. The diagnostic criteria for NF-1 are met in an individual if two or more of the following are found: six or more café-au-lait macules over 5 mm in greatest diameter in prepubertal individuals and over 15 mm in greatest diameter in postpubertal individuals;

DIAGNOSTIC CRITERIA FOR NF-1

Two or more of the following:
- Six or more café-au-lait macules >5 mm in diameter if prepubertal; >15 mm in diameter if postpubertal
- Two or more neurofibromas or one plexiform neurofibroma
- Axillary or inguinal freckling
- Optic glioma
- Two or more Lisch nodules (iris hamartomas)
- Distinctive osseous lesion such as sphenoid dysplasia or thinning of a long bone cortex with or without pseudarthrosis
- First-degree relative with NF-1

---

two or more neurofibromas of any type or one plexiform neurofibroma; axillary or inguinal freckling; optic glioma; two or more Lisch nodules (iris hamartomas); a distinct osseous lesion such as sphenoid dysplasia or thinning of a long bone cortex with or without pseudarthrosis; a first-degree relative with NF-1.[25]

Radiographic Features

Radiographic survey of a patient with neurofibromatosis should include anteroposterior and lateral views of the entire axial skeleton, to assess for cervical, thoracic, and lumbosacral deformity. Oblique radiographs are helpful in areas where dystrophic changes exist. When necessary, CT and magnetic resonance imaging (MRI) have been useful adjuncts for visualizing the spinal abnormalities in neurofibromatosis in greater detail. These abnormalities are outlined in the following discussion.

Spinal Deformities

Spinal deformities are seen in up to 60% of patients with neurofibromatosis, and include coronal and sagittal plane deformities such as scoliosis and kyphosis; spondylolisthesis; and cervical spine abnormalities and lesions related to spinal cord tumors and abnormal pressure phenomena in and around the spinal canal neuraxis, such as meningoceles, pseudomeningoceles, dural ectasia, and dumbbell lesions. The spinal deformities in neurofibromatosis have been classified into dystrophic and nondystrophic types. Dystrophic changes include rib-penciling (likely due to severe rib rotation in the anteroposterior direction), spindling of the transverse processes, vertebral scalloping, severe apical rotation, foraminal enlargement, and paravertebral neurofibromas, and have been found to be important in the prognosis and management of spinal deformity.[35]

Scoliosis

Scoliosis is the most common osseous defect associated with neurofibromatosis, characteristically presenting in the first and second decade. A single thoracic curve of fewer than six segments has been identified as the most common curve pattern, and right and left

---

SPINAL ABNORMALITIES IN NEUROFIBROMATOSIS

- Scoliosis (dystrophic, nondystrophic)
- Kyphoscoliosis
- Thoracic lordosis
- Spondylolisthesis
- Cervical anomalies
- Meningocele, dural ectasia, dumbbell lesions

RISK FACTORS FOR SUBSTANTIAL PROGRESSION OF DYSTROPHIC CURVES

- Early age at onset
- High Cobb angle at initial presentation (>26 degrees)
- Abnormal kyphosis
- Vertebral scalloping
- Severe apical rotation in upper thoracic curves
- Rib penciling on concave side, both sides, or of >4 ribs

SCOLIOSIS IN NEUROFIBROMATOSIS

- Most common spinal deformity
- Short (<6 segments) thoracic curves most common
- Nondystrophic curves similar to idiopathic scoliosis
- Nondystrophic curves may develop dystrophic features (modulation)
- Dystrophic curves have worse prognosis, different management
- Neurologic compromise uncommon if kyphosis is absent, unless intraspinal lesion is present

---

TREATMENT OF DYSTROPHIC CURVES

Nonoperative
- Bracing ineffective
- No justification for observing progressive deformity

Operative

Nonkyphotic dystrophic curves
- Posterior spinal fusion for nonkyphotic curves measuring 20 to 40 degrees (consider planned reinforcement of graft at 6 months)
- Combined anterior/posterior fusion for nonkyphotic curves greater than 50 to 60 degrees
- Segmental spinal instrumentation is recommended, but use MRI to evaluate for intraspinal pathology

Kyphotic dystrophic curves
- Combined anterior/posterior fusion if kyphosis >50 degrees
- Pseudarthrosis rate high, especially if only posterior fusion performed

---

convex thoracic curves appear to occur in equal numbers. Early identification of dystrophic curves is critical due to the different prognosis and management.

Nondystrophic curves in neurofibromatosis appear to be similar to curves seen in idiopathic scoliosis, and can be managed similarly. However, it is important to recognize that there is considerable potential for a nondystrophic curve to develop dystrophic features during childhood.[9] It is possible that such patients are too young at initial evaluation to demonstrate the osseous manifestations of vertebral dystrophy, or that modulation across a spectrum of nondystrophic to dystrophic changes occurs.[7] Funasaki et al.[13] identified four different natural histories in the development of dystrophic changes in neurofibromatosis: no dystrophic features at presentation, but development of dystrophic changes over time; no change in dystrophic features apparent at initial presentation; progression of dysplastic lesions but no spreading to adjacent areas over time; and spreading and progression of dystrophic changes over time.

There are few reports on the natural history of progression of dystrophic curves. Winter et al.[35] and Funasaki et al.[13] found that dystrophic curves progressed by a mean of 5 degrees per year. Risk factors for substantial progression of the curve were an early age at onset, high Cobb angle at initial presentation (greater than 26 degrees), abnormal kyphosis, vertebral scalloping, severe rotation at the apex of the curve in the middle or caudal thoracic region, penciling of one or more ribs on the concave side or on both sides of the curve, and penciling of four or more ribs.

Bracing for dystrophic curves in neurofibromatosis has been found to be ineffective in halting the progression of curvature.[35] There is no justification for observation of a progressively increasing spinal deformity in neurofibromatosis. Operative stabilization by spinal fusion, with or without instrumentation, is the treatment of choice for dystrophic curves; when operative stabilization is performed promptly, good results can be achieved. Nonkyphotic dystrophic curves measuring greater than 20 to 40 degrees, even in very young patients, can be treated with posterior procedures alone. Winter et al.[35] has recommended planned reinforcement of the graft at 6 months for more dystrophic curve patterns. In their study, only two pseudarthroses occurred in 34 patients with nonkyphotic dystrophic curves treated by posterior surgical procedures, both of which subsequently fused with a single posterior repair. Crawford[8] reported a pseudarthrosis rate of 13% in 46 patients with dystrophic curves treated by posterior fusion alone. Accordingly, he has recommended posterior spinal fusion with segmental spinal instrumentation for all dystrophic curves measuring greater than 20 to 40 degrees, and combined anterior and posterior procedures for dystrophic curves measuring greater than 50 to 60 degrees.

Kyphoscoliosis

Spinal deformities in the sagittal plane are commonly seen in neurofibromatosis, and have been divided into two typical patterns: (1) kyphoscoliosis with acute angulation (gibbus) and marked dystrophic changes and (2) so-called kyphosing scoliosis (a scoliosis with so much rotation [90 degrees] that progression is only evident on the lateral roentgenogram) with a more rounded kyphosis.[13] In some cases, the vertebrae at the apex of the kyphosis can be so distorted as to resemble congenital kyphosis. Kyphosis has been implicated as a cause of paraplegia in neurofibromatosis.[10,21,24,35]

Winter et al.[35] reported a pseudarthrosis rate of 64% of patients with dystrophic scoliosis associated with kyphosis greater than 50 degrees who underwent only posterior surgical procedures. Attempts at posterior pseudarthrosis repair were uniformly unsuccessful in achieving fusion. The authors recommended combined anterior and posterior procedures for all dystrophic curves associated with kyphosis greater than 50 degrees, and emphasized complete anterior disc excision along the entire structural area of the deformity, use of fibular strut grafts, and massive autogenous bone grafting. For severe deformities, preoperative halo-femoral traction proved to be a useful adjunct to anterior and posterior procedures. Crawford[9] recommended a similar approach, advocating anterior fusion one or two levels past both end vertebrae in the kyphotic region, with reexploration and augmentation of the posterior fusion mass at 6 months if radiographic studies demonstrate any evidence of weakness of the fusion mass or pseudarthrosis.

Anterior decompression is required for spinal cord compromise due to kyphosis. Laminectomy is never indicated in such circumstances. The inciting pathology is anterior, and removal of the posterior elements eliminates valuable bone stock required for posterior fusion and predisposes the spine to further kyphosis, with catastrophic outcome. Evaluation for an intraspinal lesion (tumor or meningocele) by preoperative MRI should always be undertaken as a possible causative factor of neurologic compromise and, if present, addressed accordingly.

Lordoscoliosis

Although infrequently reported, thoracic lordosis (hypokyphosis) may occur in neurofibromatosis. Winter et al.[35] described this deformity in 5 of 80 patients with dystrophic curves. Deformity correction using instrumentation is challenging in such patients, and must take into account dysplastic thinning of the posterior elements in the region to be instrumented.

Spondylolisthesis

Spondylolisthesis in association with neurofibromatosis has been infrequently reported. In most cases, the deformity has been attributed to erosions of the pedicles or pars interarticularis secondary to dural ectasia with meningoceles or foraminal neurofibroma. Instrumentation in such cases should be discouraged, due to the abnormal bone stock. Crawford[7] recommended posterior spinal fusion and prolonged pantaloon cast immobilization in hyperextension, with augmentation of the fusion mass at 6 months if necessary.

Cervical Anomalies

Cervical spine deformity in neurofibromatosis has received scant attention in the literature. Yong-Hing et al.[38] noted cervical deformity in 17 of 56 patients with neurofibromatosis, which was often associated with severe scoliosis. Cervical kyphosis or hypolordosis has been the most commonly described deformity; however, atlantoaxial or subaxial subluxation may occur. The presence of a severe scoliosis or kyphosis in the thoracic or lumbar spine may direct attention away from this important consideration. All patients with neurofibromatosis require cervical radiographs to evaluate for the presence of any cervical spine pathology, especially if surgery for scoliosis is contemplated. If any pathology is noted, even in asymptomatic patients, MRI should be considered (Figure 48-6).

Meningoceles, Dural Ectasia, and Dumbbell Lesions

Meningoceles (protrusion of the spinal meninges through an intervertebral foramen or bony defect), dural ectasia (saccular dilatations of the dura), and dumbbell lesions (intraspinal neurofibromas) result from the presence of neurofibromas or other pressure-inducing phenomena in or around the spinal neuraxis. The presence of such lesions leads to erosive changes in the vertebrae, which may appear radiographically as scalloping and indentation of vertebral bodies, pedicle deformities, widening of intervertebral foramina, instability, protrusion of ribs into the spinal canal, and even frank vertebral column dislocation (Figure 48-7). Intrathoracic meningoceles can result from protrusion of the meninges through eroded foramina, and may appear as a large density on chest radiographs (Figure 48-8). MRI has proved invaluable for the identification of intraspinal lesions and for evaluation of cord compression. Major and Huizenga[22] used CT scanning to demonstrate cord impingement due to the penetration of ribs into the spinal canal.

Because of the spinal canal widening that often accompanies such anomalies, severe angular deformities of the spine may occur without neurologic compromise. Spinal instrumentation and fusion in the presence of an unsuspected lesion can nonetheless result in neurologic catastrophe when laminar erosion or cord impingement is present. Winter et al.[34] described two cases of spinal cord injury that resulted from direct contusion by a periosteal elevator during surgical exposure of the spine. A preoperative MRI is therefore recommended for all cases where spinal fusion is planned, even in the neurologically intact patient.

When neurologic compromise exists, especially in the absence of significant kyphosis, an intraspinal lesion must be ruled out (Figure 48-9). In the series by Winter et al.,[35] cord compression in a scoliotic spine without kyphosis was always due to an intraspinal tumor. When spinal cord impingement is demonstrated, the lesion should be addressed directly, either anteriorly with

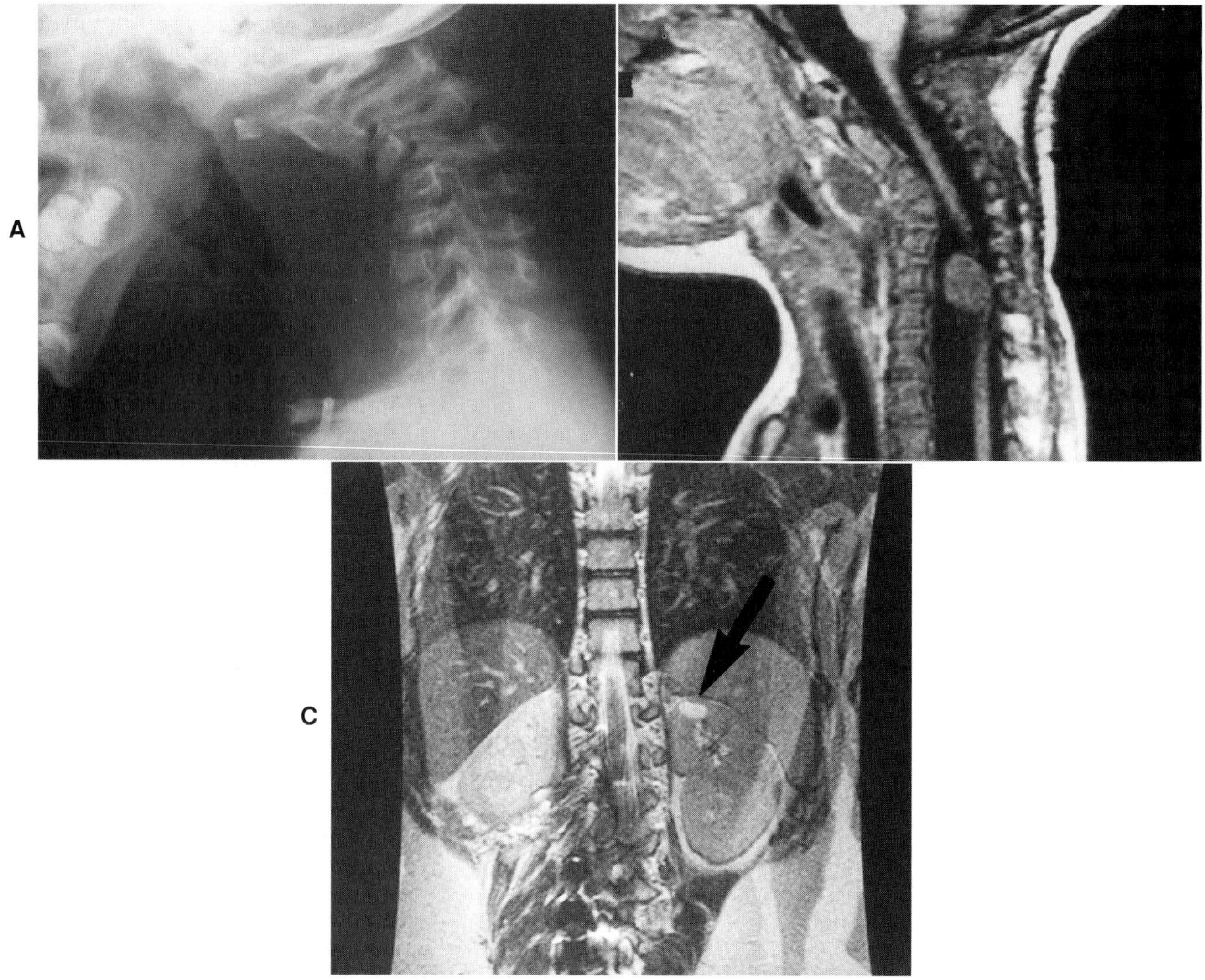

Figure 48-6. Three-year-old patient with neurofibromatosis and severe scoliosis. **A,** Detailed radiographic evaluation revealed a marked cervical kyphosis. **B,** MRI demonstrates a large cord lesion within the cervical spine. **C,** The patient died at the age of 13 years from a marked hypertensive crisis associated with renal artery stenosis. A kidney lesion is noted *(arrow).*

PATIENTS WITH NEUROLOGIC COMPROMISE

- MRI to evaluate for intraspinal lesion (meningocele, dural ectasia, dumbbell lesions)
- If secondary to tumor, approach directly; decompression without fusion *never* indicated
- If secondary to kyphosis, anterior decompression and fusion; laminectomy *never* indicated

---

partial corpectomy for anterior lesions or posteriorly with hemilaminectomy for posterior lesions. Decompression without fusion is never indicated due to the potential for the creation of severe deformity. Winter et al.[35] described six patients who underwent laminectomy without fusion for tumor removal in an area of dystrophic spinal deformity. In all six patients severe progressive deformity developed, resulting in cord compression in three of the patients.

Conclusions

Spinal anomalies are common in neurofibromatosis. Identification of dystrophic features, including abnormal kyphosis, is critical for the safe management of scoliosis in this disorder. Neurologic compromise can result from severe kyphosis or intraspinal tumor, and erosion of posterior elements or space-occupying lesions increase the chances for iatrogenic spinal cord injury when fusion and instrumentation are planned. Severe deformity can detract attention from other areas of spinal pathology, including the cervical spine. Careful preoperative assessment and planning, with judicious use of plain radiographs and MRI, can help the surgeon avoid neurologic catastrophe.

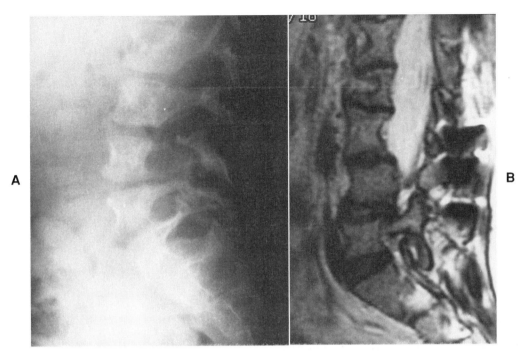

Figure 48-7. Eight-year-old patient with neurofibromatosis. **A,** Lateral radiograph of the lumbosacral spine demonstrates vertebral scalloping and foraminal enlargement. **B,** MRI demonstrates the presence of saccular dilatations of the dura (dural ectasia).

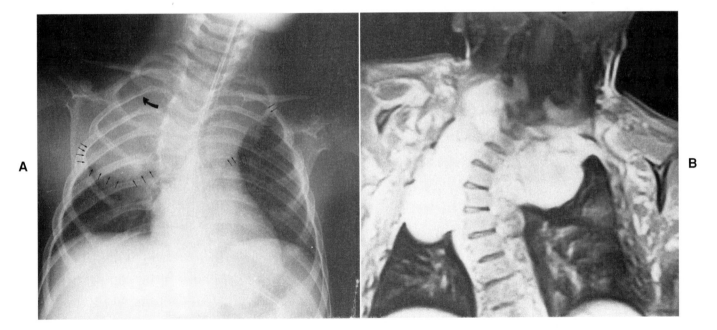

Figure 48-8. Intrathoracic meningocele in a 5-year-old patient with neurofibromatosis. **A,** Large intrathoracic densities are present on an anteroposterior chest radiograph *(small arrows)*. Dystrophic changes of the ribs are also apparent *(large arrow)*. **B,** MRI demonstrates the extent of the protruding meninges.

MUCOPOLYSACCHARIDOSES

The mucopolysaccharidoses represent a group of genetic disorders in which there is a deficiency of a specific lysosomal enzyme responsible for the degradation of the sulfated glycosamine glycans (heparan sulfate, dermatan sulfate, and keratan sulfate) (Table 48-1). The mucopolysaccharides, in conjunction with collagen, form the matrix of connective tissue. Their incomplete breakdown leads to an accumulation of a degradation product within the lysosomes of tissues such as the brain, viscera, and joints, resulting in characteristic clinical features.

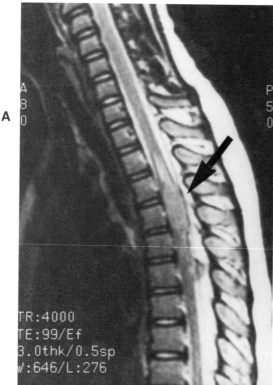

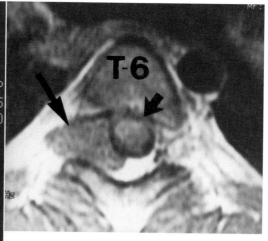

Figure 48-9.   Ten-year-old patient with neurofibromatosis and scoliosis. Acute change in her neurologic examination prompted MRI evaluation of her brain and spine. **A,** Extensive involvement by tumor is noted in the upper and middle thoracic spine on the sagittal images. **B,** Transverse image at T6 reveals both intradural and extradural tumor.

The mucopolysaccharidoses are rare disorders. They are transmitted by autosomal recessive inheritance, except for mucopolysaccharidosis (MPS) II (Hunter's syndrome), which is X-linked. The most commonly encountered forms are MPS I-H (Hurler's syndrome), MPS III (Sanfilippo's syndrome), and MPS IV (Morquio's syndrome).

Urine screening, using a toluidine blue spot test, allows early identification of a mucopolysaccharidosis, which can be further classified by specific blood testing. Chemical abnormalities can usually be detected by the age of 6 to 12 months, and the clinical appearance is usually well established by the age of 2 to 3 years.

In general, these patients exhibit coarse and thickened facial features, short stature, and stiff joints, with particularly severe involvement of the hands. Radiographs typically demonstrate pelvic and spinal anomalies, including wide, flattened ilia with large acetabula, coxa valga, ossification defects of the femoral heads, ovoid vertebral bodies with anterior projections (platyspondyly), thoracolumbar kyphosis, and odontoid hypoplasia (Figure 48-10). As in all skeletal dysplasias, careful evaluation for cervical instability is required prior to any surgical intervention.

The spectrum of involvement in the mucopolysaccharidoses is extremely variable. In some, such as MPS I-H, life expectancy is extremely short, whereas in others, such as MPS I-S (Scheie's syndrome), a normal life expectancy may be anticipated. As the prospect for treatments such as enzyme replacement therapy or bone marrow transplantation improves, significant changes in life expectancy for all of the MPS syndromes may be realized.

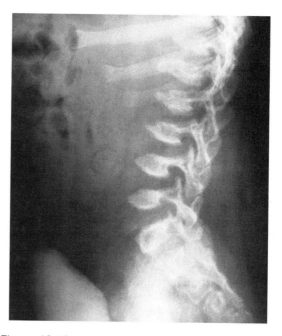

Figure 48-10.   Lateral lumbosacral radiograph of a 17-year-old patient with Morquio's syndrome demonstrating ovoid vertebral bodies with anterior projections (platyspondyly).

Thoracolumbar kyphosis has been noted in most MPS types to varying degrees, and may be progressive (Figure 48-11). In most cases, however, neurologic compromise from progressive thoracolumbar kyphosis has not been demonstrated, with the exception of MPS IV (Morquio's

Table 48-1 Mucopolysaccharidoses and Mucolipidoses

MPS	Enzyme Defect	Mucopolysacchariduria	Inheritance	Lifespan	Intelligence	Comments
I-H (Hurler)	α-L-Iduronidase	Dermatan/heparan sulfate	AR	6 to 10 yr	MR	Kyphosis, odontoid hypoplasia
I-S (Scheie)	α -L-Iduronidase	Dermatan/heparan sulfate	AR	Normal	Normal	No kyphosis
I-H/S (Hurler/Scheie)	α -L-Iduronidase	Dermatan/heparan sulfate	AR	20s	Mild MR	No kyphosis
II severe (Hunter)	Sulfoiduronide sulfatase	Dermatan/heparan sulfate	X-R	Teens	MR	Kyphosis
II mild (Hunter)	Sulfoiduronide sulfatase	Dermatan/heparan sulfate	X-R	Normal	normal	Kyphosis
III A (Sanfilippo)	Sulfoglucosamine sulfatase	Heparan sulfate	AR	Teens-20s	MR	Minimal
III B (Sanfilippo)	N-Acetyl-β-D-glusaminidase	Heparan sulfate	AR	Teens-20s	MR	Minimal
III C (Sanfilippo)	Acetyl-CoA:alpha-glucosaminide N-acetyltransferase	Heparan sulfate	AR	Teens 20s	MR	Minimal
III D (Sanfilippo)	N-Acetylglucosamine-6-sulfate sulfatase	Heparan sulfate	AR	Teens-20s	MR	Minimal
IV A (Morquio)	N-Acetylgalactosamine-6-sulfatase	Keratan sulfate	AR	20 to 40	Normal	Odontoid hypoplasia, cervical compression
IV B (Morquio) V (formerly Scheie)	β-Galactosidase		AR	20 to 50	Normal	Milder, but similar to IV A
VI severe (Maroteaux-Lamy)	Sulfogalactosamine sulfatase	Dermatan sulfate	AR	10 to 20	Normal	Cervical myelopathy, lumbar radiculopathy, dural thickening
VI mild (Maroteaux-Lamy)	Sulfogalactosamine sulfatase	Dermatan sulfate	AR	20s-normal	Normal	Milder, but similar to VI severe
VII (Sly)	β-Glucuronidase	Dermatan sulfate	AR	Shortened	MR	T-L kyphosis, kyphoscoliosis

From Kelly TE: The mucopolysaccharidoses and mucolipidoses, *Clin Orthop Rel Res* 114:116-136, 1976.
AR, Autosomal recessive; *MR*, mental retardations; *X-R*, X-linked recessive.

syndrome).[5] Whether progressive kyphosis can, or even should, be halted or reversed in the majority of these disorders is largely unknown. Published reports on the effectiveness of bracing for thoracolumbar kyphosis in the MPS syndromes are lacking. Consideration of bracing may be reasonably entertained for mild to moderate kyphosis so long as it does not impair pulmonary function. Posterior spinal fusion, with or without ante-

rior fusion, may be necessary for severe progressive thoracolumbar kyphosis. Anterior decompression would be indicated in cases of neurologic compromise from thoracolumbar kyphosis. As for all kyphotic deformities, laminectomy is *never* indicated to address spinal cord compromise from kyphosis. As prospects for systemic treatments and thus life expectancy improve for the MPS syndromes, the reasons for prevention of a progressive kyphosis may become more apparent.

Hypoplasia of the odontoid process has been reported in the MPS syndromes, and may result in atlantoaxial instability and neurologic compromise (Figure 48-12). Careful radiographic evaluation of the cervical spine is mandated in all patients with an MPS syndrome prior to any surgical intervention. As well, the progressive nature of the disorder may mandate frequent radiographic surveillance, even in the absence of any neurologic symptoms. This is especially true for MPS IV, in which acute paraparesis, progressive neuropathy, and sudden death from cord compression associated with odontoid hypoplasia are well established.[20,32] The severity of neurologic compromise has recently been attributed to the accumulation of thickened anterior extradural soft tissue rather than the atlantoaxial instability itself.[32] Several authors have recommended early prophylactic posterior cervical fusion. Lipson[20] reported on 11 patients with atlantoaxial instability associated with Morquio's syndrome, and noted poor recovery when fusion was performed after the onset of neurologic symptoms. Stevens et al.[32] proposed prompt occipitocervical fusion for patients demonstrating cord compression from anterior extradural thickening, including asymptomatic patients demonstrating reduction of spinal cord diameter approaching 50%.

Cervical and lumbar radiculopathy and cervical myelopathy have also been reported in MPS VI (Maroteaux-Lamy syndrome), resulting from odontoid

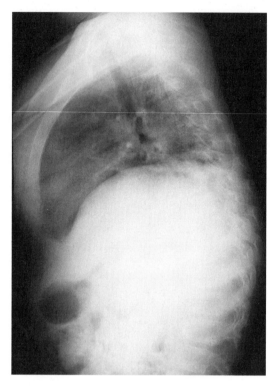

Figure 48-11.   Mild thoracolumbar kyphosis in a 16-year-old patient with Sanfilippo's syndrome.

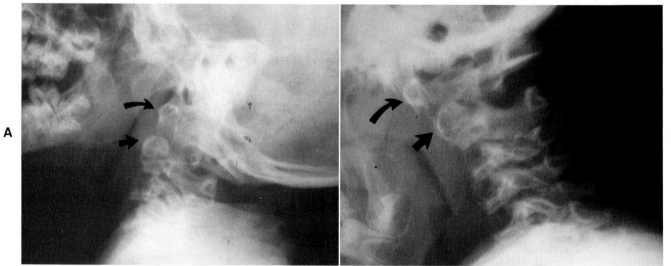

Figure 48-12.   Lateral extension, **A,** and flexion cervical, **B,** radiographs in a 3-year-old patient with Morquio's syndrome. There is odontoid hypoplasia *(straight arrow)*, resulting in increased translation of C1 on C2 *(curved arrow)*.

hypoplasia, dural thickening, narrowing of the subarachnoid space at the occipitocervical junction, protrusion of a dysplastic C1 arch into the foramen magnum, and spinal stenosis due to dural thickening at the lumbosacral junction.[29] Maroteaux-Lamy syndrome is similar clinically to MPS 1 H, except for longer survival and preservation of intelligence. Later skeletal manifestations include kyphoscoliosis and disabling contractures of the hips and knees. Neurosensory deafness, hydrocephalus with attendant visual impairment, congestive heart failure, and recurrent respiratory tract infections are late complications of the disorder.

MUCOLIPIDOSES

The term *mucolipidosis* was coined by Spranger and Weidemann[30] in 1970 to describe a group of lysosomal storage diseases in which combined features of the mucopolysaccharidoses and sphingolipidoses exist. Mucolipidoses are genetic disorders characterized by the excessive accumulation of mucopolysaccharides and sphingolipids in visceral and mesenchymal cells. Clinically and radiographically, the mucolipidoses resemble the MPS syndromes; however, urinary mucopolysaccharide levels are normal and excessive oligosaccharides are excreted in the urine.

Mucolipidosis (ML) I is a neurodegenerative disorder resulting from neuramidase deficiency, and is confirmed by thin-layer chromatography and urine and fibroblast sialic acid levels.[31] ML II (I-cell disease) is an autosomal recessive disorder that resembles Hurler's syndrome, but is clinically apparent at an earlier age with faster progression and earlier death.[18] ML II is due to a deficiency of *N*-acetylglucosaminylphosphorotransferase. Findings of dense cytoplasmic inclusions ("I-cells") in cultured skin fibroblasts are characteristic. ML III (pseudo-Hurler polydystrophy) is an autosomal recessive disorder that appears to be similar to ML II, but onset of clinical signs appears later, and survival well into adult life is possible.[16] The enzymatic defect has not been clearly elucidated. ML IV is a recessive disorder found with high frequency in Ashkenazic Jews, in which electron microscopy reveals typical storage organelles.[1]

Thoracolumbar kyphosis of varying degrees has been reported in the ML syndromes, with no published reports of significant morbidity. Goodman and Pang[14] reported on spinal cord injury from atlantoaxial instability in ML II. No specific recommendations regarding management of spinal deformity in the ML syndromes can be made from the paucity of reports in the literature. As with the MPS syndromes, as prospects for systemic treatments and thus life expectancy improve for the ML syndromes, the reasons for prevention of a progressive kyphosis may become clear.

HOMOCYSTINURIA

Homocystinuria is an autosomal recessive disorder caused by an inborn error of sulfur amino acid (methionine) metabolism, and is characterized clinically by lens dislocation (ectopia lentis), mental retardation, skeletal deformity, and thrombotic tendency. The cause appears to be related to deficiency of cystathionine β-synthetase, the enzyme that sulfurates homocysteine (a metabolite of methionine) to cystathionine, which is converted to cysteine. In the classic form of the disease, methionine and homocysteine accumulate in blood and tissues and are excreted in large amounts in the urine, while urinary cysteine levels are diminished.[3,6]

Affected individuals appear normal at birth, but motor and speech delay or regression is common by 1 year of age. The characteristic facial feature is malar flush, and the hair is often thin and light in color. With growth, the extremities appear long but deficient in muscle, and pectus excavatum or carinatum, arachnodactyly, scoliosis, and kyphoscoliosis may occur.[3]

The skeletal and ocular manifestations of homocystinuria can resemble those of Marfan syndrome, with notable differences. Patients with homocystinuria typically demonstrate inferior ectopia lentis, osteoporosis, biconcave and flattened vertebrae, mental retardation, and severe thrombotic tendencies. Early death from myocardial infarction, pulmonary embolism, mesenteric thrombosis, and cerebral vascular accidents has been reported. Venous thrombosis precipitated by illness or surgery can be fatal.[6]

The most frequent curve pattern of scoliosis in homocystinuria appears to be right thoracic and left lumbar, with the lumbar curve being greater in magnitude.[3] Recommendations for treatment of scoliosis or kyphoscoliosis in homocystinuria cannot be made from the paucity of literature available, but it is likely that surgical planning and technique can be based on principles used for idiopathic scoliosis. The role of bracing in this disorder has not been established. Consultation with a hematologist experienced in treating this disorder is strongly recommended when contemplating spinal fusion in a patient with homocystinuria, due to the risk of significant and life-threatening thrombosis. The effects of osteoporosis on fixation of spinal instrumentation in this disorder may require special consideration.

SELECTED REFERENCES

Amir N, Ziotogora J, Bach G: Mucolipidosis type IV: clinical spectrum and natural history, *Pediatrics* 79:953-959, 1987.

Beals RK: Homocystinuria, *J Bone Joint Surg Am* 51:1564-1572, 1969.

Brenton DP et al.: Homocystinuria and Marfan's syndrome: a comparison. *J Bone Joint Surg Br* 54:277-297, 1972.

Crawford AH, Bagamery N: Osseous manifestations of neurofibromatosis in childhood, *J Pediatr Orthop* 6:72-88, 1986.

Francke U, Furthmayr H: Marfan's syndrome and other disorders of fibrillin, *N Engl J Med* 330:1384-1385, 1994.

Funasaki HE et al.: Pathophysiology of spinal deformities in neurofibromatosis, an analysis of seventy-one patients who had curves associated with dystrophic changes, *J Bone Joint Surg Am* 76:692-700, 1994.

Lipson SJ: Dysplasia of the odontoid process in Morquio's syndrome causing quadriparesis, *J Bone Joint Surg Am* 59:340-344, 1977.

National Institutes of Health: *Consensus development conference statement*, 6(12), 1987.

Pyeritz RE et al.: Dural ectasia is a common feature of the Marfan syndrome, *Am J Hum Genet* 43:726-732, 1988.

Robins PR, Moe JH, Winter RB: Scoliosis in Marfan's syndrome: its characteristics and results of treatment in thirty-five patients, *J Bone Joint Surg Am* 57:358-368, 1975.

Sostrin RD et al.: Myelographic features of mucopolysaccharidoses: a new sign, *Radiology* 125:421-424, 1977.

Stevens JM et al.: The odontoid process in Morquio-Brailsford's disease: the effects of occipitocervical fusion, *J Bone Joint Surg Br* 73:851-858, 1991.

Winter RB et al.: Spine deformity in neurofibromatosis: a review of one hundred and two patients, *J Bone Joint Surg Am* 61:677-694, 1979.

REFERENCES

1. Amir N, Ziotogora J, Bach G: Mucolipidosis type IV: clinical spectrum and natural history, *Pediatrics* 79:953-959, 1987.

2. Amis J, Herring JA: Iatrogenic kyphosis: a complication of Harrington instrumentation in Marfan's syndrome, *J Bone Joint Surg Am* 66:460-464, 1984.

3. Beals RK: Homocystinuria, *J Bone Joint Surg Am* 51:1564-1572, 1969.

4. Birch JG, Herring JA: Spinal deformity in Marfan syndrome, *J Pediatr Orthop* 7:546-552, 1987.

5. Blaw ME, Langer LO: Spinal cord compression in Morquio-Brailsford's disease, *J Pediatr* 74:593-600, 1969.

6. Brenton DP et al.: Homocystinuria and Marfan's syndrome: a comparison, *J Bone Joint Surg Br* 54:277-297, 1972.

7. Crawford AH: Neurofibromatosis. In Weinstein SL, ed: *The pediatric spine: principles and practice*, New York, 1994, Raven, pp. 619-649.

8. Crawford AH: Pitfalls of spinal deformities associated with neurofibromatosis in children, *Clin Orthop* 245:29-42, 1989.

9. Crawford AH, Bagamery N: Osseous manifestations of neurofibromatosis in childhood, *J Pediatr Orthop* 6:72-88, 1986.

10. Curtis BH et al.: Neurofibromatosis with paraplegia: report of eight cases, *J Bone Joint Surg Am* 51:843-861, 1969.

11. Dietz HC et al.: Marfan syndrome caused by a recurrent de novo missense mutation in the fibrillin gene, *Nature* 352:337-339, 1991.

12. Francke U, Furthmayr H: Marfan's syndrome and other disorders of fibrillin, *N Engl J Med* 330:1384-1385, 1994.

13. Funasaki H et al.: Pathophysiology of spinal deformities in neurofibromatosis: an analysis of seventy-one patients who had curves associated with dystrophic changes, *J Bone Joint Surg Am* 76:692-700, 1994.

14. Goodman ML, Pang D: Spinal cord injury in I-cell disease, *Pediatr Neurosci* 14:315-318, 1988.

15. Hobbs WR et al.: The cervical spine in Marfan syndrome, *Spine* 22:983-989, 1997.

16. Kelly TE: The mucopolysaccharidoses and mucolipidoses, *Clin Orthop* 114:116-136, 1976.

17. Lee B et al.: Linkage of Marfan syndrome and a phenotypically related disorder to two fibrillin genes, *Nature* 352:330-334, 1991.

18. Leroy JG et al.: I-cell disease: a clinical picture, *J Pediatr* 79:360, 1971.

19. Levander B, Mellstrom A, Grepe A: Atlantoaxial instability in Marfan's syndrome: diagnosis and treatment, *Neuroradiol* 21:43-46, 1981.

20. Lipson SJ: Dysplasia of the odontoid process in Morquio's syndrome causing quadriparesis, *J Bone Joint Surg Am* 59:340-344, 1977.

21. Lonstein JE et al.: Neurologic deficits secondary to spinal deformity, *Spine* 5:331-355, 1980.

22. Major MR, Huizenga BA: Spinal cord compression by displaced ribs in neurofibromatosis: a report of three cases, *J Bone Joint Surg Am* 70:1101-1102, 1988.

23. Maslen CL et al.: Partial sequence of a candidate gene for the Marfan syndrome, *Nature* 352:334-337, 1991.

24. Miller A: Neurofibromatosis with reference to skeletal changes, compression myelitis and malignant degeneration, *Arch Surg* 32:109, 1936.

25. National Institutes of Health: *Consensus development conference statement*, 6(12), 1987.

26. Pyeritz RE et al.: Dural ectasia is a common feature of the Marfan syndrome, *Am J Hum Genet* 43:726-732, 1988.

27. Robins PR, Moe JH, Winter RB: Scoliosis in Marfan's syndrome: its characteristics and results of treatment in thirty-five patients, *J Bone Joint Surg Am* 57:358-368, 1975.

28. Savini R, Cervellati S, Beroaldo E: Spinal deformities in Marfan syndrome, *Ital J Orthop Traumatol* 6(1):19-40, 1980.

29. Sostrin RD et al.: Myelographic features of mucopolysaccharidoses: a new sign, *Radiology* 125:421-424, 1997.

30. Spranger JW, Weidemann HR: The genetic mucolipidosis: diagnosis and differential diagnosis, *Humangenetik* 9:113, 1970.

31. Staalman CR, Bakker HD: Mucolipidosis I: roentgenographic follow-up, *Skeletal Radiol* 12(3):153-161, 1984.

32. Stevens JM et al.: The odontoid process in Morquio-Brailsford's disease: the effects of occipitocervical fusion, *J Bone Joint Surg Br* 73:851-858, 1991.

33. Taylor LJ: Severe spondylolisthesis and scoliosis in association with Marfan's syndrome: case report and review of the literature, *Clin Orthop* 221:207-211, 1987.

34. Winter RB: Severe spondylolisthesis in Marfan syndrome: report of two cases, *J Pediatr Orthop* 2:51-55, 1982.

35. Winter RB et al.: Spine deformity in neurofibromatosis: a review of one hundred and two patients. *J Bone Joint Surg Am* 61:677-694, 1979.

36. Winter RB: Thoracic lordoscoliosis in Marfan syndrome: report of two patients with surgical correction using rods and sublaminar wires, *Spine* 15:233-235, 1990.

37. Yajnik VH et al.: Marfan's syndrome, ventricular septal defect and basilar impression in one patient, *J Indian Med Assoc* 64:242-244, 1975.

38. Yong-Hing K, Kalamchi A, MacEwen GD: Cervical spine abnormalities in neurofibromatosis, *J Bone Joint Surg Am* 61:695-699, 1979.

Myelomeningocele: Neurosurgical Perspectives

Bradley E. Weprin, W. Jerry Oakes

Open neural tube defects are among the most common congenital anomalies to involve the central nervous system. These malformations of the neural tube result from the failure of the neural folds to fuse in the embryo. Neural tissue is exposed at birth. A spectrum of clinical variations and dysfunctions exists. The myelomeningocele is the most common form of open neural tube defect. The term is frequently used synonymously with the terms *spina bifida aperta* and *spina bifida cystica*. The term *spina bifida* has also been used to describe a variety of occult spinal dysraphic malformations, and its use is somewhat confusing.

The myelomeningocele occurs with an incidence of approximately 4.5 per 10,000 live births, though the fetal prevalence is undoubtedly much higher. It affects between 6000 and 11,000 newborns in the United States each year. Affected individuals experience varying degrees of sensory and motor deficits in the areas served by the portions of the spinal cord below the lesion. However, myelodysplasia is not simply a deformity of the spinal cord. It is associated with multiple abnormalities and is a significant cause of serious neurologic, urologic, orthopedic, and developmental disabilities. Many of the conditions faced by these patients are potentially predictable and preventable. The care of the individual with myelomeningocele is complex and dynamic. Knowledge of the associated abnormalities and their inherent interactions is required for optimal management.

MYELOMENINGOCELE

- Incidence 4.5 per 10,000 live births
- Affects 6000 to 11,000 newborns in United States each year
- Various degrees of sensory and motor deficits below level of spinal cord lesion
- Associated with serious neurologic, urologic, orthopedic, and developmental disabilities

---

DEFINITION AND EMBRYOLOGY

The myelomeningocele is clinically obvious at birth (Figure 49-1). The lesion is characterized by the presence of exposed neural tissue, the spinal cord, usually without meningeal, bony, or cutaneous covering. The exposed neural tissue rests on the dorsal aspect of an abnormal arachnoid sac created by the fusion of the meninges to the cutaneous surface. The posterior vertebral arch is open, the dura mater is open, fused laterally to the dermis, and the pia remains fused to the epidermis.

The superficial tissue in the center of the defect is unfolded neural tissue and represents the neural placode. At its rostral pole, the placode exits from a fully formed spinal canal. The central canal terminates at this cephalic region and continues as a midline groove that is often visible. The neural tissue of the placode is often dysplastic and gliotic.[14]

The sensory and motor roots are formed primarily on the ventral surface of the placode. The dorsal roots exit from the lateral anterior half of the abnormal spinal cord, whereas the ventral roots exit from the medial anterior half. Nerve roots seem to exit at an angle that is more tangential than that of their normal rostral counterparts. In addition, aberrant nerve roots may frequently develop. They can run dorsal or lateral from the spinal cord and end blindly within the dura, paravertebral musculature, or skin. The neural placode is always abnormally low and tethered to its surrounding tissues.

Although the skin is deficient over the abnormalities, it is in continuity with the outer edges of the defect. The adjacent cutaneous layer often lacks a full thickness of skin. The dura and leptomeninges are usually open and everted over the open pedicles and hypoplastic laminae that make up the bony spina bifida. The dura frequently extends farther laterally to cover the paraspinous fascia. Anomalous blood vessels are noticeable on the inner walls of the dura and arachnoid.[14]

The location of the open defect is variable. The distal thoracic, lumbar, and sacral regions are the most common sites of abnormality. Over 85% of malformations are found at such levels. Ten percent of lesions are detected in the thoracic region, whereas less than 5% are

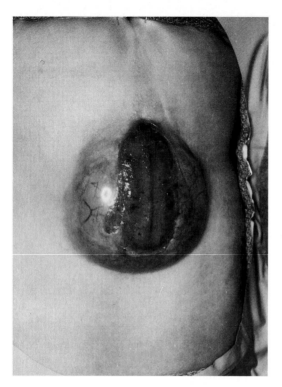

Figure 49-1. Myelomeningocele exhibiting neural placode with the midline groove representative of an open central canal. The tissue adjacent to the placode lacks a full complement of skin layers.

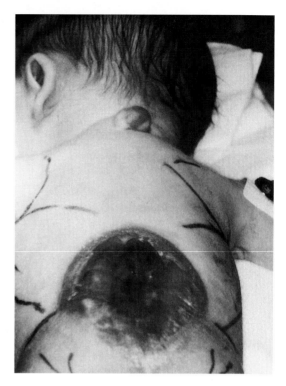

Figure 49-2. A neonate with two separate myelomeningocele lesions, cervical and lumbar.

located in the cervical area. Occasionally, more than one lesion affects the spinal axis (Figure 49-2).[17]

Most research suggests that the origin of the myelomeningocele results from a sequence of abnormalities that happen during a critical period between the end of the third week and the beginning of the fourth week of gestation, when folding and closure of the neural tube occurs. During this period, the neural groove deepens and the neural folds meet in the dorsal midline to create a tube. The site of initial tube closure is at the future cervicomedullary junction. Closure extends in both cephalic and caudal directions. Ectoderm, which is contiguous with the lateral margin of the neural folds, also closes in the midline. The cutaneous ectoderm separates from the neural tube, following which mesoderm interposes it to form fat, muscle, and skeletal structures.[17]

The exact cause for failure of the neural tube to close is presently unknown. Most cases are likely heterogeneous in origin with both genetic and environmental components. Epidemiologic studies have demonstrated an increased incidence of myelodysplasia in previously affected families. If one child is affected with a neural tube defect, a second sibling has a 2% to 5% chance of being born with a myelomeningocele. If two children have been affected, the risk further increases to approximately 10%. Myelodysplasia has also been associated with various chromosomal anomalies such as trisomy 13, 14, 15, and 18 and triploidy.[11,46]

Certain identifiable associations appear to be present. Research has provided overwhelming evidence

---

EMBRYOLOGY

- Location of neural tube defect: Distal thoracic, lumbar, and sacral regions most common (85%)
- Critical period for insult resulting in neural tube defect: End of third week and beginning of fourth week of gestation
- Causes for failure of neural tube closure: Genetic and environmental components
- Chance of second sibling being affected: 2% to 5%

---

implicating maternal diet, particularly low intake of folic acid during early pregnancy. Studies have demonstrated that high-dose folic acid supplements used by women who had prior pregnancies affected by neural tube defects reduced the risk of subsequent affected pregnancies by 70%.[33] The U.S. Public Health Service has recommended that all women of childbearing age who can become pregnant consume 0.4 mg of folate per day to reduce the risk of having children affected with neural tube defects. However, in light of such measures, the exact pathophysiology of neural tube defects is uncertain. Further investigation is needed.

ASSOCIATED ABNORMALITIES

The myelomeningocele is not simply a spinal cord malformation. A variety of additional anomalies may be associated in an individual with myelomeningocele. These abnormalities may further contribute to the disabilities of the affected individual. They may also impact the therapeutic management of such patients. Associated brain anomalies exist. Hydrocephalus, an obstruction to normal flow of cerebrospinal fluid (CSF), is present in 80% to 92% of patients. The Chiari II malformation, characterized by displacement of the cerebellum and brainstem through the foramen magnum and caudal elongation of the fourth ventricle, is almost uniformly present in varying degrees, but infrequently symptomatic. Other common anomalies of the cerebrum include heterotopias, polygyria, and corpus callosal dysgenesis or agenesis. Associated skull anomalies include craniolacunae, small posterior fossa with an enlarged foramen magnum, low-set tentorium, low-lying torcular Herophili, and anomalous dural sinuses within the posterior fossa. Additional anomalies within the spinal cord including syringohydromyelia, split cord malformations, lipomas, and defective myelinization were found in 88% of 25 autopsy cases.[12,14,17,18,31] A split cord malformation is not uncommon among such abnormalities. The presence of an asymmetric neurologic deficit should alert one to the possible presence of a diastematomyelia or diplomyelia. Both the rostral and caudal ends of the myelomeningocele defect should be inspected prior to complete closure. The location of bony spurs associated with split cord malformations is within one to two adjacent segments in approximately 70% of such cases.* A thickened filum terminale will occasionally be present in these newborns; it requires sectioning to prevent a future source of tethering.

Spinal deformities are quite common, usually progressive, and may cause further disability. The most consistent and unique abnormality is the incomplete posterior arch of the spine. The spinous processes and laminae are absent at the site of the defect. Occasionally, rudimentary laminae are present at adjacent vertebral levels. The vertebral bodies of the affected segments are almost ovoid, the result of a reduction in anteroposterior size. At the dysplastic level, the interpedicular distance is widened and the height of the pedicles is reduced. Transverse processes are displaced laterally. Hemivertebrae, partial or complete vertebral fusion, unsegmented bars, and fusion of transverse processes may occur at any level along the spine.

Systemic abnormalities are not uncommon. The gastrointestinal, cardiovascular, pulmonary, and genitourinary systems may be involved. Multiple variations in urologic anatomy and function exist. Inguinal hernias, Meckel's diverticulum, malrotation, omphalocele, and imperforate anus have been described in association with myelomeningocele. Septal defects, patient ductus arteriosus, and coarctation of the aorta have also been observed.[10]

---

* Oakes WJ: Personal communication.

ASSOCIATED ABNORMALITIES

- Brain: Hydrocephalus, Chiari II malformation, cerebral, heterotopias, polygyria, and corpus callosal dysgenesis or agenesis
- Skull: Craniolacunae, small posterior fossa with enlarged foramen magnum, low-set tentorium, low-lying torcular herophili
- Spinal cord: Syringohydromyelia, split cord malformations, lipoma, defective myelinization

PROGNOSIS
Survival

Technologic and therapeutic advances have allowed individuals with myelodysplasia to enjoy an excellent long-term survival. Prior to 1960, when left primarily untreated, only 11% of infants born with spina bifida aperta survived to adolescence. Most died as the result of either infection or hydrocephalus. With the advent of CSF diversion and early closure of the back defect, the survival rates for those affected have greatly improved. One study reported a survival rate of 60% in 1963 that improved to 90% by 1974.[25] McLone et al.[29] recorded 86% survival in a consecutive series of 100 patients observed from 5 to 9 years. The majority of deaths were presumably related to the Chiari II hindbrain anomaly. It is estimated that up to 70% of individuals born with a myelomeningocele will survive well into adulthood.[40] The most serious life-threatening problem appears to be the maintenance of a functional shunt, with 1% to 2% of the patient population dying each year from shunt-related complications. Approximately 10% to 15% of patients will die prior to reaching the first grade despite aggressive medical care.

Intellectual Development

With an improved prognosis, modern therapeutic modalities are now focused on allowing patients to become socially productive and economically independent. The intellectual development is difficult to assess for an individual infant. In most children with myelomeningocele, the ability to develop normal intelligence is present. Severe mental retardation requiring custodial care occurs in only 10% to 15%. Untreated hydrocephalus and episodes of ventriculitis have been shown to have an adverse effect on intellectual potential. Children with coexistent myelomeningocele and hydrocephalus that have been successfully managed perform within the normal range on standardized IQ testing. Hydrocephalus alone does not significantly limit the development of normal intelligence. Although McLone and Naidich[29] reported that shunt infections have an adverse impact on IQ, Steinbok et al.[42] and Sutton et al.[43] did not identify similar correlations between shunt infection and intelligence. Intelligence does not seem to be affected by the type of shunt or number of revisions.

Wide arrays of complex learning disabilities have been identified. Verbal skills develop better than nonverbal skills in affected individuals. Reduction in memory, conceptual and problem-solving difficulties, deficient linguistic ability, short attention span, difficulty comprehending abstract concepts, and visual-motor coordination abnormalities have been reported. Comprehensive neuropsychologic evaluations are necessary to maintain quality education, in spite of reasonable intelligence.

Ambulation

Factors that determine ambulatory status have been extensively reviewed. The neurologic level of the lesion is considered to be the most important factor to influence walking ability.[1,5,6,20,39] Patients with cervical and sacral myelomeningoceles have a higher rate of normal function than those with lesions in other locations. The rate of ambulation typically increases with the more caudal location of the abnormality. Age, hydrocephalus, intellectual level, syringohydromyelia, tethered spinal cord, scoliosis, pelvic obliquity, contractures, foot deformities, type of bracing, motivation, major medical events, and environment may also influence the ability to walk.* As children with myelomeningocele age, the increase in body weight may exceed the increase in motor strength, thereby impeding the ability to walk. Many will ultimately become wheelchair bound. However, with improved recognition and treatment of the tethered cord, hydrocephalus, and syringohydromyelia, with the use of orthopedic modalities to correct spinal lower extremity deformities, and with the use of adequate orthotic support, the rates of ambulation may reach 80%.

Patients are typically grouped into community ambulators, household ambulators, and nonambulators. Community ambulators are capable of walking both indoors and outdoors regardless of external supports such as crutches or braces. They may use wheelchairs for long-distance ambulation. Household ambulators do not walk outdoors. They may use a wheelchair for some activities, but use cane, crutch, or brace support during all attempts at walking. Nonambulators use a wheelchair on all occasions, but may be independent in transfers.[20] Strong hip flexors, hip adductors, and quadriceps muscles are needed to achieve community or household status. Reported rates of community ambulation vary between 43% and 68%.[40] Inconsistencies may be subject to varying interpretations of community ambulation.

Delay in achieving ambulation can be expected in most children, regardless of the neurosegmental level.[47] If patients are to become community ambulators, they usually do so by 9 years.[47] Even with high-level paralysis, ambulation has been achieved, though most adults with thoracic level function will require the use of wheelchairs to remain mobile. Mobility in a wheelchair may be more important than ambulation. Patients may choose to use the wheelchair to conserve energy for other activities of daily living. It is socially more important that

---

*References 1, 5, 6, 16, 20, 39, 47.

> ### PROGNOSIS
>
> - Survival rates have improved from 60% in 1963 to 90% by 1974
> - Majority of deaths related to Chiari II hindbrain anomaly
> - Most serious life-threatening problem: Maintenance of a functional shunt
> - Outcome in majority: Able to develop normal intelligence
> - Neurologic level is the primary factor determining ambulation potential
> - Community ambulation achieved by 43% to 68% of patients

affected individuals be able to move about the community to accomplish their business.[40]

Genitourinary Function

Only 6% to 17% of myelodysplastic patients are continent of urine. If left untreated, the remaining individuals would be incontinent of urine and/or feces. The introductions of clean intermittent catheterization and combined pharmacotherapy have improved continence rates. Social continence, defined as being dry most of the time without the need for a diaper, has been reported in 75% to 85% of cases.[40] Comprehensive urologic programs have also greatly reduced the frequency of urinary tract infections, helped to preserve normal renal function, and reduced the number of diversion procedures. Constipation is a frequent problem. Bowel habit has been significantly improved with the use of training with or without medications.

Sexual development is highly variable. Individuals with lesions below the S1 level typically have normal sexual function. Those with abnormalities between L3 and L5 have sexual function that is variable, but more common than would be expected in theory. Those with lesions at or above L2 are considered to be asexual, but may still have an interest in sex. The fertility of affected females is not affected by their neurologic condition.[40,49]

TREATMENT
Sac Closure

The initial treatment of the child with a myelomeningocele typically commences following birth whether the condition was anticipated or not. A general neonatal assessment is performed. In the absence of an associated lethal condition, early intervention is indicated. The primary goals of surgery are to preserve neural tissue, reconstitute normal anatomy, and release the tethered spinal cord in an effort to retain neurologic function and reduce the risk of infection. Additionally, closure of the defect should both facilitate future nursing and self-care and improve the cosmetic appearance. Recent data suggest that the promptness with which the defect is closed reduces the incidence of serious infection. In

GOALS OF SURGERY

- Preserve neural tissue
- Reconstitute normal anatomy
- Release tethered spinal cord

McLone and Naidich's series,[29] the rate of ventriculitis approached 37% when closures were performed later than 48 hours following birth. The infection rate was reduced to 7% in children whose repairs were completed within 48 hours of birth. Closure within the first 48 hours of life promotes the optimal preservation of function.[27,28]

Prior to surgery, a complete neurosurgical assessment is made of the multiple structural and functional abnormalities. Particular attention is focused on measurement of the head circumference and sensory and motor examination of the trunk and extremities, anal sphincter, and urinary stream. The level of the sensory impairment is usually slightly higher than the anticipated motor dysfunction. Subtle asymmetry in sensorimotor function is not uncommon. However, if the disparity in segmental level between the two sides is greater than one level, an occult neurologic problem, such as a split cord malformation, should be suspected.

The spine should be carefully examined. The size and the site of the malformation should be recorded. The location of the defect, the size of the placode, and the healthiness and laxity of the surrounding skin and soft tissues are highly variable. The presence of early spinal curvature and kyphosis should be assessed. Plain radiographs of the spine help to demonstrate the presence and degree of kyphosis that may require spinal osteotomy for closure. They may also reveal associated vertebral anomalies.

The fundamental principles and surgical goals remain the same in spite of the variable anatomy and characteristics of the different malformations. Meticulous dissection, débridement of nonviable tissue, and reconstitution of the normal tissue layers, with little manipulation of neural structures, are paramount for success. Iodinated scrubs and topical antibiotics should not contact the placode because of the potential neurotoxicity. Closure is started with the isolation of the neural elements and continues with the sequential closure of the dura mater, lumbodorsal fascia, subcutaneous tissue, and skin.

The child is positioned in a prone fashion on rolls that freely suspend the abdomen. Dissection is initially performed in a circumferential manner along the margins of the neural placode. The placode, nerve roots, proximal, and on occasion distal, spinal cord segments should be identified and isolated. The superior and inferior poles of the placode are more adherent than the lateral poles. To prevent retethering, the neural structures must be completely separated from the surrounding meningeal tissue, with care not to leave remnants of cutaneous or dermal tissue under the skin closure.

The placode is then reconstituted into a neural tube, resembling the remainder of the spinal cord. The lateral edges of the placode are approximated with microsutures. Such an artificial approximation has the potential benefit of limiting the exposure of relatively rough dorsal placode surface to the overlying dural construction. Theoretically, the maneuver will limit the incidence of placode tethering following initial closure. The placode, however, may occasionally be too bulky to approximate the lateral edges.

As mentioned above, the coexistence of a split cord malformation with or without a bony spur is not uncommon. Asymmetric motor function should alert the clinician to its possible presence. It is a potential source of tethering and should be treated at the initial closure. The rostral and caudal regions should be carefully inspected prior to dural closure. Extension of the exposure with removal of adjacent laminae may be necessary for adequate inspection.

The dura mater is then isolated and separated from the iliocostal fascia. The intact dorsal dura is identified at the rostral aspect of the exposure. The skin incision may need to be extended rostrally in the midline to appreciate the most caudal intact lamina and this normal rostral dura. With the dura isolated superiorly, dissection proceeds laterally and inferiorly to the caudal termination of the defect. The dura is then approximated in the midline. Dural grafting is rarely necessary, but fascia, cadaveric dura, and Gore-Tex have been reported in cases in which simple linear closure fails to provide adequate coverage.

Children who have defects complicated by an associated kyphosis present several problems. Difficulty in achieving primary skin closure over the kyphos presents initial concern. And, even if closure over the deformity is possible, the overlying skin is subject to recurrent ulceration. The infant may develop problems resting supine or sitting upright, making care difficult. Compression of the abdominal cavity can precipitate respiratory compromise. Kyphosis has been estimated to appear in 12% to 28% of cases.[15,24,26,33,35] The gibbus typically develops between L2 and L5. It is usually restricted to the level of the spinal defect. The angle of deformity is usually greater than 90 degrees. When the iliopsoas is present, the patient has iliopsoas function but typically has a flaccid paraplegia below that level. The iliopsoas is transposed in front of the equator of the spine to act as a spinal flexor rather than an extensor. It is often associated with a number of paralytic deformities of the lower extremities. It is often progressive. Simultaneous kyphectomy with postnatal closure has been proposed in an attempt to slow or even arrest the progression of deformity while facilitating closure and improving postoperative care of the child.[36] Reduction and internal fixation have been sporadic in the neurosurgical community. When they are performed in the newborn, the need for a complex skin flap may be lessened. The long-term effects on improved function, recurrence of deformity and nonunion, and improvement in the ability to assume an erect posture are debatable.

Finally, the superficial soft tissue layers are closed with the attempt to provide adequate full-thickness skin coverage of the defect without excessive tension

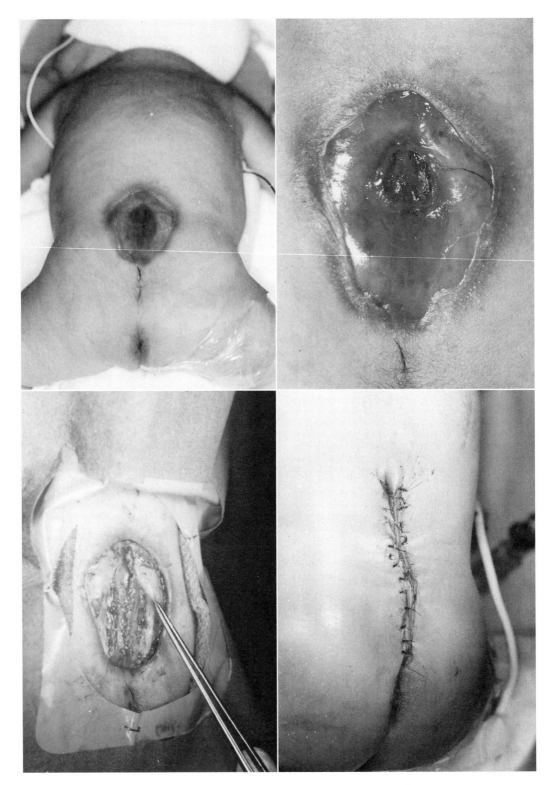

Figure 49-3.   Sequential steps in the primary closure of a myelomeningocele.

(Figure 49-3). Some will incise the lumbosacral fascia laterally off the posterior iliac crest and underlying sacrospinalis muscle. The edges of the fascial flaps are folded medially and sutured in the midline, adding to the multilayer closure. The skin is undermined surrounding the defect and approximated in two layers. A variety of surgical adjuncts, including rotation flaps, bipedicle flaps, myocutaneous flaps, and advancement flaps, have been employed when simple closure techniques have not been possible (Figure 49-4). Such procedures extend operative time and are prone to increased blood loss.

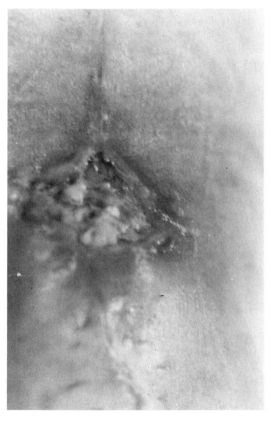

Figure 49-4. A large thoracolumbar defect that required transfer of soft tissue from the buttock for a tension-free coverage.

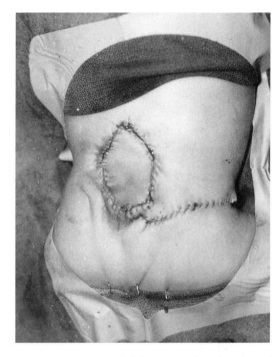

Figure 49-5. Wound dehiscence that developed in response to unrecognized hydrocephalus and shunt malfunction.

SURGICAL STEPS

- Position patient prone.
- Perform dissection in circumferential manner along margins of the neural placode.
- Identify and isolate the placode, nerve roots, proximal, and on occasion distal spinal cord segments.
- Reconstitute placode into a neural tube.
- Isolate dura mater and separate from iliocostal fascia.
- Approximate dura in midline.
- Close superficial soft tissue layers, attempting to provide adequate full-thickness skin coverage of defect without excessive tension.

The postoperative care is directed toward preserving the integrity of the wound closure without infection or CSF leakage. Hydrocephalus, which may not have been clinically apparent preoperatively, may be exacerbated by or become symptomatic following surgical closure of the myelomeningocele. Once radiographically confirmed, the hydrocephalus is treated by the placement of a shunt to divert CSF, thereby relieving the ventricular pressure and reducing any tension on the incision (Figure 49-5).

The operative mortality rate is approaching zero, inasmuch as 95% or greater survival rates for the first 2 years of life are being reported. The most common cause of death is respiratory dysfunction related to the associated Chiari II malformation. Minimal complications were reported in a series of 358 consecutive myelomeningocele closures. The average blood loss was 29 cc. Morbidity included postoperative ileus (3%), wound effusion (2.7%), pneumonia (6.3%), and wound infection (12%). There was no report of wound dehiscence. A total of 18% of patients developed ventriculitis, the risk of which increased with delayed primary closure or remote sources of infection such as the urinary tract.

The assumption that gradual deterioration of neurologic function is part of the natural history of children with myelomeningocele is incorrect. Functional deterioration should not necessarily occur, provided that conditions that may account for delayed deterioration are identified and treated. The initial search for a cause of neurologic deterioration in the patient with a myelomeningocele is directed at hydrocephalus and the shunt. Once it is determined that the shunt is functional, other causes are sought. Major late complications in this population include the symptomatic Chiari II malformation, an associated syringohydromyelia, or the tethering of the spinal cord at the site of closure, at an inclusion cyst, or from a diastematomyelia. Progressive orthopedic problems include scoliosis, pelvic obliquity, and lower limb deformities, each of which may develop or become exacerbated in the face of the associated neurologic abnormalities.

Hydrocephalus

The common coexistence of hydrocephalus with myelomeningocele is well recognized. The incidence of hydrocephalus in this population ranges from 80% to 92%. The cause is not completely understood but is likely multifactorial. Etiologic factors that have been postulated include the obstruction of the flow of CSF out of the fourth ventricle secondary to deformities of the hindbrain, impaired absorption of CSF, and blockage of CSF flow at the cerebral aqueduct. Although some reports support the presence of an association between defect level and ventricular dilatation in the postnatal period, others have concluded that the level of the spinal defect does not independently affect the degree of ventriculomegaly or severity of the posterior fossa deformity in fetuses with myelomeningoceles.[2-4]

Features of symptomatic hydrocephalus in individuals with myelomeningocele are usually present within the first 2 to 3 weeks following birth. Hydrocephalus frequently progresses following closure of the lesion. The open defect may serve as a conduit for the leakage of a substantial volume of CSF and ventricular decompression.

Many of the clinical manifestations of hydrocephalus in infants with myelomeningocele are similar to those associated with hydrocephalus from other causes. Bulging fontanelle, splaying of the cranial sutures, an enlarging head circumference, poor feeding or emesis, limitation of upward gaze, and apnea or bradycardia should alert the physician to the presence of hydrocephalus. However, the concomitant presence of the myelomeningocele and associated Chiari II malformation may alter the presentation of hydrocephalus in this population.

The child with the myelomeningocele may exhibit some unique features of symptomatic hydrocephalus. The recently closed spinal defect may bulge or leak CSF, even in the absence of overt clinical signs of intracranial hypertension. Furthermore, radiographic analysis by cranial ultrasound or computed tomography (CT) may fail to demonstrate significant ventricular enlargement because of the decompression associated with persistent leakage of fluid from the wound. Such a CSF leak may be the only evidence to the presence of hydrocephalus requiring functional treatment. Patients with worsening hydrocephalus may also develop signs of lower brainstem compromise secondary to the associated hindbrain anomaly, the Chiari II malformation. Though stridor, facial paresis, dysphonia, dysphagia, nasal regurgitation, aspiration, and upper extremity weakness are anatomically related to the Chiari II malformation and/or syringohydromyelia, these symptoms develop or become exacerbated in the face of hydrocephalus.

Insertion of a valve-regulated shunt is the standard treatment for hydrocephalus. It may be placed at the time of spinal closure or in a delayed fashion. Criteria for shunting have been suggested on the basis of head circumference, ventricular size, and the ratio of ventricular size to thickness of the brain parenchyma. Special care must be taken to ensure normal ventricular size, as the absence of overt signs does not obviate the need for shunt placement.

If adequately treated, the presence of hydrocephalus is consistent with an excellent cognitive outcome. The concept of shunt independence in children with myelodysplasia is controversial. Children with transient communicating hydrocephalus, usually following inflammatory processes and not associated with spina bifida, have been shown to function without significant deterioration in intelligence or motor function after shunt occlusion. However, such a concept is not routinely accepted in the myelodysplasia population. Respiratory arrest and death have been reported in patients with nonfunctioning shunts that were originally placed to treat hydrocephalus in association with spina bifida. The placement of a shunt should be viewed as a commitment to compulsory long-term follow-up that ensures adequate function throughout the life of the patient. The use of endoscopic third ventriculostomy has been reported in increasing frequency among individuals with myelodysplasia in the management of hydrocephalus. It can be a safe and effective means of treating a select group of patients, offering hope of long-term shunt independence.[9,45]

Over half of shunted children with myelodysplasia will require at least one shunt revision within the first 6 years following placement. Twenty percent will need multiple revisions. The possibility of shunt malfunction should be paramount in the thoughts of any clinician when evaluating the patient for any clinical change. Headache, nausea, emesis, lethargy, extraocular movement abnormalities, and poor feeding may be suggestive of intracranial hypertension and shunt failure. However, their absence does not conclusively indicate a functional shunt. Similarly, the change in ventricular size that may be witnessed with serial radiographic imaging studies may be subtle or even absent. Most patients exhibit a visible change in ventricular size with shunt malfunction. Cognitive changes manifest by a decline in school performance or worsening behavior are not infrequent. Changes in lower brainstem function, decrease in strength, increase in spasticity, alterations in ambulation, changes in urinary function, pain in the back or legs, and worsening of orthopedic deformities have been recorded in association with malfunction of the shunt.

HYDROCEPHALUS

- Incidence: 80% to 92%
- Cause: Multifactorial; obstruction of CSF flow out of fourth ventricle secondary to deformities of hindbrain, impaired absorption of CSF, and blockage of CSF flow at cerebral aqueduct
- Symptoms: Usually present within first 2 to 3 weeks after birth
- Clinical manifestations: Bulging fontanelle, splaying of cranial sutures, enlarging head circumference, poor feeding or emesis, limitation of upward gaze, apnea, bradycardia
- Treatment: Valve-regulated shunt

Chiari II Malformation

The Chiari II malformation is part of a group of abnormalities that involve the contents of the craniocervical junction. It is a complex deformity almost exclusively associated with a myelomeningocele. It is characterized by variable displacement of cerebellar tissue into the spinal canal accompanied by caudal dislocation of the lower brainstem and fourth ventricle (Figure 49-6). The spectrum of abnormalities is variable. In addition to the anatomic disturbances that occur in the posterior fossa and upper cervical spinal canal, a wide range of pathologic disturbances exists throughout the neuraxis.

Essential features of the Chiari II malformation include structural changes of the cerebellum, lower pons, and medulla. The inferior aspect of the cerebellar vermis is displaced a variable degree below the foramen magnum. It may extend as far down as the thoracic spinal canal. The lower pons and medulla are also displaced into the spinal canal. The medulla buckles backward as it descends into the spinal canal, creating a characteristic cervicomedullary kink or spur behind the spinal cord in up to 70% of patients. It is frequently positioned between the vertebral segments of C2 to C4, but may fall significantly lower. Curnes et al. reported that 75% of symptomatic patients exhibited a spur at the level of C4 or below.[13] No asymptomatic individual had a kink below the C3 to C4 level.[13] The fourth ventricle is often elongated and narrowed.

Although the bony volume of the posterior fossa is small, the opening of the foramen magnum is enlarged. The tentorium is hypoplastic and associated with an enlarged incisura through which the extent of the cerebellum towers. The insertion of the tentorium is low and may displace the transverse and sigmoid sinuses to the level of the foramen magnum.

Supratentorial anomalies are also evident. The tectum of the mesencephalon develops a beak-shaped appearance where the collicular plates fuse into a conical mass. The massa intermedia of the diencephalons is unusually large. In contradistinction to the lateral ventricles, the third ventricle is usually not enlarged. Colpocephaly, enlargement of the posterior aspects of the lateral ventricles relative to the anterior horns, is prominent. The falx may also be hypoplastic, which frequently results in interdigitations of the cerebral gyri of the occipital lobes. Agenesis or partial genesis of the corpus callosum occurs in up to one third of patients.

The prevalence of associated syringohydromyelia has been estimated to occur in 19% to 95% of cases.[12,34] It is important to point out that of the list of possible pathologic abnormalities an individual patient may express, some elements are of an extreme form whereas other aspects remain normal. The sporadic representation makes prediction of the extent of pathologic changes difficult.

Studies indicate that the hindbrain abnormality may become clinically significant in 18% to 33% of myelodysplastics, especially in those 3 months of age or younger.[8,21-23,28,32,41] Of the symptomatic children, approximately one third will not survive infancy despite aggressive attempts at surgical and medical management. The Chiari II has become the leading cause of death in patients treated with myelomeningocele during the first 2 years of life. Respiratory insufficiency is the principal cause of death. The clinical presentation and the rate and extent of neurologic deterioration of these individuals is variable and largely a function of age irrespective of the size and extent of the myelomeningocele.

The pattern of rapid neurologic decompensation in neonates and young infants differs significantly from the insidious progression observed in older children. During the infancy period, the clinical picture is dominated by rapid dysfunction of the lower cranial nerves and brainstem. The earliest symptoms frequently reflect swallowing and feeding difficulties. Poor feeding, nasal regurgitation, and emesis may lead to weight loss and episodes of aspiration pneumonia. Respiratory difficulties seem to be the most common problem and are the most lethal. Vocal cord paralysis, stridor apnea, and loss of respiratory drive are indicative of lower brainstem dysfunction. Bradycardia, opisthotonos, and sudden death are not infrequent.

The clinical presentation in older children and adults is usually slower, less severe, and more amenable to surgical therapies. Symptoms reflect dysfunction of the spinal cord and cerebellum. Progressive upper extremity weakness, spasticity, and truncal or appendicular ataxia may be witnessed in older individuals. Pain in the occiput or cervical region may also reflect hindbrain compression.

Management of the Chiari II malformation is challenging from both a therapeutic and a technical standpoint. Controversy exists regarding the natural history and the ability of surgical intervention to alter its course. There is uniform agreement that problems that develop in response to compression of the hindbrain beyond the neonatal period respond to posterior cervical decompression. The indications for operation on neonates and

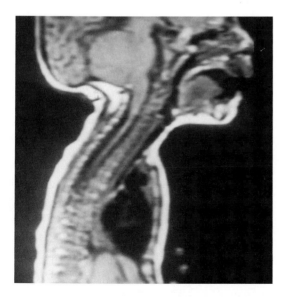

Figure 49-6.   Sagittal T1 weighted magnetic resonance image exhibiting hindbrain herniation, tectal beaking, and enlarged supracerebellar space characteristic of the Chiari II malformation.

CHIARI II MALFORMATION

- Characteristics: Variable displacement of cerebellar tissue into spinal canal accompanied by caudal dislocation of the lower brainstem and fourth ventricle
- Leading cause of death during first 2 years of life
- Treatment: Controversial—decompression of posterior cervical arches

SYRINGOHYDROMYELIA

- A cavity outside the confines of the central canal
- Prevalence associated with Chiari II ranges from 19% to 95%
- Results from abnormality in CSF dynamics and flow
- Symptoms: Upper extremity weakness, spasticity, pain, progressive scoliosis, dissociative sensory loss, and ascending motor loss in lower extremities
- Treatment: Establishment of adequate control of hydrocephalus

infants remain complicated, reflecting the variable clinical presentation, potential rapidity of deterioration, risks of intervention, and mixed results of benefit. Procedures are performed for clinical symptoms and are not based on the amount of caudal displacement of the cerebellar vermis.

Prior to decompression, there should be confirmation of adequate shunt function and control of hydrocephalus. Adequate decompression requires removal of the lowest cervical arch that overlies the herniated cerebellar tissue. A suboccipital craniectomy is rarely necessary and may be ill advised. The foramen magnum is typically generous in size, and the transverse sinuses are often displaced caudally, positioned at the lip of the foramen magnum. The need to open the dura and insert a patch graft is also controversial. In many cases, upon the removal of the posterior cervical arches, the dura bulges dorsally, creating adequate space for neural elements. Others argue that excision of intradural adhesions, identification of the fourth ventricle, and the reestablishment of outflow from the fourth ventricle are necessary for surgical success. A late consequence of Chiari II decompression is cervical instability. Cervical spine radiographs should be closely monitored.

Syringohydromyelia

The term *hydromyelia* has historically been associated with those cavities within the spinal cord lined by ependymal cells. It represents dilatation of the central canal. *Syringomyelia* is a term often used to represent those cavities outside of the confines of the central canal. Distinction between the two conditions is often not possible with either routine imaging studies or histologic review. The terms *syringohydromyelia* and *syrinx* are currently used to represent any CSF-containing cavity within the spinal cord that is associated with abnormalities of the hindbrain, irrespective of its continuity with the central canal.

The prevalence of syringohydromyelia associated with Chiari II ranges from 19% to 95%.[12,34] The wide variability reflects the degrees to which ventricular dilatation is controlled, the difficulty in making the diagnosis prior to modern neuroimaging techniques, and the effort with which the diagnosis is sought. These syrinx cavities have a propensity for the lower cervical spinal cord. The cause of development is variable. Syringohydromyelia likely develops from an abnormality in CSF dynamics and flow. The most common manifestations include

weakness of the upper extremities, spasticity, pain, progressive scoliosis, dissociative sensory loss, and ascending motor loss in the lower extremities.

Various types of surgical procedures have been proposed for the management of cavitating lesions of the spinal cord. Treatment strategies are based on findings on radiographic imaging studies and suspected cause. In the myelomeningocele population, the initial therapy involves the demonstration of adequate control of hydrocephalus. Communication between the syrinx and the fourth ventricle has been demonstrated in a small percentage. Such cases respond to ventricular shunting in the presence of ventriculomegaly. Malfunction of the shunt should be ruled out prior to any other form of surgical management. The lack of classical symptoms suggestive of elevated intracranial pressure and a normal-sized ventricular system is no guarantee of adequate CSF drainage. Effective therapy is based on the extent of syringohydromyelia, segmental versus holocord, and the associated symptoms. Magnetic resonance (MR) imaging may confirm the Chiari II malformation in association with cervical segmental or holocord cavities. An attempt at restoration of normal CSF dynamics at the cervicomedullary junction is indicated. Improvement or stabilization of function has been reported with posterior cervical decompression in individuals with symptoms referable to hindbrain compression and findings on radiographic examinations that correlate with such. Direct shunting of the syringomyelic cavity has been used as an adjunct as well. Similarly, when the cavity is felt to develop in response to tethering of the spinal cord, aggressive treatment to release the spinal cord and shunt the cavity has had success in relieving further functional deterioration.

Reduction in the size of the spinal cord cavity is usually observed within several months of surgery. Arrest or improvement in symptoms is common. There does not appear to be evidence that clinical improvement following therapy is related to a reduction in the size of the syrinx. Late recurrence has been reported.

Tethered Cord Syndrome

The tethered spinal cord consists of a group of conditions in which the conus medullaris is usually located in an abnormally low position. The spinal cord is fixed in a relatively immobile state by a variety of abnormalities.

Many of these conditions are occult: a thickened filum terminale, an intraspinal lipoma, a split cord malformation, and a dermal sinus tract and inclusion tumor. The myelomeningocele also fixes the distal spinal cord and prevents it from moving to the normal level.

Limitation of movement of the caudal aspect of the spinal cord can cause deterioration of neurologic function. Yamada et al.[50] have demonstrated significant architectural and metabolic disturbances within the spinal cord as a direct consequence of stretch under tension. The clinical result is the tethered cord syndrome, which is manifested by a variety of symptoms.

Almost all patients with myelodysplasia will exhibit caudal displacement of the conus medullaris and dorsal fixation of the neural tissue at the previous operative site.[44]

However, not all patients will develop delayed deterioration. It is estimated that only a small percentage will become symptomatic. Between 15% and 19% of these patients will develop functional decline as a result of the tethered spinal cord, the tethered cord syndrome.[7,31,44] Reasons why some develop the syndrome while others remain asymptomatic are speculative and not clear.

Radiographic studies define the pathologic anatomy rather than establish the diagnosis. Correlation between radiologic findings and physiologic function are difficult. To date, no imaging techniques have been developed to consistently predict future deterioration. Clinical criteria still define the syndrome.

Progressive loss of motor function is frequently recognized as a manifestation of a tethered cord. Changes may be reflected in muscle tone or progressive spasticity, weakness, limitation of joint range of motion secondary to muscle imbalance, and refractory contractures. Deterioration in ambulation and gait are not infrequent. Bladder dysfunction, manifest by a change in catheterization pattern, increasingly frequent urinary tract infections, and decreasing bladder capacity, can also represent the signal of a tethered cord. Progressive deformity of the lower limbs and incapacitating pain in the back and lower limbs are not uncommon symptoms.

Scoliosis may develop or worsen in response to a tethered spinal cord. The tethered cord usually causes a dorsolumbar or lumbar scoliosis with a marked increase in lumbar lordosis. Results of surgery to release the tethered cord are variable with respect to scoliosis. In cases of mild scoliosis, untethering procedures can frequently prevent progression of or even improve the deformity. If the scoliotic curve is greater than 50 degrees, however, the scoliosis will likely require internal fixation, which can often be performed at the time of the tethered cord release.[30] Sudden and precipitous deterioration in neurologic function can occur if a spine-straightening procedure is carried out in the face of a symptomatic tethered spinal cord.

The recognition and diagnosis of the tethered spinal cord are difficult. This may result from a slow rate of deterioration, the presence of preexisting fixed deficits, and trouble in assessing the natural changes due to growth and development in children. The greatest fre-

---

TETHERED CORD SYNDROME

- Conus medullaris—located in an abnormally low position
- Causes: Thickened filum terminale, an intraspinal lipoma, a split cord malformation, a dermal sinus tract, or inclusion tumor
- Symptoms: Progressive loss of motor function, worsening of scoliosis
- Treatment: Surgical release, reconstitution of capacious subarachnoid space

---

quency of onset occurs between 8 and 10 years of age, a period dominated by rapid growth.[44] Increase in stature contributes to mechanical stretch. However, patients may still deteriorate early or well into adulthood as the result of the stresses of repetitive trauma and daily activity to the spine.

The diagnosis of symptomatic tethering at the site of previous surgery is frequently a diagnosis of exclusion. Contributing causes of functional impairment continue to remain a nonfunctional cerebrospinal fluid shunt, syringohydromyelia, and symptomatic Chiari II malformation. The syndrome may be associated with other intraspinal pathology. Benign inclusion tumors may develop as a result of entrapped skin or skin appendages at the time of initial closure. Dermoid and/or epidermoid cysts were present in 16% of surgically treated tethered cord cases.[31] Previously unrecognized intraspinal lipomas or split cord malformations may also contribute to functional loss. Nevertheless, a significant difference of opinion exists concerning which problems are sufficient to warrant therapeutic intervention.

By their nature, surgical modalities of treatment are associated with a significant risk of function. Surgical release is offered to alleviate symptoms and to prevent further deterioration. Goals of treatment include attempts at the release of neural tissue from surrounding points of attachment and the reconstitution of capacious subarachnoid space. A potential site of tethering is at the caudal most intact lamina. Surgical release typically involves laminectomy at the level rostral to the original defect, lysis of intradural adhesions, excision of intradural masses (inclusion tumors, lipomas), and a search and section of a thickened filum terminale. The previously stretched spinal cord should appear relaxed upon completion. A duraplasty may be considered for further decompression of the thecal sac. Therapy frequently results in cessation of progression and improvement in symptoms. Although the surgical procedure results in stabilization for a number of patients, it likely does not address all of the causal factors associated with why the symptomatic tether occurred in the first place. Late deterioration as the result of recurrent tethering has been observed in a significant proportion of patients. As many as 50% to 66% of patients may develop recurrence of previous deficits during long-term follow-up.[30,37] And, like initial tethering, subsequent symptomatic tethering is difficult to predict. The role of surgical intervention, associated with the risks of neurologic compromise and of subsequent recurrent tethering, is also not clearly defined.

ISSUES OF SPINAL DEFORMITY AND MYELOMENINGOCELE

A major problem confronting the individual with myelomeningocele is progressive spinal deformity (scoliosis, kyphosis, and lordosis). Its development is multifactorial. The curvature is usually proximal to the level of the placode. Scoliosis affects greater than 80% of children with myelodysplasia by the tenth year of life. Deformities are often progressive and can interfere with the functional status of the individual with myelomeningocele. Progressive spinal changes lead to decline in ambulatory skills, loss of sitting ability, chronic skin breakdown, and restrictive respiratory difficulties in a percentage of myelomeningocele patients.

Spinal deformities in myelodysplasia present multiple unique features when compared with congenital and developmental deformities of other etiologies. Structural anomalies impact the natural history of the deformity and its treatment outcome. The incomplete posterior arch of the spine is the most obvious and consistent abnormality. Other associated vertebral anomalies, hemivertebrae and wedge-vertebrae, act to further complicate and accelerate the abnormal spinal curvature. Muscle imbalance, fixed from birth, contributes to the spinal deformity. The everted rudimentary laminae cause the abnormal placement of the paraspinous muscles. The erector spinae muscles are lateral and even anterior to the axis of flexion in these patients. In addition, the psoas and quadratus lumborum are displaced anterolaterally. Associated deformities of the pelvis and hips have also been demonstrated to complicate spine balance in this population.

Likewise, the associated anomalies of the brain and spinal cord may often precipitate or exacerbate scoliosis. Hydrocephalus, symptomatic hindbrain compression, syringohydromyelia, and tethered spinal cord must be adequately addressed before successful orthopedic involvement. The relationship between neurologic level of involvement and the presence of spinal deformity is significant. The higher the level of paralysis, the more common is a spinal deformity. Although patients with low-level lesions may develop severe scoliosis, those with abnormalities above the L3 level carry a considerably higher risk.[35]

The spinal deformity frequently develops at a younger age than is characteristic of most developmental abnormalities. It often is present by 2 to 3 years of age, becoming severe by age 7. The expected rate of progression varies between 2.5 and 3.5 degrees per year. These deformities continue to progress following cessation of growth, in contrast to idiopathic scoliosis. Corrective bracing is often used as the initial therapy in an effort to delay surgical intervention until the child matures. However, if spinal curvature progresses beyond 30 degrees, orthotics usually fails and fusion is required to stop progression.

The treatment of spinal deformities must be individualized. It depends upon the level, type of deformity, age of the patient, ambulatory status, and associated neurologic factors. Neurologic pathology should be sought as a potential cause for worsening scoliosis. Operative management of spinal deformities in the presence of coexisting neurologic factors may result in a number of complications. Reported adverse effects include death secondary to associated shunt failure and hydrocephalus, worsening deficits of function in the face of tethered spinal cord, and progression of spinal curvature. Coordinated interdisciplinary care is required.

Syringohydromyelia and the Chiari II malformation have been reported to cause or exacerbate scoliosis by affecting the strength of the muscles of the torso and extremities. The tethered spinal cord is another neurologic factor identified in the cause of scoliosis.[30] Scoliosis has been suggested to be a significant sign of a tethered cord in some cases. The mechanism is purely speculative. And as mentioned above, release of the tethered cord can have a significant effect on the spinal deformity of select patients, though the literature on such is sparse.

McLone et al.[30] retrospectively evaluated the courses of 30 patients with progressive loss of function and scoliosis in the absence of vertebral anomalies, hindbrain compression, and syringohydromyelia. Though the exact symptoms for each patient were not reported, tethered cord alone was considered to be the most common cause of scoliosis. It is not clear whether any of these patients had scoliosis as the sole manifestation of their tethered cord or also had additional clinical symptoms. Untethering procedures were performed on all. Of the 6 children with preoperative curves greater than 50 degrees, only one improved. Of the additional 24 patients, 96% of children with curves below 50 degrees improved or remained stable at 1-year follow-up. However, at subsequent follow-up, between 2 and 7 years, 37% of deformities began to progress. Progression beyond the first year of follow-up was concluded to represent retethering in most cases.[30]

Reigel et al.[37] had somewhat different conclusions with respect to the nature of scoliosis and the tethered cord. They retrospectively reviewed their experience with both the changes in spinal deformities following tethered cord release in 262 patients and the clinical course of 74 patients without tethered cord syndrome. Untethering procedures were not found to have benefit in the control of scoliosis of patients with thoracic level lesions. To the contrary, the authors found that tethered cord release significantly reduced the incidence and progression of scoliosis of patients with lumbar and sacral level lesions. They also found that the neurosurgical procedures altered the course of lordosis in L1 through L3 level lesions and the magnitude and progression of kyphosis.[37]

The optimal management of the myelomeningocele patient with progressive spinal deformities is not entirely clear. Orthopedic and neurologic factors can affect each individual differently. The exact role of the tethered spinal cord in scoliosis is not always clear.

Reliable data do not exist to support the routine or indiscriminate untethering of patients with scoliosis in the absence of other clinical findings to suggest a tethered cord. The role of recurrent tethering is also perplexing in the management of these individuals because its timing has not been clearly determined.

As mentioned previously, the kyphotic deformity is present in 12% to 28% of patients and progresses until the rib cage rests on the pelvis. Optimal surgical results require the resection of vertebral segments at the apex of the deformity. Timing of treatment remains controversial. As described earlier, postnatal kyphectomy can aid in closure. Its long-term effect on stabilization has been suspect. A variety of methods of internal fixation have been described.

Transection of the spinal cord and ligation of the thecal sac has become a useful adjunct in the management of kyphosis in the individual with a nonfunctional spinal cord. Cordectomy allows exposure of the posterior surface of the vertebral bodies in preparation for vertebral osteotomies. It may also relieve any associated tethering phenomenon contributing to the progression of deformity. Change in bladder capacity with subsequent alteration in catheterization schedule and acute alterations in intracranial pressure have been reported to complicate this maneuver.[19,48]

CONCLUSIONS

The management of the individual with myelodysplasia is both complex and variable. The advent of modern therapeutic advances and aggressive care has improved the long-term outcome of these patients. Whenever an individual affected with a myelomeningocele fails to achieve an expected functional outcome or deteriorates, a pathologic reason should be identified and corrected if possible. The multiple possibilities and their associated interactions require interdisciplinary cooperation. Compulsory surveillance and evaluation are necessary for optimal care.

SELECTED REFERENCES

Lindseth RE: Myelomeningocele spine. In Weinstein SL, ed: *The pediatric spine: principles and practice*, New York, 1994, Raven.

McLone DG, Naidich TP: Myelomeningocele: outcome and late complications. In McLaurin RL et al., eds: *Pediatric neurosurgery*, ed 2, Philadelphia, 1989, WB Saunders.

Partington MD, McLone DG: Hereditary factors in the etiology of neural tube defects: results of a survey, *Pediatr Neurosurg* 23:311-316, 1995.

Reigel DH, Rotenstein D: Spina bifida. In Cheek WR et al., eds: *Pediatric neurosurgery: surgery of the developing nervous system*, ed 3, Philadelphia, 1994, WB Saunders.

Steinbok P et al.: Long-term outcome and complications of children born with myelomeningocele, *Childs Nerv Syst* 8:92-96, 1992.

Yamada S, Zinke DE, Saunders D: Pathophysiology of "tethered cord syndrome," *J Neurosurg* 54:494-503, 1981.

REFERENCES

1. Asher M, Olsen I: Factors affecting the ambulatory status of patients with spina bifida cystica, *J Bone Joint Surg Am* 65:350-356, 1983.
2. Assad A et al.: Spinal dysraphism: experience with 280 cases operated upon. *Childs Nerv Syst* 5:324-329, 1989.
3. Babcock CJ, Drake CM, Goldstein RM: Spinal level of fetal myelomeningocele: does it influence ventricular size? *Am J Roentgenol* 169:207-210, 1997.
4. Badell-Ribera A, Shulman K, Paddock N: The relationship of non-progressive hydrocephalus to intellectual functioning in children with spina bifida cystica, *Pediatrics* 37:782-793, 1996.
5. Banta JV et al.: Long-term ambulation in spina bifida, *Dev Med Child Neurol* 25:110, 1983 (abstract).
6. Bartonek A et al.: Ambulation in patients with myelomeningocele: a twelve-year follow-up, *J Pediatr Orthop* 19:202-206, 1999.
7. Beeger JH et al.: Progressive neurologic deficit in children with spina bifida aperta, *Z Kinderchir* 41(suppl I):13-15, 1986.
8. Bell WO et al.: Symptomatic Arnold-Chiari malformation: review of experience with 22 cases, *J Neurosurg* 66:812-816, 1987.
9. Brockmeyer D et al.: Endoscopic third ventriculostomy: an outcome analysis, *Pediatr Neurosurg* 28:236-240, 1998.
10. Brown SF: Congenital malformations associated with myelomeningocele, *J Iowa Med Soc* 65:101-104, 1975.
11. Byrne J et al.: Multigeneration maternal transmission in Italian families with neural tube defects, *Am J Med Genet* 66:303-310, 1996.
12. Cameron AH: The Arnold-Chiari and other neuroanatomical malformations associated with spina bifida, *J Pathol* 73:195-211, 1957.
13. Curnes JT, Oakes WJ, Boyko OB: MR imaging of hindbrain deformity in Chiari II patients with and without symptoms of brainstem compression, *Am J Neuroradiol* 10:293-302, 1989.
14. Emery JL, Lendon RG: The local cord lesion in neurospinal dysraphism (meningomyelocele), *J Pathol* 110:83-96, 1973.
15. Eysel P, Hopf C, Schwarz M, Voth D: Development of scoliosis in myelomeningocele: differences in the history caused by idiopathic pattern, *Neurosurg Rev* 16:301-306, 1993.
16. Findley TW et al.: Ambulation in the adolescent with myelomeningocele. I. Early childhood predictors, *Arch Phys Med Rehabil* 68:518-522, 1987.
17. French BN: Midline fusion defects and defects of formation. In Youmans JR, ed: *Neurological surgery*, ed 2, Philadelphia, 1982, WB Saunders.
18. Gilbert JN et al.: Central nervous system anomalies associated with myelomeningocele, hydrocephalus, and the Arnold-Chiari malformation: reappraisal of theories regarding the pathogenesis of posterior neural tube closure defects, *Neurosurgery* 18:559-563, 1986.
19. Hall JE, Bobechko WP: Advances in the management of spinal deformities in myelodysplasia, *Clin Neurosurg* 20:457-463, 1973.
20. Hoffer MM et al.: Functional ambulation in patients with myelomeningocele, *J Bone Joint Surg Am* 55:137-148, 1973.
21. Hoffman HJ, Hendrick EB, Humphreys RP: Manifestations and management of Arnold-Chiari malformation in patients with myelomeningocele, *Childs Brain* 2:167-176, 1976.
22. Hoffman HJ et al.: Hydrosyringomyelia and its management in childhood, *Neurosurgery* 21:347-351, 1987.
23. Holliday PO et al.: Brain-stem auditory evoked potentials in Arnold-Chiari malformation: possible prognostic value and changes with surgical decompression, *Neurosurgery* 16:48-53, 1985.
24. Hoppenfield S: Congenital kyphosis in myelomeningocele, *J Bone Joint Surg Br* 49:276-280, 1967.
25. Laurence KM: The natural history of spina bifida cystica: detailed analysis of 407 cases, *Semin Neurol* 9:169-175, 1964.
26. Lindseth RE: Myelomeningocele spine. In Weinstein SL, ed: *The pediatric spine: principles and practice*, New York, 1994, Raven.
27. McLaughlin JF et al.: Influence of prognosis on decisions regarding the care of newborns with myelodysplasia, *N Engl J Med* 312:1389-1394, 1985.
28. McLone DG: Results of children born with myelomeningocele, *Clin Neurosurg* 30:407-412, 1983.
29. McLone DG, Naidich TP: Myelomeningocele: outcome and late complications. In McLaurin RL et al., eds: *Pediatric neurosurgery*, ed 2, Philadelphia, 1989, WB Saunders.
30. McLone DG et al.: Tethered cord as a cause of scoliosis in children with myelomeningocele, *Pediatr Neurosurg* 3:8-13, 1990.
31. Nelson MD Jr et al.: The natural history of repaired myelomeningocele, *Radiographics* 8:695-706, 1988.
32. Park TS et al.: Experience with surgical decompression of the Arnold-Chiari malformation in young infants with myelomeningocele, *Neurosurgery* 13:147-152, 1983.

33. Partington MD, McLone DG: Hereditary factors in the etiology of neural tube defects: results of a survey, *Pediatr Neurosurg* 23:311-316, 1995.

34. Peach B: The Arnold-Chiari malformation: anatomic features of 20 cases, *Arch Neurol* 12:613-621, 1965.

35. Piggot H: The natural history of scoliosis in myelodysplasia, *J Bone Joint Surg Br* 62:54-58, 1980.

36. Reigel DH, Rotenstein D: Spina bifida. In Cheek WR et al., eds: *Pediatric neurosurgery: surgery of the developing nervous system*, ed 3, Philadelphia, 1994, WB Saunders.

37. Reigel DH et al.: Change in spinal curvature following release of tethered cord associated with spina bifida, *Pediatr Neurosurg* 20:30-42, 1994.

38. Samuelsson L et al.: MR imaging of syringohydromyelia and Chiari malformation in myelomeningocele patients with scoliosis, *Am J Neuroradiol* 8:539-546, 1982.

39. Selber P, Dias L: Sacral-level myelomeningocele: long-term outcome in adults, *J Pediatr Orthop* 18:423-427, 1998.

40. Shurtleff D: Myelodysplasia: problems of long-term survival and social function, *West J Med* 122:199-205, 1975.

41. Sieben RL, Hamida MB, Shulman K: Multiple cranial nerve deficits associated with the Arnold-Chiari malformation, *Neurology* 21:673-681, 1971.

42. Steinbok P et al.: Long-term outcome and complications of children born with myelomeningocele, *Childs Nerv Syst* 8:92-96, 1992.

43. Sutton LN et al.: Myelomeningocele: the question of selection, *Clin Neurosurg* 33:371-381, 1986.

44. Tamaki N et al.: Tethered cord syndrome of delayed onset following repair of myelomeningocele, *J Neurosurg* 69:393-398, 1988.

45. Teo C, Jones R: Management of hydrocephalus by endoscopic third ventriculostomy in patients with myelomeningocele, *Pediatr Neurosurg* 25:57-63, 1996.

46. Toriello HV, Higgins JV: Occurrence of neural tube defects among first-, second-, and third-degree relatives of probands: results of a United States study, *Am J Med Genet* 15:601-606, 1983.

47. Williams E, Broughton NS, Menelaus MB: Age-related walking in children with spina bifida, *Dev Med Child Neurol* 41:446-449, 1999.

48. Winston K et al.: Acute elevation of intracranial pressure following transection of the non-functional spinal cord, *Clin Orthop* 128:41-44, 1977.

49. Woodhouse CRJ: The sexual and reproductive consequences of congenital genitourinary anomalies, *J Urol* 152:645-651, 1994.

50. Yamada S, Zinke DE, Saunders D: Pathophysiology of "tethered cord syndrome," *J Neurosurg* 54:494-503, 1981.

Scheuermann's Disease

Thomas G. Lowe

Scheuermann's disease is a common cause of structural kyphosis of either the thoracic or thoracolumbar spine. The condition has been reported to occur in 0.4% to 8.0% of the general population of the United States and is seen equally in both sexes.[2,19,20] It seldom becomes problematic in adults unless severe deformity develops. The diagnosis is usually apparent on physical examination but must be confirmed radiographically according to the criteria of Sorenson by the presence of anterior wedging greater than 5 degrees of at least three contiguous vertebral bodies.[33] There appears to be a high familial predilection but no definite mode of inheritance has been established, although it is likely to be inherited in an autosomal dominant manner with a high degree of penetrance and variable expressivity.[9,13,22]

The etiology and pathogenesis of the condition are probably related in part to biomechanical factors, but the cause remains unknown.[1,19,20,22] The condition must be differentiated from adolescent postural kyphosis, which usually runs a benign course clinically and has no structural vertebral changes radiographically.[19,20] If Scheuermann's disease is detected before skeletal maturity, it can virtually always be treated successfully by nonoperative means. However, it is frequently confused with postural kyphosis, which may lead to delayed treatment.[17] Patients in whom the disease is not recognized prior to skeletal maturity frequently have few sequelae unless severe deformity has developed.[19,20,24] When severe deformity develops and pain is unresponsive to nonoperative measures, operative treatment may be indicated.

ETIOLOGY AND PATHOGENESIS

Many theories have been proposed for the etiology of Scheuermann's disease but the true cause remains unknown. Most of the early investigation regarding the etiology of Scheuermann's disease, which included avascular necrosis of the ring apophysis, herniation of Schmorl's nodes through the growth plate, and persistence of the anterior vascular groove, have all been refuted.[1,2,6,19,20] At the present time, it is felt that there is a strong genetic factor as well as mechanical factors, such as a thickened anterior longitudinal ligament acting as a tether on the anterior column of the thoracic or thoracolumbar spine, resulting in diminished anterior growth of the vertebral bodies with wedging as a response to the Hueter-Volkmann law.[19,20] Investigators have noted that patients with Scheuermann's disease are also taller than average and have shown that their skeletal age is often ahead of their chronologic age.[31] Osteoporosis has been noted in these patients by some investigators but has been refuted by others.[6,11,15,18,30] Few data are available in the literature on the pathologic findings in patients with this disease because of the lack of postmortem specimens; however, Scoles et al.[30] has described alterations in vertebral shape in museum specimens suspected of having Scheuermann's disease.

CLINICAL FINDINGS

The onset of Scheuermann's disease usually occurs around puberty as an increased kyphosis of the thoracic or thoracolumbar spine. In adolescents, pain is frequently present and may be aggravated by standing, sitting, or heavy physical activity. The pain is usually not severe and often subsides with the cessation of growth. However, if the deformity is severe in adults with

---

OVERVIEW OF SCHEUERMANN'S DISEASE

- Common cause of structural kyphosis of either the thoracic or thoracolumbar spine
- Occurs in 0.4% to 8.0% of general population
- Confirmed radiographically by presence of anterior wedging greater than 5 degrees of at least three contiguous vertebral bodies
- If detected prior to maturity, often treated successfully nonoperatively

---

ETIOLOGY AND PATHOGENESIS

- Etiology unclear: Strong genetic influence
- Contributing factors: Thickened anterior longitudinal ligament acting as a tether
- Affected individuals: Taller than average, skeletal age ahead of chronologic age

untreated Scheuermann's disease (greater than 80 degrees), they may present with significant back pain.[19,20,24] The pain, when present, is usually located near the apex of deformity but also may be located in the lumbosacral region, especially if a marked lumbar lordosis is present. Physical examination of the patient with Scheuermann's disease usually reveals a well-circumscribed, angular thoracic or thoracolumbar kyphosis, which is accompanied by a compensatory hyperlordosis of the lumbar spine as well as the cervical spine. When viewed from the side during forward bending (Adam's test), the kyphosis appears sharply angular as opposed to postural kyphosis, where the spine assumes a normal rounded contour. On hyperextension the deformity of Scheuermann's disease remains apparent but disappears in patients with postural kyphosis. Mild or moderate scoliosis is present in approximately one third of patients with Scheuermann's disease. Patients with Scheuermann's disease also frequently have anterior bowing of the shoulder girdle, as well as tightness of the pectoral, hamstring, and hip flexor muscle groups.[16,20,32]

RADIOGRAPHIC FINDINGS

Guidelines for normal thoracic kyphosis established by the Scoliosis Research Society and other investigators include a normal range from 20 to 45 degrees (T1 to T12) in the adolescent.[3,10] The normal range of lumbar lordosis (L1 to S1) is between 50 and 70 degrees. The thoracolumbar spine (T10 to L2) is normally "neutral" or slightly lordotic (0 degrees to 10 degrees). The normal sagittal gravity line passes through the spinous process of T1 and T12, and the sacral promontory.

The diagnosis of Scheuermann's disease is based on a standing lateral 36-inch radiograph with the arms 30 to 45 degrees below the horizontal. To establish the diagnosis there must be a minimum of 5 degrees of anterior vertebral body wedging of three adjacent vertebrae.[33] Schmorl's nodes, as well as irregularity and flattening of vertebral end plates and narrowing of the intervertebral disc spaces, are frequently seen in Scheuermann's disease.* The structural nature of the deformity is determined by obtaining a lateral radiograph made with the patient placed in a supine hyperextended position over a bolster. In adults with Scheuermann's disease, severe degenerative changes are frequently seen within the deformity often at a young age.[24,26] Patients with pos-

tural kyphosis, on the other hand, have a less acutely angulated nonstructural deformity radiographically and the absence of wedging of vertebral bodies on the standing lateral radiograph. Isthmic spondylolisthesis of L5 has been noted to occur in a small percentage of patients with Scheuermann's disease, presumably related to the hyperlordosis of the lumbar spine.[25]

NATURAL HISTORY

The natural history of Scheuermann's disease is not well documented in the literature and appears to be quite variable. Occasionally it may be present throughout the adolescent growth period with little deformity and minimal symptomatology developing with growth. At other times, however, patients with untreated Scheuermann's disease develop a progressive structural kyphosis throughout the adolescent growth period, resulting in a clinically significant deformity. During adolescence, back pain and fatigue are common but they usually disappear with skeletal maturity unless the deformity is severe.

There are two distinct patterns of Scheuermann's disease based on the location of the apex of the deformity as demonstrated in Figure 50-1.[19] The most common pattern is thoracic with an apex in the midthoracic spine. The thoracic pattern has little likelihood of progression or significant pain later in life as long as the magnitude of the kyphosis is less than 75 degrees. If the deformity is greater than 80 degrees, there is a higher risk of continuing progression and significant risk of disabling pain. A study by Murray et al.[24] detailing a follow-up study of 67 patients with thoracic Scheuermann's disease for an average of 32 years noted that patients worked in jobs requiring less physical activity than age-matched controls. These patients also had more severe pain and were concerned about their appearance but did

---

*References 1, 12, 14, 20, 28, 29.

A   B   C

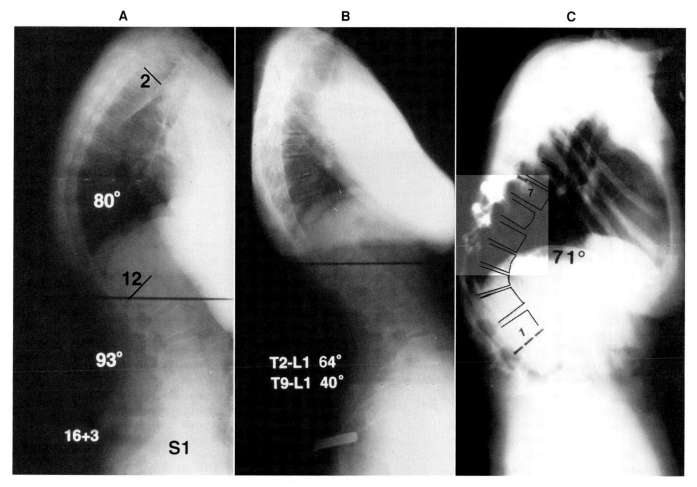

Figure 50-1. **A,** Standing lateral radiograph of a 16-year-old female demonstrates the more common thoracic pattern of Scheuermann's disease. **B,** Standing lateral radiograph of a 15-year-old male with the less common thoracolumbar pattern of Scheuermann's disease. **C,** Note severity of deformity relative to Cobb measurement.

not appear to be limited greatly by their symptoms, although there were only a few patients with thoracic kyphosis greater than 80 degrees.

The thoracic pattern of Scheuermann's kyphosis is the most common pattern present in adolescents and adults. The less common pattern has an apex at the thoracolumbar junction (T10 to L1). This region of the spine normally is straight so that any kyphosis is abnormal. This pattern of Scheuermann's disease is much more likely to progress and become painful when the magnitude of the kyphosis approaches 60 to 65 degrees. Sagittal imbalance also frequently becomes a problem in these patients later in life if degenerative disc disease limits the ability of the lumbar spine to accommodate the kyphotic deformity above it.

Neurologic complications related to either a severe kyphotic deformity or disc herniation have been reported infrequently in the literature.[4,8,35] Pain related to isthmic spondylolisthesis, which has been reported to occur in 5% of patients with Scheuermann's disease, may also contribute to low back pain experienced by these patients.[25]

NONOPERATIVE TREATMENT

The need for treatment of Scheuermann's disease is based on the severity of the deformity, the location of the deformity, the presence of pain, and the age of the patient. The treatment of Scheuermann's disease is largely nonoperative.

Adolescents in whom the kyphosis remains mild need only an exercise program to increase flexibility and periodic radiographs until skeletal maturity. Adolescent patients with Scheuermann's disease whose kyphosis is greater than 55 degrees in the thoracic spine or 40 degrees in the thoracolumbar spine should be placed in a combined brace and exercise program. Initial brace treatment should be full time (greater than 20 hours per day) until full correction of the deformity in the brace has occurred, including a partial reversal of vertebral body wedging. At that point, brace treatment can usually be reduced to 12 to 14 hours per day. Part-time brace treatment needs to be continued for 1 year after the fusion of the iliac apophysis. For kyphotic deformities with an apex at T7 or above, a Milwaukee type brace should be considered, whereas those with an apex below T7 can normally be managed with an under-arm thoracolumbosacral orthosis (TLSO) with anterior infraclavicular outriggers. Both stretching and strengthening exercises should be prescribed for trunk, as well as tight hamstring and pectoral musculature. Although the initial improvement in kyphosis may be significant, there is often a gradual loss of correction within the first few years of discontinuance of the brace with only a modest overall long-term correction of the pre-brace deformity.[23,27]

Patients with postural kyphosis can almost always be managed with an exercise program alone because of the nonstructural nature of the deformity. The majority of adults with untreated Scheuermann's disease, as long as the deformity is less than 75 to 80 degrees, will respond to a combination of physical therapy and an aerobic and torso strengthening exercise program.[19,20]

OPERATIVE TREATMENT

Indications for surgical treatment in the adolescent include (1) a progressive kyphotic deformity of 80 degrees in the thoracic spine or 65 degrees in the thoracolumbar spine, (2) a symptomatic thoracic kyphosis of greater than 75 degrees or a thoracolumbar kyphosis greater than 60 degrees not controlled by conservative measures, or (3) patients with significant sagittal imbalance secondary to the kyphotic deformity.[7,19,20]

The basic biomechanical principles for correction of kyphosis include (1) lengthening of the anterior column of the spine by means of anterior discectomy and release and providing anterior column support with structural grafting or continued growth (Hueter-Volkmann), and (2) shortening and stabilization of the posterior column usually performed by posterior rigid instrumentation using cantilever bending and compression as corrective forces.

Goals of surgical treatment include (1) maximizing safe correction of the kyphosis, (2) achieving sagittal balance, and (3) providing rigid internal fixation, which will promote a successful fusion without the use of internal support.

SURGICAL TECHNIQUES
Posterior Instrumentation and Fusion

Posterior instrumentation alone probably should be reserved for the skeletally immature patient with a very flexible kyphosis, as shown in Figure 50-2.[19] Because of

remaining anterior vertebral body growth, continued growth will frequently occur in response to Hueter-Volkmann's law, thereby resulting in a stable anterior column providing for load sharing. Levels of posterior instrumentation should include all vertebrae within the upper and lower Cobb levels of the kyphosis plus the first lordotic level distally, as shown in Figure 50-3.

The basic posterior instrumentation construct should include a minimum of eight anchors above the apex of the kyphosis and eight anchors below the apex, as shown in Figure 50-4. A minimum of two transverse connectors, one at each end of the construct, should be used for constructs longer than 12 segments. If longer constructs are required, a third transverse connector should be used near the middle of the construct. Anchors above the apex of the kyphosis would generally be hooks, although pedicle screws have also been used successfully despite the fact that their safety and strength relative to hooks have yet to be determined. When hooks are used, they should be placed in a two-level claw configuration for maximal grip strength. Two pediculo-transverse process claws bilaterally above the apex provide excellent fixation. Below the apex of the kyphosis, a pedicle hook should be used approximately two levels distal to the apex of the kyphosis on either side. Fixation distally should consist of pedicle screws in the distal two or three levels plus an optional infralaminar hook on each side of the construct caudal to the inferior pedicle screw. Following insertion of hooks and screws, facetectomies should be carried out at each level bilaterally. Correction is achieved by first under-bending the kyphosis into the rods based on the hyperextension lateral radiograph. In general a 5.5- to 6.0-mm rod is the ideal size, providing adequate strength and allowing adequate flexibility to avoid hook pullout. Next the upper end of the rods are inserted into the hooks above the apex of the deformity and compression is applied to each claw followed by tightening of the locking screws, securing the hooks to the rod. This is then followed by cantilever bending of the distal end of the rod towards the spine. The rods are first inserted into the pedicle hooks just below the apex and the rods are secured to the hooks with the locking screws. Next the distal ends of the rods are delivered into the two or three distal screws and finally, when used, the infralaminar hooks.

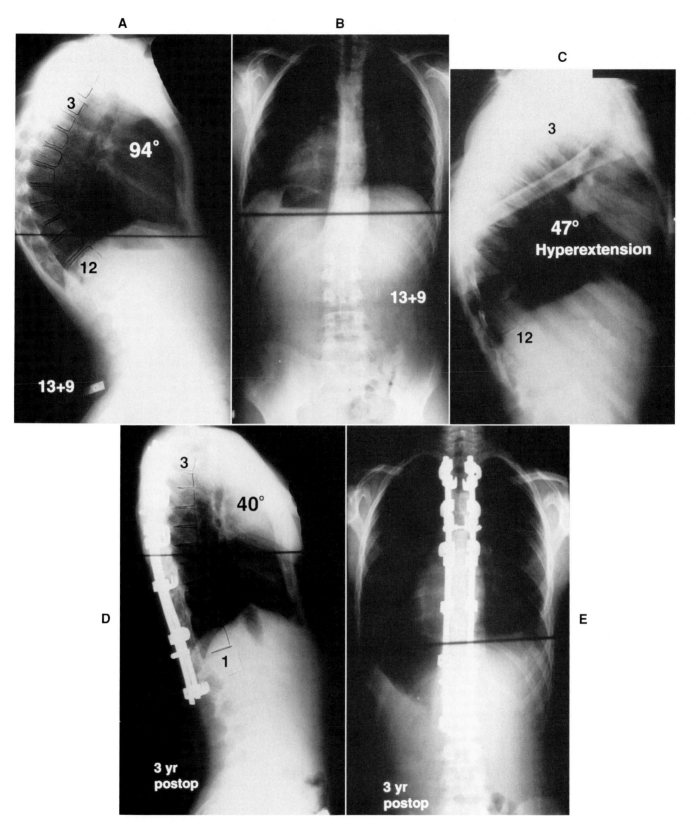

Figure 50-2. **A** to **E,** Pre- and postoperative standing radiographs of a 12-year-old male with Scheuermann's disease. Kyphosis progressed in spite of brace treatment (poor compliance), as noted in **A** and **B**. Note flexibility on hyperextension in radiographs (**C**). Treatment consisted of posterior spinal fusion/instrumentation alone. Note reversal of vertebral wedging on 3-year postoperative radiographs (**D** and **E**).

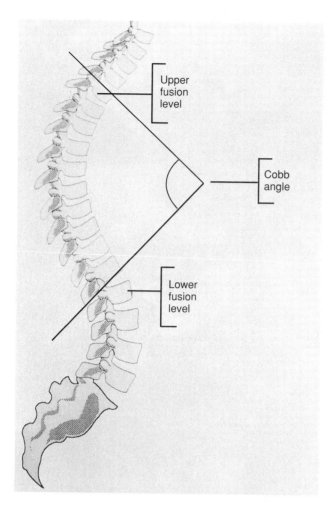

Figure 50-3. Levels for posterior instrumentation should include the upper and lower levels of kyphosis (Cobb method) plus the first lordotic level distally.

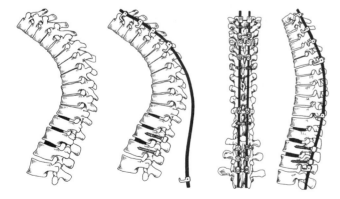

Figure 50-4. Basic posterior construct for kyphosis consisting of double pediculo-transverse claws above the apex and a pedicle hook, two pedicle screws, and an infralaminar hook below the apex. Reduction of the kyphosis by cantilever bending followed by compression toward apex.

POSTERIOR INSTRUMENTATION AND FUSION

- Levels of instrumentation include all vertebrae within upper and lower Cobb levels plus first lordotic level distally
- Next minimum of 8 anchors above apex of kyphosis and 8 anchors below the apex
- Use two transverse connectors for fusions involving >12 segments
- Initially place spinal anchors followed by facetectomies
- Correction achieved by under-bending kyphosis into rods based on hyperextension lateral radiograph
- Insert upper end of rod first, followed by compression of each claw, then cantilever the rod into the distal spinal anchors and perform compression forces to complete reduction of deformity

Further correction is achieved by the application of compressive forces to the pedicle hooks below the apex of the kyphosis as well as the distal screws and infralaminar hooks. Transverse connectors are applied near each end of the construct. Following this, iliac bone graft is packed into each of the facets, as well as along the decorticated transverse processes from the top to the bottom of the construct.

COMBINED ANTERIOR AND POSTERIOR FUSION

In skeletally mature patients there is no potential for reversal of anterior column wedging by growth and so a combined anterior and posterior approach should be considered to provide load sharing and avoid the increased risk of pseudoarthrosis.[7] These combined procedures are normally performed at the same sitting. An anterior release and fusion is usually performed first, followed by a posterior fusion with segmental spinal instrumentation. Levels for anterior release and fusion should include all "fixed" levels above and below the apex of the kyphosis based on the hyperextension lateral radiograph (usually 6 to 8 segments) and distally across the thoracolumbar junction to the distal level of the planned posterior fusion. This would generally include the distal Cobb level plus the first lordotic level. The anterior procedure should be performed first utilizing either a formal thoracotomy or a thoracoscopic approach. The author's preference is an open approach, which allows for a more thorough discectomy and end plate preparation. It is also mandatory to use a double-lumen endotracheal tube so that the ipsilateral lung can be collapsed during the anterior procedure. This greatly facilitates the exposure of the spine. Morselized rib graft is normally used above T10, whereas structural grafts or cages should be considered from T10 distally to provide anterior column support where larger discs are present. A complete discectomy should be carried out back to the posterior longitudinal ligament. Lamina spreaders are used at each level to facilitate better visualization

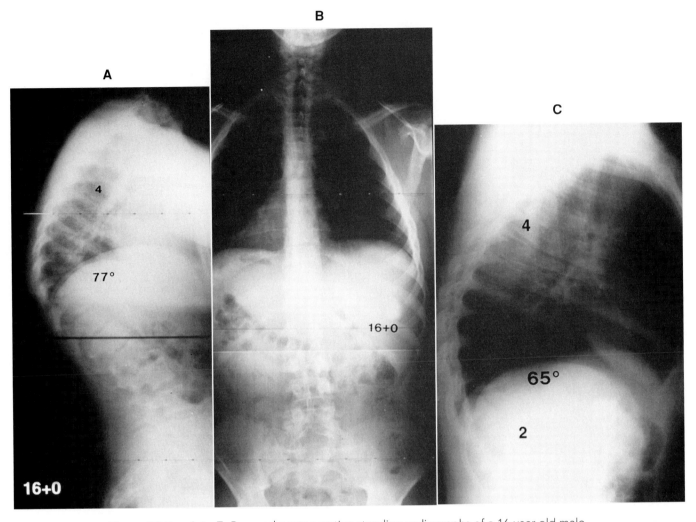

Figure 50-5.   **A** to **E,** Pre- and postoperative standing radiographs of a 16-year-old male with Scheuermann's disease. Note titanium mesh providing interbody support and standard posterior kyphosis construct.

Continued

and disc removal. The bony end plates should be preserved at each level to avoid subsidence when the cages or structural allografts are placed to provide anterior column support. At levels where structural anterior column support is being provided, morselized rib graft should be packed tightly within the disc space around the structural support. Levels above the T10 disc spaces are packed tightly with morselized rib graft, which is usually sufficient unless severe wedging is present. During the exposure, segmental vessels can be ligated and divided or they can be preserved and isolated with vessel loupes, for mobilization when necessary. Malleable narrow spatula retractors work very nicely for facilitating discectomy when segmented vessels are preserved. Following insertion of a chest tube and closure of the chest, the patient is placed on a spine frame in the prone position. It is important to place the upper chest pad proximal to the apex of the kyphosis to facilitate exposure of the proximal end of the thoracic spine.

The levels for posterior fusion and instrumentation should include the upper level of the measured kyphosis (Cobb method) and should include the distal measured

---

ANTERIOR SPINAL RELEASE AND FUSION IN COMBINED ANTERIOR AND POSTERIOR FUSION

- Levels include all "fixed" levels above and below apex of kyphosis and distally across thoracolumbar junction to distal level of planned posterior fusion (distal Cobb level plus first lordotic level)
- Structural grafts usually used below T10
- Bony vertebral end plates preserved
- Segmental vessels ligated or preserved with vessel loupes

level of kyphosis as well as the first lordotic level. Figure 50-5 represents an adolescent patient in whom the standard anterior-posterior construct was used whereas, Figure 50-6 represents another adolescent patient in whom pedicle screws were substituted for hooks above the apex of the kyphosis.

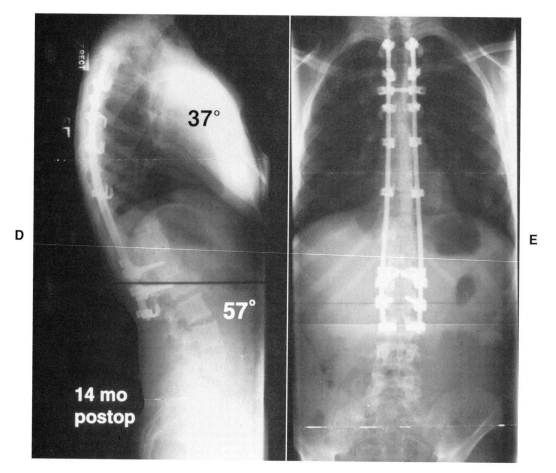

Figure 50-5, contd.

Anterior Instrumentation and Fusion

In adolescent patients with Scheuermann's disease, it is occasionally possible to correct and instrument the deformity anteriorly alone without the need for a posterior procedure. This technique also provides the added ability to save levels proximally. Indications for this procedure would include flexible thoracolumbar or thoracic deformities as long as the apex of the kyphosis is below T9. Instrumentation levels with this technique would include three levels below the upper Cobb level to the distal Cobb level. This technique requires discectomy at each of the levels to be instrumented plus structural grafts or cages at each level to be instrumented.

Following insertion of the structural grafts or cages, bicortical vertebral body screws are inserted at each level followed by insertion of a single 6.5- to 7.0-mm rod that is contoured to the adjacent vertebral bodies. During insertion of the rod, slight compression is applied to each level to provide load sharing between the cages or structural grafts and retracting the pleura between segmental vessels while the discectomies are being carried out. Notice that a larger diameter rod is required than for posterior instrumentation because the rod is loaded in compression rather than tension. The author has used this technique on selected cases during the past 2 years with good early results but a longer follow-up is needed. Figure 50-7 is an example of ante-

> ### ANTERIOR INSTRUMENTATION AND FUSION
>
> - Indications: Flexible thoracic or thoracolumbar deformity with apex of kyphosis below T9
> - Instrumentation levels: Three levels below upper Cobb level to distal Cobb level
> - Requires structural grafts at each instrumental level
> - Following graft insertion, insert bicortical vertebral body screws
> - Larger rod (6.5 to 7.0 cm) is necessary because of anticipated compressive loads
> - Apply compression to each level

rior instrumentation and fusion in an adolescent with a flexible thoracic kyphosis.

Postoperative Management

The patients are out of bed walking on the second postoperative day and are generally discharged on day 6 or 7. No postoperative orthosis is needed. Patients are on a walking program for the first 2 months and then are phased into a light aerobic exercise program that includes swimming and the use of an exercise bike or

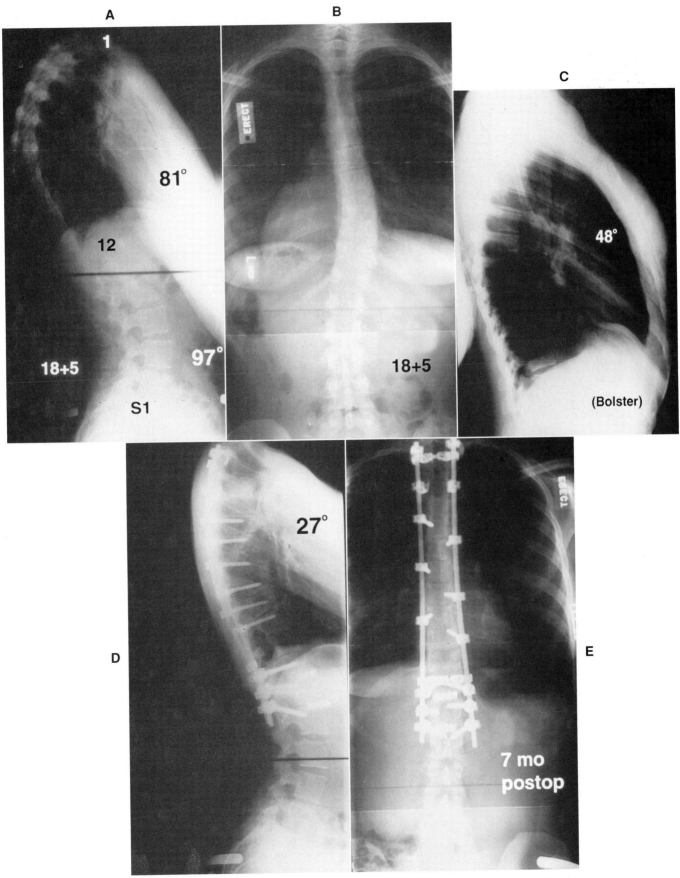

Figure 50-6. **A** to **E,** Pre- and postoperative standing radiographs of a 17-year-old female with Scheuermann's disease. Note the use of pedicle screws in place of hooks above the apex of the kyphosis. Hooks should be used at upper level.

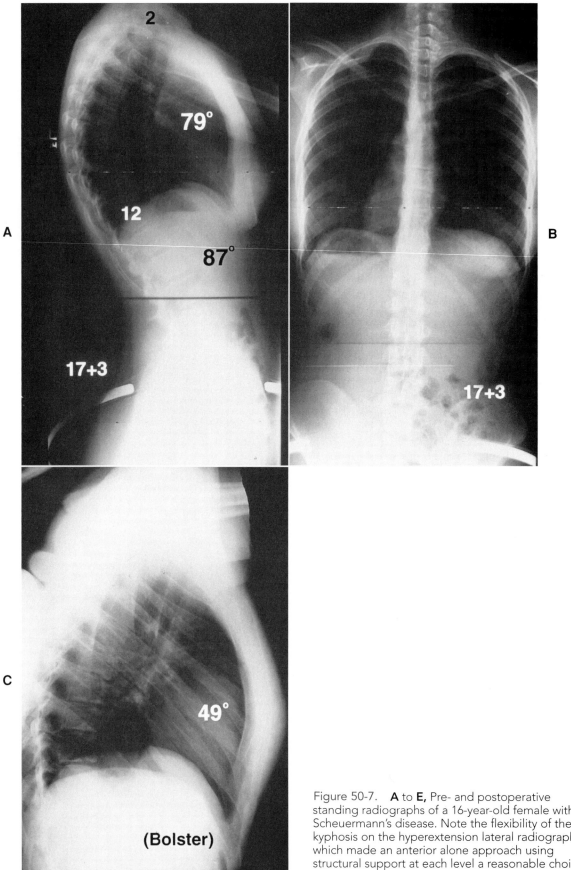

Figure 50-7. **A** to **E,** Pre- and postoperative standing radiographs of a 16-year-old female with Scheuermann's disease. Note the flexibility of the kyphosis on the hyperextension lateral radiograph, which made an anterior alone approach using structural support at each level a reasonable choice. The alternative approach would have been a combined anterior-posterior fusion/instrumentation.

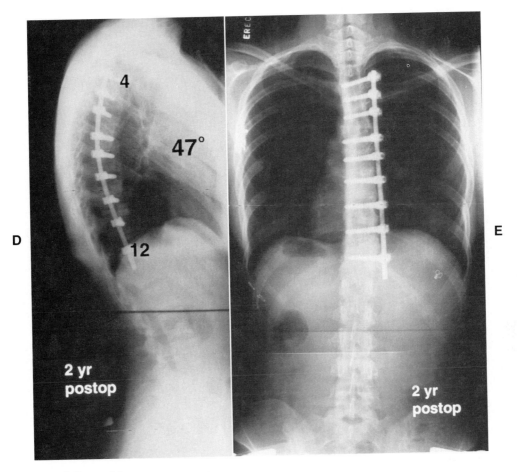

Figure 50-7, cont'd.

POSTOPERATIVE ISSUES

- No postoperative orthosis necessary
- Walking program for first 2 months followed by a light aerobic exercise program and then full activities by 6 to 12 months
- Risk of neurologic injury from surgery: <0.5%
- Junctional kyphosis possible if correction of kyphosis exceeds 50%

treadmill, and they are generally back to full activities in 6 to 12 months.

The risk of a neurologic injury following surgery for Scheuermann's disease is probably less than 0.5%. However, the use of neurologic monitoring is essential during the entire surgical procedure. Evoked potential monitoring, both motor and sensory, or a Stagnara wake-up test should be used on all patients. An increase in latency in motor or sensory evoked potentials of more than 10% or an amplitude drop of greater than 50% is an indication for an immediate wake-up test during surgery. If the patient has a motor deficit postoperatively, instrumentation should immediately be removed and emergency magnetic resonance imaging or a computed tomography-myelogram should be obtained to

rule out the presence of a compressive lesion as a possible cause of cord injury.

The incidence of postoperative wound infections in adolescents undergoing major surgery with instrumentation is approximately 1%. Prophylactic antibiotics should always be given for 48 hours postoperatively. Traffic in operative suites should be kept to an absolute minimum during surgery.

Pseudarthrosis following posterior-only surgery in adolescents and adults may approach 20% in some series and, for that reason, a combined anterior and posterior approach provides the least risk for pseudarthrosis, which should not be greater than 5%.[5,7,21,34]

Probably the major complication after the surgical correction of kyphotic deformities is the development of a junctional kyphosis occurring either above or below the primary kyphotic deformity. In patients undergoing posterior instrumentation and fusion, failure to incorporate all levels within the kyphosis as well as the first lordotic segment distally may result in a proximal or distal junctional kyphosis, as shown in Figure 50-8. Junctional kyphosis may also occur if correction of the kyphosis exceeds greater than 50%. Lowe and Kasten noted in a series of 32 patients with Scheuermann's kyphosis undergoing surgery that all but two demonstrated "negative" sagittal balance preoperatively, that is, their sagittal gravity line from T1 was more than 2 cm behind the

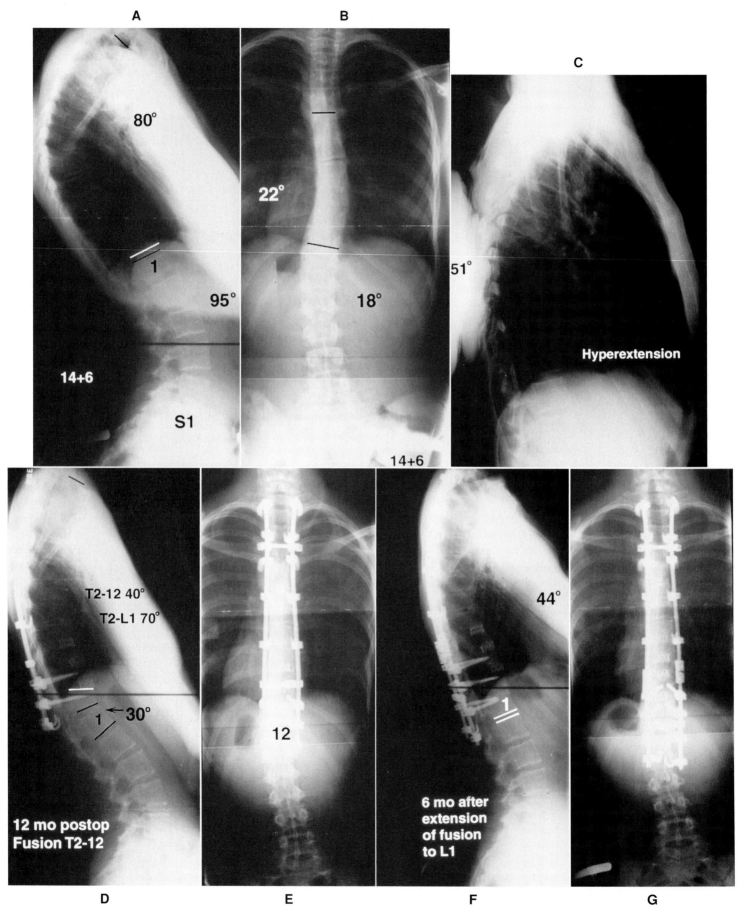

Figure 50-8. *For legend see opposite page.*

Figure 50-8.   **A** to **G**, A 17-year-old female with painful Scheuermann's thoracic kyphosis and a combined anterior/posterior fusion with instrumentation to lower Cobb level but not including the first lordotic disc. Postoperative lateral radiograph revealed a symptomatic distal junctional kyphotic deformity. The fusion and posterior instrumentation was extended by one level with correction of junctional kyphosis.

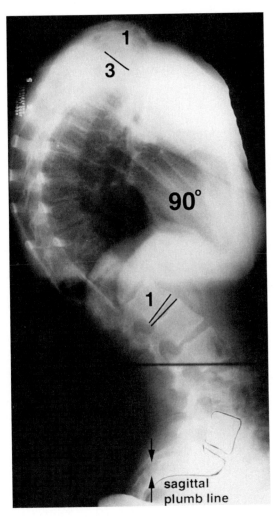

Figure 50-9.   Standing lateral radiograph of a 15-year-old female demonstrating "negative" sagittal balance seen commonly in patients with Scheuermann's disease overcorrection (>50%), which may result in junctional kyphosis.

mity is frequently attributed to "poor posture," resulting in delayed diagnosis and treatment. Indications for treatment remain highly debated because the true natural history of the disease has not been clearly defined. Brace treatment is almost always successful in patients with kyphosis of greater than 55 degrees if the diagnosis is made prior to skeletal maturity. Kyphosis greater than 80 degrees in the thoracic spine or 65 degrees in the thoracolumbar spine is almost never treated successfully without surgery. Surgical treatment in adolescents and young adults should be considered in patients with thoracic deformities greater than 75 degrees and thoracolumbar deformities greater than 60 degrees where there is documented progression, refractory pain, loss of balance, or neurologic deficit. The major complication after surgical treatment is junctional kyphosis, either proximal or distal, which is usually related to not including all levels of the deformity and/or overcorrection of the deformity (greater than 50%). With proper patient selection, excellent outcomes can be expected with either nonoperative or operative treatment in patients with Scheuermann's disease.

SELECTED REFERENCES

McKenzie L, Silence D: Familial Scheuermann's disease: a genetic and linkage study, *J Med Genet* 29:41-45, 1992.

Murray PM, Weinstein SL, Spratt KF: The natural history and long-term follow-up of Scheuermann kyphosis, *J Bone Joint Surg Am* 75:236-248, 1993.

Ogilvie JW, Sherman J: Spondylolysis in Scheuermann's disease, *Spine* 12:251-253, 1987.

Sorensen KH: *Scheuermann's juvenile kyphosis: clinical appearances, radiography, aetiology, and prognosis,* Copenhagen, 1964, Munksgaard.

REFERENCES

1. Aufdermaur M: Juvenile kyphosis (Scheuermann's disease): radiography, histology, and pathogenesis, *Clin Orthop* 154:166-174, 1981.
2. Aufdermaur M, Spycher M: Pathogenesis of osteochondrosis juvenilis Scheuermann, *J Orthop Res* 4:452-457, 1986.
3. Bernhardt M, Bridwell K: Segmental analysis of the sagittal plane alignment of the normal thoracic and lumbar spines and thoracolumbar junction, *Spine* 14:717-721, 1989.
4. Bradford DS, Garcia A: Neurological complications in Scheuermann's disease: a case report and review of the literature, *J Bone Joint Surg Am* 51:567-572, 1969.
5. Bradford DS, Moe JH, Montalvo FJ, et al.: Scheuermann's kyphosis: Results of surgical treatment by posterior spine arthrodesis in twenty-two patients. *J Bone Joint Surg Am* 57:439-448, 1975.
6. Bradford DS et al.: Scheuermann's kyphosis: a form of osteoporosis? *Clin Orthop* 118:110-115, 1976.
7. Bradford DS et al.: Scheuermann's kyphosis: results of surgical treatment by combined anterior-posterior spine arthrodesis in twenty-four patients. *J Bone Joint Surg Am* 62:705-712, 1980.
8. Chiu KY, Luk KD: Cord compression caused by multiple disc herniations and intraspinal cyst in Scheuermann's disease, *Spine* 20:1075-1079, 1995.

sacral promontory, as shown in Figure 50-9.[21] It is felt that if the preoperative kyphosis is corrected more than 50%, sagittal balance will be shifted further posteriorly, which may result in a proximal or distal junctional kyphosis as an attempt to achieve more normal sagittal balance.

CONCLUSIONS

Scheuermann's disease is the most common cause of structural kyphosis in adolescents. The kyphotic defor-

9. Findlay A, Conner AN, Conner JM: Dominant inheritance of Scheuermann's juvenile kyphosis, *J Med Genet* 26:400-403, 1989.

10. Fon GT, Pitt MJ, Thies AC Jr: Thoracic kyphosis: range in normal subjects, *Am J Roentgenol* 134:979-983, 1980.

11. Gilsanz V, Gibbeus DT, Carlson M: Vertebral bone density in Scheuermann's disease, *J Bone Joint Surg Am* 71:894-897, 1989.

12. Greene TL, Hensinger RN, Hunter LY: Back pain and vertebral changes simulating Scheuermann's disease, *J Pediat Orthop J* 5:1-7, 1985.

13. Halal F, Gledhill RB, Fraser FC: Dominant inheritance of Scheuermann's juvenile kyphosis, *Am J Dis Child* 1323:1105-1107, 1978.

14. Harreby M et al.: Are radiologic changes in the thoracic and lumbar spine of adolescence risk factors for low back pain in adults? A 25-year prospective cohort study of 640 school children, *Spine* 20:2298-2302, 1995.

15. Ippolito E, Bellocci M, Montanavo A: Juvenile kyphosis: an ultra-structure study, *J Pediatr Orthop* 5:315-322, 1985.

16. Lambrinudi C: Adolescent and senile kyphosis, *Br Med J* 2:800-804, 1934.

17. Lings S, Mikkelsen L: A Scheuermann's disease with low localization: a problem of under diagnoses, *Scan J Rehab Med* 14:77-79, 1982.

18. Lopez RA et al.: Osteoporosis in Scheuermann's disease, *Spine* 13:1099-1102, 1988.

19. Lowe TG: Scheuermann's disease. In Bridwell KH, DeWald RL, eds: *Textbook of spine surgery*, Philadelphia, 1997, Lippincott-Raven, pp. 1173-1198.

20. Lowe TG: Current concepts review: Scheuermann disease, *J Bone Joint Surg Am* 72:940-945, 1990.

21. Lowe TG, Kasten MD: An analysis of sagittal curves and balance after Cotrel-Dubousset instrumentation for kyphosis secondary to Scheuermann's disease: a review of 32 patients, *Spine* 19:1680-1685, 1994.

22. McKenzie L, Silence D: Familial Scheuermann's disease: a genetic and linkage study, *J Med Genet* 29:41-45, 1992.

23. Montgomery SP, Erwin WE: Long-term results of Milwaukee brace treatment, *Spine* 6:5-8, 1981.

24. Murray PM, Weinstein SL, Spratt KF: The natural history and long-term follow-up of Scheuermann kyphosis, *J Bone Joint Surg Am* 75:236-248, 1993.

25. Ogilvie JW, Sherman J: Spondylolysis in Scheuermann's disease, *Spine* 12:251-253, 1987.

26. Paajaanen H et al.: Disc degeneration in Scheuermann disease, *Skeletal Radiol* 18:523-526, 1989.

27. Sachs B et al.: Scheuermann kyphosis: follow-up of Milwaukee-brace treatment, *J Bone Joint Surg Am* 69:50-57, 1987.

28. Scheuermann H: Kyfosis dorsalis juvenilis, *Ugeskr Laeger* 82:385-393, 1920.

29. Schmorl G, Junghanns H: *The human spine in health and disease*, New York, 1959, Grune & Stratton, pp. 198-218.

30. Scoles PV et al.: Vertebral alterations in Scheuermann's kyphosis, *Spine* 16:509-515, 1991.

31. Skogland LB, Steen H, Trygstad O: Spinal deformities in tall girls, *Acta Orthop Scand* 56:155-157, 1985.

32. Somhegyi A, Ratko I: Hamstring tightness and Scheuermann's disease, *Am J Phys Med Rehab* 72:44, 1993 [commentary].

33. Sorensen KH: *Scheuermann's juvenile kyphosis: clinical appearances, radiography, aetiology, and prognosis*, Copenhagen, 1964, Munksgaard.

34. Strum PF, Dobson JC, Armstrong GW: The surgical management of Scheuermann's disease, *Spine* 18:685-691, 1993.

35. Yablon JS, Kasdon DL, Levine H: Thoracic cord compression in Scheuermann's disease, *Spine* 13:896-898, 1988.

Complications IX

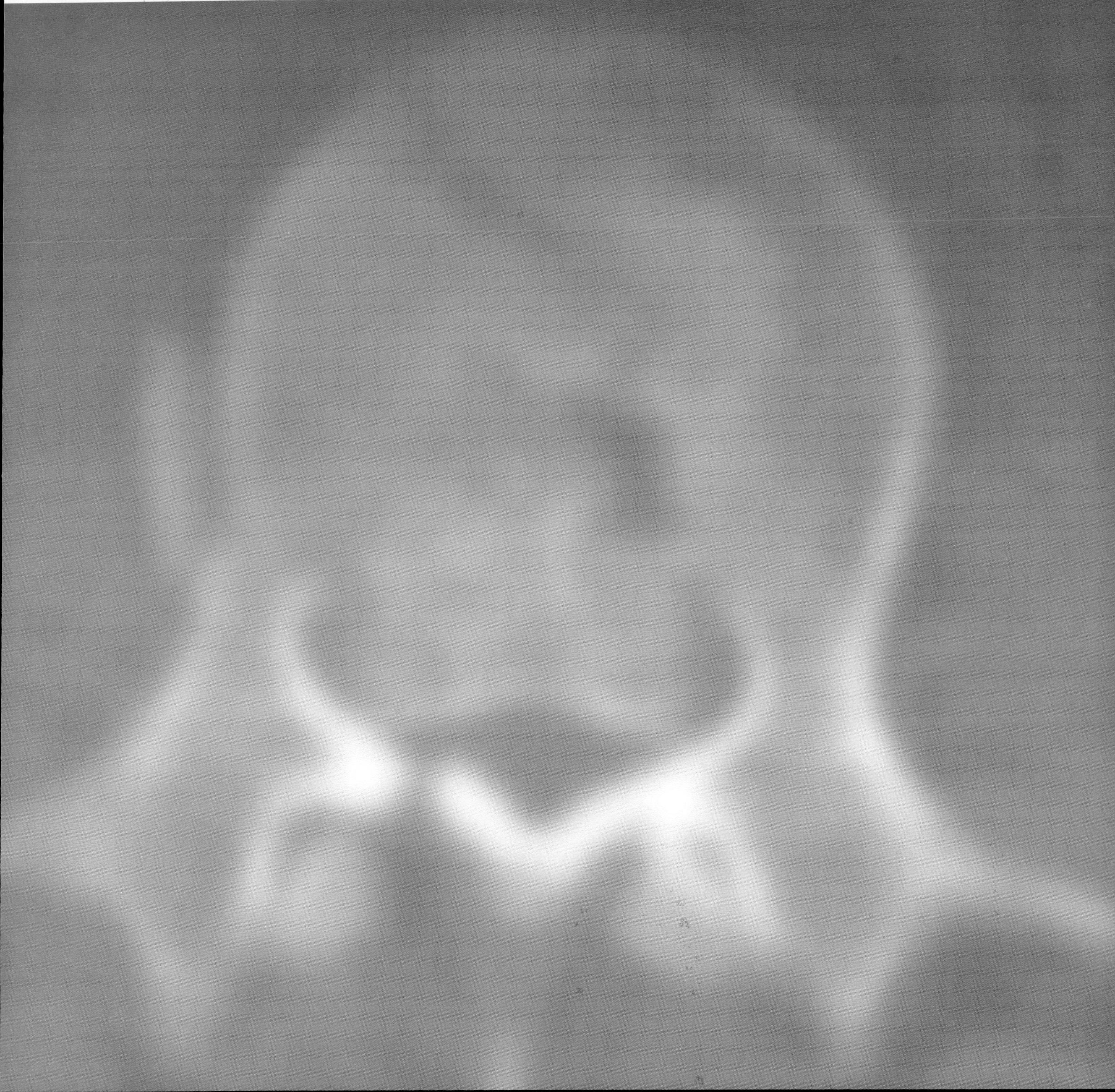

Management of Iatrogenic Neurologic Loss Due to Spinal Instrumentation

William M. Oxner, James D. Kang

Spinal surgery is a complex and demanding field. With the advent of modern spinal instrumentation and surgical technique, many patients with previously inoperable lesions can now be safely and effectively treated. For example, patients with metastatic cancer to the spine and impending neurologic deficit were once inadequately treated with laminectomy alone, and went on to dismal results, often with worsening of the neurologic deficit. Such patients can now be treated with anterior decompression and rigid instrumentation either anteriorly or posteriorly, and this has increased the likelihood of a successful outcome. However, with the increase in the rates of instrumentation, in both the cervical and thoracolumbar spine, has come an increase in serious complications such as deep wound infection, hardware failure, and iatrogenic neurologic injury. Neurologic injury is probably the most feared complication in spine surgery and is probably underreported in the medical literature, so that the exact incidence is difficult to quantify. For practical purposes, in this chapter we will discuss neurologic deficits arising from instrumentation in the cervical, thoracolumbar, and lumbosacral spine as separate topics.

CLASSIFICATION OF DEFICIT

Postoperative neurologic deficits can be classified according to the severity of the deficit. Minor deficits take the form of radiculopathy, sensory impairment without motor loss, temporary dysesthesias in the feet, or lesser degrees of neurologic deficit. Many of these lesions are transient in the postoperative course of these patients and may, at times, go unnoticed. Major deficits are considered those in which the patient suffers postoperative paraparesis, paraplegia, or a spinal cord syndrome. Paraparesis is defined as a definite weakness bilaterally in the lower extremities and paraplegia as complete lower extremity paralysis. Approximately 50% of spinal cord lesions arising from deformity correction in the thoracolumbar spine are complete deficits.[37] The

Brown-Séquard syndrome is most commonly seen with intraoperative damage caused by a surgical instrument or with the placement of a hook or wire within the spinal canal. Anterior cord syndrome is often the result of interruption of the anterior spinal artery and has been seen most commonly as the result of distraction of a kyphotic spine. In these cases, with distraction the spinal column is lengthened and the anterior aspect of the spinal cord is drawn up against the vertebral bodies at the apex of the curve. This complication has even been seen accompanying preoperative skeletal traction in kyphoscoliosis. Central cord and posterior cord syndromes are very rarely associated with spinal instrumentation. Another method of classifying postoperative deficits involves dividing into those that are transient and those that are persistent. Most deficits are transient, with only about 30% of those in a large series of scoliosis cases being persistent.[42]

ROLE OF SPINAL CORD MONITORING

The majority of surgeons performing complicated cervical and thoracolumbar spine surgery, which puts the neurologic contents as risk, use some form of spinal cord monitoring. The Stagnara wake-up test is still the

---

CLASSIFICATION OF NEUROLOGIC INJURY

MINOR
- Radiculopathy
- Sensory impairment
- Temporary dysesthesias in the feet

MAJOR
- Paraparesis
- Paraplegia (50% of deficits in scoliosis)
- Spinal cord syndrome

Note: 70% of deficits are transient

SPINAL CORD MONITORING

SSEP
- Valuable diagnostic tool
- Used by 153/173 surgeons in the United States during deformity surgery in the 1995 SRS report
- Significant change defined as follows
  - 50% decrease in amplitude of signal
  - 10% change in latency of signal
- False negatives: 1 in 787 cases
- False positives: 1 in 66 cases

NMEP
- May be better predictor of motor paralysis than SSEP
- Positive when 10% latency change or 80% amplitude

gold standard in detecting gross motor deficits.[53] If done properly, this test can be a very sensitive and reliable diagnostic tool.[43] There are two important steps in the correct and efficient use of this test. First, patients must be prepared adequately before surgery. They must be informed that they will be awakened during surgery and asked to move their arms and legs near the end of the operation. Second, the anesthesiologist must have the patient prepared by eliminating muscle relaxants and anesthetic agents over the appropriate time period to allow the test to proceed. The principal disadvantages are that it cannot be performed continuously throughout the case and it is a measure of gross motor function only. This has led to the development of other monitoring devices: somatosensory evoked potentials (SSEP) and neurogenic motor evoked potentials (NMEP).

SSEP spinal cord monitoring has been carried out during deformity correction, tumor surgery, and thoracolumbar trauma surgery for the past two to three decades. In addition to its use as a monitoring tool in thoracolumbar surgery, many surgeons in high-risk surgeries of the cervical spine now routinely use them. SSEPs are a valuable clinical tool that can monitor the function of both the spinal cord and the individual nerve roots. This ability not only makes SSEP a diagnostic tool but also allows for intraoperative differentiation of spinal cord and spinal nerve root problems. This form of monitoring is somewhat limited in those patients with neuromuscular abnormalities. Most surgeons utilize SSEPs during thoracolumbar deformity, trauma, and tumor surgery, with 153 of 173 surgeons polled in the Scoliosis Research Society (SRS) group using them routinely in a 1995 SRS report.[42] Some authors have even written that spinal cord monitoring is mandatory during scoliosis correction. If monitoring is used, it has become clear that both the latency of the signal and the amplitude should be measured routinely. Failure to follow both may result in false negative results.[11,42] A significant change in SSEP signal has been defined as one in which the signal latency changes by more than 10% or when the amplitude of the signal decreases by more than 50%.[43] Amplitude is more sensitive to the onset of the injury,[43] but should not be used in isolation.

Unfortunately no monitoring tool is perfect and some false positive results (change in SSEP with no detectable postoperative deficit) and false negative results (neurologic deficit with normal SSEP) will be obtained. In 1995 the SRS reported on spinal cord monitoring in 51,263 cases and identified the false-negative rate as 0.127% (1 in 787) and the false-positive rate as 1.51% (1 in 66).[42] It is important to note that the group of false positives includes those in which there was a change in SSEP, which caused the surgeon to alter the treatment plan in order to avoid a postoperative deficit. On occasion surgeons have ignored the change in SSEP with disastrous consequences.[5,28] Given what we know today about SSEPs, it would be inadvisable to study what the effect of leaving the instrumentation in place would be on the postoperative outcome if the SSEPs are positive during the operative case.

SSEP is a good measure of the sensory pathways of the spinal cord. One major limitation of SSEP monitoring is that it is principally a measure of posterior spinal column function and the major complication we are trying to prevent is motor paralysis, which occurs with anterior spinal cord injury. Animal studies have shown that the dorsal columns are a good measure of the entire spinal cord function but, on occasion, a significant motor deficit arises with normal dorsal column function. This may occur in kyphosis correction where the anterior spinal artery is injured, resulting in motor paralysis with preservation of posterior column function.

Some investigators have advocated the use of motor evoked potentials, (MEP) but their use has been tempered by the limitation of anesthetic medications compatible with MEPs. The development of neurogenic MEP (NMEP) has been an advantage.[43] NMEP measures action potentials in the nerves, not the contraction in the muscle, and has been shown to be a reliable measure of motor tract function. They are reliable in amplitude, latency, and morphology, and the patient can be fully relaxed. This has allowed specific criteria to be developed: a 10% change in latency and an 80% decrease in amplitude are both significant changes.[43] In several animal studies, NMEPs always correlate with postoperative motor status regardless of what is demonstrated on SSEP.[43]

Some form of spinal cord monitoring should be used during high-risk cases. Neurologic deficit can be detected as early as 2 minutes after a mechanical injury, which allows the surgeon to react immediately to the potential problem. A recent report on 22 patients with false-negative SSEP identified that the failure to detect the deficit was personnel related in each of the cases.[43] High-quality monitoring is essential, and the surgeon should have a good knowledge of the monitoring system to be used in the operating room and should work closely with the neurophysiology personnel.

There is a wide variability of surgical procedures performed in each of the different areas of the spine with a marked difference in the types of implants used. For practical purposes we have divided the rest of the discussion into neurologic deficits arising from the cervical spine instrumentation, those arising from thoracolumbar deformity correction, and those arising from instrumentation of the lumbosacral spine.

CERVICAL SPINE
Incidence

Anterior and posterior instrumentation of the cervical spine is indicated for a number of clinical conditions, which include degenerative disorders, trauma, iatrogenic instability, and neoplastic or infectious destruction. Anterior cervical plates have offered the advantage of decreased bone graft complications (e.g., graft extrusion) and enhanced fusion rates, particularly with multiple level fusions. Flynn reported neurologic deficit with anterior cervical fusion in 311 of 82,114 total cases (0.3%) in his 1974 questionnaire of 704 neurosurgeons.[18] In the 70 myelopathic complications reported in this series, 53 were noted immediately postoperatively. This report predates the widespread use of anterior plating for anterior cervical disc fusion (ACDF) and most deficits were due to hematoma or by technical mishaps, such as overpenetration with a Cloward drill, or by direct injury with a surgical instrument. Although some authors advocate bicortical purchase with anterior screws, most current techniques advocate unicortical purchase only. With this standard technique, iatrogenic neurologic injury should be unlikely because of anterior instrumentation alone.

Posterior cervical surgery is generally riskier than anterior cervical surgery with regard to potential neurologic injury. According to the Cervical Spine Research Society, the neurologic risk of posterior cervical surgery approaches 2% and is more than double the risk of anterior surgery. It is unclear how much of the increased risk results from spinal instrumentation alone. There are far more fixation techniques that are used in the posterior cervical spine compared to anterior fusion surgery. The gold standard of posterior cervical fusion has been interspinous wiring, considered a very safe technique with almost no risk of neurologic complication related to the placing of the wires themselves. Alternatives have included sublaminar wires, clamps, hook plates, and lateral mass plates. Sublaminar wires and clamps are both devices that occupy space within the spinal canal and, as such, put the neurologic contents at risk. Sublaminar wires are still routinely used in fusions at the atlantoaxial interval for posttraumatic instability and for instability secondary to inflammatory arthritis. They can be safely used there due to the large space available for the cord in most circumstances. However, passing sublaminar wires under C1 can lead to serious neurologic injury if the patient has stenosis such as may occur in certain rheumatoid patients with marked subluxation or hypertrophic retrodental pannus. Their use should be avoided in stenotic patients, and alternatives such as occiput to C2 instrumentation with or without C1 laminectomy should be used. In the subaxial spine, adverse neurologic outcomes have been reported with the placement of sublaminar wires[6] and sublaminar hooks such as a Halifax clamp into a marginally stenotic canal (Figure 51-1).

CERVICAL SPINE SURGERY AND DEFICITS

- Anterior cervical discectomy: 0.3% incidence of deficit
- Posterior cervical discectomy: 2% incidence of deficit
- Use devices that occupy space in the cervical canal with extreme caution
- Nerve root injury more common than spinal cord injury with posterior cervical surgery

---

Lateral mass screws and plates have been used for over two decades in Europe and in the last decade have become popular in North America. They have emerged as a good alternative to spinous process wiring. Lateral mass or pedicle fixation has a major advantage over interspinous wiring in that it can be used as a posterior fixation device even if the lamina are absent, such as in a postlaminectomy patient or in trauma patients with spinous process fractures. Lateral mass plates have been shown to be biomechanically superior to interspinous wiring[48,51,52] but there is a theoretically greater risk[30] of iatrogenic neurologic injury to the spinal cord and spinal nerve roots.[26] Several authors have shown good clinical results with these plates,* but the rates of neurologic injury have probably been underreported. Only four reports list adverse neurologic outcomes as one of the complications of this technique.[22,25,34,47] Heller et al.[25] reported on 78 consecutive patients who underwent posterior cervical plating with lateral mass screws using the technique described by An, Gordin, and Renner,[3] with a total of 654 screws inserted. Intraoperative fluoroscopy was used and bicortical purchase was attempted in all cases. There were a total of six cases of postoperative radiculopathy. Four cases of radiculopathy were directly attributable to screw trajectory noted on postoperative computed tomography (CT) scans (one screw in each of C5 and C7 and two in the C6 lateral mass), and two other cases of radiculopathy were attributed to iatrogenic foraminal stenosis secondary to reduction or shifting of a lateral mass with screw insertion. Graham et al.[22] found three cases of acquired radiculopathy in 21 patients with a 1.8% incidence per screw and felt the complications were due to attempts at bicortical purchase in the lateral mass.

Cervical pedicle screws are an alternative to lateral mass screws in cervical instrumentation and their use has been reported clinically in the mid to lower cervical spine since 1994.[1] They have been shown to be superior to lateral mass screws in biomechanical testing.[9,29] Their use, however, has been quite limited due to concerns about their safety both with regard to neurologic injury and to interruption of the vertebral arteries. Many surgeons routinely insert pedicle screws at C2 because the vertebral artery courses through the lateral mass at this level and the C2 pedicle is the most forgiving with regards to size and risk of pedicle perforation. There is also usually more room for the cord at this level, making

---

*References 4, 17, 23, 27, 41, 45, 54.

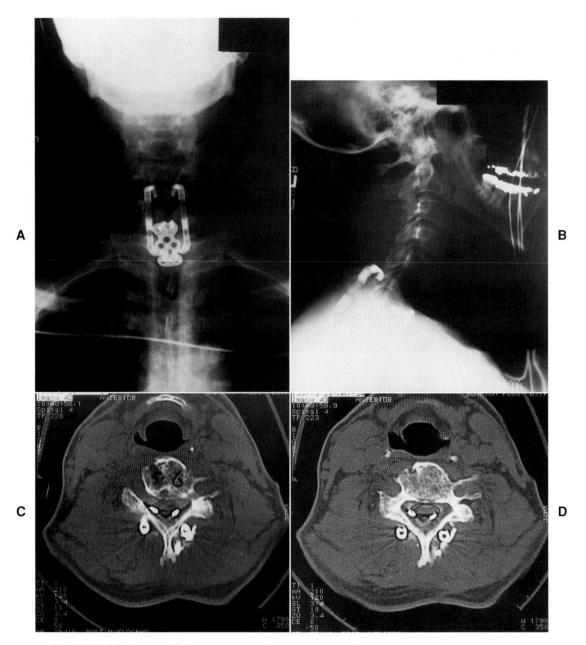

Figure 51-1. **A** and **B,** Elderly patient with cervical clamp inserted in a stenotic spine for posterior fusion. This patient awoke with evidence of myelopathy that went undetected. Several months later the patient presented in florid myelopathy. **C** and **D,** CT-myelogram shows spinal cord compression from degenerative disc disease and the laminar hooks. The patient responded favorably to repeat fusion with lateral mass plates and removal of the clamp.

LATERAL MASS SCREWS

- Spinal cord injury very rare because screws are aimed laterally
- Nerve root injury may be
  Direct: Secondary to direct injury with screw
  Indirect: Iatrogenic foraminal stenosis
- Incidence approximately 1% to 2% of screws
- Primary treatment is prevention

insertion safer. C7 pedicle screws are also commonly used at C7 after performing a foraminotomy to visualize the pedicle. This is a high-stress area, and the pullout strength of a pedicle screw is better than that of a lateral mass screw. However, most surgeons hesitate to use them in the intervening segment from C3 to C6 due to the variability in size and trajectory of the pedicle and the proximity of major neurovascular structures. Recently, Abumi et al.[1] reported on 180 patients in which 712 cervical pedicle screws were inserted. Most patients were studied with CT scans postoperatively. Forty-five

> **CERVICAL PEDICLE SCREWS**
>
> - Commonly performed at C2 and C7
> - Biomechanically superior to lateral mass screws
> - C3 to C6 pedicle morphology variable; neurovascular structures close
> - Abumi reported only two cases of radiculopathy in 180 patients with 712 screws

> **MANAGEMENT**
>
> - Key to treatment: Prevention
> - Avoid bicortical lateral mass screws
> - 14-mm screws may be the optimal length
> - An technique may be the safest
> - SSEPs should monitor ulnar nerve if screws are inserted at C6 or below
> - Remove or replace screw if a problem is detected intraoperatively

screws (6.7%) were found to penetrate the pedicle on postoperative imaging studies. There were three neurovascular complications. Two patients developed radiculopathy; one patient developed a C6 nerve root lesion that resolved without screw removal and another patient developed a C5 nerve root lesion from an inferiorly placed C4 pedicle screw that resolved to normal after removal of the screw. They reported one vertebral artery injury that did not result in neurologic deficit and one case of iatrogenic foraminal stenosis.[2] The authors note that there is variability in pedicle morphometry and orientation, and they recommend careful preoperative planning by experienced surgeons and some form of intraoperative imaging.

MANAGEMENT
Prevention

The first step in the management of iatrogenic deficit is prevention. Experienced and adequately trained spinal surgeons who have a good knowledge of spinal anatomy should carry out instrumentation of the cervical spine. The appropriate implant should be chosen, and space-occupying implants should not be placed in the spinal canal, especially in a stenotic cervical canal. Preoperative planning should include a careful assessment of the radiographs to determine appropriate screw trajectory and to determine the size of the lateral masses, because there can be some variability, particularly at the lateral mass of C7.[3] Bicortical screws probably should not be used, because there will be a higher likelihood of nerve root injury and they have not been shown to have a greater pullout strength than unicortical lateral mass screws.[46] The exception may be at C7, where engaging the second cortex can biomechanically add 20% more resistance to failure.[25] In an anatomic study, Seybold et al.[46] showed that 14-mm screws placed in a superolateral direction did not directly injure any nerve roots.[46] This study, as well as others,[22] suggests that 14 mm may be the optimal screw length if the surgeon is trying to obtain unicortical purchase with a low morbidity. Currently the spine surgeon has three trajectories to chose from—the Magerl, Anderson, and An techniques. A recent anatomic study has shown that the potential risk of nerve root violation is lowest with the An technique.[58] Intraoperative fluoroscopy can be a useful adjunct in correct placement of lateral mass screws.[14] SSEPs of the appropriate nerve territories should be used to aid in intraoperative detection of nerve violation. In Heller, Silcox, and Sutterlin's series[25]

there was one case of false-negative SSEP, in which a C7 lateral mass screw injured the C8 nerve root. This lesion was not picked up intraoperatively because only the median nerve was being monitored. The authors of that series recommend monitoring the ulnar nerve as well if the operative plan includes insertion of lateral mass screws into the C6 lateral mass or lower.

Intraoperative Detection of Deficit

Detection of a neurologic deficit intraoperatively usually is the result of a change in neurophysiologic monitoring. An attenuation of the signal of more than 50% of the baseline amplitudes and/or a latency change of 10%[60] have been shown to be very suggestive of neurologic injury.[12,19,49] Monitoring the spinal cord potentials can identify whether the changes are due to a single nerve root or a spinal cord lesion. In addition, the neurophysiologist can often identify which maneuver was temporally related to the drop in SSEP. A systematic search should then be carried out to determine the cause of neurologic deficit. If the canal has been decompressed, it should be checked to ensure that there is no hematoma or migration of a bone graft into the canal. Any space-occupying implants that have been placed into the cervical canal such as a sublaminar hook or wire should probably be carefully removed at this time. An intraoperative radiograph can help determine whether the trajectory of the screws has been appropriate. If the SSEPs suggest a unilateral nerve root deficit and the surgeon has inserted a screw into the corresponding lateral mass, this screw should be carefully investigated. The screw should be removed and the hole probed to see if there was an overpenetration of the far cortex. If this is the case, the screw should be replaced with a shorter screw or the hole redrilled in a more appropriate trajectory. If there has been a single nerve root lesion and the screw hole trajectory is adequate without overpenetration of the far cortex, the surgeon should consider the possibility of iatrogenic foraminal stenosis due to shifting of the lateral masses relative to one another. The plate could then be contoured differently or a foraminotomy of the nerve root could be performed at this time.

Postoperative Detection

All patients undergoing cervical spinal surgery should be examined in the recovery room as soon as they are

POSTOPERATIVE DETECTION

- MRI is best test if there is a spinal cord injury
- Evacuate any hematoma or bone graft in the canal urgently
- CT scan is best test for determining path of lateral mass and pedicle screws
- Symptoms usually resolved by removing or replacing screw impinging a nerve root

SCLIOSIS—INCIDENCE OF PARALYSIS

MacEwen (1975): 0.72% in 7885 cases; 50% of deficits complete[37]
SRS (1983): 0.72%
SRS (1995): 0.55%

awake enough to undergo a physical examination. When a serious neurologic deficit such as a spinal cord syndrome is detected in the early postoperative period, the patient should be emergently treated with dexamethasone intravenously and a lateral radiograph should be taken to determine the position of bone graft and plates. Although the position of lateral mass screw can be estimated from plain radiographs, other tests may be more definitive. If nothing is found on the plain radiograph, the physician should order CT myelography or magnetic resonance imaging (MRI). MRI offers the advantage of better visualization of a possible epidural hematoma and the ability to see contusion within the spinal cord. CT has a distinct advantage in detecting the exact position of lateral mass screws. If the investigation shows spinal cord impingement from bone graft, hardware, or hematoma, the patient should be taken back to the operating room urgently for decompression with removal or repositioning of hardware. Nerve root impingement secondary to iatrogenic foraminal stenosis or suboptimally positioned lateral mass screw can be detected with CT myelography. In the case of a screw that has penetrated the neural foramen, removal of the screw or replacing it with a shorter screw should provide partial or complete resolution of the radiculopathy in most cases.[22,25] The natural history of iatrogenic foraminal stenosis secondary to shifting of lateral mass with insertion of screws is unknown; however, with time the situation should resolve with conservative treatment. Strong consideration should be given to taking the patient back to the operating room for a foraminotomy in the early postoperative period. In Heller, Silcox, and Sutterlin's series,[25] both patients with foraminal stenosis eventually required foraminotomy.

THORACOLUMBAR INSTRUMENTATION

Instrumentation of the thoracolumbar spine is commonly done for trauma, tumors, and most commonly for scoliosis. The most devastating complication in spinal surgery performed on neurologically normal children and young adults is spinal cord injury. Before the development of complex spinal instrumentation, postoperative neurologic deficit was quite uncommon but not unheard of. With the increased ability to correct deformities with modern implants, more stresses are developed on the contents of the spinal canal. Neurologic injury secondary to instrumentation of the thoracolumbar spine can be the result of one of two processes: coincident or direct.

Coincidental damage occurs as the result of distraction of the spinal cord itself or due to an interruption of the blood supply to the cord such as may occur during stretching of the spinal cord. Direct injury to the cord may arise from improper placement of a hook or a sublaminar wire or from impingement on the cord secondary to a process such as a fracture of the lamina.

Incidence

The true incidence of spinal cord injury secondary to instrumentation in the thoracolumbar spine is difficult to identify because of the variety of new instruments, variability in the use of spinal cord monitoring, and the fact that there is probably a certain amount of underreporting. In 1975 MacEwen, Bunnell, and Sriram[37] reported to the SRS an incidence of 0.72% cord injury in a review of 7885 cases submitted by the SRS. Over half of the patients suffered from complete paraplegia and half from partial paraplegia, and 46% were persistent. Six patients became paraplegic following skeletal traction alone.[37] In 1983 the same group reported an incidence of 0.72% and in 1987 the Morbidity Report noted the incidence of cord injury in patients with idiopathic scoliosis was 0.26%. Sublaminar wires represented 39% of the total injuries and C-D instrumentation accounted for 33%. The Harrington rod accounted for a small percentage of the neurologic injuries, but it is unknown what percentage of the total cases they represent in this study. Nuwer et al.[42] reported on behalf of the SRS in 1995. There were 51,263 monitored cases performed by American surgeons, with a neurologic deficit rate of 0.55%. There was also a decrease in the number of persistent deficits compared with MacEwen, Bunnell, and Siram's report[37] (0.31% versus 0.46%). The incidence of neurologic complications of thoracic pedicle screw and anterior systems is unknown, but there have been reports of cord injury in the literature.[59] Numerous studies have documented the neurologic complications associated with sublaminar wires especially if used with a Harrington distraction system.[13,28,37,56] However, many of the neurologic problems with sublaminar wires are temporary sensory deficits.[56] There has been definite evidence of a learning curve associated with the use of both sublaminar wires[56] and the complex C-D system. Proper training and careful handling are imperative factors in the use of these implants (Figure 51-2).

Identification of Risk Factors

In dealing with potential complications such as paraplegia, the major emphasis should be on prevention. The

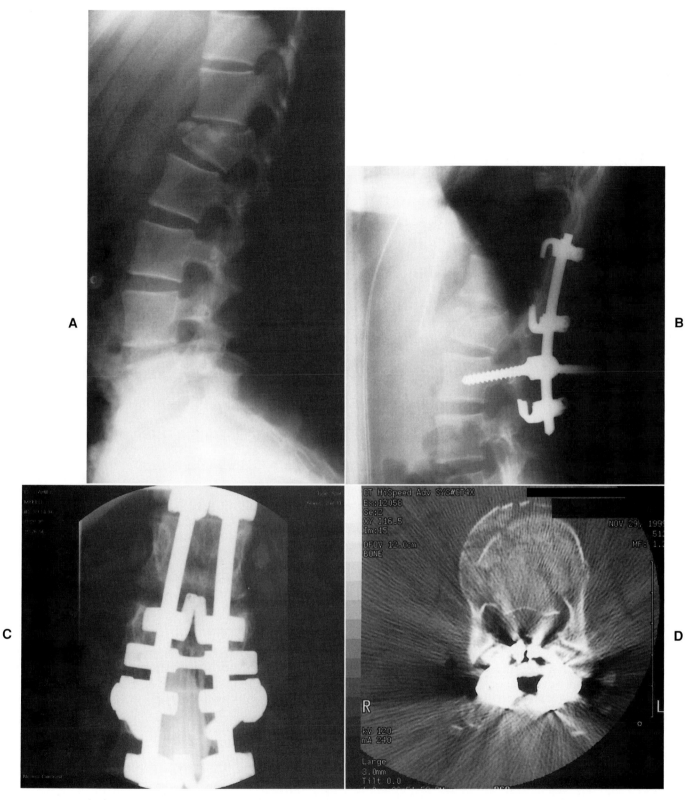

Figure 51-2. This case illustrates the dangers of inserting laminar hooks too close to the zone of injury in a thoracolumbar spine trauma. **A,** Lateral radiograph of a 22-year-old woman who suffered a lumbar burst fracture. She remained neurologically intact. **B,** She underwent operative intervention, but a hook was inadvertently inserted under the lamina at T11. **C** and **D,** Myelogram showed a block at the fracture site, and the patient awoke with a conus medullaris syndrome.

Continued

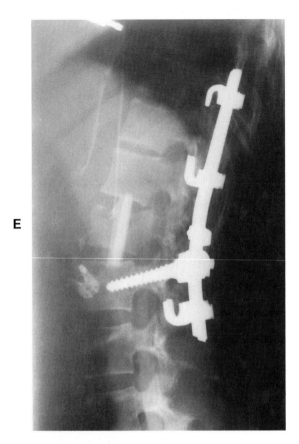

E

Figure 51-2, cont'd.   **E,** She recovered after repositioning of the hooks and anterior decompression.

key element in prevention is identification of patients who are at high risk. One group of patients at high risk is trauma patients who are neurologically intact or who already have a partial deficit. Great care must be taken to avoid placing implants within the canal near the zone of injury because there may be reduced space available for the cord due to fracture fragments and spinal cord swelling. Failure to avoid this zone with laminar hooks can be disastrous. With anterior spinal surgery, care must be taken not to ligate the segmental vessels too close to the vertebral foramen, which may put the cord at risk of ischemia and susceptible to injury at the time of spinal correction. Some surgeons advocate temporary occlusion of the segmental vessels with SSEP monitoring. Apel et al.[5] noted 7 of 44 cases of positive SSEP findings with application of surgical clips during anterior surgery for kyphoscoliosis. In each case the electrophysiologic monitoring was consistent with neurologic deficit but returned to baseline after removal of the clips and all patients awoke with no evidence of neurologic deficit. Obviously the surgeons in that series had to choose an alternative treatment plan with failure to ligate the segmental vessels. Elective patients who are at greatest risk from spinal instrumentation are those with a short segment kyphosis[57]: congenital kyphosis, neurofibromatosis, and skeletal dysplasias, and those with postinfection and postirradiation deformity. The risk is proportional to the size and rigidity of the curve.

RISK FACTORS FOR PARALYSIS

- Preoperative neurologic deficit
- Congenital kyphosis
- Neurofibromatosis
- Skeletal dysplasias
- Following infection or radiation
- Congenital scoliosis: Especially a hemivertebra with a contralateral bar
- Severe, rigid curves more risky

Several investigators have seen permanent paraplegia as the result of preoperative traction in which the spinal cord is pulled up against the apex of the curve and is felt to impinge the cord and obstruct the anterior spinal artery.[37] Intraspinal anomalies are also important to identify as they have been noted to occur in as much as 18% of patients with congenital scoliosis.[38] The most common anomalies include diastematomyelia, cysts, teratoma, tethering of the cord, lipoma, and lipofibroma, and the highest incidence of anomaly was found in unilateral unsegmented bar with a contralateral hemivertebra. Preoperative traction is contraindicated in these patients and preoperative consultation with a surgeon who specializes in these anomalies should be sought.

Another risk factor in scoliosis surgery is the severity and rigidity of the curve. A large rigid curve represents a high-risk situation in which there will be hooks placed on the apex of the curve and there may be risk of laminar fracture and subsequent spinal cord injury.[50] Correction of a curve beyond the limits of the preoperative bending films has also been shown to have a higher incidence of neurologic deficit, especially if a distraction system with sublaminar wires is to be used. Overcorrection should be avoided.[36,56] Luque[36] has stated that the maximum correction safely achieved is the number of degrees on maximum preoperative bending correction plus 10 degrees (Figure 51-3).

Preoperative Planning

Prevention of neurologic injury starts with identifying high-risk patients for surgery as mentioned earlier. Careful planning is advised to avoid overcorrection or distraction of high-risk curves,[56] and MRI is used to identify potential problems in this patient population. If the patient already has a neurologic deficit or is deemed high risk for surgery, consideration should be given to preoperative administration of intravenous steroids. In the research for drug management of spinal cord injury in dogs, it has been shown that the animals that are treated before the injury usually fare the best. This group should include those with rigid kyphosis, who are at highest risk. In no circumstances should those patients with kyphoscoliosis or congenital curves be treated with preoperative skeletal traction or with distraction instrumentation such as Harrington rods. In addition the preoperative plan should probably include avoiding putting implants such as hooks and sublaminar wires within the

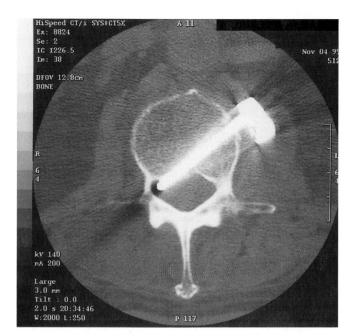

Figure 51-3. This patient awoke after anterior spinal surgery with anterior thigh pain. CT scan shown here detects a screw inserted into the spinal canal. This patient's symptoms resolved within several days of surgery.

canal at the apex of kyphotic deformities, as the canal may be small here. Finally, deformity correction in the spine should be carried out by those surgeons with adequate training and expertise in the field of deformity surgery as many of the newer instrumentation systems are complicated and have a learning curve associated with them.

Intraoperative Detection of Deficit

Even with appropriate planning and meticulous and careful surgical technique by an experienced spine surgeon, problems can still arise. Intraoperative detection of neurologic deficit occurs by either a classical wake-up test or more commonly by a drop in the amplitude of the SSEPs. Many surgeons use both tests. The limitation of the Stagnara wake-up test is that it is unreliable and is usually done only once at the end of the case. SSEP monitoring has the advantage that it is a continuous source of information on spinal cord function and provides immediate and useful information that the surgeon can use to alter the intraoperative course of surgery. A drop in the amplitude of the SSEPs by 50% or greater is considered significant as is a change in the latency by greater than 10%. In one study of 1168 consecutive cases using 50% as the cutoff produced a false-negative rate of 0%.[19] Once the SSEP drop has been verified by the neurophysiologist, the first step is to investigate whether the drop may be due to a secondary effect such as a drop in blood pressure or body temperature or to a change in anesthetic agents. If this is ruled out, a systematic inspection of the construct should be

> ### INTRAOPERATIVE CHANGE IN SSEP
> - Consult with neurophysiologist
> - Inspect entire construct for laminar fracture or abnormalities of hook placement
> - Stabilize blood pressure; avoid hypotension
> - Check anesthetic agents
> - Modify or remove instrumentation if changes persist despite management
> - Consider IV steroids if changes persist

made to rule out possible laminar fracture or hooks that may be in a suspicious position. Once other sources have been eliminated and the SSEPs are still attenuated, the universal recommendation at this time is to modify or remove the internal fixation device. It is unknown how long a period is safe after a drop in the SSEPs, but it is safest to err on the shorter side. If the SSEPs do not respond to modification of the implants, the surgeon should remove them completely and consideration should be given to administering intravenous corticosteroids. In some cases there may be false-positive SSEP changes, but most surgeons do not want to take this chance with the spinal cord in neurologically normal patients. The true rate of false positives is difficult to identify because most surgeons do alter or remove the implants if the SSEPs drop. It would be unwise to ignore these changes in monitoring given what we know about the reliability of these monitoring devices.

False-Negative SSEP

There appears to be a distinct group of patients in whom SSEP monitoring remains normal despite the development of a spinal cord injury, which is readily detectable upon the patient in the recovery room. In the 1991 report on SSEP by the SRS, there were 26 cases in 33,000 of false-negative operative cases in which the electrophysiologic monitoring remained completely normal despite the development of a neurologic deficit. This study concluded that one of the factors involved was that in many of these monitored cases both the latency response and amplitude changes were not being monitored. Despite which type of monitoring is used, if the patient is noted in the recovery room to have a neurologic deficit, the universal recommendation is to remove the rods immediately. In MacEwen, Bunnell, and Siram's 1975 report,[37] the rate of neurologic recovery was directly related to the speed at which the rods were removed. Recovery was seen in 75% of cases if the rods were removed in less than 3 hours of the index operation. If possible, an imaging study may help to detect epidural hematoma, which should be evacuated.

Postoperative Development of Deficit

There is a group of patients who have normal SSEPs and who are found to be neurologically normal in the recovery room who go on to develop a neurologic deficit in the early postoperative period.[28,33] This may happen in the first few hours to the first several days. The cause of this phenomenon is unclear but is possibly related to edema, which may reach a point that blood flow to the spinal cord is altered. Intravenous steroids should be administered when the deficit is detected. Although the initial response of the surgeon is often to go emergently to the operating room to remove the implants,[33] the rationale for doing this has not been clearly established in the literature, especially in the case of an incomplete lesion. In 1975 MacEwen, Bunnell, and Siram showed no difference in the course of incomplete lesion whether the rods were left in or removed. It must be kept in mind that there is often morbidity associated with removal of instrumentation and in fact there may be more potential harm in the removal of sublaminar wires especially if there is an incomplete deficit. The prognosis is usually better than when the paresis occurs immediately postoperatively.[33] A more rational approach may be to radiographically image the patient urgently with CT myelography, to detect possible hematoma or a definite source of cord compression. If a source can be identified, such as a screw in the spinal canal, it should be removed urgently. It is essential for nursing staff, residents, and surgeons to be aware that this problem can arise in the postoperative period so that early detection is possible.

Remote Postoperative Deficit

Late neurologic deterioration can occur after a long spinal instrumentation due to progression of the curve, nonunion, infection,[37] and problems with the instrumentation.[7,24,32,40] Traditional treatment of scoliosis involved instrumentation with a Harrington rod down to the lamina of L5. Because the Harrington rods are straight and cannot be contoured to reproduce lumbar lordosis, they exert a direct downward pressure on the L5 lamina. There have been several reports of the distal hook migrating through the lamina of L5, coming to rest within the canal at the L5 to S1 region, and causing radiculopathy. Kornberg, Herndon, and Rechtine[32] and Hales, Dawson, and Delamarter[24] reported such problems. After removal of the hardware in these cases, all patients had improvement of radicular pain and resolution of the neurologic abnormalities. Stopping a fusion short of the L5 lamina and avoiding the use of Harrington rods can avoid these complications.

POSTOPERATIVE NEUROLOGIC DEFICIT

False-negative SSEP: 1 in 767 cases
- Remove rods immediately
- MacEwen: Best results if the hardware is removed in <3 hours

Postoperative deficit several hours or days later
- Investigate with MRI or CT scan
- Role of hardware removal is unclear
- Removal of sublaminar wires may be risky in partial deficits

---

LUMBOSACRAL SPINE

Instrumentation of the lumbar spine and the lumbosacral junction has become an important adjunct in the treatment of many conditions of the spine including degenerative disease and lumbosacral spondylolisthesis. With the introduction of pedicle screws, there has been much controversy over the safety of these implants, because there have been several reports of neurologic injury with their use.[10,31,59] In the last decade has also come the introduction of posterior lumbar interbody fusion cages (PLIF); some of the problems related to their use will be discussed.

Pedicle Screws

Pedicle screws are an important part of the armamentarium of the spine surgeon and allow the surgeon to perform many complex and successful operations. Many authors have written on the complications of their insertion and misplacement, which ranges from 1% to 18%,[10,16,20,55] as well as neurologic complications associated with their use. However, in the hands of experienced spine surgeons the rate of neurologic injury appears to be relatively low.[8,10,31] Lonstein et al.[35] recently reported on 4790 screws inserted in 915 operative procedures on 875 patients. They reported 115 complications (2.4%) directly related to the insertion of pedicle screws. Neurologic problems occurred after 9 procedures (1.0%) and were caused by 11 screws (0.2%). The authors in this series were experienced spine surgeons and had performed a laminectomy prior to screw insertion in most cases and commonly performed a laminotomy to check a screw if its position was in question. Clearly, inferior and medial displacement of a screw is associated with the highest risk of neurologic injury.

Prevention

As with other aspects of spine surgery, prevention of a neurologic deficit is the key to a successful outcome. Only qualified spine surgeons with expertise in the area of pedicle screw insertion should perform such operations. Careful review of the preoperative imaging and the intraoperative radiograph can help in selecting the trajectory of the screws at each level. Great care must be taken to prevent overpenetration in the lateral sacral zone where the lumbosacral trunk is at risk.[39] Some surgeons prefer to use fluoroscopy and others use intraoperative stereotactic devices to aid in proper screw placement. Performing a laminectomy at each level the pedicle screws are inserted can help in identifying the medial and inferior aspects of the pedicle where perforation will cause the highest likelihood of neurologic injury.[35,55] When a perforation does occur and is detected intraoperatively, the screw can often be successfully replaced in a safer position within the pedicle in over 50% of cases.[35] In some cases, such as trauma, laminectomy is not feasible and reliance on fluoroscopy, plain radiographs, or some form of stereotactic device may be necessary. With the use of careful technique in the hands of an experienced spinal surgeon, the rate of neurologic injury should be so low as to make routine SSEP or intra-operative electromyography (EMG) study unnecessary.

Postoperative Detection

Occasionally despite meticulous technique, a perforation will occur and result in symptomatic neuropathy. The patient may awake with sciatic leg pain and/or weakness in a particular dermatome. Radiographs in the anteroposterior (AP) and lateral planes may detect a pedicle perforation but are unreliable as a definitive

---

PEDICLE SCREWS

- Initial concerns over safety of screws
- Neurologic problems in about 1% of patients if performed by experienced surgeons
- Key to management: Prevention
- Medial and inferior placement is riskiest
- Performing laminectomy at the time of insertion may be safest technique
- Intraoperative guidance may be of value
- Treatment: Prompt removal of screw if detected postoperatively; most patients will improve

---

diagnostic tool. A CT scan should be obtained in these cases to determine if a screw is incorrectly placed and if its location fits the clinical scenario. If the patient is having pain, definitely weak in the affected nerve distribution, and CT scan confirms the perforation of the pedicle, the patient should be taken back to the operating room as soon as is possible for removal or repositioning of the screw. Prompt diagnosis and removal of the offending screw gives the best chance of neurologic recovery. In most cases the radiculopathy will improve or resolve completely.[44,55] In Lonstein et al.'s series,[35] of the eight patients who had a screw removed for radiculopathy, only one had a marked persistent neurologic deficit. Two others had mild residual weakness. A ninth patient with radiculopathy had such a mild deficit that after careful observation the deficit resolved without removal of the screw (Figure 51-4).

Posterior Lumbar Interbody Fusion Cages

The concept of lumbar interbody fusion has been around for several decades, but the development of threaded titanium and carbon fiber PLIF cages is a relatively new advancement in spinal instrumentation. They are designed to provide anterior column support to enhance fusion rates and decrease back pain that may

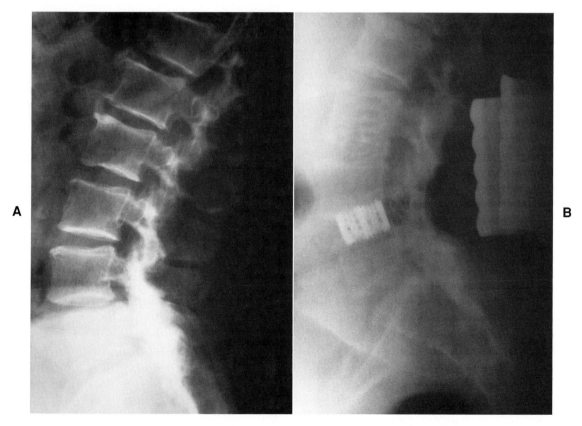

Figure 51-4.   This series of radiographs shows a patient with degenerative spondylolisthesis who had a posterior interbody fusion with titanium cages (**A** and **B**).

Continued

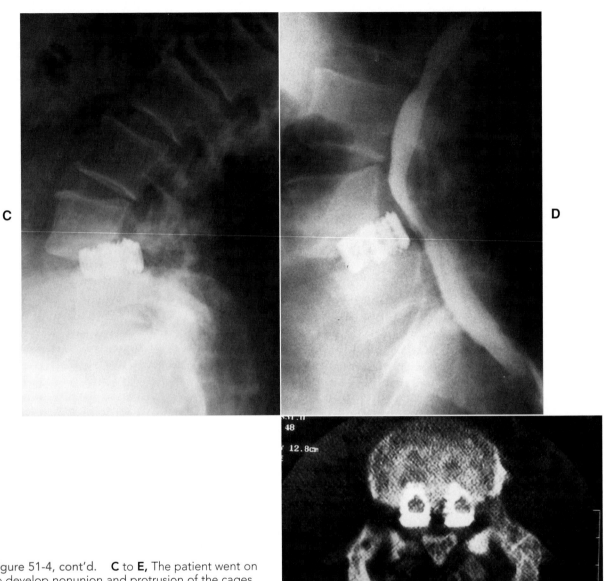

Figure 51-4, cont'd.   **C** to **E,** The patient went on to develop nonunion and protrusion of the cages into the canal. The patient developed sciatica that required posterolateral instrumented fusion and the symptoms resolved with a solid arthrodesis.

be associated with disc motion that occurs even after a solid posterolateral fusion. Initially they were advocated as a stand-alone device but subsequent biomechanical analysis has shown that, in most cases, the spine must be destabilized to insert a cage of sufficient size to provide immediate stability sufficient to provide a high rate of union. Nerve root injury can occur as the result of overzealous nerve root retraction that is sometimes necessary in order to insert the cages. This complication has been reported to be as high as 14.9% in a recent series of 67 patients, with one case of permanent motor deficit with sexual dysfunction.[15] Late neurologic complications have also been reported as a result of PLIF cages backing out into the spinal canal and causing radiculo-

pathy. Glassman et al.[21] reported a case in which the PLIF cage backed into the spinal canal, causing a neurologic deficit. Posterior removal was not attempted because of fear of injuring the neurologic elements by the amount of retraction in the scarred axilla of the nerve root that would be required to remove the cage successfully. The cage was removed from an anterior retroperitoneal approach, which required significant vertebral body resection despite the appearance of a gross nonunion. Reconstruction was performed with allograft followed by posterior instrumentation and fusion. Removal of a PLIF cage is technically demanding and requires a spine surgeon experienced in lumbar revision surgery.

PLIF CAGES

- Relatively new devices
- Can back into canal
- Neuropathic pain can be related to retraction of nerve or epidural fibrosis
- Radiculopathy may resolve with stabilization
- Only cages frankly extruded into the spinal canal need removal

CONCLUSIONS

The advent of modern spinal instrumentation has solved some major problems in spinal surgery and has been responsible for many advances in the field. Along with them have come some problems, not the least of which is iatrogenic neurologic deficit. Understanding the anatomy, experience with the various spinal implants, careful preoperative planning, and meticulous intra-operative technique can prevent many of these problems. Postoperative management should always include prompt identification of problems and initiation of appropriate investigation and treatment.

SELECTED REFERENCES

An HS, Gordin R, Renner K: Anatomic considerations for plate-screw fixation of the cervical spine, *Spine* 16(suppl 10):S548-S551, 1991.

Dawson EG et al.: Spinal cord monitoring: results of the Scoliosis Research Society and the European Spinal Deformity Society survey, *Spine* 16(suppl 8):S361-S364, 1991.

MacEwen GD, Bunnell WP, Sriram K: Acute neurological complications in the treatment of scoliosis: a report of the Scoliosis Research Society, *J Bone Joint Surg Am* 57(3):404-408, 1975.

Nuwer MR et al.: Somatosensory evoked potential spinal cord monitoring reduces neurologic deficits after scoliosis surgery: results of a large multicenter survey, *Electroencephalogr Clin Neurophysiol* 96(1):6-11, 1995.

Vauzelle C, Stagnara P, Jouvinroux P: Functional monitoring of spinal cord activity during spinal surgery, *Clin Orthop* 93:173-178, 1973.

Xu R et al.: The anatomic relation of lateral mass screws to the spinal nerves: a comparison of the Magerl, Anderson, and An techniques, *Spine* 24(19):2057-2061, 1999.

REFERENCES

1. Abumi K et al.: Transpedicular screw fixation for traumatic lesions of the middle and lower cervical spine: description of the techniques and preliminary report, *J Spinal Disord* 7(1):19-28, 1994.
2. Abumi K et al.: Complications of pedicle screw fixation in reconstructive surgery of the cervical spine, *Spine* 25(8):962-969.
3. An HS, Gordin R, Renner K: Anatomic considerations for plate-screw fixation of the cervical spine, *Spine* 16(suppl 10):S548-S551, 1991.
4. Anderson PA et al.: Posterior cervical arthrodesis with AO reconstruction plates and bone graft, *Spine* 16(suppl 3):S72-S79, 1991.
5. Apel DM et al.: Avoiding paraplegia during anterior spinal surgery: the role of somatosensory evoked potential monitoring with temporary occlusion of segmental spinal arteries, *Spine* 16(suppl 8):S365-S370, 1991.
6. Blacklock JB: Fracture of a sublaminar stainless steel cable in the upper cervical spine with neurological injury: case report, *J Neurosurg* 81(6):932-933, 1994.
7. Bowen JR, Ferrer J: Spinal stenosis caused by a Harrington hook in neuromuscular disease: a case report, *Clin Orthop* 180:179-181, 1993.
8. Brown CA et al.: Complications of pediatric thoracolumbar and lumbar pedicle screws, *Spine* 23(14):1566-1571, 1998.
9. Bueff HU et al.: Instrumentation of the cervicothoracic junction after destabilization, *Spine* 20(16):1789-1792, 1995.
10. Davne SH, Myers DL: Complications of lumbar spinal fusion with transpedicular instrumentation, *Spine* 17(suppl 6):S184-S189, 1992.
11. Dawson EG et al.: Spinal cord monitoring: results of the Scoliosis Research Society and the European Spinal Deformity Society survey, *Spine* 16(suppl 8):S361-S364, 1991.
12. Dolan EJ et al.: The effect of spinal distraction on regional spinal cord blood flow in cats, *J Neurosurg* 53(6):756-764, 1980.
13. Dove J: Segmental wiring for spinal deformity: a morbidity report, *Spine* 14(2):229-231, 1989.
14. Ebraheim NA et al.: Lateral radiologic evaluation of lateral mass screw placement in the cervical spine, *Spine* 23(4):458-462, 1998.
15. Elias WJ et al.: Complications of posterior lumbar interbody fusion when using a titanium threaded cage device, *J Neurosurg* 93(suppl 1): 45-52, 2000.
16. Esses SI: The AO spinal internal fixator, *Spine* 14(4):373-378, 1989.
17. Fehlings MG, Cooper PR, Errico TJ: Posterior plates in the management of cervical instability: long-term results in 44 patients, *J Neurosurg* 81(3):341-349, 1994.
18. Flynn TB: Neurologic complications of anterior cervical interbody fusion, *Spine* 7(6):536-539, 1982.
19. Forbes HJ et al.: Spinal cord monitoring in scoliosis surgery: experience with 1168 cases, *J Bone Joint Surg Br* 73(3):487-491, 1991.
20. Gertzbein SD, Robbins SE: Accuracy of pedicular screw placement in vivo, *Spine* 15(1):11-14, 1990.
21. Glassman SD et al.: Management of iatrogenic spinal stenosis complicating placement of a fusion cage: a case report, *Spine* 21(20):2383-2386, 1996.
22. Graham AW et al.: Posterior cervical arthrodesis and stabilization with a lateral mass plate: clinical and computed tomographic evaluation of lateral mass screw placement and associated complications, *Spine* 21(3):323-328, discussion 329, 1996.
23. Grob D et al.: The role of plate and screw fixation in occipitocervical fusion in rheumatoid arthritis, *Spine* 19(22):2545-2551, 1994.
24. Hales DD, Dawson EG, Delamarter R: Late neurological complications of Harrington-rod instrumentation, *J Bone Joint Surg Am* 71(7):1053-1057, 1989.
25. Heller JG, Silcox DH III, Sutterlin CE III: Complications of posterior cervical plating, *Spine* 20(22):2442-2448, 1995.
26. Heller JG et al.: Anatomic comparison of the Roy-Camille and Magerl techniques for screw placement in the lower cervical spine, *Spine* 16(suppl 10):S552-S557, 1991.
27. Jeanneret B et al.: Posterior stabilization of the cervical spine with hook plates, *Spine* 16(suppl 3):S56-S63, 1991.
28. Johnston CED et al.: Delayed paraplegia complicating sublaminar segmental spinal instrumentation, *J Bone Joint Surg Am* 68(4):556-563, 1986.
29. Jones EL et al.: Cervical pedicle screws versus lateral mass screws: anatomic feasibility and biomechanical comparison, *Spine* 22(9):977-982, 1997.
30. Jonsson H Jr, Rauschning W: Anatomical and morphometric studies in posterior cervical spinal screw-plate systems, *J Spinal Disord* 7(5):429-438, 1994.
31. Kinnard P et al.: Roy-Camille plates in unstable spinal conditions: a preliminary report, *Spine* 11(2):131-135, 1986.
32. Kornberg M, Herndon WA, Rechtine GR: Lumbar nerve root compression at the site of hook insertion. Late complication of Harrington rod instrumentation for scoliosis, *Spine* 10(9):853-855, 1985.
33. Letts RM, Hollenberg C: Delayed paresis following spinal fusion with Harrington instrumentation, *Clin Orthop* 125:45-48, 1977.
34. Levine AM, Mazel C, Roy-Camille R: Management of fracture separations of the articular mass using posterior cervical plating, *Spine* 17(suppl 10):S447-S454, 1992.
35. Lonstein JE et al.: Complications associated with pedicle screws, *J Bone Joint Surg Am* 81(11):1519-1528, 1999.
36. Luque ER: Segmental spinal instrumentation for correction of scoliosis, *Clin Orthop* 163:192-198, 1982.
37. MacEwen GD, Bunnell WP, Sriram K: Acute neurological complications in the treatment of scoliosis: a report of the Scoliosis Research Society, *J Bone Joint Surg Am* 57(3):404-408, 1975.

38. McMaster MJ: Occult intraspinal anomalies and congenital scoliosis, *J Bone Joint Surg Am* 66(4):588-601, 1984.
39. Mirkovic S et al.: Anatomic consideration for sacral screw placement, *Spine* 16(suppl 6):S289-S294, 1991.
40. Montane I, Engler GL: Radicular pain after Harrington instrumentation, *J Spinal Disord* 2(1):1-5, 1989.
41. Nazarian SM, Louis RP: Posterior internal fixation with screw plates in traumatic lesions of the cervical spine, *Spine* 16(suppl 3):S64-S71, 1991.
42. Nuwer MR et al.: Somatosensory evoked potential spinal cord monitoring reduces neurologic deficits after scoliosis surgery: results of a large multicenter survey, *Electroencephalogr Clin Neurophysiol* 96(1):6-11, 1995.
43. Owen JH: The application of intraoperative monitoring during surgery for spinal deformity, *Spine* 24(24):2649-2662, 1999.
44. Rose RD, Welch WC, Donaldson WF III: Correlation of late intraforaminal screw removal with somatosensory evoked potentials and neurologic improvement, *Arch Phys Med Rehabil* 79(2):226-229, 1998.
45. Roy-Camille R et al.: Treatment of lower cervical spinal injuries: C3 to C7, *Spine* 17(suppl 10):S442-S446, 1992.
46. Seybold EA et al.: Characteristics of unicortical and bicortical lateral mass screws in the cervical spine, *Spine* 24(22):2397-2403, 1999.
47. Smith SA et al.: The effects of depth of penetration, screw orientation, and bone density on sacral screw fixation, *Spine* 18(8):1006-1010, 1993.
48. Sutterlin CED et al.: A biomechanical evaluation of cervical spinal stabilization methods in a bovine model: static and cyclical loading, *Spine* 13(7):795-802, 1988.
49. Tamaki T et al.: The prevention of iatrogenic spinal cord injury utilizing the evoked spinal cord potential, *Int Orthop* 4(4):313-317, 1981.
50. Thompson GH et al.: Segmental spinal instrumentation in idiopathic scoliosis: a preliminary report, *Spine* 10(7):623-630, 1985.
51. Ulrich C et al.: Comparative study of the stability of anterior and posterior cervical spine fixation procedures, *Arch Orthop Trauma Surg* 106(4):226-31, 1987.
52. Ulrich C et al.: Biomechanics of fixation systems to the cervical spine, *Spine* 16(suppl 3):S4-S9, 1991.
53. Vauzelle C, Stagnara P, Jouvinroux P: Functional monitoring of spinal cord activity during spinal surgery, *Clin Orthop* 93:173-178, 1973.
54. Wellman BJ, Follett KA, Traynelis VC: Complications of posterior articular mass plate fixation of the subaxial cervical spine in 43 consecutive patients, *Spine* 23(2):193-200, 1998.
55. West JL, Bradford DS, Ogilvie JW: Results of spinal arthrodesis with pedicle screw-plate fixation, *J Bone Joint Surg Am* 73(8):1179-1184, 1991.
56. Wilber RG et al.: Postoperative neurological deficits in segmental spinal instrumentation: a study using spinal cord monitoring, *J Bone Joint Surg Am* 66(8):1178-1187, 1984.
57. Winter RB, Moe JH, Lonstein JE: The surgical treatment of congenital kyphosis: a review of 94 patients age 5 years or older, with 2 years or more follow-up in 77 patients, *Spine* 10(3):224-231, 1985.
58. Xu R et al.: The anatomic relation of lateral mass screws to the spinal nerves: a comparison of the Magerl, Anderson, and An techniques, *Spine* 24(19):2057-2061, 1999.
59. Yalcin S, Guven O: Reversible anterior cord syndrome due to penetration of the spinal canal by pedicular screws, *Paraplegia* 33(7):423-425, 1995.
60. York DH, Chabot RJ, Gaines RW: Response variability of somatosensory evoked potentials during scoliosis surgery, *Spine* 12(9):864-876, 1987.

Complications of Anterior and Posterior Cervical Instrumentation

Brian T. Brislin, Alan S. Hilibrand, Brett A. Taylor

Over the past 10 years there has been an increase in the use of instrumentation for the treatment of cervical spine disorders. The use of anterior cervical instrumentation to supplement established techniques of anterior interbody grafting has provided increased stability and earlier postoperative mobilization. In the setting of cervical trauma, techniques of posterior stabilization have benefited from newer devices that provide improved torsional rigidity when compared with traditional posterior wiring techniques, such as transarticular screws and lateral mass plates.[12] These new posterior systems have become the standard of care for treatment of posterior element injuries. However, there are also significant complications associated with the use of these constructs and devices.[13]

This chapter will review the indirect and direct complications of anterior and posterior cervical instrumentation. Indirect complications include those associated with the surgical approach or grafting procedure, whereas direct complications are associated with the placement of instrumentation. This chapter will briefly discuss the indirect complications and focus primarily upon the complications directly associated with the use of internal fixation, including those related to anterior screw placement, plate/screw loosening, plate kick out, and malposition of odontoid screws, as well as those related to the use of posterior wiring constructs, transarticular screws, occipitocervical screws, and lateral mass/pedicle screws.

INDIRECT COMPLICATIONS
Bone Graft Harvest Morbidity

Numerous potential complications are associated with bone graft harvest from the iliac crest. Most are uncommon and result in minimal morbidity. Hematoma and infections are the most common.[60] Other complications include cosmetic deformity, chronic pain (most commonly due to violation of the sacroiliac joint), muscle weakness with gait abnormalities, pelvic instability, iliac

---

BONE GRAFT HARVEST MORBIDITY

MOST COMMON COMPLICATIONS
- Hematoma
- Infection

ANTERIOR EXPOSURE
- Places the lateral femoral cutaneous nerve at risk.
- Harvest bone graft from anterior iliac crest through an incision beginning two fingerbreadths, or approximately 3 to 4 cm, behind the anterior superior iliac spine.

POSTERIOR APPROACH
- Harvesting bone graft through a posterior approach to the posterior superior iliac spine places the superior cluneal nerves at risk.
- Limit exposure to ≤ medial 7 cm of posterior iliac crest.

PLACEMENT OF RETRACTORS INTO THE SCIATIC NOTCH
- Places the superior gluteal artery at risk.
- Caudal limit of dissection is inferior margin of the origin of the gluteus maximus muscle at the posterior superior iliac spine.

---

wing fractures, peritoneal perforation, muscle hernia, and neurovascular and visceral injuries.[29,53]

An understanding of the local anatomy and the limits of dissection for these approaches will minimize the occurrence of complications (Figure 52A-1). The lateral femoral cutaneous nerve is at risk with an anterior exposure. An incision within 2 cm of the anterior superior iliac spine may injure this nerve, as well as the attachments of the sartorius muscle and inguinal ligament.[21] To avoid this complication anterior iliac crest bone grafts should be harvested through an incision beginning two fingerbreadths, or approximately 3 to 4 cm, behind the anterior superior iliac spine. The aponeurosis of the transversalis

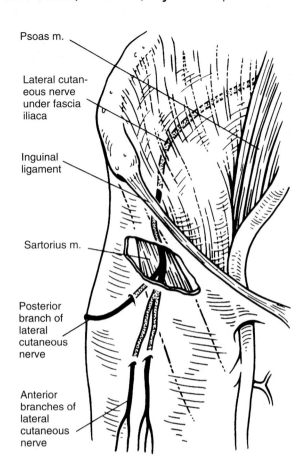

Figure 52A-1.   Relevant anatomy for anterior iliac crest bone graft harvesting. *(Redrawn from Kurz LT, Garfin SR, Booth RE: Harvesting autogenous iliac bone grafts: a review of complications and techniques, Spine 14[12]:1324-1331, 1989.)*

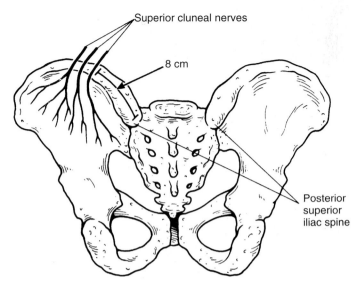

Figure 52A-2.   Relevant anatomy for posterior iliac crest bone graft harvesting. *(Redrawn from Kurz LT, Garfin SR, Booth RE: Harvesting autogenous iliac bone grafts: a review of complications and techniques, Spine 14[12]:1324-1331, 1989.)*

and external oblique muscles should be identified and preserved. Careful reapproximation of these structures during abdominal wound closure can prevent abdominal wall herniation.[60]

The harvest of bone graft from the posterior superior iliac spine places the superior cluneal nerves at risk. They cross the iliac crest approximately 8 cm from the posterior superior iliac spine (Figure 52A-2). By limiting the exposure to the medial 7 cm of the posterior iliac crest, the risk of this complication can be minimized. Placement of retractors into the sciatic notch places the superior gluteal artery at risk.[36,37] To avoid injury the caudal limit of dissection along the posterior iliac crest should be the inferior margin of the origin of the gluteus maximus muscle at the area of the posterior superior iliac spine.[37]

Fracture of the ilium at the harvest site has been reported. With the use of osteotomies and deep saw cuts there is the potential for the propagation of fracture lines.[29,32] Sudden onset of moderate to severe pain in the region of the harvest site during the first 6 to 8 weeks postoperatively is usually seen. Treatment of symptomatic fractures involves initial crutch-assisted partial weight bearing.[29]

Complications of the Surgical Approach

The most common complications of the anterior approach to the cervical spine are sore throat and dysphagia. Chronic dysphonia (hoarseness) is an uncommon complication associated with injury to one of the recurrent laryngeal nerves (RLNs). Such an injury may also cause problems with swallowing and potential aspiration.[5] The right RLN is at increased risk of injury during retraction because of its minimal redundancy and its variable course outside of the tracheoesophageal groove in the lower cervical spine.[5,59] An anatomic study of the right-sided approach to C7 showed an in situ stretch of 12% to 24% with 3 cm and 4 cm of Cloward retraction (Figure 52A-3). This was significant because the authors also demonstrated the potential for significant neurologic injury with nerve stretch greater than 12%.[59]

The complications of Horner's syndrome, esophageal perforation, and vertebral artery injury are less common. Injury to Chassaignac's ganglion in the lower cervical area can result in an ipsilateral Horner's syndrome. Subperiosteal dissection of the longus colli muscle can help avoid this complication. Esophageal injury during the perioperative period may be due to retraction and ischemia to smooth muscle or from direct penetration with sharp instruments and may lead to retropharyngeal abscess formation.[5] The use of a nasogastric tube that can be palpated in the neck and then flooded with indigo carmine dye can help identify an esophageal injury if this complication is suspected. Subcutaneous emphysema on postoperative plain films is another finding suggestive of an esophageal perforation.[5]

The approximate incidence of vertebral artery injury is 0.3%.[22] The use of the air drill was responsible for vertebral artery injury in 10 patients undergoing partial vertebral body resection.[49] Soft tissue retraction and

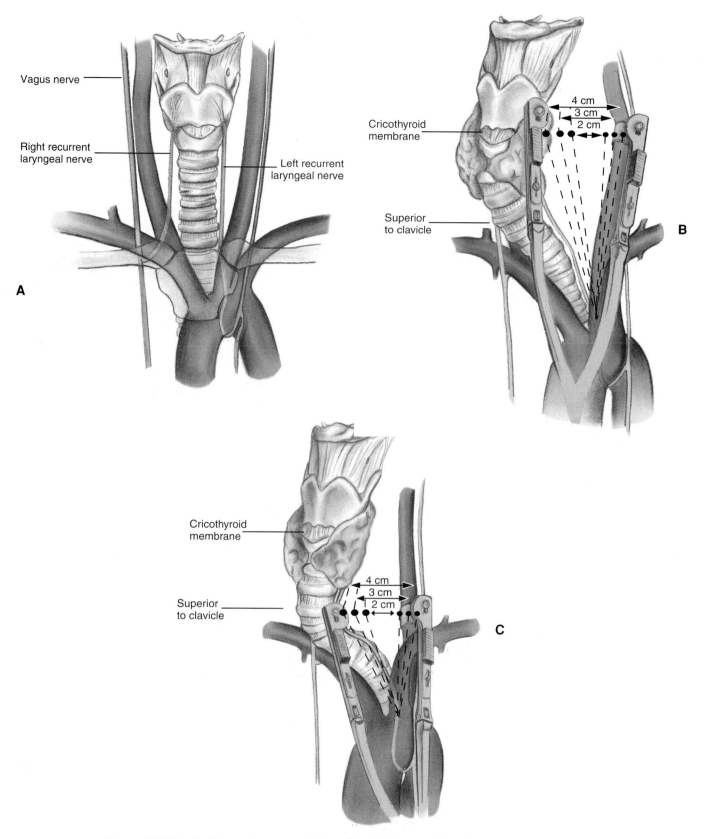

Figure 52A-3.   **A,** Normal anatomy of the neck showing the left recurrent laryngeal nerve (RLN) within the tracheoesophageal groove and the right RLN coursing obliquely in the neck. **B,** Left-sided approach at the C4 level demonstrating changes seen with increasing Cloward retraction. **C,** Left-sided approach at the C7 level demonstrating changes seen with increasing Cloward retraction.

Continued

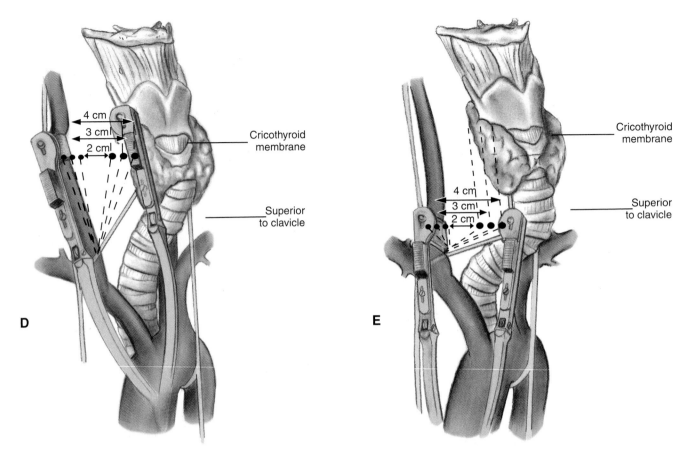

Figure 52A-3, cont'd. **D,** Right-sided approach at the C4 level demonstrating changes seen with increasing Cloward retraction. **E,** Right-sided approach at the C7 level demonstrating changes seen with increasing Cloward retraction. Note increased bowstringing of the right RLN across the inferior edge of the retractor with increasing retraction. *(From Weisberg NK, Spengler DM, Netterville JL: Stretch-induced nerve injury as a cause of paralysis secondary to the anterior cervical approach,* Otolaryngol Head Neck Surg *116[3]:317-326, 1997.)*

COMPLICATIONS OF ANTERIOR SURGICAL APPROACH

MOST COMMON COMPLICATIONS
- Sore throat
- Dysphagia

LESS COMMON COMPLICATIONS
- Chronic hoarseness
  - Associated with injury to one of the recurrent laryngeal nerves (RLNs)
- Right RLN at increased risk of injury when performing surgery at C6 to C7 and C7 to T1 levels
- Injury to Chassaignac's ganglion
  - Located in lower cervical spine
  - Can result in ipsilateral Horner's syndrome

- Esophageal injury during the perioperative period
  - Caused by retraction and ischemia to smooth muscle or by direct penetration from a sharp instrument
  - Use a nasogastric tube to assist in diagnosis of this complication
  - Flood the nasogastric tube with indigo carmine perioperatively to identify the presence of any esophageal injury
  - Also indicated by subcutaneous emphysema on postoperative radiographs

---

transfixion by malposition of unicortical screws are other causes of iatrogenic injury to the vertebral artery. Treatment by tamponade, obtaining control by direct exposure and electrocautery, or primary repair have been recommended.[22,51]

The complications of the posterior approach are primarily problems from muscle stripping and exposure (Figure 52A-4). Care should be taken to retain the attachments of the extensor muscles at C2. They are dynamic stabilizers of the head and neck, and loss of their attach-

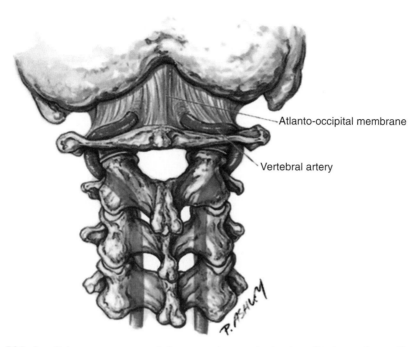

Atlanto-occipital membrane

Vertebral artery

Figure 52A-4. Relevant anatomy of the posterior cervical spine. *(Redrawn from Albert TJ, Balderston RA, Northrup BE, eds: Surgical approaches to the spine, Philadelphia, 1997, WB Saunders.)*

COMPLICATIONS OF POSTERIOR SURGICAL APPROACH

- Take care to maintain the attachments of the extensor muscles at C2 because they are dynamic stabilizers of the head and neck.
- Aggressive subperiosteal dissection for exposure of the ring of C1 can injure vertebral artery:
  - Be careful to limit dissection to within 1.5 cm of the posterior tubercle of C1 in adults and within 1 cm in children.
- Increased risk of dural injury is noted in the presence of thin dura, especially in rheumatoid arthritis patient.
- Perform careful dissection at area between C1 and C2 to avoid possible dural injury.

---

ments may result in postoperative deformity.[44,52] The vertebral artery can be injured with overzealous subperiosteal dissection for exposure of the ring of C1. Limiting the dissection to within 1.5 cm of the posterior tubercle of C1 in adults (1 cm in children) may help avert this complication.[7,10] The thin membrane of dura at this level increases the risk of a dural tear with aggressive dissection and stripping of the laminae and with passing wires under the C1 lamina. Stauffer recommends threading the wire from cranial to caudal, citing a higher risk of dural tear with wires passed beneath the spinous processes from caudal to cranial.[52] Any dural tear should be repaired in a watertight fashion, if possible.

Both anterior and posterior approaches are associated with a small risk of neurologic deficits and paralysis. In general, careful preoperative positioning, an experienced anesthesiologist, and electrophysiologic monitoring can be used to minimize the risks of surgery.

Careful monitoring of the patient to avoid hypotension, especially in the setting of myelopathy, may reduce the risk of spinal cord ischemia. Depending upon the length of surgery and the patient's overall health, overnight intubation to avoid postoperative retropharyngeal hematoma and acute respiratory distress should be considered.

Bone Graft Displacement

Anterior discectomy and fusion are associated with complications of pseudarthrosis, graft extrusion, graft collapse, and progressive deformity (Figure 52A-5).[14,56] The farthest caudal interbody graft has been reported to be the most common site for nonunion.[56] The likelihood of a nonunion may be minimized by the use of an anterior cervical plate and/or concomitant posterior stabilization. In addition, there is a higher nonunion rate with allograft fibula versus autograft fibula in multilevel cervical reconstructions.[20]

Neurologic injury can occur with graft collapse and retropulsion, with the subsequent development of cervical kyphosis and neural element compression. Anterior graft extrusion may present with dysphagia, erosion of the esophagus with infection, and loss of initial postoperative alignment on radiographs. Treatment of these patients may involve reoperation or halo vest immobilization.[19] Graft fracture and extrusion is more common with long strut grafts after multilevel procedures. Graft extrusion anteriorly may cause kyphosis and require reoperation with possible anterior plating and posterior stabilization. Posterior extrusion of the graft is associated with a high risk of spinal cord compression. In cases of

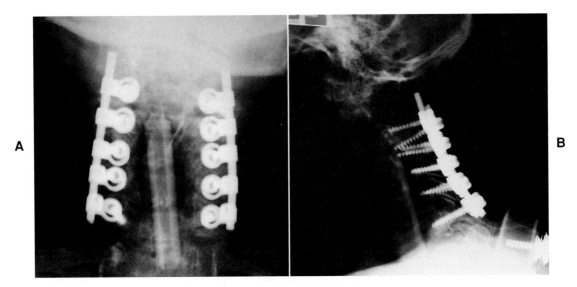

A

B

Figure 52A-5. Bone graft dislodgement. A 77-year-old woman with cervical myelopathy, treated with C4 to C6 corpectomy and fibular strut graft from C3 to C7 combined with posterior cervical instrumentation from C3 to C7, who presents with progressing kyphosis and recurrent myelopathy. **A,** Anteroposterior radiograph demonstrating dislodgement of inferior portion of graft. **B,** Lateral radiograph demonstrating displacement of graft and kyphotic deformity.

> ### BONE GRAFT DISPLACEMENT
>
> * Complications associated with anterior discectomy and fusion
>   - Pseudarthrosis
>   - Graft extrusion
>   - Graft collapse
>   - Progressive deformity
> * Most common site for a nonunion: Farthest caudal interbody graft
> * Indications of anterior graft extrusion
>   - Dysphagia
>   - Erosion of esophagus, leading to infection
>   - Loss of initial postoperative alignment on radiographs (i.e., kyphosis)
>   - Recurrent radiculopathy or myelopathy
> * Posterior graft extrusion associated with
>   - Spinal cord compression
>   - Recurrent myelopathy necessitating reoperation

posterior extrusion, reoperation is usually required to decompress the spinal cord. With fracture of either the cephalad or caudal vertebra, a new fusion that incorporates the fractured vertebra is usually required.

DIRECT COMPLICATIONS OF INSTRUMENTATION—ANTERIOR
Anterior Plating

The use of an anterior cervical plate has dramatically increased with the development of "locking plates." In two-level anterior cervical discectomy and fusion, the use of anterior cervical plating has been shown to decrease pseudarthrosis rates without increased com-plications.[14,57] It has also been shown that plated fusions have less disc space collapse and less postoperative kyphosis.[57] Many authors have also suggested that the use of an anterior plate with anterior cervical discectomy and fusion can decrease the need for postoperative immobilization.[14,42,56,57]

The development of constrained systems that lock the screws to the plate have obviated the need for bicortical screw purchase, decreasing the risk of injury to the spinal cord.[42] However, screws that are directed laterally or a plate that is positioned too laterally may injure the vertebral artery.[7] Lowery et al.[38] recently reviewed the complications associated with 70 nonconstrained plates and 39 constrained plates and found at least one mode of failure in 38 cases. There were 31 failures with the Orozco (nonconstrained) plate, 5 cervical spine locking plate (CSLP) failures, and 2 Orion plate failures. There were 10 broken and 1 settled Orozco plates, 2 broken and 2 loosened CSLP plates, and no broken or loosened Orion plates. The majority of failures in the Orozco, CSLP, and Orion plates occurred with three- to four-level procedures. The constrained systems (CSLP, Orion) had fewer failures than the nonconstrained Orozco system. The authors suggested reoperation in cases of progressive screw loosening beyond 5 mm or clinical signs of dysphagia. In their study, 4 patients with prominent hardware failure on radiographs required reoperation with removal of the plates and screws. At hardware removal, there was extensive soft tissue envelopment of the metallic implants and no damage to the neighboring anatomic structures. The authors recommended long-term follow-up in patients with plate/screw loosening or plate/screw breakage. They also advocated the use of constrained plate/screw systems to minimize hardware-related complications.[38]

In another study of revision surgery for failed anterior fusions, the authors described hardware failure in 9 of 20 patients treated with anterior plating alone. The failures were loosened or broken plates/screws that posed no risk to the esophagus or neurovascular structures. One patient had early bilateral inferior screw breakage with dislodgement of plate and graft. Two patients treated with circumferential revision had screw breakage without the need for reoperation.[38]

Multilevel cervical corpectomy and fusion requires longer anterior plates for stability. Previous studies have shown a high rate of success with this procedure when performed *without instrumentation*.[19] However, Foley et al. reported two graft displacements in patients with multilevel corpectomy and anterior cervical plating. One graft and plate dislodged in extension and required reoperation. A second graft and plate displaced due to vertebral body fracture and inferior plate pullout. This plate was removed secondary to persistent dysphagia.

Vaccaro et al. reported on 9 patients with early failure of long segment anterior cervical plating after treatment for cervical degenerative, traumatic, or neoplastic disease.[54] Three of the 33 (9%) patients who underwent two-level corpectomy and strut grafting with plating had dislodgement of the graft and plate within 3 months. Two of these patients had failure due to fracture of the inferior vertebral body that led to the hardware failure. Following a three-level corpectomy, 6 of 12 (50%) patients developed hardware failure with dislodgement of the graft and plate. Two patients with graft and plate dislodgement had screws that were incompletely tightened to the plate on initial postoperative x-ray films. One patient with a "peg-in-hole" fibula graft had dislodgement of the inferior screws and plate as a result of graft settling. Four patients (one two-level, three three-level) who had screws inadvertently placed in the adjacent disc space went on to have plate loosening and dislodgement. Failure to lock the screw to the plate and the use of a peg-in-hole bone graft technique were factors associated with failure in the three-level corpectomy and fusion.[54]

Isomi et al. applied cyclic fatigue loads to human cadaveric cervical spine to simulate the in vivo loads after surgery for one-level corpectomy (C5) with instrumentation (C4 to C6) and three-level corpectomy (C4 to C6) with instrumentation (C3 to C7).[30] The authors hypothesized that a longer plate generates greater motion at the fusion sites under physiologic loads because of its longer lever arm. After initially describing the increased stability of the anterior plate in one-level and three-level corpectomy to flexion, extension, and lateral bending, the authors applied cyclic fatigue loads to the specimens. The results demonstrated that the stability of the three-level corpectomy decreased much more rapidly in fatigue testing compared with the one-level corpectomy model. The authors concluded that the stability afforded by the long anterior plate in the three-level corpectomy is significantly reduced as a result of fatigue loading and this may account for the high rate of early instrument failure seen in multilevel fusions (Figure 52A-6).[30,54]

ANTERIOR PLATING

- In a two-level anterior cervical discectomy and fusion, use of an anterior cervical plate decreases pseudarthrosis rates without increased complications
- Screws directed laterally or a plate applied lateral to the uncovertebral joints may injure the vertebral artery
- Short buttress plates
  - Used to avoid the complications associated with long anterior plates
  - May be applied at either the inferior or superior junction of the construct
  - Used to prevent migration or extrusion of the bone graft
- Recommendation: Add posterior cervical fixation to augment anterior strut grafting and buttress plating
- Most common complications associated with anterior odontoid screw
  - Screw malposition
  - Breakout

Kirkpatrick et al. studied the in vitro biomechanical behavior of the cervical spine after multilevel corpectomy and reconstruction with fibular strut graft and supplementation with either anterior or posterior plating.[34] They tested sagittal plane flexibility and range of motion in 11 intact human cadaveric cervical spines. After three-level corpectomy (C4 to C6) and fibular strut grafting (C3 to C7), the testing was repeated. An anterior plate (Orion by Sofamor Danek, Memphis) was applied, tested, then removed. Posterior lateral mass screws were then added from C3 to C7 and the specimens tested. After testing, compressive loads were applied to simulate the graft's settling. Five specimens with anterior plates and six specimens with posterior plates were tested to failure. The range of motion after reconstruction compared with the intact spine decreased 24% with strut grafting, 43% after application of an anterior plate, and 62% after application of a posterior plate. Posterior plates tested to failure required greater compressive loads than the anterior plates. The authors concluded that the application of an anterior locking plate or posterior lateral mass screws and plates add stability to the reconstruction after multilevel cervical corpectomy. Furthermore, their results demonstrated that posteriorly applied plates provide better stability than anterior plates.[34]

Anterior Cervical Buttress Plates

In order to avoid the complications associated with long anterior cervical plates in multilevel procedures, the use of short buttress plates has been described. These plates can span either the superior or inferior junction of the construct and have been used to prevent graft migration and extrusion. Vanichkachorn et al. described the use of these plates in 11 patients, with 8 plates placed at the inferior end of the fusion mass, 2 at the superior end, and in 1 patient at both ends.[55] In the study there were

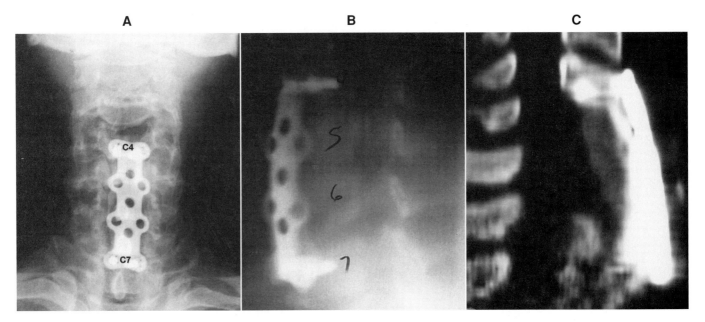

Figure 52A-6.   Failure of long anterior plate. A 43-year-old man who had undergone a C5 to C6 corpectomy with application of a long anterior plate from C4 to C7. **A,** Plain anteroposterior radiograph showing anterior plate spanning C4 to C7 levels. **B,** Postoperative lateral tomogram demonstrating graft and anterior plate in appropriate position. **C,** CT sagittal reconstruction demonstrating failure of anterior plate with graft displacement inferiorly into the C7 vertebral body.

no instances of graft extrusion or dislodgement, plate failures, or complications related to the plates. One graft fractured with the use of a locking screw penetrating the graft itself and required a revision. They further recommended the addition of posterior cervical fixation with the use of these plates. However, serious complications of buttress plating have also been described (Figure 52A-7). Riew et al. used the buttress plate in 14 patients at the inferior end of the graft.[45] One patient had graft extrusion that led to airway compromise and death. A second patient had the plate dislodge secondary to graft settling (Figure 52A-8). They also recommended posterior cervical fusion to augment the anterior strut graft and plate.

Anterior Odontoid Screws

Little has been written regarding the complications of anterior odontoid screws, which have been advocated for the early treatment of type II odontoid fractures. Indications have included a reducible fracture with an intact transverse atlantal ligament.[43] Poor outcomes have been reported with the application of odontoid screws in elderly and osteoporotic patients. Preoperatively, alignment of the cervical spine should be assessed, because this can prevent improper positioning of the screws. Screw malposition and breakout are the main complications, with incidences of 2% and 1.5%, respectively. Graziano et al. compared the stability for fixation from one anterior odontoid screw versus two anterior odontoid screws.[24] They artificially created a type II odontoid fracture in eight human cervical cadaveric spines. Four specimens received

one anterior odontoid screw, whereas the second four received two anterior screws. After testing in rotation and bending, the authors demonstrated no significant difference in bending or torsional stiffness between the one-screw and the two-screw specimens.

DIRECT COMPLICATIONS OF INSTRUMENTATION—POSTERIOR
Posterior Cervical Wiring

Stabilization with spinous process wiring, as described by Rogers[46] and McAfee et al.,[41] has been advocated for cases of posterior instability for many years. Complications associated with interspinous process wiring include wire breakage, wire pullout, nonunion, loss of reduction, and neurologic injury, especially with the use of sublaminar wires. Wire breakage can occur with excessive manipulation during wire placement or if the caliber of the wire is too small. The 20-gauge wire (0.8 mm) is most commonly used in posterior cervical wiring. Failure of the interspinous wire and bone graft may occur secondary to collapse/dislodgement of the graft, which may cause increased translational movement of C1 on C2. Weiland et al. have reported favorable results with the use of the Bohlman triple-wire technique.[58] This construct has the same biomechanical advantages as other posterior wiring methods, without the need for sublaminar wires, and provides additional fixation through the application of bilateral strut grafts. This could obviate the need for halo immobilization (except in patients with rheumatoid arthritis) and avoid halo-related complications.[58]

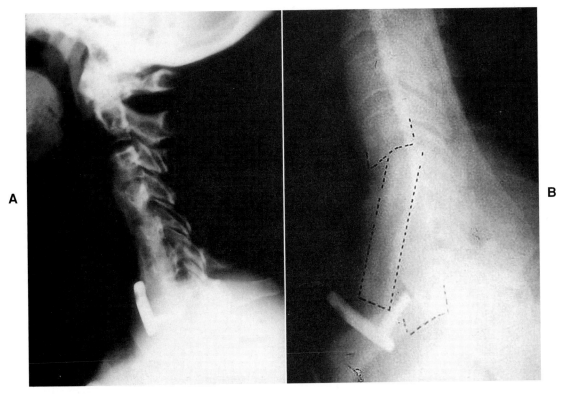

Figure 52A-7. Failure of inferior buttress plate causing airway obstruction. **A,** Anteroposterior radiograph of patient treated with strut graft and application of cervical buttress plate at inferior end of fusion segment. **B,** Lateral radiograph demonstrating failure of plate with forward dislodgement of graph that resulted in obstruction of the patient's airway.

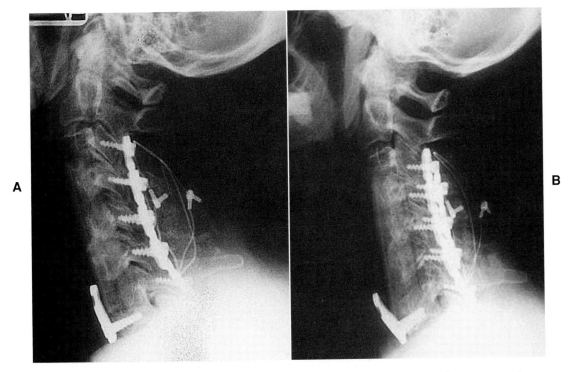

Figure 52A-8. Complications of combined anterior and posterior cervical instrumentation. **A,** Lateral radiograph after application of anterior buttress plate and posterior cervical instrumentation. **B,** Follow-up lateral radiograph demonstrating displacement of inferior buttress plate secondary to the settling of the graft into the body of C7.

Lateral Mass Screws

Posterior lateral mass screws/plates provide improved stability and decrease the need for postoperative stabilization. Biomechanical studies have shown increased rigidity when compared with posterior wiring and anterior plating[34] and may be used regardless of the integrity of the posterior structures. There are several established techniques used for the placement of lateral mass screws into the posterior cervical spine, including those described by An et al.,[8] Magerl,[26] Anderson et al.,[9] and Roy-Camille.[26]

Heller et al. retrospectively studied 78 patients to describe the perioperative complications of posterior cervical lateral mass screws and plates.[28] Six hundred fifty-four screws (averaging 8.4 screws per patient) were placed according to the technique described by An et al.[8] The complication rate as a function of the number of screws inserted included nerve root injury (0.6%), facet violations (0.2%), vertebral artery injury (0%), broken screws (0.3%), screw avulsion (0.2%), and screw loosening (1.1%). Complications as a percentage of the number of cases performed (78) included spinal cord injury (2.6%), iatrogenic foraminal stenosis (2.6%), broken plate (1.3%), lost reduction (2.6%), adjacent segment degeneration (3.8%), infection (1.3%), and pseudarthrosis (1.4%). There were no injuries to the spinal cord related to screw insertion in their study. There is little chance of this type of injury with strict adherence to the established techniques.[28]

An anatomic study comparing the Magerl and Roy-Camille techniques found an increased incidence of nerve root injury with the former technique (7.3% vs 0.8%).[26] Xu et al. measured the distances from the superficial posterior center of the lateral mass to the nerve roots superiorly and inferiorly.[62] They reported superior and inferior distances of 5.7 ± 1.5 mm and 5.5 ± 0.8 mm. Heller et al. reported on six patients with acquired radiculopathy after posterior cervical plating. In four of the six patients the deficits resulted from

screws that were too long and protruded through the ventral cortex of the lateral mass. These patients had partial or complete recovery with additional surgery to remove or replace the screws. The remaining two were the result of iatrogenic foraminal stenosis induced by a lag effect with placement of the screws. When a gap existed between the lateral mass plate and a subluxed lateral mass, the lateral mass was pulled dorsally against the plate as the screw was tightened. To avoid any significant foraminal stenosis or radiculopathy from this effect, the authors suggested placing a bone graft into the gap between the plate and the lateral mass (Figure 52A-9).[28]

Graham et al. prospectively reviewed the clinical and radiographic outcomes for 21 consecutive patients that were treated with lateral mass plating and reported a

---

POSTERIOR COMPLICATIONS

COMPLICATIONS OF LATERAL POSTERIOR MASS SCREWS

- Nerve root injury
- Facet violations
- Vertebral artery injury
- Broken screw
- Screw avulsion
- Screw loosening
- Pseudarthrosis
- Spinal cord injury

- Iatrogenic foraminal stenosis
- Broken plate
- Lost reduction
- Adjacent segment degeneration
- Infection

RISK FOR SURGERY

- Vertebral artery at risk from a screw placed too medially
- Spinal cord at risk from a screw placed too medially
- Screws with greater cephalad angulation at increased risk of injuring the nerve root that exits at the anterolateral portion of the superior facet
- Facet joints at risk with screws directed perpendicular to the posterior cortex to the lateral mass

---

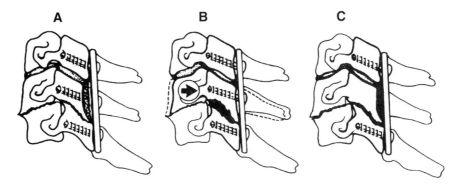

Figure 52A-9. Technique to avoid complication of iatrogenic foraminal stenosis. **A,** A gap exists between the lateral mass plate and the lateral mass secondary to degenerative changes or subluxation. **B,** When the screw is tightened, a lag effect pulls the lateral mass dorsally against the plate. Clinically significant foraminal stenosis and radiculopathy may result. **C,** The lag effect can be avoided with the placement of bone graft into the gap between the plate and the lateral mass before the screw is tightened. (Redrawn from Heller JG, Silcox DH III, Sutterlin CE: Complications of posterior cervical plating, Spine 20[22]:2442-2448, 1995.)

1.8%-per-screw risk of radiculopathy.[23] Computed tomography (CT) scans were used to evaluate patients, with thin slices (2 mm) parallel to the vertebral end plates. The cervical lateral masses were divided into three zones in the sagittal plane according to Heller et al.[26] The authors devised a similar system to divide the lateral masses into three zones in the axial plane. This allowed for the location of the screw tip in relation to the neurovascular structures at risk in the transverse plane. At C3 to C6, screws placed into the medial zone place the spinal cord at risk. The central axial zone represents the area of vertebral artery and nerve root. Five screws placed in this zone were malpositioned, placing these structures at risk. Five screws placed in the lateral zone had penetrated the cortical margin, placing the nerve root at risk. Three patients had radiculopathy, two sensory and one motor and sensory.

Safe screw lengths for the Roy-Camille and Magerl techniques at C3 to C6 are 14 to 15 mm and 15 to 16 mm, respectively (Table 52A-1).[15] A lateral angulation of at least 10 degrees is needed to avoid the neuroforamina, with the screw's trajectory running from posteromedial to anterolateral. The nerve root exits the neuroforamina at the anterolateral portion of the superior facet; therefore screws with a more cephalad angulation place the nerve roots at greater risk of injury.

The vertebral artery travels cephalad within the foramen transversarium beginning at the C6 vertebra. The vertebral artery is at risk of injury from a screw that is placed too medially. The foramen is located medial to the center of the lateral mass from C3 to C5. At C6 the foramen may at times be located directly in front of the center of the lateral mass.[18,62] The incidence of vertebral artery injury is rare, yet it represents a potentially devastating complication. Heller et al. reported no vertebral artery injuries with the placement of 654 screws.[28] Ebraheim et al. recommend directing the screw perpendicular to the posterior aspect of the lateral mass at C3 to C5 and 10 degrees lateral to the center of the C6 lateral mass in the sagittal plane to avoid the vertebral artery.[18]

The Roy-Camille screws are directed perpendicular to the posterior cortex to the vertebral body and may violate the inferior facet. The techniques of An, Magerl, and Anderson avoid this complication by cephalad angulation of the screws 25 to 30 degrees, which is almost parallel with the parasagittal angle of the superior articular facet.[26] In a cadaver study, Choueka et al. showed that 53% of screws placed using the Roy-Camille technique violated the inferior facet joint, compared with 0% utilizing the Magerl technique.[11]

Hardware failures related to lateral mass plating include broken screws, broken plates, screw loosening, and screw avulsion. In a study by Heller et al. there were two broken screws and one broken plate. One patient required additional surgery for a broken screw, whereas the one patient with the broken plate was asymptomatic.[28] Ebraheim et al. had six patients with loose screws, with one patient developing postoperative deformity that required anterior fusion for a successful outcome.[15] In the study by Choueka et al., lateral mass fracture on screw insertion occurred in 6% of Roy-Camille screws and in 7% of the Magerl screws.[11] The three cases of radiculopathy after lateral mass screw insertion reported by Graham et al. were believed to be the direct result of bicortical purchase.[23] Bicortical purchase may place the vertebral artery and the nerve root at additional risk of injury from the drill bit, tap, depth gauge, and the screw itself. However, unicortical screws are at greater risk for pullout than bicortical screws.[33]

Cervical Pedicle Screws

Several authors have reported the use of cervical pedicle screws as a more appropriate means of achieving posterior fixation of C2 or C7. Pedicle screws have also been shown to have a higher resistance to pull-out than lateral mass screws.[33]

According to An et al., the C2 pedicle screw is directed 15 degrees medially and 35 degrees cephalad.[8] At the C2 level a laterally deviated screw may injure the vertebral artery, whereas a screw with excessive medial angulation places the spinal cord at risk. Smith et al. described a starting point for screw insertion as 3 to 5 mm above the center of the C2 to C3 facet, angled 10 to 25 degrees medially and 25 degrees cranially.[49] The authors reported no neurovascular complications with this procedure. Ebraheim et al. compared two techniques for placing C2 pedicle screws. In the first the pedicle screws were placed 5 mm inferior to the superior border of the lamina and 7 mm lateral from the lateral border of the spinal canal. The screws were angled 30 degrees medial in the sagittal plane and 20 degrees cephalad. A 3.5-mm screw was placed bilateral into the C2 pedicles of eight cadavers. In another group of eight specimens, they placed 3.5-mm pedicle screws after intraoperative identification of the superior and medial aspects of the pedicle with a nerve root retractor. Four violations of the lateral wall occurred with the first method and two with the second. There were no superior, inferior, or medial wall violations in their study. The authors believe that identification of the superior and medial aspects of the pedicle allows safe placement of pedicle screws at C2.[17]

Abumi et al. retrospectively studied the use of pedicle screw fixation in 45 patients with nontraumatic lesions of the cervical spine. Thirty-nine patients underwent

Table 52A-1	Recommendations for Lateral Mass Screw Placement	
Technique	Cephalad Angulation (Inferior to Superior) (degrees)	Lateral Angulation (Medial to Lateral) (degrees)
An et al.[8]	33	17
Anderson et al.[9]	30-40	10
Magerl[26]	Parallel to superior facet in sagittal plane	25
Roy-Camille[26]	0	10

CERVICAL PEDICLE SCREWS

- Direct the C2 pedicle screw 15 degrees medially and 35 degrees cephalad.
  - A laterally deviated C2 pedicle screw may injure the vertebral artery.
  - Excessive medial angulation of the screw places the spinal cord at risk.
- There is less risk of violating lateral wall of the C2 pedicle if superior and medial aspects of the pedicle are identified.
- The technique of laminoforaminotomy and direct palpation of pedicle improves accuracy and safety when used in lower cervical spine.

---

cervical or cervicothoracic fixation, 1 patient underwent occipitocervical and cervicothoracic fixation, and 5 patients underwent occipitocervical fixation. The authors placed 183 screws. By radiography 11 of 13 screws (6.0%) placed into the pedicles from C3 to C7 were determined to violate the pedicle and to be at risk for causing injury to the spinal cord, nerve root, or vertebral artery. Although there was one case of radiculopathy from screw threads perforating superiorly, no other neurovascular complications were reported.[2] Recently Abumi et al. reported on an injury to the vertebral artery after placement of a pedicle screw at the C6 to C7 level. The artery was injured during tapping of a fractured pedicle. In a prospective study by the same authors, 45 of 669 pedicle screws (189 patients) perforated the pedicle wall. The medial wall was perforated in 21 screws, inferior in 10, lateral in 10, and superior in 4. There were no cases of vertebral artery injury in the 10 screws that perforated laterally. The highest incidence was at the C4 level with the lowest incidence at the C2 level. Two of the 45 screws caused radiculopathy. A C6 radiculopathy in one patient caused by a superiorly angulated C6 screw resolved without screw removal. Another patient had a C5 nerve root lesion from an inferiorly angulated C4 screw that required screw removal. The authors believe that the incidence of clinically significant complications could be minimized by careful evaluation of appropriate preoperative studies and strict attention to screw insertion and placement.[3]

Albert et al. have also described the safe use of pedicle screws at the cervicothoracic junction. They retrospectively reviewed 21 patients who were treated with C7 pedicle screws. The pedicle screws were placed after direct palpation of the pedicle, with a right angle nerve hook, after a laminoforaminotomy at C7. There were no neurovascular complications related to pedicle screw placement. The authors concluded that placement of pedicle screws through the use of the laminoforaminotomy and direct palpation of the pedicle was safe and effective with excellent results.[6] Although the technique of laminoforaminotomy and palpation has been shown to improve accuracy and safety, the development of new frameless stereotactic systems may provide added protection and safety for these important neurovascular structures.[35]

C1 to C2 Transarticular Screws

Transarticular screws spanning the C1 to C2 lateral mass articulation have been advocated for patients with instability at C1 to C2. The C1 to C2 transarticular screw can provide for greater stability and allow earlier postoperative ambulation. However, several complications are possible with the use of transarticular screws, including injury to the vertebral artery, upper cervical nerve roots, and the spinal cord.

Preoperative evaluation with CT scan and sagittal reconstruction allows measurement of the dimensions of the C2 isthmus. Mandel et al. in an anatomic study found mean isthmus width was 8.2 ± 1.5 mm for males and 7.2 ± 1.3 mm for females. Mean isthmus height was 8.6 ± 2 mm in males and 6.9 ± 1.5 mm in females. The authors noted that an isthmus diameter of less than 4 mm makes accurate screw placement completely within the C2 isthmus technically impossible. They also found that the left C2 isthmus is generally larger, possibly due to the dominance of the left vertebral artery in most patients.[40]

The vertebral artery occupies the superior lateral quadrant of the C2 lateral mass and passes anterior to posterior and medial to lateral to enter the transverse foramen of C1. The transarticular screw travels posterior to anterior and slightly medially to reduce the chance of injury to the artery. Ten percent of patients are at risk of vertebral artery injury because of either a narrow isthmus height or width. Female patients may also be at higher risk for vertebral artery injury because of smaller isthmus dimensions.[40] Sasso et al. reported a case of massive bleeding around the C2 isthmus prior to placement of a transarticular screw, most likely due to laceration of the vertebral artery by the drill.[48] A retrospective survey of the American Association of Neurologic Surgeons/Congress of Neurologic Surgeons identified a 4.1% incidence of vertebral artery injury.[61] Their study also reported a 0.2% incidence of neurologic deficit with C2 transarticular screw placement. The low incidence of neurologic compromise is most likely due to adequate collateral flow up the contralateral uninjured artery circulation. We strongly recommend preoperative assessment of the vertebral arteries with axial and sagittal CT images to identify an anomalous artery or a narrow C2 isthmus before placing the transarticular screws at C1 to C2 joints.

Jeanneret et al. recommend a screw insertion point 3 mm cephalad and 2 mm lateral to the border of the inferior C2 articular process. The screw path is angled 60 to 65 degrees cephalad and 0 to 5 degrees medially. The drill is aimed towards the anterior arch of the atlas and is confirmed by the use of lateral fluoroscopic guidance. Care should be taken to keep the cephalad angulation sufficient to penetrate the C1 lateral mass. The drill hole is tapped to avoid possible anterior dislocation of the atlas during screw insertion. In their prospective study, one patient experienced transient bilateral hypoglossal nerve paresis from a screw that was too long. The paresis resolved when the screw was exchanged for the proper size.[31]

Grob et al. reported no injury to the vertebral artery or medulla in a study of 161 patients treated with trans-

> ## TRANSARTICULAR SCREWS SPANNING THE C1 TO C2 LATERAL MASS ARTICULATION
>
> - Advocated for patients with instability at C1 to C2 where an anterior procedure is contraindicated
> - Can provide greater stability and allow earlier postoperative mobilization than traditional wiring techniques
> - Potential complications
>   - Injury to vertebral artery
>   - Spinal cord injury
>   - Injury to upper cervical nerve roots
>   - Hypoglossal nerve paresis
> - Vertebral artery
>   - Occupies superior lateral quadrant of C2 lateral mass
>   - 10% of patients at risk of vertebral artery injury because of either a narrow isthmus height or width
>   - Do preoperative CT scan to confirm isthmus diameter of ≥4 mm
>   - Female patients at higher risk for vertebral artery injury because of smaller isthmus dimensions
>   - Left C2 isthmus generally larger in most patients
>   - Perform preoperative assessment of vertebral arteries with axial and sagittal CT images to identify an anomalous artery or a narrow C2 isthmus before placing a transarticular screw

> ## OCCIPITOCERVICAL INSTRUMENTATION
>
> **INDICATIONS**
> - Decompressive procedures at the cervicomedullary junction and upper cervical spine associated with removal of midline posterior structures
> - Occipitocervical fusion with plates and screws increases stability over wiring/bone graft alone
>   - Less rigid postoperative immobilization necessary
>
> **COMPLICATIONS**
> - Perforation of inner cortical table into the transverse sinus places patient at risk for "posterior fossa syndrome"
> - Cerebrospinal fluid leak and/or fistula

articular screw fixation. Ideal screw position was evaluated with anteroposterior (AP) and lateral radiographs; 273 screws (85%) were found in the ideal position, with both screws lying entirely within the bone and crossing the joint space on the AP view. Twenty-five screws (7.7%) were positioned too far laterally, and 7 (2.1%) too far medially. Eleven screws (3.4%) were too short or inserted at the wrong angle and did not cross the joint. Six screws (1.8%) were too long and protruded through the lateral mass of the atlas ventrally. In 1 patient a right-sided screw was too long and caused erosion of the right atlanto-occipital joint. The patient required reoperation to extend the fusion to the occiput and for relief of pain. Another patient developed a unilateral paresis of the hypoglossal nerve secondary to a long screw projecting anterior to the occipital condyle. The symptoms improved when the screw was exchanged for an appropriately sized screw.[25]

Occipitocervical Instrumentation

Decompressive procedures at the cervicomedullary junction and upper cervical spine may require removal of the arch of the atlas, enlargement of the foramen magnum with resection of the inferior occipital bone, and laminectomy of C2.[49] In such patients, sublaminar and spinous process wiring may not be possible. Occipitocervical fusion with plates and screws may be performed in patients without midline posterior structures and provides increased stability with the need for less rigid postoperative immobilization.[4]

Ebraheim et al. defined the relevant clinical anatomy of the occiput. The external occipital protuberance (EOP) overlies the thickest portion of bone. This region measures 11.5 to 15.1 mm in males and 9.7 to 12 mm in females. The thickness of the occipital bone is 8 mm up to 2 cm lateral and inferior from the EOP. The confluence (Torcula) of the superior sagittal sinus and transverse sinuses lies directly behind the inner occipital protuberance. An excessively long screw placed 1 cm lateral to the midline at the level of the EOP and 1 cm inferior places the transverse sinus at risk for penetration. Also, a screw that penetrates the inner cortical table will enter the cerebellar fossa and may lead to a potential "posterior fossa syndrome" if the contents of this cavity are injured.[16]

Cerebrospinal fluid (CSF) leaks with subsequent development of a CSF fistula may result as a complication of occipital screw insertion. When CSF is encountered, bone wax can be used as a sealant and the screw advanced in the usual manner. Smith et al. reported no neurovascular injuries, CSF fistulas, or infections in their study of 14 patients treated with occipitocervical plate fixation.[50]

CONCLUSIONS

The cervical spine is a common site of symptomatic degenerative disease, often resulting in radiculopathy or myelopathy. In addition, traumatic injuries to the cervical spine may be associated with significant neurologic injury and require surgical stabilization. The ability of surgeons to treat these pathologies has greatly improved over the past decade with the development of newer instrumentation techniques. However, many of these newer techniques have the potential for significant complications, in addition to the well-established complications related to the surgical approaches and bone grafting.

In general, these procedures can be used to improve patient care when the risks of the operation are recognized and respected by the surgeon. Also, the potential for complications decreases as the surgeon gains experience with these techniques. It should also be noted that the U.S. Food and Drug Administration has not formally approved the application of screws or wires specifically into the posterior elements of the cervical spine.

SELECTED REFERENCES

An HS, Gordin R, Renner K: Anatomic considerations for plate-screw fixation of the cervical spine, *Spine* 16(suppl. 10):S548-S551, 1991.

Anderson PA et al.: Posterior cervical arthrodesis with AO reconstruction plates and bone graft, *Spine* 16(suppl. 10):S72-S79, 1991.

Connolly PJ, Esses SI, Kostuik JP: Anterior cervical fusion: outcome analysis of patients fused with and without anterior cervical plates, *J Spinal Disord* 9(3):202-206, 1996.

Fernyhough JC, White JI, LaRocca H: Fusion rates in multilevel cervical spondylosis comparing allograft fibula with autograft fibula in 126 patients, *Spine* 16(suppl. 10): S561-S564, 1999.

Golfinos JG et al.: Repair of vertebral artery injury during anterior cervical decompression, *Spine* 19(22):2552-2556, 1994.

Heller JG, Silcox DH, Sutterlin CE: Complications of posterior cervical plating, *Spine* 20(22):2442-2448, 1995.

Heller JG et al.: Anatomic comparison of the roy-camille and magerl techniques for screw placement in the lower cervical spine, *Spine* 16(suppl. 10): S552-S557, 1991.

Isomi T et al.: Stabilizing potential of anterior cervical plates in multilevel corpectomies, *Spine* 24(21):2219-2223, 1999.

Lowery GL, McDonough RF: The significance of hardware failure in anterior cervical plate fixation: patients with 2- to 7-year follow-up, *Spine* 23(2):181-186, 1998.

McMullen GM, Garfin SR: Spine update: cervical spine internal fixation using screws and screw-plate constructs, *Spine* 25(5):643-652, 2000.

Stauffer ES: Wiring techniques of the posterior cervical spine for the treatment of trauma, *Orthopedics* 11(11):1543-1548, 1998.

Vaccaro AR et al.: Early failure of long segment anterior cervical plate fixation, *J Spinal Disord* 11(5):410-415, 1998.

Weiland DJ, McAfee PC: Posterior cervical fusion with triple-wire strut graft technique: one hundred consecutive patients, *J Spinal Disord* 4(1):15-21, 1991.

Weisberg NK, Spengler DM, Netterville JL: Stretch-induced nerve injury as a cause of paralysis secondary to the anterior cervical approach, *Otolaryngol Head Neck Surg* 116(3):317-326, 1997.

REFERENCES

1. Abumi KA et al.: Transpedicular screw fixation for traumatic lesions of the middle and lower cervical spine: description of the techniques and preliminary report, *J Spinal Disord* 7(1):19-28, 1994.
2. Abumi KA, Kaneda K: Pedicle screw fixation for nontraumatic lesions of the cervical spine, *Spine* 22(16):1853-1863, 1997.
3. Abumi KA et al.: Posterior occipitocervical reconstruction using pedicle screws and plate-rod systems, *Spine* 24(14):1425-1434, 1999.
4. Abumi KA et al.: Complications of pedicle screw fixation in reconstructive surgery of the cervical spine, *Spine* 25(8):962-969, 2000.
5. Albert TJ: Anterior middle and lower cervical exposures. In Albert TJ, Balderston RA, Northrup BE, eds: *Surgical approaches to the spine*, Philadelphia, 1997, WB Saunders, pp. 9-24.
6. Albert TJ et al.: Use of cervicothoracic junction pedicle screws for reconstruction of complex cervical spine pathology, *Spine* 23(14):1596-1599, 1998.
7. An HS, Cooper M: Cervical spine instrumentation. In An HS, ed: *Principles and techniques of spine surgery*, Philadelphia, 1998, Willliams & Wilkins, pp. 653-673.
8. An HS, Gordin R, Renner K: Anatomic considerations for plate-screw fixation of the cervical spine, *Spine* 16(10S):S548-S551, 1991.
9. Anderson PA et al.: Posterior cervical arthrodesis with AO reconstruction plates and bone graft, *Spine* 16(suppl. 10):S72-S79, 1991.
10. Andreshak TG, An HS: Posterior cervical exposures. In Albert TJ, Balderston RA, Northrup BE, eds: *Surgical approaches to the spine*, Philadelphia, 1997, WB Saunders, pp. 81-113.
11. Choueka J et al.: Flexion failure of posterior cervical lateral mass screws: influence of insertion technique and position, *Spine* 21(4):462-468, 1996.
12. Coe JD et al.: Biomechanical evaluation of cervical spinal stabilization methods in a human cadaveric model, *Spine* 14(10):1122-1131, 1989.
13. Conant RF, Vaccaro AR, Albert TJ: Complication of posterior occipital and cervical screw placement, *Semin Spine Surg* 10(3):228-236, 1998.

14. Connolly PJ, Esses SI, Kostuik JP: Anterior cervical fusion: outcome analysis of patients fused with and without anterior cervical plates, *J Spinal Disord* 9(3):202-206, 1996.
15. Ebraheim NA, Xu R, Yeasting RA: The location of the vertebral artery foramen and its relation to posterior lateral mass screw fixation, *Spine* 21(11):1291-1295, 1996.
16. Ebraheim NA et al.: Anatomic consideration of C2 pedicle screw placement, *Spine* 21(6):691-695, 1996.
17. Ebraheim NA et al.: An anatomic study of the thickness of the occipital bone: implications for occipitocervical instrumentation, *Spine* 21(15):1725-1730, 1996.
18. Ebraheim NA et al.: Safe lateral-mass screw lengths in the Roy-Camille and Magerl techniques, *Spine* 23(16):1739-1742, 1998.
19. Emery SA et al.: Anterior cervical decompression and arthrodesis for the treatment of cervical spondylotic myelopathy: two to seventeen-year follow-up, *J Bone Joint Surg Am* 80(7):941-951, 1998.
20. Fernyhough JC, White JI, LaRocca H: Fusion rates in multilevel cervical spondylosis comparing allograft fibula with autograft fibula in 126 patients, *Spine* 16(suppl. 10):S561-S564, 1991.
21. Fischgrund JS, Kurz LT, Herkowitz HN: Techniques of bone graft harvesting for cervical fusions, *Semin Spine Surg* 7(1):27-32, 1995.
22. Golfinos JG et al.: Repair of vertebral artery injury during anterior cervical decompression, *Spine* 19(22):2552-2556, 1994.
23. Graham AW et al.: Posterior cervical arthrodesis and stabilization with a lateral mass plate: clinical and computed tomographic evaluation of lateral mass screw placement and associated complications, *Spine* 21(3):323-329, 1996.
24. Graziano G et al.: A comparative study of fixation techniques for type II fractures of the odontoid process, *Spine* 18(16):2383-2387, 1993.
25. Grob D et al.: Atlanto-axial fusion with transarticular screw fixation, *J Bone Joint Surg Br* 73(6):972-976, 1991.
26. Heller JG, Silcox DH, Sutterlin CE: Complications of posterior cervical plating, *Spine* 20(22):2442-2448, 1995.
27. Heller JG et al.: Anatomic comparison of the Roy-Camille and Magerl techniques for screw placement in the lower cervical spine, *Spine* 16(suppl. 10):S552-S557, 1991.
28. Heller JG et al.: Biomechanical study of screws in the lateral masses: variables affecting pullout resistance, *J Bone Joint Surg Am* 78(9):1315-1321, 1996.
29. Hu RW, Bohlman HH: Fracture at the iliac bone graft harvest site after fusion of the spine, *Clin Orthop* 309:208-213, 1994.
30. Isomi T et al.: Stabilizing potential of anterior cervical plates in multilevel corpectomies, *Spine* 24(21):2219-2223, 1999.
31. Jeanneret B, Magerl F: Primary posterior fusion C1/2 in odontoid fractures: indications, technique, and results of transarticular screw fixation, *J Spinal Disord* 5(4):464-475, 1992.
32. Jones AAM et al.: Iliac crest bone graft: osteotome versus saw, *Spine* 18(14):2048-2052, 1993.
33. Jones EL et al.: Cervical pedicle screws versus lateral mass screws: anatomic feasibility and biomechanical comparison, *Spine* 22(9):977-982, 1997.
34. Kirkpatrick JS et al.: Reconstruction after multilevel corpectomy in the cervical spine: a sagittal plane biomechanical study, *Spine* 24(12):1186-1191, 1999.
35. Kramer DL et al.: Placement of pedicle screws in the cervical spine: comparative accuracy of cervical pedicle screw placement using three techniques, *Orthop Trans* 21:496, 1997.
36. Kurz LT, Garfin SR, Booth RE: harvesting autogenous iliac bone grafts: a review of complications and techniques, *Spine* 14(12):1324-1331, 1989.
37. Lim EV, Lavadia WT, Roberts JM: Superior gluteal artery injury during iliac bone grafting for spinal fusion: a case report and literature review, *Spine* 21(20):2376-2378, 1996.
38. Lowery GL, McDonough RF: The significance of hardware failure in anterior cervical plate fixation: patients with 2- to 7-year follow-up, *Spine* 23(2):181-186, 1998.
39. Ludwig SC et al.: Transpedicle screw fixation of the cervical spine, *Clin Orthop* 359:77-88, 1999.
40. Mandel IM et al.: Morphologic considerations of C2 isthmus dimensions for the placement of transarticular screws, *Spine* 25(12):1542-1547, 2000.
41. McAfee PC, Bohlman HH, Wilson WL: The triple wire fixation technique for stabilization of acute fixation: a biomechanical analysis, *Orthop Trans* 9:142, 1985.

42. McMullen GM, Garfin SR: Spine update: cervical spine internal fixation using screws and screw-plate constructs, *Spine* 25(5):643-652, 2000.

43. Morone MA et al.: Anterior odontoid screw fixation: indications, complication avoidance, and operative technique, *Contemp Neurosurg* 18(18):1-6, 1996.

44. Nolan JP, Sherk HH: Biomechanical evaluation of the extensor musculature of the cervical spine, *Spine* 13(1):9-11, 1988.

45. Riew DK et al.: Complications of buttress plate stabilization of a cervical corpectomy, *Spine* 24(22):2404-2410, 1999.

46. Rogers WA: The treatment of fractures and dislocations of the cervical spine, *J Bone Joint Surg Am* 24:245-250, 1942.

47. Roy-Camille R et al.: Treatment of lower cervical spinal injuries: C3 to C7, *Spine* 17(suppl. 10):S442-S446, 1992.

48. Sasso RC et al.: Occipitocervical fusion with posterior plate and screw instrumentation: a long-term follow-up study, *Spine* 19(20):2364-2368, 1994.

49. Smith MD, Anderson P, Grady MS: Occipitocervical arthrodesis using contoured plate fixation: an early report on a versatile fixation technique, *Spine* 18(14):1984-1990, 1993.

50. Smith MD et al.: Postoperative cerebrospinal fluid fistula associated with erosion of the dura: findings after anterior resection of ossification of the posterior longitudinal ligament in the cervical spine, *J Bone Joint Surg Am* 74(2):271-277, 1992.

51. Smith MD et al.: Vertebral artery injury during anterior decompression of the cervical spine: a retrospective review of ten patients, *J Bone Joint Surg Br* 75(3):410-415, 1993.

52. Stauffer ES: Wiring techniques of the posterior cervical spine for the treatment of trauma, *Orthopedics* 11(11):1543-1548, 1998.

53. Taylor BA, Vaccaro AR, Albert TJ: Complications of anterior and posterior surgical approaches in the treatment of cervical degenerative disc disease, *Semin Spine Surg* 11(4):337-346, 1999.

54. Vaccaro AR et al.: Early failure of long segment anterior cervical plate fixation, *J Spinal Disord* 11(5):410-415, 1998.

55. Vanichkachorn JS et al.: Anterior junctional plate in the cervical spine, *Spine* 23(22):2462-2467, 1998.

56. Wang JC et al.: The effect of cervical plating on single-level anterior cervical discectomy and fusion, *J Spinal Disord* 12(6):467-471, 1999.

57. Wang JC et al.: Increased fusion rates with cervical plating for two-level anterior cervical discectomy and fusion, *Spine* 25(1):41-45, 2000.

58. Weiland DJ, McAfee PC: Posterior cervical fusion with triple-wire strut graft technique: one hundred consecutive patients, *J Spinal Disord* 4(1):15-21, 1991.

59. Weisberg NK, Spengler DM, Netterville JL: Stretch-induced nerve injury as a cause of paralysis secondary to the anterior cervical approach, *Otolaryngol Head Neck Surg* 116(3):317-326, 1997.

60. Whitecloud TS, Ricciardi JE, Werner JG: Bone graft, hardware, and halo fixator-related complications. In Cervical Spine Research Society: *The cervical spine*, ed 3, Philadelphia, 1998, Lippincott-Raven, pp. 903-921.

61. Wright NM, Lauryssen C: Vertebral artery injury in C1-2 transarticular screw fixation: results of a survey of the AANS/CNS section on disorders of the spine and peripheral nerves, *J Neurosurg* 88(4):634-640, 1998.

62. Xu R et al.: The location of the cervical nerve roots on the posterior aspect of the cervical spine, *Spine* 20(21):2267-2271, 1995.

Complications of Anterior and Posterior Thoracic and Lumbar Instrumentation

Keith H. Bridwell

The complications to be discussed in this chapter are pseudarthrosis; implant fatigue and pull-out; neurologic deficits relative to the spinal cord and lumbar and sacral nerve roots; sagittal and coronal imbalance; acute and delayed infection; vascular problems; implant prominence; sacropelvic fixation issues; visceral impingement; and the effect of nutrition on adjacent discs and instrumented unfused segments.

PSEUDARTHROSIS

Many factors affect whether a spinal fusion solidifies underneath instrumentation. Therein pseudarthrosis is not directly a complication of the instrumentation. Rather, it is a complication of either the bed not being appropriately prepared for the fusion, an inadequate quantity or quality of bone graft, inadequate use of the instrumentation (e.g., inappropriate placement of hooks and pedicle screws or inadequate number of fixation points above and below), or patient factors such as noncompliance, smoking, diabetes, a connective tissue disorder, or a dysplastic bed.

If pseudarthrosis occurs, usually the implants will fatigue in some way by either fracture, pull-out, or loosening. Occasionally a pseudarthrosis can coexist with instrumentation and only become apparent after the instrumentation has been removed (Figure 52B-1).

Detection of pseudarthrosis is complicated. Bone scans, oblique x-ray films, spiral computed axial tomography scan studies, and tomograms all provide some information. A 3- to 5-year period after surgery without implant fatigue or failure is good evidence of a stable fusion. If the implants break or pull out or if a deformity progresses, a pseudarthrosis probably exists.

FATIGUE OF THE IMPLANTS

The attainment of a solid fusion is a race between either the fusion becoming solid or the implants failing. If the implants fail first, then one is usually dealing with a

> ### PSEUDARTHROSIS
> - Is more common in kyphotic than lordotic deformities
> - Increases with advancing age
> - Often leads to progression of deformity

> ### IMPLANT FATIGUE
> - Usually occurs late (i.e., between 1 and 5 years after surgery)
> - Usually signals a pseudarthrosis
>
> Pull-out of implants
> - More likely to occur early (in the first postoperative year)
> - Usually leads to progression of the deformity and pseudarthrosis

pseudarthrosis. Implant fatigue not only demonstrates a pseudarthrosis but frequently results in a progressive deformity. It is uncommon for implant fracture to injure adjacent structures.

PULL-OUT OF THE IMPLANTS

Fatigue of implants usually occurs late, from 1 to 10 years after surgery. However, pull-out of implants is more likely to occur within the first postoperative year. Implants pull out if they are in essence "overpowering" the bone. Kyphotic deformities and high-grade spondylolisthesis are known to have a high incidence of implant pull-out, usually at either the proximal or distal fixation points. Protective measures include multiple fixation points, reduction in the cantilever force on any one implant fixation point, and structural grafting anteriorly.

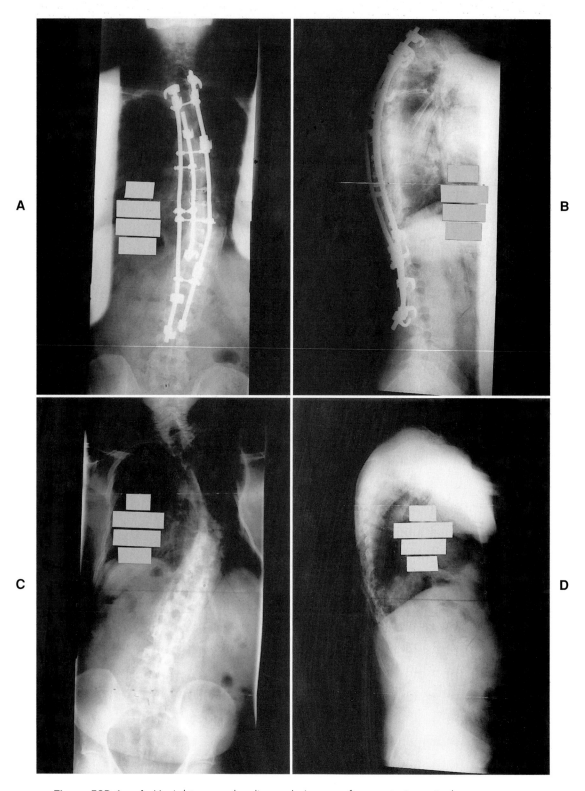

Figure 52B-1.   **A,** Upright coronal radiograph 4 years after posterior spinal fusion/posterior segmental spinal instrumentation (PSF/PSSI). **B,** Upright sagittal radiograph 4 years after PSF/PSSI. **C,** Upright coronal radiograph 6 months after PSSI removal. **D,** Upright sagittal radiograph 6 months after PSSI removal.

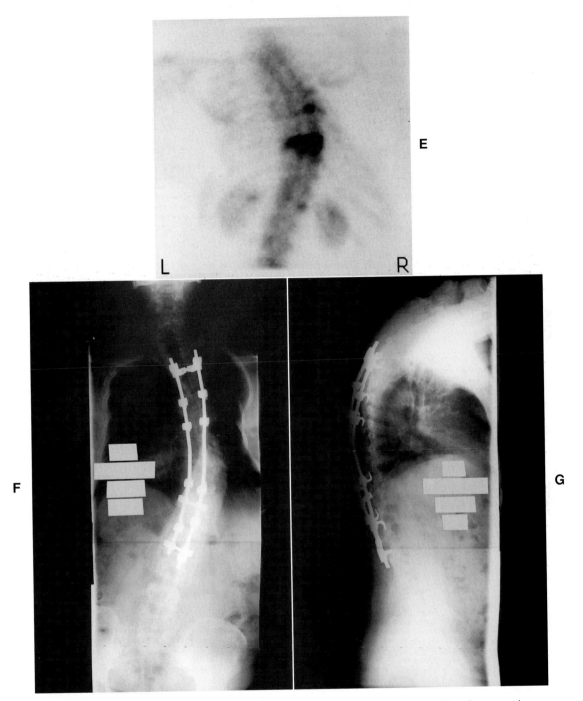

Figure 52B-1, cont'd.   **E,** Bone scan showing apical pseudarthrosis(es). **F,** Upright coronal radiograph 14 months after pseudarthrosis repair. **G,** Upright sagittal radiograph 14 months after pseudarthrosis repair.

SACROPELVIC ISSUES

Fixation of the sacrum has been an ongoing problem. For short-segment pathology, such as one-segment disc degeneration at L5 to S1, fixation posteriorly with two pedicle screws in L5 and two pedicle screws in S1 may be sufficient. But for high-grade spondylolisthesis, it is clear that the screws should either be coupled with either a second set of fixation points distally (e.g., sacral alar or iliac screws) or with anterior column structural support. Longer fusions to the sacrum, such as for adult scoliosis fusions, should be coupled with both anterior structural grafting at L5 to S1 and multiple fixation points of the sacrum and pelvis.[9] Options include bicortical S1 pedicle screws with long iliac screws, and the Jackson intrasacral technique coupled with sacral screws.[6] Long fusions to the sacrum in older adults may result in sacral stress fractures, iliac stress fractures, and stress fractures of the pubic rami.

NEUROLOGIC DEFICITS INVOLVING THE SPINAL CORD AND NERVE ROOTS

Kyphosis cases and revision deformities are at higher risk for perioperative neurologic deficits. Also, cases with both anterior and posterior exposure of the spine, as well as cases associated with significant blood loss, increase the risk. Causes of neurologic deficits include material imploding into the spinal canal (disc, bone, or portions of the implants) or lengthening of the spinal canal. Any anterior or posterior distractive force will lengthen the spinal canal. Our institution is presently engaged in a study to assess the effect of translational and rod rotational forces on spinal canal length, but it appears that those maneuvers lengthen the spinal canal. It would appear that neurologic deficits to the spinal cord are detected on a reliable basis by spinal cord monitoring if both somatosensory and motor-evoked potential methods are used. However, somatosensory potentials alone do not always detect problems.[3]

Deficits to specific lumbar roots are not always picked up by somatosensory potential monitoring, spontaneous electromyelograms (EMGs), or dermatomal potential monitoring. Pedicle stimulation and spontaneous EMG techniques are helpful for alerting the surgeon to medial pedicle perforation and/or irritation of nerve roots by pedicle screw placement.

With pedicle screws, inadvertent perforation of the medial pedicle wall can irritate the traversing nerve root. In other words, if the L4 pedicle is perforated medially, this can irritate and/or injure the L4 root. The placement of S1 pedicle screws can be technically difficult if the patient is muscular and has a narrow pelvis. In this circumstance, it becomes difficult to angulate the S1 pedicle screw medially. Rather than coming out the promontory anteriorly, the surgeon might inadvertently perforate laterally along the anterior ala and thus disturb the L5 root.

Reduction of high-grade spondylolisthesis poses a significant risk of traction on the L5 nerve roots.[13] With reduction of a spondyloptosis, traction on the cauda equina is a risk. With any high-grade spondylolisthesis surgery, the sacral roots also may be at risk. Some surgeons advocate pudendal spontaneous EMG monitoring techniques.

If a neurologic deficit occurs, the surgeon must decide whether to remove the implants. If the implants or bone or disc implode into the canal, this should be addressed. If the spinal canal has been lengthened, then the implants should be removed. At times, a neurologic etiology may be entirely vascular, in which case the implants can be retained. The other option is temporary removal of the implants and replacement at a later date if the deformity is unstable.

FIXED SAGITTAL IMBALANCE

The classic cause of fixed sagittal imbalance (FSI) is Harrington distraction instrumentation in the lumbar spine. It is also seen with anterior compression instrumentation done without structural grafting. Other causes are positioning the patient in a lumbar flexed position rather than a lumbar extended position when doing a lumbar fusion, high-grade spondylolisthesis, a breakdown adjacent to previous fusion, widespread degenerative disc disease, osteoporosis, and systemic conditions such as ankylosing spondylitis.[2,8,10]

Management of FSI involves removal of old implants, performing an osteotomy or osteotomies, and reinstrumenting the spine. Options include Smith-Petersen osteotomies and/or a pedicle subtraction osteotomy, depending upon the circumstances and the amount of correction needed (Figure 52B-2).

CORONAL IMBALANCE

When correcting a scoliosis in which the patient has several curves and one curve is more fixed than the others, it is possible to worsen the coronal balance. Common circumstances include patients with oblique take-offs from the sacrum, false double major curves, and double thoracic curves. Occasionally these conditions occur with true double major curves, because the lumbar deformity is usually more flexible than the thoracic deformity.[4]

It is helpful to obtain long-cassette coronal x-ray films when the patient is still on the operating table

---

CAUSES OF NEUROLOGIC DEFICIT

- Lengthening the spinal canal
- Intrusion into the spinal canal by either bone, disc, or metal
- A vascular problem with the spinal cord

Often the true cause is a combination of all three.

METAL INSTRUMENTATION CAUSES OF NEUROLOGIC DEFICIT

All forms of metal instrumentation have the potential to intrude on the spinal canal and thereby create neurologic deficits. These include the following:
- Hooks
- Dublaminar wires
- Anterior vertebral screws
- Posterior pedicle screws

CAUSES OF FIXED SAGITTAL IMBALANCE

- The classic cause of iatrogenic sagittal imbalance is posterior column distraction.
- Recent causes are surgeries on middle-age and older individuals that result in multiple pseudarthroses and multiple implant failures associated with either osteoporosis or widespread disc degeneration.

For fixed deformities, Smith-Petersen osteotomies or a pedicle subtraction osteotomy may be the solution.

and/or with the patient turned supine, for analysis before the patient leaves the operating room. That long-cassette coronal x-ray film should be put up with the pelvis in the same inclination as it is when the patient stands. These radiographs can still be confusing, and the surgeon may not know for sure whether the patient's coronal balance has been maintained until the patient stands at the bedside. With the combination of long-cassette coronal x-ray examination of the patient on the operating table, long-cassette coronal x-ray examination

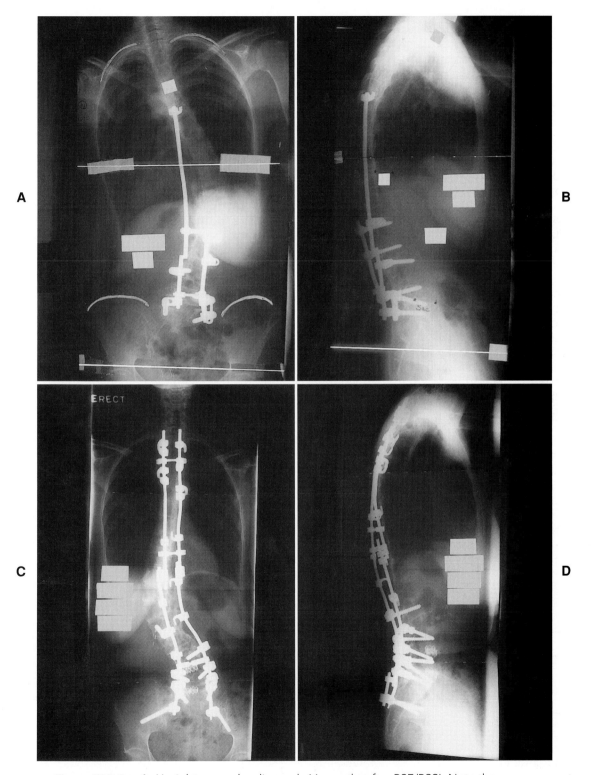

Figure 52B-2.   **A,** Upright coronal radiograph 16 months after PSF/PSSI. Note the coronal imbalance and broken implant. **B,** Upright sagittal radiograph 16 months after PSF/PSSI shows a sagittal imbalance. **C,** Upright coronal radiograph 3 years after revision. **D,** Upright sagittal radiograph 3 years after revision.

of the patient turned supine on the bed immediately after surgery, and standing the patient at the bedside the day after the surgery, the surgeon should know the status of coronal balance.

The other source of imbalance presents later if the implants pull out at junctional levels or if curves above or below progress.

ACUTE INFECTION

Usually, acute infection is accompanied by increasing pain, fever, and drainage within the first month postoperatively.[14] The sedimentation rate usually will be elevated and the white count may be elevated, although the latter is not always the case. Appropriate treatment is to return the patient to the operating room to débride the soft tissues and close the wound over drains, leaving the drains in for an extended period and administering intravenous antibiotics. In most cases, this treatment will preserve the implants for at least a year. The exception is if the patient has poor soft tissues around the implants. Posterior wound infection is more common than anterior infection.

DELAYED INFECTION

Delayed infection usually appears between 1 and 3 years after surgery and a several-week history of intermittent fevers and malaise without an elevated white count but with an elevated sedimentation rate. Sometimes there are no localizing signs. At other times, the wound opens and starts to drain. In this circumstance, the most likely causative bacteria is of low virulence. The treatment for a delayed wound infection is implant removal. The concomitant use of intravenous antibiotics may be of some help, but removal of the implants is the key. If a pseudarthrosis is present beneath the implants, it may be necessary to replace the instrumentation and bone graft at a later date. Therefore some consideration for preservation of critical fixation points may be in order[5] (Figure 52B-3).

VASCULAR CONSIDERATIONS

With Dunn anterior segmental spinal instrumentation, there have been reports of erosion into the aorta if the implant was placed on the left side of the spine.[7] Subsequently, anterior segmental spinal instrumentations have been placed anterolaterally without bulk along the anterior aspects of the vertebral body to reduce the incidence of this complication. To my knowledge, implants such as the Kaneda device for fractures,

the Kaneda device for scoliosis, and the Z-plate for fracture and tumor have not been associated with a similar complication. Obviously, exposing the spine to place such implants introduces a potential for disturbing vessels, more so veins than arteries. In placing posterior systems, in particular pedicle screws, there is some potential for disturbing an anterior vascular structure if the pedicle screws are too long or if the preparation for the pedicle screws has included tapping or drilling beyond the anterior cortex of the vertebral body. On a lateral x-ray film of the spine, considering the anterior shape of the vertebral body, the anterior cortex of the vertebral body is usually two-thirds of the way from the posterior to anterior view.

IMPLANT PROMINENCE

In thin individuals, posterior implants can be prominent under the skin. Also, a partial pull-out adds to the prominence. This is one reason why surgeons have recently considered anterior instrumentation for thoracic curves in thin patients.

Certain implants have a proclivity for being prominent, such as iliac screws. Also, junctional kyphosis next to a fusion will make the instrumentation more prominent at that segment.[11]

VISCERAL IMPINGEMENT

Placement of implants anterior to the sacral ala risks irritating or compressing the ureters, which has occurred with the extremely valuable Dunn-McCarthy technique.[12] Anterior instrumentation is obviously in contact with lung tissue, although this does not seem to cause a problem. Anterolateral instrumentation may contact the kidney, but I have never seen or heard of hematuria being caused by the implants themselves.

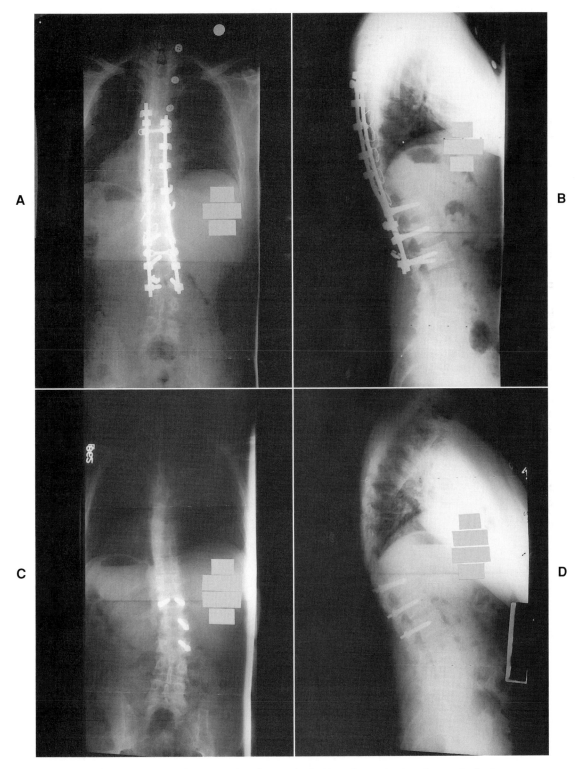

Figure 52B-3. **A,** Upright coronal radiograph. **B,** Upright sagittal radiograph. Patient had pain and a high sedimentation rate. **C,** Upright coronal radiograph after PSSI removal. **D,** Upright sagittal radiograph after PSSI removal. The implants were infected.

ROD LONG/FUSE SHORT TREATMENT

Rod long/fuse short treatment was more popular in the days before pedicle screw implants.[1] It may still have a role today for certain conditions, such as unusual revision cases and fractures in the middle and distal lumbar spine.

It is clear that the segments that are instrumented without a fusion should be "liberated," perhaps as early as 6 months and no later than a year after the instrumentation. Immobilization of segments without fusion reduces their nutrition and leads to accelerated disc degeneration.

ROD LONG/FUSE SHORT TREATMENT

- This treatment is not as popular as it was many years ago.
- If lumbar segments are instrumented without fusion, implants are ideally removed as early as 6 months after surgery to avoid altered nutrition and accelerated degeneration of instrumented/unfused segments.

SELECTED REFERENCES

Akbarnia BA et al.: Use of long rods and a short arthrodesis for burst fractures of the thoracolumbar spine: a long-term follow-up study, *J Bone Joint Surg Am* 76(11):1629-1635, 1994.

Booth KC et al.: Complications and predictive factors for the successful treatment of flatback deformity (fixed sagittal imbalance), *Spine* 24(16):1712-1720, 1999.

Bridwell KH et al.: Major intraoperative neurologic deficits in pediatric and adult spinal deformity patients: incidence and etiology at one institution, *Spine* 23(3):324-331, 1998.

Clark CE, Shufflebarger HL: Late developing infection in instrumented idiopathic scoliosis, *Spine* 24(18):1909-1912, 1999.

Theiss SM, Lonstein JE, Winter RB: Wound infections in reconstructive spine surgery, *Orthop Clin North Am* 27(1):105-110, 1996.

REFERENCES

1. Akbarnia BA et al.: Use of long rods and a short arthrodesis for burst fractures of the thoracolumbar spine: a long-term follow-up study, *J Bone Joint Surg Am* 76(11):1629-1635, 1994.

2. Booth KC et al.: Complications and predictive factors for the successful treatment of flatback deformity (fixed sagittal imbalance), *Spine* 24(16):1712-1720, 1999.

3. Bridwell KH et al.: Major intraoperative neurologic deficits in pediatric and adult spinal deformity patients: incidence and etiology at one institution, *Spine* 23(3):324-331, 1998.

4. Bridwell KH et al.: Coronal decompensation produced by Cotrel-Dubousset "derotation" maneuver for idiopathic right thoracic scoliosis, *Spine* 16(3):769-777, 1991.

5. Clark CE, Shufflebarger HL: Late developing infection in instrumented idiopathic scoliosis, *Spine* 24(18):1909-1912, 1999.

6. Jackson RP, McManus AC: The iliac buttress: a computed tomographic study of sacral anatomy, *Spine* 18(10):1318-1328, 1993.

7. Jendrisak MD: Spontaneous abdominal aortic rupture from erosion by a lumbar spine fixation device: a case report, *Surgery* 99(5):631-633, 1986.

8. Kostuik JP et al.: Combined single stage anterior and posterior osteotomy for correction of iatrogenic lumbar kyphosis, *Spine* 13(3):257-266, 1988.

9. Kuklo TR et al.: Minimum 2-year analysis of sacropelvic fixation and L5/S1 fusion using S1 and iliac screws, *Spine* 26(18):1976-1983, 2001.

10. LaGrone MO et al.: Treatment of symptomatic flatback after spinal fusion, *J Bone Joint Surg Am* 70(4):569-580, 1988.

11. Lee GA et al.: Proximal kyphosis after posterior spinal fusion in patients with idiopathic scoliosis, *Spine* 24(8):795-799, 1999.

12. McCarthy RE, Dunn H, McCullough FL: Luque fixation to the sacral ala using the Dunn-McCarthy modification, *Spine* 14(3):281-283, 1989.

13. Petraco DM et al.: An anatomic evaluation of L5 nerve stretch in spondylolisthesis reduction, *Spine* 21(10):1133-1138, 1996.

14. Theiss SM, Lonstein JE, Winter RB: Wound infections in reconstructive spine surgery, *Orthop Clin North Am* 27(1):105-110, 1996.

Treatment of Cerebrospinal Fluid Leaks

K. Daniel Riew, Nitin Khanna

Dural tears are a relatively common complication of spinal surgery. Reported rates of dural tears range from less than 1% to 17%.[2,3,6,7,12]

As expected, the risk of dural tears is higher in revision surgery secondary to scar formation and adhesions.[2] Also, an increased rate of dural tears is noted in decompression for ossification of the posterior longitudinal ligament and the use of a high-speed drill.[4,8,11] In primary procedures, meticulous technique is essential to avoid durotomies. However, the presence of thin dura, adhesions in the dura, and redundant dura in patients with tight spinal stenosis may all lead to unintended incidental dural tears.

Both Wang et al.[12] and Jones et al.[6] reported on the long-term sequelae of appropriately managed dural tears.[3,6,12] Jones et al.[6] retrospectively reviewed 450 patients undergoing spine surgery. In their study there was a 4% incidence of dural tears (17 patients). These dural tears were recognized intraoperatively and repaired primarily. The matched controlled patients were followed for an average of 25.1 months postoperatively. No statistically significant difference could be found between the outcomes of the two groups. They concluded that an unintended incidental durotomy, if identified and repaired intraoperatively, did not increase morbidity or influence long-term outcome.

In the largest reported series in the literature Wang et al.[12] reviewed Bohlman's experience with lumbar dural tears. They reviewed 641 consecutive patients undergoing lumbar spine surgery and found a 14% incidence of dural tears (88 patients). The majority of these patients had one or more previous lumbar decompressions. These dural tears were identified and repaired at the time of surgery. The average follow-up was 4.3 years. They concluded that a dural tear recognized and repaired at the time of surgery does not have any long-term deleterious effects on outcome. Specifically, there was no increase in the risk of postoperative infection, neural damage, or arachnoiditis.

An effective dural repair will reduce the likelihood of untoward sequelae, including meningitis, pseudomeningocele, nerve root entrapment with resultant neurologic compromise, arachnoiditis, and durocutaneous fistulas.

PHYSIOLOGY OF CEREBROSPINAL FLUID

Cerebrospinal fluid (CSF) is considered an ultrafiltrate of plasma, which provides an ideal protective chemical and mechanical environment for the central nervous system (CNS).[13] In its normal state it is an acellular, clear, colorless fluid.

The production of CSF is primarily from the choroid plexus in an energy-dependent secretory process. This occurs in the lateral, third, and fourth ventricles of the brain. CSF is also formed by the flow of extracellular fluid in the brain across the ependymal lining of the ventricular system.

The normal total volume of CSF is 150 ml. There is 75 ml in the cisterns, 50 ml in the subarachnoid space, and 25 ml in the ventricles. Its rate of production is about 0.5 ml/min. This results in the production of 450 to 600 ml of CSF each day. The total volume of CSF is turned over about three to four times a day.

DURAL TEARS

- Relatively common complication of spine surgery (1% to 17%)
- Higher risk with revision surgery, tight spinal stenosis, ossification of the posterior longitudinal ligament
- No long-term sequelae if appropriately managed
- Effective dural repair reduces the likelihood of meningitis, pseudomeningocele, nerve root entrapment with resultant neurologic compromise, arachnoiditis, and durocutaneous fistula

---

PHYSIOLOGY OF CSF

- Acellular, clear, colorless, fluid
- Produced in choroid plexus
- Total volume: 150 ml—turned over 3 to 4 times/day
- Rate of production: 0.5 ml/min

The chemical content of CSF varies depending on its location in the CNS. For example, CSF sampled from the ventricles contains 15 mg/100 ml of protein and 75 mg/100 ml of glucose, whereas lumbar CSF contains 45 mg/100 ml protein and 60 mg/100 ml glucose.

SIGNS AND SYMPTOMS OF A DURAL LEAK

The diagnosis of a dural leak often can be made from clinical information. Persistent drainage of clear or serosanguinous fluid from the wound is suggestive of a dural tear. The patient will classically complain of a spinal headache. The headache increases in severity when the patient is erect and is relieved by lying flat. Other possible symptoms include photophobia, tinnitus, vertigo, dizziness, blurred vision, neck stiffness, nausea, and vomiting. The symptoms are believed to be due to a decrease in the CSF pressure, which leads to traction on the supporting structures in the CNS.[5] Bed rest is theorized to alleviate the symptoms by decreasing both the hydrostatic pressure intradurally and traction on the CNS.

If the patient presents with a fluctuant mass over the surgical site, the diagnosis of a pseudomeningocele must be considered. The formation of a pseudomeningocele is a mechanical process. The durotomy is kept patent by intradural pressure, which causes a constant outflow of CSF. The pseudomeningocele is connected to the subarachnoid space by a stalk of variable length. The diagnosis can be confirmed by myelography or magnetic resonance imaging (MRI) (Figure 53-1).

> ### SIGNS AND SYMPTOMS OF DURAL LEAK
>
> - Persistent drainage of clear fluid from wound
> - Spinal headache
> - If fluctuant mass present, must consider pseudomeningocele

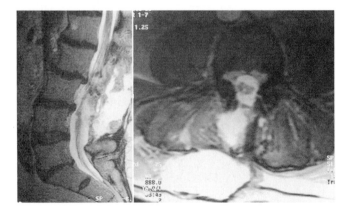

Figure 53-1 MRI of pseudomeningocele. T2 weighted sagittal and axial images demonstrating the communicating stalk between the subdural space and the pseudomeningocele.

REPAIR OF DURAL TEARS
Intraoperative Dural Tears

The literature supports the immediate repair of dural leaks noted at the time of surgery before proceeding with the remainder of the surgical procedure.[2] There is a loss of the tamponade effect on the epidural veins as the CSF leaks out of the durotomy site. Excessive bleeding in conjunction with CSF can obscure the operative field for the remainder of the procedure. For this reason it is preferable to repair the dura as soon as possible. If the durotomy site is not immediately accessible (e.g., persistent lateral recess stenosis), it can be covered with a paddy until the stenosis has been decompressed. During the repair, the patient should be positioned to decrease the hydrostatic pressure at the durotomy site. For a lumbar durotomy, this involves placing the patient in a Trendelenburg position. For a cervical spine case, it is helpful to place the patient in a reverse Trendelenburg position.

Once a durotomy has been repaired, it can be tested by both the Valsalva maneuver and tilting the table to increase the dependent position of the durotomy site (i.e., reverse Trendelenburg positioning for lumbar tears and Trendelenburg positioning for cervical spine tears). This allows for the adequacy of the repair to be evaluated under direct visualization intraoperatively.

Bed rest alone is often insufficient treatment for most dural tears. The use of Gelfoam alone or placement of fat, muscle, or fascia at the site of the tear, without a direct repair, is not an adequate seal for dorsal or lateral tears. Occasionally, ventral tears may tamponade and seal themselves without direct repair.

Cervical Dural Tears

Dural tears in the cervical spine most commonly occur in the presence of an ossified posterior longitudinal ligament and/or dura.[11] Following the removal of the ossified ligament or dura, a patch is often necessary to close the defect. Occasionally, the dural defect is so large that one cannot completely sew a patch in place. In such cases the patch can be sewn onto as much of the remaining dura as possible and the remainder can be sealed with a small amount of fibrin glue. The bone graft is then placed into the corpectomy site and fibrin glue is used to seal the edges of the bone graft. Putty forms of demineralized bone matrix can also be used to seal the bone in place and simultaneously enhance bone fusion.

> ### INTRAOPERATIVELY NOTED DURAL TEARS
>
> - Repair dura as soon as possible.
> - To ease repair, position patient to lower hydrostatic pressure at durotomy site (i.e., Trendelenburg position for lumbar tears/reverse Trendelenburg for cervical tears).
> - Under direct visualization in the operating room, test the repair with Valsalva maneuver performed under anesthesia.

Dural tears in the cervical spine are often easier to deal with than those in the lumbar spine. Usually the durotomy has been made in the midline, and there are no nerve roots evaginating through the dural defect. Small dural leaks in relatively inaccessible areas can be often be left alone, unlike in the lumbar spine, where small dural leaks are often more problematic than larger ones. In the lumbar spine the high hydrostatic pressure at the bottom of the water column tends to keep small leaks open. CSF at the level of the cervical spine is at the top of the water column and is under significantly less hydrostatic pressure. By keeping the patients sitting or standing postoperatively, one can often get small leaks to close up spontaneously. If the defect is irreparable or inadequately repaired, a lumbar drain can be placed to divert the CSF so as to lower the cervical hydrostatic pressure.

Techniques of Dural Repair
Suture

Direct repair of the dura has historically been the gold standard. It is essential to have excellent visualization of the dural tear. This includes meticulous hemostasis, adequate exposure, and either microscope or loupe magnification. We have a separate dural repair set that consists of a Castro-Viejo micro needle holder, microforceps, and microscissors (Aesculap, Germany) (Figure 53-2).

We prefer a 5-0 or 6-0 silk suture on a reverse cutting or taper, one half circle needle. Alternatively a Prolene suture can be used. An innovative suture used primarily by the vascular and cardiac surgeons can also be used. Gore-Tex suture (Figure 53-3) (Gore, AZ), polytetrafluoroethylene nonabsorbable monofilament, uses a

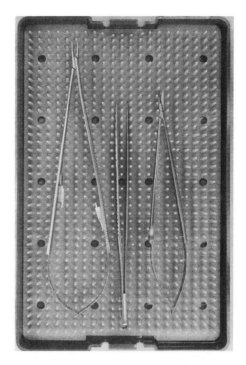

Figure 53-2 Dural repair kit *(left to right)* includes Castro-Viejo needle driver, microforceps, microsuture scissors (Aesculap, Germany). The use of microinstruments facilitates repair of the dura.

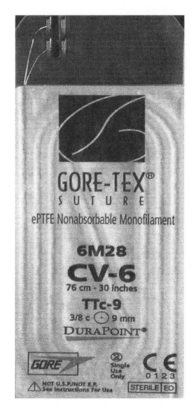

Figure 53-3 Gore-Tex suture (Gore, AZ). The suture is larger than the needle. Once the needle punctures the dura, the hole created by the needle is overstuffed by the suture.

CERVICAL DURAL TEARS

- Cervical dural tears commonly after an ossified posterior longitudinal ligament.
- A patch graft may be used to close the defect augmented with fibrin glue or putty forms of demineralized bone matrix around bone graft.
- Cervical dural tears are typically easier to treat than lumbar tears because no nerve roots are evaginating.
- If patients are kept sitting upright or standing, small leaks may close up.
- If tear is inaccessible and cannot be repaired, place a lumbar drain to divert the CSF, thereby lowering cervical hydrostatic pressure.

TECHNIQUES OF DURAL REPAIR

- Simple stitch
- Running locked stitch
- Patch graft
  ○ Local source: thoracodorsal fascia
  ○ Remote source: Fascia lata, muscle
  ○ Cervical spine: Platysma

swage technique, which allows the suture to closely approximate the diameter of the needle. Because the suture is the same size or slightly larger than the needle, it will "overstuff" the hole created by the needle. The package insert claims reduced needle hole fluid leakage when tested on cadaver dura mater.

Different suture techniques have been reported in the literature. Eismont et al.[2] recommended the use of a running locked stitch (Figure 53-4). Most of the studies that compare suture to other modes of dural repair use simple interrupted sutures placed 2 to 3 mm apart (Figure 53-5, *A*).

Graft

For tears that cannot be closed without undue tension, the use of a patch graft is recommended. Different grafts have been reported including fascia lata, thoracodorsal fascia, fat, or muscle. For the thoracolumbar spine, our preference is the use of thoracodorsal fascia because it is a local source of tissue (Figure 53-5, *B*). For cervical spine cases, one can use allograft fascial or dural patches, or synthetic materials. We prefer using a small piece of platysma along with its underlying fascia. This is usually less time consuming than locating and preparing a packaged substitute and has the added advantage of

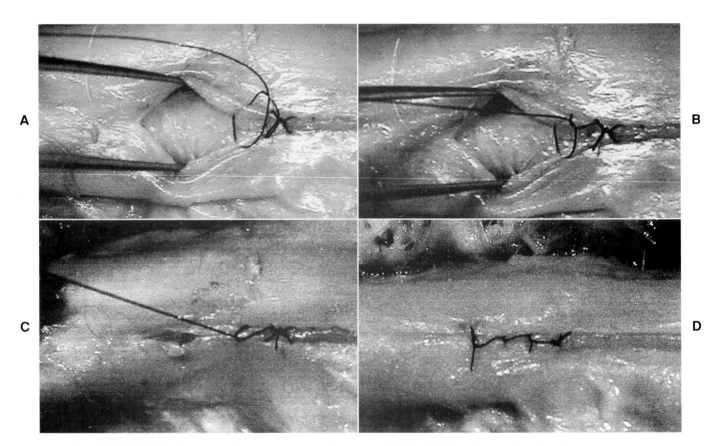

Figure 53-4 Running locked stitch. **A,** The durotomy site. **B,** The running stitch is being locked. **C,** The suture is tensioned, sealing the durotomy site. **D,** The final closure.

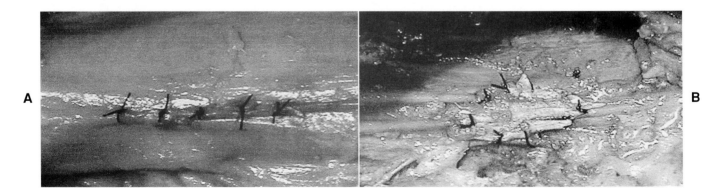

Figure 53-5 **A,** Simple interrupted stitch. 6-0 silk suture is placed approximately 2 to 3 mm apart. **B,** Thoracodorsal fascial patch graft with circumferential simple interrupted sutures placed 2 to 3 mm apart.

being less expensive. Both a simple and a running locked suture technique can be used to secure the graft.

A tear in the ventral or ventral lateral sac makes direct repair technically difficult. Eismont et al.[2] described an innovative method of creating an intentional central durotomy to visualize the difficult-to-reach defect. An indirect method of repair through the intentional durotomy site is used. A fat graft is obtained from a local source and a simple suture is tied to the graft. The suture is passed from the intentional central durotomy to the dural defect. The graft is then pulled into place so as to plug the dural defect from within (Figure 53-6). There are no reports in the literature detailing the effectiveness of this method of treatment.

Fibrin Glue

Fibrin glue is made from cryoprecipitate, which is coagulated by mixing with thrombin. In the first syringe, one draws up the cryoprecipitate, which is composed of human fibrinogen, factor XIII, fibronectin, and plasminogen. In the second syringe, thrombin powder is mixed with calcium chloride solution (Figure 53-7). The two solutions are injected onto the dural repair site simultaneously. The benefits of the fibrin glue are that it pro-

vides an immediate seal to the dura. The glue invokes a minimal inflammatory response and has been reported to reabsorb in the healing phase because it is a purely biologic substance. The potential drawback to the use of fibrin glue relates to its possibility of transmitting viral disease. There have been no reported cases of virally transmitted disease with the use of this technique to date, but the possibility still exists. This can be solved by using autologous fibrin. However, the processing of autologous fibrin glue takes 3 days, making it a less practical modality.

Cain et al.[1] demonstrated the comparative advantage of suture reinforced with fibrin glue over either of these modalities alone. They demonstrated in vitro that with human physiologic pressures, the suture alone, regardless of technique, did not maintain a watertight seal. However, when this primary suture line was reinforced with fibrin glue, it yielded a sevenfold increase in bursting pressure. This was sufficiently above physiologic intradural pressures.

Dural Stapler

A dural stapler can facilitate the closure of a simple dorsal tear (Figure 53-8). It is not effective for a lateral

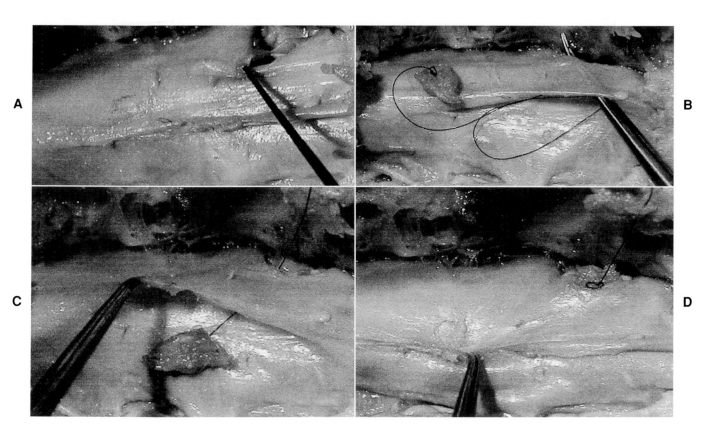

Figure 53-6 Intentional durotomy technique to repair far lateral or ventral defects. **A,** The ventral lateral defect is demonstrated with a nerve hook. **B,** A suture is anchored to a fat plug. The intentional dorsal durotomy is used to pass the suture from inside to outside. The suture enters under the dura and exits through the ventral lateral dural defect. **C,** The suture anchored to the fat plug is slowly advanced subdurally. **D,** The fat plug is pulled halfway through the dural defect. Care must be taken to fashion an appropriately sized fat plug. If the plug is too large, it may lead to neural compression. If the plug is too small, it will not close the defect. The graft may be secured in place with simple interrupted sutures.

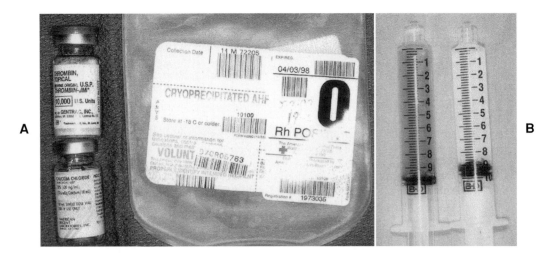

Figure 53-7 Fibrin glue. **A,** Separate bottles of thrombin in powder form and calcium chloride. Packet containing cryoprecipitate. **B,** The syringe on the left contains calcium chloride and thrombin mixed together. The syringe on the right contains the cryoprecipitate. The two syringes are to be injected simultaneously onto the dural repair site.

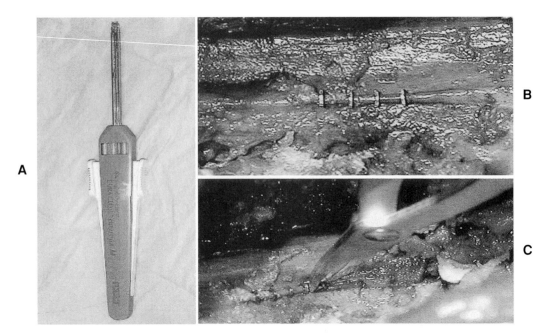

Figure 53-8 **A,** Disposable dural stapler (Surgical Dynamics, Norwalk, Conn). **B,** Example of dural staples in place 2 to 3 mm apart. **C,** Demonstration of removing dural staples.

tear where nerve roots may get entrapped. It is quick and easy to place and remove staples. There have not been any reported studies in the literature comparing its use alone or in conjunction with other methods of closure.

Subfascial Drains

The subfascial drain is not a treatment for a dural tear. However, it is worth mentioning because many spine surgeons favor the use of subfascial drains in their standard closure of a spine wound. The literature has been relatively clear on the concern of developing a durocuta-neous fistula with the use of a subfascial drain in the presence of a dural tear. Wang et al.,[12] however, demonstrated that the use of subfascial drains after definitive closure of dural tears was not associated with increased problems.

Postoperatively Noted Dural Tears

If necessary, the clinical diagnosis can be confirmed by MRI or computed tomography (CT)-myelogram. Once confirmed, these postoperative dural tears should be addressed expeditiously. There are four treatment alter-

---

CLOSURE

FIBRIN GLUE
- Cryoprecipitate and thrombin mixed together form an immediate seal of the dura.
- Suture reinforced with fibrin glue had a 7-fold increase in bursting pressure compared with suture alone.
- There is still a remote possibility of viral disease transmission from donor cryoprecipitate.

DURAL STAPLER

SUBFASCIAL DRAINS
- Used in standard closure.
- Not associated with durocutaneous fistulas in the presence of a dural tear.

POSTOPERATIVELY NOTED DURAL TEARS

- Patient's own blood can be percutaneously injected into epidural space, forming a blood patch to seal a dural tear, preventing reoperation
- May inject fibrin glue percutaneously to seal a dural tear and avoid reoperation
- Placing an epidural drain to reduce hydrostatic pressure at the durotomy site can also induce nonoperative healing of a dural tear
- Definitive treatment: Reoperation and closure of the dura

---

natives: (1) blood patch; (2) percutaneous fibrin glue; (3) subarachnoid drain; and (4) reoperation with direct repair.

Blood Patch

Maycock et al.[9] reported on the use of percutaneous injection of an epidural blood patch. The procedure, which is usually performed by an anesthesiologist or the pain service, involves the injection of the patient's own blood into the epidural space. The concept is based on animal studies that demonstrated that blood injected into the epidural space forms a clot that plugs a needle hole breach in the dura. The recommendation is to place the blood patch at an interspinous space at or above the level of the dural breach because the blood tends to migrate in a caudal rather than cephalad direction. If the patient has a high lumbar dural leak, then the blood patch can be administered caudally with the patient maintained in a Trendelenburg position.

The controversy regarding the blood patch revolves around how much blood to inject. The literature reports effective treatment ranging from 2 ml to 20 ml. Regardless of the volume injected, the procedure should be stopped if the patient feels pain at any time during the procedure. Some anesthesiologists prefer to perform the procedure under fluoroscopic guidance with a small amount of contrast mixed with the blood. This prevents an inadvertent intradural injection, which can lead to headaches and bilateral buttock and leg pain. If present, these symptoms usually subside spontaneously after a few weeks.

Percutaneous Injection of Fibrin Glue

Fibrin glue may also be used postoperatively by the percutaneous approach described by Patel et al.[10] They reported three of six patients successfully treated by this technique. The patient was placed in the prone position in the CT scanner and the site of the CSF leak was located. The overlying skin was marked, and an 18- to 20-gauge spinal needle was introduced under CT guidance

adjacent to the dural tear. A preprocedure MRI was used to identify the exact location of the dural leak. Once the needle was felt to be in an acceptable position, a syringe with 3 ml of cryoprecipitate (either the patient's own blood or donor blood/plasma) was connected to a three-way stopcock. The second port was connected to a syringe with calcium chloride and thrombin. The two syringes were injected simultaneously into the extradural space in the vicinity of the dural leak. The fibrin plug set up in vivo. The total volume injected ranged from 4 to 18 ml. Following the procedure the patient was restricted to overnight bed rest.

Subarachnoid Drain

A subarachnoid drain may be placed at the time of surgery if the repair is felt to be inadequate or tenuous. It can also be used to treat a dural leak discovered in the postoperative period. The use of a subarachnoid drain proximal to the durotomy site is an effective method of reducing the intradural pressure, thereby decreasing the outflow of CSF through the dural defect. If the dural tear is high up in the lumbar spine, the catheter should be placed caudal to the dural tear and threaded cephalad to the defect. The procedure is performed under sterile conditions at the patient's bedside. A Teflon epidural catheter is placed into the subarachnoid space and then connected to a sterile collection bag, creating a closed collection system (Figures 53-9 and 53-10). The bag is moved up or down in reference to the patient in order to maintain a steady flow of CSF into the bag. The goal is to drain approximately 10 to 20 ml of fluid each day. Kitchel et al.[7] recommended 4 days of bed rest after placement of the catheter. They reported an 82% success rate with this approach. We have found that 2 to 3 days of bed rest is usually adequate. The catheter is clamped after 2 days and the patient is allowed to sit upright for 4 to 6 hours. If the symptoms of a dural leak recur, the patient is kept down another 2 days with the drain open. The advantage of this system is that surgical intervention may be avoided. The drawbacks are that the presence of an indwelling catheter does increase the risk of infection. Kitchel et al.[7] recommended daily cultures, cell counts, and protein and glucose CSF measurements to detect any signs of infection. We have not found this to be necessary, but we keep our patients on antibiotics.

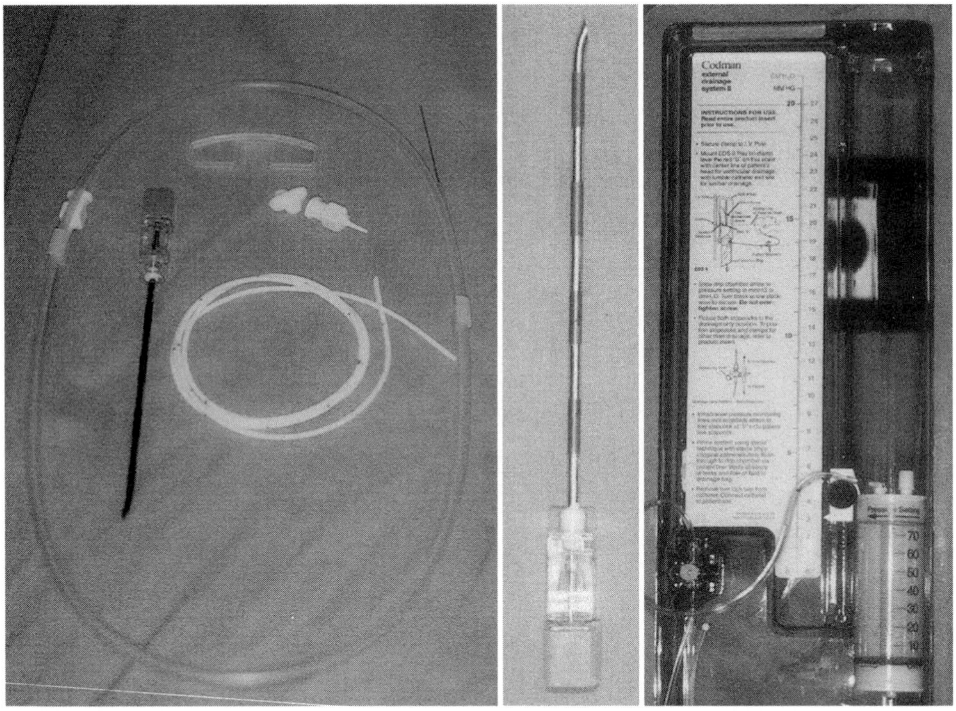

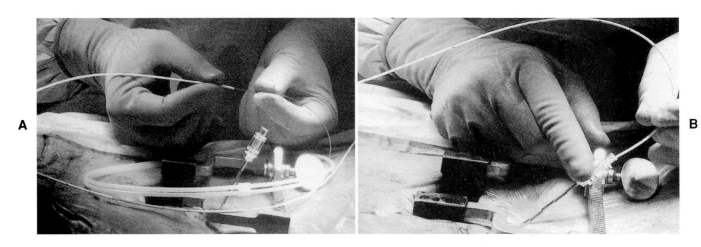

Figure 53-9 **A,** Subdural catheter kit includes *(center-left)* large-bore introducer needle, *(center-right)* Silastic catheter, and *(outside)* wire used to stiffen the catheter to ease insertion. **B,** Large-bore needle used to introduce catheter. **C,** Closed system to reduce infection risk (Codman).

Figure 53-10 **A,** The catheter is stiffened with a small wire in its lumen. The end of the catheter is capped to prevent the wire from protruding past the catheter tip. This prevents inadvertent perforation of neural structures with the wire during its introduction. The perforations in the catheter are peripheral to allow for drainage of the CSF. **B,** Technique of placing a subdural drain: The drainage catheter is introduced through the large-bore needle into the subdural space. The introducer needle is removed first, followed by the stiffening wire, taking care not to pull out the drain. The drain is then sutured into place.

POSTOPERATIVE CARE

After a dural tear is adequately repaired intraoperatively, the amount of time a patient should remain flat in bed is controversial. Eismont et al.[2] recommended placing patients on 4 days of bed rest postoperatively. Wang et al.[12] reported resolution of dural leaks after watertight closure with silk interrupted suture in 86 of 88 patients treated with an average of 3 days of bed rest. The 2 remaining patients who persisted with a leak after 3 days were taken back to the operating room for definitive

---

POSTOPERATIVE CARE

LUMBAR TEAR
- Typically, the patient should remain flat for 24 to 48 hours after a repaired dural tear to decrease the pressure at the repair site.
- The patient can then sit up in bed to check for resolution of the spinal headache, indicating effective dural closure.

CERVICAL TEARS
- Keep the head of bed >30 degrees at all times for the first 24 hours.
- The patient is to remain sitting or standing to decrease hydrostatic pressure in the cervical spine.

---

closure of the dural defect. Hodges et al.[5] recently studied 20 patients retrospectively. Nineteen of the patients had a dural tear that was noted at the time of surgery and repaired with suture in conjunction with fibrin glue. All of their patients had the integrity of their repairs tested with both the Valsalva and reverse Trendelenburg tests. They allowed their patients to ambulate immediately after surgery. They found 75% of the patients with no symptoms related to their dural tear. Five patients had symptoms such as headaches, nausea, and vomiting; however, in only one patient (5%) was there noted to be stitch loosening requiring revision surgery.

Based on the aforementioned findings, we recommend the following: For small tears that are easily repaired with a watertight seal, we typically keep the patients on bed rest overnight only. They are then mobilized as per our normal routine. For larger tears that are again adequately repaired, we keep the patients on bed rest for 24 hours and then mobilize them normally. For tears that have only tenuous repair and that we are concerned about, we will typically keep the patient on bed rest for 48 hours.

In the cervical spine, we do not advocate bed rest because sitting and standing decrease the hydrostatic pressure in the cervical area. We therefore mobilize these patients immediately and keep the head of their bed up at greater than 30 degrees at all times for the first 24 hours.

SELECTED REFERENCES

Cain JE Jr, Dryer RF, Barton BR: Evaluation of dural closure techniques: suture methods, fibrin adhesive sealant, and cyanoacrylate polymer, *Spine* 13:720-725, 1988.

Eismont FJ, Wiesel SW, Rothman RH: Treatment of dural tears associated with spinal surgery, *J Bone Joint Surg Am* 63:1132-1136, 1981.

Hodges SD et al.: Management of incidental durotomy without mandatory bed rest, *Spine* 24:2062-2064, 1999.

Jones AA et al.: Long term results of lumbar spine surgery complicated by unintended incidental durotomy, *Spine* 14:443-446, 1989.

Smith MD et al.: Postoperative cerebrospinal fluid fistula associated with erosion of the dura, *J Bone Joint Surg Am* 74:270-277,1992.

Wang JC, Bohlman HH, Riew KD: Dural tears secondary to operations on the lumbar spine, *J Bone Joint Surg Am* 80:1728-1732, 1998.

REFERENCES

1. Cain JE Jr, Dryer RF, Barton BR: Evaluation of dural closure techniques: suture methods, fibrin adhesive sealant, and cyanoacrylate polymer, *Spine* 13:720-725, 1988.
2. Eismont FJ, Wiesel SW, Rothman RH: Treatment of dural tears associated with spinal surgery, *J Bone Joint Surg Am* 63:1132-1136, 1981.
3. Finnegan WJ et al.: Results of surgical intervention in the symptomatic multiply-operated back patient: analysis of sixty-seven cases followed for three to seven years, *J Bone Joint Surg Am* 61:1077-1082, 1979.
4. Graham JJ: Complications of cervical spine surgery, *Spine* 14;1046-1050, 1989.
5. Hodges SD et al.: Management of incidental durotomy without mandatory bed rest, *Spine* 24:2062-2064, 1999.
6. Jones AA et al.: Long term results of lumbar spine surgery complicated by unintended incidental durotomy, *Spine* 14: 443-446, 1989.
7. Kitchel SH, Eismont FJ, Green BA: Closed subarachnoid drainage for management of cerebrospinal fluid leakage after an operation on the spine, *J Bone Joint Surg Am* 71:984-987, 1989.
8. Marshall LF: Cerebrospinal fluid leaks: etiology and repair. In Herkowitz HN et al., eds.: *The spine*, Philadelphia, 1992, WB Saunders, pp. 1982-1989.
9. Maycock NF, van Essen J, Pfitzner J: Post-laminectomy cerebrospinal fluid treated with an epidural blood patch, *Spine* 19:2223-2225, 1995.
10. Patel MR, Louie W, Rachlin J: Postoperative cerebrospinal fluid leaks of the lumbosacral spine: management with percutaneous fibrin glue, *Am J Neuroradiol* 17:495-500, 1996.
11. Smith MD et al.: Postoperative cerebrospinal fluid fistula associated with erosion of the dura, *J Bone Joint Surg Am* 74:270-277, 1992.
12. Wang JC, Bohlman HH, Riew KD: Dural tears secondary to operations on the lumbar spine, *J Bone Joint Surg Am* 80:1728-1732, 1998.
13. Young PA, Young PH: *Basic clinical neuroanatomy*, Philadelphia, 1997, Williams & Wilkins.

Postlaminectomy Cervical Kyphosis

Todd J. Albert, Alexander R. Vaccaro, Brian T. Brislin

There is an abundance of literature regarding surgical treatments for disorders of the cervical spine. Posterior approaches that include laminectomy were the earliest to be described and have had varied success in the treatment of patients with cervical spondylotic myelopathy, infection, and spinal cord tumors. However, there are a number of complications related to the performance of a cervical laminectomy. Cervical deformity as a result of iatrogenic instability has resulted after laminectomy for the removal of spinal tumors in children and in several reports of adults (Figure 54-1). The causes of this instability are the result of disruption of the posterior cervical supporting elements, which at times may be further exaggerated by a lack of appreciation of preoperative sagittal malalignment of the spinal column (i.e., preoperative kyphosis) before the performance of a posterior decompressive procedure.[2,18,19,24] The patient with pain and myelopathy due to postlaminectomy kyphosis represents a significant treatment challenge because of the triad of deformity, neurologic compromise, and incomplete soft-tissue restraints.[2]

POSTLAMINECTOMY KYPHOSIS IN CHILDREN

The incidence of postlaminectomy kyphosis varies in the literature. Several factors regarding its etiology have been studied: age at the time of surgery, preoperative alignment, preoperative instability, preoperative diagnosis, aggressiveness of the laminectomy, the number and location of the laminae removed at the time of surgery, and the degree and number of facets resected.[1,2,18,33,39] Unfortunately, children have the highest incidence of postlaminectomy deformity.* Bell et al.[5] reported an incidence of 37%, whereas Aronson et al.[4] noted an incidence of 95% when a suboccipital decompression is combined with a cervical laminectomy. Lonstein[19] reported an incidence of an average of 49% in children

treated with cervical laminectomy for spinal cord tumors. It has often been debated whether this deformity is actually a complication of the surgical procedure or a result of instability related to the presence of tumor.

There is an increased incidence of kyphosis in younger patients and in patients with laminectomy of the more cephalad cervical levels. Yasouka et al.[39] reported in their study of 26 patients younger than 15 years who were treated with laminectomy that a postlaminectomy cervical kyphosis developed in 12 of the 26 patients. The authors noted the development, after surgery, of anterior vertebral body wedging as the cause of the kyphosis. They also found that a postoperative deformity developed in 100% of patients after a cervical laminectomy compared with 36% of those after a thoracic laminectomy. In a second study, Yasouka et al.[38] postulated that incomplete ossification of the cervical vertebral bodies and the increased viscoelasticity of the intervertebral ligaments of children could be responsible for the development of this deformity even in the absence of facet injury. These authors concluded that the incidence of postoperative instability or deformity is related to the age at time of surgery and the level of the laminectomy.[38,39] In an analysis of risk factors, Katsumi et al.[18] also showed that age at surgery, a neutral preoperative curvature, number of laminae removed, a C2 laminectomy, and the addition of facetectomy were important predictors of postoperative instability. This

> ### POSTLAMINECTOMY KYPHOSIS: RESULTS FROM POSTOPERATIVE INSTABILITY IN THE CERVICAL SPINE
>
> - Presents significant challenge in treatment based on triad of deformity, neurologic compromise, and incomplete soft tissue restraints
> - Anterior procedures to correct the deformity remove the anterior supporting structures and give the patient 360 degrees of instability

*References 4, 9, 18, 19, 38, 39.

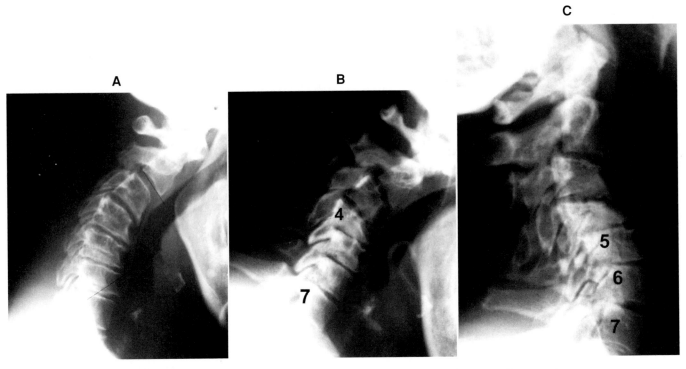

Figure 54-1. Examples of sagittal cervical deformities. **A,** Kyphotic. **B,** Swan neck. **C,** Meandering.

was further supported by Cattell et al.,[7] who also noted the association of skeletal and ligamentous deformities after cervical laminectomy.

POSTLAMINECTOMY CERVICAL KYPHOSIS IN ADULTS

The literature has not supported the potential occurrence of postlaminectomy cervical kyphosis in adults when there is normal preoperative sagittal alignment with no evidence of instability. The normal cervical sagittal alignment is lordotic with an average angle of −14.4 degrees.[41] To maintain this lordosis, the weight-bearing axis of the cervical spine lies posterior to the vertebral bodies.[28,29] Pal and Sherk,[27] in a human cadaver study, demonstrated that axial compressive forces were normally distributed among three columns (one anterior and two posterior) of the cervical spine. The anterior column contains the vertebral bodies and the intervertebral disc, whereas the two posterior columns are made up of the articular facets. The anterior column receives 36% of axial compressive force, and each posterior column receives 32% (64% total). These compressive forces in the posterior column are distributed among the lamina of C2 to C7 and their articular processes.[27] Loss of integrity of the posterior neural arch transfers the resting compressive loads to the anterior spinal column, potentially compromising preservation of the normal cervical lordotic posture.[28,31] Tensile forces are now applied to the facets instead of the compressive forces that are normally found there. In their experimental model of spinal instability, White et al. reported that any disruption of either the anterior or posterior cervical structures could result in instability.[35] Panjabi et al.[28,29] experimentally demonstrated a progressively increasing degree of cervical instability to flexion-compression loads with the sequential removal of the posterior supporting ligaments and structures. Most significant was the degree of instability that resulted from the removal of the posterior facet joints in flexion testing.

In a finite element analysis study by Saito et al.,[33] the authors cited that the primary cause of postlaminectomy deformity was the resection of one or more of the spinous processes and/or ligaments. They found that after removal of these structures, tensile forces that were preoperatively distributed through the posterior columns were transferred to the facets. This imbalance of forces, especially in the middle cervical spine, may lead to the wedging deformity seen in the anterior vertebral bodies.[33] According to studies by Mikawa et al.,[22] Sim et al.,[34] and Kamioka et al.,[17] the presence of any preoperative kyphosis or instability significantly increases the risk of increasing deformity after laminectomy. Due to less-than-successful results with laminectomies in patients with spondylotic myelopathy, Miyazaki et al.[23] began to include a posterolateral fusion in all such cases to improve the degree of postlaminectomy cervical stability. Although they reported improved clinical results with this approach and emphasized the tendency for malalignment to progress when fusion was not performed, 5% of their patients continued to develop either a new deformity or worsening of preexisting malalignment in spite of attempted fusion.

The contribution of facet resection to postlaminectomy instability has also been well documented.[20,29,32,43] Originally, Scoville stated that partial or complete face-

POSTLAMINECTOMY CERVICAL DEFORMITY

- Normal cervical curvature: Lordotic with an average angle of −14.4 degrees
- Anterior column of cervical spine (vertebral bodies and intervertebral discs) receives 36% of axial compressive forces
- Posterior columns (facet joints) receive 64% of axial compressive forces
  - Results of inadequacy of normal posterior supporting structures
  - Loss of normal cervical sagittal alignment
  - Shift of the weight-bearing axis anteriorly
- Tensile forces instead of compressive forces applied to the facet joints
- Destruction of posterior tethering elements
- Transfers tensile forces to facet joints and vertebral bodies
- Imbalance of forces leading to anterior wedging deformity of vertebral bodies
- Stabilizers of head and neck

Dynamic: semispinalis cervicis and capitis; static: posterior ligaments and structures.

FACET RESECTION AND POSTLAMINECTOMY KYPHOSIS

- Resection of facet joints associated with increased incidence of postlaminectomy kyphosis
- Kyphosis induced by facetectomy of as little as 25% added to laminectomy
- With disruption of posterior ligaments and facets, increased horizontal translation of vertebral bodies
- Exposure of 3 to 5 mm of nerve root requires 50% facetectomy
- Exposure of 8 to 10 mm of nerve root requires 75% facetectomy

tectomy added no risk of instability to the cervical spine.[13] This has been refuted by the results of many observational clinical series and basic science research. Nowinski et al.[26] reported that kyphosis was induced by a facetectomy of as little as 25% when combined with a laminectomy and suggested a prophylactic fusion after a multilevel laminectomy. Epstein[10] noted the importance of the facet joint in retaining stability after laminectomy and warned against the removal of more that one fourth to one third of the joint during cervical laminectomy. Fager[11] also emphasized the importance of retaining facet integrity when performing a cervical laminectomy. In a primate model, Munechika[25] demonstrated that a laminectomy of five or more levels was not the cause of postoperative kyphosis but that resection of even one facet increased the likelihood of a gibbous formation. Cusick et al.,[9] in their study of cervical motion segments subjected to increasing flexion-compression loads, also showed increased instability after unilateral or bilateral facet resection.

Zdeblick et al.[43] studied the effect of progressive cervical facet resection with laminectomy in a human cadaver model. The specimens were tested in axial load, flexion-extension, and torque with physiologic loading. The authors found that a facetectomy of 50% or greater caused statistically significant loss of stability in flexion and torsion. They further found that the remaining facet capsule played a role in the limitation of rotation and flexion. In a similar study, they reported on the stability of the cervical spine after progressive facet capsule resection and showed that significant hypermobility did occur with rotation and flexion testing after 50% or greater resection of the facet capsule.[41] Raynor et al.[30] showed that 3- to 5-mm exposure of the nerve root required a 50% facetectomy and 8- to 10-mm exposure required a facetectomy of 70%. The authors also showed

that a facetectomy of 50% significantly reduced the resistance to shear stresses. Herkowitz[15] reported a 25% incidence of postlaminectomy kyphosis in patients with bilateral facetectomy. Callahan et al.[6] also demonstrated a significant association between foraminotomy added to a laminectomy and postlaminectomy kyphosis.

SURGICAL PREVENTION OF IATROGENIC CERVICAL KYPHOSIS

Given the potential for iatrogenic instability after a posterior cervical decompressive procedure, the surgeon must take into account several factors when deciding to perform a cervical laminectomy.[18,23] The need for a multilevel decompression or the addition of facet resection, the degree of preoperative sagittal instability, the presence of anterior structural instability, and the presence of skeletal immaturity all necessitate strong consideration for an adjunctive reconstructive fusion in these clinical scenarios.[22] In patients with a neutral sagittal alignment, consideration for a posterior stabilization procedure should strongly be considered to prevent the morbid consequence of postoperative instability and deformity formation. In the setting of preexisting kyphosis, the spinal cord does not have the ability to migrate posteriorly after a laminectomy and often is further draped over the anterior kyphotic vertebral elements, potentially exasperating any preoperative neurologic deficits (Figure 54-2). These patients are best managed with an initial anterior decompressive and reconstructive procedure.

In the patient selected for a posterior cervical stabilization procedure after a laminectomy, the patient's sagittal alignment may be adjusted by manipulating the Mayfield pin holder to recreate the desired degree of cervical lordosis before the fusion procedure. Laminoplasty has also been developed as a surgical alternative to the degree of bony and ligamentous resection required with a formal laminectomy. However, in studies by Yonenobu et al.,[40] in patients treated with laminoplasty for cervical spondylotic myelopathy, kyphosis developed later in 10% and anterolithesis of greater than 3 mm developed later in 5%, even with the articular facets/capsules left intact.

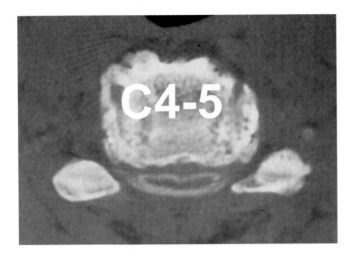

Figure 54-2. Postmyelogram computed tomography scan demonstrating spinal cord draped over an area of kyphosis. Note flattening and atrophy.

POSTOPERATIVE DEFORMITY

- If the preoperative sagittal alignment is not lordotic or at least neutrally aligned, cord may become draped over a kyphotic deformity and a posterior procedure may not adequately resolve the cord compression.
- Laminoplasty is an alternative to laminectomy in patients with neutral preoperative sagittal alignment, but it is best performed in a lordotic cervical spine.

CLINICAL EVALUATION OF POSTLAMINECTOMY KYPHOSIS

- With progressing kyphosis and increasing forward decompensation of the head on the torso, the patient may complain of
  - Increasing neck pain
  - Muscle spasm
  - Steadily progressive neurologic dysfunction

RISK FACTORS FOR POSTLAMINECTOMY KYPHOSIS

- Factors
  - Young age at time of initial surgery
  - Abnormal preoperative sagittal alignment
  - Presence of preoperative instability
  - Aggressiveness of laminectomy
  - Number and location of the laminae removed
  - Degree and number of facets resected
- Children
  - Highest incidence
  - Incidence related to age at initial operation and level of laminectomy
- Adult
  - Clinical reports: No significant incidence when preoperative alignment is normal and no preoperative instability is present
  - Presence of preoperative kyphosis or instability: Significant increase in risk of postoperative deformity after cervical laminectomy

---

CLINICAL AND RADIOLOGICAL EVALUATION OF POSTLAMINECTOMY CERVICAL KYPHOSIS

Patients in whom a postlaminectomy cervical deformity develops often experience initial relief of their presenting symptoms (the "honeymoon period") after their index surgical procedure.

Initially, they may be symptom free. However, with progressing cervical kyphosis and increasing forward decompensation of the head on the torso, the patient often complains of increasing neck pain and muscular spasm and steady progressive neurologic dysfunction. The patient may have difficulty in holding the head upright volitionally, and often the visual horizon is lost (implying fixed downward angulation). A thorough neurologic evaluation must be conducted to evaluate the patient's neurologic status, including bowel, sexual, and motor and sensory function.

Plain radiographs, including flexion-extension views, are important to measure the degree of cervical kyphosis in the sagittal plane. The presence of ankylosis must be assessed due to its implications for future surgical management. Although facet ankylosis often can be ruled out with oblique plain radiographic films, computed tomography with sagittal and coronal reconstructions is very useful. Magnetic resonance imaging is invaluable in assessing spinal cord compression and cord changes, including myelomalacia, syrinx formation, and cord atrophy (Figure 54-3). These findings significantly affect the degree of risk of any future surgical correction. Magnetic resonance imaging is also useful in assessing the degenerative status of the discs at the end of a proposed posterior reconstructive fusion, and when combined with computed tomography, magnetic resonance imaging is valuable in discerning specific anatomic variants such as the location of the vertebral artery within the C7 foramen transversarium and whether a pedicle is large enough to accept a screw. Angiography is occasionally necessary to assess the patency of the vertebral system, especially in the presence of tumor, as well as to evaluate the ability of the extracranial vasculature to serve as conduits for vascularized fibular grafts in cases that involve multiply operated graft beds.

SURGICAL CONSIDERATIONS IN POSTLAMINECTOMY KYPHOSIS

The goals of surgery for postlaminectomy kyphosis are to correct and stabilize the existing deformity while relieving neural compression.[16,36] Deformity correction should never compromise neurologic function, which is often tenuous in this clinical setting. In the majority of cases, neural decompression and deformity correction can be attained simultaneously.[2] Herman and Sonntag[16] thought that regardless of the cause, kyphosis is commonly associated with instability and results in an anterior compression of the spinal cord or nerve roots. The biomechanics of surgical correction involve anterior column lengthening and posterior column shortening, with the axis of rotation centered around the posterior longitudinal ligament.[1,2] Using the posterior longitudinal ligament as a hinge helps to prevent undue traction on the neural elements. In the setting of objective anterior cord compression, an initial anterior decompression is necessary and further facilitates deformity correction. The surgical strategy chosen (posterior correction of deformity with fusion and instrumentation, anterior decompression and fusion with instrumentation, anterior fusion followed by posterior correction with instrumentation, or a combination of anterior and posterior procedures) depends in large part on the degree and rigidity of the spinal deformity.[1,2,13]

Zdeblick et al.[42] reported on the use of anterior corpectomy and strut grafting to treat 14 patients with severe kyphosis resulting in anterior cord compression and myelopathy. In 8 of the 14 patients, kyphosis was the result of a prior laminectomy of three to five cervical vertebrae. The average preoperative kyphosis was 52 degrees (22 to 80 degrees). Surgery involved an anterior decompression of all compressed cervical levels. Seating holes for a future bone graft were created in the inferior and superior ends of the trough. Skeletal tong traction, with or without the use of a roll placed behind the patient's shoulders, was used to reduce the deformity and facilitate placement of the graft. After radiographic documentation of cervical reduction, a strut

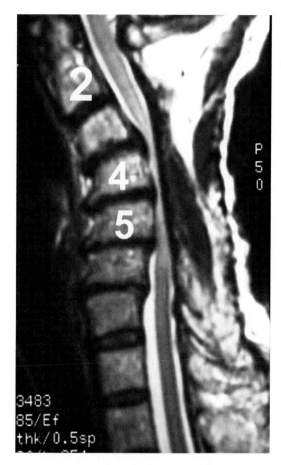

Figure 54-3. Myelomalacia and spinal cord atrophy in the setting of postlaminectomy kyphosis.

graft was placed, followed by traction release to secure the graft. A corticocancellous iliac graft was used for one- to two-level corpectomies, whereas a fibular strut graft was used for three- to five-level corpectomies. Four patients required an additional posterior arthrodesis for enhanced stability. Patients who received a fibular strut graft or had prior laminectomy were treated with halo vest immobilization. Patients treated with iliac graft and anterior-posterior arthrodesis were managed with a two-post cervical orthosis. Overall, the mean amount of kyphosis decreased from 45 degrees before surgery to 13 degrees immediately after surgery with 17 degrees of residual kyphosis at follow-up. No patient lost neural function and nine patients had complete recovery of neural function. Three patients had dislodgment of their anterior graft in the immediate postoperative period (Figure 54-4); two patients required reoperation to lengthen the graft, and the third patient was treated successfully with halo traction. All 14 patients had solid fusion. The authors demonstrated that in patients with cervical kyphosis and myelopathy, adequate decompression of neural elements and correction of deformity can be achieved with anterior corpectomy and strut grafting.[42]

Herman et al.[16] treated 20 patients with postlaminectomy kyphosis and anterior compressive pathology with anterior decompression, bone grafting, and anterior instrumentation. The mean degree of preoperative kyphosis was 38 degrees. A trial of preoperative skeletal traction was used without reduction of the kyphosis or relief of neurologic symptoms in 15 of the 20 patients. Decompression consisted of an anterior discectomy in one patient with pathology limited to the disc space and corpectomies for the other patients. A mean of two or

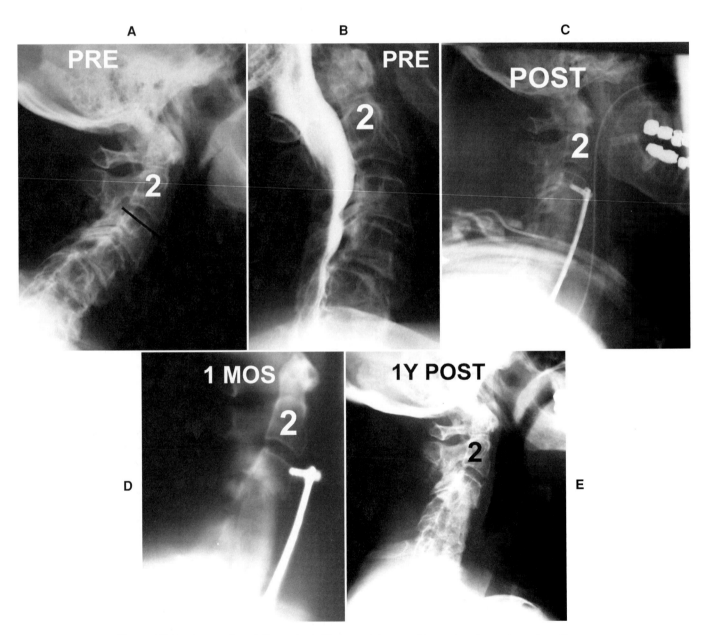

Figure 54-4. Long plate failure. **A,** A 63-year-old man with neck pain and myelopathy after cervical laminectomy. **B,** Preoperative myelogram demonstrating severe stenosis at level of kyphotic deformity. **C,** Patient treated with posterior cervical arthrectomy, anterior corpectomy and strut-graft with anterior plate spanning corpectomy defect. **D,** After 1 month, the plate failed secondary to the settling of the graft. **E,** Solid fusion at 1 year after removal of anterior plate.

more levels were involved in the majority of patients. All patients received autologous iliac bone graft or allograft supplemented by either the Caspar (85%) or Synthes (15%) anterior plating system. Two patients were immobilized in a halo vest, whereas the 18 remaining patients wore a hard cervical orthosis for 6 to 8 weeks after surgery. Two patients had complete resolution of symptoms, 11 patients had substantial improvement in neurologic function, and 6 patients continued to have persistent neurologic dysfunction. One patient had initial improvement in neurologic function with late development of mild progressive myelopathy and paresthesias. All patients had solid osseous union with a mean of 16 degrees of residual kyphosis at follow-up.[16]

McAfee et al.[21] described the use of a one-stage combined anterior-posterior approach in a patient with 70 degrees of postlaminectomy cervical kyphosis and neurologic dysfunction. The patient was treated with anterior osteotomies of the fourth and fifth and the fifth and sixth cervical levels, as well as with posterior wiring and arthrodesis. The kyphosis was reduced, and neurologic function returned to normal. Heller et al.[14] reported on the use of anterior and posterior cervical decompression and reconstruction with instrumentation in a patient with cervical kyphosis and worsening neurologic deficit. After discharge from the hospital, the patient experienced acute neurologic deterioration caused by pullout of the lower posterior cervical screws. The patient's posterior fixation was then revised and extended to T4 with resultant neurologic improvement. Recently, Abumi et al.[1] reported on the use of cervical pedicle screws for the correction of kyphosis in 30 patients. Three of the 30 patients were treated for postlaminectomy kyphosis. Two patients had a flexible kyphosis and were managed with a posterior procedure alone, whereas the third had a rigid kyphosis and was treated with a combined anterior and posterior procedure. In the patients with flexible kyphosis, the lower parts of the inferior articular processes were resected for improved deformity correction. After pedicle screw insertion, the application of compression between the inserted screws allowed segmental correction of the kyphosis through shortening of the posterior column and lengthening of the anterior column. The preoperative flexible kyphosis of 43 and 30 degrees improved to 7 and −6 degrees, respectively, after surgery and was 7 and −5 degrees at final follow-up. In the patient with the rigid kyphosis, a circumferential osteotomy that included a corpectomy, bilateral uncinectomies, and bilateral facetectomies was performed to loosen the bony fusion. Segmental posterior correction with pedicle screws and anterior strut grafting were then used to correct the deformity. This patient's rigid kyphosis improved from 46 degrees before surgery to 16 degrees after surgery with 16 degrees of residual kyphosis at follow-up. All patients wore a short neck collar for 2 to 3 weeks after surgery.

AUTHORS' PREFERRED TREATMENT

Before surgery, gentle axial traction is performed to assess the flexibility of the decompression, as well as to improve overall sagittal alignment. This is carefully monitored due to the ischemic nature of the deformity and the potential for worsening neurologic dysfunction with excessive axial traction. The patients are placed in skeletal traction during the surgical procedure with starting weights of approximately 10 to 15 lb. Our personal practice has evolved toward the use of internal fixation both anteriorly and posteriorly in the face of 360 degrees of instability created when a postlaminectomy patient undergoes an anterior corpectomy. Our surgical management of the patient with postlaminectomy kyphosis with myelopathy without ankylosis includes maximal postural correction, anterior corpectomies, and strut grafting with a junctional buttress plate, followed by sequential posterior segmental fixation and facet fusions with morselized autograft (Figure 54-5). When ankylosis is present, a posterior osteotomy that includes removal of the inferior portion of the facet is required to allow for maximal correction.

At C2, C7, and T1, pedicle fixation is preferred given the improved biomechanical properties compared with those of lateral mass screws.

Graft selection depends on the length of fusion. For three or fewer disc levels, we prefer iliac crest autograft. For longer fusions, a fibular graft is ideal in the cervical spine.[12,37] Although some investigators have shown better healing potential with autograft, we use allograft if a posterior stabilization with autograft and instrumentation is planned. If substantial deformity correction is to be attempted, with increased loads on the fibular graft, preference is given to an autogenous fibula. If cord compression and myelopathy are caused primarily by the kyphotic deformity with draping of the cord over the gibbous, consideration is given to segmental correction with interbody grafts[3,8] (Figure 54-6). The healing potential of this type of construct given the multiple junctions is less than that of a fibular strut. However, intersegmental correction can provide better deformity correction with less acute lengthening of the neural elements.

SURGICAL TREATMENT OF CERVICAL POSTLAMINECTOMY KYPHOSIS

- Gentle preoperative traction
- Intraoperative skeletal traction
- Surgical options
  - Anterior corpectomy and strut grafting with iliac crest or fibula graft followed by halo placement
  - Anterior corpectomy, bone grafting, and application of an anterior plate
  - Anterior segmental correction with interbody grafting and instrumentation
  - Anterior corpectomy, fusion, and instrumentation (possible junctional plate) followed by a posterior arthrodesis with instrumentation
  - Posterior decompression and segmental instrumentation
  - With ankylosis: Posterior osteotomy, removing inferior portions of facet followed by anterior decompression and fusion and final posterior segmental stabilization

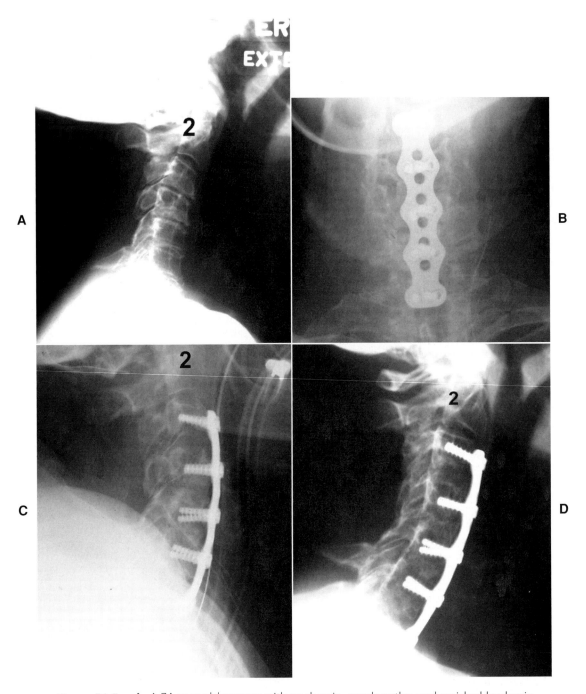

Figure 54-5.   **A,** A 74-year-old woman with neck pain, myelopathy, and residual kyphosis in extension after cervical laminectomy. **B,** Postoperative anteroposterior radiograph. **C,** Lateral radiograph after treatment with segmental fusion and anterior plating. **D,** Follow-up lateral radiograph showing solid fusion and maintenance of established cervical lordosis.

CONCLUSIONS

Postlaminectomy kyphosis is a rare entity. A combination of strict attention to deformity principles, respect for the compromised state of the spinal cord, and an understanding of the presence of 360 degrees of insta-bility created after an anterior release will help the spine surgeon render appropriate surgical care. The potential for neurologic and graft complications is higher than in other types of surgically treated myelopathy, even with strict attention to these principles.

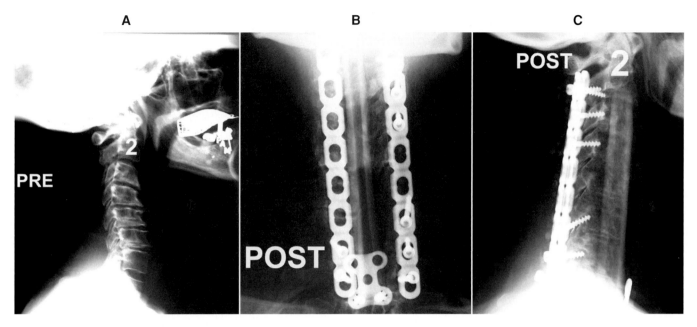

Figure 54-6. Anterior-posterior correction of postlaminectomy kyphosis. **A,** Preoperative radiograph showing residual kyphosis in extension in a patient with severe myelopathy after cervical laminectomy. **B,** Anteroposterior radiograph. **C,** Lateral radiograph after anterior corpectomy, strut grafting, and anterior buttress plating combined with posterior cervical plating.

SELECTED REFERENCES

Albert TJ, Vaccaro AR: Postlaminectomy kyphosis, *Spine* 23:2738-2745, 1998.

Lonstein JE: Postlaminectomy kyphosis, *Clin Orthop Rel Res* 128:93-100, 1977.

Nowinski GP et al.: A biomechanical comparison of cervical laminoplasty and cervical laminectomy with progressive facetectomy, *Spine* 18:1995-2004, 1993.

Panjabi MM, White AA, Johnson RM: Cervical spine biomechanics as a function of transection of components, *J Biomech* 8:327-336, 1975.

White AA et al.: Biomechanical analysis of clinical stability in the cervical spine, *Clin Orthop Rel Res* 109:85-96, 1975.

REFERENCES

1. Abumi K et al.: Correction of cervical kyphosis using pedicle screw fixation systems, *Spine* 24:2389-2395, 1999.
2. Albert TJ, Vaccaro AR: Postlaminectomy kyphosis, *Spine* 23:2738-2745, 1998.
3. Aronson DD, Filtzer DK, Bagan M: Anterior cervical fusion by the Smith-Robinson approach, *J Neurosurg* 29:397-404, 1968.
4. Aronson DD, Kahn RJ, Canady A: Cervical spine instability following suboccipital decompression and cervical laminectomy for Arnold-Chiari syndrome (abstract). Presented at the 56th annual meeting of the American Academy of Orthopaedic Surgeons, Las Vegas, Nev, 1989.
5. Bell DF et al.: Spinal deformity after multiple-level cervical laminectomy in children, *Spine* 4:406-411, 1994.
6. Callahan RA et al.: Cervical facet fusion for the control of instability following laminectomy, *J Bone Joint Surg Am* 59:991-1002, 1977.
7. Cattell HS, Clark GL: Cervical kyphosis and instability following multiple laminectomy in children, *J Bone Joint Surg Am* 49:713-720, 1967.
8. Connolly E, Seymour R, Adams J: Clinical evaluation of anterior cervical fusions for degenerative cervical disc disease, *J Neurosurg* 23:431-437, 1965.
9. Cusick JF et al.: Biomechanics of cervical spine facetectomy and fixation techniques, *Spine* 13:808-882, 1988.
10. Epstein JA: The surgical management of cervical spinal stenosis, spondylosis, and myeloradiculopathy by means of the posterior approach, *Spine* 13:864-869, 1988.
11. Fager CA: Results of adequate posterior decompression in relief of spondylotic cervical myelopathy, *J Neurosurg* 8:684-692, 1973.
12. Fernyhough JC, White JI, Larocca H: Fusion rates in multilevel cervical spondylosis comparing allograft with autograft fibula in 126 patients, *Spine* 16:S561-S564, 1991.
13. Heller JG, Silcox DH III: Postlaminectomy instability of the cervical spine: etiology and stabilization technique. In Frymoyer JW, ed.: *The adult spine: principles and practice,* ed 2, Philadelphia, 1997, Lippincott-Raven, pp. 1413-1434.
14. Heller JG, Silcox DH III, Sutterlin CE: Complications of posterior plating, *Spine* 20(22):2442-2448, 1995.
15. Herkowitz HN: A comparison of anterior cervical fusion, cervical laminectomy, and cervical laminoplasty for the surgical management of multiple level spondylitic radiculopathy, *Spine* 13:774-780, 1988.
16. Herman JM, Sonntag VKH: Cervical corpectomy and plate fixation for postlaminectomy kyphosis, *J Neurosurg* 80:963-970, 1994.
17. Kamioka Y et al.: Postoperative instability of cervical OPLL and cervical radiculopathy, *Spine* 14:1177-1183, 1989.
18. Katsumi Y, Honma T, Nakamura T: Analysis of cervical instability resulting from laminectomy for removal of spinal tumor, *Spine* 14:1172-1176, 1989.
19. Lonstein JE: Postlaminectomy kyphosis, *Clin Orthop Rel Res* 128:93-100, 1977.
20. Mayfield FH: Cervical spondylosis: a comparison of the anterior and posterior approaches, *Clin Neurosurg* 13:181-188, 1965.
21. McAfee PC et al.: One-stage anterior cervical decompression and posterior stabilization: a study of one hundred patients with a minimum of two years follow-up, *J Bone Joint Surg Am* 77:1791-1800, 1995.
22. Mikawa Y, Shikata J, Tammamuro T: Spinal deformity and instability after multilevel cervical laminectomy, *Spine* 12:6-11, 1987.
23. Miyazaki K et al.: Posterior extensive simultaneous multi-segment decompression with posterolateral fusion for cervical instability and kyphotic and/or S-shaped deformities, *Spine* 14:1159-1170, 1989.

24. Morgan TH, Wharton GW, Austin GN: The results of laminectomy in patients with incomplete spinal injuries, *J Bone Joint Surg Am* 52:822 (abstract), 1970.

25. Munechika Y: Influence of laminectomy on the stability of the spine: an experimental study with special reference to the extent of laminectomy and the resection of the intervertebral joint, *J Jpn Orthop Assoc* 47:111-125, 1973.

26. Nowinski GP et al.: A biomechanical comparison of cervical laminoplasty and cervical laminectomy with progressive facetectomy, *Spine* 18:1995-2004, 1993.

27. Pal GP, Sherk HH: The vertical stability of the cervical spine, *Spine* 13:1447-1449, 1988.

28. Panjabi MM et al.: Three dimensional load-displacement curves due to forces on the cervical spine, *J Orthop Res* 4:151-152, 1986.

29. Panjabi MM, White AA, Johnson RM: Cervical spine biomechanics as a function of transection of components, *J Biomech* 8:327-336, 1975.

30. Raynor BB, Pugh J, Shapiro I: Cervical facetectomy and its effect on spine strength, *J Neurosurg* 63:278-282, 1985.

31. Raynor RB et al.: Alterations in primary and coupled neck motions after facetectomy, *Neurosurgery* 21:681-687, 1987.

32. Rogers L: The surgical treatment of cervical spondylitic myelopathy. mobilization of the complete spinal cord into an enlarged canal, *J Bone Joint Surg Br* 43:3-6, 1961.

33. Saito T et al.: Analysis and prevention of spinal column deformity following cervical laminectomy. I. Pathogenesis of postlaminectomy deformities, *Spine* 16:494-502, 1991.

34. Sim FH: Swan neck deformity following extensive cervical laminectomy: a review of twenty-one cases, *J Bone Joint Surg Am* 56:564-580, 1974.

35. White AA et al.: Biomechanical analysis of clinical stability in the cervical spine, *Clin Orthop Rel Res* 109:85-96, 1975.

36. Whitecloud TS III, Butler JC: Postlaminectomy kyphosis of the cervical spine. In Rothman-Simeone HH, *The spine*, ed 4, Philadelphia, 1999, WB Saunders, pp. 1687-1694.

37. Whitecloud TS III, LaRocca H: Fibular strut graft in reconstructive surgery of the cervical spine, *Spine* 1:33-43, 1976.

38. Yasouka S et al.: Pathogenesis and prophylaxis of postlaminectomy deformity of the spine after multiple level laminectomy: difference between children and adults, *Neurosurgery* 9:145-152, 1985.

39. Yasouka S, Peterson HA, MacCarty CS: Incidence of spinal deformity after multilevel laminectomy in children and adults, *J Neurosurg* 57:441-445, 1982.

40. Yonenobu K et al.: Laminoplasty versus subtotal corpectomy: a comparative study of results in multi-segmental cervical spondylitic myelopathy, *Spine* 17:1281-1284, 1992.

41. Zdeblick TA et al.: Cervical stability after sequential capsule resection, *Spine* 18:2005-2008, 1993.

42. Zdeblick TA, Bohlman HH: Myelopathy: cervical kyphosis and treatment by anterior corpectomy and strut grafting, *J Bone Joint Surg Am* 71:170-182, 1989.

43. Zdeblick TA et al.: Cervical stability after foraminotomy: a biomechanical in vitro analysis, *J Bone Joint Surg Am* 74:22-27, 1992.

Management of Postoperative Spinal Infections

Lee H. Riley, III

The incidence of postoperative spine infections varies widely, from less than 1% to 25%. The type of procedure, local conditions at the operative site, and the patient's underlying condition all affect the overall rate. Prolonged hospitalization, additional surgery, and an extended course of antibiotics due to infection have been estimated to add an additional $100,000 to patient care costs. A higher rate of nonunion has also been demonstrated. Because infection is such a potentially devastating complication, every effort should be made to minimize its occurrence. This includes a careful preoperative evaluation, meticulous surgical technique, and careful monitoring in the postoperative period for signs and symptoms suggestive of infection. If an infection does develop, early and aggressive treatment is the key to minimizing the impact on outcome.

RISK FACTORS

Local conditions at the operative site, such as an underlying infection or prior history of infection, prior surgery or radiation, and fibrosis and atrophy of the surrounding soft tissues due to myelodysplasia, have been shown to contribute to an increased rate of infection. Patient conditions that increase the risk of infection include diabetes, malnutrition, immunosuppression, rheumatoid arthritis, obesity, smoking, steroid use, and preoperative hospitalization exceeding 7 days.[28] The magnitude and length of surgery also influence the infection rate.

> ### BASICS OF POSTOPERATIVE SPINE INFECTIONS
>
> - Incidence: 1% to 25%
> - Adds $100,000 to overall costs
> - Compromises outcome
> - Important to recognize and treat aggressively

Diabetes is associated with a higher rate of infection in patients undergoing spine surgery. This is felt to be due in part to microangiopathic changes associated with the disease. Simpson et al.[21] studied 62 patients with diabetes mellitus and lumbar disc disease or spinal stenosis managed with a posterior spinal decompressive procedure. They found a 24% incidence of persistent drainage and delayed wound healing suggestive of a superficial infection that were culture negative. There were six culture-positive wound infections, for an incidence of 10%. Five patients grew *Staphylococcus aureus* and one *Escherichia coli*. One patient with a staphylococcal infection died of an associated myocardial infarction. In an age- and sex-matched control group undergoing similar procedures there were no wound complications or infections.[21]

Malnutrition and a subsequent loss of immunocompetence are associated with a higher incidence of postoperative complications. A total lymphocyte count of less than 2000 and an albumin of less than 3.5 g/100 ml[23] were found in a retrospective study of patients with postoperative spinal infections to increase the risk of infection in patients undergoing spinal surgery. Mandelbaum et al.[13] studied 37 patients undergoing staged anterior and posterior spinal reconstructive procedures and found that 31 (84%) became malnourished during hospitalization. In the malnourished group there were 15 patients with urinary tract infections, 4 with bacterial sepsis, 4 with pneumonia, and 4 with postoperative wound infections. The postoperative stay following the second operation was nearly 4 days longer in the malnourished group.[13] In a prospective, randomized study of patients undergoing staged anterior-posterior spinal reconstructive procedures, comparing the benefits of receiving total parenteral nutrition (TPN) or no TPN, there was a significant decrease in the albumin and prealbumin depletion of patients who did receive TPN compared with those who did not. Patients who were nutritionally depleted were more likely to develop complications such as pneumonia and urinary tract infections. The study did not demonstrate statistically

<table>
<tr><td colspan="2">

RISK FACTORS

HOST
- Diabetes
- Malnutrition
- Immunosuppression
- Steroid use
- Obesity
- Smoking

LOCAL
- Prior surgery
- Infection
- Local tissue damage

SURGICAL
- Instrumentation
- Extent of dissection
- Operative time
- Posterior approach
</td></tr>
</table>

CAUSATIVE ORGANISMS

- Most common: *Staphylococcus* species
- Gram-negative organisms
- Multiple organisms
- Anaerobic organisms

significant differences in the incidence of postoperative wound complications, but this was thought to be due to the small study size.[8]

The type of procedure performed also influences the risk of infection. Anterior procedures have a much lower risk of infection than posterior procedures. In one review of 276 anterior spinal procedures there were no documented infections. The rate of infection for posterior procedures in the same study was 3.8%.[28] Posterior procedures requiring minimal soft tissue dissection and limited exposure, such as lumbar discectomy, have an infection rate of less than 1%.[7] Posterior spinal fusions without instrumentation have an infection rate of 2%. Spinal fusion with instrumentation increases the rate of infection of 4% to 6%.[11,28] Higher rates have been reported in instrumented fusions involving multiple segments.[28] This was felt to be due to both the increased size of the surgical exposure and to the increased operative time. Blood loss of greater than 1000 ml and operative time greater than 3 hours have also been found to increase the risk of infection.[28]

CAUSATIVE ORGANISMS

Staphylococcus species remain the most common organism found in postoperative infections, occurring in over half of reported cases in several series.[7,11,28] Gram-negative organisms such as *E. coli*, *Pseudomonas aeruginosa*, and *Salmonella*, *Haemophilus*, *Klebsiella*, *Proteus*, and *Acinetobacter* species are also found. Infections from these opportunistic organisms commonly cultured from the feces, mouth, and skin of healthy individuals can occur either as a result of direct contamination at the time of surgery or as a result of septicemia from a variety of sources, but most commonly from a urinary tract infection existing at the time of surgery or developing in the postoperative period. Infections with multiple organisms and anaerobic organisms can also occur and can lead to a more complicated treatment regimen, including multiple debridements, prolonged antibiotic therapy, and a poorer ultimate outcome.[24]

MINIMIZING INFECTION RISK

Every effort should be made to minimize the risk of wound inoculation at the time of surgery. A preoperative

evaluation to identify preexisting infection either at the operative site or distant locations should be performed. A history and physical examination should include auscultation of the lungs, inspection of the operative site for signs of local infection, and complete blood count (CBC), electrolytes, and urinalysis. An erythrocyte sedimentation rate needs to be ordered when there is sufficient suspicion of a preexisting infection. Preoperative admission should be avoided or minimized because this increases the rate of postoperative infection.[14,15] In one large study of over 23,000 surgical patients, the risk of infection doubled with each week of hospitalization prior to surgery.[4]

The selection of the appropriate prophylactic antibiotic should take into account the nature of the surgical procedure, the condition of the patient (allergies, immunocompetence, and preexisting medical conditions) and the pharmocologic characteristics of the antibiotic.[12] Prophylactic intravenous (IV) antibiotics should be administered prior to skin incision. A first- or second-generation cephalosporin provides good coverage of gram-positive organisms. Cefazolin, a first-generation cephalosporin, has been found to have good penetration of muscle, bone, and hematoma. Polly et al.[16] found that tissue levels well above the minimum inhibitory concentration were maintained in spinal surgery cases with blood loss up to 1200 ml. They recommended redosing no sooner than every 6 hours based on their study. Antibiotics need to be present in sufficient levels at the start of surgery and maintained throughout surgery and into the postoperative period. The appropriate duration of postoperative antibiotics remains controversial, with recommendations ranging from 24 hours to continuing antibiotics until drain removal. Fitzgerald and Thompson[5] showed no benefit of continuing antibiotics beyond 24 to 48 hours. Aminoglycosides may be added in cases involving spinal instrumentation and for patients with sickle cell anemia, immunocompromised patients, patients with IV drug use, and patients who have been hospitalized for a long period of time in order to widen aerobic gram-negative coverage.[12]

Sterile technique must always be maintained, and all recognized breaks in sterility should be addressed immediately. Operative room traffic and personnel should be kept at a minimum. In a review of postoperative infections following instrumented fusion for scoliosis, Lonstein et al.[11] speculated that the rate of infection was related to the number of personnel and observers present during surgery. Ritter et al.[19] have demonstrated that an average of 13 colony-forming units (CFUs)/ft²/hr were present in an empty operating room. This increased to 447 CFU/ft²/hr when five people were present in the room. Greater movement within and traffic through

---

MINIMIZING RISK

- Identify preexisting infections
- Minimize preoperative hospitalization
- Administer prophylactic antibiotics
- Maintain sterility
- Irrigate, débride, and drain

EVALUATION

- Signs and symptoms unreliable
- Deviation from expected course of recovery
- C-reative protein
  ○ Peak: Day 2 to 3
  ○ Normalize: Day 5 to 14
- Erythrocyte sedimentation rate (ESR)
  ○ Peak: Day 4 to 5
  ○ Normalize: Day 21 to 42
- Cultures mandatory before antibiotics

---

the room were also found to significantly increase the potential inoculum within the surgical environment.[18] Operative time should also be minimized to reduce the risk and volume of wound inoculation. People routinely shed bacteria. Although most individuals shed fewer than 1000 bacteria per minute, a subset of individuals routinely shed substantially more bacteria.[2] Operative technique that minimizes soft tissue trauma should be employed. Retractors should be periodically released to minimize soft tissue necrosis and the wound irrigated to reduce the overall bacterial contamination load within the wound. Before closure, devitalized soft tissue should be débrided, hemostasis obtained, and layered closure over drains performed to minimize dead space and hematoma formation.

SIGNS AND SYMPTOMS

The clinical symptoms of a postoperative infection are muscle spasm, back pain, and lethargy. Because these symptoms are common after uncomplicated spinal surgery, distinguishing between routine postoperative complaints and symptoms suggestive of infection is difficult in the early postoperative period. However, routine postoperative symptoms generally resolve with a predictable pattern after surgery. This pattern is not followed in patients with infection, who have pain and spasm that continue longer than expected. Anxiety is also a common distinguishing feature that is often unrecognized but frequently associated with postoperative infection. This was highlighted by Thibodeau,[26] who reported 14% of patients with discitis following discectomy had been referred for psychiatric evaluation before the correct diagnosis was established.

Because deviation from a predictable pattern of recovery is one of the hallmarks of postoperative infection, the time to diagnosis after surgery is related to the magnitude of the surgery performed. Following lumbar discectomy, the diagnosis can often be made within 1 week of surgery.[17,22] Following spinal fusion with instrumentation, the diagnosis is made on average from 2 to 4 weeks postoperatively.[10,23] These differences appear to reflect the different pace of recovery from discectomy versus spinal fusion surgery and the masking of symptoms of infection after major spinal surgery due to routine postoperative pain. Fever is not a reliable indicator of infection and is present in 30% to 80% of cases.[17] This is also true of local signs of infection such as erythema, warmth, swelling, or neurologic deficit, which are not predictably present. However, erythrocyte sedimentation rate and C-reactive protein follow a predictable pattern after spinal surgery and are useful tests to detect postoperative infections and to monitor recovery after treatment.[9,25] The erythrocyte sedimentation rate peaks at postoperative day 4 to 5. With a discectomy the average value is 75, and with lumbar fusion it is 102.[9] There is a downward trend with normalization at 21 to 42 days. Although an elevated sedimentation rate is a sensitive test for infection, the value can be normal in the presence of infection when patients are on chronic steroids.[17] C-reactive protein generally peaks at postoperative day 2 or 3 and normalizes within 5 to 14 days.[25] Because the C-reactive protein value reaches its peak earlier and declines more rapidly than the erythrocyte sedimentation rate, it can be more useful in the early detection of an infection and in demonstrating response to treatment. Although routinely ordered as part of the initial evaluation, a white blood cell count is not a reliable indicator of infection. Rawlings et al. found no elevation of the white blood cell count in 8 of 27 patients with postoperative infection.[17] Jonsson et al. could not demonstrate any characteristic trend in the total white cell count in the postoperative period.[9]

Once infection is suspected, an aggressive work-up must ensue. Deep cultures need to be obtained in order to both establish a diagnosis and guide treatment. At the very least, deep percutaneous aspiration below the fascia in the operative site must be obtained. In instances where the need for open irrigation and débridement is apparent, culture and Gram stain can be performed in the operating room at the time of surgery prior to the administration of antibiotics. Aerobic, anaerobic, fungal, and acid-fast bacillus (AFB) cultures and a Gram stain need to be obtained.

TREATMENT

A variety of treatment protocols have been demonstrated to be effective in the treatment of postoperative infections. No single treatment protocol is useful in all cases. Treatment needs to be tailored to the individual patient in all cases and depends on the underlying medical condition of the patient, type of infection, response to initial treatment, and degree of soft tissue necrosis and débridement necessary to control the infection locally. Adequate débridement of the infected and nonviable tissues may create a large dead space not amenable to primary closure. Organisms that do not respond to aggressive antibiotic treatment may require multiple irrigations and débridement, as well as delayed healing by secondary intention or delayed closure with muscle-flap coverage.

A classification scheme for postoperative infections with instrumentation was developed by Thalgott et al. to help guide treatment.[24] This was based on the clinical staging system proposed by Cierny et al.[3] for adult osteomyelitis. Treatment guidelines were based on the severity of infection, which was divided into three groups. Group 1 is a superficial or deep single-organism infection. Thalgott et al.[24] reported good results with

single irrigation and debridement followed by closure over suction drainage tubes. Group 2 is a multiple-organism, deep infection. This group required an average of three irrigations and debridements. There were also a higher number of successful closures with closed inflow-outflow suction irrigation systems (Figure 55-1) compared with simple suction drainage. This group used 1 L of normal saline solution with 500 mg of vancomycin and 1000 units of heparin at a rate of 125 ml/hr for 3 to 4 days with conversion to a pure suction system and drain removal on day 6. Group 3 patients had multiple organisms with myonecrosis. This group required six surgeries and flap closure. These patients were routinely given hyperalimentation.

Rawlings et al. demonstrated that postoperative disc space infections can be treated with immobilization and IV antibiotics followed by oral antibiotics. They found that there was a 93% relief of pain, and a 70% spontaneous fusion rate in patients treated in this manner. This study also recommended percutaneous Craig needle biopsy for culture before initiation of antibiotics to determine the appropriate antibiotic regimen. Discectomy and anterior fusion were necessary in cases that failed antibiotic treatment.[17] Levi et al.[10] treated postoperative infections following instrumented fusions with irrigation and debridement of all necrotic tissue of the wound in the operating room and layered closure of the incision over inflow-outflow drains with a 1- to 6-week course of IV antibiotics followed by a course of oral antibiotics. Nafcillin (1 g/L normal saline) or vancomycin (500 mg/L normal saline) was infused at a rate of 25 to 50 ml/hr for 5 to 7 days followed by discontinuation of the inflow system for 1 day before removal of drains. Instrumentation was maintained in all cases, and one patient required a muscle-flap coverage.[10]

TREATMENT

- Individualize to patient
- Evaluate factors
  - Organism type
  - Host response to treatment
- Irrigate and débride, close over drains
- Irrigate and débride, use inflow-outflow system
- For muscle-flap coverage
  - Trapezius: Upper thoracic and cervical
  - Latissimus dorsi: Midthoracic and thoracolumbar
  - Gluteus maximus: Lower lumbar and sacral
  - Combination: Large defects, overlap zones
- Use antibiotics based on culture results
- Monitor nutritional status
- Offer nutritional supplementation
  - Oral
  - Feeding tube
  - Total parenteral nutrition (TPN)
- Monitor erythrocyte sedimentation rate (ESR), complete blood count (CBC)

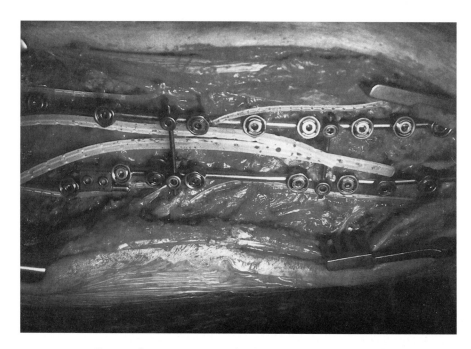

Figure 55-1.   Inflow-outflow system using ⅛-inch drain for inflow and ¼-inch drain for outflow.

Muscle flaps play an important role in the treatment of postoperative infections (Figure 55-2). They provide coverage of exposed hardware and other vital structures, fill dead spaces created by wound débridement, and provide fresh blood supply to the area through the vascularity of the muscle.[20] This allows delivery of oxygen, antibiotics, and other factors directly to the wound, promoting eradication of the infection and wound healing. The specific muscle used will depend upon the location of the wound needing coverage. The trapezius myocutaneous flap is useful in covering wounds in the upper thoracic and cervical region. The latissimus dorsi muscle can be used as a muscle or myocutaneous flap in the midthoracic and thoracolumbar regions. The gluteus maximus muscle can be used as a muscle or myocutaneous flap in the lower lumbar or sacral region.

Combination flaps may be necessary to cover large wounds that spread across the margins of different flap coverage areas. Frank reported use of local latissimus dorsi–gluteus maximus rotational flap coverage of deep lumbar spine infections.[6] Indications for the procedure were postoperative infections of the thoracic or lumbar spine with soft tissue loss or soft tissue retraction that prevented wound closure. Contraindications to the procedure were anaerobic infections with extensive, ongoing tissue necrosis; mixed aerobic and anaerobic infections; and infections unresponsive to serial débridements and culture-specific antibiotic treatment.

Broad-spectrum antibiotics, including an aminoglycoside and penicillinase-resistant antibiotic, should be started only after obtaining deep cultures. The culture results and response of the patient to treatment will determine the definitive antibiotic. Response should be documented with declining serial erythrocyte sedimentation rate and white count. C-reactive protein is useful in the early stages to demonstrate a therapeutic response. Four to six weeks of antibiotic treatment with longer courses of IV and oral antibiotic coverage may be

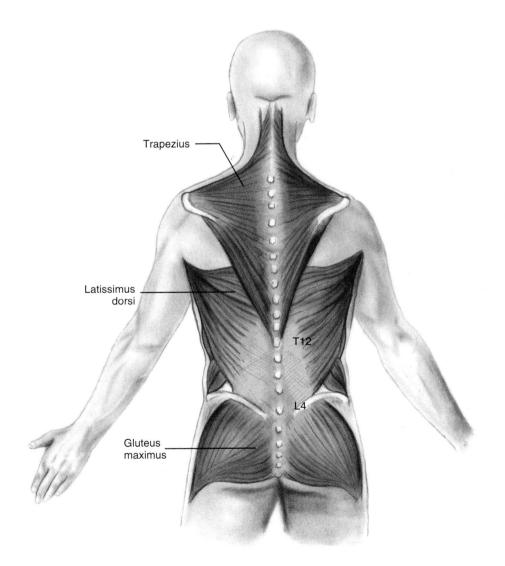

Figure 55-2. Muscles commonly used for local flap coverage of posterior spinal infections. *(Redrawn from Rubayi S: Wound management in spinal infection,* Orthop Clin North Am *27[1]:137-153, 1996.)*

necessary to eradicate the infection or suppress the infection long enough to obtain a solid fusion.[1] Every effort should be made to maintain spinal hardware until solid fusion has been obtained. Late hardware removal followed by a 4- to 6-week course of antibiotic treatment may be necessary in some cases of persistent infection.[1]

Nutritional assessment and supplementation is critical in the successful management of a postoperative infection.[20] Nutritional requirements increase above baseline in the face of infection, and it is important to maintain a positive nitrogen balance during the healing period. Requirements of 2 g of protein per kilogram of body weight per day and 3000 to 3500 calories per day are not unusual. Nutritional supplementation using health shakes, feeding tubes, or hyperalimentation need to be considered if these requirements cannot be met by diet alone. Serum albumin needs to be monitored and maintained in the normal range.

Even when postoperative infections are recognized and treated, the final outcome is adversely affected. Weiss et al. retrospectively reviewed 29 patients with postoperative infections following fusion surgery.[27] Eighteen of 29 patients (62.1%) had successful fusion. Patients fused to the sacrum had an overall fusion rate of 36%, whereas 87% of fusions not involving the sacrum led to solid arthrodesis. The rate for allograft fusions was 17.2% compared with 83.3% for autogenous grafting. Interestingly, female patients also had a lower incidence of union (33.3% versus 82.4%).

CONCLUSIONS

Postoperative infection following spinal surgery is often difficult to diagnose in its early stages. Back pain, spasm, malaise, the appearance of the wound, fever, and elevated white blood cell count are all unreliable indicators of infection. However, an infection should be suspected when there is any deviation from the anticipated clinical course. Once an infection is suspected, an aggressive work-up that includes a sedimentation rate, C-reactive protein, and deep culture of the wound should be performed. Early recognition and aggressive management of the infection are the key to obtaining the best outcome following postoperative infection. Cultures and sensitivities need to be obtained to guide antibiotic therapy. Aggressive irrigation and débridement of the wound needs to be performed to halt progression of the infection. The success of treatment needs to be monitored with serial laboratory testing, including sedimentation rate, to determine if the treatment plan is working to eradicate the infection. Instrumentation removal may be necessary to control or eradicate the infection, but every effort should be made to maintain instrumentation until a solid fusion has been obtained. Treatment needs to be tailored to the individual patient and is affected by the condition of the surgical wound, the patient's medical condition, infection type, and response to therapy.

SELECTED REFERENCES

Abbey DM: Treatment of postoperative wound infections following spinal fusion with instrumentation, *J Spinal Disord* 8(4):278-283, 1995.

Cruse PJE, Foord RA: A five-year prospective study of 23,649 surgical wounds, *Arch Surg* 107:206-209, 1973.

Rubayi S: Wound management in spinal infection, *Orthop Clin North Am* 27(1):137-153, 1996.

Thalgott JS et al.: Postoperative infections in spinal implants: classification and analysis—a multicenter study, *Spine* 16(8):981-984, 1991.

Wimmer C et al.: Predisposing factors for infection in spine surgery: a survey of 850 spinal procedures, *J Spinal Disord* 11(2):124-128, 1998.

REFERENCES

1. Abbey DM et al.: Treatment of postoperative wound infections following spinal fusion with instrumentation, *J Spinal Disord* 8(4):278-283, 1995.
2. Bethune DA et al.: Dispersal of *Staphylococcus aureus* by patients and surgical staff, *Lancet* 1:480-483, 1965.
3. Cierny G, Mader JT, Penninck JJ: A clinical staging system for adult osteomyelitis, *Contemp Orthop* 10:17-37, 1985.
4. Cruse PJE, Foord RA: A five-year prospective study of 23,649 surgical wounds, *Arch Surg* 107:206-209, 1973.
5. Fitzgerald RH, Thompson RL: Cephalosporin antibiotics in the prevention and treatment of musculoskeletal sepsis, *J Bone Joint Surg Am* 65:1201-1205, 1983.
6. Frank CJ, Brantigan J, Cronan J: Bilateral interconnected latissimus dorsi–gluteus maximus musculocutaneous flaps for closure of subfascial infections of the lumbar spine: a technical note, *Spine* 22:564-567, 1997.
7. Horwitz NH, Curtin JA: Prophylactic antibiotics and wound infections following laminectomy: a retrospective study, *J Neurosurg* 43:727-731, 1973.
8. Hu SS et al.: Nutritional depletion in staged spinal reconstructive surgery: the effect of total parenteral nutrition, *Spine* 23(12):1401-1405, 1998.
9. Jonsson B, Soderholm R, Stromqvist B: Erythrocyte sedimentation rate after lumbar spine surgery, *Spine* 16:1049-1050, 1991.
10. Levy ADO, Dickman CA, Sonntag VKH: Management of postoperative infections after spinal instrumentation, *J Neurosurg* 86:975-980, 1997.
11. Lonstein J et al.: Wound infection with Harrington instrumentation and spine fusion for scoliosis, *Clin Orthop* 96:222-233, 1973.
12. Mader JT, Cierny G III: The principles of the use of preventive antibiotics, *Clin Orthop* 190:75-82, 1984.
13. Mandelbaum BR et al.: Nutritional deficiencies after staged anterior and posterior spinal reconstructive surgery, *Clin Orthop* 234:5-11, 1988.
14. Nichols RL: Techniques known to prevent postoperative wound infection, *Infect Control* 3:34-37, 1982.
15. Polk HC Jr et al.: Guidelines for prevention of surgical wound infection, *Arch Surg* 118:1213-1217, 1983.
16. Polly DW et al.: The effect of intraoperative blood loss on serum cefazolin level in patients undergoing instrumented spinal fusion: a prospective, controlled study, *Spine* 21(20):2363-2367, 1996.
17. Rawlings CE et al.: Postoperative intervertebral disc space infection, *Neurosurgery* 13(4):371-375, 1983.
18. Ritter MA: Surgical wound environment, *Clin Orthop* 190:11-13, 1984.

SUMMARY

- Difficult to diagnose and treat
- Maintain high index of suspicion
- Treat aggressively
- Tailor treatment to individual patient
  - Nature of infection
  - Response to treatment
- Affects outcome

19. Ritter MA, French ML, Hart JB: Microbiologic studies in a horizontal wall-less laminar air-flow operating room during actual surgery, *Clin Orthop* 97:16, 1973.

20. Rubayi S: Wound management in spinal infection, *Orthop Clin North Am* 27(1):137-153, 1996.

21. Simpson JM et al.: The results of operations on the lumbar spine in patients who have diabetes mellitus, *J Bone Joint Surg Am* 75:1823-1829, 1993.

22. Spiegelmann R et al.: Postoperative spinal epidural empyema: clinical and computed tomography features, *Spine* 16(10):1146-1149, 1991.

23. Stambough JL, Berringer D: Postoperative wound infection complicating adult spine surgery, *J Spinal Disord* 5:277-285, 1992.

24. Thalgott JS et al.: Postoperative infections in spinal implants: classification and analysis—a multicenter study, *Spine* 16(8):981-984, 1991.

25. Thelander U, Larsson S: Quantitation of C-reactive protein levels and erythrocyte sedimentation rate after spine surgery, *Spine* 17:400-404, 1992.

26. Thibodeau AA: Closed space infection following removal of lumbar intervertebral discs, *J Bone Joint Surg Am* 50:400-410, 1968.

27. Weis LE et al.: Pseudarthrosis after postoperative wound infection in the lumbar spine, *J Spinal Disord* 10(6):482-487, 1997.

28. Wimmer C et al.: Predisposing factors for infection in spine surgery: a survey of 850 spinal procedures, *J Spinal Disord* 11(2):124-128, 1998.

Failed Back Surgery Syndrome

Seth M. Zeidman

Failed back surgery syndrome (FBSS), or the "failed back syndrome," is a clinical condition in which patients who undergo one or more surgical procedures for lumbosacral disease obtain unsatisfactory long-term relief of symptoms, with persistent or recurrent low back pain.[1-3]

FBSS is characterized by a constellation of pain, psychologic disturbances, and incapacitation from low back and/or leg pain secondary to lumbar spinal disease. The major causes of FBSS include inappropriate patient selection, diagnosis, poor operative technique, iatrogenic instability, and surgical complications. FBSS most often occurs in those patients inappropriately selected for surgery who are then left with residual pain and neurologic deficits. Most FBSS patients have undergone multiple surgical procedures in attempts to relieve intractable and incapacitating sciatica and/or low back pain. Appropriate therapeutic decision making in FBSS patients depends on two factors: (1) establishment of an accurate diagnosis that considers underlying medical problems and related comorbidities and (2) a rational, individualized therapeutic regimen that addresses the diagnosed abnormalities.

Prevention of FBSS is more important and helpful than any available treatment. It requires an understanding of the natural history of spinal traumatic and degenerative disease as well as the complications from psychologic, social, and economic factors. In this chapter, we will define FBSS, detail the causes of failure in patients who have had lumbosacral spine surgery, and outline the clinical presentations of FBSS patients. We will also delineate the therapeutic regimens available when specific failures have occurred, and provide an algorithm for the evaluation and treatment of this complex clinical entity (Box 56-1).

HISTORY AND EPIDEMIOLOGY

Mixter and Barr first recognized lumbar disc herniation as a distinct surgical entity in 1934. Operations to correct disc herniation rapidly gained acceptance, and by the early 1950s, reports of the first series of reoperations on the lumbar spine were published.[29] Each year

| Box 56-1 | Algorithm for the Treatment of Failed Back Surgery Syndrome |

Diagnosis—history and physical examination
  History
    Number of previous back operations
    Length of pain-free interval(s)
    Distribution of pain
    Exacerbating/relieving factors
  Physical examination
    Neurologic examination
    Tension signs
    Functional signs
    Thorough general medical examination and review of systems
  Determine if pain has nonspinal cause—diabetes, abdominal aortic aneurysm, pancreatitis
    Psychiatric evaluation (if any hint of psychosocial abnormality)
    Radiographic evaluation
  Plain radiographs
  Flexion-extension films
  CT myelogram
  MRI with gadolinium
Therapeutic intervention
  Nonsurgical
    Rehabilitation
    Detoxification as needed
    Multidisciplinary pain treatment center
  Surgery
    Reoperation (minority)
    Ablative procedures other than facet denervations are not helpful
    Spinal cord stimulation (particularly for radicular pain)

more than 250,000 patients undergo lumbosacral operative procedures.[24,63] The response of 207 patients to a questionnaire indicates that success rates from lumbosacral surgery depend on the design of the questionnaire, with satisfactory results ranging from 97% to 60%.[31] Burton et al.[15] report that conservative treatment including complete bed rest with analgesics or gravity traction is frequently inadequate in patients with low

763

back pain. Failure to identify and treat patients with lateral spinal stenosis could increase the high incidence of FBSS.[15] Statistically, 10% of patients who undergo lumbar disc surgery are permanently disabled and unable to work, and 25% never return to their original occupation.

ETIOLOGY AND PATHOGENESIS

Multiple factors that contribute to the failure of lumbar surgery to relieve symptoms and effect a favorable outcome from surgery include incorrect preoperative diagnosis, improper patient selection, inadequate surgical decompression, complications from the procedure, and psychosocial factors. Biologic and iatrogenic factors also contribute to FBSS. Spinal stenosis, recurrent disc herniation, fusion overgrowth, development of mechanical pain, pseudarthrosis, and neuropathic pain all may follow lumbar spine surgery. Neuropathic pain may result from nerve root injury, pseudomeningocele formation, adhesive arachnoiditis, epidural fibrosis, and reaction to a retained foreign body. Patient populations and author biases are often poorly defined, which increases the problem of identifying FBSS.

Complaints of pain are subjective phenomena, and clinicians can only observe pain-related behavior. Pain does not necessarily denote active tissue damage or injury, and chronic pain behaviors rarely correlate with active tissue irritation or damage. In general, FBSS patients are not malingerers. Many of the factors that contribute to the chronicity and incapacity are on a subconscious level, and failure is likely when inadequate preoperative assessment is combined with incomplete comprehension of the impact of psychosocial problems on outcome.

Most clinicians gain insight into a patient's psychologic status during the history and physical examination. Personality dysfunction is the most common psychologic problem complicating FBSS. Over 50% of patients referred to the Johns Hopkins chronic pain treatment center suffer from substantial personality dysfunction.[43] Questions relating to interactions with family and friends, marital history, military and vocational history, problems with the law, and substance abuse, including misuse of narcotics and psychotropics, often provide relevant information.

The role of psychologic factors in FBSS is difficult to assess, but these factors, which include unresolved compensation issues, should be considered in patient selection. Many patients who present with intractable back pain are incapacitated by personality and psychosocial factors. The degree of incapacitation should reflect demonstrated pathology and the degree of physical impairment. Patients should be carefully observed for signs of exaggerated pain and disability during the history and physical examination. Skilled clinicians learn to recognize these behaviors, which other patients do not display and which are always related to psychosocial dysfunction. Several studies indicated that patients diagnosed with psychologic problems have poor outcomes for reoperation.[14,26] Psychologic testing

> ## CHARACTERISTICS AND CAUSES OF FAILED BACK SURGERY SYNDROME
>
> - Characteristics of failed back surgery syndrome (FBSS)
>   - Persistent or recurrent pain
>   - Psychologic disturbances
>   - Incapacitation from low back and/or leg pain
> - Causes
>   - Inappropriate patient selection
>   - Incorrect preoperative diagnosis
>   - Poor operative technique
>   - Iatrogenic instability
>   - Surgical complications
>   - Psychosocial factors
> - 10% of patients who undergo lumbar disc surgery are permanently disabled and unable to work; 25% never return to their original occupation
> - Role of psychosocial factors difficult to assess but should be considered in patient selection
>   - FBSS patients are not generally malingerers
>   - Personality dysfunction commonly complicates FBSS
>   - Do not deny patients with drug habituation necessary therapy, but encourage them to seek assistance with substance abuse before performing direct intervention

may be affected by organic disease, reflecting the underlying diagnosis. Standardized psychologic testing explains only a portion of the variance in treatment outcome and should be used as one of several patient-selection criteria.

Before selection for any procedure, FBSS patients with drug habituation problems should undergo a behavioral program with an emphasis on detoxification. Patients with substance "addiction" should not be denied necessary therapy because of psychosocial symptomatology; however, they should be encouraged to seek assistance with their substance abuse before direct intervention is initiated.[43]

CLINICAL FINDINGS AND CRITERIA
Criteria of the American Association of Neurological Surgeons and the American Academy of Orthopedic Surgeons

The American Association of Neurological Surgeons and the American Academy of Orthopedic Surgeons developed criteria for the selection of patients for lumbosacral spine surgery that include (1) failure of extended conservative therapy; (2) abnormal myelograms, computed tomography (CT) scan, and/or magnetic resonance imaging (MRI) study that demonstrates nerve root compression and/or segmental instability consistent with the patient's symptoms and signs; (3) conformity of radicular pain complaints to physiologic, dermatomal, or sclerotomal patterns; and (4) one or more of the following: sensory loss, motor loss, and deep tendon reflex abnormalities in corresponding segment(s). These criteria apply to both reoperation and

AMERICAN ASSOCIATION OF NEUROLOGICAL SURGEONS AND AMERICAN ACADEMY OF ORTHOPEDIC SURGERY CRITERIA FOR THE SELECTION OF PATIENTS FOR LUMBOSACRAL SPINE SURGERY

- Failure of extended conservative therapy
- Abnormal myelogram, CT scan, and/or MRI study that demonstrates nerve root compression and/or segmental instability consistent with the patient's symptoms and signs
- Conformity of radicular pain complaints to physiologic, dermatomal, or sclerotomal patterns
- One or more of the following:
  - Sensory loss
  - Motor loss
  - Deep tendon reflex abnormalities in corresponding segments

EXTRASPINAL CAUSES OF PAIN
- Abdominal aortic aneurysm
- Gynecologic disease
- Prostate tumor
- Renal disease
- Rectosigmoid disease

primary procedures. Analyses of the initial preoperative imaging studies of patients with FBSS commonly fail to meet standard criteria for surgical intervention.[15,56] The probability of a successful outcome is small in these circumstances even if criteria for reoperation are met.

PATIENT HISTORY AND PHYSICAL EXAMINATION

Clinical evaluation of FBSS patients does not differ substantially from that of other patients who suffer from intractable and incapacitating low back pain. It is important to obtain the complete details of the patient's original presentation, previous examinations, prior neurodiagnostic imaging studies, and reports of interventional therapy. These data should be reviewed before the patient's initial visit because these provide technical details of which the patient may be unaware as well as an overview of prior interactions with the health care system. They also make the initial appointment more directed and revealing. Pain behavior, postural abnormalities, impairment of range of motion, and elements of neurologic deficit are often evident even before formal examination begins.

A general medical history and physical examination can rule out extraspinal causes of pain that include abdominal aortic aneurysm, gynecologic disease, prostate tumor, renal disease, or rectosigmoid disease. Entities such as meralgia paresthetica, acetabular pain, and sacroiliac joint pain should form part of a working differential diagnosis. Patients should be examined for evidence for local myositis, fasciitis, or bursitis, and also indications of arthritic or autoimmune disease. The possibility of undiagnosed disease, including Paget's

disease, metastatic neoplasia, and rheumatoid/acromegalic spondylitis, should also be considered.

The combination of history and physical examination often provides a reasonable idea of both instability and nerve root compression. Straight leg raising can be useful to identify root compression. The interpretation of neurologic findings may be difficult because of residual deficits from prior surgery. Long-term follow-up studies have shown that 40% to 50% of patients with prior successful disc excision have residual alterations in deep tendon reflexes and sensation corresponding to the original level of root involvement.[25,53] Fixed neurologic deficits suggest root injury but may result from ongoing compression, although nerve root tension signs rarely persist after surgery and are very useful when positive.[27] It is unlikely that surgical intervention will be useful in the absence of symptoms suggesting nerve root compression or instability.[80] One goal of examination is to determine physical impairment as well as exaggeration of impairment. Waddell et al.[79] proposed the use of clinical tests that provide a simple means of identifying patients who have inappropriate pain responses.

DIAGNOSIS

The physician must distinguish between the patient with a mechanical lesion such as recurrent disc herniation, spinal instability, or spinal stenosis, and one with nonmechanical conditions including intradural scar tissue and systemic medical disease. Surgery benefits patients with mechanical lesions, but surgical intervention rarely helps patients with nonmechanical lesions.

The clinical history is critical to assessing the probable reasons for the patient's symptoms, particularly when radiculopathy is predominant because surgical candidates have a history of radicular pain. The pain from instability is worsened by sitting, standing, and normal activity, and bracing often lessens the pain. Neurogenic claudication, which is characterized by increasing lower extremity pain from walking even short distances, continues for a brief period upon cessation of the activity. The pain is reduced by bending forward to expand the spinal canal.

The probability of a favorable outcome diminishes with each procedure, regardless of diagnosis. Finnegan et al.[21] emphasized the importance of the postoperative pain-free interval and identified three typical syndromes: (1) no initial relief or symptoms immediately worse; (2) initial relief followed by increased numbness or weakness; and (3) patient receives complete relief but develops recurrent radiculopathy months or years later. Persistent radicular pain in the immediate postoperative period suggests inadequate nerve root decompression, irreversible nerve root injury, or improper patient selection.[32] If the pain-free interval is between 1 and 6 months and the recurrent symptoms occur gradually, scar tissue may be responsible. Recurrent pain 6 months postoperatively may result from disc herniation at the same or a different level. Frymoyer et al.[25] stressed the importance of long-term failures, which are usually the manifestation of an ongoing degenerative process. Predominant

PAIN IN FAILED BACK SURGERY SYNDROME

- Persistent radicular pain in immediate postoperative period suggests the following:
  - Inadequate nerve root decompression
  - Irreversible nerve root injury
  - Improper patient selected
- Suspect scar tissue if pain-free interval between 1 and 6 months and recurrent symptoms develop gradually
- Recurrent pain 6 months postoperatively: Possible disc herniation of same or different level

leg pain suggests disc herniation or spinal stenosis, although scar tissue can also produce this. Instability, infection, and scar tissue are all possible causes if back pain is the major component.

Physical examination should include attention to functional findings, which may have alternative explanations. Some apparently nonphysiologic findings can result from arachnoid fibrosis, including nondermatomal sensory loss and nerve injury producing superficial lumbosacral spine tenderness with hyperalgesia; such syndromes often predict a poor response to therapy on a physiologic rather than a behavioral basis, suggesting the need for alternative treatments. New neurologic deficits occurring after the last surgery or positive tension signs as on straight-leg raising may indicate pressure on the neural elements though these deficits are not pathognomonic.

IMAGING AND DIAGNOSTIC STUDIES

Precise correlation of clinical findings with diagnostic imaging studies is necessary because of the high incidence of clinically false-positive myelograms, discograms, CT scans, and MRI scans in asymptomatic individuals or at asymptomatic levels.* Studies of asymptomatic postoperative patients often reveal significant abnormalities. Frymoyer et al.[27] reported that 40% of CT scans, myelograms, and discograms show abnormalities in asymptomatic individuals. The combination of clinical history, physical examination, and radiologic imaging studies should provide an excellent correlation between anatomic abnormalities and the patient's complaints. Nonspecific spondylotic changes do not necessarily correlate with pain, and these changes do not always indicate the need for surgery. Anatomic abnormalities must be consistent with the patient's complaints and disabilities, and their relative importance must be assessed. The specificity of diagnostic imaging in FBSS is not yet established; in patients diagnosed with the latest imaging techniques, long-term clinical correlations with radiographic findings are unavailable.

Modern diagnostic imaging techniques have improved the definition of both primary and postsurgical lumbosacral spine disease. Radiologic evaluation is particularly

*References 9-12, 30, 72, 75, 76, 81, 82.

IMAGING

- Precise correlation of clinical findings with diagnostic imaging studies needed because of high incidence of clinically false-positive myelograms, discograms, CT scans, and MRI scans in asymptomatic levels
- Imaging studies confirm possible cause deduced from history and physical examination rather than providing dominant basis for diagnosis
- Plain radiographs: Initial study
  - Determine extent and level of previous surgery
  - Obtain lateral flexion-extension radiographs
    - Abnormal motion and instability
    - Primary bone tumors
  - Note degree of disc degeneration, facet joint arthritis, spinal misalignment, and spondylolisthesis with or without motion

MYELOGRAPHICALLY ENHANCED CT
- Permits determination of canal size, bony defects, hypertrophic bony changes, bony encroachment on neural elements, and evaluation of lateral recesses and neural foramina
- Use of intrathecal contrast allows evaluation of cauda equina

MRI
- Very sensitive to inflammatory and neoplastic conditions

important in excluding surgically correctable lesions, including retained or recurrent disc herniation, spinal stenosis, instability, and pseudarthrosis. However, imaging studies should confirm the probable cause deduced from the history and physical examination rather than providing the dominant basis for diagnosis.

Plain Radiographs

Radiographic evaluation should begin with plain radiographs to determine the extent and level of previous surgery. Lateral flexion-extension radiographs may demonstrate abnormal motion and instability and may also detect the presence of primary bone tumors. The degree of disc degeneration, facet joint arthritis, spinal misalignment, and spondylolisthesis with or without motion can all be identified from plain radiographs. MRI and/or CT is usually satisfactory and plain myelography is generally unnecessary for patients who have had a single surgical procedure.

Myelographically Enhanced Computed Tomography Scan

Oil-based myelography, which were the only radiographs of the spinal cord available in the past, showed large recurrent disc protrusions but frequently overlooked more subtle lesions. Myelography with water-soluble contrast media is a significant improvement but can miss a number of lesions, including far lateral disc herniations.[11-12,54]

The first improvement over conventional myelography was high-resolution CT scanning and computed tomography with myelographic enhancement (CT myelography). CT myelography is perhaps the most important diagnostic technique in evaluating the patient with FBSS. Patients who have undergone previous operations are often difficult to evaluate without intrathecal contrast. However, CT myelography permits determination of canal size, bony defects, and hypertrophic bony changes as well as bony encroachment on the neural elements and evaluation of the lateral recesses and neural foramina. Contrast allows evaluation of the cauda equina by demonstrating the presence or absence of nerve root compression and the relationship of the nerve roots to the lateral recesses, foramina, and discs.

Myelography with enhanced multiplanar CT provides the most powerful modality to assess the possibility of lateral or central stenosis as a cause of continued nerve root symptomatology after lumbar decompression. CT with three-dimensional reconstruction is a significant advancement that benefits examinations of the neural foramina and the remainder of the bony anatomy.

Magnetic Resonance Imaging Scan

The enhanced MRI scan is very sensitive to inflammatory and neoplastic conditions and is the most sensitive technique for differentiating scar tissue from recurrent pathology. In the immediate postoperative period, the area of bone and ligament resection shows edematous soft tissues isointense to muscle on T1 weighted images that increase on T2 weighted images and replace normal tissue signal. In the absence of postoperative hematoma, significant mass effect on the thecal sac is unusual. Gradual replacement of the immediate postoperative changes from scar tissue occurs 6 months postsurgery.[15,16] The signal intensity of posterior scar tissue is variable on T2 weighted images.

Changes from discectomy are visible immediately after surgery. T1 weighted images show increased signal anterior to the thecal sac, with an indistinct posterior annular margin. This soft tissue signal may blend smoothly into the disc space and may increase on T2 weighted images. Anterior epidural edema combined with posterior annular disruption caused by disc incision and curettage can mimic preoperative disc herniation and produce mass effect. These changes within the anterior epidural space involute in the months after surgery, with a corresponding normalization of the thecal margin.

Sagittal T2 weighted images can define the site of annular disruption and disc curettage in the immediate postoperative period by high signal in the nucleus pulposus extending posteriorly in the area of annular disruption. Annular perforation, which is not clearly seen on T1 weighted images, resolves within 6 months.

The interpretation of MRI within the first 6 weeks postoperatively requires caution because of the tremendous changes in the epidural soft tissues and intervertebral disc after surgery. Tissue disruption and edema can impinge on the thecal sac. MRI in the immediate post-operative period provides a gross overview of the thecal sac and epidural space and can often exclude significant hemorrhage, pseudomeningocele, or disc space infection. Small posterior fluid collections are common after laminectomy. Signal intensities depend upon whether the collections are serous [cerebrospinal fluid (CSF)] or serosanguinous (increased signal on T weighted images); MRI cannot distinguish between benign and infected collections on the basis of morphology or signal intensity.

ELECTROPHYSIOLOGY, THERMOGRAPHY, AND SPINAL EVOKED POTENTIALS

Electromyography (EMG), thermography (TMG), and spinal evoked potentials are of limited use in the evaluation of the patient with FBSS. The major benefit of these diagnostic tools is in differentiating cauda equina compression from peripheral nerve entrapment syndromes. Electromyography will corroborate root injury but cannot differentiate injury from compression. Thermography may help diagnose a secondary sympathetic dystrophy syndrome and can be useful in differentiating root from peripheral nerve injury. Both electrophysiologic studies and TMG have a role in certain clinical settings, though their sensitivity is limited. Equivocal neurologic deficits may be objectively demonstrated and quantitated clinically. Paraspinous EMG typically demonstrates nonspecific postsurgical changes in the patient with FBSS.

LUMBAR DISCOGRAPHY

Lumbar discography has undergone a resurgence as a physiologic rather than an anatomic study. Injection of fluid into the disc is postulated to reproduce pain originating in the same disc. Subsequent injection of local anesthetic provides relief. Pain provocation by injection and relief with local anesthetic constitutes a positive study. However, no controlled study has verified the hypothesis underlying this procedure.

CT discography may be useful when low back pain predominates, particularly in light of additional information derived from pain provocation. Although standard lumbar discography has been abandoned for diagnosing disc herniation, CT discography may have a role in the evaluation of recurrent disc herniations. Grenier et al.[30] postulate that extravasation of contrast medium from the disc space 3 to 6 months after surgery indicates a persistent rent in the annulus, which may be consistent with a recurrent herniated disc. Conversely, if dye does not escape, it suggests an intact annulus and that any epidural mass represents fibrosis. In their study, 21 of 23 patients with positive discograms had recurrent disc herniations at surgery, but 2 of 3 patients with negative discograms also had herniated discs.[30]

FACET AND NERVE BLOCKS

Facet blockade has been unsatisfactory for defining the role of anatomic structures that cause pain, although in one series it did prove useful.[20] Selective nerve root injections under radiographic control are helpful in more difficult cases in which radiculopathy predominates.[36] No definitive scientific evidence exists that peripheral blockade that produces pain relief predicts a successful outcome from surgery. The role of blockade of the lumbar zygapophyseal joints remains unproven.

Some patients suffer from intractable back pain because of zygapophyseal joint arthritis. Specific blockade of these joints by intraarticular blockade, or blocking the medial branch of the posterior primary rami that supply the joint, relieves back pain in some individuals. It is less predictable whether percutaneous facet denervation can relieve pain for a prolonged period of time. Patients selected for facet blockade should have back pain that is exacerbated by rotation and lateral bending and improved with bracing. The block technique described by Bogduk and Long[8] includes blocking the medial branch of the posterior primary ramus on the transverse process or the sacrum with a small amount of local anesthetic. A positive block provides total pain relief for the duration expected from the procedure. Patients with radicular pain and those with partial pain relief from blockade rarely respond satisfactorily to permanent neurotomy.[8]

INCORRECT DIAGNOSIS
Inappropriate Surgery

Incorrect diagnosis may cause continued pain after discectomy with an incidence of 0.3% in these cases.[42,63] Metastatic carcinoma, diabetic radiculopathy, neurofibroma, sacral cyst, and lumbar spondylosis can all mimic disc rupture. In the subset of patients with suspected lumbar disc herniations, neural tumors are reported to be present in 1%.

Inappropriate surgery that results from inaccurate diagnosis or incomplete comprehension of the involved pathologic processes is one of the major causes of FBSS. It is often difficult for the surgeon experienced in the evaluation and management of these types of cases to find objective clinical data that support the initial decision for operative intervention. As many as 50% of patients with FBSS are found on review of their original history, physical examination, and diagnostic studies not to have met generally accepted criteria for the primary surgical procedure. Despite the absence of physical findings in 80% of patients with low back pain, in one large series, 30% of these patients underwent lumbar spine surgery.

Inappropriate stabilization procedures in patients with mechanical causes for their pain are another source of FBSS. Although inadequate surgery is often cited, inappropriate surgery is the major factor. Operations at the wrong level, on the wrong side, and for the wrong pathology are rare but often quite dramatic and memorable.[46]

PSYCHOSOCIAL CAUSES

Psychogenic factors are the single most common cause of failure to relieve pain by discectomy. Long[42] states that "patients suffering from failed back syndrome are incapacitated by psychiatric, psychologic and social/vocational factors which relate to the back complaint only indirectly." In a study of 266 patients with FBSS, 15% of these patients were diagnosed with psychiatric disorders before the onset of low back pain.[8,42] Sorenson et al.[72] attempted to predict the outcome of disc surgery by preoperative testing with a modification of the Minnesota Multiphasic Personality Inventory (MMPI). Some patients can be expected to do poorly for reasons unrelated to the surgery. The important factors in predicting failure are workers' compensation, job dissatisfaction, low education and income, heavy job requirements, cigarette smoking, psychologic disturbances, and litigation.[26,74]

DISCOGENIC PAIN/INTERNAL DISC DISRUPTION

Internal disc disruption (IDD) is a condition marked by alterations in the internal structure and metabolic functions of one or more discs, usually after significant trauma. The clinical syndrome includes axial and extremity pain exacerbated by any physical activity that compresses affected discs. The pain is typically deep, does not rapidly abate with rest, and worsens over time. Profound energy loss occurs, sometimes in conjunction with significant weight loss and psychologic disturbances. It is not associated with herniation of the disc fragment. Disc degeneration with loss of disc height and osteophyte formation is rare.

Discography, which was the principal diagnostic tool for IDD, has been supplanted by MRI. Patients with IDD show changes in the signal generated from the affected intervertebral disc and often from adjacent vertebral levels. Once the diagnosis of disc disruption is made and surgical intervention is considered appropriate, disc excision with anterior interbody fusion is the most effective operation for persistent disabling symptoms. Disc excision is also indicated for patients who do not respond to nonoperative therapies, including analgesics, nonsteroidal antiinflammatory drugs, and psychotropic agents.

MISSED LEVEL OR LEVELS

Surgery on the wrong interspace may be discovered either intraoperatively or afterward when the patient has no relief from pain. The incidence from this rare surgical error ranges from 0.14% to 2.7%. The highest incidence was reported with a microsurgical series because the limited exposure used with microsurgery may increase the occurrence of the error. Intraoperative recognition permits redirection to the proper interspace. Neither nontraumatic exploration nor violation of a nonpathologic interspace is associated with appreciable morbidity.

Wide exposure with identification of the sacrum and intraoperative radiographic localization are effective but not foolproof methods to avoid operating on the wrong interspace. Discovery of the disc herniation is the best

SURGICAL CONSIDERATIONS

- Up to 50% of patients with FBSS are found on review of their original history, physical examination, and diagnostic studies not to have generally accepted criteria for the primary surgical procedure
- Psychogenic factors are the single most common cause of failure to relieve pain by discectomy
- Incidence of surgery on the wrong interspace ranges from 0.14% up to 2.7%
  - Consider this possibility if patient complains of lower extremity pain persisting 2 days postsurgery
- Inadequate decompression
  - Common pitfall: Failure to recognize contribution of lateral foraminal or extraforaminal compression to the patient's radiculopathy with initial disc removal without adequate decompression of bony component
- Consider surgery only if patient suffers from either compression and/or instability, particularly if disease is progressive or associated with major neurologic deficits
- Note that surgery will be ineffective and may lead to FBSS if patient's underlying problem is not a neural compressive lesion or incapacitating mechanical instability
- Be aware that decompressive surgery is indicated when patient's complaints of pain are compatible with demonstrated compression or in cases of overt instability

way to identify the correct interspace and avoid this complication. Obese patients often prevent adequate intraoperative radiographic confirmation of the level of disc herniation.

Segmentation abnormalities can produce a neurologic level of involvement different from the motion segment level. A sacralized L5 or lumbarized S1 can disorient even an experienced spine surgeon. Review of anteroposterior (AP) and lateral plain radiographs and correlating them with more sophisticated imaging modalities are essential to avoid surgery at the wrong level. The possibility that the wrong disc was operated upon should be considered if the patient complains of lower extremity pain that persists 2 days postsurgery. In a patient with a missed level or side, scarring is not a problem if reoperation is performed immediately.

INADEQUATE SURGERY

Inadequate surgery (i.e., inadequate decompression) has been suggested as a frequent cause of FBSS. Lateral recess stenosis and persistent disc herniation are usually cited as the responsible pathologies for inadequate decompression. One of the most common pitfalls is failure to recognize the contribution of lateral foraminal or extraforaminal compression to the patient's radiculopathy, with initial disc removal without adequate decompression of the bony component. Burton[14] analyzed the data of 800 FBSS patients and reported concomitant lateral recess and/or central stenosis

account for 71% of failures. MacNab[48] concluded that lateral recess stenosis was the most common source of failure after lumbar disc surgery. Spengler et al.[74] reported a 30% incidence of lateral recess stenosis that required medial foraminotomy at surgery in his series of discectomy patients. Nerve root decompression should provide an excursion of at least 5 mm, so that a blunt probe can be easily passed into the foramen. Further bony decompression to uncover a laterally herniated disc or hypertrophic superior facet in the foramen should be necessary if nerve root decompression is not accomplished. In some cases, the entire joint or even the pedicle must be sacrificed. Fusion is indicated in these patients with a destabilized spine.

RETAINED DISC FRAGMENT

A retained disc fragment can cause continued postoperative pain. In one large series, 13 retained fragments accounted for 29 failures, representing an incidence of 0.2%. When the patient awakens from anesthesia with unrelieved lower extremity pain, the possibility should be considered that one or more fragments of disc have been left behind. The presence of multiple free fragments of disc at the initial surgery increase the chances that retained fragments were overlooked. Reexploration is indicated if other causes of pain have been excluded. Adequate operative exposure provides the best means of avoiding the complication. The increased possibility of overlooking a retained fragment is one of the inherent problems with microsurgical discectomy.

CONJOINED NERVE ROOT

A conjoined nerve root is present in 2% to 14% of patients. Surgical decompression in patients with a conjoined root is associated with a significant incidence of failure. Failure to recognize the conjoined nerve root at the time of the initial surgery may have three consequences: (1) the conjoined nerve root is avulsed, which produces a neurologic deficit; (2) the conjoined nerve root is battered, which causes increased perineural scanning; or (3) the compressed portion of the nerve root is overlooked, which allows continued symptoms. The first two conditions are more common than the third, which is the only one amenable to further surgical intervention.

TEMPORARY RELIEF (DAYS TO WEEKS) WITH EARLY FAILURE OF RELIEF OR DEVELOPMENT OF INFECTION

In 1936 Milward[52] described the clinical and radiographic characteristics of interspace infection after the inadvertent introduction of microorganisms into a disc space during lumbar puncture. Ramirez and Thisted[65] reported an infection rate of 0.3% in an analysis of 28,395 patients who underwent lumbar laminectomy for radiculopathy in the United States in 1980. Patients with aseptic necrosis of interspace infection are typically asymptomatic immediately after surgery but within 2 weeks begin to experience excruciating spasms in the lower back with or without radiation into the legs. The white blood cell count and temperature of these patients are often normal but the sedimentation rate is elevated, often higher than 100 mm/hr. Lumbosacral radiographs may reveal erosion of the cartilaginous plates as the disease progresses. Needle aspirations of the interspace may reveal the offending organisms, although such aspirations are often negative.[28] Patients with a clear-cut infectious syndrome should be given intravenous antibiotics. The persistence of an elevated temperature for several days postoperatively may indicate an infection. The wound should be examined for erythema, swelling, tenderness, and drainage. Management of the infection should include Gram's stain and culture with antibiotics if the clinical indication is strong. The patient should be returned to the operating room, and the wound reopened, thoroughly débrided, and irrigated if the infection continues despite antibiotic treatment. The wound can be managed open with frequent dressing changes.

DISCITIS

Postoperative intervertebral disc space infection (discitis) is uncommon, with reports of infection rates ranging from 0.1% to 3.8%.* The presence of the microscope over the open wound may account for the higher incidence of disc space infection from microsurgery. Postoperative discitis typically produces persistent intense back pain with unremarkable associated physical findings 2 weeks to 3 months after discectomy.

Patients with discitis often have elevated erythrocyte sedimentation rates. Bone scan, CT, and MRI are sensitive for detecting discitis and can identify changes associated with discitis earlier than plain radiographs. CT is effective in the early diagnosis of discitis; hypodensity of the affected disc space may be detected as early as 10 days postoperatively. The responsible bacteria are identified in fewer than 50% of cases with *Staphylococcus* species, the most common organism cultured.

Early diagnosis and prompt treatment are important to prevent chronic infection. Immobilization is often effective for pain relief, and 4 to 6 weeks of intravenous antibiotic therapy is recommended. Uncomplicated discitis should not require surgery, and most patients undergo spontaneous interbody fusion. Paresis may develop from lumbar epidural abscesses, which then require immediate decompressive laminectomy.

POSTOPERATIVE OSTEOMYELITIS

Infection may be introduced directly into the intervertebral disc space during surgery and can spread to the adjacent vertebral bodies, producing osteomyelitis. Surgery for protruding or herniated discs is the most frequent cause of infection introduced directly into the intervertebral disc space. This complication from disc surgery occurs in less than 1% of patients. Organisms

may be inadvertently inoculated during surgery, and residual hematoma, necrotic tissue, and foreign bodies provide an environment conducive to bacterial proliferation. Weeks, months, or even years may elapse before the diagnosis of a disc space infection is established. Symptoms of an infection may not be apparent immediately after surgery, and often initial pain relief is followed by recurrence several days to weeks later. Fever may be transient, intermittent, or nonexistent, and frequently no evidence of infection exists when symptoms develop. The degree of pain may appear to be out of proportion to the objective findings and may erroneously be attributed to hysteria, malingering, or even psychoneurosis.

The typical radiologic changes of vertebral osteomyelitis may not be apparent for several months. Radionuclide bone scans are sensitive and often demonstrate evidence of infection before plain films of the spine show any changes. However, they are not specific; surgical edema and disc changes may yield false-positive results. The bone scan may be negative in a significant percentage of patients early in the course of disc space infection.[76] CT may show destructive changes of the vertebral bodies before these are evident on plain films. However, end plate irregularities on CT are not specific for discitis, and normal curettage changes in vertebral end plates may mimic erosions of discitis.[14] MRI may show changes of discitis long before any changes are present radiologically.[15] MRI and CT may be negative early in the course of postoperative or posttraumatic discitis, and the risk of infection is always a possibility. Any patient with increasing back pain more than 2 weeks postoperatively and an erythrocyte sedimentation rate greater than 50 mm/hr should be considered to have discitis until proven otherwise. Percutaneous disc biopsy can be helpful in the diagnosis of postoperative discitis but is often falsely negative. A 1990 study[70] compared MRI, plain radiographs, and radionuclide studies in the evaluation of vertebral osteomyelitis. MRI and combined bone and gallium scans were equally accurate and sensitive, whereas MRI was more sensitive than plain films. MRI is a rapid, noninvasive method for the detection of vertebral osteomyelitis and its complications, including epidural abscess, because of the characteristic appearance of pyogenic infection on MRI. Infected disc material on T1 weighted images shows decreased signal intensity from the intervertebral disc space and contiguous vertebral bodies relative to the normal vertebral signal, while on T2 weighted images, these infected tissues show increased signal. MRI provides more anatomic detail than radionuclide scanning and allows differentiation of neoplasm and degenerative disease from osteomyelitis. The disc space is nearly always spared in neoplastic disease, whereas degenerative disease with nucleus desiccation produces decreased disc signal on T2 weighted images. Gallium scans may be positive earlier than MRI in the course of infection and are more sensitive to changes due to treatment and decreasing inflammation.

Spontaneous resolution does occur in many patients with postoperative discitis and vertebral osteomyelitis.

---

*References 6, 22, 23, 55, 58, 62, 65, 68.

Intermittent antibiotic therapy obscures the diagnosis of postoperative vertebral osteomyelitis. Turnbull[77] described a patient who developed postoperative staphylococcal lumbar vertebral osteomyelitis 3 years after successful surgery for a herniated disc. The patient required three operations before a psoas abscess was successfully treated.

EPIDURAL ABSCESS

Epidural abscess after decompression is rare but should be considered in a patient with increasing neurologic symptoms and signs in the early postoperative period. It may be difficult to differentiate from an expanding hematoma in the absence of systemic evidence of infection.

MRI can localize the site of infection and provide more information than CT regarding the extent of abscess involvement and degree of cord compromise.

Decompression and aggressive antibiotic management are the cornerstones of therapy. Epidural abscess often arises in association with vertebral osteomyelitis and is an indication for early decompression.

MENINGEAL CYST/PSEUDOMENINGOCELE

Meningeal cysts rarely cause early recurrent radiculopathy after disc excision and are reported in less than 1% of patients. Incidental durotomy during disc excision does not compromise later results if the dural leak is recognized and closed; durotomy that is unrecognized or incompletely repaired can produce a slowly expanding mass. Nerve roots can become trapped in the meningeal cyst and cause pain. Physical examination occasionally reveals soft tissue bulging that may or may not be recognized as fluctuant, but often increases when the patient stands. Myelography and MRI are important diagnostic studies to identify meningeal cysts. Removal of the meningeal cyst requires careful dissection around the cyst and identification of the dural opening. The cyst should be opened to avoid injury to involved nerve roots prior to excision. Closure can be accomplished by closing the dura with or without duroplasty.

MIDTERM FAILURES (WEEKS TO MONTHS)
Herniated Intervertebral Disc

There are many explanations for persistent pain caused by disc herniation. An inadequate discectomy produces pain because of continued nerve root irritation. Patients do not report any pain-free interval and sometimes awaken from surgery complaining of their preoperative pain. Recurrent intervertebral disc herniation at the previously decompressed level may also occur. Patients with this problem often have a pain-free interval of more than 6 months. Those patients with a herniated disc that ruptures at a different level usually benefit from a repeat operation. Patients may describe persistent severe pain and paresthesias in a radicular distribution after unsuccessful lumbar disc surgery. The pain is superimposed on an area of residual numbness that is constant and described as either burning or ice cold. It is often more distressing than the original disc herniation pain. These patients with pain of nerve injury or deafferentation sometimes respond to spinal cord stimulation (SCS).[40,56]

RECURRENT DISC FRAGMENT

The incidence of recurrent rupture after laminectomy has been reported to range from a low rate of 0.26% for ruptures that occur within the first 6 weeks after surgery (on the same side and level) to a rate of 18% for recurrences that take place at any time or any level after the initial operation. Recurrent disc herniation may occur on the same side and at the same level as the prior operation, on the opposite side at the same level, or at an entirely new level. Vigorous disc space evacuation does not prevent recurrent disc herniation. In some cases, the patient is pain free for years after surgery, and then back and sciatic pain suddenly returns. MRI with gadolinium-DTPA (Gd-DTPA) and CT myelography can confirm a diagnosis of disc herniation but may be difficult to interpret because of postoperative changes.[81] Physical examination reveals signs of disc herniation with positive tension signs. Once the diagnosis is established and nonsurgical treatment fails, surgery is indicated for intractable pain. Previous back surgery does not preclude an excellent result: Some patients feel better after the second operation than the first. Frymoyer et al.[24] have shown that the outcome of surgery after recurrent disc herniation and the outcome following primary disc excision are identical.[25]

Ikko et al.[34] analyzed the spine 1 week postoperatively and reported a soft tissue mass composed of blood and early scar tissue on the posterior aspect of the disc space is always present in both symptomatic and asymptomatic patients. Teplick and Haskin[75,76] reviewed 750 patients with persistent postoperative symptoms and found that recurrent disc problems can be distinguished from epidural fibrosis. Fibrosis is characterized by thecal sac retraction toward the soft tissue lesion, a location above or below the disc space, an indistinct border, and a shape that conforms to rather than compresses the dural sac.

Scar tissue is generally less dense than recurrent disc fragments. In contrast, recurrent disc compresses rather than conforms to the sac, has a sharp border, and has a density of 90 to 120 Hu. Postoperative CT appearance normalizes over time with a decrease of hyperdense fibrotic material, which is difficult to distinguish on CT in symptomatic from asymptomatic patients.

BATTERED-ROOT SYNDROME OR PERINEURAL SCARRING

Perineural scarring is a common occurrence after spinal decompression, although clinical failure from perineural scarring occurs in only 1% to 2% of patients who undergo disc excision.[25] Nerve root scarring may be caused by excessive bleeding, conjoined nerve roots, and the use of cottonoid patties. The immediate postoperative course is generally benign but may be associated with incomplete resolution of sciatica, sometimes accompanied by an increased sensory or even motor deficit. Sciatica and back pain gradually increase over 3 to 6 months. Various surgical therapies have been advocated, including scar removal with membrane interposition, radical decompression, longitudinal sectioning of scar over nerve root, spinal fusion, and electrical stimulator implantation.[9]

EPIDURAL SCARRING

Scar tissue around the dura and nerve roots can cause recurrent sciatica. Prevention is essential owing to the lack of effective surgical therapy for epidural fibrosis. In this difficult patient population, the differentiation of recurrent disc herniation from scar is critical because reoperation on scar often produces a poor surgical result and additional scarring. CT with intravenous contrast that has an accuracy of 67% to 100% in distinguishing scar tissue from disc is technically demanding, involves a large contrast load, and includes only single-plane imaging. Intravenous contrast increases the diagnostic accuracy of CT from 43% to 74%, which makes differentiating between recurrent herniated disc fragments and postsurgical scar tissue more likely.[10,81] Recurrent disc fragments are avascular and enhance only at the periphery, whereas postsurgical scar tissue demonstrates uniform enhancement after infusion of intravenous contrast material. The peripheral enhancement observed in recurrent disc herniation is thought to be due to a thin layer of surgical scar tissue or to vascularity in the annulus fibrosus or epidural venous plexus.

MRI allows differentiation of recurrent disc herniation from epidural scar. MRI has 100% sensitivity, 71% specificity, and 89% accuracy in distinguishing recurrent disc herniation from epidural scar. Bundschuh[11] evaluated 20 patients with MRI, 14 of whom underwent exploration. MRI diagnosis was confirmed in 12 patients at surgery. Eight of nine of these patients also had CT findings confirmed at surgery.

Epidural fibrosis can be differentiated from disc by signal intensity and the configuration and margination of the extradural mass on unenhanced MRI scans. Recurrent disc herniations are seen at or near the disc space, exhibit mass effect, and on T1 weighted image are slightly hyperintense compared to fibrosis. Free fragments are hyperintense on T2 weighted images. Unenhanced epidural scar that lacks mass effect is not contiguous with the disc space and is hypointense or isointense on T1 weighted images. On T2 weighted images, fibrotic scar has higher signal intensity than disc material or annulus. Sotiropoulos[73] compared the diagnostic accuracy of contrast CT to unenhanced MRI in 25 patients and found that unenhanced MRI is equivalent to contrast-enhanced CT for identifying scar from disc. Anterior epidural scars are slightly hypointense to isointense relative to intervertebral disc on T weighted images. Anterior epidural scars show increased signal on T2 weighted images. Scar generally conforms to the dural margin with retraction of the thecal sac toward the scar. Lateral and posterior scar exhibits similar charac-

teristics, but not as consistently. Increased signal intensity at the operative sites is often noted laterally, posteriorly, and within the paraspinal musculature, whereas low signal intensity on T2 weighted images is not unusual for lateral and posterior scar.

Herniated discs, except free fragments, are often in contiguity with the parent disc space. Small protruded discs are low in signal intensity on T2 weighted images. Larger protruded, extruded, and free fragments can show central high intensity on T2 weighted images that creates a problem in differentiating the herniated material from scar tissue and the high-signal-intensity CSF. A rim of low signal intensity surrounds these larger disc herniations, allowing for good contrast between the CSF and the herniated material. This low signal intensity may reflect the remnants of the outer annular fibers and the posterior longitudinal ligament.

MRI with intravenous Gd-DTPA administration is the most accurate technique to distinguish scar from disc. Hueftle et al.[33] analyzed the role of Gd-enhanced MRI in the differentiation of scar tissue versus disc. Enhanced MRI was able to predict operative findings with 100% accuracy in 30 patients evaluated with MRI before and after administration of 0.1 mmol/kg Gd. Hueftle et al.[33] reported uniform scar enhancement on early postcontrast T weighted images, whereas recurrent discs exhibited peripheral enhancement on delayed postcontrast images.

Injection of Gd-DTPA consistently enhances anterior epidural scar irrespective of the time since surgery. Three components are necessary for contrast enhancement of any tissue: vascular supply, route for contrast material out of the vasculature, and some amount of interstitial space to sequester the contrast. Disc material does not enhance on early postinjection images because of its avascular nature. Disc material may enhance on delayed images (greater than 30 minutes after injection) owing to diffusion of contrast into the disc from adjacent vascularized tissue. In cases with a mixture of scar and disc material, scar will enhance and the disc material will not enhance on early postinjection images.[4,5] Problems can occur when the volume of nonenhancing herniated disc is small relative to the volume of enhancing scar where partial volume averaging might obscure the disc. The disc material will enhance if sufficient time elapses for contrast material to diffuse into the disc material from the surrounding vascular scar. It is important to obtain both sagittal and axial T weighted images before and after contrast. Patients should not be moved between the precontrast and postcontrast scans to assure precise comparison between the same regions of interest. Postinjection images should be completed within 20 minutes of contrast administration. In one study of 44 patients at 50 reoperated levels,[12] 96% accuracy was reported in differentiating scar from disc with precontrast and postcontrast MRI in the postoperative lumbar spine.

Although limited data are available on the use of contrast in the immediate postoperative period, enhancement is visible in the epidural space within the first 4 days of surgery. Pathologic changes are difficult to differentiate from the tremendous changes that normally occur after any surgical procedure, which creates a problem in identifying enhancement.

Careful hemostasis and gentle handling of the neural tissue will decrease scar tissue formation, and use of fat grafts at the time of the initial surgery can diminish scarring. A free or pedicled fat graft is superior to materials such as Gelfoam. Free fat grafts should be less than 5 mm in thickness to prevent cauda equina compression and enhance graft vascularization.

ARACHNOIDITIS

Although arachnoiditis was originally described as a complication of infection, we prefer the term *chronic adhesive arachnoiditis*, derived from the descriptions of Horsley and Stookey.[43] A dramatic increase in surgery for spondylotic diseases of the spine occurred after the introduction of myelography and once infection was ruled out as the cause of arachnoiditis.[13,17,44]

The Imaging Diagnosis of Arachnoiditis

Much confusion exists over what constitutes *arachnoiditis*. Some radiologists have used the term to describe minor inflammatory changes that occur with the injection of any intrathecal agent. Arachnoiditis is characterized by (1) partial or complete block of spinal fluid flow; (2) narrowing of the subarachnoid space; (3) obliteration of nerve root sheaths; (4) apparent thickening or clumping of nerve roots; (5) irregular distribution of contrast agents, with loculation being common; (6) formation of cysts; and (7) immobility of oil-based contrast agents. Myelography remains the standard method to diagnose the problem because MRI can be misinterpreted.

The Clinical Syndromes of Arachnoiditis

Most patients diagnosed with arachnoiditis have low back and lower extremity symptoms; recurrent symptoms are often similar to those that occurred originally. A neurogenic claudication syndrome has been diagnosed in some patients who complain of leg weakness and burning pain that is affected by sitting or standing. Bowel or bladder dysfunction is common in these patients. The burning character of the pain, associated with hyperpathia and claudication, suggests arachnoiditis but cannot be differentiated from other forms of spinal stenosis.

Causes of Arachnoiditis

Any agent injected into the lumbar subarachnoid space has the potential to cause arachnoiditis. All of the contrast agents cause a severe inflammatory reaction in the subarachnoid space. Oil-based agents were used for years with minimal problems. Although early water-soluble contrast agents were extremely noxious, improvements to these agents have reduced the potential for inflammation. Little evidence is available that use of the common clinical contrast materials causes a significant incidence of arachnoiditis. Traumatic or repeated myelography, particularly with multiple surgeries, may affect the incidence of arachnoiditis.

All authors[13,17,44] stress the fact that the new syndrome of chronic adhesive arachnoiditis is quite different from the rapidly progressive arachnoiditis that complicates infection. The patients are stable, neurologic deterioration occurs but is rare, and pain is the predominant issue.

Diagnosis and Treatment of the Disease

The diagnosis of arachnoiditis usually occurs in the course of repeat myelography.[69] In our experience, clear-cut abnormalities that would otherwise be candidates for reparative surgery should be treated even if arachnoiditis is diagnosed. The arachnoiditis will not detract from the potential success of reparative surgery. Direct surgery on the arachnoiditis should not be considered unless the patient has a progressive neuralgic deficit. Surgery to correct arachnoiditis is a delicate and dangerous operation, and the surgeon must be very familiar with this highly technical procedure. Pain relief occurs in less than half of the patients, and the risk of a substantial new neurologic deficit is high.

Alternatives to Direct Therapy

SCS is the most effective therapy to relieve the pain in those patients with arachnoiditis and FBSS who are not candidates for any other procedure. Brain stimulation and intrathecal narcotic pumps have both successfully reduced pain in severely disabled patients. The use of chronic oral narcotic administration is undergoing investigation in a select group of patients.[44] Improved myelographic techniques, the newest water-soluble agents, and improved surgical techniques may all contribute to reduce the incidence of this difficult complication.

SPINAL STENOSIS

Multiple operations can produce both axial and radicular pain in the patient with spinal stenosis. The cause may be progression of degenerative disease, previous inadequate decompression, or overgrowth of a previous posterior fusion. Spinal stenosis and scar often coexist. Bony compression is an indication for laminectomy; in the presence of substantial scar tissue, however, pain relief may be minimal.

LONG-TERM FAILURES (MONTHS TO YEARS)

Instability is defined as abnormal or excessive movement of one vertebra on another, which may cause pain. The patient's intrinsic back disease or excessively wide bilateral laminectomies may be responsible for the instability. Patients complain predominantly of back pain, and physical examination is often unremarkable. Relative flexion-sagittal plane translation of more than 8% of the AP diameter of the vertebral body or a relative flexion-sagittal plan rotation of more than 9% or degrees between adjacent segments are the most commonly cited radiographic guidelines for instability of the lumbar spine.[55] Spinal fusion should be considered for symptomatic patients with evidence of instability.

The incidence of post-decompression spondylolisthesis ranges from 2% to 10% whereas the incidence of progressive slippage after decompressive laminectomy in patients with preoperative degenerative spondylolisthesis is even higher.[71] The factors that contribute to post-decompression slippage include patients younger than 40 years of age with normal disc heights, who have undergone extensive surgery. The extent of surgery is an important contributor in the development of postoperative instability. Discectomy at the time of laminectomy may cause additional instability. Complete laminectomy and bilateral facetectomies will also create spinal instability.

Symptoms sufficient to require later stabilization occur in only 3% of patients following simple discectomy. It is possible to excise 50% of both facets or 100% of one facet without significantly altering the stiffness of human intervertebral segments. After extensive spinal decompression, accentuation of preexistent deformity occasionally occurs but is often asymptomatic. Radical facetectomy for degenerative spondylolisthesis always produces increased deformity but is frequently asymptomatic. Greater disc space height at the time of decompression, the absence of osteophytes, discectomy at the time of decompression, and a younger age may predispose the patient to later deformity. Presence of any or all of these factors can indicate the need for fusion at the time of decompression. Younger patients who undergo multilevel decompressive laminectomies for congenital or mixed spinal stenosis commonly develop a new deformity after the laminectomy.

PSEUDARTHROSIS OF PRIOR FUSION

Pseudarthrosis is a complication that may stem from technical faults by the surgeon or from biologic deficiency of the patient. The incidence of pseudarthrosis depends on the number of levels fused, the techniques involved, and whether the patient smokes. The overall rate of pseudarthrosis is higher in two-level compared with one-level fusion, with the lumbosacral junction presenting a special challenge. The variety of therapeutic options for FBSS emphasizes the lack of a uniform method of treatment. The majority of conditions producing low back or sciatic pain are nonlethal and can be successfully managed without further surgery. Nonsurgical therapy can be effective at minimal risk and cost. Recognition of the "failed back" as a syndrome has resulted in the development of algorithms for its management.* Treatment options include physiologic, behavioral, and rehabilitative measures and a number of surgical procedures. The literature on the treatment of FBSS and its results encompasses many different outcome measures, obtained in a number of ways, at variable follow-up intervals.[42,56] Lack of uniformity in the treatment and outcome measures makes comparison of therapies difficult.

Treatment of the FBSS should include surgery for only a small minority of patients. In reported series on reoperation,[57,60,64] success has been defined most commonly by patient self-reports of pain relief and satisfaction with treatment results. Fifty percent estimated that relief of pain is a common criterion for "success." Return to work is an outcome measure that is given particular emphasis by rehabilitation programs. Analgesic requirements are commonly considered, as are the ability to engage in activities of daily living, preservation of strength, sensation, and bladder and bowel function.

The source of follow-up information is of fundamental importance in interpreting outcomes. Reports from physicians' and surgeons' offices and hospital records commonly overestimate results and are substantially more favorable than patient interviews by disinterested third parties.[57,60,64] Reports of outcome of reoperation and behavioral/rehabilitation programs have with few exceptions been based upon the former.[60] Third-party interview is the most objective evaluation mechanism for obtaining follow-up of pain therapies.

TREATMENT OPTIONS
Nonsurgical Treatment

Certain general principles should be followed in treating FBSS, irrespective of the pathologic process. Rehabilitation is an important component in the management of FBSS patients, and programs specializing in this are proliferating. The ultimate goal of rehabilitation is restoration of the patient to a functional status. Psychiatric and psychosocial comorbidities must be identified and treated. The effect of economic issues must be addressed. Psychologic dysfunction affects the patient's ability to cope as well as the rehabilitation process. Detrimental pain behaviors can be modified by appropriate therapies, and it is important to use these psychotherapeutic techniques within the context of an overall program.

The psychologic needs of each patient must be identified and treated specifically because stereotyped programs are generally of little value. Professional assessment of patients' physical therapy needs and an individualized regimen of graduated exercise are essential. Formal evaluation and treatment sessions allow the patient to understand the techniques and rationale for physical therapy. Patients with FBSS must be urged to translate the short-term pain relief resulting from effective application of therapies into increased productive activity.

In some cases, hospitalization in a multidisciplinary pain treatment program may be necessary. Abuse of medications, including narcotics and benzodiazepines, must be curtailed. Pain management centers focus on increasing the quality of life and physical function in spite of residual pain that maximal therapy cannot relieve. The pain treatment center also educates the patient about physical and nonphysical factors in chronic pain and the realistic expectations from therapy.

*References 14, 19, 24, 29, 42, 56.

Patients initially require therapy to stretch muscles back to a functional length; they also need coordinated muscle activity with intensive physical reconditioning to improve strength and endurance. Some patients require specific therapy to address myofascial pain and careful instruction in body biomechanics to prevent further insults.

The concept of productive rehabilitation or work hardening with worksite-style conditioning has been both practical and popular. Work-hardening programs specify when patients are fit to return to work and what practical work restrictions are necessary. Patients should gain the physical capacity and confidence to do their jobs, and lead a more normal life once they have completed the program.

Surgical Treatment and Reoperation

The physician is obliged to rule out a persistent surgical problem as part of the surgical history. Surgery should be viewed as part of a continuum of care rather than as the sole event leading to functional restoration of the patient.

An ongoing complaint of pain in the absence of defined pathology is not an indication for an operative procedure. The majority of patients are not surgical candidates; they should be protected from ineffective surgical procedures and treated with measures to improve back function. Surgery should only be considered if the patient suffers from either compression and/or instability, particularly if the disease is progressive or associated with major neurologic deficits. Stereotyped procedures applied without considering the physical and psychologic components of each patient are virtually guaranteed to fail. Patients with spondylotic disease characterized by disc herniation, canal and foraminal stenosis, and instability benefit the most from surgery. Radicular pain, back pain related to activity and relieved by rest, improvement with stabilization, and neurogenic claudication will improve with surgical intervention.

The first reoperations on the lumbar spine were reported less than 20 years after the original description of lumbar disc surgery.[47] A variety of procedures have been reported,[57] with a wide range of "success" rates. The reported success rate for reoperation for FBSS has varied from 12% to 100%.[60] Loss of neurologic function is rare after reoperation. The presence of positive tension sign, focal and correlative neurologic deficit, and a positive confirmatory radiographic study are strong indications that mechanical nerve root compression will be found at surgery. Surgical results under these circumstances are generally excellent provided that complications are avoided. It is important to recognize the limitations and benefits of interventional therapy. Appropriate and definitive decompression and/or stabilization procedures should be done in conjunction with an intensive low back rehabilitation effort in patients with pathology amenable to surgery. The residual effects of abnormalities already treated definitively (e.g., disc herniation causing root injury before its removal) from untreated and iatrogenic abnormalities are sometimes difficult to distinguish when a patient needs reoperation. Repeat surgery may be the only way to relieve the patient's pain if a correctable lesion exists. Another operation will not help and may have an adverse effect if such a lesion is not present. Patients with pathology amenable to surgical intervention should be offered reoperation, usually decompression or stabilization.

The initial decision to operate is most important; once recurrent pain occurs after surgery, the potential for relief is limited at best.[3] It is no longer acceptable to consider exploratory surgery of the lower back when objective criteria are not met.[1] The residual effects of abnormalities already treated definitively (e.g., disc herniation causing root injury before its removal) may be difficult to differentiate from untreated and iatrogenic abnormalities in patients considered for reoperation.[45]

If the surgeon is convinced that a disc protrusion was originally present, surgery may be necessary to exclude persistent root compression from retained disc fragments or unrelieved lateral recess stenosis. Statistics from several studies[19,29,42] show that 57% to 66% of patients with persistent symptoms after lumbar spine surgery suffered from root compression within the lateral recess. These series failed to account for patients in whom adequate central and foraminal decompression did not relieve low back pain.

Prior to reoperation, the surgeon should review the contrast studies to be certain of the location of the original disc injury. Fragments that are lateral or in the axilla of the nerve root are often overlooked. Repeat surgery is relatively easy within days of the first operation but is more difficult several weeks later, when adhesions are present. We prefer to extend the bone removal above and below the original laminotomy, which increases the exposure and allows identification of normal structures prior to removing epidural scar at the original operative site. A foraminotomy is necessary to expose the axilla of the root, and a portion of the facet joint must be removed to obtain lateral exposure. Tactile exploration using a blunt nerve hook to palpate in all directions is also most important. An experienced surgeon can often sense the presence of a fragment by the absence of root or dural pulsations, or a sense of fullness at the end of the nerve hook. The root must be completely mobilized and retracted to confirm the presence of a disc fragment.

A complete laminectomy may have to be considered to adequately expose the surgical site if canal stenosis is present. Osseous compression most often occurs in the lateral recess but may occur at the pedicle or in the foramen. Dural erythema can frequently be identified at the site of compression after bone removal.

Careful repeat exposure is mandatory because dural tears, anomalous nerve roots, and other abnormalities may be overlooked or not recorded in the operative note. The patient will do well if definite correctable pathology is found at early reoperation. The prognosis is guarded, however, if no pathology is found and surgical indications were marginal at the beginning.

Interventional or surgical therapy can only achieve two objectives: neural decompression and spinal stabilization. Interventional therapy will be ineffective and may lead to FBSS if the patient's underlying problem is not a neural compressive lesion or incapacitating mechanical instability. Of the degenerative processes where reparative surgery is the only reasonable alternative to leaving the patient untreated, neurogenic claudication cannot be treated by any other technique.

Decompressive surgery is indicated when the patient's complaints of pain are compatible with demonstrated compression. The other problem for which surgery is generally indicated is overt instability. Although the patient may be temporarily relieved by bracing, nothing will correct the problem except stabilization. Spinal fusion is used to stabilize segments that have been damaged to such a degree that normal physiologic forces will cause damage to neural structures or progressive loss of biomechanical integrity.

Loss of stability may occur following operative decompression and destabilization of a spinal motion segment. *Stability* is a mechanical term that is often used without a clear or precise definition. Clinical instability does not necessarily indicate mechanical instability. Patients with clinical instability have abnormal symptomatic motion, whereas patients with mechanical instability do not necessarily have to be symptomatic. Patients with symptomatic instability are able to function, although minor changes in motion may precipitate severe symptomatic back and/or leg pain. Symptoms and signs that may be indicative of clinical instability include low back pain exacerbated with standing and lifting and relieved by lying down. A sudden catch when extending from the flexed to the straight posture as well as a feeling of disconnection in the lumbar spine accentuated by motion is helpful in identifying instability. Lumbar bracing may provide some relief in these patients. Clinical instability is frequently present in patients who have had previous surgery for back disorders.[49]

Patients who respond well to bracing can be treated satisfactorily with fusion of the involved segments. Objective criteria that suggest local instability exists include demonstrated motion on flexion-extension films and progressive spinal deformity in any direction including an unstable spondylolisthesis. Iatrogenic surgical destruction of greater than one complete zygapophyseal joint and obvious pseudarthrosis with motion within the prior fusion site are other signs of instability. Definite radiographic instability exists in the lumbar spine from L1 to L5 when there is greater than 4 mm of translatory motion and greater than 10 mm of angulatory motion as compared with adjacent levels. The translatory limit at the lumbosacral junction is 4 mm and the angular limit is 20 mm. Values that exceed these limits often indicate instability. MacNab[48] analyzed the causes of nerve root involvement and showed that traction osteophytes often indicate instability of a motion segment. Careful exploration of the integrity of the zygapophyseal joints, the status of the pars interarticularis, and the articular processes is necessary at the time of spinal surgery.

North et al.[64] conducted a retrospective review of their experience with reoperation on the lumbosacral spine in an effort to identify patient characteristics and treatment methods associated with the most successful outcomes. Surgical techniques and strategies for repeat operation included decompression with aggressive removal of extruded disc and hypertrophic scar, generous lateral decompression, and foraminotomy (but not facetectomy except in cases of spondylolysis). Spondylolysis, spondylolisthesis, or gross instability on dynamic flexion-extension films were corrected with intertransverse and facet fusion with autologous bone graft. The operative procedures in this study included discectomy (24%), foraminotomy (50%), laminectomy (80%), excision and/or lysis of epidural scar (28%), and fusion (27% including repair of pseudarthrosis in 4%). One hundred two patients were interviewed at an average of 5.05 years postoperatively by disinterested third parties. Thirty-four percent of the surgeries were successful, with 50% of patients reporting pain relief at a follow-up of 2 years. Twenty-one patients who were disabled before surgery returned to work postoperatively; 15 who worked preoperatively became disabled and/or retired. Patients reported loss of neurologic function (strength, sensation, bowel and bladder control) more often than improvement in daily activities. A majority reduced or eliminated their intake of analgesics after reoperation. Outcomes were better for younger and female patients. Favorable outcomes were associated with a history of good results from prior surgeries, a small number of prior operations, the absence of epidural scar requiring surgical lysis, employment before surgery, and predominance of radicular (as opposed to axial) pain. No relationship between outcome and inclusion of a fusion in the operative procedure was found.

Ablative Procedures

Ablation of the involved primary afferent neurons is expected to provide pain relief whether pain originates in a joint, disc, or ligament due to mechanical nociceptive stimulation or from an irritated injured peripheral nerve, root, or dorsal root ganglion. Large myelinated afferents, which do not normally conduct pain sensation, may transmit postinjury hyperalgesia. Primary afferent ablation should address any of these mechanisms.

Dorsal rhizotomy may reduce persistent radicular pain after lumbosacral surgery. More proximal radiofrequency thermocoagulation of the primary spinal nerve trunk and ganglion has been described. Dorsal

---

INSTABILITY

- Clinical instability: Abnormal symptomatic motion
- Mechanical instability: May not be symptomatic
- Objective criteria suggesting local instability include
  - Demonstrated motion on flexion-extension films
  - Progressive spinal deformity in any direction, including an unstable spondylolisthesis
  - Iatrogenic surgical destruction of more than one complete zygapophyseal joint
  - Obvious pseudarthrosis with motion within the prior fusion site

rhizotomy does not interrupt all afferent input because numerous ventral root afferents with cell bodies in the dorsal root ganglia exist, and these convey pain from peripheral receptors even after dorsal rhizotomy. Dorsal root ganglionectomy has also not been effective for FBSS.[58] One study of 13 patients reported no "successes" in the mean follow-up period of 5.5 years.[58]

Incomplete primary afferent ablation after dorsal root ganglionectomy could be the cause of disappointing results of dorsal rhizotomy. Authors for a century have described cell bodies in the ventral root and peripheral nervous system that escape ganglionectomy. The central pathophysiology of pain after nerve injury and deafferentation may be another reason for the failure of primary afferent ablation to relieve pain.

Percutaneous radiofrequency lumbar facet denervation (medial branch posterior primary ramus neurotomy) is a simple peripheral ablative procedure for patients with mechanical low back syndrome. North et al.[61] reported that facet denervations are successful on a long-term basis in just under one half of the patients interviewed. These results compare favorably with that of reoperation, with the advantage that the morbidity of facet denervation is negligible.

The problem may lie in the pathophysiology of pain following nerve injury and deafferentation.[7] The effectiveness of ablative procedures to relieve pain may be limited by a number of anatomic and physiologic changes occurring after primary afferent ablation. Nerve fibers sprout into denervated areas in the peripheral nervous system. After dorsal rhizotomy, intact axons from dorsal roots above and below the lesion form new central synapses in the dorsal horn. Dorsal horn recordings show confirmatory receptive field expansion and abnormal bursting activity. Single unit recordings during thalamic electrode implantation to treat the pain from deafferentation show abnormal bursting activity and somatotopic map reorganization.

Attempts to screen patients and improve outcomes for these procedures have used diagnostic paravertebral nerve root blocks preoperatively.[8] Nerve root blocks can be misleading and do not reliably predict the results of ablative or decompressive procedures. Nerve blocks distal to painful root or peripheral nerve lesions may provide temporary relief. These nonspecific results may reflect the systemic effects of lidocaine but are probably related to a central mechanism that interrupts pain sensation after blockade of major afferent input to the painful segment. Permanent interruption of the same input does not necessarily afford lasting relief.

Many fusion patients experience minimal postoperative pain following posterolateral fusion of the transverse processes and facet joints. Rees[66] suggests that the early postoperative absence of pain results from denervation of the facet joints during the fusion. Percutaneous procedures to denervate the facet joints were devised, using a modified tenotomy knife with posterior ramus section, that yielded a 99% success rate; the success rate was associated with a 20% incidence of subcutaneous hematomas. Fluoroscopically guided temperature-controlled radiofrequency thermocoagulation of

the articular nerve branches has since been added to percutaneous procedures.[61] Low-voltage stimulation at the proper site reproduces the patient's pain without eliciting a motor response. One study[61] of low-voltage stimulation showed significant improvement in 88 of 100 unoperated patients with low back pain and/or sciatica with no motor weakness.

Percutaneous lumbar facet denervation is a simple ablative procedure for patients with mechanical low back pain. Patients with prior lumbar surgery respond less well to facet injections or denervations than unoperated patients. In our experience, previously operated and unoperated patients show minimal differences in response to nerve blocks, and no difference to denervations.[56] Facet denervations are successful on a long-term basis in just under half the patients, which is comparable to the results of reoperation, but facet denervations have the advantage of negligible morbidity. Coagulation can produce a motor or sensory deficit if the electrode is placed too close to the primary spinal root or articular ramus (below the intertransverse ligament). Deafferentation procedures are also irreversible and have the potential to alter the substrate for alternative procedures such as electrical stimulation devices. Ganglionectomy destroys primary afferents that ascend in the dorsal columns, which renders SCS ineffective.

Dorsal Column or Spinal Cord Stimulation

In 1965, Shealy et al.[40] and coworkers introduced electrical stimulation of the spinal cord to treat patients with intractable chronic pain. Before 1980, surgeons used arachnoid, subdural, or intradural electrode systems, with a laminectomy required for permanent placement of the electrode. Contemporary programmable systems with multiple electrodes are more reliable, and clinical outcome is significantly better than the older single-channel devices. SCS provides an effective reversible technique for the management of chronic intractable pain, and FBSS has been the most common indication for this procedure. The current epidural electrodes avoid much of the morbidity associated with the earlier systems that included problems with CSF leakage and lead migration. The most frequent complications of the electrode systems are technical or equipment related. Infection is infrequent but does occur in about 5% of procedures.[59] Epidural electrode placement has eliminated spinal fluid leakage and arachnoid scarring.

SCS should be considered only for patients who have exhausted standard surgical therapy and in whom inoperable arachnoid fibrosis and/or nerve root injury is the major pathologic condition. Percutaneous placement of electrodes involves potential morbidity and discomfort to the patient comparable to diagnostic nerve blocks, myelography, and denervation procedures. The two types of epidural electrodes in use are a narrow Silastic strip containing four electrode discs, and a single or multicontact insulated wire electrode. The electrode is tunneled into the dorsal epidural space by percutaneous or semipercutaneous techniques with the patient under local anesthesia and with mild intravenous sedation. Intraoperative stimulation must produce reproducible paresthesias covering the area of the patient's pain. All electrodes are inserted through a Touhy-style needle placed in the dorsal epidural space. A 2- to 7-day period of trial stimulation using percutaneous extension wires and an external pulse generator is recommended to determine the optimal parameters for pain relief. The surgeon can then calculate when the patient receives worthwhile stimulation-induced analgesia and which electrode poles deliver optimal analgesia.

After successful trial stimulation, a second operation is necessary to implant the lead. A passively driven radiofrequency-coupled receiver is placed in a subcutaneous pocket with the battery and adjustable pulse generator contained in a unit equipped with a detachable antenna disc. The fully implantable pulse generator is a recent innovation to the implant system. Programmable multicontact devices that permit noninvasive selection of stimulating anodes and cathodes facilitate selection of an effective stimulation combination.[63] Correspondence of stimulation paresthesias with the topography of the pain is important for the patient to obtain pain relief.

Researchers[50,51] have attempted to understand the physiologic and pharmacologic mechanisms involved in the analgesic effects of SCS. Meyerson et al.[51] showed that SCS caused an increase in extracellular gamma-aminobutryric acid (GABA) in the dorsal horn of rats. Stimulation affects the firing pattern of neurons, and increased GABA concentration reduces the release of excitatory amino acids in the dorsal horn.[50,51]

Kumar et al.[38] analyzed the effects of SCS on 114 patients with FBSS. Long-term pain relief was reported in 52 patients and failure in 49 patients, after follow-up periods that averaged 5 years; 13 patients did not receive permanent implants because of failure during the trial stimulation period. No significant differences were found in the success rates of males and females to SCS, although better results in women patients have been reported previously in the literature. North et al.[59] followed 50 patients with SCS implants for 5 years postoperatively. The outcome was considered successful in 53% of patients after 2 years, whereas 47% of patients called the implant a success after 5 years. An important benefit of SCS is the significant reduction in drug usage reported by most patients.

Patients with radicular pain have better results from SCS and reoperation for FBSS than patients with axial (low back) pain.[64] Technical improvements in SCS have increased the physician's ability to treat axial pain that is mechanical or nociceptive rather than neuropathic, for which SCS is a less effective procedure.[63] Although the original physiologic rationale for dorsal column stimulation (based on the gate-control theory of spinal cord pain processing) has come into question,[64] the technique satisfactorily relieves pain in selected patients.

A prospective, randomized study is necessary even though SCS has superior results in patients with a history of problems with pain management. The natural history of neural compression and/or instability or pseudarthrosis managed conservatively with pain relieving techniques such as SCS is unknown. The condition of many of these reoperated patients may have deteriorated postoperatively, but their deterioration may have been worse without surgery. Long[42] states that "effective use requires a thorough understanding of the pain states to be treated, appreciation of the comorbidities that accompany chronic pain, an infrastructure to support the patient and the surgeon, and a dedication to lifelong care for the patient with the implant."

Deep Brain Stimulation

Deep brain stimulation (DBS) provides an effective, reversible, nondestructive technique for surgical management in selected patients with intractable nociceptive and/or central deafferentation pain states, including FBSS. The two principal DBS sites are the periaqueductal/periventricular gray region of the midbrain and caudal thalamus, and the ventroposterior medial/ventroposterior lateral thalamic somatosensory relay nuclei including the posterior limb of the internal capsule. The mechanisms, pathways, and neurotransmitters involved in stimulation-produced analgesia remain an area of active investigation and have been effective in some patients with low back or lower extremity pain that is refractory to peripheral nerve stimulation or SCS. Research[83] has shown that the periaqueductal periventricular gray area is the most effective stimulation site. In three studies of patients with DBS implants,[37,39,67] 58 (72%) had the system internalized and 42 of these (72%) experienced substantial long-term pain relief. Although severe complications are rare, greater risks are associated with DBS than with other neuromodulatory modalities.

Intraspinal Narcotics

Intraspinal narcotic therapy has been reported in small series of FBSS patients with encouraging results.[2] None have extended follow-up or disinterested third-party assessment, making comparison with other therapies difficult. Chronic subarachnoid narcotic infusion in patients with arachnoiditis, with a demonstrated propensity to react adversely, is problematic.[62]

REHABILITATION PROGRAMS AND FAILED BACK SURGERY SYNDROME

Because rehabilitation is an important part of the management of FBSS, rehabilitation programs specializing in this area are proliferating. Patients who completed such programs have a high rate of reported functional improvement and return to work although pain ratings are not reduced.[1] These programs complement surgical management for selected patients, but the roles of these different therapies await prospective study.

CONCLUSIONS

Because FBSS comprises a wide range of primary pathologies, the determination of precise treatments and outcomes is difficult. It is difficult to assess treatment options or outcomes accurately until clarification with subsets of diagnoses is achieved. The FBSS diagnosis is too broad to be meaningful and should be eliminated.

The overall goal in the management of the patient with FBSS is to maximize quality of life, using a treatment program that is highly effective yet poses the smallest amount of risk. The diagnosis and management of FBSS often requires sophisticated diagnostic imaging and multidisciplinary input. Many patients are best served by a comprehensive pain treatment program. The cornerstone of any successful program for patients with FBSS is accurate diagnosis, allowing precisely targeted therapy. The inherent complexity of these cases necessitates a diagnostic and therapeutic protocol that is precise and cost efficient.

The initial decision for surgery must be based on valid criteria and a clear anatomic diagnosis, with imaging studies that can confirm the clinical diagnosis rather than provide the primary indication for operation. The best solution for recurrent symptoms after spine surgery is a preventive one that avoids inappropriate surgery. Criteria for surgical intervention must be strictly applied, and postoperative emphasis on rehabilitation must be maintained. The patient with persistent or recurrent symptoms forces the surgeon to reassess the original indications for surgery. With the lack of strong indications for surgical intervention, together with psychosocial issues, the possibility exists that repeat surgery will not solve the problem. The treating physician has to determine the cause of the pain with history, physical examination, and confirmatory studies even with clear indications for the initial surgery. If the second operation is well founded, the probability of success is high and approaches the success rate of the primary procedure.

The surgical treatment options for FBSS include re-operation, but this applies to few patients. Ablative procedures, with the exception of facet neurotomy, have a low yield and high morbidity. Reversible, minimally invasive treatments such as SCS have a more favorable benefit-risk ratio. In the assessment of FBSS, the goals and expectations of both the patient and physician must be clear. Expectations of surgical procedures are often unrealistic and beyond what could be expected from any form of therapy. Recognition of the patient's needs, goals, and expectations will provide a more successful outcome. Prospective comparisons of treatment methods and continued research into the pathologic basis of pain in FBSS should lead to better selection criteria and more effective therapy.

SELECTED REFERENCES

Barrios C et al.: Clinical factors predicting outcome after surgery for herniated lumbar disc: an epidemiological multivariate analysis, *J Spinal Disord* 3:205, 1990.

Bogduk N, Long DM: The anatomy of the so-called "articular nerves" and their relationship to facet denervation in the treatment of low back pain, *J Neurosurg* 51:172-177, 1979.

Braun I, Hoffman J, David P: Contrast enhancement in CT differentiation between recurrent disc herniation and postoperative scar: prospective study, *Am J Radiol* 145:785, 1985.

Bundschuh CV et al.: Distinguishing between scar and recurrent herniated disc in postoperative patients: value of contrast-enhanced CT and MR imaging, *Am J Neuroradiol* 11:949, 1990.

Burton CV: Causes of failure of surgery on the lumbar spine: ten-year follow-up, *Mt Sinai J Med* 58:183, 1991.

Meyerson BA et al.: Modulation of spinal pain mechanisms by spinal cord stimulation and the potential role of adjuvant pharmacotherapy, *Stereotact Funct Neurosurg* 68(1-4 Pt 1):129-140, 1997.

Ross JS et al.: MR imaging of lumbar arachnoiditis, *Am J Radiol* 149:1025, 1987.

Spengler DM et al.: Low-back pain following multiple lumbar spine procedures: failure of initial selection? *Spine* 5:356, 1980.

REFERENCES

1. Anderson SR: A rationale for the treatment algorithm of failed back surgery syndrome, *Curr Rev Pain* 4(5):395-406, 2000.
2. Angel IF, Gould HJ Jr, Carey ME: Intrathecal morphine pump as a treatment option in chronic pain of nonmalignant origin, *Surg Neurol* 49(1):92-98, 1998.
3. Barrios C et al.: Clinical factors predicting outcome after surgery for herniated lumbar disc: an epidemiological multivariate analysis, *J Spinal Disord* 3:205, 1990.
4. Bems DH, Blaser SI, Modic MT: Magnetic resonance imaging of the spine, *Clin Orthop* 244:78, 1989.
5. Bobman SA et al.: Postoperative lumbar spine: contrast-enhanced chemical shift MR imaging, *Radiology* 179:557, 1991.
6. Bircher M et al.: Discitis following lumbar surgery, *Spine* 13:98, 1988.
7. Bogduk N, Long DM: The anatomy of the so-called "articular nerves" and their relationship to facet denervation in the treatment of low back pain, *J Neurosurg* 51:172-177, 1979.
8. Bogduk N, Long DM: Percutaneous lumbar medial branch neurotomy: a modification of facet denervation, *Spine* 5:193, 1980.
9. Braun I, Hoffman J, David P: Contrast enhancement in CT differentiation between recurrent disc herniation and postoperative scar: prospective study, *Am J Radiol* 145:785, 1985.
10. Brodsky AE, Kovalsky ES, Khalil MA: Correlation of radiologic assessment of lumbar spine fusions with surgical exploration, *Spine* 16:S261-S265, 1991.
11. Bundschuh CV: Imaging of the postoperative lumbosacral spine, *Neuroimaging Clin North Am* 3(3):499-516, 1993.
12. Bundschuh CV et al.: Distinguishing between scar and recurrent herniated disc in postoperative patients: value of contrast-enhanced CT and MR imaging, *Am J Neuroradiol* 11:949, 1990.
13. Burton CV: Lumbosacral arachnoiditis, *Spine* 3(1):24-30, 1978.
14. Burton CV: Causes of failure of surgery on the lumbar spine: ten-year follow-up, *Mt Sinai J Med* 58:183, 1991.
15. Burton CV et al.: Causes of failure of surgery on the lumbar spine, *Clin Orthop* 157:191, 1981.
16. Crock HV: Anterior lumbar interbody fusion: indications for its use and notes on surgical technique, *Clin Orthop* 165:157, 1982.
17. Dolan RA: Spinal adhesive arachnoiditis, *Surg Neurol* 39(6):479-484, 1993.
18. Esses SI, Moro JK: The value of facet joint blocks in patient selection for lumbar fusion, *Spine* 18:185, 1993.
19. Fager CA, Freidberg SR: Analysis of failures and poor results of lumbar spine surgery, *Spine* 5:87, 1980.
20. Fairbank J, Park W, McCall I: Apophyseal injection of local anesthetic as a diagnostic aid in primary low-back pain syndromes, *Spine* 6:598, 1981.
21. Finnegan W et al.: Results of surgical intervention in the symptomatic multiply-operated back patient: analysis of sixty-seven cases followed for three to seven years, *J Bone Joint Surg Am* 61:1077-1082, 1979.
22. Ford L, Key I: Postoperative infection of the intervertebral disc space, *South Med J* 48:1295, 1955.
23. Fraser R, Osti O, Vernon-Roberts B: Discitis after discography, *J Bone Joint Surg Br* 69:26, 1987.
24. Frymoyer JW, Cats-Barfl BW: An overview of the incidences and costs of low back pain, *Orthop Clin North Am* 22:263, 1991.
25. Frymoyer JW et al.: Failed lumbar disc surgery requiring second operation: a long-term follow-up study, *Spine* 3:7-11, 1978.
26. Frymoyer JW et al.: Psychologic factors in low-back-pain disability, *Clin Orthop* 195:178, 1985.

27. Frymoyer JW et al.: Clinical tests applicable to the study of chronic low-back disability, *Spine* 16:681, 1991.
28. Gieseking H: Lokalisierte Spondylitis nach operiertern Bandscheibenvorfall. *Zenti-albi Chir* 76:1470, 1951.
29. Greenwood J, McGuire T, Kimball F: A study of causes of failure in the herniated disc operation: an analysis of 67 repeated cases, *J Neurosurg* 9:15, 1952.
30. Grenier N, Vital J, Greselle J, Richard O: CT discography in the evaluation of the postoperative lumbar spine, *Neuroradiology* 30:232, 1988.
31. Howe J, Frymoyer JW: The effects of questionnaire design on the determination of end results in lumbar spinal surgery, *Spine* 10(9):804-805, 1985.
32. Hudgins W: The role of microdiscectomy, *Orthop Clin North Am* 14:589, 1983.
33. Hueftle MG et al.: Lumbar spine: postoperative MR imaging with Gd-DTPA, *Radiology* 167:817, 1988.
34. Ikko E et al.: Computed tomography after lumbar disc surgery, *Acta Radiol* 29:179, 1988.
35. Kim SS, Michelsen CB: Revision surgery for failed back surgery syndrome, *Spine* 17(8):957-60, 1992.
36. Krempen J, Smith B: Nerve root injection: a method for evaluating the etiology of sciatica, *J Bone Joint Surg Am* 56:1435, 1974.
37. Kumar K, Toth C, Nath RK: Deep brain stimulation for intractable pain: a 15-year experience, *Neurosurgery* 40(4):736-746, 1997.
38. Kumar K et al.: Epidural spinal cord stimulation for treatment of chronic pain: some predictors of success—a 15-year experience, *Surg Neurol* 50(2):110-120, 1998.
39. Levy RM, Lamb S, Adams JE: Treatment of chronic pain by deep brain stimulation: long term follow-up and review of the literature, *Neurosurgery* 21(6):885-893, 1987.
40. Long DM: Stimulation of the peripheral nervous stem for pain control, *Clin Neurosurg* 31:323, 1983.
41. Long DM: Nonsurgical therapy for low back pain and sciatica, *Clin Neurosurg* 35:351, 1989.
42. Long DM: Failed back surgery syndrome, *Neurosurg Clin North Am* 2:899, 1991.
43. Long DM: Decision making in lumbar disc disease, *Clin Neurosurg* 39:36, 1992.
44. Long D: Chronic adhesive spinal arachnoiditis: pathogenesis, prognosis, and treatment, *Neurosurg* 2:296, 1992.
45. Long DM et al.: Clinical features of the feedback syndrome, *J Neurosurg* 69:61, 1988.
46. Love J, Rivers M: Spinal cord tumors simulating protruded intervertebral discs, *JAMA* 179:878, 1962.
47. Mayfield F: Complications of laminectomy, *Clin Neurosurg* 23:435, 1976.
48. MacNab I: Negative disc exploration: an analysis of the causes of nerve root involvement in 68 patients, *J Bone Joint Surg Am* 53:891, 1971.
49. Markwalder TM, Reulen HJ: Diagnostic approach in instability and irritative state of a "lumbar motion segment" following disc surgery: failed back surgery syndrome, *Acta Neurochir (Wien)* 99(1-2):51-57, 1989.
50. Meyerson BA, Linderoth B: Mechanisms of spinal cord stimulation in neuropathic pain, *Neurol Res* 22(3):285-292, 2000.
51. Meyerson BA et al.: Modulation of spinal pain mechanisms by spinal cord stimulation and the potential role of adjuvant pharmacotherapy, *Stereotact Funct Neurosurg* 68(1-4 Pt 1):129-140, 1997.
52. Milward F: Changes in the intervertebral discs following lumbar puncture, *Lancet* 2:183, 1936.
53. Nashold BJ, Hrubec A: *Lumbar disc disease: a twenty-year clinical follow-up study*, St. Louis, 1971, Mosby.
54. Neill S: Computed tomography in failed back syndrome, *Radiogr Today* 57:9, 1991.
55. Nizard RS, Wybier M, Laredo JD: Radiologic assessment of lumbar intervertebral instability and degenerative spondylolisthesis, *Radiol Clin North Am* 39(1):55-71, 2001.
56. North R, Zeidman S: Failed back surgery syndrome, *Cont Neurosurg* 16:1, 1993.
57. North RB, Kidd DH, Piantadosi S: Spinal cord stimulation versus reoperation for failed back surgery syndrome: a prospective, randomized study design, *Acta Neurochir Suppl* 64:106-108, 1995.
58. North et al.: Dorsal root ganglionectomy for failed back surgery syndrome: a 5-year follow-up study, *J Neurosurg* 74:236, 1991.
59. North RB et al.: Failed back surgery syndrome: 5-year follow-up after spinal cord stimulator implantation, *Neurosurgery* 28(5):692-699, 1991.
60. North RB et al.: Failed back surgery syndrome: 5-year follow-up in 102 patients undergoing repeated operation, *Neurosurgery* 28:685, 1991.
61. North RB et al.: Radiofrequency lumbar facet denervation: analysis of prognostic factors, *Pain* 57(1):77-83, 1994.
62. North RB et al.: Spinal cord compression complicating subarachnoid infusion of morphine: case report and laboratory experience, *Neurosurgery* 29:778, 1991.
63. North RB et al.: Spinal cord stimulation for chronic, intractable pain: superiority of "multi-channel" devices, *Pain* 44:119, 1991.
64. North RB et al.: Spinal cord stimulation versus reoperation for the failed back surgery syndrome: a prospective, randomized study design, *Stereotact Funct Neurosurg* 62(1-4):267-272, 1994.
65. Ramirez L, Thisted R: Complication and demographic characteristics of patients undergoing lumbar discectomy in community hospitals, *Neurosurgery* 25:226, 1989.
66. Rees WS: Comparision of reported results of various treatments for relief of benign intractable pain, *Med J Aust* 1(17):642-643, 1977.
67. Richardson DE: Deep brain stimulation for the relief of chronic pain, *Neurosurg Clin N Am* 6(1):135-144, 1995.
68. Roberts M: Complications of lumbar disc surgery, *Spinal Surg* 2:13, 1988.
69. Ross JS et al.: MR imaging of lumbar arachnoiditis, *Am J Radiol* 149:1025, 1987.
70. Ross JS et al.: MR imaging of the postoperative lumbar spine: assessment with gadopentetate dimeglumine, *Am J Roentgenol* 155:867-872, 1990.
71. Sienkiewicz PJ, Flatley TJ: Postoperative spondylolisthesis, *Clin Orthop* 221:172-180, 1987.
72. Sorenson L, Mors O, Skorlund O: A prospective study of the importance of psychological and social factors for the outcome after surgery inpatients with slipped lumbar disc operated on for the first time, *Acta Neurochir* 88:119, 1987.
73. Sotiropoulos S et al.: Differentiation between postoperative scar and recurrent disc herniation: prospective comparison of MR, CT, and contrast enhanced CT, *Am J Neuroradiol* 10:639, 1989.
74. Spengler DM et al.: Low-back pain following multiple lumbar spine procedures: failure of initial selection? *Spine* 5:356, 1980.
75. Teplick JG, Haskin ME: Review: computed tomography of the postoperative lumbar spine, *Am J Radiol* 141:865, 1983.
76. Teplick JG, Haskin ME: Intravenous contrast-enhanced CT of the postoperative lumbar spine: improved identification of recurrent disc herniation, scar, arachnoiditis, and discitis, *Am J Radiol* 143:845, 1984.
77. Turnbull F: Postoperative inflammatory disease of lumbar discs, *J Neurosurg* 10:469, 1953.
78. Waddell G et al.: Failed lumbar disc surgery and repeat surgery following industrial injuries, *J Bone Joint Surg Am* 61:201, 1979.
79. Waddell G et al.: Objective clinical evaluation of physical impairment in chronic low back pain, *Spine* 17:617, 1992.
80. Walsh T, Weinstein J, Sprath K: Lumbar discography in normal subjects: a controlled prospective study, *J Bone Joint Surg Am* 72:1081-1088, 1990.
81. Weiss T, Treisch J, Krazner E: CT of the post-operative lumbar spine: the value of intravenous contrast, *Neuroradiology* 28:241, 1986.
82. Wilkinson LS et al.: Defining the use of gadolinium enhanced MRI in the assessment of the postoperative lumbar spine, *Clin Radiol* 52(7):530-534, 1997.
83. Young RF et al.: Release of beta-endorphin and methionine-enkephalin into cerebrospinal fluid during deep brain stimulation for chronic pain: effects of stimulation locus and site of sampling, *J Neurosurg* 79(6):816-825, 1993.

X

After Treatment

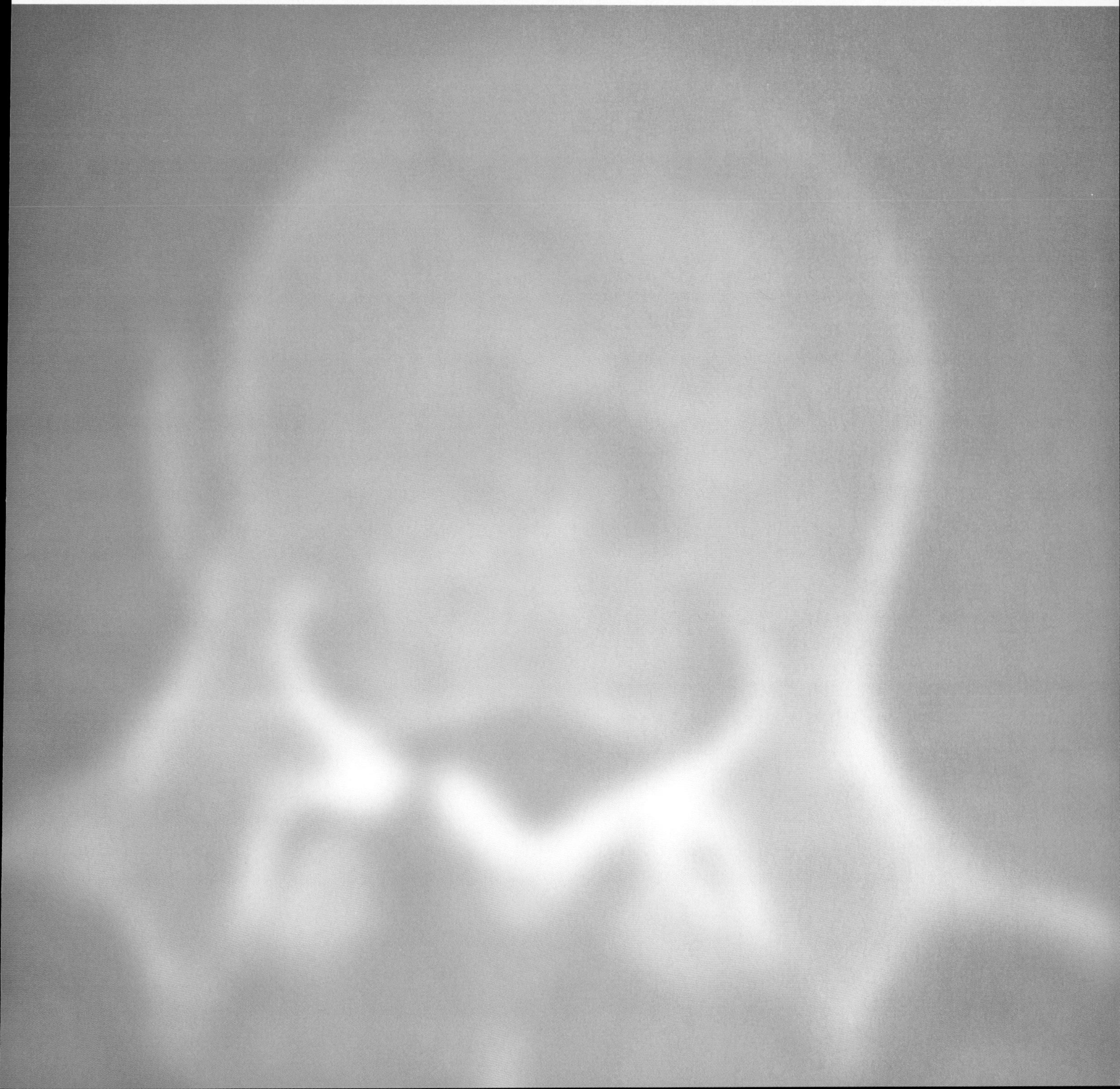

Spinal Orthoses

David Gregory Anderson, Alexander R. Vaccaro,
Kenneth F. Gavin, Amy Fromal

Spinal orthoses are externally applied devices designed to restrict motion of the spinal column. Forces are indirectly applied to the spine by contacting the soft tissue envelope of the head, neck, chest, trunk, and pelvis. Spinal orthoses are divided into categories depending on the region of the spine immobilized. These categories include cervical orthoses (COs), cervicothoracic orthoses (CTOs), cervicothoracolumbosacral orthoses (CTLSOs), thoracolumbosacral orthoses (TLSOs), lumbosacral orthoses (LSOs), and sacral orthoses (SOs). Spinal orthoses are generally useful for treating spinal deformities, trauma, pain, and instability and providing postoperative spinal protection.

The earliest documented use of cervical orthoses for restricting neck motion and correcting deformities comes from the fifth Egyptian dynasty (2750-2625 BC). The biomechanical principles of modern cervical orthoses can be traced to the devices used by Hippocrates and his successors. Ambrose Pare (1509-1590 AD) is considered to be the first to widely use lumbar bracing. Professor Nicholas Andry (1704-1756 AD), at the University of Paris, improved the understanding of biomechanical bracing principles and invented a number of orthoses.[76]

Today a wide variety of spinal orthoses are available. Spinal orthoses are often named for their inventor (e.g., Benjamin-Taylor, Jewett, Guilford), the locality where they were designed (e.g., Philadelphia collar, Boston brace, Milwaukee brace), or by a description of the brace (e.g., two-poster, TLSO).

Spinal orthoses may be prescribed by specifying the type of orthosis (e.g., Philadelphia collar) or the orthosis category (e.g., lumbosacral orthosis). It is important for the prescribing physician to understand the biomechanical principles of orthosis usage and to communicate to the fitting orthotist the degree and type of instability that is anticipated. Equally important is patient education in the donning, care, and precautions of the prescribed orthosis and close follow-up.

In a biomechanical review Chase et al. concluded that orthoses may be divided into three categories based on the purpose of the orthosis.[18] First, an orthosis may have a dynamic function, in which the purpose is to actively correct an existing deformity. This type of brace is used to treat idiopathic scoliosis or adolescent kyphosis.

Second, an orthosis may limit spinal motion, thus relieving pain related to disc disease or osteoporosis. This category of brace is also useful in providing protection of a postoperative spinal construct. Third, an orthosis may support the spine against the effects of gravity. Such a brace would be used to support the spine following a fracture or support the spine in the setting of weak spinal musculature. In clinical usage an orthosis may combine these functions to achieve a clinical goal.

Advances in materials science and engineering have revolutionized the bracing industry in recent years. Traditional plaster body casts have been replaced by modern thermoplastic braces that are lightweight, relatively comfortable, and durable. Magnetic resonance imaging (MRI)–compatible materials such as graphite and titanium are now commonly used in braces such as the halo vest orthoses. Synthetic brace liners made of sheepskin and Orthowick increase patient comfort and compliance. In spite of the advances in orthosis design, many newer braces remain unproven in a clinical setting. Therefore it is important to thoroughly evaluate an orthosis before using the device.

The comfort and motion restriction provided by spinal braces vary widely. When choosing an orthosis for a given condition, the degree and direction of potential instability must be considered along with the level of compliance that is required. Although studies have documented the level of motion restriction of many orthoses in normal spines, the ability of braces to restrict motion in unstable spines has not been well studied. In this chapter we will review the biomechanical and clinical features of the commonly used spinal orthoses and discuss the appropriate application of spinal bracing in a clinical setting. Due to the unique biomechanics of various spinal regions, bracing of the cervical spine will be discussed separately from the thoracolumbar spine.

CERVICAL BIOMECHANICS

Cervical motion in biomechanical cadaver studies is generally measured by establishing exact movement of joints within six degrees of freedom reference system (translation and rotation in the X, Y, and Z planes). For clinical studies, however, measurements of neck flexion-extension, lateral bending, and rotation have proven to be more useful.[80] The flexibility of intervertebral discs, shape and inclination of the facets, integrity of capsular structures, and ligamentous laxity help to determine the overall motion of the cervical spine, as well as the intersegmental motion of an individual cervical articulation.

Normal cervical motion has been evaluated by Kottke and Mundale and found to average 70 ± 10 degrees of flexion, 45 ± 10 degrees of side bending, and 75 ± 10 degrees of axial rotation.[47] Using radiographs to study motion, Bhalla and Simmons found the C4 to C5 articulation to be the most flexible,[11] whereas Kottke and Mundale recorded the most mobility at the C5 to C6 level.[47] Using cineradiography, Fielding noted that flexion caused a slight anterior shift in the upper vertebral bodies, whereas extension resulted in a posterior shift.[26]

SPINAL MOBILITY IN CERVICAL ORTHOTICS

The first author to report studying cervical motion in cervical orthoses was Jones.[39] Using cineradiography, he was able to evaluate the relative motion of normal subjects wearing soft and rigid collars. Although specific measurements were not made, he concluded that rigid collars restricted motion more than soft collars but noted that all the collars tested allowed significant motion of the cervical spine.

Various authors have measured cervical motion while wearing orthoses using both goniometry[28,41,54,71] and radiography.* Fisher et al. measured cervical motion using both goniometry and radiography and concluded that goniometry provided an adequate clinical tool to assess the overall sagittal plane motion of the cervical spine.[28] Generally motion control is better for flexion-extension than for lateral bending and axial rotation with the use of external orthoses.†

Fisher et al. studied cervical motion in 10 normal subjects using the Camp collar, Philadelphia collar, four-poster brace, and the sternal occipital mandibular immobilizer (SOMI) brace. Overall the SOMI brace provided the best restriction to flexion of the upper cervical spine, whereas the four-poster brace provided the best immobilization of the mid and lower cervical spine. The Philadelphia collar, which was rated the most comfortable, was found to provide the least immobilization at all levels, particularly the occiput to C2 region. The Camp collar provided the best immobilization of the C1 to C2 region but was noted to be extremely uncomfortable.[27,28]

Johnson et al.[38] used radiography and photographs to evaluate cervical motion in normal subjects using the soft collar, Philadelphia collar, four-poster brace, cervicothoracic brace, and SOMI brace. In addition, similar techniques were used to measure motion in the halo vest orthosis applied following cervical surgery or trauma. The orthoses were ranked according to their ability to limit flexion-extension as follows (most to least stable): halo > cervicothoracic brace > four-poster brace > SOMI = Philadelphia > soft collar. Only the halo vest orthoses provided good control of sagittal plane motion for the occiput to C2 region. Cervical collars were noted to increase motion at the occiput to C1 articulation. The halo vest orthosis provided the best immobilization of the subaxial cervical spine but still allowed segmental motion at each level. The SOMI orthosis effectively limited C1 to C2 flexion (but not extension) and thus was recommended for isolated atlantoaxial flexion instability.[38]

Kaufman et al.[41] compared cervical motion in 10 normal subjects wearing either the Philadelphia collar or the Nec-Loc collar. The Nec-Loc collar was found to be more restrictive, limiting 62% of flexion-extension, 43% of lateral bending, and 62% of axial rotation. The Philadelphia collar limited flexion-extension by 46%, lateral bending by 25%, and axial rotation by 29%.

Podolsky et al.[72] evaluated collars for trauma extrication and transport in normal subjects comparing the soft collar, hard collar, Philadelphia collar, extrication collar, bilateral sandbags with tape, and Philadelphia collar with sandbags and tape. Sandbags and tape provided excellent motion restriction except in extension. Adding the Philadelphia collar to sandbags and tape provided a further limitation of extension. The use of collars without sandbags and tape did not provide rigid restriction of cervical motion.

Lunsford et al.[54] measured cervical motion and skin contact pressure in normal subjects wearing the Philadelphia collar, Miami J collar, Malibu collar, and Newport Extended Wear collar (now called the Aspen collar). The more contemporary collars were found to provide motion control that was similar to or better than the Philadelphia collar. Overall the Malibu collar provided the best immobilization, restricting lateral bending 41%, extension 40%, flexion 57%, and axial rotation 61%.[54]

Koch and Nickel[43] studied cervical spine segmental motion in six patients with unstable injuries immobilized in a halo orthosis. Lateral radiographs were taken in positions chosen to replicate normal daily activities including lying supine, sitting with a forward or backward lean, and recumbent in a transport sling. The halo uprights were instrumented with strain gauges to determine the compression or distraction forces on the neck in each position. The authors noted significant motion of the cervical spine with changes in position. They described a phenomenon of "snaking," where some spinal segments assumed a flexed posture and other regions assumed an extended posture. Overall C4 to C5 experienced the greatest mobility, averaging 7.2 degrees, whereas C2 to C3 demonstrated the highest percentage (42%) of normal motion. Axial forces measured at the halo uprights varied from 5 pounds compression to 17 pounds traction and were noted to change dramatically with changes in position or when patients abducted their arms.[43]

Anderson et al.[3] also studied intersegmental motion of the cervical spine in 42 patients immobilized in a halo vest orthosis for unstable trauma. Lateral radiographs

---

*References 20, 21, 26, 28, 39, 72.
†References 9, 21, 28, 38, 41, 80.

MOBILITY IN CERVICAL ORTHOSES

- No available orthosis provides complete motion control of the cervical spine.
- The halo vest orthosis provides the best motion restriction of the occiput–C1 to C2 articulation.
- Cervicothoracic orthosis generally provides better motion restriction of the mid and lower cervical spine compared with cervical collars.
- The halo vest orthosis may allow significant "snaking" of the mid and lower cervical spine.
- Cervical collar generally restricts flexion and extension better than lateral bending.

COMFORT OF ORTHOSES

- Orthosis comfort is an important factor improving compliance with brace wear.
- Brace contact pressures may exceed capillary closing.
- Orthosis usage with comatose or insensate patients is a special challenge, requiring close supervision of skin integrity.
- Weaning from a cervical orthosis should begin when immobilization is no longer needed.

---

were taken in an upright and supine position within 5 days of injury. Noninjured levels demonstrated an average 3.9 degrees of angulation, whereas injured levels demonstrated 7 degrees of angulation and 1.7 mm of translation. Overall, motion greater than 3 degrees of angulation or 1 mm of translation was observed at 77% of injured levels. Lateral radiographs in a supine and upright position were recommended by the authors to determine the "personality" of a cervical injury, allowing unstable injuries to be treated by an alternate method.[3]

ORTHOSIS COMFORT

An external orthosis controls cervical motion by force application to the soft tissue envelope surrounding the spine. The forces necessary to control motion vary depending on the level of injury and degree of instability. In addition, individual variations in anatomy will significantly affect the ability of an orthosis to provide immobilization.

Therefore a cervical orthosis should be carefully matched to the patient's anatomy. Ideally the contact area should be maximized to lower contact pressures. Soft or semirigid materials should be used at the sites of skin contact. When possible, breathable materials should be used to minimize perspiration beneath the orthosis.

Comatose and insensate patients provide a special challenge with orthosis utilization. Due to the loss of protective sensory input, skin breakdown beneath the orthosis is a significant risk. Frequent inspection of skin contact areas is mandatory when using an orthosis for patients with altered sensory function. In addition, braces with low intrinsic contact pressures should be chosen. Finally, trimming or shaving hair beneath the brace and maintaining good skin hygiene can lower the risk of skin compromise.

Off-the-shelf orthoses, which are available in a wide range of sizes, can be fit to the majority of patients. However, some situations require a custom-fabricated orthosis to accommodate unusual patient anatomy. Using modern thermoplastic technology, brace fabrication has become a more rapid process. Another option for noncompliant patients or those requiring intimate control of neck motion is a plaster or fiberglass body cast connected to a halo ring.

Fisher studied skin contact pressures in eight normal subjects fitted with the SOMI brace. Contact pressures well in excess of the capillary closing pressure (CCP) were observed with the SOMI applied in the "usual" fashion. The SOMI braces were then reapplied using a pressure-sensing device to maintain the contact pressure at 20 mm Hg (below CCP). When comparing cervical motion in the "usual" and "low pressure" fittings of the SOMI, no degradation of the motion control was observed. The author concluded that with the use of a pressure-sensing device, cervical braces could be applied with lower pressures without a loss of motion control.[27]

Plaisier et al.[71] studied craniofacial pressures in 20 normal subjects wearing the Stiffneck collar, Philadelphia collar, Miami J collar, and Newport collar (now called the Aspen collar) in an upright and supine position. The Stiffneck collar was noted to exceed CCP in both the upright and supine positions. The Philadelphia collar exceeded CCP only in the supine position. Both the Newport and Miami J collars demonstrated skin contact pressures below the CCP in the upright and supine positions, which correlated with improved subjective comfort reported by the test subjects.[71]

Weaning from a collar is preferable to simply removing the orthosis at the end of a period of immobilization. This allows the patient an opportunity to gradually regain normal muscle strength and proprioception and lessens the psychologic fear many patients have regarding removal of brace protection. During this transition a program of physical therapy and use of a soft collar may help to hasten the return of physiologic neck mobility.

SELECTED ORTHOSES

The soft cervical collar has gained popularity for treating cervical strains and "whiplash" syndromes (Figure 57-1). Soft collars are inexpensive and comfortable but provide minimal motion restriction. Soft collars promote muscle relaxation and provide a kinesthetic reminder to patients following minor cervical strains.

The Philadelphia collar is a two-piece semirigid Platazote orthosis reinforced with anterior and posterior plastic struts (Figure 57-2). The Philadelphia collar provides better motion control than the soft collar and is an excellent choice for use during bathing due to the water-resistant Platazote construction. Due to the absence of a removable liner, the Philadelphia collar is not as optimal

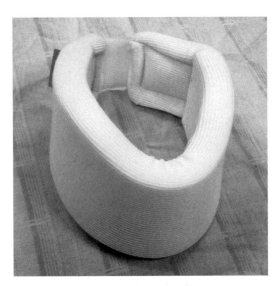

Figure 57-1.   Soft cervical collar. *(Courtesy D. Anderson)*

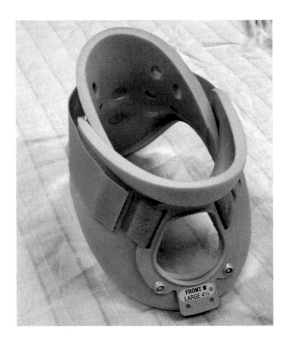

Figure 57-2.   Philadelphia collar.

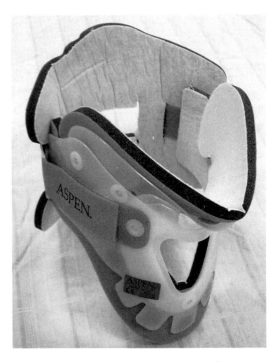

Figure 57-3.   Aspen cervical collar.

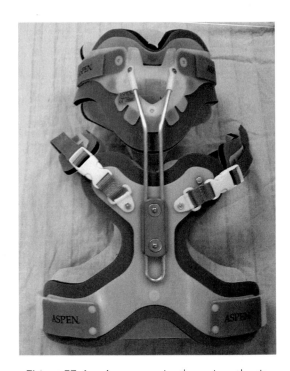

Figure 57-4.   Aspen cervicothoracic orthosis.

for hygiene or comfort with long-term use as the Miami J or Aspen collars.

The Aspen collar (formerly the Newport collar) is a semirigid, two-piece cervical orthosis utilizing an adjustable plastic shell with removable foam pads. The Aspen collar also includes a relief area for posterior incisions. Although the Aspen collar is more expensive, it provides greater motion control and is more comfort-

able than the Philadelphia collar. A version of the Aspen collar has a thoracic extension and therefore is more appropriate when motion control of the lower cervical spine and cervicothoracic junction is required (Figures 57-3 and 57-4).

The Miami J collar is a similar semirigid two-piece cervical orthosis utilizing a firm plastic shell with removable foam pads. The Miami J orthosis provides slightly

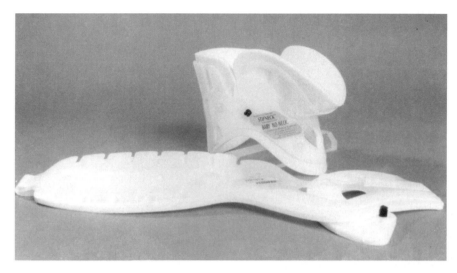

Figure 57-5. Stiffneck collar.

Table 57-1	Motion Restriction of Cervical Orthoses					
	PERCENT MOTION RESTRICTION					
Orthosis	Flexion	Extension	Total Sagittal Motion	Lateral Bending (1 direction)	Axial Rotation (1 direction)	Cost*
Soft collar	26	26	10	8	17	$19.00
Philadelphia collar	74	59	46	25	29	$94.00
Aspen collar	59	64	62	31	38	$94.00
Miami J collar	85	75	73	51	65	$94.00
Malibu collar	57	40	NT	41	61	$229.00
Nec-Loc collar	NT	NT	62	43	62	$94.00
Stiffneck collar	73	63	70	50	57	$94.00
SOMI	93	42	87	66	66	$264.00
Minerva	NT	NT	NT	NT	NT	$398.00
Halo	NT	NT	96	96	99	$1916.00

*Prices are based on Medicare allowables year 2001 (region A).
NT, Not tested.

better motion restriction than the Aspen collar without the optional thoracic extensions.

The Malibu brace is a semirigid two-piece orthosis utilizing a firm plastic shell with incorporated inner padding. The Malibu brace projects farther on the chest and back compared with the Miami J and Aspen collars to improve motion restriction in the sagittal plane.

The motion restriction and estimated cost of each collar are detailed in Table 57-1. The semirigid cervical collars described above are similar in concept, but each has unique features that may prove useful in a particular setting. Each of these collars may be used to treat stable cervical fractures and provide postoperative protection. Our preference is to use a semirigid cervical collar with removable pads for patients requiring more than 2 to 3 weeks of immobilization. These collar provide superior comfort and allow cleaning or exchange of the pads for optimal patient hygiene. Patients are also provided with a Philadelphia collar for use during bathing (Table 57-1).

Rigid cervical collars are routinely used during pre-hospital extrication and transport of accident victims. In this setting the ideal collar is inexpensive, provides rigid motion control, is compact for storage, and is easy to apply. The Nec-Loc and Stiffneck collars fulfill these goals and are commonly used by paramedics and ambulance personnel (Figure 57-5). The motion restriction provided is detailed in Table 57-1. These collars exert relatively high skin contact pressures and thus should only be used on a short-term basis.

The SOMI orthosis has a rigid anterior chest piece attached to curved, rigid shoulder supports (Figure 57-6). Straps cross the patient's back and attach the shoulder supports to the lower section of the chest piece. Mandibular and occipital supports project from the anterior yolk to control the head. During mastication, the mandibular component can be removed and replaced with a separate headpiece employing a forehead strap. The SOMI orthosis can be easily applied to a patient in

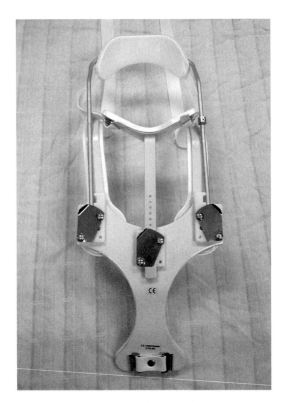

Figure 57-6.   SOMI orthosis.

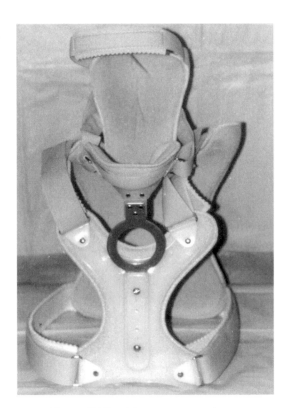

Figure 57-7.   Minerva vest orthosis.

the supine position. As shown in Table 57-1, the SOMI orthosis provides good restriction to flexion, especially in the upper cervical spine, but is less optimal for control of neck extension.[37]

The original Minerva brace was a molded CTO that provided fairly rigid control of mid and lower cervical motion at the expense of comfort. A modern version of the Minerva jacket orthosis, however, incorporates a padded, plastic vest component similar to a halo vest and padded extensions to the mandibular region and posterior head, yielding a more comfortable fit (Figure 57-7). Such a Minerva jacket orthosis has been compared to the halo orthosis by Benzel et al. in 10 patients following cervical surgery or a cervical fracture.[10] The Minerva jacket orthosis was found to allow less sagittal plane segmental motion compared with the halo at all levels except C1 to C2. This phenomenon is attributed to the "snaking" of the cervical vertebrae within the halo as described above. Patients preferred the comfort of the Minerva jacket orthosis compared with the halo orthosis.

Selecting the appropriate treatment for an injury to the cervical spine involves many considerations, including injury type, severity, neurologic status, risk of displacement, patient body habitus, and patient compliance. The treatment for each cervical injury should be individualized after considering these factors. The most commonly used orthoses for treatment of various cervical spine injuries are listed in Table 57-2.

COMPLICATIONS OF CERVICAL ORTHOSES

Complications of cervical orthoses may include inadequate immobilization, skin rash or breakdown, psy-

chologic dependence, muscle atrophy, soft tissue contracture, pain, and decreased pulmonary function.[77] Nearly all cervical orthoses can be modified or adjusted to increase comfort and decrease skin pressure. In general the risk of complications can be minimized by proper brace selection and fitting and close follow-up.

THE HALO SKELETAL FIXATOR

Perry and Nickel[70] first described the halo orthosis for immobilization of the cervical spine in patients with poliomyelitis. The original halo consisted of a complete metal ring that curved upward posteriorly to allow surgical access to the neck. Holes in the ring allowed the placement of metal pins that pierced the outer table of the skull, providing secure fixation of the head. Two upright posts attached the ring to a molded body cast. Since the original description, the indications for the halo orthosis have been expanded to include stabilization in cases of trauma, tumor, infection, inflammatory arthritis, fusion surgery, and congenital deformities involving the cervical spine in both children and adults.*

Modern halo rings are generally made of radiolucent and nonferromagnetic materials such as carbon fiber and titanium. This allows radiographic and MRI studies to be performed in the halo device. Body casts have been largely replaced by molded plastic body jackets with padded inserts. These body jackets are available in a wide variety of sizes and are easier to apply and more comfortable than a body cast. However, casting continues to be useful in rare situations of abnormal body

*References 14, 16, 22, 44, 46, 50, 51, 59, 67-70.

Table 57-2	Cervical Injuries and Methods of Treatment
Diagnosis	**Orthosis**
Occipitalocervical dislocation and subluxation	Surgery plus halo
Fractures of the atlas	
Posterior arch	Rigid collar
Jefferson fractures	
<7-mm displaced	Rigid collar or SOMI
>7-mm displaced	Halo
Rupture mid transverse ligament	Surgery
Odontoid fractures	
Type I	Rigid collar
Type II	Halo
If: >4-mm translation	
>10-degree angulation	
>40 years of age	Consider surgery
Type III	Halo
Atlantoaxial rotatory deformities	
Reducible	Rigid collar/SOMI
Unreducible	Traction or surgery
Hangman's fracture	
Type I	Rigid collar
Type II	Rigid collar/halo
Type III	Surgery
C3 to C7 flexion-compression fractures	
Stable (intact posterior ligamentous complex)	Rigid collar/halo
Unstable	Surgery
C3 to C7 burst fracture	
Neurologically intact/stable fracture pattern	Halo/Minerva/Yale
Neurologic deficit/unstable fracture pattern	Surgery
Facet dislocations	
Unilateral	Halo then surgery
Bilateral	Halo then surgery
Distraction-extension injuries	
Intact ligaments/disc	
Without spinal cord compression	Halo/surgery
With spinal cord compression	Surgery
Ruptured ligaments/disc/fracture	Surgery
C3 to C7 compression-extension injuries	
No displacement	Rigid collar/Minerva/Yale
Displaced	Surgery

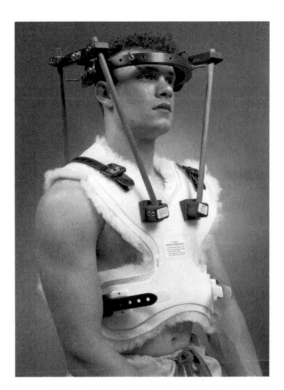

Figure 57-8. Halo vest orthosis.

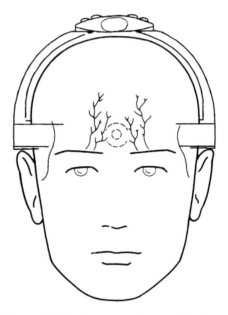

Figure 57-9. Diagram of supraorbital and supratrochlear nerves.

habitus. In spite of advances in halo materials, the basic principles and halo application techniques have changed little since their original description (Figure 57-8).

Application of the Halo Ring

The optimal position for the anterior halo pins is in the anterolateral skull, approximately 1 cm above the orbital rim, below the greatest circumference (equator) of the skull and cephalad to the lateral two thirds of the eyebrow. This region has been described as the "safe-zone" because it lies lateral to the supraorbital and supra-

trochlear nerves and the frontal sinus and medial to the temporal fossa (Figure 57-9). In addition, the halo pin is protected from displacement into the orbit by the supraorbital rim and lies on a relatively flat portion of the skull, preventing superior migration. Posterior halo pin placement is less critical due to the uniform thickness of the skull and lack of critical anatomic structures. The optimal posterior location is at the 4 o'clock and 8 o'clock positions (12 o'clock is the anterior midline), thus lying behind the ears and opposite the anterior pins. With the pins in these positions, the halo ring should lie just above the eyebrows and the upper helix of the ear.[14,15]

Garfin et al.[30] studied skull osteology in cadavers and noted that the anterolateral and posterolateral skull had the most optimal bone for halo pin placement. The temporal fossa, in contrast, was noted to have much thinner cortical bone and little space between the bony tables.[30] Pin placement in the temporal fossa may also tether the temporalis muscle, which can cause pain and impede mastication.

Halo pins should be inserted perpendicular to the skull (at the equator) to improve the mechanical strength of the bone-pin interface.[7,78] Pin insertions up to 10 inch pounds (1.13 newton-meters) have been shown to minimally penetrate the outer table of the skull.[12] Mechanical testing of the pin-bone interface with cyclic loading and load-to-failure have shown that 8 inch pounds (0.9 newton-meters) of torque significantly improves the mechanical quality of the bone purchase compared with 6 inch pounds (0.68 newton-meters).

Children and infants may require modification of the halo application technique due to softer, thinner calvaria bone. Patients less than 2 years of age should be treated with six to eight halo pins with a reduced torque in the range of 2 to 5 inch pounds.[44,59]

Generally application of a halo device in an unstable cervical condition requires at least three individuals. One person immobilizes the head while the second and third persons apply the halo ring. Proper sizing of the ring and vest should be completed prior to starting the application process. The ring should allow 1 to 2 cm of clearance around the perimeter of the head. Vest sizes are determined by measuring the patient's chest circumference. All materials should be assembled prior to beginning halo application. A list of the suggested materials is provided in Box 57-1. A resuscitation crash cart should be available during the procedure.

The patient should be placed in a supine position. Folded towels are placed under the head and shoulders to provide access for halo ring placement. Alternatively the patient's head may be supported beyond the edge of a gurney. The head should be manually immobilized throughout the halo application process.

Box 57-1	Materials List for Halo Vest Application

Halo ring (1 to 2 cm larger than head)
Sterile halo pins
Torque wrench or "breakaway" wrenches
Halo vest (sized to chest)
Upright connecting rods
Rod-to-ring connector blocks
Wrenches to tighten nuts on halo pins
Razor
Povidone-iodine solution
Sterile gloves
Sterile gauze
Syringe/needle
Local anesthetic
Crash cart

Hair is shaved at the posterior pin sites, and the skin is prepared with povidine-iodine solution. The halo ring is placed around the skull in the optimal location and held with positioning pins or by a fourth assistant. The skin is then anesthetized with local anesthetic at the site selected for the halo pin insertion. The anesthetic should be injected deep to the level of the galea.

The pins should be threaded through the halo ring holes and advanced to the point of skin contact. Diagonally opposing pins should then be advanced in small (2 inch pounds) increments to allow all the pins to seat evenly. The pins are tightened with a torque screwdriver to the appropriate torque (6 to 8 inch pounds). Skin incisions are not required for the halo pins.[13] During tightening of the anterior pins, the patient should be asked to close his or her eyes and relax the forehead to prevent tethering of the skin. Any area of skin tenting around the halo pins after final tightening should be released with a scalpel.

The halo vest should be applied by rolling the patient or elevating the patient's trunk while maintaining in-line traction of the cervical spine. After the posterior portion of the halo vest has been applied, the patient may return to a supine position. The anterior vest is secured, and then the uprights are assembled to attach the vest and halo ring. Final tightening of all components should be performed. Radiographs of the cervical spine should then be taken to confirm a satisfactory position of the spine. Halo screwdrivers and wrenches should be maintained at the patient's bedside or taped to the halo vest to be used in an emergency.

The pins should be retorqued 24 to 48 hours after the initial halo application. The pin sites should be cleaned every 1 to 2 days with a dilute solution of hydrogen peroxide. Periodic radiographic studies should be taken to ensure that an appropriate position of the cervical spine is maintained.

After halo removal, the use of a comfortable, semirigid cervical orthosis such as a Philadelphia, Aspen, or Miami J collar is useful to allow the patient to gradually regain muscle strength and confidence. Physical therapy to improve muscle strength, proprioception, and range of motion is beneficial in restoring cervical function and lessening neck pain.

Halo Complications

Complications of halo usage include pin loosening, pin-site infections, loss of reduction, severe pin discomfort, swallowing difficulties, dural puncture, pin-site bleeding, nerve injury, severe scaring, skin breakdown under the halo vest, and intolerance by patients.[29]

Pin loosening may occur during the course of halo treatment and may precipitate pain at the pin site. New-onset pain at a pin site should lead the physician to suspect pin loosening or infection. Pin loosening may be managed by retightening the pin one time. Resistance should be met within the first two complete rotations of the pin. If no resistance is met, the pin should be replaced. In this case, the new pin should be seated before removal of the loose pin.

Rizzolo et al.[75] evaluated pin torque in a clinical series of patients treated in the halo device. Complications, including pin-tract infections and pin loosening, were compared using a torque protocol of either 6 inch pounds or 8 inch pounds. No significant differences between the groups were identified.[75]

Pin-tract infections are relatively common in patients treated with long-term halo immobilization. Aggressive pin care and oral antibiotic medication should be initiated to treat minor pin-site erythema or drainage. If the patient fails to rapidly respond to this treatment or if cellulitis develops, the pin should be replaced and systemic antibiotics should be administered. New pins should be placed through an adjacent hole in the ring, as long as it will not result in placement of the pin through an area of cellulitis. The new pin should be placed prior to removing the infected pin to prevent shift of the head within the halo ring.

Swallowing difficulties may be encountered with excessive neck flexion, extension, or translation of the head in a posterior or anterior direction. Adjustment of the head position in the halo device will usually resolve the dysphagia symptoms.

Dural puncture is a potentially severe complication of halo usage and may result from a fall while wearing a halo orthosis.[29] Dural puncture may lead to an intracranial abscess and should be suspected in a patient who presents with symptoms of headache, photophobia, nausea, and fever. Aggressive treatment is indicated, including head computed tomography (CT) scanning, neurosurgical consult, appropriate débridement, and antibiotics. Dural puncture in the absence of infection should be treated with pin removal, prophylactic antibiotics, and upright positioning. If cerebrospinal fluid (CSF) drainage is a continued problem, a lumbar subarachnoid drain may be considered.

Five patients who developed a subdural abscess in connection with halo traction were reviewed by Garfin et al.[31] All infections resolved with pin removal, drainage and débridement of the abscess, and parenteral antibiotics. The use of long-term halo traction was discouraged due to the risk of an intracranial infection.[31]

Anticoagulation therapy may lead to pin-site bleeding in patients immobilized in a halo device. Packing and pressure dressing of the pin sites has been reported to be ineffective. Therefore tapering or discontinuation of anticoagulation medications may be necessary to control the bleeding.[14]

Many miscellaneous complications, including nerve injury, should be avoidable with proper halo application technique. The risk of skin compromise under a halo vest may be minimized by applying a well-fitting vest with ample padding. Older patients with severe thoracic kyphosis or insensate patients present an elevated risk for skin breakdown and mandate close skin monitoring (Figure 57-10).

Glaser et al. reviewed the complications of halo vest usage in 248 patients treated for cervical spine instability following trauma (203 patients) or after surgery (45 patients). Complications included 1 death, 23 lost reductions, 24 cases of late instability, 14 pin-tract problems, 2 displacements of an anterior strut graft, 5 premature halo removals, and 7 miscellaneous problems. There were no cases of neurologic deterioration in the halo device. The authors noted that ligamentous cervical injuries had a high incidence of late instability in spite of halo treatment.[32]

THORACIC AND LUMBOSACRAL BIOMECHANICS

White and Panjabi[80] have described the spine as a series of semirigid bodies (vertebrae) separated by viscoelastic linkages (ligaments and discs). This mobile column is suspended in a viscoelastic cylinder (the body). Braces generally attempt to control motion of the vertebral

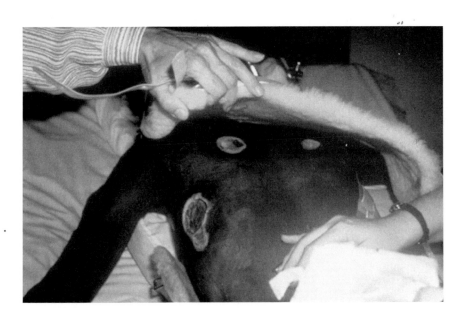

Figure 57-10. Skin breakdown under halo vest.

column indirectly by applying forces to the viscoelastic cylinder containing the spine.[77]

The thoracic spine is significantly more rigid than the cervical or lumbar spine due to the supporting rib cage. The effects of the rib cage have been shown to increase the stiffness of the thoracic spine by 200%.[4] Motion of the lumbar spine is greater in the sagittal plane (flexion-extension) than in a transverse plane (rotation) due to the orientation of the facet joints. In addition, flexion mobility is greater than extension mobility in this region of the spine.[77]

Biomechanical stresses are often concentrated at the junctions between the mobile and rigid portions of the spine, and thus the cervicothoracic, thoracolumbar, and lumbosacral junctions are subject to high mechanical stresses. In addition, during lifting activities the compressive forces in the thoracolumbar spine are enormous. For instance, a force-body diagram analysis of a 170-pound man bending to lift a 200-pound weight demonstrates a compressive load on the thoracolumbar spine of 1568 pounds. To lessen these stresses, some have theorized that abdominal muscle contraction during lifting converts the abdominal cavity into a rigid cylinder, limiting the forces on the spine to 791 pounds in the above example.[58]

Albrook, using radiographic measurements, found that the flexion-extension arc of lumbar motion (L1 to S1) in healthy subjects ranged from 52 to 83 degrees. In addition, the range of motion was noted to decrease with age, degenerative spinal disease, and back pain but not with race or sex. The greatest sagittal plane mobility was noted at the L4 to L5 and L5 to S1 levels with gradually decreasing motion noted at higher lumbar levels.[1]

Thoracolumbosacral orthoses function by contact with the trunk, especially at the bony prominences, including the iliac crest, thoracic cage, sternum, and posterior spine. Although difficult to quantitate, the degree of immobilization provided to obese patients with bracing is significantly less than that provided to slender patients using the same brace.[80] The lumbar spinal motion restriction provided by bracing has been evaluated in terms of gross body motions[48] and intersegmental motion.[5] Overall, braces in the lumbar spine are more effective at providing gross immobilization than segmental immobilization.[48]

MOTION, MUSCLE ACTIVITY, AND PRESSURE STUDIES

The effectiveness of thoracolumbosacral orthoses has been investigated by studying motion restriction, muscle activity, and intradiscal pressure while wearing various braces. Each method of evaluation has certain limitations. This section will review the available studies evaluating brace effectiveness.

Norton and Brown[65] published the first quantitative evaluation of spinal motion in lumbar braces. In their study four LSO braces (three rigid, one soft) and a TLSO brace were evaluated in normal subjects. Motion from L3 to S1 was evaluated by measuring the angular change of Kirschner wires placed in the spinous processes and by performing lateral radiographs of the spine. Motion at the lumbosacral junction was noted to increase with

use of rigid braces compared with the unbraced state. Motion restriction was noted to be better for the upper and mid lumbar spine than for the lower lumbar spine and lumbosacral junction.

Lumsden and Morris[53] studied the clinical and radiographic motion of the lumbosacral spine in axial rotation by placing Steinmann pins into the posterior superior iliac spine of test subjects. Motion restriction of a chairback brace and a corset were compared to the unbraced state. The authors found that use of either brace increased the rotational motion of the lumbosacral joint.

Lantz and Schultz[48] studied gross motion restriction (flexion-extension, lateral bending, and torsion) in five healthy men wearing a chairback brace, a molded TLSO, and a lumbosacral corset. Active motion in both a standing and sitting position was evaluated using end-point photography. Although each orthosis limited motion compared to the unbraced state, all braces allowed significant motion. Overall the corset provided the least motion restriction, whereas the TLSO provided the most motion restriction. The TLSO was found to limit overall mobility by one third to one half of normal.

Fidler and Plasmans[25] studied the effect of a canvas corset, Raney jacket, Baycast jacket, and Baycast spica on segmental mobility of the lumbosacral spine in five healthy men using lateral radiographs. The canvas corset was noted to reduce angular movement at each level by approximately one third, whereas the Raney and Baycast jackets limited motion of the mid lumbar spine by about two thirds. Braces without leg extension (corset and jacket braces) were unable to immobilize the L4 to S1 region. However, the Baycast spica was noted to limit motion at L4 to L5 and L5 to S1 to 12% and 8% of the unbraced state, respectively.

Axelsson et al.[5,6] studied the effect of bracing on lumbosacral motion in an erect and supine position 1 month following a lumbosacral fusion using stereophotogrammetric analysis. In this study, subjects were instructed to limit active motion of the spine. The authors measured vertebral translation after soft tissue healing but prior to bony consolidation. In an initial study a canvas corset and a molded, rigid TLSO brace were compared with the unbraced state. In a subsequent study a molded, rigid TLSO and a TLSO with a unilateral leg extension immobilizing one hip were compared with the unbraced state. None of the braces were effective in limiting sagittal, vertical, or transverse translation at the lumbosacral junction compared with the unbraced state. The authors concluded that lumbosacral braces provided minimal segmental immobilization but rather functioned primarily to limit gross motion of the trunk.

In addition to evaluating motion restriction, measurements of muscle activity are also used to assess the effectiveness of orthoses. Morris and Lucas[57] studied myoelectric activity and intraabdominal pressure in subjects wearing lumbar braces during static lifting postures. The authors reasoned that decreased myoelectric activity in a brace should correlate with decreased loads in the lumbar spine. The investigators found that the use of lumbar braces was associated with decreases in the myoelectric activity of abdominal muscles but did not appear to change intraabdominal pressure.

Waters and Morris[79] studied 10 subjects wearing a corset, a chairback brace, or no brace. Subjects were evaluated at rest and while walking on a treadmill by attachment of multiple electromyography (EMG) leads to back and abdominal muscles. Abdominal muscle activity was noted to be decreased at rest and with moderate activity when wearing either brace compared with the unbraced state. In contrast, the erector spinae activity was unaffected by brace wear at rest but was increased with use of the chairback brace during high-level activities.

A conflicting result was noted by Lantz and Schultz,[49] who studied oblique abdominal and erector spinae myoelectric muscle activity in five healthy men who performed 19 isometric tasks. Each subject was examined unbraced and wearing a lumbosacral corset, a chairback brace, and a molded TLSO. Muscle activity while wearing each brace was compared with the unbraced state. Muscle activity while performing isometric tasks in each brace demonstrated marked variability, leading the authors to conclude that bracing did not consistently reduce myoelectric activity and therefore failed to provide a consistent reduction in lumbar spinal loads.

Intradiscal pressure analysis has also been used to assess the effectiveness of lumbosacral bracing. Nachemson and Morris[60] measured intradiscal pressure in subjects fitted with an inflatable lumbar corset. When not inflated, intradiscal pressure was about the same as in the unbraced state. However, when the corset was inflated, the intradiscal pressure was decreased by about 25%.

Nachemson et al.[62] evaluated intradiscal and intragastric pressures and myoelectric trunk muscle activity in four subjects wearing the Camp corset, Raney flexion jacket, and the Boston brace. Intradiscal pressure and myoelectric muscle activity were not consistently affected by wearing any of the braces. Generally, intradiscal pressure was increased by flexion tasks while wearing the braces and decreased by extension tasks.

In conclusion, lumbar orthoses are able to restrict gross lumbar motion better than intersegmental motion. TLSO and LSO braces provide better immobilization of the upper and mid lumbar spine than the lower lumbar spine. Segmental immobilization of the L4 to S1 segments requires the use of a thigh extension to control the position of the pelvis. Lumbar orthosis seems to have minimal effect on the muscle activities of the trunk muscles during normal activities. Intradiscal pressure is not greatly affected by the use of a lumbar orthosis without an inflatable bladder.

EFFECTS OF TLSO AND LSO BRACES

- Decreased gross motion of the upper lumbar spine
- Increased motion of the L4 to S1 region unless a thigh extension is added
- Decreased intradiscal pressure and myoelectric activity not consistent with use of LSO braces
- Intradiscal pressure decreased with use of LSO braces with an inflatable bladder

---

DEFORMITY ORTHOSES

Scoliosis and kyphosis are spinal deformities commonly treated by spinal bracing. The natural history of adolescent idiopathic scoliosis (AIS) has been well documented and demonstrates a high risk of curve progression in younger patients, higher magnitude curves, and thoracic and thoracolumbar curve patterns.[81] Spinal bracing has shown efficacy for improving the natural history of AIS in several large, well-controlled studies.[24,52,61] In a more recent study Korovessis et al.[45] demonstrated that treatment of scoliosis with a TLSO brace maintained a number of radiographic parameters at prebrace levels at an average of 3.5 years after termination of brace wear and reduced the incidence of surgery in the study population.

In spite of this, some investigators have found that bracing has not provided superior results to the unbraced natural history. Goldberg et al.[33] compared 32 patients treated in Boston with bracing to 32 patients treated without bracing in Ireland. All curve parameters at the start of bracing were comparable in the two groups. At the latest follow-up, curve progression was noted to be similar in both groups regardless of whether or not bracing was utilized. Noonan et al.[64] evaluated the use of the Milwaukee brace in 111 patients with AIS at an average of 6 years 4 months after cessation of brace wear. Overall 48% of the patients progressed in the brace 5 or more degrees, and 42% met the criteria for surgical intervention. The authors suggested that the outcome of bracing in this study failed to support the conclusion that bracing improved the natural history of untreated AIS. Goldberg et al.[34] reviewed the results of 153 patients with AIS who were not treated by bracing. The rate of surgery in this group was noted to be 28.1% and thus not different from the rate of surgery at centers where bracing of AIS is performed. Thus, although bracing remains a well-accepted treatment, the exact role of spinal bracing continues to evolve.

Classic recommendations are that a spinal brace for AIS should be worn 20 to 23 hours per day as supported by large, well-controlled studies showing efficacy of this length of treatment.[24,52,61] Some authors have suggested that part-time bracing for AIS may be an effective alternative to full-time brace wear.[35,73,74] Allington et al.[2] compared full-time and part-time brace wear with electrical stimulation in 188 patients. Curve progression of more than 5 degrees was seen in 36% of full-time braced patients, 41% of part-time braced patients, and 70% of the patients treated with electrical stimulation. Both forms of bracing showed statistical improvement compared with electrical stimulation; however, the differences between the part-time and full-time bracing programs failed to show a significant difference. Wiley et al.[81] evaluated 50 patients treated with the Boston brace for curves of 35 to 45 degrees. Three groups of patients were identified based on compliance with brace wear. Group 1 wore the brace 18 hours or more per day, group 2 wore the brace 12 to18 hours per day, and group 3 wore the brace 0 to 18 hours per day. Significant differences were seen between the groups in the initial amount of curve correction, as well as the amount of curve progression. Results favored the use of the brace for 18 or more hours per day.[81]

Bracing is generally recommended for progressive scoliosis with a curve magnitude of 25 to 40 degrees in patients with remaining growth. Lonstein and Winter[52] reported that the risk of curve progression is related to curve pattern, magnitude, age of the patient at the time of presentation, Risser grade, and menarchal status.

Scoliosis orthoses utilize transverse forces to correct coronal plane curves. Sagittal plane forces are also important to analyze, because malposition of brace contact points can worsen the sagittal alignment of the spine.[52,82] Mathematical modeling has shown that the optimal pad position in a scoliosis construct is at the apex of the curve or below.[23] Pad position can be evaluated clinically and radiographically to ensure that maximal corrective forces are utilized.

Generally bracing of AIS is able to correct a coronal deformity by as much as 50% in the first 6 to 9 months of brace treatment. There is often a gradual loss of correction so that at the end of bracing the curve magnitude may be 15% less than the prebrace deformity. Five years following the brace removal, the deformity is often about the same as the initial deformity. Thus the goals of bracing are to halt progression in a curve that would likely worsen and to maintain good spinal balance, resulting in a well-balanced curve with a magnitude of 40 degrees or less at skeletal maturity.[82]

The Milwaukee brace (a CTLSO) was developed by Blount and Schmidt for use in paralytic scoliosis following a spinal fusion. This brace was the first to be widely used for the nonoperative treatment of AIS. The results of scoliosis treatment using the Milwaukee brace continue to be the standard to which other forms of bracing are compared.[52,56]

The Milwaukee brace has a pelvic molded section with two posterior and one anterior upright connecting to a neck ring that has a throat mold and two occipital pads (Figure 57-11). Lateral thoracic and lumbar pads are attached to the brace frame depending on the curve pattern. In the presence of thoracic hyperkyphosis the thoracic pads are adjusted to provide some sagittal correction, whereas in thoracic hypokyphosis the pad is positioned to produce only a coronal plane force vector.[82] The Milwaukee continues to be used by many centers for high thoracic curves with an apex above T6 to T8.[36]

Underarm braces (TLSOs) have gained popularity in certain centers for treating AIS. Underarm bracing has demonstrated good results in curves with an apex at T6 to T8 and below.[8,17,35,55] Cosmesis and comfort are better with TLSO braces compared with the Milwaukee brace. Examples of underarm TLSOs include the Boston brace,[19] Wilmington brace,[8] and the Charleston bending brace.[74] The Charleston bending brace is designed for use while the patient is sleeping.

The Boston brace and Charleston bending brace have been compared by Katz et al.[40] in 319 patients with AIS. All patients were at least 10 years of age with a curve magnitude of 25 to 40 degrees and a Risser grade of 0 to 2. The Boston brace was noted to be significantly more effective than the Charleston bending brace in preventing progression and the need for surgery. This finding was especially significant in the patients with a curve magnitude of 36 to 40 degrees, where the Charleston bending brace demonstrated failure in 83%, compared with 43% of the patients wearing the Boston brace.[40] Howard et al. reported a retrospective review of 170 patients with AIS treated in either the TLSO, Charleston bending brace, or the Milwaukee brace. The TLSO and the Charleston bending brace were used in similar patients, whereas the Milwaukee brace was used for higher thoracic curves. The TLSO brace was found to be significantly more effective than the Charleston bending brace in reducing curve progression and the need for surgery.[36]

Contraindications to bracing for AIS include severe thoracic hypokyphosis or lordosis (<0 degrees of thoracic kyphosis) and severe obesity.[82] In some cases, brace modifications can be used to improve mild to moderate

---

BRACING

- May improve the natural history of untreated adolescent idiopathic scoliosis.
- Wearing scoliosis braces for longer periods each day more effective than short periods of brace wear.
- Treat scoliosis curves with an apex above T6 to T8 with a CTLSO brace.
- Best results with scoliosis braces when transverse forces contact the trunk at or below the apex of the deformity.
- Contraindication to bracing of idiopathic scoliosis: Thoracic lordosis.

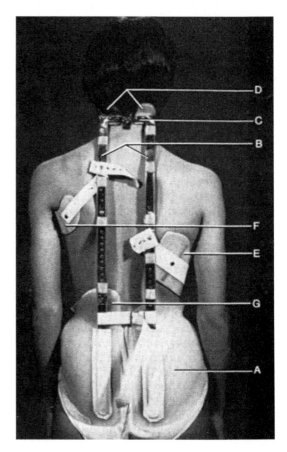

Figure 57-11. Milwaukee brace.

thoracic hypokyphosis. In addition, brace wear can be psychologically difficult for adolescents. Support groups are often helpful in introducing scoliosis patients to other teens with their condition.

SELECTED RIGID THORACOLUMBAR ORTHOSES

Body casts and custom-molded, plastic orthoses (TLSO) have traditionally been utilized to provide maximal stability to the thoracolumbar spine. Rigid orthoses can be fabricated from polyethylene (semiflexible plastic),

copolymer (rigid plastic), and polypropylene (very rigid plastic) (Figures 57-12 and 57-13). TLSO braces are able to restrict vertebral motion from T7 to L4. Thoracic lesions above T7 require purchase of the head and neck with a cervical extension. Alternately, upper thoracic lesions may be immobilized with a halo ring and long vest attachment. Unstable lumbar lesions at the L4 or L5 levels require the addition of a thigh extension to control pelvic mobility (Figure 57-14). The thigh extension should be positioned with the leg in extension or slight flexion to obtain the best control. Stable conditions can be treated with a drop-lock thigh extension

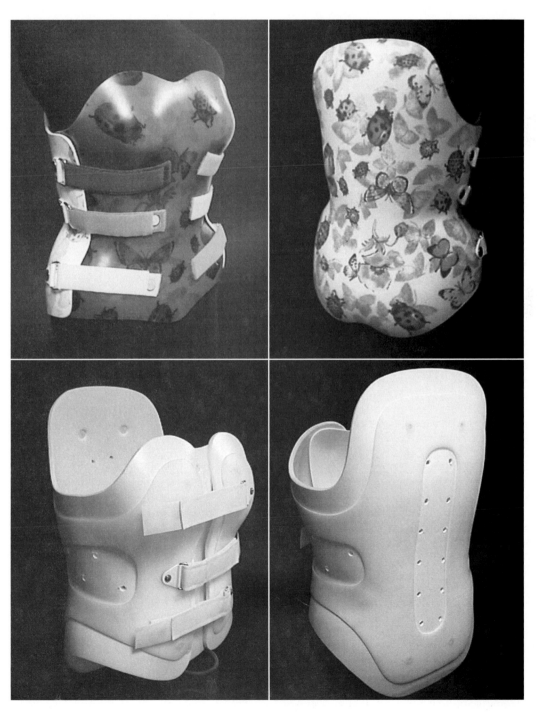

Figure 57-12. Anterior and posterior views of TLSO braces with various closing mechanisms.

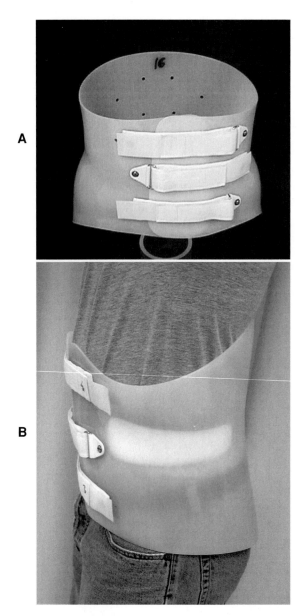

Figure 57-13. LSO brace. **A,** Anterior view. **B,** Lateral view in place on a patient.

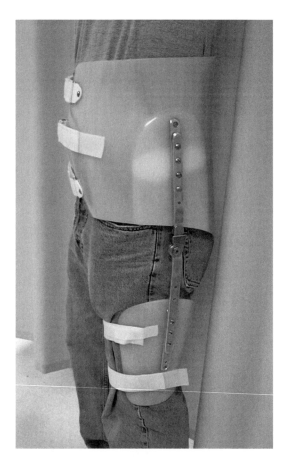

Figure 57-14. LSO with thigh extension.

allowing the patient to lock the thigh extension during ambulation and unlock the thigh extension to facilitate sitting.

The use of rigid bracing after lumbosacral fusion for spondylolisthesis has received attention by several authors. Kim et al.[42] reviewed 65 patients with isthmic spondylolisthesis who underwent a spinal fusion. In this study, patients were managed surgically with various fusion techniques, including posterolateral fusion or an anterior and posterior fusion. Only 15 patients were treated with instrumentation. Overall 72% of the patients achieved a solid fusion and 72% of patients had a good or excellent result following surgery. Due to the small number of patients with instrumentation, it was not possible to draw any conclusions regarding the efficacy of instrumentation in terms of fusion success

rate. A combined anterior and posterior fusion had a trend toward better clinical results compared with a posterolateral fusion but did not reach statistical significance. The use of a single-leg or double-leg spica cast rather than a TLSO brace was associated with a statistically significant improvement in the fusion rate and clinical outcome.

Johnsson et al.[38] divided patients with spondylolisthesis into two groups following an uninstrumented lumbar fusion. The first group (11 patients) was treated with a rigid, molded TLSO for 3 months, whereas the second group (11 patients) was treated with the same brace for 5 months postoperatively. All the patients were instructed to minimize active motions of the lumbar spine during the period of brace wear. Using x-ray stereophotogrammetric analysis, the time to fusion and rate of pseudarthrosis was determined. Decreased motion at the fusion site was noted to begin 3 to 6 months following fusion, and full rigidity of the fusion mass was complete by about 1 year postoperatively. The group wearing the brace for only 3 months had a statistically higher rate of pseudarthrosis compared with the 5-month bracing group.

Use of a rigid TLSO brace in the postoperative period may require specific modifications for patient comfort such as an incisional relief along the length of the incision, as well as soft interface padding to decrease skin irritation. Brace measurements should be taken in the

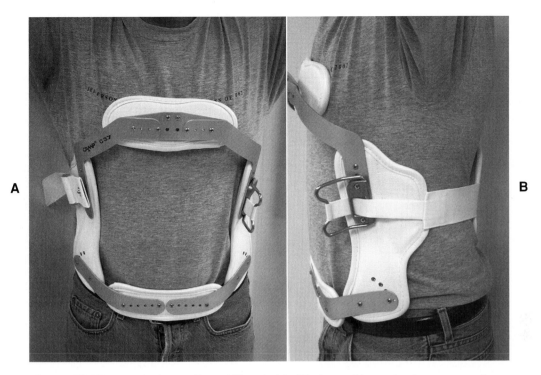

Figure 57-15. Jewett brace. Front **(A)** and side **(B)** views of brace in place on a patient.

early postoperative period so that brace fitting will not delay mobilization of the patient.

Rigid braces are also used frequently to treat patients with thoracolumbar fractures. The Jewett hyperextension orthosis uses a three-point system of pads to control sagittal plane motion of the thoracolumbar junction (Figures 57-15 and 57-16). Anterior pads contact the sternum and pubis while a posterior adjustable pad is placed over the spine at the apex of the injury or deformity. Tightening of the posterior pad will apply significant corrective forces to the apex of an injury to counteract the kyphosing tendency of an anterior column deficiency. The Jewett hyperextension brace has been successfully used to treat stable compression and burst fractures at the thoracolumbar junction. However, due to the skin pressure generated by the pads, this brace may not be tolerated in some patients.

Patwardhan et al.[68] performed a biomechanical evaluation of the Jewett brace, concluding that it was best for treating injuries at the T11 to L1 levels where the loss of segmental stiffness was not greater than 50%. Nagel et al.[63] studied the effectiveness of the Jewett brace for the treatment of seat-belt injuries (flexion-distraction injuries) at the L1 to L2 region, concluding that the Jewett brace provided fair limitation of flexion-extension motion but had minimal ability to control lateral bending or axial rotation.

Mild compression fractures in elderly adults are common and are often treated with bracing for comfort or to prevent progressive deformity. However, the need to brace these injuries remains controversial, and many physicians recommend early mobilization without a brace. Ohana et al.[66] reviewed the results of patients

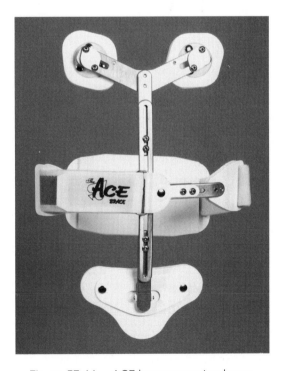

Figure 57-16. ACE hyperextension brace.

with up to 30% compression of the vertebral body who underwent brace treatment or mobilization without a brace. No differences were observed in these two groups with regard to deformity, healing, or pain. The authors recommended early mobilization without an orthosis and close clinical follow-up in treating these injuries.

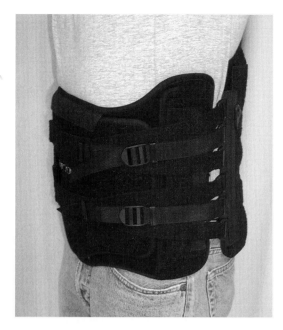

Figure 57-17. Ortholign brace.

> ## MOTION CONTROL
>
> - TLSO braces control spinal motion in the T7 to L4 region.
> - Motion control above T7 and below L3 is achieved by adding cervical extension or thigh extension, respectively.
> - Odds of obtaining a successful fusion of lumbosacral spine when instrumention is not used are improved by lumbosacral bracing with a thigh extension.
> - Effect of bracing for instrumented lumbosacral fusions is unknown.
> - Jewett orthosis is used to treat stable compression fractures at T11 to L1 levels.

SEMIRIGID BRACES

The chairback brace has a firm, plastic lumbar support with a soft, compressive abdominal component. The chairback brace has been commonly used to provide symptomatic relief for patients with low back pain and to provide limited postoperative support. The chairback brace is easy to don and is well tolerated by patients; however, it is not comfortable for use in bed due to the posterior firm shell.

The Knight-Taylor brace is similar to the chairback brace but has the addition of posterior uprights extending to the medial scapular area. Shoulder straps connect the upper section of the brace and assist with flexion control. Nagel et al.[63] evaluated the effectiveness of the Knight-Taylor in stabilizing the L1 to L2 segment. The Knight-Taylor brace was found to be effective in limiting lateral bending and provided fair restriction of flexion-extension, but had little effect on axial rotation. The Knight-Taylor brace is also simple to don and generally well tolerated by patients, although some patients complain of discomfort from the shoulder straps.

Newer prefabricated braces, available from companies such as Atlanta International Inc. (Atlanta, Ga.), have gained popularity in recent years. A full line of products, including prefabricated LSOs and TLSOs, is available. These braces are manufactured in a variety of models but incorporate a rigid, plastic shell and total contact foam liner. Velcro straps secure the front and back portion of the brace when in use. Cervical and thigh extensions are available to allow immobilization of the upper thoracic and lumbosacral areas. Another type of LSO brace called the Ortholign is made of lightweight, breathable material that is more comfortable than a standard plastic LSO brace and yet seems to offer the advantage of semirigid motion control (Figure 57-17). Although these newer prefabricated bracing systems seem to function well in clinical usage, they have not yet been fully evaluated by scientific testing.

Cybertech (Pasadena, Calif.) also manufactures prefabricated LSO and TLSO braces that are well tolerated by patients due to the incorporation of a pulley system that allows a patient to alter and adjust the fit of the orthosis, making these braces comfortable and easy to don (Figure 57-18). This brace provides a breathable nylon-mesh abdominal component with adjustable compression. The brace can be fit over clothing and is available with optional lordotic pads. The TLSO version of this brace has a sternal extension with shoulder straps to improve control of the upper lumbar or lower thoracic spine.

FLEXIBLE ORTHOSES

Various lumbar corsets and abdominal binders are available primarily for symptomatic relief of lumbar pain and to provide a kinesthetic reminder to patients. These orthoses provide minimal restriction of motion and are not indicated for treatment of potentially unstable spinal conditions. Flexible orthoses may provide increased hydrostatic pressure within the abdominal cavity but have not been shown to alter intradiscal pressure. Modern devices often include stays and plastic molded inserts that may be inserted in either the anterior or posterior aspect of the brace, depending on the specific direction of motion control that is desired. Table 57-3 lists the immobilization characteristics of various categories of braces.

COMPLICATIONS OF THORACOLUMBAR BRACING

Complications of thoracolumbar orthoses usage include skin breakdown, weakening of axial spinal musculature, local pain, symptom aggravation, loss of reduction, and psychologic dependence.[76] To minimize these effects, frequent inspection of skin and proper hygiene are important. In addition, fractures treated with bracing should undergo periodic radiographic examination to

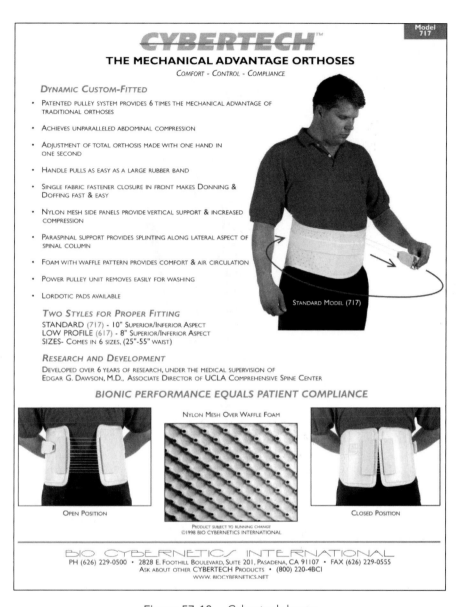

Figure 57-18. Cybertech brace.

ensure that loss of position has not occurred. Finally, long-term brace usage should be accompanied by active trunk exercises to minimize the loss of muscle strength (Table 57-3).

CONCLUSIONS

Spinal orthoses usage continues to be more of an art than a science because data on the treatment of most conditions using spinal bracing are limited. However, under-standing the biomechanics of a spinal condition allows the treating health-care provider to make a rational decision regarding brace usage. The available studies demonstrate that complete immobilization of the spine is not possible with any orthosis. Orthoses are able to augment other forms of treatment in many spinal conditions. Avoidance of complications with brace usage is best achieved by proper brace fitting and close clinical follow-up. In the future more scientific studies are needed to further quantify spinal bracing for specific conditions.

Table 57-3	Biomechanical Immobilization Characteristics of Various Brace Categories
Brace	**Motion Restriction**

Cervical thoracic orthosis (CTO)
  Lerman Minerva
  Yale orthosis
  Aspen
	Restricts motion from C3 to T3 in all planes

Halo vest orthosis	Restricts motion of occiput to T3 in all planes; may extend restriction to T7 with the use of a long vest

TLSO with neck extension
  Minerva attachment
  SOMI attachment
	Restricts motion from lower cervical spine to L4 in all planes

Thoracic lumbar sacral orthosis (TLSO)	Restricts motion from T7 to L4 in allplanes
Thoracic lumbar sacral orthosis with thigh extension	Restricts motion from T7 to sacrum in all planes
Lumbar sacral orthosis with thigh extension	Restricts motion from L3 to S1 in all planes
Lumbar sacral orthosis (LSO)	Restricts motion L3 to L4 in all planes; some restriction L2 to L3

Hyperextension TLSO
  Jewett
  ACE
  CASH
	Restricts flexion-extension from T11 to L1

Cloth semirigid LSO/TLSO
  Ortholign
  Cybertech
	Increased comfort, decreased restriction compared with standard LSO/TLSO

Corset or elastic lumbar support	Minimal motion restriction; acts as proprioceptive reminder of injury

REFERENCES

1. Allbrook D: Movements of the lumbar spinal column, *J Bone Joint Surg Br* 39:339-345, 1957.
2. Allington NJ, Brown RJ: Adolescent idiopathic scoliosis: treatment with the Wilmington brace: a comparison of full-time and part-time use, *J Bone Joint Surg Am* 78:1056-1062, 1996.
3. Anderson PA et al.: Failure of halo vest to prevent in vivo motion in patients with injured cervical spines, *Spine* 16:S501-S505, 1991.
4. Andriacchi T et al.: A model for students of the mechanical interaction between the human spine and the ribcage, *J Biomech* 7:497, 1974.
5. Axelsson P, Johnsson R, Stromqvist B: Effect of lumbar orthosis on intervertebral mobility: a roentgen stereophotogrammetric analysis, *Spine* 17:678-681, 1992.
6. Axelsson P, Johnsson R, Stromqvist B: Lumbar orthosis with unilateral hip immobilization: effects on intervertebral mobility determined by roentgen stereophotogrammetric analysis, *Spine* 18:876-879, 1993.
7. Ballock RT et al.: The effect of pin location on the rigidity of the halo pin-bone interface, *Neurosurgery* 26:238-241, 1990.
8. Bassett GS, Bunnell WP: Influence of the Wilmington brace on spinal decompensation in adolescent idiopathic scoliosis, *Clin Orthop* 223:164-169, 1987.
9. Beavis A: Cervical orthoses, *Prosthet Orthot Int* 13:6-13, 1989.
10. Benzel EC, Hadden TA, Saulsbery CM: A comparison of the Minerva and halo jackets for stabilization of the cervical spine, *J Neurosurg* 70:411-414, 1989.
11. Bhalla SK, Simmons EH: Normal ranges of intervertebral motion of the cervical spine, *Can J Surg* 12:181-187, 1969.
12. Botte M J et al.: Halo skeletal fixation: techniques of application and prevention of complications, *J Am Acad Orthop Surg* 4:44-53, 1996.
13. Botte MJ, Byrne TP, Garfin SR: Application of the halo device for immobilization of the cervical spine utilizing an increased torque pressure, *J Bone Joint Surg Am* 69:750-752, 1987.
14. Botte MJ, Byrne TP, Garfin SR: The use of skin incisions in the application of halo skeletal fixator pins, *Clin Orthop* 246:100, 1989.
15. Botte MJ et al.: The halo skeletal fixator: principles of application and maintenance, *Clin Orthop* 239:12-18, 1989.
16. Bucci MN et al.: Management of post-traumatic cervical spine instability: operative fusion versus halo vest immobilization: analysis of 49 cases, *J Trauma* 28:1001-1006, 1988.
17. Bunnell WP, MacEwen GD, Jayakumar S: The use of plastic jackets in the non-operative treatment of idiopathic scoliosis: preliminary report, *J Bone Joint Surg Am* 62:31-38, 1980.
18. Chase AP et al.: The biomechanical effectiveness of the Boston brace in the management of adolescent scoliosis, *Spine* 14:636-642, 1989.
19. Chase A, Pearcy M, Bader D: *Biomechanical basis of orthotic management*, Butterworth & Heinemann, 1993, Oxford.
20. Colachis SC Jr, Strohm BR: Radiographic studies of cervical spine motion in normal subjects: flexion and hyperextension, *Arch Phys Med Rehabil* 46:753-760, 1965.
21. Colachis SC Jr, Strohm BR, Ganter EL: Cervical spine motion in normal women: radiographic study of effect of cervical collars, *Arch Phys Med Rehabil* 54:161-169, 1973.
22. Cooper PR et al.: Halo immobilization of cervical spine fractures: indications and results, *J Neurosurg* 50:603-610, 1979.
23. Emans J: In Rowe DE, ed: SRS bracing manual, Section 5, Chicago, 1998, Scoliosis Research Society.
24. Fernandez-Filiberti R et al.: Effectiveness of TLSO bracing in the conservative treatment of idiopathic scoliosis, *J Pediatr Orthop* 15:176-181, 1995.
25. Fidler MW, Plasmans CM: The effect of four types of support on the segmental mobility of the lumbosacral spine, *J Bone Joint Surg Am* 65:943-947, 1983.
26. Fielding JW: Normal and selected abnormal motion of the cervical spine from the second cervical vertebra to the seventh cervical vertebra based on cineradiography, *J Bone Joint Surg Am* 46:1779, 1964.
27. Fisher SV: Proper fitting of the cervical orthosis, *Arch Phys Med Rehabil* 59:505-507, 1978.
28. Fisher SV et al.: Cervical orthoses effect on cervical spine motion: roentgenographic and goniometric method of study, *Arch Phys Med Rehabil* 58:109-115, 1977.
29. Garfin SR et al.: Subdural abscess associated with halo-pin traction, *J Bone Joint Surg Am* 70:1338-1340, 1988.
30. Garfin SR et al.: Complications in the use of the halo fixation device, *J Bone Joint Surg Am* 68:320-325, 1986.
31. Garfin SR et al.: Skull osteology as it affects halo pin placement in children, *J Pediatr Orthop* 6:434-436, 1986.
32. Glaser JA et al.: Complications associated with the halo-vest: a review of 245 cases, *J Neurosurg* 65:762-769, 1986.
33. Goldberg CJ et al.: A statistical comparison between natural history of idiopathic scoliosis and brace treatment in skeletally immature adolescent girls, *Spine* 18:902-908, 1993.

34. Goldberg CJ et al.: Adolescent idiopathic scoliosis: the effect of brace treatment on the incidence of surgery, *Spine* 26:42-47, 2001.

35. Green NE: Part-time bracing for adolescent idiopathic scoliosis, *J Bone Joint Surg Am* 68:738-742, 1986.

36. Howard A, Wright JG, Hedden D: A comparative study of TLSO, Charleston, and Milwaukee brace for idiopathic scoliosis, *Spine* 23:2404-2411, 1998.

37. Johnson RM et al.: Cervical orthoses: a study comparing their effectiveness in restricting cervical motion in normal subjects, *J Bone Joint Surg Am* 59:332-339, 1977.

38. Johnsson R et al.: Influence of spinal immobilization on consolidation of posterolateral lumbosacral fusion: a roentgen stereophotogrammetric analysis, *Spine* 17:16-20, 1992.

39. Jones MD: Cineradiographic studies of the collar-immobilized cervical spine, *J Neurosurg* 17:633-637, 1960.

40. Katz DE et al.: A comparison between the Boston brace and the Charleston bending brace in adolescent idiopathic scoliosis, *Spine* 22:1302-1312, 1997.

41. Kaufman WA et al.: Comparison of three prefabricated cervical collars, *Orthot Prosthet* 39:21-28, 1986.

42. Kim SS et al.: Factors affecting fusion rate in adult spondylolisthesis, *Spine* 15:979-984, 1990.

43. Koch RA, Nickel VL: The halo vest: an evaluation of motion and forces across the neck, *Spine* 3:103-107, 1978.

44. Kopits SE, Steingass MH: Experience with the "halo-cast" in small children, *Surg Clin North Am* 50:935-943, 1970.

45. Korovessis P: Effects of thoracolumbosacral orthosis on spinal deformities, trunk asymmetry, and frontal lower rib cage in adolescent idiopathic scoliosis, *Spine* 25:2064-2071, 2000.

46. Kostuik JP: Indications for the use of the halo immobilization, *Clin Orthop* 154:46-50, 1981.

47. Kottke FL, Mundale, MO: Range of mobility of the cervical spine, *Arch Phys Med Rehabil* 40:379-382, 1959.

48. Lantz SA, Schultz AB: Lumbar orthosis wearing. I. Restriction of gross body motions, *Spine* 11:834-837, 1986.

49. Lantz SA, Schultz AB: Lumbar spine orthosis wearing. II. Effect on trunk muscle myoelectric activity, *Spine* 11:838-842, 1986.

50. Lind B, Nordwall A, Sihlbom H: Odontoid fractures treated with halo-vest, *Spine* 12:173-177, 1987.

51. Lind B, Sihlbom H, Nordwall A: Halo-vest treatment of unstable traumatic cervical spine injuries, *Spine* 13:425-432, 1988.

52. Lonstein JE, Winter RB: Milwaukee brace treatment of adolescent idiopathic scoliosis: review of 1020 patients, *J Bone Joint Surg Am* 76:300-311, 1994.

53. Lumsden RM, Morris JM: An in vivo study of axial rotation and immobilization at the lumbosacral joint, *J Bone Joint Surg Am* 50:1591-1602, 1968.

54. Lunsford TR, Davidson M, Lunsford BR: The effectiveness of four contemporary cervical orthoses in restricting cervical motion, *J Prosthet Orthot* 6:93-99, 1994.

55. Michel CR et al.: The placement of a four piece spinal support in the conservative treatment of 700 cases over 10 years, *Orthop Trans* 7:131, 1983.

56. Moe JH, Kettleson DN: Idiopathic scoliosis: analysis of curve patterns and the preliminary results of Milwaukee-brace treatment in one hundred sixty-nine patients, *J Bone Joint Surg Am* 52:1509-1533, 1970.

57. Morris JM, Lucas DB: Physiologic considerations in bracing of the spine, *Orthop Prosthet Appl*, 1963, pp. 37-44.

58. Morris JM, Lucas DB, Bresler MS: Role of the trunk in stability of the spine, *J Bone Joint Surg Am* 43:327-349, 1961.

59. Mubarak SJ et al.: Halo application in the infant, *J Pediatr Orthop* 9:612-614, 1989.

60. Nachemson A, Morris JM: In vivo measurements of intradiscal pressure, *J Bone Joint Surg Am* 46:1077-1092, 1964.

61. Nachemson A, Peterson L: Effectiveness of treatment of a brace in girls who have adolescent idiopathic scoliosis: a prospective, controlled study, *J Bone Joint Surg Am* 77:815-822, 1995.

62. Nachemson A, Schultz A, Andersson G: Mechanical effectiveness studies of lumbar spine orthoses, *Scand J Rehabil Med Suppl* 9:139-149, 1983.

63. Nagel DA et al.: Stability of the upper lumbar spine following progressive disruptions and the application of individual internal and external fixation devices, *J Bone Joint Surg Am* 63:62-70, 1981.

64. Noonan KJ et al.: Use of the Milwaukee brace for progressive idiopathic scoliosis, *J Bone Joint Surg Am* 78:557-567, 1996.

65. Norton PL, Brown T: The immobilizing efficiency of back braces, *J Bone Joint Surg Am* 39:111, 1957.

66. Ohana N et al.: In there a need for lumbar orthosis in mild compression fractures of the thoracolumbar spine? A retrospective study comparing the radiographic results between early ambulation with and without lumbar orthosis, *J Spinal Disord* 13:305-308, 2000.

67. Parry H, Delargy M, Burt A: Early mobilisation of patients with cervical cord injury using the halo brace device, *Paraplegia* 26:226-232, 1988.

68. Patwardhan AG et al.: Orthotic stabilization of thoracolumbar injuries: a biomechanical analysis of the Jewett hyperextension orthosis, *Spine* 15:654-661, 1990.

69. Perry J: The halo in spinal abnormalities: practical factors and avoidance of complications, *Orthop Clin North Am* 3:69-80, 1972.

70. Perry J, Nickel VL: Total cervical spine fusion for neck paralysis, *J Bone Joint Surg Am* 41:37-43, 1959.

71. Plaisier B et al.: Prospective evaluation of craniofacial pressure in four different cervical orthoses, *J Trauma* 37:714-720, 1994.

72. Podolsky S et al.: Efficacy of cervical spine immobilization methods, *J Trauma* 23:461-465, 1983.

73. Price CT et al.: Nighttime bracing for adolescent idiopathic scoliosis with the Charleston bending brace: long-term follow-up, *J Pediatr Orthop* 17:703-707, 1997.

74. Price CT et al.: Nighttime bracing for adolescent idiopathic scoliosis with the Charleston bending brace: preliminary report, *Spine* 15:1294-1299, 1990.

75. Rizzolo SJ et al.: The effect of torque pressure on halo pin complication rates: a randomized prospective study, *Spine* 18:2163-2166, 1993.

76. Smith GE: The most ancient splints, *Br Med J* 1:732-734, 1908.

77. Sypert GW: External spinal orthotics, *Neurosurgery* 20:642-648, 1987.

78. Triggs KJ et al.: The effect of angled insertion on halo pin fixation, *Spine* 14:781-783, 1989.

79. Waters RL, Morris JM: Effect of spinal supports on the electrical activity of muscles of the trunk, *J Bone Joint Surg Am* 52:51-60, 1970.

80. White AA, Panjabi MM: *Clinical biomechanics of the spine*, Toronto, 1978, JB Lippincott.

81. Wiley JW et al.: Effectiveness of the Boston brace in treatment of large curves in adolescent scoliosis, *Spine* 25:2326-2332, 2000.

82. Winter RB, Lonstein JE: Juvenile and adult scoliosis. In Herkowitz NH et al., eds: *The spine*, Philadelphia, 1999, WB Saunders.

CHAPTER 58

Outcomes Assessment in Spine Surgery

Rocco R. Calderone, Louise Toutant

Outcomes studies of patients undergoing treatment for spinal disorders are essential. Wide variations in treatment practices for spinal disorders, escalating cost of health care, and deficiencies within the clinical literature have revealed the need for outcomes-based treatment. Assessments of the process of care such as radiographic results or physical signs do not always coincide with improved quality of life. Generic and disease-specific measures exist for assessing the patient-oriented results of treatment for patients with spinal disorders. Wide geographic variation of interventions of the spine, especially lumbar fusion surgery, has been noted in studies from large databases. This indicates a need to study the efficacy of various treatments. Randomized controlled trials (RCTs) are the best method of assessing treatment alternatives and new technologies. RCTs are rare in the evaluation of spinal surgery; prospective cohort studies are a substitute when RCTs are not possible. Meta-analysis is an increasingly important and useful tool for outcomes research. Cost-benefit and cost-effectiveness analyses (CBA and CEA, respectively) are being used increasingly to examine the value of treatment choices. Decision analysis is applied to data from outcomes studies. Clinical practice guidelines formulated from these data aim at disseminating the knowledge of appropriate and effective treatment with optimal patient outcomes.

INTRODUCTION: THE OUTCOMES MOVEMENT

As far back as 1930, surgeon Ernest Codman recommended systematic follow-up of the end results of surgical treatments.[28] In the 1970s, Ellwood coined the term "outcomes management" with the goal of achieving quality health care for every patient.[11] In 1988 the *New England Journal of Medicine* editorialized outcomes research as the "third revolution" in health care.[31] Outcomes assessment is a preeminent issue in medicine today. Three major factors brought this issue to the forefront of medicine: practice-pattern variations, deficiencies in clinical literature, and the rising cost of health care.

EVOLUTION OF THE OUTCOMES MOVEMENT

- 1930, Codman: "End results" of treatment
- 1970, Ellwood: Termed "outcomes management"
- 1973, Wennberg and Gittelsohn: Geographic variation in practice
- 1988, Relman: "Third revolution" in health care, *New England Journal of Medicine*
- 2000, Outcomes assessment: Universal concern

Practice-pattern variation refers to the unexplained variation of utilization rates for similar diagnoses in different geographic locations per population base. In 1973, Wennberg and Gittelsohn published a landmark article on small area variations in treatment based on geographic location.[43] These variations in utilization of medical care were unexplained.

Information on *clinical treatment* is based on scientific literature. The medical literature, including orthopedic and spine literature, is lacking in standard definitions, measures, and randomized controlled studies. Deficiencies in methodology and analysis have produced varying and inaccurate results as to the best treatment methods.[41] This lack of definitive knowledge contributes to practice variations.

Varied utilization has raised the suspicion of overutilization of resources in an environment of increased health plan provider competition. *Cost* is also a concern in a country that spends nearly 14% of its gross domestic product (GDP) on health care. The increase in this sector has been rapid and greater than that of other sectors of the economy. It also exceeds the percentage of GDP that other countries spend on health care without a comparably superior health status. In addition, the annual rate of increase in medical costs has exceeded the rate of inflation, often without a measurable increase in the quality and end result of treatment.

Outcomes summarize and standardize results in the context of the patient's well-being. Outcomes seek to answer questions regarding relief from pain, recovery of

---

FACTORS LEADING TO OUTCOMES MOVEMENT

- Geographic practice pattern variation
- Deficiencies in existing clinical literature
- Escalating health care costs

OUTCOMES RESEARCH

- View patient's perspective
- Standardize research
- Eliminate bias
- Define clinical terminology (e.g., spinal instability)
- Measure health-related quality of life
- Report satisfaction with treatment
- Quantify relief of pain
- Assess daily functioning
- Assess role functioning
- Assess psychosocial functioning

---

function, return to work, patient satisfaction, and cost of resources used to attain such results. Outcomes management means controlling contributing factors and accomplishing a successful end result of delivered health care for the patient. Outcomes research has become a central feature of medical practice today. Results of outcome studies are being used in treatment guidelines and policies in today's cost-managed health care environment.

OUTCOMES MOVEMENT IN TREATMENT OF SPINAL DISORDERS

Outcomes research asks the question, "Is the patient satisfied?" The goal of treatment of spinal disorders is the enhancement or improvement of the quality of life. This is accomplished when a patient has less pain as well as improved function in daily activities and work. This may or may not correspond to the appearance of successful fusion on radiographs, the removal of an extruded disc fragment, or even reduction in a spinal deformity.

Wide variations in spine surgery rates have been reported between different geographic areas, and geographic variations in spinal fusion are prevalent.[23] Widely differing opinions of treatment are held in national conferences regarding a particular spinal disorder, and a plethora of new treatments and implants are introduced on a yearly basis. These procedures, technologies, and treatment alternatives are increasing, ranging from basic exercise therapy to spinal manipulations, intermittent axial traction, spinal arthrodesis, pedicle screw fixation, interbody prosthetic cage implants, intradiscal electrotherapy, artificial discs, and vertebroplasty. The development of less-invasive techniques, enabling outpatient and office procedures, also expands the list of treatment alternatives and health care providers who are performing spinal interventions. Outcomes studies in spine treatments must assess the true benefits as well as the risk of complications associated with new spinal procedures if practice-pattern variation in spinal procedures is to become more uniform.

Outcomes studies in treatment of the spine are also needed to control cost relative to effectiveness in the face of new technologies. Positive outcomes and effective treatment do not necessarily correspond with smaller incisions and less-invasive techniques or new technology. A positive outcome means that surgery or intervention on the spine significantly and consistently improves a patient's quality of life.

Outcomes analysis in the treatment of spinal disorders is aimed at improving the quality of clinical research and is a necessary step toward appropriate and quality medical care for the spine. Outcomes assessment is the attempt to refine, remove bias, and standardize research on the results of medical treatment. It is an evaluation of treatment from the patient's perspective, which includes increased functioning, pain relief, improved quality of life, and satisfaction with treatment. Decision analysis can be applied to the results of this research. This leads to the construction of algorithms and the development of clinical guidelines. This approach differs from that adopted in the majority of existing orthopedic and spine literature.

Traditionally, orthopedic and neurosurgical literature includes many retrospective studies on the results of spinal surgery. Fusion rates, techniques, and implants are compared in a retrospective nonrandomized fashion. Many of these data, although important, fail to add to the clinical knowledge of our patients' outcome and well-being. Literature of this sort lacks adequate outcomes assessment and contains biased, anecdotal information. The nature of surgical treatment often precludes randomized and blinded studies.

Another common difficulty with the spine literature is a lack of standard definitions and measures, which precludes comparison of different studies. For example, how do we define and quantify spinal instability? Existing literature is relied on for critical thinking and formulation of standards of care. How can we justify our treatment standards to patients when such essential elements are missing from our knowledge base? Do the current treatment standards improve our patients' quality of life? These are issues that outcomes research addresses.

Treatment of spinal disorders is diverse, costly, and often extensive. Back pain is one of the most prevalent reasons patients seek medical care today. What course will best benefit the patient? Will patients with degenerative disc disease benefit from spinal arthrodesis compared with those treated nonoperatively? Choosing and justifying the best treatment course in today's health care climate are increasingly important issues. Patients demand and deserve knowledge of the expected outcome to an increasing variety of spinal interventions. Payers demand positive outcomes for costly treatments. The spine literature is not definitive on many of the current treatment courses for spinal disorders. Outcomes research seeks to refine the answers to these questions.

GEOGRAPHIC VARIATIONS IN SPINE SURGERY RATES

Disparities exist among areas in the rate of health care intervention that is provided. This geographic variation has been documented among countries, regions, and counties, as well as hospitals.[4,36,38,39] This is true for spinal disorder treatments as well as for other types of medical care. Widespread variation in the surgical treatment of lower back pain has been illustrated in studies among hospital regions in Washington State, as well as in other areas.[38,39,42]

Disparity of treatment rates among geographic areas is not unique to spine surgery.[43] Can these rate variations be explained? Wennberg[44] disposes the implausible explanation that treatment rates vary because illness rates are different in that geographic region. No scientific data support the suggestion that illness rates such as back pain vary in correspondence to spinal surgery rates. More likely, clinical practices, such as surgery rates for back pain, vary because of lack of outcomes data. In addition, treatment decisions regarding back pain are not uniform among practitioners; physician training and clinical experience differ, and community standards, which may have developed over many years, differ. This is all the result of deficient reliable outcomes data to promote conformity of practice patterns.

These geographic variations raise the issue of quality, appropriateness, and cost-effectiveness of spinal surgery. In an era of health care cost containment, there is great interest in reducing high rates of utilization and cost. Health care utilization is under constant scrutiny by government agencies, insurance companies, and third-party payers. Treatment plans for various spinal disorders require submission to payers for authorization. Hospitalization for spinal surgery is accompanied by standard recommendations on length of stay. Extended inpatient treatment requires justification for longer than "average" stay for that type of treatment. Analysis of practice variation serves as a basis for these recommendations.

Some of the studies documenting variation in practice do not correspond to discreet areas of individual practice. Although this is helpful in illustrating practice variation, it falls short of usefulness in addressing those variations. With more availability of data, areas of study are becoming more defined. Local level data and individual physician data can be obtained with advancing computer and Internet technology. Individual physician practice patterns are under scrutiny. Third-party payers, insurance companies, and health care policy analysts look at these data with the goal of decreasing high utilization rates. Should underutilization be correspondingly increased? What is the correct rate of utilization? In the hands of third parties, this goal to decrease practice variation is removed from clinical decision making and patient treatment. Physicians must take an active role to influence the future direction of health care and decisions on optimal treatment of spinal disorders.

Studies of geographic variation and small area analysis must be examined more critically than expected by third parties. Volinn et al.[39] note potential flaws in data examining rate variance studies in spinal treatment. Analyses based on individual diagnosis-related groups (DRGs) may inadvertently collect heterogeneous events into the same category. Specific events and diagnoses being analyzed must be considered. The DRGs used for spine surgery in some data include cervical, thoracic, and lumbar regions and elective and emergency procedures within one group. As a result, data indicating a high rate of spinal surgery compared with other regions would not provide sufficient specific detail.

Proper outcome evaluation for spine surgery requires data on specific procedures for each diagnosis in particular regions of the spine. Algorithms are needed to create homogeneous comparisons of similar groups of diagnoses and treatments. In addition, geographic units of analysis must be appropriately defined. Ideal units consist of small areas of one or more hospitals that treat patients from a defined population. Regions defined by treatment centers are skewed by major treatment centers that treat patients referred from other areas.

Accuracy of the data on area rates is important. The denominator of the equation can be accurately assessed through census data in the defined region. The actual treatment population, however, may also depend on travel patterns and referral patterns in the region. Changes in disease or diagnosis codes affect rates, and hospital data can be inaccurate or nonspecific. There have been recent changes in spinal surgery International Classification of Diseases (ICD) as well as Current Procedural Terminology (CPT) codes. As technology creates new procedures for the spine, new codes are devised.

Statistical analysis of the rate data must show that the rate differences are not a chance event. The coefficient of variation in analysis of variance is recommended to describe the distribution and dispersion of rates. Confidence levels must show that rate variance is the result of more than chance alone. This must be adjusted for multiple comparisons as the rates of more areas are compared.

Although high rates are more likely to attract attention in a cost-conscious environment, area analysis must address both high and low rates. Increasing certain rates of health services may result in improved quality of care. Katz et al.[21] documented a clear example in comparing mammography rates between British Colombia and Washington State; the authors found rates inappropriately low in British Columbia. The low rate of a particular practice does not determine appropriateness.[45] Unfortunately, in spine surgery, answers to appropriate intervention rates are deficient. This is where outcomes data can be helpful in defining the varied rate as too high or too low.

Variance is often difficult to explain. Precise explanations of rate variance are elusive. Explanations focus on both supply and demand characteristics of a region. Hypotheses include supply factors such as hospital bed or physician per capita, demand variables involving education and socioeconomic factors, and physician practice styles developed as a result of training or within the local medical community.

GEOGRAPHIC VARIATIONS IN PRACTICE PATTERN

- Variation documented between:
  - Country
  - Region
  - County
  - Hospital
- Factors in variation
  - Variation in physician training
  - Variation in clinical experience
  - Variation in community standards
  - Lack of outcomes data

DEFICIENCIES IN CLINICAL LITERATURE

- Lack of randomized prospective studies
- Faulty experimental design
- Erroneous statistical analysis
- Lack of patient-oriented outcomes

ELEMENTS OF META-ANALYSIS

- Aggregate of randomized controlled trials into one large cohort
- Inclusion and exclusion criteria
- Data pooling criteria
- Blinded data extraction
- Evaluation of statistical error and confidence intervals
- Evaluation of individual study design and methodology
- Sensitivity analysis of end result of meta-analysis

Finally, geographic variation studies must address "presentation styles." This is particularly important in evaluating treatment variance for back and neck pain. Patients present or express themselves in a highly variable way regarding symptoms of back and neck pain. Area health care utilization depends on seeking care, expectations of care, and subjective disabilities of back or neck pain symptoms, which may vary according to locale.[39] Local level data are important to have an impact on and to change styles of local practitioners.[39] Many published results performed at research institutions may not be relevant to local practice. The search for reasons for geographic variance in rates of care has fueled the study of outcomes in orthopedics. There remain many unanswered questions in the rates of spine intervention.

QUALITY OF CLINICAL RESEARCH IN SPINE CARE

Knowledge in the practice of medicine is based on clinical research. Journals and medical texts embody the major source of information. Without a basic core of validated medical knowledge, clinical medicine remains deficient. Without scientific research, much of what is done in the treatment of spinal disorders becomes the practice of folk medicine.

Gartland et al.[13] pointed out the deficiencies that exist within the orthopedic literature. Significant flaws include faulty experimental design, erroneous statistical analysis, and lack of focus on patient-oriented outcomes of treatment. Statistical deficiencies were noted in 54% of studies examined in the spine literature.[41]

Meta-analysis is a tool of outcomes research and was described in the literature in 1976.[14] It is the statistical analysis of results from a collection of studies on the same topic. A meta-analysis aggregates existing literature in an attempt to construct one large cohort from several smaller cohorts. Traditionally, a meta-analysis includes only RCTs. The use of meta-analysis in the field of spine surgery is made difficult because there are few RCTs reported in the spine literature.

Properly performed, a meta-analysis includes a thorough search with specific inclusion and exclusion protocol. Readers must be presented the criteria by which the data were pooled. Extraction of data from studies should be performed in a blinded fashion. Statistical error and confidence intervals are evaluated. Individual studies need to be evaluated qualitatively for methodology and study design. Finally, the end result of the meta-analysis requires a sensitivity analysis. The cost of a proper meta-analysis has been documented at $30,000 to $50,000.[16,23]

One example from the spine literature is Turner et al.'s[37] meta-analysis of surgery for lumbar spinal stenosis. Their review found a deficiency of RCTs in lumbar surgery for spinal stenosis. Satisfaction rates of surgical treatment averaged around 68% but varied widely, from 16% to 95%. Outcomes included complication rates of 14% for pseudarthrosis and 9% for painful donor site.

Literature reviews have taken many forms. A *structured literature review* is an attempt at meta-analysis when the literature is deficient of RCTs. *Narrative literature reviews* summarize existing clinical studies on a particular topic; however, the author picks and chooses studies, which invites significant bias.

The requirements for a true meta-analysis avoid reader bias through inclusion and exclusion criteria. A meta-analysis is useful when existing literature presents conflicting results of treatment. It is also helpful in evaluating small effects and low rates of occurrences that require larger populations. The goal of meta-analysis is to assemble existing literature and to subject it to quantitative and qualitative analysis.[16]

RCTs control bias and represent the strongest scientific evidence. RCTs are the ideal; however, they are not always possible. RCTs are a standard within the pharmaceutical industry for the study of prescription medication. They are not the standard for spinal interventions or new spine technology. It is difficult and often impossible to evaluate surgical treatment in a blinded, randomized, controlled fashion. Retrospective studies are replete with methodologic problems; often the records were not set up for a particular evaluation, and

---

USEFULNESS OF META-ANALYSIS

- Forms consensus over conflicting literature
- Constructs larger subject base
- Examines low occurrence rate phenomenon
- Performs qualitative and quantitative review of existing literature

---

CRITICAL EVALUATION OF LITERATURE

- Compare patients in study with patients in your practice.
- Make treatment description sufficiently detailed to replicate.
- Choose a clinically relevant end point.
- Identify the time frame of relevant end point.
- Choose an appropriate comparison group.
- Address sources of bias: Compliance, contamination, cointervention of treatment groups.
- Keep loss to follow-up less than 20%.
- Identify clinical significance as well as statistically significant results.

STATISTICAL ANALYSIS

- Type I error
  - Chance probability
  - $P < .05$
  - False-positive less than 1 in 20
- Type II error
  - Significant sample size
  - Statistical power greater than 80%
  - False-negative rate less than 20%

---

the data were not originally collected with this purpose in mind. This raises significant doubt about the accuracy and validity of the study conclusions.[2]

Prospective clinical trials often substitute for RCTs in the evaluation of surgical treatment. This represents a closer approximation to the gold standard of RCTs. Randomization of surgical treatment is difficult to achieve, and alternating treatment of patients does not always result in true randomization. Attempts at randomization of surgical treatment are complicated by bias and ethical concerns.

One solution to the ethical concerns surrounding randomization of treatment is to randomize patients to physicians preferring alternative treatments. The study by Herkowitz et al.[17] is an example of randomized prospective research on surgical treatment. This study details the outcomes of patients undergoing lumbar decompression and attempted arthrodesis for spinal stenosis with spondylolisthesis compared with those decompressed without fusion.

The application of clinical findings in the literature to one's own practice pattern requires careful consideration.[33] The patients included in a particular study must be described in sufficient detail to allow comparison with the patients within one's particular practice. Likewise, the treatment must be described in sufficient detail. The end point assessed in the study should be clinically relevant. For example, assessing spinal flexion as an end point may not be relevant. The correlation between degree of spinal flexion and daily functioning is weak. Also, *when* an end point is measured matters. Assessing back pain at 2 years may not be as clinically relevant an end point as is assessing results of treatment at 1 or 3 months for a therapeutic modality, because most back pain will be better at 2 years regardless of therapy. Assessment of an end point of spinal fusion, on the other hand, would be more relevant at 2 years as opposed to 3 months. The study requires an appropriate comparison group.

Potential sources of bias should be eliminated or accounted for within the study methodology. Compliance of patients with treatment, contamination by patients seeking alternative treatment, and cointervention by patients receiving other treatment all represent potential biases. Loss to follow-up of greater than 20% raises concern about the validity of the findings. The Food and Drug Administration requires less than 15% loss to follow-up when evaluating research data. Results of the study should be clinically significant and not just statistically significant; clinically significant results require adequate sample sizes for statistical significance.[9,18]

Comprehensive and well-designed clinical studies require a team approach. Through power analysis, research methodologists determine `the number of patients required for statistical significance. Survey methodologists develop and test questionnaires and determine how to obtain the data needed in the study. The expertise of epidemiologists, health economists, and sociologists is often needed, as well as the skill and evaluation of biostatisticians.[23]

Statistical analysis includes evaluation for a type I error. This is referred to as the α level or probability (P). This is a statement as to the probability that an observed difference is due to chance alone. Conventionally, an acceptable α level or P value should be .05 or less. This means that the false-positive rate or type I error is less than 1 in 20. If the risk is less than 1 in 20 that the observed difference is due to chance alone, then the observed difference is considered statistically significant.[18]

A type II error deals with sample size. The sample size must be sufficiently large to demonstrate a statistically significant difference. A type II error is known as a *false-negative result*. The risk of a type II error should not be greater than 20%. Also known as *statistical power*, a power of 80% is required to avoid a type II error of greater than 20%.

Power calculations are needed in the planning phase of a study. Statistical power calculations depend on sample size, size of treatment effects or measured occurrences, and variability of outcomes assessed. Reasonable accuracy and small confidence intervals for case series require a sufficient sample size, which generally means more than 30 participants.[18,20]

Use of Large Database Analysis

Large computerized databases exist for billing purposes and hospital data. Examples of these databases include hospital discharge registries, Medicare claims data, national health surveys, and insurance claims databases. This large quantity of data makes possible the comparison of geographic practice patterns. Use of these data is increasing in evaluating patterns of medical care and examining the outcomes of different medical treatments.[10]

An example includes the evaluation of lumbar fusion rates across the United States. Through analysis of the database from the National Center for Health Statistics, a 56% greater rate of spinal fusion was noted for the Midwestern region as opposed to the Northeastern region of the United States.[36] Large database analyses are also used in evaluating complications. Analysis of a statewide database in Washington State revealed a complication rate of 5.4% for discectomy versus 12% for discectomy plus fusion.[7]

Large databases offer the opportunity to evaluate data based on thousands and even millions of patients. These databases, however, are limited; the information contained within them is primarily gathered for billing purposes or other reasons often unrelated to the planned study. For evaluation of issues concerning costs, length of stay, and population-based treatment, large databases are extremely helpful. For evaluation of other issues, such as comorbidity or patient satisfaction, such databases are often deficient. Claims databases and discharge databases require skill and attention to interpret. Areas of limited outcomes analysis from these databases include well-defined and recorded data such as mortality, length of stay, complications, and reoperation rates.[8]

Large databases complement other research methods. Most importantly, they focus the direction of needed outcomes investigations. With advancing computer technology, increasing employer-supported computers, and Internet access for employees and patients, these databases will continue to grow with detailed data that are useful for outcomes assessment.

COST ANALYSIS

The percentage of the GDP that is being spent on health care in the United States, along with its annual rate of increase, is under scrutiny. Medical resources are finite, and economic analysis of clinical decisions in health care has become an integral part of outcomes research. Maximizing health care quality and minimizing costs are inseparable goals.

Allocations of health care resources reflect on microeconomic and macroeconomic societal concerns. The microeconomics of health care delivery address the treatment option that is most cost effective. The macroeconomics of health care delivery must look at the allocation of health care resources for widespread availability of treatment whose benefits exceed their costs.[5]

Cost analysis in health care is *perspective dependent*, meaning that the results of an analysis vary depending on the perspective used to focus the evaluation. Third-party payer, patient, and provider all value outcomes differently. The relevant cost of surgery is defined as the *additional cost*, compared with no treatment or performing alternative nonsurgical treatment.

The methodology of economic decision analysis has included both CBA and CEA. CBA requires the assignment of monetary value to health outcomes and benefits. It asks how much the benefits exceed the costs of a particular treatment in terms of dollars. CEA seeks the cost of treatment per unit of effectiveness. It defines cost in nonmonetary terms such as lives saved or persons cured.[5]

Placing value on the benefit of pain relief or increased quality of life is difficult and controversial. The cost-effectiveness can be ascertained only in comparison with other therapies. The least expensive route is not always the most cost-effective, especially if the outcome is poor. Perspective of cost must remain consistent within an analysis. Cost analysis, however, varies widely depending on perspective. The payer or insurance company sees the costs that they pay and does not value a patient's time spent waiting or seeking care. Patients see their deductible or copayment amounts, as well as the time costs, whereas society sees lost productivity, disability compensation, and medical costs. Studies must clarify the perspective and illustrate only one perspective at a time and consistently value costs in the context of that perspective.

Finally, it remains with the analyst to set parameters with which to judge values that support treatment decisions. Values, such as amount of cost savings or per-

---

COSTS OF HEALTH CARE

- Health care 14% of gross domestic product
- Rate of increase greater than rate of inflation
- Direct medical costs
- Indirect opportunity costs
- Societal costs: Disability, lost productivity

LARGE DATABASE

- Hospital discharge registries
- Statewide databases
- Insurance billing information
- HCFA/Medicare claims data
- National databases

COST ANALYSIS

- Cost-benefit, confounding factors
  - Monetary value of outcome
- Cost-effectiveness
  - Units of benefit, persons cured, nonmonetary terms
- Varied perspectives

centage improvement in function, serve to quantify clinical decisions beyond a physician's practice style. Thus cost analysis, despite limitations, offers help in improving the delivery of quality spine care in the context of clinical intuition, varying patient circumstances, and patient preferences.

SPINE AND MUSCULOSKELETAL OUTCOMES MEASUREMENT

Spinal disorders are associated with considerable disability and high economic costs. Pain relief and physical function are important outcomes of treatment of spinal disorders. *Physical function* refers to general daily activity functioning, social functioning, role functioning, and general well-being. Many patients with spinal disorders that cause neck or back pain fail to return to their previous level of functioning. Many studies fail to properly assess general functioning and well-being after treatment.[13]

Clinical studies frequently evaluate the results of the *process* of treatment. Treatment *processes* include the results of diagnostic tests such as radiographic studies, laboratory findings, or clinically objective "hard" data such as range of motion, diagnostic tests, or surgeon-defined criteria of technical success rather than subjective patient criteria and physical functioning. These objective clinical end points are important but may not always be significant to well-being and functioning of the patient.

Evaluation of "soft" data such as improvement in the quality of life, patient utilities or the usefulness of a specific outcome in the life of a given patient, day-to-day functioning, role functioning, and relief from pain have been lacking or have been assessed in a nonstandardized way with assessment methods that lack validity. Valid and standardized instruments have been developed for assessing these "softer" results of treatment. Improvement in these factors correlate with improved health-related quality of life for the patient. *Quality of life* measured by validated instruments and self-administered questionnaires has been shown to be as reproducible and valid as the assessment of more traditional anatomic and physiologic measures.[7] From a patient's perspective, quality-of-life measurements are the most important type of outcome. Outcomes assessment and evidence-based medicine are in demand. Valid and reliable measures to assess the effectiveness and outcomes of spinal treatment are essential to a complete evaluation.

Assessment Tests

Instruments have been developed to assess symptoms and function, including both general and region-specific assessments.[29] Development of these assessment instruments involves the planning of wording and layout, as well as the development of scales that are clear and reliable. Cultural differences must be taken into account as to avoid biased assessments. Finally, validation of the instrument with reliability and sensitivity testing is required.

Validation must be established for a particular study of a group of patients. *Validity* is the extent to which the measure is able to assess what it claims to assess, such as back pain and physical function. *Validity* also refers to the ability to correlate with other outcome measures. *Reliability* signifies that a measure produces consistent results each time. Reliability requires internal consistency and reproducibility.[10]

Other necessary characteristics of measurements include responsiveness, feasibility, and sensibility. *Responsiveness* is the ability of an assessment to detect subtle but relevant clinical change. Measurements must be *feasible* in terms of time and expense of administration and ease of use and interpretation. In addition, it should be *sensible* in that it is appropriate for patient use in the intended setting and well suited for the study.[10]

The three components to validity are content, criterion, and construct. *Content validity* is also known as *face validity*. It refers to the appropriateness of content or questions as assessed by the patient and practitioner. The content needs to assess all relevant areas. *Criterion validity* refers to the ability to show that the scores are systematically related to one or more outcome criteria. *Construct validity* refers to the ability of the measure to relate to other measures or data in a plausible way.[19]

There are many musculoskeletal and spinal outcomes measures within the literature. The basis of many of these measures began as assessments of activities of daily living (ADL). Early published studies on ADL assessment detailed physical requirements.[21,25] From these general functioning assessments, region- and disease-specific assessments have been developed. In addition, the American Academy of Orthopedic

---

OUTCOMES MEASURES

- Process-oriented outcome measures
  - Anatomic
  - Physiologic
  - Physical examination signs
  - Complications
  - Mortality
- Patient-oriented outcome measures
  - Health-related quality of life
    - Symptoms/pain
    - Functional status: Activities of daily living, social, psychologic
    - Role status/employment
  - Satisfaction
  - Costs

OUTCOMES MEASURES

- Validity: Measures what it claims to measure
- Reliable: Consistent and reproducible
- Responsive: Detects subtle change
- Feasible: Easy to use, interpret, not cost prohibitive
- Sensible: Relevant, appropriate, well suited

Surgeons (AAOS) along with the North American Spine Society (NASS) and other musculoskeletal specialty societies have sought through committee to develop standard definitions and measurements. This project was behind the development of AAOS Outcomes Questionnaires.[6]

For a comprehensive outcome evaluation, one should include an assessment of symptoms and an assessment of functional status. Furthermore, functional status should include general overall assessment of functional well-being as well as being disease or region specific. Disease- and region-specific assessments focus on function of the neck or back in the setting of a spinal disorder. Functional status can focus on general status or role status. General functioning includes ADLs and recreation. Role status evaluates functioning in an employment or work setting.[3,10]

Generic measures assess physical, mental, and psychosocial domains of health. Generic measures provide a broad picture of health and quality of life as affected by a range of diseases and disorders. Disease-specific measures focus on particular domains. These specific domains are concentrated on symptoms and complaints specific to a particular disorder. Measures for spinal assessment usually consist of a section of questions that deal with back and leg pain or neck and arm pain, physical functioning, and psychosocial functioning.[3,29]

Symptom Assessment

Symptom assessment can be measured with instruments that assess symptoms alone or with sections of more complete instruments that assess function as well. Symptoms are subjective, and the patient is the sole guide. In spinal care, we seek to quantify the intensity, frequency, and duration of pain as well as pain location, associations of depression, anxiety, perceived weakness, numbness, and paresthesias. Current instruments include the NASS Questionnaire, the McGill Pain Questionnaire, Dallas Pain Score, VonKorff Chronic Pain Grade, visual analog scales, and the AAOS Musculoskeletal Outcomes Data Evaluation and Management (MODEM) instruments.

The *NASS Outcomes Questionnaire* assesses role function as well as symptoms. It consists of 12 questions regarding pain and requires approximately 3 minutes to complete the symptom section. It distinguishes back pain from leg pain, for frequency, severity, and duration, along with numbness and weakness.

OUTCOMES INSTRUMENTS AND HEALTH-RELATED QUALITY OF LIFE

- Symptom assessment
- Functional status assessment: Generic or region/disease-specific
  - General, activities of daily living
  - Role, employment
  - Social, recreational, psychologic

The *McGill Pain Questionnaire* evaluates pain severity and affective response. It is the most extensive symptom evaluation of those listed. It consists of 26 items, requiring on average 15 minutes to complete.[27] The McGill Pain Questionnaire consists of three major classes or word descriptors that are used by patients to specify subjective pain experience.[3]

The *Dallas Pain Questionnaire*, developed and published in 1989, focuses on spinal pain and its impact on behavior. This is a 16-item visual analog scale with an average completion time of 5 minutes. Issues addressed include the influence of pain severity on daily activities, work and social or leisure involvement, and anxiety and depression. The Dallas Pain Questionnaire combines functional and psychologic capacities.[24] The instrument developed by Von Korff et al.[40] addresses the severity of chronic pain. The perceived impact of chronic pain requires about 5 minutes for evaluation through seven items. Other visual analog scales are also used for symptom assessment. They vary in length but generally require the least amount of time to complete: about 1 minute.

Spine *MODEMS* questionnaires developed by the AAOS, NASS, and other specialty societies consists of more than 60 items for the cervical or lumbar spine. The scoliosis assessment has 90 items. About one third of the assessment addresses symptom severity and its impact. These sections require about 5 minutes to complete.

Unfortunately, the MODEMS program was terminated March 1, 2000, because of lack of financial viability. The AAOS was successful in developing these validated instruments, which are still available. The AAOS Functional Outcome Questionnaires also assess symptoms of spinal disorder.[6]

Generic Functional Status Assessments

General assessments of the health status of the individual patient include the Short Form 36 Health Survey Questionnaire (SF-36), the Short Form 12 Health Survey Questionnaire (SF-12), the Musculoskeletal Function Assessment Instrument (MFA), the Short Musculoskeletal Function Assessment Questionnaire (SMFA), and the Sickness Impact Profile (SIP).

The SMFA was designed for office-based assessment of patients with musculoskeletal disorders. It is a shortened version of the MFA. This assessment instrument consists of 46 questions. It represents a tool for assessing musculoskeletal care in general delivered in a community-based setting. It has been found to give a reliable, valid, and responsive assessment of the health status of individual patients.[35]

The SF-36 consists of 36 questions requiring 15 to 20 minutes to complete. It assesses eight health areas or scales, including physical, role, emotional, and social functioning, pain, mental health, vitality, and general health. The SF-12 consists of 12 questions requiring 6 minutes to complete. It is a validated shortened version of the SF-36.[10]

The SIP consists of 136 questions and requires 30 minutes to complete. The 12 categories that it covers include sleep and rest, work, home management, recreation, ambulation, mobility, bodily care and movement, social interaction, alertness, behavior, emotional behavior, and communication.[1]

Region- or Disease-Specific Assessments

Outcomes assessment of patients with spinal disorders is challenging. For spine care physicians, region-specific measures of the neck or back give a more responsive assessment of spinal treatment. Many interrelated factors affect a patient's response to treatment, such as pain, neurologic deficit, functional limitation, psychologic impairment, and complicating social circumstances. A multidimensional disease-specific assessment is needed. However, using a spine-specific measure in conjunction with a generic measure will avoid missing complications in areas unrelated to the spine. Examples of region-specific instruments include the Oswestry low back pain disability questionnaire, the Roland-Morris Disability scale, the Prolo scale, and the AAOS MODEMS questionnaires and NASS instruments.

The Oswestry disability and Roland-Morris disability scales focus on the impact on role function evaluation. They are useful in assessment of outcomes in relation to work status.[12,32] The Prolo scale is a paradigm designed to provide uniformity in evaluating the results of lumbar spine operations. It uses an anatomic, economic, and functional rating system. With this scale, overall results are quantitatively rated as excellent (10, 9), good (8, 7), fair (6, 5), or poor (4, 3, 2).[30] The economic status ranges from a category of E1, which is defined as a complete invalid, to category E5, which is equivalent to working the previous occupation with no restrictions. Functional status includes an F1, which is total incapacity or worse than before the operation, to a category of F5, which is complete recovery with no recurrent episodes of low back pain and able to perform all previous sport activities. An anatomic scale was also proposed; however, the economic and functional rating scale that has a possible numerical range from 2 to 10 is the portion of the scale that is most commonly used.[3]

The NASS and AAOS instruments have become the most predominant, prevalent, and extensively tested of region-specific assessments for the spine. The NASS Lumbar Spine Outcome Assessment Instrument, known as the "NASS instrument," was developed based on studies by NASS as well as other spine societies beginning in 1991. In 1993, the AAOS developed a set of outcomes questionnaires covering the musculoskeletal areas of spine, lower extremity, upper extremity, and pediatrics. These efforts were aimed at collecting quality data and measuring clinical outcomes.

In 1994 the NASS instrument was presented to the AAOS as the prototype for other musculoskeletal societies to develop similar region-specific instruments. By 1996 this joint project involved the Council of Musculoskeletal Specialty Societies (COMSS), Council of Spine Societies (COSS), including NASS, Scoliosis Research Society, Cervical Spine Research Society, Orthopedic Rehabilitation Association, and American Spinal Injury Association. The instrument is known as the

AAOS/COMMS/COSS Spine Outcomes Data Collection Questionnaire (MODEMS) Questionnaire. These societies participated in the development of this instrument with more than 100 surgeons.*,†

The NASS instrument was tested in 1996 for acceptability, reliability, and validity. It was found to be acceptable in that it requires about 20 minutes to complete and was practical for patients. It was reliable in that it was consistent on repeated testing and correlated on a sufficient number of items within scales so that random errors would not unacceptably distort results. It was valid as measured by comparing results with judgments made by patients and experts. Results of individual scales were similar to scales on other tests and were able to discriminate between varying clinical circumstances.[6] It addresses the multidimensional effects on patients with a spinal disorder. The instrument assesses a pain disability score, neurologic impairment score, expectation score, and expectation-met score. This instrument can be used as a tool to compare individual databases through these core scores.

The goal of these ongoing efforts remains the development of reliable measures to assess the quality of care and well-being of patients in response to treatment. The joint effort with COSS is expanding the NASS instrument to include cervical, myelopathic, and cosmetic assessment. The evaluation of these instruments remains a continual process for various diagnoses and diverse groups of patients. The applicability, reliability, and validity testing of these instruments must be repeated for

---

OUTCOME INSTRUMENTS

- Symptom assessment
  - Dallas Pain Score
  - McGill Pain Questionnaire
  - Von Korff Chronic Pain Grade
  - Visual analog scales
- Generic functional assessment
  - Sickness Impact Profile
  - Musculoskeletal Functional Assessment (MFA)
  - Short Musculoskeletal Functional Assessment (SMFA)
  - Short Form 36 Health Survey Questionnaire (SF-36)
  - Short Form 12 Health Survey Questionnaire (SF-12) Sickness Impact Profile (SIP)
- Region or disease specific
  - NASS Lumbar Spine Outcomes Instrument
  - AAOS/COMMS/COSS: Lumbar, cervical, scoliosis
  - Roland-Morris Disability Scale
  - Oswestry Low Back Pain Disability Questionnaire
  - Prolo Scale

---

* www.aaos.org/wordhtml/outcomes/outguide.htm and
  www.modems.org/AAOS/COMMS/COSS
  Spine Data Collection Questionnaire and AAOS Musculoskeletal Outcomes Data Evaluation and Management System (MODEMS) Baseline and Follow-up Instruments: Cervical Spine Questionnaire, Lumbar Spine Questionnaire, and Scoliosis Spine Questionnaire.
† www.spine.org
  The NASS outcomes instrument.

each differing study application. Current evaluations include patient benefit from surgical and nonsurgical treatment for painful degenerative disc disease, using the NASS instrument as the assessment tool.*,†

DECISION ANALYSIS AND CLINICAL GUIDELINES

Decision analysis has been used in both business and military strategies. It has been adopted for medical decision making. Decision analysis is useful in making decisions in the face of uncertainty. Probabilities are assigned based on statistical results from clinical research. The analysis presents a series of probabilities of occurrences. Outcomes are weighted differently according to desirability. Combining probabilities and values yields strategies for maximum results. Through decision analysis, it is possible to estimate the outcome of various treatment alternatives. It translates statistical results into a series of probabilities of patient outcomes given various conditions. This method also shows where information is missing and where additional data through clinical research are needed. Decision analysis leads to the formation of algorithms or decision trees.[28,34]

Algorithms and clinical guidelines have become more important and prevalent in health care. The health care environment demands efficacious and cost-effective treatment. Accountability of care with the need to explain practice variation has created a demand for developing evidence-based algorithms. There is a need to define what is reasonable and what works. Clinical guidelines are being used by physicians, government agencies, and insurance companies. Algorithms and clinical guidelines develop both as a product and as a tool of outcomes research. Through this tool, knowledge from studies is disseminated into clinical practice.

Clinical guidelines are not standards of care. Clinical guidelines present a very narrow view of a topic, whereas standards of care cover a much broader area. These practice guidelines help define areas of standards of care, especially because only a very small percentage of today's standards of surgery and medical intervention

are supported by evidence. Developing clinical guidelines leads the standards of care of a community toward the practice of evidence-based medicine.[26]

Clinical guidelines are written as algorithms as well as pathways or matrices or even in narrative form. Guidelines include those developed, written, and used in individual practices. Formal guidelines draw on the literature, including outcomes studies and meta-analyses. They are also developed by a consensus of experts in a particular field based on clinical experience and knowledge. Guidelines from the literature require strong scientific evidence. Frequently, there are gaps in evidence in regard to surgical treatment due to a lack of randomized controlled studies. Expert consensus is often drawn on to supplement the formulation of an algorithm. Guideline development is a continuous process and requires repeated revision and refinement as new data become available.

NASS and AAOS have developed and continue to refine algorithms on clinical care of the spine. These algorithms represent reasonable guides to clinical decision making. The clinical algorithms on low back pain are divided into three phases. The guidelines address the diagnosis and treatment of adult low back pain not associated with infection, trauma, or neurologic deficit. They outline reasonable information-gathering and decision-making processes used in the management of low back pain. The first two phases were developed jointly by AAOS and NASS in 1996. The third phase is being developed and refined by NASS.*,†

Phase I of the NASS Low Back Pain algorithm addresses back pain in the first 4 to 6 weeks as presented to the treating physician. Phase II is oriented toward musculoskeletal specialists. It is intended for patients with back pain persisting beyond the first 4 to 6 weeks and addresses unremitting low back pain with the potential diagnosis of disc herniation, spinal stenosis, and spondylolisthesis.*,†

Phase III is intended for multidisciplinary spine care specialists and expands on the information in the first two phases. It is intended to coordinate and refine common clinical definitions and definitions of treatment success as well as treatment failure. Phase III addresses treatment time frame, end points of treatment, and other planned areas of focus.

The algorithms are intended to be educational tools to improve care for practicing physicians in the multidisciplinary field of spine care.*,† The process involves limited use testing, refinement, finalization, and dissemination.

NASS has taken a leading position in the development of guidelines for spine care. The NASS guidelines are

---

┌───┐
│   **DECISION ANALYSIS**   │
│ ─────────────────────────────────────   │
│ • Presents a series of probabilities of occurrences │
│ • Estimates outcomes of treatment alternatives │
│ • Allows decision making in face of uncertainty │
│ • Illustrates areas of data deficiency │
│ • Constructs algorithms   │
└───┘

---

* www.aaos.org/wordhtml/outcomes/outguide.htm and
   www.modems.org/AAOS/COMMS/COSS
   Spine Data Collection Questionnaire and AAOS Musculoskeletal
   Outcomes Data Evaluation and Management System (MODEMS)
   Baseline and Follow-up Instruments: Cervical Spine Questionnaire,
   Lumbar Spine Questionnaire, and Scoliosis Spine Questionnaire.
† www.spine.org
   The NASS outcomes instrument.

* www.aaos.org/wordhtml/outcomes/outguide.htm and
   www.modems.org/AAOS/COMMS/COSS
   Spine Data Collection Questionnaire and AAOS Musculoskeletal
   Outcomes Data Evaluation and Management System (MODEMS)
   Baseline and Follow-up Instruments: Cervical Spine Questionnaire,
   Lumbar Spine Questionnaire, and Scoliosis Spine Questionnaire.
† www.spine.org
   The NASS outcomes instrument.

developed by and are intended for multidisciplinary health care professionals. The NASS methodology uses the existing literature as well as expert consensus. The multidisciplinary approach uses both specialists and primary care providers. Specialists include orthopedists, neurosurgeons, physiatrists, neurologists, anesthesiologists, radiologists, rheumatologists, and psychiatrists. Consultation with family practitioners, managed care specialists, and third party payers is also included.*

Currently, NASS guidelines on the herniated disc are in draft version. Guidelines on unremitting low back pain, spinal stenosis, and spondylolisthesis are in progress. These guidelines will be helpful educational tools. The goal of guidelines is to disseminate clinical information gathered through outcomes research for improved patient care. Guidelines are not edicts. As medicine is not exact, room for variation and preferences is necessary.

There exist separate and distinct guidelines from various parties. Guidelines are used to authorize or deny treatment. The potential for misuse of guidelines by third party payers exists. Physician expert and clinical specialist involvement is a necessary part of the development process. Many individualized guidelines exist in health care, some with political and business objectives. With a particular set of treatment guidelines, it is necessary to know who developed the guidelines, the purpose for which they were developed, and the methods on which they were based.

IMPLEMENTATION

Implementation of an outcomes program within one's clinical practice is becoming common and essential. Examination of the outcomes of patients affords opportunity to improve the quality of health care. The steps involved in performing outcomes assessment are multiple. A complete assessment requires a team working together on the various aspects. Decisions need to be made regarding the treatment that one wants to study. High-cost and high-volume procedures are suitable for study. These treatments have the necessary volume for assessment and are in need of evaluation due to high utilization of resources. The appropriate questionnaire and timeline need to be chosen. Data collection must be coordinated with simplified and organized data entry. Technology and software decisions determine ease of data collection. Data will need appropriate analysis along with the aid of a biostatistician. Discussion of the results, determination of clinical relevance, and decisions of future treatment practices also require a team approach. Considerable expense and time devoted to such a project will require large groups of participating practitioners who are part of the same team.[9,23]

Assembling quality data is an ongoing process with a long learning curve. Requirements include compliance to a practical, easy process with a good project design. Handheld computers, workable software, and forms that can be scanned help ensure compliance. Comorbidity must be recorded; underreporting of comorbidity will diminish the quality of data. Comorbidity and severity must be stratified. Follow-up needs to be addressed appropriately by office visits, e-mail, or telephone. Analysis of data requires spreadsheet and software programs. Standardized instruments are available for participation with large groups or for comparison with other pools of data. Alternatively, one can design and validate questionnaires to answer questions about one's practice. Another option includes hiring an outside professional company from which you can purchase the level of service desired.

Costs for an outcomes program is estimated at $30,000 to $60,000 for the first year, including setup. Each year thereafter is estimated at $15,000 to $30,000 per year to run. There are many variables, however, including the personnel need, software and technology chosen, available office space, and committed time.

Questions to answer through outcomes research of spine surgery include length of stay, pain level, patient satisfaction (would the patient have had the surgery again?), functional status, return to work, and complications of treatment. Ultimately, it is not how many procedures were performed but how many were successful that is important. Eliminate that which does not work well. Outcomes assessment allows one to practice evidence-based medicine. Outcomes assessment can be used to demonstrate effective clinical practice. Outcomes data help the clinician to educate the patient on expectations and improve patient satisfaction. The gratification

---

CLINICAL GUIDELINES

- Disseminate outcomes information.
- Formation of algorithms, pathways, matrices, and narrative protocols.
- Use clinical experience, literature, and expert consensus.
- Continuous revision and refinement.
- Guidelines help define standards of care.
- Guidelines lead to practice of evidence-based medicine.

PATIENT ASSESSMENT USED IN PRACTICE

- Demonstrate effective practice.
- Educate patient on expectations.
- Improve patient satisfaction.

OUTCOMES DATA

- Clinical: Complications, reoperation, readmission rate
- Functional: Physical, quality of life, patient derived
- Financial: Length of stay, total cost reimbursement

---

* www.spine.org
The NASS outcomes instrument.

PHYSICIAN DIRECTION IN OUTCOMES ASSESSMENT

- Physician-patient relationship strongest
- Closest to patient interests
- Directly accountable for health care decision
- Comprehensive medical knowledge
- Extensive training in delivery of health care

---

derived from outcomes assessment lies in verification that the way you do it works well!

CONCLUSIONS

Assessing the outcomes of individual patients receiving a treatment for the spine is essential in today's health care environment. Quality results are complex, highly personal, and difficult to determine without standardized and validated instruments. Many individual issues exist independent of and diverse to each patient and physician. Physicians need to include patients in the assessment process. Health care requires greater patient understanding and selection of treatment alternatives. The physician who understands outcomes beyond an in-depth knowledge of spinal disorders is best positioned to improve the quality of life of patients through surgical as well as nonsurgical treatment.

In summary, to assess the benefits and effectiveness of his or her treatment approach with patients, the spine specialist can use these assessment instruments and methods. Appropriate data will guide the direction of future treatment. The existence of national databases, online instruments via the Internet, and private assessment companies serves to assemble and interpret these data to be used by consumers and purchasers of health care services. The leaders and specialty providers of health care services for the spine cannot avoid influencing and directing this process. Third party entities that control assessment will direct the outcomes process toward self-interest perspectives. Physicians are closest to the patients' interests and are directly accountable for the health care decisions. We must involve ourselves in outcome assessments that emphasize the patient's perspective.

WEBSITES AND QUESTIONNAIRES

- www.aaos.org/wordhtml/outcomes/outguide.htm and www.modems.org/AAOS/COMMS/COSS
  Spine Outcomes Data Collection Questionnaire and AAOS Musculoskeletal Outcomes Data Evaluation and Management System (MODEMS) Baseline and Follow-up Instruments: Cervical Spine Questionnaire, Lumber Spine Questionnaire, and Scoliosis Spine Questionnaire
- www.med.umn.edu/ortho/clinoutres.htm
  Musculoskeletal Function Assessment Instrument (MFA)

- www.ncqa.org/pages/communications/publications/hedispub.htm
  NCQA Health Plan Employer Data and Information Set (HEDIS) Includes HEDIS-2000, SF-12, and HEDIS-3000
- www.outcomes.org/thkr/womac.html
  Interpretation guide to The Western Ontario and McMaster Universities (WOMAC) Osteoarthritis Index
- www.sf-36.com/
  Short Musculoskeletal Function Assessment Questionnaire (SMFA), SF-36 and SF-12 Health Surveys
- www.spine.org
  The NASS outcomes instrument

Outcomes Web Sites

- www.aaos.org
- www.med.umn.edu
- www.modems.org
- www.ncqa.org
- www.outcomes.org
- www.sf-36.com
- www.spine.org

SELECTED REFERENCES

Calderone RR et al.: Outcome assessment in spinal infections, *Orthop Clin North Am* 27(1):201-205, 1996.

Daltroy LH et al.: The North American Spine Society Lumbar Spine Outcome Instrument; Reliability and Validity Tests, *Spine* 21(6):741-749, 1996.

Haselkorn JK et al.: Meta-analysis: a useful tool for the spine researcher, *Spine* 19(18S):2076S-2082S, 1994.

Keller RB: Outcomes research in orthopaedics, *JAAOS* 1(2):122-129, 1993.

Relman AS: Assessment and accountability: the third revolution in medical care, *N Engl J Med* 319:1220-1222, 1988.

Volinn E et al.: Why does geographic variation in health care practices matter? (And seven questions to ask in evaluating studies on geographic variation), *Spine* 19(18S):2092S-2100S, 1994.

Vrbos LA et al.: Clinical methodologies and incidence of appropriate statistical testing in orthopaedic spine literature: are statistics misleading? *Spine* 18(8):1021-1029, 1993.

REFERENCES

1. Bergner M et al.: The sickness impact profile: development and final revision of a health status measure, *Med Care* 19:787-805, 1981.
2. Bombardier C et al.: A guide to interpreting epidemiologic studies on the etiology of back pain, *Spine* 19(18S):2047S-2056S, 1994.
3. Calderone RR et al.: Outcome assessment in spinal infections, *Orthop Clin North Am* 27(1):201-205, 1996.
4. Cherkin DC et al.: An international comparison of back surgery rates, *Spine* 19:1201-1206, 1994.
5. Conrad DA, Deyo RA: Economic decision analysis in the diagnosis and treatment of low back pain: a methodologic primer, *Spine* 19(18S):2102S-2106S, 1994.
6. Daltroy LH et al.: The North American Spine Society Lumbar Spine Outcome Instrument; Reliability and Validity Tests, *Spine* 21(6):741-749, 1996.
7. Deyo RA, Cherkin DC, Loeser JD: Morbidity and mortality in association with operations on the lumbar spine: the influence of age, diagnosis and procedure, *J Bone Joint Spine Am* 74:536-543, 1992.
8. Deyo RA et al.: Analysis of automated administrative and survey databases to study patterns and outcomes of care, *Spine* 19(18S):2083S-2091S, 1994.
9. Deyo RA et al.: Designing studies of diagnostic tests for low back pain or radiculopathy, *Spine* 19(18S):2057S-2065S, 1994.

10. Deyo RA et al.: Outcome measures for studying patients with low back pain, *Spine* 19(18S):2032S-2036S, 1994.

11. Ellwood PM: Shattuck Lecture: outcomes management, *N Engl J Med* 318(23):1549-1557, 1988.

12. Fairbank JC et al.: The Oswestry low back pain disability questionnaire, *Physiotherapy* 66(8):271-273, 1980.

13. Gartland JJ: Orthopaedic clinical research: deficiencies in experimental design and determinations of outcome, *J Bone Joint Surg Am* 70:1357-1364, 1988.

14. Glass GV: Primary, secondary, and meta-analysis of research, *Educ Res* 5:3-8, 1976.

15. Guyatt G, Walter S, Norman G: Measuring change over time: assessing the usefulness of evaluative instruments, *J Chronic Dis* 40:171-178, 1987.

16. Haselkorn JK: Meta-analysis: a useful tool for the spine researcher, *Spine* 19(18S):2076S-2082S, 1994.

17. Herkowitz HN, Kurz LT: Degenerative lumbar spondylolisthesis with spinal stenosis: a prospective study comparing decompression with decompression and intertransverse process arthrodesis, *J Bone Joint Surg Am* 73(6):802-808, 1991.

18. Hoffman RM et al.: Therapeutic trials for low back pain, *Spine* 19(18S):2068S-2075S, 1994.

19. Jaglal S, Lakhani Z, Schatzker J: Reliability, validity, and responsiveness of the lower extremity measure for patients with a hip fracture, *J Bone Joint Surg Am* 82(7):955-962, 2000.

20. Kahn HA, Sempos CT: *Statistical methods in epidemiology,* New York, 1989, Oxford University Press.

21. Katz S et al.: Studies of illness in the ages: the index of ADS and standardized measure of biological and psychosocial function, *JAMA* 185:914-919, 1963.

22. Katz SJ, Larson EB, LoGerfo JP: Trends in the utilization of mammography in Washington State and British Columbia, *Med Care* 30:320-328, 1992.

23. Keller RB: Outcomes research in orthopaedics, *JAAOS* 1(2):122-129, 1993.

24. Lawlis GF et al.: The development of the Dallas Pain Questionnaire: an assessment of the impact of spinal pain on behavior, *Spine* 14(5):511-516, 1989.

25. Lawton MP, Brody EM: Assessment of older people: self-maintaining and instrumental activities of daily living, *Gerontologist* 9:179-186, 1969.

26. Lomas J: Words without action? The production, dissemination, and impact of consensus recommendations, *Annu Rev Public Health* 12:41-65, 1991.

27. Melzack R: The McGill pain questionnaire: major properties and scoring methods, *Pain* 1:277-299, 1975.

28. Orthopedic Knowledge Update 4, Frymoyer JW, ed: *Outcomes studies in orthopedic surgery,* Rosemont, Ill, 1993, American Academy of Orthopedic Surgeons.

29. Patrick DL, Deyo RA: Generic and disease-specific measures in assessing health status and quality of life, *Med Care* 27(suppl 3):S217-S232, 1989.

30. Prolo DJ, Oklund SA, Butcher M: Toward uniformity in evaluating results of lumbar spine operations, *Spine* 11(6):601-606, 1990.

31. Relman AS: Assessment and accountability: the third revolution in medical care, *N Engl J Med* 319:1220-1222, 1988.

32. Roland M, Morris R: A study of the natural history of low back pain, *Spine* 8(2):145-150, 1983.

33. Shekelle PG et al.: A brief introduction to the critical reading of the clinical literature, *Spine* 19(18S):2028S-2031S, 1994.

34. Sox HC et al., eds: 1988 Decision making when the outcomes have several dimensions. In *Medical decision making,* New York, Butterworth Publishers.

35. Swiontkowski MF et al.: Short musculoskeletal function assessment questionnaire: validity reliability, and responsiveness, *J Bone Joint Surg Am* 81(9):1245-1260, 1999.

36. Taylor VM et al.: Low back pain hospitalization: recent U.S. trends and regional variations, *Spine* 19:1207-1212, 1994.

37. Turner JA et al.: Surgery for lumbar spinal stenosis: attempted meta-analysis of the literature, *Spine* 17(1):1-8, 1992.

38. Volinn E et al.: Small area analysis of surgery for low back pain, *Spine* 17:575-581, 1992.

39. Volinn E et al.: Why does geographic variation in health care practices matter? (And seven questions to ask in evaluating studies on geographic variation), *Spine* 19(18S):2092S-2100S, 1994.

40. Von Korff M: Studying the natural history of back pain, *Spine* 19(18S):2041S-2046S, 1994.

41. Vrbos LA et al.: Clinical methodologies and incidence of appropriate statistical testing in orthopaedic spine literature: are statistics misleading? *Spine* 18(8):1021-1029, 1993.

42. Walsh K, Cruddas M, Coggon D: Low back pain in eight areas of Britain, *J Epidemiol Commun Health* 46:227-230, 1992.

43. Wennberg A, Gittelsohn A: Small area variations in health care delivery, *Science* 182:1102-1108, 1973.

44. Wennberg JE: Population illness rates do not explain population hospitalization rates, *Med Care* 25:354-359, 1987.

45. Wennberg JE, Freeman JL, Culp WJ: Are hospital services rationed in New Haven or over-utilized in Boston? *Lancet* 1:1185-1189, 1987.

Outpatient Rehabilitation of the Spine Patient

Vert Mooney

LUMBAR SPINE REHABILITATION
Subacute Evaluation and Treatment

The value of rehabilitation for the patient suffering from first-time back and/or leg pain is not clear. Several extensive studies have offered some guidelines, but none have provided a scientifically based rationale. The most recent major report is from the U.S. Department of Health and Human Services Agency Report of Health Care Policy and Research, published in 1994.[1]

The government guidelines failed to recommend a specific treatment program because of the perceived lack of scientific evidence or the political need to avoid controversy. The report emphasizes that commonly used modalities such as ultrasound, massage, bracing, and traction have no scientific evidence to support the benefit for the subacute back or leg pain sufferer. The guidelines recommended swimming and other aerobic exercises, although no evidence exists to support the benefit of aerobic exercises for back pain. The guidelines opposed specific exercises such as stretching, without providing evidence why stretching would not be helpful (or why stretching would be harmful). The report also includes the statement that "exercises for trunk muscles are more mechanically stressful to the back than aerobic exercises." Although conditioning exercises for the cardiovascular system are recommended, conditioning exercises for the musculoskeletal system are not.

Even the Quebec guidelines, the predecessor to the U.S. Department of Health and Human Services report, offered no specific recommendations for exercise or physical treatment.[48] No apparent rationale for exercise was proposed in this extensive survey of 769 articles published in 1987. The Quebec study stated that "a series of prescribed therapeutic exercises or activities taught to the patient and done at home or work following a given schedule may be appropriate."

The purpose of this chapter is to propose a rationale for an exercise program for the spine. Rational rehabilitation of the spine should be an active process and correspond to principles that are used with the rest of the musculoskeletal system. The rehabilitation available to an injured professional athlete is the best demonstration of how a spinal injury should be treated. The athlete's recovery is supervised by a trainer employed by the professional team; he/she also has access to a fully equipped training room funded and staffed by the professional team. The rehabilitation program incorporates a progressive training schedule using equipment that measures progress and identifies deviation from normal.

Spine rehabilitation will be more effective if it includes some measurement of progress. A patient's change in subjective pain response to treatment is a way of measuring progress, although the character of that change should correspond to some conceptual framework. The McKenzie program is the only system that identifies a conceptual framework for the treatment of spinal pain secondary to disc abnormality. In addition, the McKenzie program is the only spinal physical therapy program with postgraduate training for the therapist leading to eventual credentialing. The McKenzie system includes the important concept that the composition of disc material can be changed to reduce peripheral irritation from repeated end-range movements.

LUMBAR SPINE

McKenzie spinal physical therapy program
- Only system that:
  - Identifies a conceptual framework for the treatment of spinal pain secondary to disc abnormality
  - Includes postgraduate training for the therapist leading to eventual credentialing
- Aims to reduce peripheral irritation via repeated end-range movements
- Progress measured by centralization, peripheralization, and range of motion with repeated end-range movements
  - Centralization: Pain moves from the leg into center of the low back and is associated with a favorable outcome
  - Peripheralization: Pain progresses more distally in the extremity
  - Extension: Range-of-motion activity most affected in back injuries

These therapeutic movements, which include extension or side gliding, are instituted through a standardized series of physical tests performed in a standard algorithm manner by a therapist.

Phenomena known as centralization and peripheralization are inherent to the measurement of progress. Centralization occurs as the pain moves from the leg into the center of the low back. Peripheralization occurs when the pain cannot retreat to the low back with repeated end-range movements but instead progresses more distally in the extremity. In 1990 Donelson et al.[10] predicted the successful outcome from physical therapy based on the centralization factor. In this study of 87 patients with back and leg pain, 87% centralized and had a good outcome, whereas only 4 patients peripheralized their pain following repeated end-range movements and required surgery.

Progress can also be measured by range of motion. The McKenzie algorithm helps to demonstrate that extension is the range-of-motion activity most affected in back injuries. Kopp et al.[27] reported that 90% of patients achieved normal lumbar extension with conservative treatment, whereas only 6% of patients demonstrated significantly improved spinal extension after lumbar disc surgery. Range and pain movements therefore constitute an important measure of treatment for the lumbar spine.

Symptom magnification is one of the most complex issues related to the treatment of back and leg pain. Although the Waddell[56] test is a reliable method to confirm this problem, the physician or therapist must assess whether there is a relationship between symptom magnification, a psychologic phenomenon, and the centralization phenomenon that is related to anatomic and chemical abnormalities. Karas et al.[24] compared the centralization phenomenon and Waddell scores in 17 patients from the Canadian Back Institute. This study demonstrated that rate of return to work in patients who centralized their symptoms and had low Waddell scores was 51% higher than in patients who centralized their symptoms and had high Waddell scores. On the other hand, with low Waddell scores, the rate of return to work was 30% higher for patients who centralized their symptoms than patients who did not. The Waddell score predicted return to work better than centralization, although both had excellent predictive value. Based on this study, return to work and response to mechanical therapy were most unlikely for patients who did not centralize their symptoms after two treatments and had high Waddell scores.

We need to determine the relationship between the centralization phenomenon and structural abnormalities because of their effect on the rehabilitation process. A physical therapist using the McKenzie algorithm on patients with severe back and leg pain put them through active end-range activities to observe the change in pain pattern. On the basis of the location of their pain and response to end-range activity, he predicted the location of the disc tear on a drawing of an axial view of the disc. The test included a discogram with computed tomography (CT) scan evaluation. A third observer with no addi-

tional information reviewed the therapist's drawing of the location of the tear within the disc and the CT scan of the discogram. The pictures of the disc correlated with the discogram in terms of level, location, and character 85% of the time, indicating significant reliability of the McKenzie evaluation system.[11]

In 1994 Rath[43] published data that examined the McKenzie method on 319 patients with subacute back pain. He reported a 95% success rate if patients were treated within the first month; the success rate dropped to 86% if the patients were treated in the first 7 weeks, whereas the success rate fell to 65% if treatment was delayed beyond 7 weeks. This study suggests that factors related to duration are involved in the recovery process that do not benefit from an active, progressive ranging-exercise program. Cherkin et al.[8] analyzed the effectiveness and costs of common treatment programs on patients with low back pain. They randomly assigned 321 adults whose back pain had persisted for 7 days to chiropractic care (40%), the McKenzie method (40%), and a third group who were given an instructional booklet as the only form of treatment (20%). Patients received manipulation for 1 month, and all groups were followed for 2 years. "Differences in the extent of dysfunction among the groups were small and approached significance only at 1 year, with greater dysfunction in the booklet group than in the other two groups ($P = 0.05$). For all outcomes, there were no significant differences between the physical therapy and chiropractic group and no significant difference among the groups in the number of days of reduced activity or missed work or in recurrences of back pain."

Evaluation and Treatment of Chronic Recurrent Lumbar Pain

Most of the problems of chronic recurrent back and leg pain are disc related or occur in the facet joint. Occasionally the sacroiliac joint can be the source of the problem in a small percentage of patients. Physicians should strive to address the problem of unresolved soft tissue injury and the impact of such an injury on back pain. The lack of predictability of radiographic degeneration seen in plain films, magnetic resonance imaging (MRI), or even discograms is a major concern for the physician treating a patient with an injured back. Although mechanical deterioration can occur, as reflected by these studies, it is not necessarily painful. Chemical analysis of the painful disc has shown increased concentrations of phospholipase A_2 and the spontaneous production of matrix metalloproteinases, nitric oxide, interleukin-6, and prostaglandins.[16,23] Kitano et al.[25] demonstrated that the pH of painful degenerative discs is more acidic than degenerative discs that are asymptomatic. Neurophysiologists have concluded that the increased concentration of all these chemicals creates noxious stimuli that the human cortex perceives as pain. The frequent end-range exercises carried out in the McKenzie program represent the physical component needed to enhance fluid exchange and return biochemical homeostasis in the disc to preinjury levels.

The physiotherapy department at the University of Queensland in Brisbane, Australia, provided additional research into the neurologic response of the soft tissue to back pain. They used real-time ultrasound and wire-electrode electromyography (EMG) analysis of specific muscles. It was possible to identify the location of the electrode in various muscles of the torso and also to determine the size of the muscles at various points in time with ultrasound.

Hides et al.[18] examined the lumbar multifidus muscle in 26 patients with acute low back pain. All patients showed a significant reduction in the size of the multifidus muscle ipsilateral to the painful side, whereas normal subjects with no history of back pain demonstrated no comparable change in size or shape of the multifidus musculature. Another study confirmed that the multifidus muscle recovered more rapidly in patients who received medical treatment combined with specific exercise therapy, compared with patients given medical treatment as the only option.[14] The investigators showed that the multifidus muscle was still reduced at 10 weeks in this group of patients.[17]

Hodges and Richardson[20,21] analyzed the importance of postinjury inhibition and facilitation on trunk muscle activity. They monitored instantaneous muscle activity using fine-wire electrode technology and myoelectric analysis when the subjects were involved in normal functional activity. It was apparent that stabilization was being used before the position of the torso was changed; the transversus muscle together with the multifidus was active 7 milliseconds before arm activity or torso activity occurred. The data indicate that the transversalis and multifidus muscles function as torso stabilizers before physical mechanical activity occurred. The onset of back pain eliminated the torso-stabilizing function and delayed the myoelectric activity of these muscles, and in addition initial torso stabilization was hindered. The lack of protection for the unguarded moment provided by these muscles may explain repeated soft tissue injury.

All these studies emphasize the importance of exercise in the recovery process. A reasonable therapeutic approach would be to include a strengthening program

---

TREATMENT ADJUNCTS

- Exercises: Important during the recovery process
- Maintenance of muscle strength: Correlates with improvement of chronic recurrent back pain in patients who have failed previous physical therapy and chiropractic treatment
- Epidural steroid injections: Successfully coupled with exercise training; the steroids reduce reactive inflammation associated with disc herniation or flare-up of inflammation secondary to excessive exercise
- Lumbar stabilization: Effective treatment program that requires a sophisticated patient and guidance from an appropriate physical therapist and lacks the potential for graded measurement of progress

---

with the demonstration that muscle inhibition resulting in muscle atrophy occurred after injury. Hodges and Richardson et al.[44] did not use exercise equipment to objectively measure initial muscle strength and monitor strength training as the exercises progressed, although they evaluated myoelectric function with a sophisticated system. They also included a calisthenics exercise program for some of the patients with demonstrable muscle atrophy. In the 1-year follow-up 30% of patients whose treatment included the exercise program reported a recurrence of back pain compared with 80% for patients not participating in any exercise activity.

This finding confirms our study with MRI and surface-electrode myography that illustrates the effect of muscle inhibition following deterioration of the disc.[41] We evaluated the effects of an exercise treatment program on 8 patients with chronic back pain and 8 normal controls. The treatment consisted of a twice-weekly exercise program that lasted for 8 weeks. The patients were assessed by evaluating myoelectric activity, lumbar extensor strength, and cross-sectional MRI of the lumbar extensor muscles. A 65% improvement and 41% reduction in pain occurred in the 8 study patients, including a decrease in fatty infiltration in 4 patients with severe fatty infiltration in the multifidus muscle. A significant amount of fatty infiltration and muscle atrophy did not develop in the other muscles of the torso, such as the oblique muscles, or even the iliopsoas muscle. The amplitude of the monitored activity of the multifidus reduced about half after 8 weeks of training (Figure 59-1). The myoelectric changes did not correlate with the changes seen on the axial view of the MRI. Complaints were significantly reduced from patients involved in the general exercise program, as well as a specific exercise program on equipment that isolated the lumbar extensors and placed the strength training into both a concentric and eccentric mode. This study used MedX equipment that measures isometric strength at various points in the range but also allows dynamic exercises with variable resistance similar to Nautilus in a concentric/eccentric manner with weight of the body removed.

Leggett et al.[29] compared the rehabilitation of 412 patients with chronic back pain at two different centers using the same protocols. Patients were evaluated at intake, on discharge, and after 1-year follow-up. The effectiveness of treatment at the two centers was based on Short Form-36 scores, the participants' self-assessment of their improvement, and their use of health care services after discharge. The authors found that over 85% of the patients with chronic recurrent back pain had improved; all had failed previous physical therapy and chiropractic treatment, and previous surgery had failed in 12%. Patients who had a good response had returned to normal strength when tested, whereas those who had poor response did not demonstrate similar improvement in strength. When tested a year later, those who did well had maintained muscle strength. The treatment program for chronic leg and back pain used a standardized protocol regardless of the diagnostic labels presented by the patient. Strength training was

A Pre-Training Lumbar Exercise Dynamic EMG

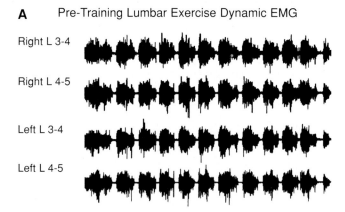

B Post-Training Lumbar Exercise Dynamic EMG

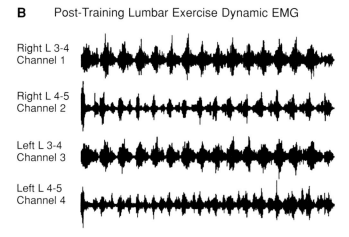

Figure 59-1. **A,** Myoelectric activity from surface electrodes in the paraspinal muscles for 11 cycles of flexion/extension resistance exercise on MedX equipment. **B,** Myoelectric activity of the same patient after 16 training sessions (8 weeks) using the same resistance that was used at the start of the training program. This record now represents 16 exercise cycles in the same time duration as in **A.**

started at 50% of their maximum isometric strength and progressed 5% on the occasion when they could do 20 repetitions with a specific resistance. Similar results were reported from both centers on all three measures used to demonstrate the benefit of these treatment programs.

A standardized protocol with a specific piece of equipment is not the only way to conduct a rehabilitation program for chronic recurrent disc problems. Saal[45,46] described a nonoperative program to treat patients with herniated nucleus pulposus and radiculopathy that incorporated aggressive physical rehabilitation methods, epidural steroid injections, and exercise training. Successful outcomes were reported in 50 out of the 52 patients participating in the treatment program. This study also demonstrated the benefit of using steroid injections to reduce reactive inflammation associated with a disc herniation or flare-up of inflammation secondary to excessive exercise.

Inflammation is an important factor when considering the sources of pain. A prospective study of conservatively treated patients who underwent CT scans after resolution of symptoms showed that 23% of the disc herniations resolved, 36% improved, and 21% remained unchanged.[13] Based on this study, no correlation appears to exist between a successful treatment program and the size of the herniation.

Lumbar stabilization is an effective treatment program and is advocated by many physicians in this country. Although lumbar stabilization requires intelligence on the part of the patient and guidance from an appropriate physical therapist, it lacks the potential for graded measurement of progress. Koes et al.[26] demonstrated the role that measurement of progress plays in rehabilitation. General practitioners were involved in this study, which included instructions to patients provided by physical therapists. Because it was a home-based program, the physicians were unable to document compliance or measure changes in muscle strength and range of motion. Despite the incomplete data, this study is often quoted as an example of the comparable results achieved from exercises and passive manual therapy for chronic back problems. An effective rehabilitation program must include equipment to identify and measure progress in the range, endurance, or resistance of the injured muscles.

The roman chair, which is a simpler piece of equipment than the MedX device, is available at some health clubs. Biering-Sorensen[6] demonstrated that the incidence of back injury was reduced in those patients who had sufficient endurance to hold the torso unsupported parallel to the ground for a minute using the roman chair. The predictive value of the roman chair was suggested because patients who were unable to complete that amount of lumbar extensor endurance had a higher incidence of back injury. The standard roman chair is extremely demanding for an individual with severe back pain or who is nonathletic and fearful of additional injury. A variable-angle Roman chair has been designed that allows the adjustment of torso position in six different angles ranging from 75 degrees to 0 degrees, parallel to the floor (Figure 59-2). In a series of studies on normal subjects the use of the variable-angle Roman chair was evaluated as the unsupported torso position moved the plates along the various angles from nearly standing erect (75 degrees) to fully parallel (0 degrees). If hand positions were changed from alongside the body to the chest and then to the head, this change in body position increased the lever arm of the body due to the arm's distance from the center axis of rotation. This maneuver increased the stresses on the lumbar extensors, and it was reported that even changing the orientation of hip rotation would challenge various muscles. The hip extensors were activated in myoelectric activity with external rotation, whereas internal rotation activated the lumbar extensors.[52] Patients benefit from this tool in a rehabilitation setting, where gradual and subtle increases in stresses are necessary to activate appropriate musculature without creating additional harm.

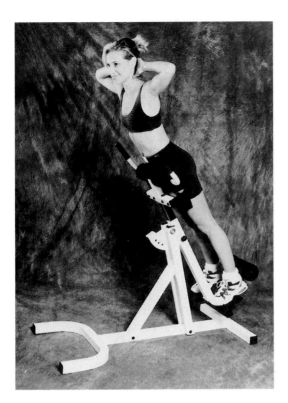

Figure 59-2. A variable-angle roman chair (BackStrong, Brea, Calif), which can be adjusted to various positions and thus allow increasing stress to the lumbar extensor muscles.

Postoperative Rehabilitation of the Lumbar Spine

Data suggest that inhibition of lumbar extensor activity and probably other torso muscles occurs in the postoperative state. Previous studies demonstrated that the lumbar extensor musculature undergoes extensive atrophy after surgery, which is reflected in diminished strength.[36] A gradual, progressive exercise program will help the patient if the postsurgery recovery program incorporates earlier mobilization of the musculature without causing additional destruction to the surgical site.

An exercise program is initiated within 2 or 3 weeks after laminotomy surgery when the incisions are comfortable. Because posterior surgery involves a defect in the annulus, patients should avoid flexion exercises but include progressive extensor exercises. A gradual introduction to various exercise programs is possible with the variable-angle roman chair, instead of the more restrained MedX equipment. Modalities such as hot packs, cold packs, massage, and ultrasound are appropriate to reduce reactive inflammation. Abdominal exercises to strengthen the transversus abdominis muscle provide an additional phase of the strengthening program, although a progressive aerobic exercise program that includes walking, treadmill, and so on should be combined with abdominal exercises. It is important to monitor the perceived exertion of the patient, and during the first phase exertion should be

REHABILITATION EXERCISES FOR THE LUMBAR SPINE

- Gradual, progressive exercise program is best with earlier mobilization of the musculature without causing additional destruction to the surgical site.
- Exercise is initiated within 2 to 3 weeks after laminectomy surgery, focusing on progressive extensor exercises while avoiding flexion exercises, because posterior surgery involves a defect in the annulus.
- Flexion exercises are appropriately introduced 4 to 5 weeks after surgery.
- The principle of postsurgical rehabilitation is first to achieve comfortable range with frequent repetitions. It is hoped that enhanced fluid exchange within the disc can occur during this period. Progressive resistance exercises are appropriate after the patient achieves functional ranging.

rated 2 to 4 out of a 10-point scale. The treatment should include ranging of the lumbar spine with minimum resistance if a pool program is available, although specific equipment to isolate the extremities for strengthening is also beneficial.

Phase II of the rehabilitation program begins 4 or 5 weeks after surgery when it is appropriate to introduce flexion exercises, and at this stage the resistance should be increased in extension exercises. Discomfort and fatigue may occur after 20 to 25 repetitions of resistance exercises. The patient should be permitted to do vigorous resistance exercises only twice a week with the exertion rate measured at 5 or 6 out of a possible 10-point scale. Phase III of a functional reconditioning program starts 6 to 8 weeks after surgery, and the exercise rate should measure 7 or 8 out of 10. The goal of exercises during Phase III should include standardized progression of resistance using specific equipment. The principle of postsurgical rehabilitation is first to achieve comfortable range with frequent repetitions. It is hoped that enhanced fluid exchange within the disc can occur during this period. Progressive resistance exercises are appropriate after the patient is capable of functional ranging.

Our studies have shown that no significant change in the protocol is necessary in cases of spinal fusion surgery. Ideally the patient is sufficiently stable after surgery to carry out the gradual, progressive exercise program, although destructive forces to the fusion can occur with sudden overload. A well-controlled, guided rehabilitation program that includes gradual, progressive ranging and resistance exercises with the assistance of equipment is not destructive to the fusion. A gradual progressive stimulus is the best physiologic force to achieve rapid bony consolidation, which is a situation similar to cases of fracture repair.

Before the patient returns to work, test maneuvers should confirm that the patient has sufficient strength and range to prevent reinjury. Some form of functional capacity evaluation is valuable because it gives the patient assurance and documentation about readiness and limits in the workplace. If deficits are present, the functional capacity evaluation will determine the kind of adjustments in lifestyle that are necessary.

FUNCTIONAL CAPACITY EVALUATION

The effects of spinal rehabilitation sometimes have administrative and legal consequences in addition to the physiologic progress of the patient. It is often difficult to settle personal injury claims, back-to-work issues, and long-term disability payments if response to rehabilitation efforts is defined purely by subjective statements on the part of the patient. The evaluation and treatment of soft tissue injuries constitute the most undefinable element of workers' compensation medical care. The lack of objective measurement has lead to the varied methodologies of treatment that have little scientific validation of one treatment method versus another. An attempt has been made in this chapter to offer some justification for the validity of rehabilitation maneuvers. However, administrative issues related to the workplace disability and personal injury often require documentation of the extent of the deficits.

In the workers' compensation arena, much of the insurance cost is used for the medical care of soft tissue injuries. With that in mind the California state legislature in 1993 asked the California Industrial Medical Council to determine the "technical feasibility of requiring objective medical findings for evaluation of soft tissue injuries." The way the legislation phrased their conclusions indicated an awareness that "medical findings" are not reliable in defining the extent of soft tissue injuries, which is also not a problem unique to California. A functional test known as the California Functional Capacity Protocol was developed and submitted in December of 1994.[40] Leonard Matheson designed the two main components of the functional test: (1) a perception-of-function test, and (2) a lift-capacity test. The perception of function includes a series of 50 pictures depicting graduated physical tacks. The system, which is known as spinal function sort (SFS), requires the patients to rate their ability to complete a specific task[32] (Figure 59-3). The patient works in a self-paced manner and, if necessary, requests help from the evaluator. Several physical functions are exactly the same but portrayed differently in different pictures. The physical demands of each picture are specifically identified and ultimately allow rating of the individual's perceived physical capacity based on a mathematical formula.

The lift-capacity test uses an isoinertial progressive lifting-capacity test known as EPIC Lift Capacity (ELC). The validity of the test is based on a comparison of age-matched controls and gender equalization controls for variations in height[35] (Figure 59-4). Standardized test circumstances are essential for a test that is dependable, and a comprehensive database should include large numbers of subjects/patients and multiple tests. The ELC method has standardized retest circumstances even to the point of using standardized instructions to achieve this reliable data.[32] The ELC uses blinded weight

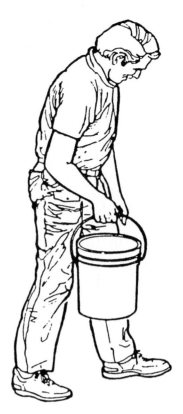

Figure 59-3. Typical pictures of the spinal function sort. The patient is asked on a scale of 5 whether he/she can or cannot do this activity, which depicts carrying a 25-pound bucket of water.

FUNCTIONAL CAPACITY EVALUATION

- Soft tissue injuries frequently very complex to treat because the severity of the injury cannot be precisely defined
- The California Functional Capacity Protocol includes:
  - A perception-of-function test
  - A lift-capacity test

---

in a standardized protocol of vertical and frequent lifting over three vertical ranges; the vertical ranges are varied according to the evaluee's height. Four repetitions of lifting are used in a 30-second cycle at three test heights. In a recent study of the reliability of the ELC based on 687 test batteries in 358 subjects, the correlation coefficient r = 0.90. The investigators reported no incidence of injury from testing.[33] These tests enable a patient to be rated according to the U.S. Department of Labor Physical Demand Characteristics System (PDC).[32] They can also be rated according to the California Disability Rating, which requires a physician to identify the percentage loss from preinjury functional capacity.

Another important phase of functional capacity testing is to recognize the validity of the patient/worker's effort. Jay et al.[22] evaluated the reliability and validity of an ELC test based on the sincere effort of a previously

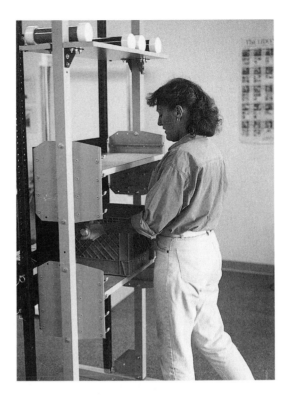

Figure 59-4. The EPIC Lift Capacity demonstrating variable positions of the shelves and blinded weights lifted in a standardized milk crate. The lifts are carried out in a standardized protocol.

SACROILIAC REHABILITATION

- Multiple clinical tests applied to identify sacroiliac disorders, including:
  - Faber: Flexion, abduction, and external rotation
  - Gaenslen: Fully flexed, the asymptomatic hip is extended over the side of the table
  - Posterior shear: Supine position with both hip and knee flexed 90 degrees while the knee receives a sharp impact
- Sacroiliac dysfunction
  - Caused by abnormal anterior rotation of the ileum on the sacrum
  - Approaches to therapy
    - Displace the ileum posteriorly through hyper-flexion of the hip
    - Stabilize the joint with sacroiliac belts or self-stabilize with muscle-strengthening exercises

injured population. This study evaluated 41 volunteers with a previously diagnosed musculoskeletal problem of the spine. Volunteers were randomized to either the control group, instructed to give a sincere maximum effort, or to the experimental group, instructed to give an insincere effort of 50% of perceived maximum effort. The results gave an overall accuracy of 87% in identifying participants' level of effort. The indicators of valid effort accounted for 95% of the total variation in the determination of the subjects' overall effort level.

It is essential for a functional capacity test to be both useful and profitable. The testing equipment and instructions must be standardized, and some relationship to normal function must be understood. A heart rate monitor is used to assess the physiologic effort in all of the leading tests in our clinic, although rating of effort is difficult. Based on this type of testing, we have been successful in identifying patients who were unfortunately trying to mislead the examiner.

SACROILIAC JOINT REHABILITATION

No reliable evidence exists that dysfunction of the disc versus the facet joint should require different strategies. There is no clinical picture that consistently separates primary pain generator in the facet joint from the pain generator in the disc. The ELC and PDC protocols provide reliable tests for either of these two generators.

The sacroiliac joint, however, presents a different problem because there is no clear-cut clinical syndrome

that clearly identifies the diagnosis. Although multiple clinical tests are applied to clarify the sacroiliac joint as the pain generator, physicians disagree about the most reliable test. No common clinical picture has emerged that fusion was necessary in a study of patients with severe pain unresponsive to conservative care.[42] A positive Faber test (flexion, abduction, and external rotation) was the most common physical finding. A positive result may be possible with the Gaenslen test, which requires the patient to fully flex the asymptomatic hip while the symptomatic side is extended over the side of the table. The posterior shear test is another common test that can predict sacroiliac problems; the test requires the patient to lie in a supine position with both hip and knee flexed at 90 degrees while the knee receives a sharp impact.[28] Schwarzer et al.[47] demonstrated that 2% lignocaine injected into the sacroiliac joint significantly reduced pain in 13 out of 43 patients (30%).

It is clear that a small amount of motion remains in patients with sacroiliac disorders. In a definitive study Sturesson et al.[50] showed that radiographic evaluation of the relative change between metal pellets on various functional activities (Selvik) demonstrates an average of 2 degrees of motion. The amount of translation on individuals with sacroiliac dysfunction was approximately 1.6 mm. Because the authors could not show any difference in motion between symptomatic and asymptomatic patients, we can conclude that tests that depend on evaluation of change of motion to the sacroiliac are probably unreliable.

It is useful to differentiate sacroiliac strain from common back pain. The patient should complain of tenderness at the long dorsal sacroiliac ligament, which is just caudal to posterior iliac spine. In a study of 300 medical practitioners only 10% recognized that the large dorsal sacroiliac ligament is so easily palpable, an indication that this physical finding is relatively unknown.[53]

Two anatomic approaches are possible to resolve the physical treatment of an incompetent or dysfunctional sacroiliac joint. The traditional approach involves a manipulative maneuver, which can be done either as a self-manipulation or with assistance. In the experience of physical therapist R. L. Don Tigny,[9] every incidence of sacroiliac dysfunction was caused by abnormal anterior rotation of the ileum on the sacrum. Don Tigny maintains that hyperflexion of the hip is necessary to displace the ileum posteriorly into its normal relationship. Other clinicians have also endorsed the effectiveness of manipulation. Cassidy et al.[7] described excellent results in 258 of 336 patients from daily manipulations for 2 to 3 weeks, but these results have not been replicated. The exact physiologic changes occurring with manipulation are unclear.

Because incompetence occurs with sacroiliac pain, it seems reasonable that stabilization of the joint would be helpful. Sacroiliac belts are successful in controlling incompetence, especially with the instability of a joint in pregnancy.[54]

Self-stabilization with muscle-strengthening exercises offers an alternative therapeutic maneuver. Mooney et al.[41] analyzed the role of the gluteus maximus and the contralateral latissimus dorsi with EMG analysis. In this study, torso rotation in a sitting position normally used the latissimus dorsi as the major force, although in individuals with sacroiliac dysfunction, the gluteus maximus was hyperactive while the contralateral latissimus dorsi was inhibited. Previous studies have demonstrated the presence of a fascial attachment from the latissimus of one side to the gluteus on the other side.[55]

When patients with sacroiliac dysfunction were placed into a progressive torso rotation–strengthening program, reversal of the EMG activity occurred. A reasonable alternative for patients with apparent sacroiliac dysfunction is for them to receive both manipulation and torso rotation–strengthening exercises. We have found that lumbar extensor strengthening in these particular individuals is a source of pain and not productive if forced into hyperextension.

THORACIC SPINE REHABILITATION

The thoracic spine is a particular area of spinal rehabilitation that seldom receives much attention, especially for patients with scoliosis. We have developed an effective approach to managing the painful thoracic spine in patients with adolescent idiopathic scoliosis that includes equipment capable of measuring a specific function.

Patients with thoracolumbar scoliosis that results from a degenerative or idiopathic basis had asymmetric strength in rotation on one side versus the other when carrying out rehabilitation programs. Although elite single-arm athletes are an exception, studies show that individuals without scoliosis are equal in rotation strength right to left and left to right. A MedX torso rotation machine, which allows isometric testing over various points in range, was used for the strength testing (Figure 59-5).

THORACOLUMBAR SCOLIOSIS

- Patients with thoracolumbar scoliosis (either degenerative or idiopathic in origin) have asymmetric strength in rotation on one side versus the other.
- Evidence that paraspinal muscle imbalance can create scoliosis in young athletes supports rehabilitation exercise regimens focusing on torso rotation strengthening to correct mild thoracolumbar scoliosis.

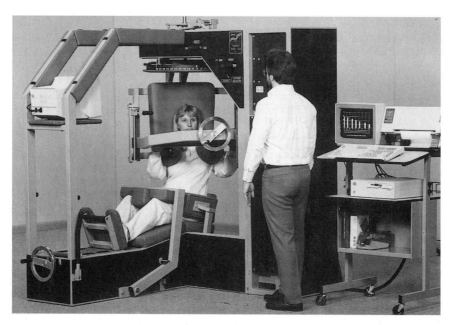

Figure 59-5. The computerized MedX torso rotation machine allows isometric testing over various points in range. The isometric strengths are depicted on the screen, as well as on a printout for comparison from one session to another.

Several studies suggest that scoliosis can develop in adolescents from vigorous single-arm activity. A Scandinavian study found that among elite athletes such as javelin throwers with asymmetric strength in their trunk and shoulders, a small thoracic curve of approximately 10 degrees occurs in more than 80% of these individuals.[51] In another study of 336 Junior Olympic swimmers, 16% had a mild scoliotic curve with the convex curvature on the side of hand dominance.[4] These data are surprising and suggest that if muscle imbalance can create scoliosis, then perhaps the reverse is also possible.

Because of these findings, we started an exercise program with torso rotation–strengthening for adolescents with scoliosis less than 45 degrees. In the torso rotation machine the pelvis is fixed with the individual sitting, and he/she rotates the torso against resistance that is varied by a weight stack. The mechanism has a rotatory axis attached to a cam so that a constant resistance can be achieved through the full arc of rotation, which is a feature typical of Nautilus type of devices. When the individual can achieve 20 repetitions with one amount of resistance, the resistance is increased about 5% at the next exercise session. The participants in this study initially exercised twice a week, but when their rotation strength became equal, it was reduced to once a week.

We also tested the myoelectric function of the paraspinal muscles and the abdominal obliques; it was clear that the paraspinal muscles were inhibited, but after an exercise program they functioned normally (Figure 59-6). Avikainen et al.[3] also described this asymmetry in the paraspinal muscles, especially the multifidus, when the thoracic and lumbar musculatures of adolescents with scoliosis were tested with electromyograms. We also found significant differences in the lumbar myoelectric activity during isometric strength testing in the standing position during sudden acts of exertion. The lumbar muscles were inhibited even when the curves were purely in the thoracic spine and did not involve the lumbar spine. This research suggests that asymmetric spinal function activation may not be caused by the curvature itself but may be caused by central nervous system dysfunction. In a limited study of 12 adolescent patients with scoliosis, asymmetries were completely corrected with torso rotation, resulting in strength gains that ranged from 12% to 40%.[39] Only 1 girl in the study progressed and required surgery, whereas 4 patients showed reductions in their curvatures.

Similar results with this program are possible in middle-age adults who develop a slight increase in their spinal curvature associated with back pain. Our data also indicate that the use of specialized computerized torso rotation equipment is unnecessary; we are

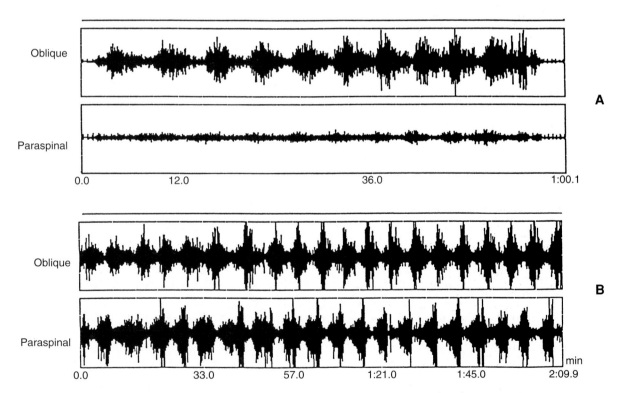

Figure 59-6.   Posttraining lumbar exercise dynamic EMG tracing. **A,** This demonstrates myoelectric activity from surface electrodes on the external abdominal oblique muscles. It also demonstrates the inhibited myoelectric activity on the lumbar paraspinal muscles during rotational activity. **B,** This demonstrates cycles of rotational activity against resistance with the surface electrodes in the same position as in **A.** It should be noted that now the paraspinal muscles are fully active and demonstrate symmetric function with the abdominal oblique muscles.

presently using an exercise-only rotation device with impressive results. Compliance on the part of the young teenagers has not been a problem, and the parents are pleased that something other than "watch and wait" is possible.

It seems appropriate to consider torso rotational strengthening on certain equipment that can measure baseline and monitor progress in a gradual specific manner. In the past scoliosis patients have not benefited from exercise programs because of the difficulty of measuring strength, progress, and compliance and also not having access to any equipment. It is appropriate to transfer the benefits of physical training available in sports medicine to spinal care. Change should come from an active exercise program and motivation provided by feedback of performance.

REHABILITATION OF THE CERVICAL SPINE

Soft tissue injuries frequently defined as whiplash injuries and degenerative disc disease are two areas of concern associated with presurgical and postsurgical care. Soft tissue injuries are frequently very complex to treat because the severity of the injury cannot be precisely defined. A relationship to litigation is frequently present that makes the duration of pain complaint sometimes suspect in terms of secondary gain. Sudden hyperextension/flexion injury, usually from a motor vehicle accident, can cause a specific injury. In a recent study of 100 patients at the Reykjavik Hospital in Iceland, where litigation does not exist, 90% of the patients had headaches, 50% had low back pain, 87% had sleep disturbances, 50% had arm pain, 47% had lack of concentration in visual disturbances, and 45% had a history of previous whiplash type of injury.[31]

Whether the pain comes from the facet joint or the disc is not clear, because a wide and varied distribution of pain in patients with whiplash symptoms exists. The referral pattern from various segments has been specifically defined with radiographic studies.[12] This same group demonstrated the resolution of segmental or sclerotomal pain by local anesthetic injections in patients suffering from whiplash complaints.[2] In the early 1950s, Ralph Cloward demonstrated similar distribution patterns with injections of the cervical disc before proceeding with an anterior cervical fusion (Figure 59-7).

There is frequently disagreement whether the trauma of the injury was severe enough to cause soft tissue injury. The reaction time after perception, which is the sudden change in tension of the cervical musculature to muscular reaction, occurs within 200 microseconds, whereas peak acceleration or deceleration occurs between 100 and 150 microseconds.[15] It is not surprising that cervical soft tissue damage can occur even with a relatively minor impact at a speed of 8 km/hr.[49]

With all this information, what is the appropriate treatment for patients with significant complaints that appear to continue even with minor injury? Studies do not support the benefits of treating whiplash with manipulation, or that immobilization with collars and rest is as effective as alternatives.[49] McKinney[37] com-

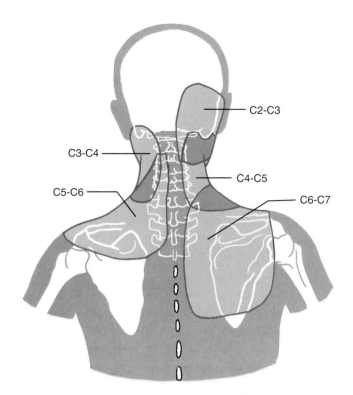

Figure 59-7. Referral patterns of pain from various levels of the zygapophyseal joints. (Redrawn from Aprill C, Dwyer A, Bogduk N: Cervical zygapophyseal joint pain patterns. II. A clinical evaluation, Spine 15:458-461, 1990.)

pared mobilization by self-directed exercise according to the McKenzie protocol with analgesic rest and collars. This study showed that early mobilization with specific active exercises is better than soft collar and rest at short-term and 2-year follow-up. Traction is less successful when compared with early mobilization.[57] No studies have supported the benefits of ultrasound, diathermy, ice, and massage as the only treatment. All the evidence indicates that self-mobilization is the most effective treatment program for the soft tissue injuries typical of whiplash. The various modalities may benefit pain perception, but no evidence supports the concept that a change in structure occurs.

It should be assumed after a period of time that some deficits in cervical strength occur with degenerative disc disease or postsurgical neck problems. The study by Leggett et al.[30] is the only one that evaluated the strength of cervical extensors in normal individuals. Tests have revealed that patients with degenerative disc disease have significant deficits. In a study of 90 patients with degenerative problems and chronic cervical strain, deficits were present in all patients compared with normal controls, using isometric testing over various ranges (MedX cervical extension machine).[19] When the patients were placed in an active, dynamic exercise program, significant increase in strength occurred, correlating with significant reduction in pain, including an improvement in their range of motion. The same type of progressive exercise program using other equipment has also been documented.[5] Both of these studies demonstrate that without equipment it is very difficult to evaluate strength and compliance with the strengthening program and to measure progress. Early motion and active exercise is supported by clinical trials.[49]

After bony union has occurred in the postsurgical patient, it is appropriate to use the same protocols of progressive strengthening exercises in the sagittal plane. The patient should be encouraged to avoid extremes of flexion/extension during the earliest phase of the program. Progressive increase in range is possible once the patient shows flexibility in midrange.

Although many exercise programs are advocated for either soft tissue strain or degenerative cervical disc disease, few of these programs have proved effective. On the other hand, no regimen of passive care has ever been shown to be more effective than the natural history of the disease process. The only justification for incorporating a particular program in the rehabilitation process is a standardized systematic program that includes a patient's measurement of progress.

SELECTED REFERENCES

Don Tigny RL: Anterior dysfunction of the sacroiliac joint as a major factor in the etiology of idiopathic low back pain, *Phys Ther* 70:250-265, 1990.

Donelson R et al.: A prospective study of centralization of lumbar and referred pain: a predictor of symptomatic discs and annular competence, *Spine* 22:1115-1122, 1997.

Matheson LN, Matheson M, Grant J: Development of measure of perceived functional ability, *J Occup Rehabil* 3:15-30, 1993.

Matheson LN et al.: A test to measure lift capacity of physically impaired adults. I. Development and reliability testing, *Spine* 20:2119-2129, 1995.

Matheson L et al.: A test to measure lift capacity of physically impaired adults. II. Reactivity in a patient sample, *Spine* 20:2130-2134, 1995.

REFERENCES

1. Agency for Health Care Policy and Research: Acute low back problems in adult treatment. AHCPR Publication 95-0643, Washington, DC, 1994, US Government Printing Office.
2. Aprill C, Dwyer A, Bogduk N: Cervical zygapophyseal joint pain patterns. II. A clinical evaluation, *Spine* 15:458-461, 1990.
3. Avikainen VJ, Rezasoltani A, Kauhanen HA: Asymmetry of paraspinal EMG-time characteristics in idiopathic scoliosis, *J Spinal Disord* 12:61-67, 1999.
4. Becker TJ: Scoliosis in swimmers, *Clin Sports Med* 5:149-158, 1986.
5. Berg HE, Berggren G, Tesch PA: Dynamic neck strength training effect on pain and function, *Arch Phys Med Rehabil* 75:661-665, 1994.
6. Biering-Sorensen F: Physical measurements as risk indicators for low-back trouble over a one year period, *Spine* 9:106-119, 1984.
7. Cassidy JB, Kirkaldy-Willis WH, MacGregor M: Spinal manipulation for the treatment of chronic low back and leg pain: an observational study. In Buerger AA and Greenman PD, eds: *Empirical approaches to the validation of spinal manipulation*, Springfield, Ill, 1985, Charles C Thomas, pp. 199-148.
8. Cherkin DC et al.: A comparison of physical therapy, chiropractic manipulation, and provision of an educational booklet for the treatment of patients with low back pain, *N Engl J Med* 339:1021-1029, 1998.
9. Don Tigny RL: Anterior dysfunction of the sacroiliac joint as a major factor in the etiology of idiopathic low back pain, *Phys Ther* 70:250-265, 1990.
10. Donelson R, Murphy K, Silva G: Centralization phenomenon: its usefulness in evaluating and treating referred pain, *Spine* 15:211-213, 1990.
11. Donelson R, Aprill C, Medcalf R, Grant W: A prospective study of centralization of lumbar and referred pain: a predictor of symptomatic discs and annular competence, *Spine* 22:1115-1122, 1997.
12. Dwyer A, Aprill C, Bogduk N: Cervical zygapophyseal joint pain patterns. I. A study in normal volunteers, *Spine* 15:453-457, 1990.
13. Ellenberg MR et al.: Prospective evaluation of the course of disc herniations in patients with proven radiculopathy, *Arch Phys Med Rehabil* 74:3-8, 1993.
14. Flicker PL et al.: Lumbar muscle usage in chronic low back pain: magnetic resonance image evaluation, *Spine* 18:582-586, 1993.
15. Foreman SM, Croft AC: Soft tissue injuries: long and short term effects. In Foreman SM and Croft AC, eds: *Whiplash injuries: the cervical acceleration/deceleration syndrome*, Baltimore, 1988, Williams & Wilkins, pp. 60-64.
16. Franson RC, Saal JS, Saal JA: Human disc phospholipase A2 is inflammatory, *Spine* 17:S129-S132, 1992.
17. Hides J, Richardson C, Jull G: Multifidus muscle recovery is not automatic after resolution of acute first episode low back pain, *Spine* 21:2763-2769, 1996.
18. Hides J et al.: Evidence of lumbar multifidus muscle wasting ipsilateral to symptoms in patients with acute/subacute low back pain, *Spine* 19:165-172, 1994.
19. Highland TR et al.: Changes in isometric strength and range of motion of the isolated cervical spine after eight weeks of clinical rehabilitation, *Spine* 17:S77-S82, 1992.
20. Hodges P, Richardson C: Relationship between limb movement speed and associated contraction of the trunk muscles, *Ergonomics* 40:1220-1230, 1997.
21. Hodges P, Richardson C: Delayed postural contraction of transversus abdominis in low back pain associated with movement of the lower limb, *J Spinal Disord* 11:46-56, 1998.
22. Jay MA et al.: Sensitivity and specificity of the indicators of sincere effort of the EPIC lift capacity test on a previously injured population, *Spine* 25:1405-1412, 2000.
23. Kang JD et al.: Herniated lumbar intervertebral discs spontaneously produce matrix metalloproteinases, nitric oxide, interleukin-6, and prostaglandin E2, *Spine* 21:271-277, 1996.
24. Karas R et al.: The relationship between nonorganic signs and centralization of symptoms in the prediction of return to work for patients with low back pain, *Phys Ther* 77:354-369, 1997.
25. Kitano T et al.: Biochemical changes associated with the symptomatic human intervertebral disk, *Clin Orthop* 293:372-377, 1993.
26. Koes BW et al.: The effectiveness of manual therapy, physiotherapy, and treatment by the general practitioner for nonspecific back and neck complaints: a randomized clinical trial, *Spine* 17:28-35, 1992.
27. Kopp JR et al.: The use of lumbar extension in the evaluation and treatment of patients with acute herniated nucleus pulposus: a preliminary report, *Clin Orthop* 202:211-218, 1986.
28. Laslett M, Williams M: The reliability of selected pain provocation tests for sacroiliac joint pathology, *Spine* 19:1243-1249, 1994.
29. Leggett S et al.: Restorative exercise for clinical low back pain: a prospective two-center study with 1-year follow-up, *Spine* 24:889-898, 1999.
30. Leggett SH et al.: Quantitative assessment and training of isometric cervical extension strength, *Am J Sports Med* 19:653-659, 1991.
31. Magnusson T: Extracervical symptoms after whiplash trauma, *Cephalagia* 14:223-227, 1994.
32. Matheson L et al.: Effect of computerized instructions on measurement of lift capacity: safety, reliability and validity, *J Occup Rehabil* 3:65-81, 1993.
33. Matheson L et al.: A test to measure lift capacity of physically impaired adults. II. Reactivity in a patient sample, *Spine* 20:2130-2134, 1995.
34. Matheson LN, Matheson M, Grant J: Development of measure of perceived functional ability, *J Occup Rehabil* 3:15-30, 1993.
35. Matheson LN et al.: A test to measure lift capacity of physically impaired adults. I. Development and reliability testing, *Spine* 20:2119-2129, 1995.
36. Mayer TG et al.: Comparison of CT scan muscle measurements and isokinetic trunk strength in postoperative patients, *Spine* 14:33-35, 1989.
37. McKinney LA: Early mobilization and outcome in acute sprains of the neck, *Br Med J* 299:1006-1008, 1989.
38. Mooney V, Matheson L: *Final report: objective measurement of soft tissue injury*, San Diego, 1994, The OrthoMed Foundation.

39. Mooney V, Gulick J, Pozos R: A preliminary report on the effect of measure strength training in adolescent idiopathic scoliosis, *J Spinal Disord* 13:102-107, 2000.

40. Mooney V et al.: Coupled motion contralateral latissimus dorsi and gluteus maximus: its role in sacroiliac stabilization. In Vleeming A et al., eds: *Movement stability and low back pain: the essential role of the pelvis*, New York, 1997, Churchill Livingstone, pp. 115-122.

41. Mooney V et al.: Relationships between myoelectric activity, strength, and MRI of lumbar extensor muscles in back pain patients and normal subjects, *J Spinal Disord* 10:348-356, 1997.

42. Moore MR: Diagnosis and surgical treatment of chronic painful sacroiliac dysfunction. In Vleeming A et al., eds: *Second Interdisciplinary World Congress on Low Back Pain: the integrated function of the lumbar spine and sacroiliac joint*. San Diego, 1995, Rotterdam ECO, pp. 339-345.

43. Rath WA: A retrospective review of the McKenzie approach in a consecutive case series. In McKenzie R, ed: The McKenzie approach, Syracuse, 1994, McKenzie Institute USA, pp.19-22.

44. Richardson C et al.: Effect of exercises compared to inactivity. In Richardson C, ed: *Therapeutic exercise for spinal segmental stabilization in low back pain: scientific basis and clinical approach*, Edinburgh, 1999, Churchill Livingston.

45. Saal JA: Dynamic muscular stabilization in the non operative treatment of lumbar pain syndromes, *Orthop Rev* 19:691-700, 1990.

46. Saal JA, Saal JS: Non operative treatment of herniated lumbar intervertebral disc with radiculopathy: an outcomes study, *Spine* 14:431, 1989.

47. Schwarzer AC, Aprill CN, Bogduk N: The sacroiliac joint in chronic low back pain, *Spine* 20:31-37, 1995.

48. Spitzer WO: Scientific approach to the assessment and management of activity related spinal disorders: a monograph for clinicians—report of the Quebec Task Force, *Spine* 12:S8-S59, 1987.

49. Spitzer WO, Skovron ML, Salmi LR, Cassidy DJ, et al.: Scientific monograph of the Quebec Task Force on whiplash-associated disorders: redefining "whiplash" and its management, *Spine* 20:1S-73S, 1995.

50. Sturesson B, Selvik G, Uden A: Movements of the sacroiliac joints: a roentgen stereophotogrammetric study, *Spine* 14:162-165, 1989.

51. Sward L: The thoracolumbar spine in young elite athletes: current concepts on the effects of physical training, *Sports Med* 13:357-364, 1992.

52. Verna JL et al.: Electromyographic activity of the trunk extensor muscles: effect of hip position and lumbo-pelvic rhythm during roman chair exercise, *Arch Phys Med Rehabil* (in press).

53. Vleeming A et al.: The posterior layer of the thoracolumbar fascia: its function in load transfer from spine to legs, *Spine* 20:753-758, 1995.

54. Vleeming A et al.: An integrated therapy for peripartum pelvic instability: a study of the biomechanical effects of pelvic belts, *Am J Obstet Gynecol* 166:1243-1247, 1992.

55. Vleeming A, Stoeckart R, Snijders CF: The sacrotuberous ligament: a conceptual approach to its dynamic role in stabilizing the sacroiliac joint, *J Clin Biomech* 4:201-203, 1989.

56. Waddell G et al.: Nonorganic physical signs in low back pain, *Spine* 5:117-125, 1980.

57. Zylbergold RS, Piper MC: Cervical spine disorders: a comparison of three types of traction, *Spine* 10:867-871, 1985.

Index